Clinical Education for the Health Professions

Debra Nestel • Gabriel Reedy •
Lisa McKenna • Suzanne Gough
Editors

Clinical Education for the Health Professions

Theory and Practice

Volume 2

With 128 Figures and 94 Tables

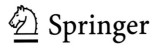

Editors
Debra Nestel
Monash University
School of Clinical Sciences
Clayton, VIC, Australia

University of Melbourne
Department of Surgery (Austin)
Melbourne, VIC, Australia

Lisa McKenna
La Trobe University
School of Nursing and Midwifery
Melbourne, VIC, Australia

Gabriel Reedy
King's College London
London, UK

Suzanne Gough
Bond University
Faculty of Health Sciences and Medicine
Gold Coast, QLD, Australia

ISBN 978-981-15-3343-3   ISBN 978-981-15-3344-0 (eBook)
https://doi.org/10.1007/978-981-15-3344-0

© Springer Nature Singapore Pte Ltd. 2023
This work is subject to copyright. All rights are reserved by the Publisher, whether the whole or part of the material is concerned, specifically the rights of translation, reprinting, reuse of illustrations, recitation, broadcasting, reproduction on microfilms or in any other physical way, and transmission or information storage and retrieval, electronic adaptation, computer software, or by similar or dissimilar methodology now known or hereafter developed.
The use of general descriptive names, registered names, trademarks, service marks, etc. in this publication does not imply, even in the absence of a specific statement, that such names are exempt from the relevant protective laws and regulations and therefore free for general use.
The publisher, the authors, and the editors are safe to assume that the advice and information in this book are believed to be true and accurate at the date of publication. Neither the publisher nor the authors or the editors give a warranty, expressed or implied, with respect to the material contained herein or for any errors or omissions that may have been made. The publisher remains neutral with regard to jurisdictional claims in published maps and institutional affiliations.

This Springer imprint is published by the registered company Springer Nature Singapore Pte Ltd.
The registered company address is: 152 Beach Road, #21-01/04 Gateway East, Singapore 189721, Singapore

Preface

The education and training of health professionals is fundamental to the success of health services. Philosophies, approaches, and practices vary internationally. We frame clinical education as any activities that prepare health professionals to learn and work effectively in clinical settings. We believe this major reference work, *Clinical Education for the Health Professions*, represents, supports, and advances scholarship and practice in this field. It assembles accessible and evidence-based content, on what is known about many facets of clinical education.

Clinical Education for the Health Professions is divided into eight parts. We start with the contemporary context of health professions education; shift focus to theoretical underpinnings, curriculum considerations, and approaches to supporting learning in clinical settings; a specific focus to assessment approaches; and then to evidence-based educational methods and content. Governance and other formal processes associated with the maturation of education programs are also considered, including the increasing professionalization of clinical education. Finally, we look to the future drawing upon much of what has surfaced in the past and present.

The development of multi-authored international work can be complex. We outline the development process in the introduction. We are grateful for the generosity of contributors – researchers, educators, and clinicians – who have given their time, especially coinciding with the COVID-19 pandemic.

Melbourne, Australia	Debra Nestel
London, UK	Gabriel Reedy
Melbourne, Australia	Lisa McKenna
Gold Coast, Australia	Suzanne Gough
July 2023	Editors

Acknowledgments

We are grateful to all the contributors to this major reference work.
We thank Ms. Shameem Aysha S. of Springer Nature for coordinating the editorial process.

Contents

Volume 1

Part I The Contemporary Context of Health Professions Education 1

1. Medical Education: Trends and Context 3
    Jennene Greenhill

2. Surgical Education: Context and Trends 29
    David J. Coker

3. General Practice Education: Context and Trends 49
    Susan M. Wearne and James B. Brown

4. Anesthesia Education: Trends and Context 69
    S. D. Marshall and M. C. Turner

5. Clinical Education in Nursing: Current Practices and Trends ... 87
    Marilyn H. Oermann and Teresa Shellenbarger

6. Nursing Education in Low and Lower-Middle Income Countries: Context and Trends 107
    Christine Sommers and Carielle Joy Rio

7. Obstetric and Midwifery Education: Context and Trends 121
    Arunaz Kumar and Linda Sweet

8. Allied Health Education: Current and Future Trends 135
    Michelle Bissett, Neil Tuttle, and Elizabeth Cardell

9. Dental Education: Context and Trends 153
    Flora A. Smyth Zahra and Sang E. Park

10. Interprofessional Education (IPE): Trends and Context 167
    Lyn Gum and Jenn Salfi

11	Global Surgery and Its Trends and Context: The Case of Timor-Leste	181
	Sean Stevens	
12	Surgical Training: Impact of Decentralization and Guidelines for Improvement	201
	Christine M. Cuthbertson	
13	Mental Health Education: Contemporary Context and Future Directions	217
	Christopher Kowalski and Chris Attoe	
14	Dental Education: A Brief History	251
	Andrew I. Spielman	
15	Surgical Education and Training: Historical Perspectives	267
	John P. Collins	
16	Nursing and Midwifery Education: Historical Perspectives	285
	Lisa McKenna, Jenny Davis, and Eloise Williams	
17	Health Sciences and Medicine Education in Lockdown: Lessons Learned During the COVID-19 Global Pandemic	303
	Suzanne Gough, Robin Orr, Allan Stirling, Athanasios Raikos, Ben Schram, and Wayne Hing	

Part II Philosophical and Theoretical Underpinning of Health Professions Education **333**

18	Cognitive Neuroscience Foundations of Surgical and Procedural Expertise: Focus on Theory	335
	Pamela Andreatta	
19	Mastery Learning in Health Professions Education	347
	Raymond Yap	
20	Threshold Concepts and Troublesome Knowledge	361
	Sarah E. M. Meek, Hilary Neve, and Andy Wearn	
21	Social Semiotics: Theorizing Meaning Making	385
	Jeff Bezemer	
22	Communities of Practice and Medical Education	403
	Claire Condron and Walter Eppich	
23	Activity Theory in Health Professions Education Research and Practice	417
	Richard L. Conn, Gerard J. Gormley, Sarah O'Hare, and Anu Kajamaa	
24	Reflective Practice in Health Professions Education	441
	Jennifer M. Weller-Newton and Michele Drummond-Young	

25	**Transformative Learning in Clinical Education: Using Theory to Inform Practice** .... Anna Jones	463
26	**Self-Regulated Learning: Focus on Theory** .... Susan Irvine and Ian J. Irvine	481
27	**Critical Theory** .... Nancy McNaughton and Maria Athina (Tina) Martimianakis	499
28	**Focus on Theory: Emotions and Learning** .... Aubrey L. Samost-Williams and Rebecca D. Minehart	521
29	**Ecological Systems Theory in Clinical Learning** .... Yang Yann Foo and Raymond Goy	537
30	**Philosophy for Healthcare Professions Education: A Tool for Thinking and Practice** .... Kirsten Dalrymple and Roberto di Napoli	555

Part III Curriculum Considerations in Health Professions Education 573

31	**Health Profession Curriculum and Public Engagement** .... Maree O'Keefe and Helena Ward	575
32	**Teaching and Learning Ethics in Healthcare** .... Selena Knight and Andrew Papanikitas	587
33	**Simulation as Clinical Replacement: Contemporary Approaches in Healthcare Professional Education** .... Suzie Kardong-Edgren, Sandra Swoboda, and Nancy Sullivan	607
34	**Teaching Simple and Complex Psychomotor Skills** .... Delwyn Nicholls	625
35	**Developing Professional Identity in Health Professional Students** .... Kathleen Leedham-Green, Alec Knight, and Rick Iedema	645
36	**Hidden, Informal, and Formal Curricula in Health Professions Education** .... Lisa McKenna	667
37	**Arts and Humanities in Health Professional Education** .... Pam Harvey, Neville Chiavaroli, and Giskin Day	681
38	**Debriefing Practices in Simulation-Based Education** .... Peter Dieckmann, Rana Sharara-Chami, and Hege Langli Ersdal	699

39	**Written Feedback in Health Sciences Education: "What You Write May Be Perceived as Banal"** .... Brian Jolly	717
40	**Technology Considerations in Health Professions and Clinical Education** .... Christian Moro, Zane Stromberga, and James Birt	743
41	**Role of Social Media in Health Professions Education** .... Victoria Brazil, Jessica Stokes-Parish, and Jesse Spurr	765
42	**E-learning: Development of a Fully Online 4th Year Psychology Program** .... F. J. Garivaldis, S. P. McKenzie, and M. Mundy	777
43	**Teaching Diversity in Healthcare Education: Conceptual Clarity and the Need for an Intersectional Transdisciplinary Approach** .... Helen Bintley and Riya E. George	795
44	**Planetary Health: Educating the Current and Future Health Workforce** .... Michelle McLean, Lynne Madden, Janie Maxwell, Patricia Nanya Schwerdtle, Janet Richardson, Judith Singleton, Kristen MacKenzie-Shalders, Georgia Behrens, Nick Cooling, Richard Matthews, and Graeme Horton	815

Volume 2

Part IV Supporting Learning in Clinical Settings **845**

45	**Learning and Teaching in Clinical Settings: Expert Commentary from an Interprofessional Perspective** .... Debra Kiegaldie	847
46	**Learning and Teaching at the Bedside: Expert Commentary from a Nursing Perspective** .... Michelle A. Kelly and Jan Forber	869
47	**Learning and Teaching in Clinical Settings: Expert Commentary from a Midwifery Perspective** .... Linda Sweet and Deborah Davis	891
48	**Learning and Teaching in the Operating Room: A Surgical Perspective** .... V. Chao, C. Ong, Debra Kiegaldie, and Debra Nestel	909

49	**Learning and Teaching in the Operating Theatre: Expert Commentary from the Nursing Perspective** .... Rachel Cardwell, Emmalee Weston, and Jenny Davis	933
50	**Learning and Teaching in Pediatrics** .... Ramesh Mark Nataraja, Simon C. Blackburn, and Robert Roseby	955
51	**Optimizing the Role of Clinical Educators in Health Professional Education** .... Simone Gibson and Claire Palermo	985
52	**Well-Being in Health Profession Training** .... Andrew Grant	999
53	**Embedding a Simulation-Based Education Program in a Teaching Hospital** .... Rebecca A. Szabo and Kirsty Forrest	1017
54	**Targeting Organizational Needs Through the Development of a Simulation-Based Communication Education Program** .... J. Sokol and M. Heywood	1039
55	**Effective Feedback Conversations in Clinical Practice** .... C. E. Johnson, C. J. Watling, J. L. Keating, and E. K. Molloy	1055
56	**Supervision in General Practice Settings** .... James Brown and Susan M. Wearne	1073
57	**Conversational Learning in Health Professions Education: Learning Through Talk** .... Walter J. Eppich, Jan Schmutz, and Pim Teunissen	1099
58	**Underperformance in Clinical Education: Challenges and Possibilities** .... Margaret Bearman	1119
Part V	**Assessment in Health Professions Education**	**1133**
59	**Approaches to Assessment: A Perspective from Education** ...... Phillip Dawson and Colin R. McHenry	1135
60	**Measuring Attitudes: Current Practices in Health Professional Education** .... Ted Brown, Stephen Isbel, Mong-Lin Yu, and Thomas Bevitt	1149
61	**Measuring Performance: Current Practices in Surgical Education** .... Pamela Andreatta, Brenton Franklin, Matthew Bradley, Christopher Renninger, and John Armstrong	1177

| 62 | Programmatic Assessment in Health Professions Education 1203
Iris Lindemann, Julie Ash, and Janice Orrell

| 63 | Entrustable Professional Activities: Focus on
Assessment Methods 1221
Andrea Bramley and Lisa McKenna

| 64 | Workplace-Based Assessment in Clinical Practice 1235
Victor Lee and Andrea Gingerich

| 65 | Focus on Selection Methods: Evidence and Practice 1251
Louise Marjorie Allen, Catherine Green, and Margaret Hay

| 66 | Practice Education in Occupational Therapy: Current Trends
and Practices 1277
Stephen Isbel, Ted Brown, Mong-Lin Yu, Thomas Bevitt,
Craig Greber, and Anne-Maree Caine

| 67 | Practice Education in Lockdown: Lessons Learned During the
COVID-19 Global Pandemic 1303
Luke Robinson, Ted Brown, Ellie Fossey, Mong-Lin Yu,
Linda Barclay, Eli Chu, Annette Peart, and Libby Callaway

**Part VI Evidence-Based Health Professions Education: Focus
on Educational Methods and Content 1323**

| 68 | Team-Based Learning (TBL): Theory, Planning, Practice, and
Implementation 1325
Annette Burgess and Elie Matar

| 69 | Learning with and from Peers in Clinical Education 1355
Joanna Tai, Merrolee Penman, Calvin Chou, and Arianne Teherani

| 70 | Simulation for Procedural Skills Teaching and Learning 1375
Taylor Sawyer, Lisa Bergman, and Marjorie L. White

| 71 | Simulation for Clinical Skills in Healthcare Education 1395
Guillaume Alinier, Ahmed Labib Shehatta, and Ratna Makker

| 72 | Screen-Based Learning 1417
Damir Ljuhar

| 73 | Artificial Intelligence in Surgical Education and Training 1435
Melanie Crispin

| 74 | Coaching in Health Professions Education: The Case of
Surgery 1447
Martin Richardson and Louise Richardson

75	Developing Health Professional Teams John T. Paige	1463
76	Developing Care and Compassion in Health Professional Students and Clinicians Karen Livesay and Ruby Walter	1485
77	Developing Patient Safety Through Education David Pinnock	1501
78	Supporting the Development of Professionalism in the Education of Health Professionals Anne Stephenson and Julie Bliss	1519
79	Supporting the Development of Patient-Centred Communication Skills Bernadette O'Neill	1535
80	Contemporary Sociological Issues for Health Professions Curricula Margaret Simmons	1553
81	Developing Clinical Reasoning Capabilities Joy Higgs	1571

Part VII Governance, Quality Improvement, Scholarship and Leadership in Health Professions Education **1589**

82	Professional Bodies in Health Professions Education Julie Browne	1591
83	Scholarship in Health Professions Education Lisa McKenna	1611
84	Developing Educational Leadership in Health Professions Education Margaret Hay, Leeroy William, Catherine Green, Eric Gantwerker, and Louise Marjorie Allen	1627
85	On "Being" Participants and a Researcher in a Longitudinal Medical Professional Identity Study Michelle McLean, Charlotte Alexander, and Arjun Khaira	1657
86	Health Care Practitioners 'Becoming' Doctors: Changing Roles and Identities Michelle McLean and Carla Pecoraro	1671

Part VIII Future Directions for Health Professions Education 1691

87 Health Professional Education in 2020: A Trainee Perspective ... 1693
Karen Muller and Savannah Morrison

88 Future of Health Professions Education Curricula 1705
Eric Gantwerker, Louise Marjorie Allen, and Margaret Hay

89 Competencies of Health Professions Educators of the Future 1727
Louise Marjorie Allen, Eric Gantwerker, and Margaret Hay

Index 1737

About the Editors

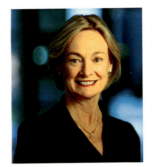

Debra Nestel has worked at the University of Hong Kong, China, Imperial College, United Kingdom, the University of Melbourne and Monash University, Australia, for over 35 years. Her first degree was in sociology, and her doctorate was in program evaluation and communication skills education in medicine and dentistry. Currently, her education and research activities focus on faculty development for health professional, surgical, and simulation educators. Dr. Debra is an experienced editor-in-chief (EIC) and has edited several books. She was the foundation EIC of *Advances in Simulation* and is EIC of the *International Journal for Healthcare Simulation*. Dr. Debra is a Fellow of the Academy of the Society for Simulation in Healthcare (United States) and is also a Fellow of the Academy of Medical Educators (United Kingdom). In 2021, Dr. Debra was appointed as Member of the Order of Australia for her service to medical education and simulation. She has received the Ray Page Lifetime Simulation Service Award and a Presidential Citation from the Society for Simulation in Healthcare.

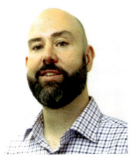

Gabriel Reedy has led the interprofessional postgraduate program in health professions education at King's College, London, the largest health sciences university in Europe, for most of his academic career. His research focuses on how healthcare professionals and emergency responders learn, how to support and train them more effectively, with a focus on the power of simulated environments, and how they can help train individuals, teams, departments, organizations, and inter-agency systems. He is a Principal Fellow of the Higher

Education Academy (United Kingdom), a Fellow of the Academy of Medical Educators (United Kingdom), and a Fellow of the Academy of the Society for Simulation in Healthcare (United States). He has served on the Scientific Committee of the Society for Simulation in Europe (SESAM) and the Research Committee for the Society for Simulation in Healthcare (United Kingdom). He is Editor-in-Chief of *Advances in Simulation*.

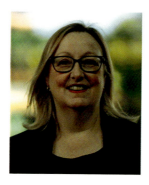

Lisa McKenna has worked at Monash University and La Trobe University, Australia, for over 30 years. Her initial qualifications were hospital-based nursing and midwifery certificates with her first degree in education. She has since completed postgraduate degrees in education, business administration, and history, and a PhD in nursing. Lisa is currently the Dean of the School of Nursing and Midwifery at La Trobe, and EIC of *Collegian: The Australian Journal of Nursing Practice, Scholarship and Research* from 2014 to 2022. Prof. Lisa has published extensively on nursing, midwifery, and health professions education. Her recent research has focused on health workforce development and competence. In 2022, Prof. Lisa was inducted into the Sigma International Nurse Researcher Hall of Fame.

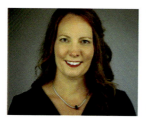

Suzanne Gough is an Associate Professor of Physiotherapy and Associate Dean of Learning and Teaching at Bond University, Australia. She is a member of the Bond Translational Simulation Collaborative team, with national and international experience in healthcare simulation education. Suzanne transitioned from clinical to academic practice in 2004, as a Senior Lecturer at Manchester Metropolitan University. She is a Principal Fellow of the Higher Education Academy (United Kingdom). As Principal Investigator, she has led international project teams to develop simulated patient governance frameworks and training resources for use across the United Kingdom, on behalf of Health Education England. Suzanne's current research interests include the use of virtual reality across diverse patient groups, simulation and technology-enhanced learning, stress and burnout, and curriculum design.

Contributors

Charlotte Alexander Emergency Department, Gold Coast University Hospital, Gold Coast, QLD, Australia

Guillaume Alinier Hamad Medical Corporation Ambulance Service, Doha, Qatar
School of Health and Social Work, University of Hertfordshire, Hatfield, UK
Weill Cornell Medicine Qatar, Doha, Qatar
Faculty of Health and Life Sciences, Northumbria University, Newcastle upon Tyne, UK

Louise Marjorie Allen Monash Centre for Professional Development and Monash Online Education, Monash University, Clayton, VIC, Australia

Pamela Andreatta The Norman M. Rich Department of Surgery, Uniformed Services University & the Walter Reed National Military Medical Center "America's Medical School", Bethesda, MD, USA

John Armstrong University of South Florida Morsani College of Medicine, Tampa, FL, USA

Julie Ash Prideaux Centre for Health Professions Education, Flinders University, Adelaide, SA, Australia

Chris Attoe Maudsley Learning, South London and Maudsley NHS Foundation Trust, London, UK

Linda Barclay Department of Occupational Therapy, Monash University – Peninsula Campus, Frankston, VIC, Australia

Margaret Bearman Centre for Research in Assessment and Digital Education (CRADLE), Deakin University, Melbourne, VIC, Australia

Georgia Behrens School of Medicine, Sydney, University of Notre Dame, Sydney, NSW, Australia

Lisa Bergman The Office of Interprofessional Simulation for Innovative Clinical Practice, University of Alabama at Birmingham, Birmingham, AL, USA

Thomas Bevitt Faculty of Health, The University of Canberra Hospital, Canberra, Bruce ACT, Australia

Jeff Bezemer Institute of Education, University College London, London, UK

Helen Bintley Barts and The London, School of Medicine and Dentistry, Queen Mary University of London, London, UK

James Birt Faculty of Society and Design, Bond University, Gold Coast, QLD, Australia

Michelle Bissett Discipline of Occupational Therapy, Griffith University, Gold Coast, QLD, Australia

Simon C. Blackburn The Learning Academy, Great Ormond Street Hospital for Children, London, UK

Julie Bliss Florence Nightingale Faculty of Nursing, Midwifery & Palliative Care, King's College London, London, UK

Matthew Bradley The Norman M. Rich Department of Surgery, Uniformed Services University & the Walter Reed National Military Medical Center "America's Medical School", Bethesda, MD, USA

Andrea Bramley Department of Dietetics and Human Nutrition, La Trobe University, Melbourne, VIC, Australia

Victoria Brazil Faculty of Health Sciences and Medicine, Bond University, Gold Coast, QLD, Australia

James B. Brown Eastern Victoria GP Training, Churchill, VIC, Australia

Gippsland Medical School, Monash University, Churchill, VIC, Australia

James Brown Royal Australian College of General Practice, East Melbourne, VIC, Australia

Gippsland Medical School, Monash University, Churchill, VIC, Australia

Ted Brown Department of Occupational Therapy, School of Primary and Allied Health Care, Faculty of Medicine, Nursing and Health Sciences, Monash University – Peninsula Campus, Frankston, VIC, Australia

Julie Browne Centre for Medical Education, Cardiff University School of Medicine, Cardiff, UK

Annette Burgess Faculty of Medicine and Health, Sydney Medical School, Education Office, The University of Sydney, Sydney, NSW, Australia

Faculty of Medicine and Health, Sydney Health Professional Education Research Network, The University of Sydney, Sydney, NSW, Australia

Anne-Maree Caine School of Allied Health Sciences – Occupational Therapy, Griffith University, Nathan, QLD, Australia

Libby Callaway Department of Occupational Therapy, Monash University – Peninsula Campus, Frankston, VIC, Australia

Elizabeth Cardell Discipline of Speech Pathology, Griffith University, Gold Coast, Australia

Rachel Cardwell Austin Health, La Trobe University, Melbourne, VIC, Australia

V. Chao National Heart Centre, Singapore, Singapore

Neville Chiavaroli Department of Medical Education, University of Melbourne, Melbourne, VIC, Australia

Calvin Chou Department of Medicine, University of California, San Francisco and Veterans Affairs Health System, San Francisco, CA, USA

Eli Chu Department of Occupational Therapy, Monash University – Peninsula Campus, Frankston, VIC, Australia

David J. Coker Department of Surgery, Royal Prince Alfred Hospital, Camperdown, NSW, Australia

Discipline of Surgery, University of Sydney, Camperdown, NSW, Australia

John P. Collins University Department of Surgery, University of Melbourne, Melbourne, Australia

Nuffield Department of Surgical Sciences, University of Oxford, Oxford, UK

Green Templeton College, Oxford, UK

Claire Condron RSCI University of Medicine and Health Sciences, Dublin, Ireland

Richard L. Conn Centre for Medical Education, Queen's University Belfast, Belfast, UK

Nick Cooling School of Medicine, College of Health & Medicine, University of Tasmania, Hobart, TAS, Australia

Melanie Crispin Monash Health & The University of Melbourne, Melbourne, Australia

Christine M. Cuthbertson Monash Rural Health, Bendigo, Monash University, North Bendigo, VIC, Australia

Kirsten Dalrymple Department of Surgery and Cancer, Imperial College London, London, UK

Deborah Davis University of Canberra and Canberra Hospital and Health Services, Canberra, ACT, Australia

Jenny Davis School of Nursing and Midwifery, La Trobe University, Melbourne, VIC, Australia

Phillip Dawson Centre for Research in Assessment and Digital Learning (CRADLE), Deakin University, Geelong, VIC, Australia

Giskin Day Imperial College London, London, UK

Roberto di Napoli Centre for Innovation and Development for Education, St. George's University of London, London, UK

Peter Dieckmann Copenhagen Academy for Medical Education and Simulation (CAMES), Center for Human Resources and Education, Herlev and Getofte Hospital, Herlev, Denmark

Department of Quality and Health Technology, Faculty of Health Sciences, University of Stavanger, Stavanger, Norway

Department of Clinical Medicine, University of Copenhagen, Copenhagen, Denmark

Michele Drummond-Young School of Nursing, McMaster University, Hamilton, ON, Canada

Walter J. Eppich RCSI SIM Centre for Simulation Education and Research, RCSI University of Medicine and Health Sciences, Dublin, Ireland

Hege Langli Ersdal Department of Quality and Health Technology, Faculty of Health Sciences, University of Stavanger, Stavanger, Norway

Department of Anaesthesiology and Intensive Care, Stavanger University Hospital, Stavanger, Norway

Yang Yann Foo Office of Education, Duke-NUS Medical School, Singapore, Singapore

Jan Forber School of Nursing and Midwifery, University of Technology Sydney, Sydney, NSW, Australia

Kirsty Forrest Faculty of Health Sciences and Medicine, Bond University, Gold Coast, QLD, Australia

Ellie Fossey Department of Occupational Therapy, Monash University – Peninsula Campus, Frankston, VIC, Australia

Brenton Franklin The Norman M. Rich Department of Surgery, Uniformed Services University & the Walter Reed National Military Medical Center "America's Medical School", Bethesda, MD, USA

Eric Gantwerker Northwell Health, Lake Success, NY, USA

Zucker School of Medicine at Northwell/Hofstra, Hempstead, NY, USA

F. J. Garivaldis School of Psychological Sciences, Monash University, Melbourne, VIC, Australia

Riya E. George Barts and The London, School of Medicine and Dentistry, Queen Mary University of London, London, UK

Simone Gibson Deparment of Nutrition, Dietetics and Food, Medicine, Nursing and Health Sciences, Monash University, Clayton, VIC, Australia

School of Clinical Sciences, Medicine, Nursing and Health Sciences, Monash University, Clayton, VIC, Australia

Andrea Gingerich Northern Medical Program, University of Northern British Columbia, Prince George, BC, Canada

Gerard J. Gormley Centre for Medical Education, Queen's University Belfast, Belfast, UK

Suzanne Gough Faculty of Health Sciences and Medicine, Bond University, Gold Coast, QLD, Australia

Raymond Goy KKH Women and Children's Hospital, Singapore, Singapore

Andrew Grant Emeritus Professor Swansea University, Swansea, UK

Craig Greber Faculty of Health, University of Canberra, Canberra, ACT, Australia

Catherine Green Royal Victorian Eye and Ear Hospital, East Melbourne, VIC, Australia

Jennene Greenhill Rural Clinical School, University of Western Australia, Perth, WA, Australia

Lyn Gum College of Nursing and Health Sciences, Flinders University, Adelaide, SA, Australia

Pam Harvey La Trobe Rural Health School, La Trobe University, Bendigo, VIC, Australia

Margaret Hay Faculty of Education, Monash Centre for Professional Development and Monash Online Education, Monash University, Clayton, VIC, Australia

M. Heywood The Royal Children's Hospital Simulation Program, Department of Medical Education, The Royal Children's Hospital, Melbourne, VIC, Australia

Joy Higgs Professional Practice and Higher Education, Charles Sturt University, Sydney, NSW, Australia

Wayne Hing Faculty of Health Sciences and Medicine, Bond University, Gold Coast, QLD, Australia

Graeme Horton Faculty of Health and Medicine, University of Newcastle, Newcastle, NSW, Australia

Rick Iedema Centre for Team-Based Practice & Learning in Health Care, King's College London, London, UK

Ian J. Irvine University of Newcastle, Newcastle, NSW, Australia

Susan Irvine Victoria University, Melbourne, VIC, Australia

Stephen Isbel Faculty of Health, University of Canberra, Canberra, ACT, Australia

C. E. Johnson Monash Doctors Education, Monash Health and Faculty of Medicine, Nursing and Health Sciences, Monash University, Melbourne, VIC, Australia

Brian Jolly Faculty of Health and Medicine, University of Newcastle, Newcastle, NSW, Australia

School of Rural Medicine, University of New England, Armidale, NSW, Australia

Anna Jones School of Medical Education, King's College London, London, UK

Anu Kajamaa Faculty of Education, University of Oulu, Oulu, Finland

Suzie Kardong-Edgren Nursing Operations, Texas Health Resources Harris Methodist Hospital, Ft. Worth, TX, USA

J. L. Keating Department of Physiotherapy, School of Primary and Allied Health Care, Faculty of Medicine Nursing and Health Science, Monash University, Melbourne, VIC, Australia

Michelle A. Kelly Curtin School of Nursing, Curtin University, Perth, Australia

Arjun Khaira Psychiatry Department, Canberra Hospital, Canberra, ACT, Australia

Debra Kiegaldie Faculty of Medicine, Nursing and Health Sciences, Monash University; Faculty of Health Sciences and Community Studies, Holmesglen Institute and Healthscope Hospitals, Melbourne, VIC, Australia

Alec Knight School of Population Health and Environmental Sciences, King's College London, London, UK

Selena Knight School of Population Health and Environmental Sciences, King's College London, London, UK

Christopher Kowalski Oxford Health NHS Foundation Trust, Oxford, UK

Arunaz Kumar Monash University, Melbourne, VIC, Australia

Victor Lee Centre for Integrated Critical Care, The University of Melbourne, Melbourne, VIC, Australia

Austin Health, Melbourne, VIC, Australia

Kathleen Leedham-Green Medical Education Research Unit, Imperial College London, London, UK

Iris Lindemann Prideaux Centre for Health Professions Education, Flinders University, Adelaide, SA, Australia

Karen Livesay School of Health and Biomedical Sciences, College of Science, Engineering and Health, RMIT University, Melbourne, VIC, Australia

Damir Ljuhar Department of Surgical Simulation, Monash Children's Hospital, Clayton, VIC, Australia

Department of Paediatrics, School of Clinical Sciences, Faculty of Medicine, Nursing and Health Sciences, Monash University, Melbourne, VIC, Australia

Kristen MacKenzie-Shalders Master of Nutrition & Dietetic Practice, Faculty of Health Sciences & Medicine, Bond University, Gold Coast, QLD, Australia

Lynne Madden School of Medicine, Sydney, University of Notre Dame, Sydney, NSW, Australia

Ratna Makker Consultant Anaesthetist, Clinical Tutor, Clinical Director of the WISER (West Herts Initiative in Simulation Education and Research), West Herts Hospitals NHS Trust, Watford, Hertfordshire, UK

S. D. Marshall Department of Anaesthesia and Perioperative Medicine, Monash University, Melbourne, VIC, Australia

Maria Athina (Tina) Martimianakis Department of Paediatrics, Faculty of Medicine, University of Toronto, Toronto, Canada

Elie Matar Faculty of Medicine and Health, Sydney Medical School, Education Office, The University of Sydney, Sydney, NSW, Australia

Faculty of Medicine and Health, Sydney Medical School, Central Clinical School, The University of Sydney, Sydney, NSW, Australia

Richard Matthews Faculty of Health Sciences & Medicine, Bond University, Gold Coast, QLD, Australia

Janie Maxwell Nossal Institute of Global Health, University of Melbourne, Melbourne, VIC, Australia

Colin R. McHenry School of Medicine and Public Health, University of Newcastle, Newcastle, NSW, Australia

Lisa McKenna School of Nursing and Midwifery, La Trobe University, Melbourne, VIC, Australia

S. P. McKenzie School of Psychological Sciences, Monash University, Melbourne, VIC, Australia

Michelle McLean Faculty of Health Sciences & Medicine, Bond University, Gold Coast, QLD, Australia

Nancy McNaughton Wilson Centre for Research in Education, University of Toronto and University Health Network, Toronto, Canada

Sarah E. M. Meek School of Medicine, Dentistry and Nursing, University of Glasgow, Glasgow, UK

Rebecca D. Minehart Department of Anesthesia, Critical Care and Pain Medicine, Massachusetts General Hospital, Boston, MA, USA

Harvard Medical School, Boston, MA, USA

Center for Medical Simulation, Boston, MA, USA

E. K. Molloy Department of Medical Education, Melbourne Medical School, University of Melbourne, Melbourne, VIC, Australia

Christian Moro Faculty of Health Sciences and Medicine, Bond University, Gold Coast, QLD, Australia

Savannah Morrison General Medicine, John Hunter Hospital, Newcastle, NSW, Australia

Karen Muller Orthopaedic Surgery, John Hunter Hospital, Newcastle, NSW, Australia

M. Mundy School of Psychological Sciences, Monash University, Melbourne, VIC, Australia

Ramesh Mark Nataraja Monash Children's Hospital, Clayton, VIC, Australia

Department of Paediatrics, School of Clinical Sciences, Faculty of Medicine, Nursing and Health Sciences, Monash University, Clayton, VIC, Australia

Debra Nestel Monash University Institute for Health & Clinical Education, Monash University, Clayton, VIC, Australia

Department of Surgery (Austin), University of Melbourne, Parkville, VIC, Australia

Hilary Neve Peninsula Medical School, Faculty of Medicine and Dentistry, University of Plymouth, Plymouth, UK

Delwyn Nicholls College of Nursing and Health Sciences, Flinders University, Adelaide, SA, Australia

Sydney Ultrasound for Women, Sydney, NSW, Australia

Sarah O'Hare Centre for Medical Education, Queen's University Belfast, Belfast, UK

Maree O'Keefe Faculty of Health and Medical Sciences, The University of Adelaide, Adelaide, SA, Australia

Bernadette O'Neill GKT School of Medical Education, King's College London, London, UK

Marilyn H. Oermann Duke University School of Nursing, Durham, NC, USA

C. Ong KK Women's and Children's Hospital, Singapore, Singapore

Robin Orr Faculty of Health Sciences and Medicine, Bond University, Gold Coast, QLD, Australia

Janice Orrell Prideaux Centre for Health Professions Education, Flinders University, Adelaide, SA, Australia

John T. Paige Department of Surgery, Louisiana State University (LSU) Health New Orleans School of Medicine, New Orleans, LA, USA

Claire Palermo Deparment of Nutrition, Dietetics and Food, Medicine, Nursing and Health Sciences, Monash University, Clayton, VIC, Australia

Monash Centre for Scholarship in Health Education, Medicine, Nursing and Health Sciences, Monash University, Clayton, VIC, Australia

Andrew Papanikitas Nuffield Department of Primary Care Health Sciences, University of Oxford, Oxford, UK

Sang E. Park Office of Dental Education, Harvard School of Dental Medicine, Boston, MA, USA

Annette Peart Department of Occupational Therapy, Monash University – Peninsula Campus, Frankston, VIC, Australia

Carla Pecoraro Faculty of Health Sciences & Medicine, Bond University, Gold Coast, Australia

Merrolee Penman Work Integrated Learning, The University of Sydney, Camperdown, NSW, Australia

David Pinnock School of Health Sciences, University of Nottingham, Nottingham, UK

Athanasios Raikos Faculty of Health Sciences and Medicine, Bond University, Gold Coast, QLD, Australia

Christopher Renninger The Norman M. Rich Department of Surgery, Uniformed Services University & the Walter Reed National Military Medical Center "America's Medical School", Bethesda, MD, USA

Janet Richardson School of Nursing and Midwifery, University of Plymouth, Plymouth, UK

Louise Richardson Epworth Hospital, Melbourne, Australia

Martin Richardson Epworth Clinical School, University of Melbourne, Melbourne, Australia

Carielle Joy Rio Faculty of Nursing, Universitas Pelita Harapan, Karawaci, Tangerang, Indonesia

Luke Robinson Department of Occupational Therapy, Monash University – Peninsula Campus, Frankston, VIC, Australia

Robert Roseby Monash Children's Hospital, Clayton, VIC, Australia

Department of Paediatrics, School of Clinical Sciences, Faculty of Medicine, Nursing and Health Sciences, Monash University, Clayton, VIC, Australia

Jenn Salfi Nursing, Brock University, St. Catharines, ON, Canada

Aubrey L. Samost-Williams Department of Anesthesia, Critical Care and Pain Medicine, Massachusetts General Hospital, Boston, MA, USA

Harvard Medical School, Boston, MA, USA

Taylor Sawyer Division of Neonatology, Department of Pediatrics, Seattle Children's Hospital, University of Washington School of Medicine, Seattle, WA, USA

Jan Schmutz Department of Psychology, University of Zurich, Zurich, Switzerland

Ben Schram Faculty of Health Sciences and Medicine, Bond University, Gold Coast, QLD, Australia

Patricia Nanya Schwerdtle Nursing and Midwifery, Faculty of Medicine, Nursing and Health Sciences, Monash University Melbourne, Melbourne, VIC, Australia

Institute of Global Health, Heidelberg University, Heidelberg, Germany

Rana Sharara-Chami Department of Pediatrics and Adolescent Medicine, American University of Beirut, Beirut, Lebanon

Ahmed Labib Shehatta Medical Intensive Care Unit, Hamad General Hospital, Hamad Medical Corporation, Doha, Qatar

Clinical Anaesthesiology, Weill Cornell Medicine, Qatar, Doha, Qatar

Teresa Shellenbarger Department of Nursing and Allied Health Professions, Indiana University of Pennsylvania, Indiana, PA, USA

Margaret Simmons Monash Rural Health, Monash University, Churchill, VIC, Australia

Judith Singleton School of Clinical Sciences (Pharmacy), Faculty of Health, Queensland University of Technology, Brisbane, QLD, Australia

Flora A. Smyth Zahra Faculty of Dentistry, Oral & Craniofacial Sciences, King's College London, London, UK

J. Sokol The Royal Children's Hospital Simulation Program, Department of Medical Education, The Royal Children's Hospital, Melbourne, VIC, Australia

University of Melbourne Department of Paediatrics, Melbourne, VIC, Australia

Christine Sommers Universitas Pelita Harapan, Jakarta, Indonesia

Andrew I. Spielman New York University College of Dentistry, New York, NY, USA

Jesse Spurr Intensive Care Unit, Redcliffe Hospital, Redcliffe, QLD, Australia

Anne Stephenson School of Population Health & Environmental Sciences, Faculty of Life Sciences and Medicine, King's College London, London, UK

Sean Stevens Department of Surgery, Austin Health, University of Melbourne, Melbourne, VIC, Australia

Allan Stirling Faculty of Health Sciences and Medicine, Bond University, Gold Coast, QLD, Australia

Jessica Stokes-Parish Hunter Medical Research Institute, Hunter New England Local Health District, Newcastle, NSW, Australia

Zane Stromberga Faculty of Health Sciences and Medicine, Bond University, Gold Coast, QLD, Australia

Nancy Sullivan Johns Hopkins University School of Medicine and Nursing, Baltimore, MD, USA

Linda Sweet Deakin University and Western Health Partnership, Melbourne, VIC, Australia

Sandra Swoboda Johns Hopkins University School of Medicine and Nursing, Baltimore, MD, USA

Rebecca A. Szabo Department of Obstetrics & Gynaecology and Department of Medical Education, Gandel Simulation Service The Royal Women's Hospital, University of Melbourne, Melbourne, VIC, Australia

Joanna Tai Centre for Research in Assessment and Digital Learning, Deakin University, Geelong, VIC, Australia

Arianne Teherani Department of Medicine and Center for Faculty Educators, School of Medicine, University of California, San Francisco, CA, USA

Pim Teunissen Faculty of Health Medicine and Life Sciences (FHML), School of Health Professions Education (SHE), Maastricht University, Maastricht, The Netherlands

M. C. Turner School of Clinical Medicine, The University of Queensland, St Lucia, QLD, Australia

Neil Tuttle Discipline of Physiotherapy, Griffith University, Gold Coast, QLD, Australia

Ruby Walter School of Nursing and Midwifery, College of Science, Health and Engineering, LaTrobe University, Melbourne, VIC, Australia

Helena Ward Faculty of Health and Medical Sciences, The University of Adelaide, Adelaide, SA, Australia

C. J. Watling Centre for Education Research and Innovation, Schulich School of Medicine and Dentistry, Western University, London, ON, Canada

Andy Wearn Medical Programme Directorate, Faculty of Medical and Health Sciences, University of Auckland, Auckland, New Zealand

Susan M. Wearne Health Workforce Division, Commonwealth Department of Health, Canberra, ACT, Australia

Academic Unit of General Practice, Australian National University, Canberra, ACT, Australia

Jennifer M. Weller-Newton Department of Rural Health, Melbourne University, Melbourne, VIC, Australia

School of Nursing, McMaster University, Hamilton, ON, Canada

Nursing and Midwifery, Monash University, Melbourne, VIC, Australia

Emmalee Weston Austin Health, Melbourne, VIC, Australia

Marjorie L. White The Office of Interprofessional Simulation for Innovative Clinical Practice, University of Alabama at Birmingham, Birmingham, AL, USA

Departments of Pediatric Emergency Medicine and Medical Education School of Medicine, University of Alabama at Birmingham, Birmingham, AL, USA

Department of Health Services Administration School of Health Professions, University of Alabama at Birmingham, Birmingham, AL, USA

Leeroy William Eastern Health Clinical School, Monash University, Box Hill, VIC, Australia

Eloise Williams Northern Health, La Trobe University, Melbourne, VIC, Australia

Raymond Yap Department of Surgery, Cabrini Hospital, Cabrini Monash University, Malvern, Melbourne, VIC, Australia

Mong-Lin Yu Department of Occupational Therapy, School of Primary and Allied Health Care, Faculty of Medicine, Nursing and Health Sciences, Monash University, Frankston, VIC, Australia

Introduction

We believe *Clinical Education for the Health Professions* represents, supports, and advances scholarship and practice in the field of health professions education. The development process of this major reference work (MRW) is important to appreciate the contents. In this introduction, we outline the process of development, our editorial practices, and characteristics of the contributors and then provide an overview of each part.

The Development Process

One editor (Debra Nestel) was approached by the publisher to propose an MRW for clinical education. The Springer MRWs are intended to provide a "foundational starting point for students, researchers, and professionals needing authoritative, expertly validated summaries of a field, topic or concept." (1) The MRW concept is also attractive because it enables individual chapters to be updated by authors as required. Some fields move more quickly than others, and so we believe that the MRW gives authors more flexibility in revising their work to maintain currency, rather than the traditional single volume with one publication date.

One aim of the MRW was to present accessible and evidence-based content, on *what is known* about many facets of clinical education. While we acknowledged the proposed audience outlined in the Springer MRW, our main target audience was anticipated to be individuals involved in the design and delivery of educational activities for health professionals and students. Additionally, the likely audience will include researchers, policy makers, and others involved in any facet of health professional practice.

In initial development, DN identified a small editorial team with diverse experiences of working in clinical education. While a slightly daunting prospect, once the editorial team was assembled and the proposal and specific aims were outlined, the project quickly shifted to one of honor and excitement as the editorial team reached out to our networks for contributions.

The development process was fluid, with the initial proposal comprising 122 chapters across 9 parts. As we consulted with prospective authors, the proposal was adjusted to further reflect their expertise, and this meant some ideas initially proposed as independent chapters were combined (and, on some occasions, chapters were omitted). The COVID-19 pandemic also occurred during the commissioning process, which meant that some new chapters were added, and the entire project took longer than we had originally planned.

We were keen to promote chapters with multiple authors facilitating diverse perspectives and, sometimes even within a chapter, to have authors from different parts of the world. Our editorial team typically appointed a senior author and, with support and guidance, agreed that final decisions about author team were for the senior author to make.

We were also excited by the management of chapters through the Springer Meteor system, which is like online peer review systems for academic journals. This greatly assisted the management of the review process. All reviews were undertaken by the editorial team, with at least two reviewers for each chapter.

The depth of content varies across chapters. This was intentional, as it reflects the diversity of topics we selected for inclusion, as well as the dynamic nature of the field of health professions education. Some topics are already well established in both scholarship and practice (e.g., feedback, supervision), while others have a very wide scope (e.g., history and trends chapters), or are relatively new contributions to the field (e.g., ecological systems theory, planetary education, etc.). Among other things, these different reasons for inclusion accounted for the varying levels of depth.

The editorial team felt strongly that the final, published chapters in this MRW should reflect the professional and scholarly voices of the authors. While this is easy to claim, our experience as authors ourselves has been that editors can impose their own vision on the work so strongly that the voices of individual authors disappear. Instead, we saw our task as ensuring there was a consistent narrative to the overall MRW, as well as to each part within it, and to remind authors of what we thought would be valuable to the broad readership of the MRW. We hope that our editorial efforts have been successful, allowing authors' voices to come through in individual chapters that fit together across the work.

We are conscious of international differences in the terms used to describe health professions and their education and training. Rather than mandating language, or seeking to "standardize" terms, we left author teams to decide what was most appropriate. Our feedback encouraged authors to invite readers to consider how the terms might relate to their contexts, and to make connections across geographical, linguistic, and other contexts.

The Editorial Team

While as editors we had previously variously worked with each other, assembling as an editorial team was an exciting opportunity to bring our networks together. We have briefly sketched our profiles (see editor biographies). Our experiences are diverse, together with the places that we have worked. The institutions in which our networks have developed include large, long-established world-leading research-intensive universities associated with academic health sciences centers and teaching hospitals and those that are relatively new, privately funded, and vocationally focused.

Contributors to the MRW

As editors, we looked at this MRW as a chance to help broaden the diversity of voices represented in the literature, and to provide opportunities to a range of scholars at various stages in their careers and from both clinical and academic backgrounds. This is an effort that we as individuals are committed to continuing – it is never complete, of course, due to the dynamic nature of the field. We surveyed our authors near the completion of the project and found that, based on those who responded, we have contributions from scholars and researchers representing 13 countries, a near balance of clinical and other backgrounds, more than a dozen health professions, and a near balance of gender identification.

Within our author community are early-career scholars and long-time experts in their fields, and they are highly educated: over 80% of contributors reported having master's qualifications, and over 60% reported having doctoral qualifications.

While we sought a diverse mix of contributors, we had hoped to have an even more international group of authors. Especially missing were voices from the southern Americas, Africa, and Asia. This continues to be an area of weakness for the field, impoverishing our shared conversation and negatively impacting our work as educators.

About the Major Reference Work

The final version of the MRW is divided into eight parts, reflecting our attempts to meaningfully map the terrain of health professions education. Some chapters will only appear in an online version since they were unavailable at the time of publication. We focus first on the contemporary context of health professions education; shift focus to theoretical underpinnings, curriculum considerations, and approaches to supporting learning in clinical settings; a specific focus to assessment approaches; and then to evidence-based educational methods and content. Governance and other formal processes associated with the maturation of education programs are considered, including the increasing professionalization of clinical education. Finally, we look to the future drawing upon much of what has surfaced in the past and present.

Part I: The Contemporary Context of Health Professions Education

Part I comprises 17 chapters that examine the contemporary contexts of health professions education. Making meaning of contemporary practice is sometimes achieved by authors examining the origins of their practice, which is illustrated for education and training in surgery, nursing, midwifery, and dentistry. While there are similarities across professions, there are also many differences and particularities that justify the range of chapters offered. Even within medicine, the trends and contexts for specialties vary (e.g., general practice, surgery, anesthesia, etc.). We also wanted to promote health professions that are often less well represented in mainstream literature; this led to chapters on mental health and allied health. There are sometimes very specific drivers for change in the structure and process of professional education. One chapter addresses structural issues in the provision of specialty training (e.g., decentralization of surgical training), while another chapter describes the provision of education in low- and middle-income countries. Part I finishes with a chapter outlining what is likely to become mainstream in educational approaches that were developed in response to the COVID-19 pandemic.

Part II: Philosophical and Theoretical Underpinning of Health Professions Education

There are frequent calls to improve the theoretical underpinnings of health professions education. While there are many classifications of educational theories (or theories that inform educational design and practice), we sought here to include theories that are either commonly cited in educational design or research studies, and that were most likely to inform readers' practices. The theories vary in their focus on individuals or the settings in which the learning occurs and emphasize cognitive, behavioral, or constructivist approaches to learning. Each theory is likely to have most relevance to educational design and practice. From the 13 chapters, selected examples include: *mastery learning*, which has been popularized in simulation-based education for supporting the development of procedural skills; *threshold concepts and troublesome knowledge*, which has become a powerful influence in framing curriculum content; a framework from *social semiotics*, which fosters reflection of the ways in which clinicians make sense of, and the meanings they ascribe to, all facets of their work; the theoretical notion of *communities of practice*, including the role of professional identify development; *reflective practice*, such that it has become the essence of professional practice; and *ecological systems theory*, which that provides a lens to examine individuals' development within the complex and dynamic systems of clinical learning and practice. Part II ends with a critical reflection on the *philosophy of health professions education*, offering a tool for readers to deepen their thinking and practice about education.

Part III: Curriculum Considerations in Health Professions Education

Conceptually, *curriculum considerations* could cover any amount of content, so in this part of the MRW, we have had to be selective. There is also some overlap between Parts III, IV, and V, meaning that in some cases we had to make editorial decisions about where to locate the chapter content within the broader scope of the MRW. While authors developed their chapters based on our brief, we respected the authors' expertise to take the chapter in the directions they thought most appropriate. We have 14 chapters with an exciting range of considerations, such as: the role of public engagement in curricula; using simulation as substitution for clinical placements; how social media can inform curriculum design; exploring nuances in the educational design for teaching simple and complex psychomotor skills; debriefing practices in simulation-based education; and effective written feedback. Another important thread is the development of professional identity among students and trainees in the health professions. There are also explorations of contemporary issues, including the role of technology in health professions education; teaching about the role of diversity; and planetary health in health curricula. Other chapters cover diverse topics such as learning and teaching ethics in healthcare; the hidden curriculum and its variants; and the role of the arts and humanities.

Part IV: Supporting Learning in Clinical Settings

In Part IV, comprising 14 chapters, the authors explore ways in which learning can be supported in various settings. While principles to support learning may be similar, their application can manifest in different ways derived from many factors. A key factor is that learning in clinical settings usually takes place alongside, or as part of, healthcare service delivery. There is expert commentary provided from an interprofessional perspective, from a nursing perspective relative to learning "at the bedside" and in "the operating theater." Based on a scoping review, learning and teaching in the operating theater from a surgeon perspective is provided. The patient population can also influence opportunities to learn and teach, and we include an example from pediatrics. For clinical educators to function effectively, there are considerations for their development too. One chapter outlines the qualities of clinical educators, especially in their capacity to support learning in clinical settings, alongside care delivery. Another chapter considers well-being in health professions training. While simulation is not strictly a *clinical* setting, we have included it in this part, because the opportunity to learn using simulation often prepares healthcare professionals to optimize their learning in clinical practice. One chapter illustrates a process for setting up a simulation service in a healthcare institution, and another provides a specific example of a simulation program to promote the development of communication skills across a health service. Three chapters consider the role of interpersonal relationships and conversation in clinical settings – specifically, targeting feedback, supervision, and the ways in which trainees learn and develop through their telephone conversations. The final chapter considers underperformance, its recognition, and approaches to management.

Part V: Assessment in Health Professions Education

We have a focused part dedicated to assessment. We consider assessment as any form of measurement of individuals – and for purposes of entering, progressing, or completing professional training; final qualification within specialties; or ongoing professional registration. Nine chapters cover foundational and contemporary approaches to assessment in health professions education. There are specific examples from occupational therapy, surgery, and the impact of COVID-19 on assessment practices.

Part VI: Evidence-Based Health Professions Education: Focus on Educational Methods and Content

The 14 chapters in Part VI target evidence-based educational methods and content in health professions education. There is evidence of human-based strategies: team-based learning, peer learning, and coaching. Core practices for all health professionals are examined – patient-centered communication skills and clinical reasoning. Staying with the human focus, a chapter looks at key sociological concepts for health professions education. Contemporary technology-mediated educational methods are also explored and include examples from teaching procedural and other clinical skills, screen-based learning, and artificial intelligence.

Part VII: Governance, Quality Improvement, Scholarship, and Leadership on Health Professions Education

In Part VII, the eight chapters cover governance in health professions education. This necessarily includes considerations of quality and improvement. The role of professional bodies is explored, as well as that of scholarship in professional education. This part reflects the maturation of the profession of clinical education, and of clinical educators.

Part VIII: Future Direction for Health Professions Education

In our educational practice, we value the importance of being future-focused. Embedded in many of the earlier chapters are hints at future directions. However, in this part, it becomes the sole focus. The first chapter reflects a future world in which junior doctors will learn. The chapter offers two contrasting scenarios, and what is key to success is the importance of productive human relationships, of which one form is mentoring. While not a new concept itself, the authors describe its prominence, potentially shifting career directions for individuals based on single encounters. In an era of workforce shortages and maldistribution, human relationships become even more important to nurture trainees. If the authors' thoughtfulness reflects the future of the medical workforce, then we have much to look forward to. We also wish the authors success with their own specialty training. Two chapters are written by the same author team – first focusing on curriculums for healthcare professionals and the second on the competencies of those involved in education, in designing curriculums, and in their implementation. Technology is a focus in both chapters with implications for the curriculum itself and those who provide it.

In summary, this MRW consists of almost 90 chapters of research and scholarship, which we and the authors hope will inspire your practice, expand your thinking, support your learners and trainees, and help you to create the future of health professions education. We are already using the chapters in our own teaching, having been inspired and impressed by the quality of the authors' contributions.

When we took on this project, we had high hopes for the MRW. Those hopes have been exceeded, as we were astounded by the quality, breadth, and depth of the contributions from our colleagues around the world. Although it has been a challenge, and the project has taken longer than we originally planned, it has been our pleasure and privilege to curate this MRW.

Part IV

Supporting Learning in Clinical Settings

Learning and Teaching in Clinical Settings: Expert Commentary from an Interprofessional Perspective

45

Debra Kiegaldie

Contents

Introduction	848
Historical Context, Political Climate, and Drivers for Interprofessionalism	850
Benefits of IPL in Relation to IPCP	851
Characteristics of IPL Delivery in Clinical Settings	851
Types of Teaching and Learning Approaches Used in IPL	853
An Exchange-Based IPL Approach	853
An Action-Based IPL Approach	854
A Blended IPL Approach	854
A Simulation-Based Education IPL Approach	855
Practice-Based Learning Approaches	855
Challenges of Interprofessional Learning	856
Outcomes from Reviews of the Literature	856
Getting Started on IPL in Clinical Practice Settings	857
Build on Existing Links	858
Build Opportunities in Clinical Settings	858
Benefits Demonstrated to all Stakeholders	858
Based on Best Evidence Approaches	858
Conclusion	863
Cross-References	863
Glossary	863
References	864

Abstract

Interprofessional learning is "... when two or more professions learn with, from and about each other to improve collaboration and quality of care..." (CAIPE 2002, p 2). Interprofessional learning in the context of clinical settings is aimed at

---

D. Kiegaldie (✉)
Faculty of Medicine, Nursing and Health Sciences, Monash University; Faculty of Health Sciences and Community Studies, Holmesglen Institute and Healthscope Hospitals, Melbourne, VIC, Australia
e-mail: debra.kiegaldie@holmesglen.edu.au

© Springer Nature Singapore Pte Ltd. 2023
D. Nestel et al. (eds.), *Clinical Education for the Health Professions*,
https://doi.org/10.1007/978-981-15-3344-0_59

ensuring health professional teams demonstrate effective interprofessional collaborative practice. Interprofessional collaborative practice is when "healthcare workers from different professional backgrounds work together with patients, carers, families and communities to deliver the highest quality of care (WHO 2010, p 13). Inherent in this definition is a common purpose, commitment and mutual respect" (L-TIPP 2009, p iv).

This chapter provides commentary on interprofessional learning (IPL) in the context of interprofessional collaborative practice (IPCP). It focuses on the IPL that takes place in clinical settings across the continuum of healthcare and social care education. Key terminology is described along with the historical and political drivers for interprofessional practice and IPL. The characteristics, benefits, and challenges of introducing IPL into complex clinical environments are explored using a range of evidence-based IPL initiatives. An Implementation framework and education design model are introduced as a practical way to support interprofessional teams wanting to establish IPL in their own clinical education contexts.

Keywords

Interprofessional learning · Interprofessional education · Interprofessional collaborative practice · Intraprofessional learning

Introduction

The international IPL community has developed several competency frameworks to describe IPCP (WHO 2010; CIHC 2010; IPEC 2011). These domains, principles, and competencies represent the knowledge, skills, and attitudes (professional behavior) needed for collaborative practice. Example domains include teamwork, roles and responsibilities, interprofessional communication, patient- and family-centered care, ethical practice and values, collaborative leadership, and conflict resolution (Weinstein et al. 2018). The competencies for IPCP generally fall into three learning domains – interprofessional knowledge, interprofessional skills, and interprofessional attitudes – all of which are required when undertaking a collaborative task or to achieve a desired patient-focused goal. It should be noted, however, that some of these competencies span across these categories, particularly patient-centered care. A summary of these competencies can be seen in Table 1.

When interpreting or assessing many of these competencies, caution is advised. IPL competencies are dependent on a number of contextual, learner, and teacher factors. By using a competency-based approach, there is a risk of reducing complex tasks to simple checklists that oversimplify the concepts involved (Thistlethwaite 2016).

Nevertheless, if IPCP is the desired outcome, then IPL is the means to achieve this. IPL that occurs in the clinical workplace can either include clinical placement learning for preregistration students or practice-based learning for health

Table 1 Competencies for interprofessional collaborative practice and learning domains (Weinstein et al. 2018; Barr 2002; Braithwaite et al. 2005a; Patterson and McMurray 2003; Pearson and Pandya 2006; Thistlethwaite 2012; Watts et al. 2007; O'Keefe et al. 2017; Reeves et al. 2018)

Competencies for interprofessional collaborative practice
Interprofessional knowledge
Awareness of professional role boundaries
Knowledge of other team members' expertise, background, knowledge, and values
Knowledge of individual roles and processes required to work collaboratively
Interprofessional skills
Team working skills (negotiation, delegation, time management, assessment of group dynamics)
Communication skills including interpersonal skills and effective social interaction
Conflict resolution skills
Collaboration skills
Collaborative leadership skills
Skills in providing accurate and timely information to those who need it at the appropriate time
Skills in coordinating and integrating care processes to ensure excellence, continuity, and reliability of the care provided including networking skills
Interprofessional attitudes
Ethical conduct
Deals with complexity and uncertainty
Respects, understands, and supports the roles of other professionals
Adaptive and flexible
Able and willing to share goals
Tolerant of differences

professionals in postgraduate studies or continuing professional development. Either way, it poses particular challenges as often the patient is the central feature and the highest priority.

The World Health Organization (WHO) in their seminal publication outlining a framework for action on interprofessional education and collaborative practice in the health professions describes IPL as "the process by which a group of students or workers from the health related occupations with different backgrounds learn together during certain periods of their education, with interaction as the important goal, to collaborate in providing promotive, curative, rehabilitative, and other health related services" (WHO 1988).

There are, however, problems associated with terminology in the IPL field. Barr et al. (2005) describes this as a "sinking in the semantics" with the field being "bedevilled by competing terms" (p. 31). In the health workforce context, IPL is often erroneously referred to as either interdisciplinary, multidisciplinary, or transprofessional. In relation to IPL in clinical practice settings, using the correct suffixes and prefixes is therefore important to clarify.

Suffixes: The suffix discipline refers to "subject," "discipline," or "field of study." Profession refers to a type of health professional worker such as a doctor or nurse, that is, an individual who has attained specialized knowledge after academic preparation (Oandasan and Reeves 2005).

Prefixes: The prefix multi- refers to "side by side," inter- is "collaborative," and "trans-" refers to role blurring or "transprofessional" (Oandasan and Reeves 2005), e.g., a nurse who takes on some of the roles of a doctor when delivering healthcare in developing countries where multiskilling is necessary. "Intra"-is a newer prefix that refers to collaborative learning that involves multiple members of the same profession working together to deliver quality care (CNO 2014). For a full list of definitions, refer to the glossary of terms at the end of this text.

IPL is consequently different than other forms of learning. Although the focus is still on subject content, there is another multifactorial layer of learning introduced such as learning about professional roles and the interactions that occur. Implicit in IPL is the notion of joint active learning. This adds greater complexity to the learning experiences and outcomes. This also makes it challenging to introduce.

Historical Context, Political Climate, and Drivers for Interprofessionalism

The history of IPCP and IPL is a rich one. According to Zwarenstein and Reeves (2000), the modern concern with interactions between doctors and nurses began with an opinion piece in a 1967 psychiatric journal. The authors likened the relationship to a game, a power struggle. The two professions were occupying the same patient care "space," but they communicated indirectly and manipulatively, with little warmth or mutual support – like a bad marriage. They argued that for this problem to be resolved, more radical approaches to collaborative working needed to be explored.

The Interprofessional Education (IPE) movement, having begun in the early 1960s, acquired greater prominence in the late 1970s when the World Health Organization (WHO), in the Declaration of Alma Ata: The Vision, sought "urgent action by all governments, development workers and the world community to train and work socially and technically as healthcare teams" (WHO 1978, p.1). The Bristol Royal Infirmary Inquiry in the UK was another significant turning point in the history of IPL. It examined the tragic deaths of children undergoing heart surgery between 1991 and 1995 and concluded that these children would probably have survived if treated elsewhere. The inquiry found poor organization, failure of communication, lack of leadership, paternalism, and a failure to put patients at the center of care were all contributors to the deaths of these children (Kennedy 2001).

Another watershed moment came with the *To Err is Human* report in which Kohn, Corrigan, and Donaldson (1999) declared that the "decentralized and fragmented nature of the health care system contributed to an epidemic of medical errors" (p.1) with failure of communication and lack of collaboration across disciplines a major contributor. Internationally, the WHO continued to add to the IPE agenda by convening a study group on IPE and Collaborative Practice in 2007. The product of this group was the 2010 Framework for Action on IPE and IPCP. This penultimate piece of work describes actions to advance IPE and IPCP and the actions to support this at the systems level. It has now become known as the call for action for policy-makers, decision-makers, educators, health workers, community leaders, and global health advocates to take action and move toward embedding IPE and IPCP in all aspects of healthcare service delivery. It provides ideas on how to contextualize existing health systems, how to commit to implementing principles of IPE and IPCP, and how to champion the benefits of IPCP with partners, educators, and health workers (WHO 2010).

The evidence supporting the implementation of IPL stretches across more than four decades with the drivers having emerged from multiple imperatives including rapid workforce changes, the need for a coordinated approach to the complexity of patient care, and the rise of the quality movement (Braithwaite et al. 2005a; Reeves 2016). The underpinning premise in all the drivers for IPL is that if individuals learn together, they will work better together, thus improving the delivery of care.

Benefits of IPL in Relation to IPCP

From a clinical practice perspective, the reported benefits of IPL and IPCP fall into three broad categories: benefits to the patient, benefits to the healthcare system, and benefits to the health professional. The claims about the benefits of IPL suggested in Table 2 are based on reported opinions, evaluation outcomes, and results of a small number of high-quality, more empirically oriented, research studies. Benefits to the patients are more difficult to substantiate in a clinical context and are based on only a handful of studies.

Characteristics of IPL Delivery in Clinical Settings

Most reported IPL initiatives in clinical settings involve nurses and doctors, as these are the two largest health professional groups in healthcare and social care (Abu-Rish et al. 2012). The learning preferences of learners and their past experiences of teamwork are also important considerations when designing learning activities. IPL teaching has the potential to move teachers out of their comfort zone and away from their area of subject expertise. To be effective, facilitators need to role model interprofessional attributes and have confidence in working in interprofessional groups (Reeves 2016). In a systematic review of IPL, Hammick et al. (2007) found that the quality of IPL supervision was the most important contribution to learner satisfaction and a key determinant to educational processes and outcomes. Skilled, knowledgeable interprofessional facilitators are integral for successful implementation of IPL initiatives (Botma 2019).

The clinical context for IPL activities varies and can be broadly categorized according to hospital- or community-based settings, settings that deal with acute or chronic clinical conditions or specific specialist areas (Barr et al. 2005). Clinical settings where there is evidence of effective IPL delivery include acute/critical care, aged care, community, rehabilitation, mental health, rural medicine, and palliative care (Reeves et al. 2010, 2017; Braithwaite et al. 2005b). The premise underpinning

Table 2 Benefits of IPL

Benefits to the patient	Benefits to the healthcare system	Benefits to the health professional/health professional student
Enables quality, holistic, safe, patient-centered care
Improves clarity of objectives for the patient
Enhances patient-family-community center goals and values
Enhances patient compliance
Meets patient's functional status needs
Supports the management of complex healthcare needs
Meets multiple patient needs
Improves health outcomes (decreased hospitalizations, shorter stays, less medical error[a])
Increases patient access to choice of provider
Delivers higher rates of patient satisfaction
Reduces patient mortality and morbidity[a]	Greater healthcare efficiency (reduces duplication and hospitalizations)
Ensures less fragmented care
Facilitates more creative and integrative responses in healthcare (diversity of team)
Common curricula develops a common world view (common values, language, and perspectives)
Enables care to be delivered across healthcare settings
Increases accountability
Integrates specialist and holistic care
Enables greater focus on preventative care
Less medical error[a]
Reduces healthcare costs[a]	Reduces the "silo" effect in education
Less hierarchy, competition, and conflict between professions
Modifies negative attitudes and perceptions of others
Remedies failures in trust and communication (provides for continuous communication)
Empowers all health professions
Enhances professional relationships (fosters respect)
Improves working/learning environment
Provides for greater job satisfaction
More positive impact on student learning, professional practice
Increases knowledge of other professions and their contributions/skills
Develops interpersonal and team working skills and collaborative competence

Adapted from (Braithwaite et al. 2005a; Thistlethwaite 2012; O'Keefe et al. 2017; Abu-Rish et al. 2012; Reeves et al. 2013; Thistlethwaite and Moran 2010; Welsch et al. 2018; Lim and Noble-Jones 2018; Lapkin et al. 2013; Kangas et al. 2018; Hammick et al. 2007; Clifton et al. 2006; Guck et al. 2019; Reeves et al. 2017
[a]less substantiated claims reported in the literature

most of these settings is the view that IPL works best where interprofessional teams exist.

One of the big debates about IPL is when should it be introduced to learners. There are two schools of thought. Some say it should be introduced early in the preregistration years (Barr et al. 2005). Others argue it would be more effective when students have not become "socialized" into their own professions and developed negative attitudes and stereotypes toward other healthcare and social care professions (Oandasan and Reeves 2005). A systematic review of IPL found that it is more effective at improving patient care if it is of longer duration (over a number of weeks) and delivered in the workplace, particularly in the acute care sector (Koppel et al. 2001). This review also found evidence to suggest that IPL, as continuing professional development, effects more change to learner behavior and patient care than in the preregistration setting (Koppel et al. 2001, p. 47).

Types of Teaching and Learning Approaches Used in IPL

A number of underpinning principles have been proposed to guide the educational planning process. All IPL approaches require detailed planning, involvement of all stakeholders, and articulation of clear learning objectives linked to curriculum and assessment outcomes (Weinstein et al. 2018). Balanced membership between professions, in terms of number, size, and stability, is also helpful to achieve the shared goal of improved patient care. Selection of subject matter must also be targeted toward generic topics and content clinically relevant to all participants with a common curriculum across all involved professions. Not only should the focus be on patient care but there should also be an explicit focus on learning about, and demonstrating the dynamics of IPCP and the skills of communication, teamwork, and conflict resolution. Often an equal emphasis on learning about a clinical topic as well as learning about the attributes of IPCP is required. Learners reportedly value both (Kiegaldie 2015).

The teaching approaches selected should be integrated, interactive, and inclusive. As such, IPL should be seen as collaborative, not competitive. Theory must be easily transferable to practice; learner-centered interactive learning activities must be considered; there should be opportunities for informal learning to take place to enable social interaction, and there is a need for establishing an inclusive, welcoming learning environment. The use of icebreakers is recommended to establish a comfortable environment, encourage initial interaction, and establish a culture of trust and openness (Kiegaldie 2015).

A variety of educational approaches work best, with a combination of didactic, clinical instruction observation and discussion all being useful approaches. Multiple IPL formats were used in the studies reviewed by Abu-Rish et al. (2012) such as small group learning, case-based learning, problem-based learning, reflective exercises, clinical teaching, direct interaction with patients, simulation, and community-based projects.

In his seminal work on the early developments of interprofessional education, Barr et al. (2005) first described five types of approaches, which are presented in Table 3. Examples that apply to the clinical context are provided.

The following presents some specific evidence-based vignettes of how these have been applied in clinical settings.

An Exchange-Based IPL Approach

Most exchange-based approaches report findings that increase knowledge about the roles and responsibilities of other professions. A postgraduate study from Canada using a case-based approach was trialed with a group of physicians, nurses,

Table 3 Classification of IPL teaching/learning approaches

Exchange-based learning	Methods that encourage participants to express views, exchange experience, compare perspectives, and expose prejudice *(e.g., shared case studies)*
Action-based learning	Methods of investigation and co-working such as collaborative enquiry (e.g., problem-based learning on clinical scenarios, continuous quality improvement projects, action research)
Observation-based learning	Psychodynamic observation (e.g., for students on placement, this could include joint patient visits, shadowing other, usually more experienced students, shadowing clinicians)
Simulation-based learning	The replication of a real clinical situation to enable relationships between professions to be explored and to receive feedback on performance as participants take different parts in realistic situations *(e.g., shared practice-based role-plays, technical skills training with part-task trainers, immersive* in situ *clinical scenarios with mannikins or simulated participants)*
Practice-based learning	Students or health professionals learning together on work-based care *(e.g., for student interprofessional training wards, interprofessional community placements, for health professionals team-based meetings, ward rounds)*

Adapted from (Barr et al. 2005)

pharmacists, physiotherapists, respiratory technicians, and kinesiologists. Following a description of the IPL literature and action research, participants were given time to create an interprofessional team approach to specific patient cases. The outcomes of this intervention were a greater understanding of others' viewpoints, enhanced interprofessional teamwork, and a recognition of the need for improved communication and collaboration (Verma et al. 2006).

An Action-Based IPL Approach

An action-based initiative focused on quality improvement and interprofessional practice was introduced into a US primary health curriculum. Participants included internal medicine residents, nurse practitioner students, pharmacy residents, and postdoctoral psychology fellows. Trainees worked in interprofessional teams to select, design, implement, evaluate, and present a project as part of a 9-month curriculum. In addition to learning about and applying quality improvement knowledge and skills, the trainees developed interprofessional skills including an appreciation of diverse perspectives and expertise (Dulay et al. 2020).

A Blended IPL Approach

The Vanderbilt Program in Interprofessional Learning based in the USA provides an excellent example of a blended approach to IPL. It places first and second year students from four professional degree programs (medicine, nursing, pharmacy, and social work) into authentic clinical environments over a 2-year period. The team spends one afternoon each week in clinic together seeing patients, creating personalized care plans, and working under the direction of a preceptor. It includes an immersion experience, seminar-based classroom teaching, simulations, and clinical experience. Students complete a capstone quality improvement project (Davidson et al. 2020). Aside from being a highly rated program from a learner perspective, 69 quality improvement projects have addressed aspects of care delivery processes and produced durable materials to contribute important innovations to the healthcare system (Davidson et al. 2020).

A Simulation-Based Education IPL Approach

Simulation-based education examples include role-play exercises, learning with simulated participants, and the use of part-task trainers and fully immersive manikin-based scenarios. It should be noted that despite many published studies in simulation investigating teamwork and communication across members of different health professions, the majority of the published research fail to measure interprofessional competencies.

A study based at the University of California examined the impact of an interprofessional standardized patient exercise on attitudes of learners from five different professions toward working in interprofessional teams. The context of learning was chronic illness management in ambulatory settings, and participants included nurse practitioners, doctors, pharmacists, physical therapists, and dentists. Perceived benefits included learning about the roles of healthcare professionals, working collaboratively, and educating other learners about their profession's role. Attitudes toward interprofessional teams showed small but significant improvements in team value and team efficiency post the experience (Wamsley et al. 2012).

Practice-Based Learning Approaches

Numerous practice-based examples are cited in the literature such as interprofessional ward rounds, community-based interprofessional clinics, and interprofessional team meetings. From a preregistration perspective, the introduction of interprofessional training wards (ITWs) provides one of the most enduring examples. In an ITW, students from different professions (nursing, medicine, allied health) collaboratively perform patient care with the goal of improving patient care. Having commenced in Sweden, ITWs have now been reported in over 12 different institutions throughout the world and show promising results in relation to patient satisfaction rates and student learning outcomes (Oosterom et al. 2019). The practical organization of ITW programs is generally based on the Scandinavian model and has the following common elements:

- An introductory session in which goals of the program are introduced
- Learners are often in the final stage of study and have a high degree of self-reliance and autonomy
- Most rotations last 2–3 weeks
- Learning objectives generally consist of profession-specific learning goals and interprofessional learning goals (Oosterom et al. 2019).

Many practice-based models likewise exist in the postgraduate context and include similar examples of positive outcomes. Examples cited in the literature include trainee general practitioners working with advanced nurse practitioners (O'Connor et al. 2018), pharmacists placed in an interprofessional training program within a primary health setting (Hazen et al. 2018), and academic-practice partnerships to foster IPCP and improve patient care outcomes in acute care hospital units (Hendricks et al. 2018).

Challenges of Interprofessional Learning

The path of introducing IPL into modern health profession education and clinical practice has not been smooth. Criticisms of IPL have focused on the need to respect and maintain the specialist's intellectual and practice base of each distinct profession (Braithwaite et al. 2005a). Overall, the reported challenges and barriers to introducing IPL are multifactorial and often relate to structural, personal, cultural, professional, organizational, and educational obstacles. The barriers that are common when undertaking IPL in clinical practice settings whether that be student placements, postgraduate learning, or continuing professional development are summarized in Table 4.

In relation to enablers for IPL in the clinical workplace, factors to consider include the presence of strong active leadership, clinical site readiness, a culture open to interprofessional clinical learning, and demonstrating the added value generated by having IPL in the clinical setting for continuous quality improvement (Hageman et al. 2017).

Outcomes from Reviews of the Literature

There has been no shortage of literature reviews about IPL. The first published systematic review was in 1999. Since then, there have been an excess of 40 published reviews across the spectrum of review types. In 2000, a UK-based team of interprofessional researchers published a Cochrane Review of IPL focused entirely on evidence for IPL interventions and limited to studies that employed randomized controlled trials, controlled before and after studies, and interrupted time series design. This was repeated in 2008 and 2013. Positive outcomes were reported in the following clinical contexts:

Table 4 Barriers to IPL in clinical contexts

Structural barriers	Cultural barriers	Educational barriers
Disproportionate numbers of learners and ensuring parity
Insufficient learning spaces
Alternate clinical placements
Availability of facilitators
Arranging meeting times
Education timing
Matching ratio of learners to facilitators	Profession differences in history, values, culture, race, gender, power dynamic, social class, and language
Perceived threat to professional identity
Mistrust between professions
Staff skepticism, unwillingness to experiment with new ways of teaching
Learners entrenched stereotypical views of other professions
Perception that clinical skills training is being diluted and that sharing of roles is to reduce costs and edge toward a generic health worker
The need to maintain the specialist intellectual and practice base of each profession	Differences in academic level of content and demands
Poor selection of professions/disciplines and team members
Institutional constraints
Lack of agreed goals that educators, learners, and professionals understand
No globally accepted core competencies of ICP
Varying practice demands
Distinctive assessment approaches of performance
Dealing with facilitator mindset barriers

Adapted from (Thistlethwaite 2012; Braithwaite et al. 2005b; Hall and Weaver 2001; Glen 2004; McKinlay and Pullon 2007; McNair et al. 2001)

- Emergency department culture and patient satisfaction
- Collaborative team behaviors and reduction of clinical error rates for emergency department teams
- Management of care delivered to domestic violence victims
- Mental health practitioner competencies related to the delivery of patient care
- Diabetes care
- Collaborative team behavior in operating rooms (Reeves et al. 2013).

In 2009, an additional review was conducted to assess the impact of practice-based interventions designed to change IPCP. The interventions included interprofessional rounds, interprofessional meetings, and externally facilitated interprofessional audits. Three of the studies had interventions that led to improvements in patient care such as drug use, length of stay, and total hospital charges (Zwarenstein et al. 2009).

Key findings from a synthesis of review evidence of interprofessional education that was first undertaken in 2010 and later updated in 2017 revealed that IPL can nurture development of knowledge, skills, and attitudes and enhance collaborative practice and patient outcomes noting that continued conduct of more quality research was needed in this field (Reeves et al. 2017).

Getting Started on IPL in Clinical Practice Settings

Given the complexity of IPL, particularly in clinical environments, it is reasonable to suggest that the use of a theoretical framework and education design model be considered. The WHO framework (WHO 2010) is useful to contemplate as an overarching framework. It outlines four critical components important to have in place before embarking on designing an IPL program in clinical settings:

Build on Existing Links

Before commencing, consider the current clinical context and the existing team environment. Questions to ask include:

- How many health professions could be involved?
- How are these members currently linked in terms of healthcare delivery?
- Is the learning program a small- or large-scale initiative?
- What ability is there to grow the program into the future?

Build Opportunities in Clinical Settings

This focuses on embedding the experience into a relevant contextual setting. Questions to ask include:

- What is the clinical context and setting for the potential IPL program, course or activity? (Is it a classroom, acute, subacute context, or is it in a community, regional, rural, or remote setting?)
- What clinical topic(s) should be considered and why? Remember learners often value the clinical topic just as much as the opportunity for IPL.

Benefits Demonstrated to all Stakeholders

Before planning the program, it is critically important to clearly identify how the program aims to benefit each stakeholder group because without their support the educational initiative is unlikely to succeed. Stakeholders include learners; the healthcare system, organization, or health service; and, most importantly, patients. Describing the benefits to each stakeholder group is integral to success.

Based on Best Evidence Approaches

It is not enough just to surmise that IPL is a good idea; educational designers need to be armed with the evidence of its efficacy to persuade the skeptics and convince stakeholders of its growing evidence base and why it should be included. As a systems-based theoretical model of learning, Biggs 3P model lends itself to work-based learning situations (Biggs 1989) and has been used extensively in the IPL field. It is comprised of three main components: presage, process, and product.

Presage factors	These factors exist prior to learning and relate to the student and the teaching context.
Process factors	This is the approach that learners use to process tasks. Biggs refers to it as either a deep or surface approach to learning (Biggs 1989).
Product factors	The product phase is related to qualitative differences in learning outcomes. In other words, deep approaches produce high-quality learning outcomes, while surface approaches result in lower-quality outcomes.

The 3P model offers an easy-to-understand approach to how all factors may affect the delivery of a program which in turn may impact on its outcomes (Baker et al. 2010). It also provides an excellent analytical tool for understanding the diversity of complex research about work-relevant learning (Tynjala 2013). Freeth and Reeves (2004) found that the 3P model was often overlooked, under-analyzed, and undermanaged in past IPL initiatives. They elaborated on this system, applied it specifically to IPCP, and presented a range of choices open to the IPL designer, particularly in the process variable section by placing more emphasis on teacher characteristics and the product section to include interprofessional competencies.

This model has been further extended to enhance the teaching and learning process by including an extra "P" for planning to emphasize the essential requirement for careful preparation and planning of all IPL interventions (Kiegaldie 2015). Presage and planning in fact go "hand in hand' with presage used to identify the issues and items and planning seen as the way to determine what is needed to ensure the presage is addressed. IPL creates a unique and complex learning environment. It is therefore important to add the "P" for planning to ensure that significant attention is given to this in the education development process. Presage relates to the "what," and planning is the "how" as in the action plan to address the political climate, regulatory frameworks, funding, management support, relationships to stakeholders, learner and teacher characteristics, administration and organization elements, space and time constraints, and competing curricula demands.

For the product components, it is essential to utilize a known evaluation framework. Kirkpatrick's hierarchy of outcomes modified for IPL that was first described by Barr et al. (2000) and later used in a number of systematic reviews of the IPL evaluation literature is suggested. Barr et al.'s (2000) framework adapts Kirkpatrick's four levels of educational outcomes to fit the IPL setting. This was later adapted to include two additional classification categories (see Table 2.3 – Levels 2a and 2b) (Hammick et al. 2007). This helps in overcoming criticisms of the Kirkpatrick model such as the propensity for educators and researchers to focus on Level 1 outcomes at the expense of others (Reio et al. 2017). A later adaptation by Payler, Myer, and Humphris (2007) added two further stages to incorporate pre-program data collection (Table 5).

Table 5 Modified Kirkpatrick evaluation for IPL evaluation (Payler et al. 2007)

Stage	Outcome measures
Literature review	Pedagogic processes in IPL
Preliminary level	Preprogram data collection
Level 1: reaction	Learners' views on the learning experience and its interprofessional nature
Level 2a modification of attitudes/perceptions	Changes in reciprocal attitudes or perceptions between participant groups. Changes in perception or attitude toward the value and/or use of team approaches to caring for a specific client group
Level 2b: acquisition of knowledge and skills	Including knowledge and skills linked to interprofessional collaboration
Level 3: behavioral change	Identifies individuals' transfer of interprofessional learning to their practice setting and changed professional practice
Level 4a: change in organizational practice	Wider changes in the organization and delivery of care
Level 4b: benefits to patients/clients	Improvements in health or well-being of patients/clients

A realist evaluation is another form of theory-driven evaluation (Pawson and Tilley 1997). It explores "what works in which circumstances and for whom" (as opposed to "does this work"). It was originally developed to explore complex social interventions and has recently emerged in health profession education, particularly in the IPL setting due to its complexity. Thistlethwaite, however, argues that due to its in-depth nature and time-consuming approach, it is rarely done without funding (Thistlethwaite 2016).

There is a wide range of validated and nonvalidated instruments measuring the impact of IPL on learners, organizations, and patients with most focusing on learner outcomes. A scoping review of instruments measuring interprofessional collaboration in healthcare found 29 instruments relevant to a variety of healthcare settings (Peltonen et al. 2020). While useful to see an expansion of instruments relevant to the clinical practice environment, the psychometric properties of these instruments are often unsystematic and in need of further testing and validation.

In summary, the 4Ps describe the educational context, the learner and teacher characteristics, the planning processes, the teaching and learning design, and the methods used to measure outcomes of an IPL program. Table 6 provides a practical guide for IPL teams designing an IPL education program in clinical practice environments using this 4P approach. It includes key questions to ask yourself and is also useful to consider when conducting research on IPL interventions. The planning components in this table are left blank as the actions required are context-dependent.

With the WHO framework (4B) as the starting point and the extended 4P as the educational model, a new educational paradigm called the 4B–4P approach to IPL education design can be considered when designing an IPL initiative (Kiegaldie 2015) (see Fig. 1). It should be noted that the 4B and 4P approach is not sequential or

Table 6 The 4B and 4P approach to IPL educational design

Items	Presage components (What are the issues?) Key questions to ask yourself	Planning components: the action plan (What do you need to do?)
The context		
Political climate	At the local level, in what way is the political climate right for introducing IPL?	
Regulatory framework	Are there any hindrances or considerations from accreditation or regulatory authorities?	
Funding	How much will it cost to deliver and where will the funds come from?	
Management support	What is your current organizational structure? Have you got management support?	
Relationship with stakeholders	Who are your stakeholders and how will they be informed of the program (e.g., learners, health service, teachers, patients)?	
What is the learning environment?	Where will the learning take place? What challenges will the environment pose (clinic, community practice, hospital ward, simulated clinical environment)?	
What resources do you have?	What resources will you need (technical, physical)?	
Competing interests	Are there any competing educational demands? Who will you manage this?	
The learners		
Learner characteristics	How many learners will be involved? Where are they located? Are the demographics similar (age, gender, culture)? Will this be compulsory or optional? What is their prior knowledge, skills attitudes, and conceptions of collaboration and learning? Are there competing learning needs? Are there social factors that might impact delivery?	
The teachers		
Teacher characteristics	Who will be your teachers/facilitators? What is their prior experience of IPL? How will you select them? Will they need training? How will this be managed? Who will be your IPL local champions?	
Process (the education program)		
What is the overall direction of the program? What are the anticipated learning objectives?		
What topics will you include in the teaching? What is the rationale for their selection?		
What teaching approaches and activities will you select (interprofessional case-based discussion, working in pairs in a community health center identifying roles, leading a grand round on collaborative management of a clinical problem, developing joint care plans, participating in immersive simulations, quality improvement projects, etc.)?		

(continued)

Table 6 (continued)

Items	Presage components (What are the issues?) Key questions to ask yourself	Planning components: the action plan (What do you need to do?)
	Are the learning activities constructively aligned to the learning objectives? What will the learners and teachers be doing?	
	What additional resources will you need (scenarios, case studies, simulated participants, facilitator training materials, videos, role-plays, written learning activities)?	
Product (evaluation of outcomes)		
	What theory-based evaluation framework will you use (e.g., Kirkpatrick, realist, other)? What aspects will you evaluate (e.g., learner perceptions of their ability to work collaboratively in clinical practice; learner perceptions of their development in knowledge, skills, and attitudes; learners' perceptions of the learning experience (process), behavior outcomes, organizational outcomes, patient-related outcomes, patient satisfaction)? What instruments will you use to measure outcomes?	

Adapted from Freeth and Reeves (2004); Kiegaldie (2015)

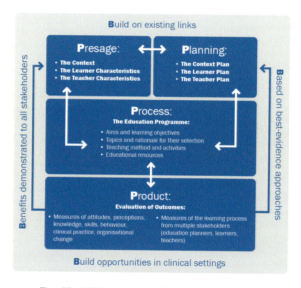

Fig. 1 The 4B–4P approach to educational design (adapted from Kiegaldie 2015) (to check citation This is an original diagram which I have created for this chapter but its adapted from content from my thesis which is the Kiegaldie 2015 citation)

linear. Educational designers could start with a vision or simply a bright idea and then revisit other aspects to ensure all components of the 4B and 4P have been addressed. It is therefore an iterative, multidirectional process with equal attention needed on every component. Ignoring any could very well make the difference between failure and success.

Conclusion

This chapter has provided commentary on teaching and learning in clinical practice settings from an interprofessional perspective. It has revealed evidence to demonstrate the value of healthcare professionals learning how to work together to develop their interprofessional competencies.

It is clear that IPL is complex to design and deliver, particularly in the clinical setting. The structural, cultural, and educational challenges create barriers that need to be overcome with multiple factors to consider. Learner and teacher characteristics, the stage and duration of the teaching, the type of teaching approach to use, and the outcomes to measure all need due diligence and planning. Ensuring that key stakeholder input is achieved and sustained is likewise just as important for ongoing sustainability. To design highly effective IPL, it is important to consider a comprehensive framework and educational model such as the 4B–4P approach to educational design with equal attention needed on every component to ensure success.

Spanning over 40 years, the WHO has been urging IPL to be embedded in all aspects of healthcare service delivery. There is a critical need for health professionals to have a shared understanding of this and a need for their actions and communication to always be directed at the best care possible, care that collaboratively, compassionately, and holistically meets the needs of patients and their families.

Cross-References

- ▶ Developing Patient Safety Through Education
- ▶ Developing Professional Identity in Health Professional Students
- ▶ Interprofessional Education (IPE): Trends and Context
- ▶ Team-Based Learning (TBL): Theory, Planning, Practice, and Implementation

Glossary

Interprofessional Education (IPE) "Occasions where two or more professions learn with, from and about each other to improve collaboration and the quality of care" (CAIPE, 2002).

Interprofessional Learning (IPL) "Learning arising from interaction between members (or students) of two or more professions. This may be a product of IPE or happen spontaneously in the workplace or in education sessions" ((Freeth et al. 2005), p. xv).

Interprofessional Collaborative Practice (ICP) "Two or more professions working together as a team with a common purpose, commitment and mutual respect" ((L-TIPP 2009), p. iv).

Interprofessionalism "an approach to team-working which emphasises highly collaborative practice and problem-solving" (Bromage 2009).

Multiprofessional Learning (MPL) "where members (or students) of two or more professions learn side by side; in other words, parallel rather than interactive learning" (Barr et al. 2005, p.32).

Multidisciplinary Education (MDE) "education between different branches of the same profession or between academic disciplines" (Barr and Low 2013, p.4), for example: a physician and a surgeon.

Uniprofessional Learning (UPL) "where members of a single profession learn together" (Freeth et al. 2005, p.xvii).

Transprofessional Learning (TPL) An emerging term not fully explained nor analysed in the literature. "A framework for professionals which allows for the sharing and integration of expertise among team members where members of a single profession learn together" (Bell et al. 2010, p.143) or, "...teamwork that includes non-professional health workers that might be of even greater importance for health-system performance, especially the teamwork of professionals with basic and ancillary health workers, administrators and managers, policymakers, and leaders of the local community" (Frenk et al. 2010, p.1944).

Intraprofessional Learning (IntraPL) "Multiple members of the same profession working together to deliver quality care" (CNO 2014).

References

Abu-Rish E, Kim S, Choe L, Varpio L, Malik E, White A, et al. Current trends in interprofessional education of health sciences students: a literature review. J Interprof Care. 2012;26:444–51.

Baker L, Egan-Lee E, Karen L, Silver I, Reeves S. Exploring an IPE faculty development program using the 3-P model. J Interprof Care. 2010;24(5):597–600.

Barr H. Interprofessional education today, yesterday and tomorrow: a review. London: LTSN for Health Sciences and Practice; 2002.

Barr H, Low H. Introducing interprofessional education. CAIPE: Fareham; 2013. Available from: http://caipe.org.uk/silo/files/introducing-interprofessional-education.pdf

Barr H, Freeth D, Hammick M, Koppel I, Reeves S. Evaluations of interprofessional education: A United Kingdom review of health and social care. London: CAIPE and the British Educational Research Association; 2000.

Barr H, Koppel I, Reeves S, Hammick M, Freeth D. In: Barr H, editor. Effective interprofessional education: argument, assumption & evidence. Oxford, UK: Blackwell Publishing; 2005.

Bell A, Corfield M, Davies J, Richardson N. Collaborative transdisciplinary intervention in early years – putting theory into practice. Child Care Health Dev. 2010;36:142–8.

Biggs J. Approaches to the enhancement of tertiary teaching. High Educ Res Dev. 1989;8(1):7–25. https://doi.org/10.1080/0729436890080102.

Botma. Consensus on interprofessional facilitator capabilities. J Interprof Care. 2019;33(3):277–9.

Braithwaite J, Travaglia J. In: Health A, editor. Inter-professional learning and clinical education: an overview of the literature. Braithwaite and Associates and the ACT Health Department: Canberra; 2005a.

Braithwaite J, Travaglia J. In: Department. AH, editor. Inter-professional learning and clinical education: an overview of the literature. Canberra: ACT Health Department; 2005b.

Bromage A. Interprofessional Education Birmingham: Higher Education Resources; 2009. Available from: Available http://highereducationresources.atspace.com/interprofessional.htm

CAIPE, Defining IPE: Centre for the Advancement of Interprofessional Education. 2002. Available from: http://caipe.org.uk/resources/defining-ipe/

CIHC. A National Interprofessional Competency Framework; 2010 [1–18]. Available from: www.cich.ca/files/CICH_IPCompetencies_Feb1210.pdf.

Clifton M, Dale C, Bradshaw C. The impact and effectiveness of inter-professional education in primary care: a literature Review. London: Royal College of Nursing; 2006.

CNO. RN and RPN practice: the client, the nurse and the environment: college of Nurses of Ontario; 2014. Available from: https://www.cno.org/globalassets/docs/prac/41062.pdf

Davidson H, Hilmes MA, Cole S, Waynick-Rogers P, Provine A, Rosenstiel D, et al. The Vanderbilt program in interprofessional learning: sustaining a longitudinal clinical experience that aligns practice with education. Acad Med. 2020;95(4):553–8.

Dulay M, Saxe JM, Odden K, Strewler A, Lau A, O'Brien B, Shunk R. Promoting quality improvement in primary care through a longitudinal, project-based, interprofessional curriculum. MedEdPORTAL. 2020;16:10932. https://doi.org/10.15766/mep_2374-8265.10932. PMID: 32934977; PMCID: PMC7485912

Freeth D, Reeves S. Learning to work together: using the presage, process, product (3P) model to highlight decisions and possibilities. J Interprof Care. 2004;18(1):43–56.

Freeth D, Hammick M, Reeves S, Koppel I, Barr H. In: Barr H, editor. Effective Interprofessional education: development, delivery & evaluation. Oxford: Blackwell Publishing; 2005.

Frenk J, Chen L, Bhutta Z, Cohen J, Crisp N, Evans T, et al. Health professionals for a new century: transforming education to strengthen health systems in in interdependent world. Lancet. 2010;376:1923–58.

Glen S. Interprofessional education: the evidence base influencing policy and policy makers. Nurse Educ Today. 2004;24(3):157–9.

Guck TP, Potthoff MR, Walters RW, Doll J, Greene MA, DeFreece T. Improved outcomes associated with interprofessional collaborative practice. Ann Fam Med. 2019;17(nSuppl 1):S82.

Hageman HL, Huggett KN, Simpson D, SHasbrouck CS, Stuber ML, Luk J, et al. Operationalizing interprofessional education in the clinical workplace. Med Sci Educators. 2017;27:753–8.

Hall P, Weaver L. Interdisciplinary education and teamwork: a long and winding road. Med Educ. 2001;35:867–75.

Hammick M, Freeth D, Koppel I, Reeves S, Barr H. A best evidence systematic review of interprofessional education: BEME guide no. 9. Med Teach. 2007;29(8):735–51.

Hazen A, de Groot E, de Gier H, Damoiseaux R, Zwart D, Leendertse A. Design of a 15 month interprofessional workplace learning program to expand the added value of clinical pharmacists in primary care. Curr Pharm Teach Learn. 2018;10:618–26.

Hendricks S, LaMothe VM, Halstead JA, Taylor J, Ofner S, Chase L, Dunscomb J, Chael A, Priest C. Fostering interprofessional collaborative practice in acute care through an academic-practice partnership. J Interprof Care. 2018;32(5):613–20. https://doi.org/10.1080/13561820.2018.1470498.

IPEC. Core competencies for interprofessional collaborative practice: report of an expert panel. Washington, DC: Interprofessional Education Collaborative; 2011. Available from: www.aacn.nche.edu/education-resources/ipecreport.pdf

Kangas S, Rintala T, Jaatinen P. An integrative systematic review of interprofessional education on diabetes. J Interprof Care. 2018;32(6):706–18.

Kennedy I. Learning from Bristol: the report of the public inquiry into children's heart surgery at the Bristol Royal Infirmary 1984–1995. London: The Stationary Office; 2001. http://docs.scie-socialcareonline.org.uk/fulltext/bristolresponsefull.pdf

Kiegaldie D. Learning about delirium in a simulated clinical environment: an interprofessional learning intervention for final year medical and nursing students. Melbourne: Monash University; 2015.

Kohn LT, Corrigan JM, Donaldson MS. To err is human. Washington, DC: National Academy Press/Institute of Medicine; 1999.

Koppel I, Barr H, Reeves S, Freeth D, Hammick M. Establishing a systematic approach to evaluating the effectiveness of interprofessional education. Issues Interdiscip Care. 2001;3(1):41–9.

Lapkin S, Levett-Jones T, Gilligan C. A systematic review of the effectiveness of interprofessional education in health professional programs. Nurse Educ Today. 2013;33:90–102.

Lim AFN, Noble-Jones R. Interprofessional education (IPE) in clinical practice for pre-registration nursing students: a structured literature review. Nurse Educ Today. 2018;68:218–25.

L-TIPP. Interprofessional health education in Australia: the way forward. In: University of Sydney and the University of Technology S, editor. 2009.

McKinlay E, Pullon S. Interprofessional learning – the solution to collaborative practice in primary care. Nurs N Z. 2007;13(10):16–8.

McNair R, Brown R, Stone N, Sims J. Rural interprofessional education: promoting teamwork in primary health care education and practice. Aust J Rural Health. 2001;9(Suppl 1):S19–26.

O'Connor L, Carpenter B, O'Connor C, O'Driscoll J. An interprofessional learning experience for trainee general practitioners in an academic urban minor injuries unit with advanced nurse practitioners. Int J Emerg Nurs. 2018;41:19–24.

O'Keefe M, Henderson A, Chick R. Defining a set of common interprofessional learning competencies for health profession students. Med Teach. 2017;39(5):463–8.

Oandasan I, Reeves S. Key elements for interprofessional education. Part 1: the learner, the educator and the learning context. J Interprof Care. 2005;19(Suppl 1):21–38.

Oosterom N, Floren LC, ten Cate O, Westerveld HE. A review of interprofessional training wards: enhancing student learning and patient outcomes. Med Teach. 2019;41(5):547–54.

Patterson E, McMurray A. Collaborative practice between registered nurses and medical practitioners in Australian general practice: Moving from rhetoric to reality. Aust J Adv Nurs. 2003;20(4):43–8.

Pawson R, Tilley N. Realist evaluation. London: Sage; 1997.

Payler J, Meyer E, Humphris D. Theorizing interprofessional pedagogic evaluation: framework for evaluating the impact of interprofessional continuing professional development on practice change. Learn Health Soc Care. 2007;6(3):156–69.

Pearson D, Pandya H. Shared learning in primary care: Participants' views of the benefits of this approach. J Interprof Care. 2006;20(3):302–13.

Peltonen J, Leino-Kilpi H, KHeikkila H, Rautava P, Tuomela K, Siekkinen M, et al. Instruments measuring interprofessional collaboration in healthcare – a scoping review. J Interprof Care. 2020;34(2):147–61.

Reeves S. Why we need interprofessional education to improve the deliver of safe and effective care. Interface. 2016;20(56):185–97.

Reeves S, Goldman J, Sawatzky-Girling B, Burton A. A synthesis of systematic reviews of interprofessional education. J Allied Health. 2010;39(Suppl1):S198–203.

Reeves S, Perrier L, Goldman J, Freeth D, Zwarenstein M. Interprofessional education: effects on professional practice and healthcare outcomes (update). Cohrane Database Syst Rev. 2013;2013(3):1–41.

Reeves S, Palaganas J, Zierler B. An updated synthesis of review evidence of interprofessional education. J Allied Health. 2017;46(1):56–61.

Reeves S, Xyrichis A, Zwarenstein M. Teamwork, collaboration, coordination, and networking: why we need to distinguish between different types of interprofessional practice. J Interprof Care. 2018;32(1):1–3.

Reio TG, Rocco TS, Smith DH, Chang E. A critique of Kirkpatrick's evaluation model. New Horiz Adult Educ Human Resource Dev. 2017;29(2):35–53. https://doi.org/10.1002/nha3.20178.

Thistlethwaite J. Interprofessional education: a review of context, learning and the research agenda. Med Educ. 2012;46:58–70.

Thistlethwaite JE. Collaboration, cooperation, communication, contact and competencies. GMS J Med Educ. 2016;33(2):1–11.

Thistlethwaite J, Moran MC. Learning outcomes for interprofessional education (IPE): literature review and synthesis. J Interprof Care. 2010;24(5):503–13.

Tynjala P. Toward a 3-P model of workplace learning: a literature review. Vocat Learn. 2013;6:11–36.

Verma S, Medves J, Paterson M, Patteson A. Demonstrating interprofessional education using a workshop model. J Interprof Care. 2006;20(6):679–81.

Wamsley M, Staves J, Kroon L, Topp K, Hossaini M, Newlin B, et al. The impact of an interprofessional standardized patient exercise on attitudes toward working in interprofessional teams. J Interprof Care. 2012;26:28–35.

Watts F, Lindqvist S, Pearce S, Drachler M, Richardson B. Introducing a post-registration interprofessional learning programme for healthcare teams. Med Teach. 2007;29(5):457–63.

Weinstein AR, Reidy AP, Simon L, Makosky A, Williams R, Collin C, et al. Creating interprofessional learning in practice. Clin Teach. 2018;17:22–30.

Welsch LA, Hoch J, Poston RD, Parodi A, Akpinar-Elci M. Interprofessional education involving didactic TeamSTEPPS and interactive healthcare simulation: a systematic review. J Interprof Care. 2018;32(6):657–65.

WHO, editor Declration of Alma-Ata. International conference on primary health care; 1978; USSR: World Health Organisation.

WHO. Learning together to work together for health. Geneva: World Health Organization; 1988, pp 6–7.

WHO. Framework for action on interprofessional education & collaborative practice. Geneva: World Health Organization; 2010.

Zwarenstein M, Reeves S. What's so good about collaboration? Br Med J. 2000;320(7241):1022–3. Available from: http://www.ncbi.nlm.gov/pmc/articles/PMC117929

Zwarenstein M, Reeves S, Goldman J. Interprofessional collaboration: effects of practice-based interventions on professional practice and healthcare outcomes. Cochrane Database Syst Rev. 2009;3:CD000072.

Learning and Teaching at the Bedside: Expert Commentary from a Nursing Perspective

46

Michelle A. Kelly and Jan Forber

Contents

Introduction	870
The Roles: Who Is Teaching and Who Is Learning from Whom?	871
Privacy and Respect	872
Safety and Quality	874
Considerations Influencing Learning and Teaching at the Bedside: Nursing Perspectives	875
The Environment and Culture of the Ward	875
Organizational Structures and Policies	877
Education and Communication Experience	879
Sociocultural Characteristics of Patients, Families, and Clinicians	881
The Patient, Learner, and Teacher	881
Personal Characteristics and Experience	882
Future Considerations for Learning and Teaching at the Bedside: The Nursing Context	883
The Learner	884
The Teacher	885
The Patient	885
Conclusion	886
Cross-References	886
References	887

Abstract

Interactions between nurses and patients are unique and personalized and often described as privileged encounters. The holistic nature of nursing practice centered on a health-based platform differs from the medicalized (disease-based) model of healthcare. These foundational aspects of nursing practice influence learning and teaching encounters at the bedside. In this chapter, a teacher-learner-

M. A. Kelly (✉)
Curtin School of Nursing, Curtin University, Perth, Australia
e-mail: Michelle.Kelly@curtin.edu.au

J. Forber
School of Nursing and Midwifery, University of Technology Sydney, Sydney, NSW, Australia
e-mail: Jan.Forber@uts.edu.au

© Springer Nature Singapore Pte Ltd. 2023
D. Nestel et al. (eds.), *Clinical Education for the Health Professions*,
https://doi.org/10.1007/978-981-15-3344-0_61

patient triad is presented as it represents the interrelatedness and fluidity of the roles, which should always be considered within the broader contexts of safety and quality (patient care) and privacy and respect.

In this chapter, the increasing resolve from safety and quality organizations globally to enable health consumer involvement in their own and others' care is acknowledged in relation to their engagement in learning and teaching encounters at the bedside.

Communication, modelling practice, health literacy, and the broader arrangements for how undergraduate nursing students attain clinical practice experience form a large part of discussions. However, focus is also given to postgraduate nursing students who concurrently work in addition to studying. This chapter seeks to offer an international perspective, while recognizing that the context of the authors' practice in Australia is a strong influence on this work.

Keywords

Teacher · Learner · Patient triad · Preparation · Experience and expectations · Safety and quality · Privacy and respect · Health literacy · Communication · Clinical facilitator · Role modelling · Mentoring

Introduction

From the outset, there are two important concepts to clarify from the title of this chapter – these are "learning and teaching" and "at the bedside." Within the context of this major work, and being mindful of articulations with other chapters, we believe these concepts are important to define.

The reference to teaching and learning has often, in more recent years, been flipped to *learning and teaching,* with greater awareness that learning should be facilitated and based on individuals' learning needs, acknowledging peoples' life and work experiences (Hager 2005). Cultural diversity, from both the learner and teacher perspective, is an equally important factor to consider as expectations, based on school and life experiences, shape what is anticipated from learning opportunities (Mikkonen et al. 2016). Taking a broader perspective on who might be the "teacher" and who the "learner" is also an important factor.

The next concept, "at the bedside," raises several contexts or situations; the one which may most readily come to mind is a patient in a bed in an acute hospital setting. However, the bedside could be in all manner of health service settings, for example, dedicated mental health facilities, primary, community health, or transitional settings. The points raised in this chapter we believe should be applicable to other health service contexts beyond acute care, with relevant adaptations to suit the situation.

Specific focus on a nursing perspective in this chapter affords opportunity to make overt the particular holistic approach central to the discipline, reflecting a socially focused philosophy where close relationships often develop between nurses and patients and their carers (Benner et al. 2009). In addition, the role of the nurse and contributions made to the multidisciplinary team (MDT) are unique in a number of ways, arising from nurses having a constant presence at the bedside and in the clinical setting. A central domain of nursing practice is patient advocacy, often involving translation of medical discourse around treatment options and concepts (Benner et al. 2009). Patients' understandings of their health issues are interconnected with their level of health literacy and can influence their capacity for self-management (Health Literacy Hub 2018).

In this chapter, we introduce a triad of persons involved in learning and teaching at the bedside – the teacher, the learner, and the patient. These nominated "roles" are not static as outlined in our discussion. While the learner is often thought of as an undergraduate student or new graduate nurse, postgraduate nursing students as practicing clinicians and nursing peers can also belong in the "learner" category. Indeed, broadening and emphasizing this concept of "learner" reflect the expectations of lifelong learning for professional practice particularly in the rapidly changing healthcare landscape. Interactions between the learner, the teacher, and the patient are usually adjusted in recognition of level of knowledge and understanding about practice and the context at hand (Tanner 2006). For novice nursing students and new graduate nurses, understanding and embodying professional discourses, including medical and specialist terminology, are central to developing practice and creating a sense of belonging within healthcare teams (Dahlke and Hunter 2020). However, medical terminology often needs to be tempered to ensure patient and learners understand the issues at hand.

While the context of this chapter is offered from an Australian perspective, consideration of country-specific and cultural nuances in learning and teaching at the bedside is offered. However, internationally, where there are particular differences in approaches, enablers, or challenges which influence learning and teaching at the bedside, points raised here will need to be adapted for the local context.

The Roles: Who Is Teaching and Who Is Learning from Whom?

To start, we pose the question, who is teaching and who is learning from whom? Those typically involved in learning and teaching at the bedside include nurses, students, patients, and, at times, carers. Other members of the multidisciplinary team may be co-opted at various stages, so clarity of information and knowing what information has previously been discussed is important to avoid confusion or conflicting opinion or advice. Figure 1 reflects the interrelatedness of those involved and the nexus of learning and teaching at the bedside.

The roles of teacher, learner, and patient will likely to be dynamic as the situation demands. The teacher role in this chapter context would most likely be the registered nurse (RN), while the learner may be a nursing (or other health professions) student

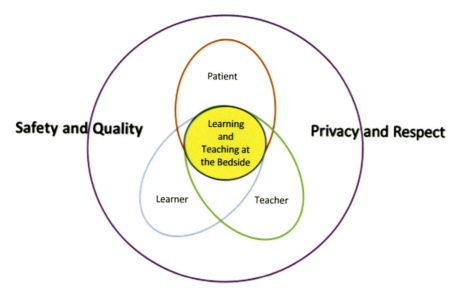

Fig. 1 The interrelatedness of participants and concepts involved with learning and teaching at the bedside (Kelly and Forber 2020)

or enrolled nurse (EN). Role changes may, for instance, see the patient become the teacher, or the learner, in partnership with others in the triad; the teacher may become the learner gaining new information from the patient and/or the (other) learner; and the learner may become the teacher as prior experiences emerge as beneficial to the situation at hand. Being mindful and open to such changing dynamics is important and fosters inclusiveness and respect.

The dynamics just described should be considered within two other broad domains – privacy and respect and safety and quality. The overall context, situation, and environment are likewise important for determining how learning and teaching at the bedside can or should proceed. Being attuned to privacy and respect, as well as safety and quality, is as important as the information or messages relayed during bedside learning and teaching encounters.

Privacy and Respect

Often, opportunities for learning and teaching are serendipitous, so taking advantage "of the moment" is paramount. Complete privacy may not always be possible on such occasions, and all need to be mindful that bedside curtains are not soundproof! However, a level of privacy, at the bedside or in private rooms or other spaces, should be considered relative to the anticipated interactions or nature of the information to be relayed. Privacy can be challenging to maintain, for instance, when unexpected, sometimes bad, news enters the conversation which triggers strong emotions. Similarly, conflicting information or delays in investigations or treatments can leave patients – and health workers – confused or conflicted. Acknowledging patients', peers', or learners' views, even when there are differences in understanding or opinions, reflects a level of respect and professionalism.

Health literacy is a central consideration applicable to all aspects of learning and teaching at the bedside. Determining others' levels of health literacy and shaping the learning and teaching discussions or demonstrations to match will likely enhance knowledge and understanding for patient self-care (Currie et al. 2015) and learner progression. Explanation of clinical management strategies helps contextualize and consolidate meaning for learners, while promoting self-care for patients often leads to higher engagement, satisfaction, and control and potentially improved health outcomes (Wong et al. 2018).

Cultural beliefs about health and illness also need to be acknowledged and incorporated into bedside learning and teaching encounters. Considerations relating to gender, age, religion, and hierarchy are different across cultures particularly in relation to the type of information discussed, by whom and whether other family members are required to be present (Hong 2018) during learning and teaching encounters. For example, beliefs about mental health or mental illness are taboo topics in many Arabic, Asian, and some Greek cultures (Tzouvara et al. 2016; Zolezzi et al. 2018). Similarly, inherent cultural beliefs are likely to influence practices and opinions of teachers and learners (Brooks et al. 2019).

In their concept analysis of culturally sensitive communication in healthcare, Brooks, Manias, and Bloomer (Brooks et al. 2019) identified numerous antecedents, attributes, and consequences that could enhance learning and teaching at the bedside. The five antecedents included the environment and culture of the ward; organizational structures and policies; education and communication experience of clinicians; sociocultural characteristics of patients, families, and clinicians; and personal characteristics and professional experience of clinicians (Brooks et al. 2019). Core recommendations from the concept analysis were that (1) the recipient of care should determine how communication proceeds relative to their individual cultural beliefs and (2) clinicians need to understand and reflect on their own cultural beliefs, values, attitudes, and practices as a key first step in learning about others' culture (Brooks et al. 2019). Being attuned to and teachers modelling such approaches may further learners' understanding and application of nuanced communication styles when engaging in learning and teaching. Observing or participating in these professional practices may help to mitigate some of the moral distress, ethical conflicts, or dilemmas nursing students have reported during clinical encounters (Albert et al. 2020).

Although clinicians should be upholding their respective professional practice standards, there are times when differences, particularly in religious beliefs or moral values, arise which may complicate learning and teaching encounters. In relation to respect, a common oversight by health professionals is not "formally" seeking patients' permission to provide care. So too, when engaging in learning and teaching at the bedside, patients, and their carers if present, should be given the opportunity to agree or not, for students to be present and part of conversations, care delivery, or skills demonstrations.

Safety and Quality

Safety and quality are global concerns with the aims of reducing medical errors and improving patient outcomes. A number of national bodies highlight the importance of the inclusiveness of health consumers at all levels of health policy and service delivery. The National Safety and Quality Health Services Standards (second edition) of the Australian Commission on Safety and Quality in Health Care exclusively dedicates one of the eight standards on Partnering with Consumers (Australian Commission on Safety and Quality in Health Care 2017). Similarly in the UK, the National Institute for Clinical Excellence (NICE), which transitioned to the National Institute for Health and Care Excellence in 2013, features policy and programs to involve patients and the public in healthcare delivery (National Institute for Health and Care Excellence 2013). In the USA, the Agency for Healthcare Research and Quality features information for the service sector on how to engage patients and their families in their healthcare (Agency for Healthcare Research and Quality 2020). The ideal level of consumer engagement however takes time to be incorporated into clinical practice settings. One element that influences consumer engagement is the perceived (or real) power differentials. Similarly, power differentials exist to varying degrees between the learner and teacher – and the patient. A workplace culture that upholds the central tenants of safety and quality may "give permission" to learners and patients to engage with clinician teachers more fully.

In addition to the above contexts, health consumers' awareness of medical ailments and treatment options from a myriad of social and online sources may influence their expectations of care. This may lead to a higher level of scrutiny or willingness to partake in learning and teaching at the bedside. Ensuring a level of aptitude and competence in clinical practice prior to learners providing care is paramount. The holism of practice, rather than competence in discrete motor skills, should be the aim of preparing learners to provide nursing care (Fagerström 2019). Contemporary learning approaches, such as simulation-based education (SBE), have been embraced as ways to prepare learners for practice (Nestel et al. 2018). When appropriately developed and delivered, SBE has been shown to support and enhance practice (Nestel et al. 2018). Following episodes of learning and teaching at the bedside, SBE can also be used as remediation to clarify or enhance learners' knowledge, skills, and attitudes. Working with simulated participants (SPs) as patients provides a more realistic and synchronous learner experience (Nestel and Bearman 2015). SP feedback to learners about the level of engagement and interaction during SBE may improve therapeutic communication and highlight the importance of consumer engagement in learning and teaching at the bedside (Nestel and Bearman 2015).

Brooks, Manias, and Bloomer's (Brooks et al. 2019) five antecedents for culturally sensitive communication provide an appropriate framework for drawing into focus key considerations that influence learning and teaching at the bedside. Given the cultural diversity of health consumers and the health workforce globally and that effective, therapeutic communication is a core component of practice, discussion continues under the following areas:

- The environment and culture of the ward
- Organizational structures and policies
- Education and communication experience
- Sociocultural characteristics of patients, families, and clinicians
- Personal characteristics and professional experience (Brooks et al. 2019)

To reflect the wider applicability of Brooks et al.'s framework, acknowledging learners and patients in learning and teaching at the bedside, we have removed "clinicians" from the subheadings. We are also mindful that some aspects overlap within these antecedent categories, so we have taken an arbitrary decision to align aspects within a "best fit" grouping.

Considerations Influencing Learning and Teaching at the Bedside: Nursing Perspectives

The Environment and Culture of the Ward

Many would maintain that the core business within the clinical setting is the delivery of safe, effective, quality patient care. Yet, the provision of clinical learning experiences is fundamental to the education of future health professionals. Hence, the two are not mutually exclusive but rather exist in a symbiotic relationship where both are interdependent. Consideration, therefore, needs to be given to how the clinical environment and culture of the workplace support both the pursuit of excellence in care delivery while also embracing the learner as integral to that dynamic milieu. Quality learning experiences arise from environments that are conducive to learning and being aware of the "... .the nuances of the workplace as a learning environment" (Newton et al. 2009a). Healthcare students typically have to navigate and sometimes individually promote their anticipated learning experiences, in university and clinical settings – each with their own unique physical, social, and practice contexts (Newton et al. 2009b). So too, the learning needs of postgraduate students and practicing nurse clinicians' ongoing development are either enabled or hampered by the tensions between the priorities of patient care and constraints on available time and opportunity.

The physical nature of the clinical environment needs to be considered, as to how it affords opportunities for both care provision and learning. Gregory et al. (2014) noted that the physical spaces and spatial aspects of the workplace need to be recognized and understood, to identify where "learning" can take place. Nursing students work alongside and under the supervision of registered nurses. At the bedside, students will engage directly with care delivery; however, subsequent informal or unplanned conversations away from the bedside are equally important for preparation, explanation, or clarification of clinical care. Havery (2019) identified multiple learning spaces in the clinical setting, each associated with and enabling particular learning activities between teacher and learner. Learning at the bedside should be considered as one of the spaces, balanced with opportunities for learning in other quiet spaces where discussions, debriefing, and personalized feedback can be undertaken. In addition to bedside learning experiences where RNs perhaps unconsciously model clinical practices, these "other" spaces also support socialization into the workforce, facilitating the novice's connection, and understanding of nurses' work (Havery 2019).

Examining the impact of the culture or pedagogical atmosphere within clinical environments on the learner's experience has been explored through both qualitative and quantitative approaches. Two prominent quantitative tools are the Clinical Learning Environment Inventory (CLEI) (Chan 2002) and the Clinical Learning Environment, Supervision and Nurse Teacher Evaluation Scale (CLES+T) (Saarikoskia and Leino-Kilpib 2002). The CLES+T scale measures students' perceptions of the learning environment and supervision during clinical experiences and is considered a reliable tool (Gustafsson et al. 2015). The scale has been used in multiple studies and examines five dimensions of the learning environment: (1) pedagogical atmosphere on the ward, (2) leadership style of the ward manager, (3) premises of nursing on the ward, (4) supervisory relationship, and (5) role of the nurse teacher (Gustafsson et al. 2015; Mikkonen et al. 2020).

Studies using the CLES+T tool have consistently identified environmental and relationship aspects of the clinical setting as important contributors to positive learning experiences. A hospitable, supportive culture, where learners feel welcome, valued, and part of the team, has consistently shown to be important for quality learning. For the learner to have a sense of belonging has been established for some time (Levett-Jones and Lathlean 2008) and is regularly reinforced (Doyle et al. 2017). Perry et al. (2018) also emphasized "belonging" as part of building partnerships and that students need to feel valued, respected, and have opportunities to be able to contribute to practice. These points are equally applicable for graduating nurses as they transition to professional practice and for any newcomer to the respective clinical setting. Materne et al. (2017) noted that the leadership within a clinical setting is an important driver of a positive culture to ensure student assimilation and engagement in the workplace. Leadership, which actively and positively drives the workplace and acknowledges and supports social capital, open communication, and a culture of shared contributions toward optimal patient care, enhanced students' learning experiences (Materne et al. 2017).

Collaborative educational models emphasize the importance of a shared workplace, positive culture, and attitudes regarding the relationships between practice, care delivery, and learning. In 2014, Edgecombe and Bowden (Edgecombe and Bowden 2014) identified the Dedicated Education Unit (DEU) model of collaborative clinical learning as originating in Adelaide, Australia, in 1997. DEUs have been adopted in several countries including the USA, New Zealand, and Sweden and are described by Gonda (2014) as "a small community where everyone (students, clinicians and academics) is continually learning from each other" (p. 168). The DEU is based on a number of learning philosophies – Wenger's (Wenger 1998) community of practice, Vygotsky's zone of proximal development (Vygotsky 1978), Lave and Wenger's situated learning (Lave and Wenger 1991), and Kolb's experiential learning (Kolb 1984). Highly collaborative in nature, the DEU involves all stakeholders in developing centers for patient care into nurturing environments that support both nursing students and staff in teaching and learning activities alongside, and complementary to, the core business of high-quality patient care delivery (Moscato et al. 2007). Outcome studies have demonstrated benefits and improved satisfaction to staff and students alike (Moscato et al. 2007). A further advantage of the DEU is seen in their "flexibility and agility" (Edgecombe and Bowden 2014) which promotes interpretation of concepts in diverse and differing contexts and aims to optimize informal learning from both intentional and incidental opportunities (Kelly and Hager 2015).

Organizational Structures and Policies

As noted earlier, the main business for healthcare providers is patient care delivery with a shared commitment to the development of the next generation of healthcare professionals. Historically however, there have been tensions between healthcare providers and universities resulting from the transition of nurse education to the higher education sector (in Australia) throughout the 1980s. A greater emphasis was afforded to students as learners due to their supernumerary role within the workplace.

Contractual agreements for undergraduate student supervision comprise some of the current organizational structures and policies influencing access. Attaining further qualifications facilitates nurses' promotional and job prospects. Postgraduate nursing students are generally employees studying part time while often working full time, and study fees may be subsidized by the employer. Completing course-related clinical assessment tasks is more independently negotiated, complemented by peer mentoring supervision. Depending on course requirements, nurse practitioner (NP) students are required to negotiate advanced practice experiences under the supervision of medical practitioners or other NPs. As illustrated, the conditions for learning and teaching at the bedside differ for each level of learner and are based on clinical governance processes.

In undergraduate nurse education, the notion of learning and teaching at the bedside differs from other disciplines, such as medical education. The organizational structures and policies within the nursing context are such that the term "placement" predominates when referring to clinical-based learning, and as Roxburgh et al. (2012) suggest, a "clinical placement" implies that learning is contained within the boundaries of a physical location, specific team, or time. It is common within nursing programs for students to experience a series of rotational placements in a range of clinical or community settings to meet a prescribed number of clinical hours within accredited courses, to gain registration.

Globally, the requirements for teaching nursing students at the bedside vary widely, and organizational structure and policy are influenced by national or state governance. In Australia, the typical 3-year Bachelor of Nursing program requires students to have a minimum of 800 supervised clinical placement hours (Australian Nursing and Midwifery Accreditation Council 2020). In contrast, nursing degree programs in European Union countries mandate 2300 hours of clinical placement across 3 years of study (World Health Organization 2009). The Nursing Council of New Zealand takes a flexible approach, requiring a minimum of 1100 clinical hours with opportunity for additional time (up to 1500 hours) for students to demonstrate competence (Nursing Council of New Zealand 2017). The duration of each episode of clinical experience (or placement) also varies, with reported duration between 1 and 42 weeks (Nursing Council of New Zealand 2017).

Within the clinical experience structure, local organization and policy determine the ways in which learners are supported in clinical environments. Studies consistently indicate that the nursing student-supervisor relationship is a key driver in student satisfaction with learning experiences (Papastavrou et al. 2016). Yet, there is a variety of approaches to how student supervision is achieved and how these are defined. Broadly, there are three main approaches. A one-to-one approach centers on a registered nurse-learner partnership and is typically referred to as *mentorship* in undergraduate education or *preceptorship* when referring to new graduates transitioning into practice. Other prominent approaches are group supervision models and collaborative models. Descriptions of these three main models are given in Box 1. Approaches to student supervision each have their challenges. In many models, the roles of supervisor and assessor are combined giving the potential for power differentials to be exaggerated.

Box 1 Prominent Models of Clinical Education/Student Supervision in the Nursing Context

Traditional group facilitation model: managed and funded by the education sector, an RN is employed on a sessional/contractual basis as supervisor/instructor to approximately 8–10 students. Student may be based across several wards/units, in one or more facilities, necessitating the "roving" nature of the CF model. Students are "buddied" with registered nurses on a shift-to-shift basis.

Mentorship or preceptorship model: a one-to-one relationship with a health facility registered nurse and student. Students work alongside their mentor on a shift-by-shift basis and may include weekend and night shifts. The mentor/preceptor is also responsible for their patient load.

Collaborative models: for example, the Dedicated Education Unit (DEU) model is one example of collaborative model in action where education-industry/service partnership support student learning. Each student is typically "based" in one healthcare organization for their program of study, and all staff engage in teaching and learning supported by academic counterparts (Spence et al. 2019; Forber et al. 2016).

Gustafsson et al. (2015) and Spence et al. (2019) cite examples from New Zealand and Australia where alternate models may be required for differing contexts. For example, clinical facilitation may be best suited to acute care settings, whereas a one-to-one mentorship approach may be suited to community settings, a consideration that will become more applicable as health service delivery diversifies. Other trends are toward coaching or team-based approaches to support learners. As an example, the UK recently adopted revised standards for student support in the clinical setting with a philosophical move away from traditional mentorship model to an approach which incorporates supervision, coaching, and peer-to-peer learning (Nursing and Midwifery Council 2018). While students continue to remain supervised at all times, the functions of supervisor and assessor have also been separated (Nursing and Midwifery Council 2018).

In response in the UK context, several centers have implemented and evaluated Collaborative Learning in Practice (CLIP) models, and although not specifically endorsed in the UK standards, the approach supports the philosophical underpinnings and roles required (Williamson et al. 2020). In coaching, Hill et al. (2020) explain that the coach engages students by questioning and using their knowledge to find solutions to patient-centered care. Learners are supported in small groups (3–6 students) to work collaboratively and are expected to take responsibility for their own learning (Hill et al. 2020). The CLIP approach is considered to have potential to better prepare students for real-world practice but requires a balanced availability of patients for staff and students per shift and sufficient preparation to execute the model effectively (Hill et al. 2020). The distribution of responsibility for student learning is also seen as an advantage, compared to the at times onerous burden in one-to-one facilitation models (Williamson et al. 2020).

Education and Communication Experience

An outstanding question in the field remains – is it better to have someone with a high level of expertise mentoring and teaching novices or someone who is closer in experience to the learner? In the end, decisions are based on the workforce present and available at the time, irrespective of advanced planning. However, those in the teacher role need to be aware of the ways in which novices operationalize their learning, that is, the predominant focus for novices is toward more concrete thinking and skill acquisition (Benner 1984). Higher-level thinking and application of knowledge through reflection on and about practice should be tempered according to the contexts and opportunities. Awareness of these pedagogical principles and how to communicate with and provide positive, and constructive, feedback to learners are acquired skills. The expectations of all involved in learning and teaching at the bedside are explored below.

The Teacher
Effective learning and teaching at the bedside is dependent on the educational preparation and experience of the teacher, most likely a registered nurse with varying skills and attributes. However, the preparedness of the learner and the patient's willingness or capacity to participate in the education process also influence each interaction. In the clinical facilitator model of student supervision, prominent in

Australia, the education and experience of both the facilitator and registered nurses* (RNs) who are "buddied" with a student day-to-day will be relevant.

In clinical facilitation, RNs are engaged in sessional, contract-based employment with one or more universities to support students in practice (Andrews and Ford 2013). Nationally, in Australia, there is no formally recognized qualification for preparation for the role clinical facilitator. Indeed, as Needham et al. (2016) note, little has been reported in the literature that describes best practice for clinical facilitation or examines the requirements in terms of education and preparation and ongoing support to sustain the role in practice.

In addition, with the clinical facilitation model, students are buddied on a shift-by-shift basis with a registered nurse to provide supervision and potentially facilitate access to learning opportunities. The ability of the buddy RN to engage in learning and teaching is influenced not only by their own education and experience but also the ebb and flow dynamics in the clinical setting, patient care priorities, skill mix, and time pressures (Spence et al. 2019).

The Learner

Preparedness of the learner, educationally, socially, and emotionally, is necessary for students to negotiate their place, and be able to work on relationship development, in the clinical setting (Cooper et al. 2015). The degree of learner engagement is influenced by prior life experiences, cultural background, and communication skills. Havery (2019), for example, found that students for whom English was an additional language (EAL), with a developed sense of self-agency and confidence in their English language skills, were better able to negotiate the required relationships with both buddy RN and facilitator in the clinical facilitator model to access learning opportunities. Communicating for patient safety resides in the domain of the learner as well as the teacher and patient (Australian Commission on Safety and Quality in Health Care (ASQHS) 2017). Tensions arise when the learner may witness less than ideal practices and the real or perceived power differentials inhibit "speaking up for patient safety" despite systems and governance processes in place to encourage shared responsibility (Australian Commission on Safety and Quality in Health Care (ASQHS) 2017).

Beyond formal university and healthcare provider partnerships, at an operational level, there is the potential for differing approaches to learning in each respective setting. In Newton et al.'s (2015) study, students wanted to feel trusted and be able to negotiate their place to learn by doing and "get the work done." In part, this requires that students be able to fit in and accept existing practices (Newton et al. 2015). However, in their university-based education, students may be encouraged via their formal curriculum to engage with frameworks that provide a systematized approach to help them develop skills in reflection and overall clinical judgment – as Tanner (2006) describes, to *think like a nurse*. However, as Smith et al. (2018) caution, learner expectations may be at odds with the clinical setting if a more traditional and rigid approach to nursing care delivery dominates or the pressures to meet government metrics dominate clinical care. McKenna (▶ Chap. 36, "Hidden, Informal, and Formal Curricula in Health Professions Education") reminds us of the "hidden curricula," where the behavioral and interactional aspects of applying theory to practice in the health setting facilitate unintended yet equally important learning outcomes. The collaborative models already noted such as DEU and CLIP may well be means to bridge this divide.

The Patient

The role of the patient or client as a contributor to learning and teaching at the bedside has received limited attention. Stockhausen (2009) considers how the patient, while not necessarily formally prepared, can engage with students and clinicians to become a "broker" of learning during teaching encounters. Patients can come to see themselves as a valuable and unique resource for learning and teaching and also someone who can offer encouragement to the learner to build their understanding of the patient experience (Stockhausen 2009). Patients and their families are increasingly engaging in speaking up for patient safety and should be encouraged to ask questions at any time during their hospitalization, including during learning and teaching encounters at the bedside. Teachers and learners need to be attuned to, and adapt conversations dependent on, patients' level of health literacy (Australian Commission on Safety and Quality in Health Care (ASQHS) 2017).

Sociocultural Characteristics of Patients, Families, and Clinicians

Episodes of bedside learning and teaching are open to the influence of the sociocultural characteristics of all involved – patients, their families or carers, nurses, other clinicians, and the learner.

The Patient, Learner, and Teacher

The sociocultural background of patients and their families may determine which interactions are considered to be culturally accepted practices, including who can deliver care based on gender and who in the family takes the lead in communication with clinicians, particularly receiving and relaying information and making decisions (Seidlein and Salloch 2020). A further consideration is when the patient knows more about their condition than the teacher or the learner. How this type of interaction is accommodated is important for the learner, and the patient, to experience. The role of patients in learning and teaching interactions is ill-defined, and traditionally patients feel they cannot speak for themselves, interrupt, or question "learned" clinicians (Seidlein and Salloch 2020).

Considering the learner, Havery (2019) identifies three facets that influence student access to learning opportunities – cultural differences, language ability, and the "teachers" pedagogical practices. Philibert et al. (2019) examined how the sociocultural characteristic of learners can influence their access to learning in the workplace, considering how gender, race, ethnicity, sexual orientation, or disability may contribute to unequal access to learning opportunities. If there is exclusion from privileged or social settings, this may distance the learner from professional socialization and opportunity to share experiences as part of learning (Philibert et al. 2019).

Personal Characteristics and Experience

In this section, the focus of discussion extends beyond the clinician, to the personal characteristics, and prior life and healthcare experiences of the learner and the patient. What each participant collectively "brings to the table" is as important as the "role" they assume.

The Teacher

The beneficial personal characteristics of the teacher regardless of whether this is a registered nurse, nurse educator, clinical facilitator, or other member of the multidisciplinary team are consistently described in the literature. Echoing the commentary on the overall environmental culture, nurses who are initially welcoming of students, maintain a continued positive attitude toward students, and provide them with ongoing support are prominent (Cooper et al. 2015). The capacity of the teacher to assist learners through engaging with patients and reflecting on practice (Benner et al. 2009) requires establishment of mutual trust. Once clinicians get to "know the learner" and are satisfied they are "safe" in their practices, increasing independence can ensue, resulting in higher satisfaction for the learner, particularly when individual needs are met (Papastavrou et al. 2016). Jack et al. (2017) remind us of the influence role models and modelling practice has on learners, not only in relation to clinical practices but the values and attitudes pertinent to the holistic nature of nursing. Teachers need to be cognizant of these factors, as both ideal and substandard practices can influence, or lead to tensions in, leaners' understanding and embodiment of practice.

The Learner

The personal characteristics and preparedness of the learner are also factors that influence learning dynamics. Billett (2015) states that "what individuals know, can do and value" enables them to engage and learn from activities and interactions" [p. 368]. The level of guidance students require will vary. As Havery (2019) found, students with higher confidence in their English language ability, and higher sense of self agency, could manage a more ad hoc approach to learning, whereas less confident students benefited from more directed learning activities and more pre-negotiated activities with the nurse they were working with. Students' preparedness, readiness, and willingness to learn have been considered important factors in successful mentorship relationships and essential for learning in the clinical setting (Papastavrou et al. 2016). Cooper et al. (2015) note that students need to have a comprehension of the relationships they will be engaged in with staff in the clinical setting and be sufficiently prepared for this.

The Patient

Stockhausen (2009) refers to the patient as pivotal in the educational context in being able to bring a different perspective on their health condition and their lived experience to enrich the learning that occurs. Globally, there is increasing expectation that service users' views are considered in all aspects of healthcare service provision, and this includes the education of health professionals. McMahon-Parkes et al. (2016) undertook a study into stakeholders' experiences of patients' and carers' involvement with the assessment of nursing students using a feedback tool. They found that patients wanted to be involved in providing feedback and felt comfortable doing so as they were best placed to comment on particular aspects of care delivered by students. Service user feedback was considered valuable by both staff and students especially in areas of developing student confidence and competence in areas of professionalism, communication, and interpersonal skills (McMahon-Parkes et al. 2016).

Suikkala et al.'s (2018) review of the literature found that whether patients engaged in student learning was determined by previous positive experiences, attitudes toward students, and existence of a caring environment. Care being provided by someone of a different gender can cause angst to the patient, family, and student. Suikkala et al. (2018) concluded that nursing curricula needed to be more explicit in ensuring students learn from and with patients, by valuing patients as active partners in the teaching and learning process.

Future Considerations for Learning and Teaching at the Bedside: The Nursing Context

The interrelatedness of the learner, teacher, and patient involved in learning and teaching at the bedside was introduced earlier in the chapter (Fig. 1). Given the centrality of this relationship, future developments in healthcare and education have the potential to impact the surrounding tenants of safety and quality and privacy and respect and are, we believe, worthy of consideration. In the nursing context, care at the "bedside" involves all the visible activities such as patient assessments, physical care, or communication. Importantly, however, embedded in these interactions are the emotional, attitudinal, and critical thinking skills at developmental levels in the learner, and these expected at competent levels in registered nurses.

This section reflects on selected indicative influences that from a nursing perspective, warrant consideration for learning and teaching at the future "bedside." While the discussion is framed as the learner, teacher, and patient triad, threads emerge that relate to demand for, and the type of future healthcare professionals, population changes, chronic disease, and lifestyle factors, technological advances and availability of health-related information.

The Learner

Globally, there is an increasing demand for healthcare workers, particularly nurses. The factors driving this demand are numerous but include the diversification of healthcare provision for aging populations, gaps in supply and demand of staff, and in many countries, loss of an aging nursing workforce to retirement (Marc et al. 2019). One strategic response to increase supply of staff has been to increase student enrollments into nursing programs, and in Australian universities, government initiatives for widening participation have also driven up student numbers and contributed to diversification of the student population. As a result, managing such large numbers of nursing students, and their access to in situ clinical learning opportunities, has notable impact on bedside or clinical education for this discipline. Capacity building, in preparation for the anticipated shortage of nurses, will be required to facilitate the clinical component of nurse education (Williamson et al. 2020). Increasing student numbers, however, affects the ability of the healthcare system and registered nurses at the bedside to support the student learning experience. Competing clinical demands and potential for staff shortages as nurses retire from the workforce puts pressure on clinical placements and risks impacting the quality of clinical learning (Spence et al. 2019). Regardless of the capability of the teacher, with factors such as increasing demands on clinical learning, there is a risk for mentor fatigue.

Cultural diversity within cohorts of nursing students and heterogenicity with mature students, school leavers, and international and local students are emergent factors in bedside learning and teaching. For example, Salamonson et al. (2012) surveyed 540 (67%) students from a cohort of 806 year-one students enrolled in New South Wales, Bachelor of Nursing Program. The study found 56% of students were born overseas, with 18% being international students and 38% were local, overseas-born students, originating from 55 different countries. Three distinct groups of students were identified in this study, (i) international; (ii) local, overseas-born; and (iii) local, Australian-born, and each was predicted to have their own specific needs, expectations, challenges, and motivators for success in their studies (Salamonson et al. 2012).

Consequently, developing ways of optimizing differing students' preparedness for bedside learning and teaching will be an important focus. The incorporation of contemporary learning strategies such as simulation-based education (SBE) is well established as a way to prepare learners for clinical practice, through skill development, critical thinking, and communication. The use of simulation also has a role in helping learners to understand their role and engagement with practice and with their "teachers" and "patients." Cooper et al. (2015) examined how to better prepare students to develop their capacity for improved relationships and understanding that the patients' needs are the clinician's priority. James and Chapman (2009) argue that preparation for clinical experience needs to be detailed and focused on the patient experience of illness to help students understand patients' responses in terms of coping or not coping. Increasingly, students need to be empowered to speak up, question practice, and manage the power differentials that can be evident, and may be encountered, between novice and senior nurses (Hartin et al. 2018).

The Teacher

The effectiveness of learning and teaching at the bedside is influenced by the preparedness and capability of the healthcare professional in the teacher role, but also the extent to which there is support and recognition of the role. While studies have identified that there is an expectation both at a professional nursing level and by local management for nurses to adopt supervisory and teaching roles, there is not always formalized recognition or preparation. In Smith and Sweet's (2019) study, novice nurse teachers found the role both challenging yet rewarding, which provided opportunities for their own learning and growth. However, as other studies reveal for effective clinical learning and teaching, there needs to be sufficient preparation (Doyle et al. 2017), ongoing guidance, support and recognition (Ratta 2018), and time for engagement between teacher and learner (Papastavrou et al. 2016).

Tensions between the primary responsibility of the teacher for providing patient care, in addition to supervising and supporting learners while ensuring safety and quality, will remain and likely become more complex. In the acute care setting, patient acuity influences how and when the learner is able to be supported to engage in active care delivery. A challenge for clinicians is getting to know the capabilities of each learner, particularly undergraduate students. Adding to the challenge is simultaneously having students who are at different stages of their course or students from multiple universities in the clinical setting. Ratta (2018) studied nurses supervising novice nurses while caring for deteriorating patients. Nurses relied on their clinical expertise to ensure patient safety and adopted techniques such as role modelling to facilitate the development of the novice nurse. With finite learning opportunities available, a further challenge is knowing when to prioritize or balance the needs of new or transitioning qualified staff with those of student nurses, which further increases competition for learning opportunities.

As healthcare diversifies and the roles, responsibilities, and classification of staff, including the nursing workforce, change, variation may be seen in who the learner is and who the teacher is as represented in Fig. 1. In the nursing context, assistants in nursing (also known as healthcare assistants) function in non-registered roles yet may find themselves engaging in teaching at the bedside. Given the many ways in which novice nurses are supervised in the clinical setting (see Box 1), and potential for greater adoption of team-based approaches, there is greater scope for non-nursing members of the multidisciplinary team to have more active roles as teachers.

The Patient

In the continued evolution of healthcare, our understanding of the term "at the bedside" can be expected to reflect the diversification of service provision predicted into the future. Historically "at the bedside" has been a literal concept, and the main approaches to learning and teaching at the bedside have developed in many disciplines, including nursing, within a traditional hospital, ward-based context. Healthcare is predicted to expand into primary care, community care, and the "hospital in the home" settings. Coupled with demand for elderly healthcare and the influence of lifestyle factors and chronic illness on well-being, preventative and long-term care will come more into focus, transforming the future concept of "at the bedside" (Gopal et al. 2019). However, the fundamental core of learning and teaching and interaction/relationship of the nurse (teacher) and the learner with the patient will retain the personal, respectful, caring, and empathic ways of engaging and building relationships.

Another area of development and change will be the continued impact of the availability of information and digital and technological adjuncts to healthcare provision. Gopal et al. (2019) note that more knowledgeable patients and their families are becoming increasingly empowered, as their access to information is unprecedented in the history of healthcare. Hence patients can be far more engaged in their own health and informed on decision-making around treatment options, "challenging" the status quo, though they may not always be discriminatory in information they source.

Conclusion

These are both exciting and challenging times for healthcare clinicians, healthcare consumers, and learners at a time of evolving and dynamic change in the nature of healthcare service provision. The education sector too faces change in response to local, national, and global influences and policy adjustments.

Learning and teaching at the bedside from a nursing perspective is reflected in a triad partnership of the teacher, learner, and patient. Within this chapter, the antecedents for effective communication, a core concept of learning and teaching, were explored. The complexity and interrelatedness of the environment and culture of the ward; organizational structures and policies; education and communication experience (of clinicians); sociocultural characteristics of patients, families, and clinicians; and personal characteristics and professional experience (of clinicians) were examined in detail. Future considerations for learning and teaching and the concept of "the bedside" were also offered.

Cross-References

- ▶ Clinical Education in Nursing: Current Practices and Trends
- ▶ Developing Clinical Reasoning Capabilities
- ▶ Developing Professional Identity in Health Professional Students
- ▶ Effective Feedback Conversations in Clinical Practice
- ▶ Health Profession Curriculum and Public Engagement
- ▶ Hidden, Informal, and Formal Curricula in Health Professions Education
- ▶ Learning with and from Peers in Clinical Education
- ▶ Nursing and Midwifery Education: Historical Perspectives
- ▶ Optimizing the Role of Clinical Educators in Health Professional Education

▶ Supporting the Development of Professionalism in the Education of Health Professionals
▶ Transformative Learning in Clinical Education: Using Theory to Inform Practice

References

Agency for Healthcare Research and Quality: Engaging patients and their families in their health care. https://www.ahrq.gov/patient-safety/resources/patient-family-engagement/index.html (2020). Accessed 16 Feb 2020.

Albert JS, Younas A, Sana S. Nursing students' ethical dilemmas regarding patient care: an integrative review. Nurse Educ Today. 2020;88 https://doi.org/10.1016/j.nedt.2020.104389.

Andrews CE, Ford K. Clinical facilitator learning and development needs: exploring the why, what and how. Nurse Educ Pract. 2013;13(5):413–7. https://doi.org/10.1016/j.nepr.2013.01.002.

Australian Commission on Safety and Quality in Health Care. National Safety and Quality Health Service Standards guide for hospitals. In: ACSQHC, editor. 2nd ed. Sydney: ACSQHC; 2017.

Australian Commission on Safety and Quality in Health Care (ASQHS). Communicating for Safety standard. National Safety and Quality Health Service Standards. 2nd ed. Sydney: Australian Commission on Safety and Quality in Health Care 2017; 2017. p. 47–54.

Australian Nursing and Midwifery Accreditation Council.: https://www.anmac.org.au/. Accessed 2020.

Benner P. From novice to expert: excellence and power in clinical nursing practice. Menlo Park: Addison-Wesley Pub; 1984.

Benner P, Tanner C, Chesla CA. Expertise in nursing practice: caring, clinical judgment and ethics. 2nd ed. New York: Springer; 2009.

Billett S. Readiness and learning in health care education. Clin Teach. 2015;12:367–72.

Brooks LA, Manias E, Bloomer MJ. Culturally sensitive communication in healthcare: a concept analysis. Collegian. 2019;26(3):383–91. https://doi.org/10.1016/j.colegn.2018.09.007.

Chan D. Associations between student learning outcomes from their clinical placement and their perceptions of the social climate of the clinical learning environment. Int J Nurs Stud. 2002;39:517–24.

Cooper J, Courtney-Pratt H, Fitzgerald M. Key influences identified by first year undergraduate nursing students as impacting on the quality of clinical placement: a qualitative study. Nurse Educ Today. 2015;35(9):1004–8. https://doi.org/10.1016/j.nedt.2015.03.009.

Currie K, Strachan PH, Spaling M, Harkness K, Barber D, Clark AM. The importance of interactions between patients and healthcare professionals for heart failure self-care: a systematic review of qualitative research into patient perspectives. Eur J Cardiovasc Nurs. 2015;14(6):525–35. https://doi.org/10.1177/1474515114547648.

Dahlke S, Hunter KF. How nurses' use of language creates meaning about healthcare users and nursing practice. Nursing Inquiry. 2020;27(3) https://doi.org/10.1111/nin.12346.

Doyle K, Sainsbury K, Cleary S, Parkinson L, Vindigni D, McGrath I, et al. Happy to help/happy to be here: identifying components of successful clinical placements for undergraduate nursing students. Nurse Educ Today. 2017;49:27–32. https://doi.org/10.1016/j.nedt.2016.11.001.

Edgecombe K, Bowden M, editors. Clinical learning and teaching innovations in nursing: dedicated education units building a better future. Dordrecht: Springer; 2014.

Fagerström L. Caring, health, holism and person-centred ethos – common denominators for health sciences? Scand J Caring Sci. 2019;33(2):253–4. https://doi.org/10.1111/scs.12732.

Forber J, DiGiacomo M, Carter B, Davidson P, Phillips J, Jackson D. In pursuit of an optimal model of undergraduate nurse clinical education: an integrative review. Nurse Educ Pract. 2016;21:83–92. https://doi.org/10.1016/j.nepr.2016.09.007.

Gonda J. Voices from the coalface: the impact of dedicated education units in nursing. In: Edgecombe K, Bowden M, editors. Clinical learning and teaching innovations in nursing: dedicated education unitsbBuilding a better future. Dordrecht: Springer; 2014.

Gopal G, Suter-Crazzolara C, Toldo L, Eberhardt W. Digital transformation in healthcare – architectures of present and future information technologies. J Clin Chem Lab Med. 2019;57(3):328–35. https://doi.org/10.1515/cclm-2018-0658.

Gregory LR, Hopwood N, Boud D. Interprofessional learning at work: what spatial theory can tell us about workplace learning in an acute care ward. J Interprof Care. 2014;28(3):200–5. https://doi.org/10.3109/13561820.2013.873774.

Gustafsson M, Kullen Engstrom A, Ohlsson U, Sundler AJ, Bisholt B. Nurse teacher models in clinical education from the perspective of student nurses-a mixed method study. Nurse Educ Today. 2015;35(12):1289–94. https://doi.org/10.1016/j.nedt.2015.03.008.

Hager P. New approaches in the philosophy of learning. Educ Philos Theory. 2005;37(5):633–4.

Hartin P, Birks M, Lindsay D. Bullying and the nursing profession in Australia: an integrative review of the literature. Collegian. 2018;25(6):613–9. https://doi.org/10.1016/j.colegn.2018.06.004.

Havery C. The effects of clinical facilitators' pedagogic practices on learning opportunities for students who speak English as an additional language: an ethnographic study. Nurse Educ Today. 2019;74:1–6. https://doi.org/10.1016/j.nedt.2018.12.004.

Health Literacy Hub. (2018). https://healthliteracyhub.org.au/. Accessed 2020.

Hill R, Woodward M, Arthur A. Collaborative learning in practice (CLIP): evaluation of a new approach to clinical learning. Nurse Educ Today. 2020;85:104295. https://doi.org/10.1016/j.nedt.2019.104295.

Hong SJ. Gendered cultural identities: the influences of family and privacy boundaries, subjective norms, and stigma beliefs on family health history communication. Health Commun. 2018;33(8):927–38. https://doi.org/10.1080/10410236.2017.1322480.

Jack K, Hamshire C, Chambers A. The influence of role models in undergraduate nurse education. J Clin Nurs. 2017:n/a–n/a. https://doi.org/10.1111/jocn.13822.

James A, Chapman Y. Preceptors and patients – the power of two: nursing student experiences on their first acute clinical placement. Contemp Nurse. 2009;34(1):34–47. https://doi.org/10.5172/conu.2009.34.1.034.

Kelly M, Hager P. Informal learning: relevance and application to health care simulation. Clin Simul Nurs. 2015;11(8):376–82. https://doi.org/10.1016/j.ecns.2015.05.006.

Kolb D. Experiential learning: experience as the source of learning and development. Englewood Cliffs: Pearson Education; 1984.

Lave J, Wenger E. Situated learning: legitimate peripheral participation. Cambridge: Cambridge University Press; 1991.

Levett-Jones T, Lathlean J. Belongingness: a prerequisite for nursing students' clinical learning. Nurse Educ Pract. 2008;8(2):103–11. https://doi.org/10.1016/j.nepr.2007.04.003.

Marc M, Bartosiewicz A, Burzynska J, Chmiel Z, Januszewicz P. A nursing shortage – a prospect of global and local policies. Int Nurs Rev. 2019;66:9–16.

Materne M, Henderson A, Eaton E. Building workplace social capital: a longitudinal study of student nurses' clinical placement experiences. Nurse Educ Pract. 2017;26:109–14. https://doi.org/10.1016/j.nepr.2017.07.007.

McMahon-Parkes K, Chapman L, James J. The views of patients, mentors and adult field nursing students on patients' participation in student nurse assessment in practice. Nurse Educ Pract. 2016;16(1):202–8. https://doi.org/10.1016/j.nepr.2015.08.007.

Mikkonen K, Elo S, Kuivila H-M, Tuomikoski A-M, Kääriäinen M. Culturally and linguistically diverse healthcare students' experiences of learning in a clinical environment: a systematic review of qualitative studies. Int J Nurs Stud. 2016;54:173–87. https://doi.org/10.1016/j.ijnurstu.2015.06.004.

Mikkonen K, Merilainen M, Tomietto M. Empirical model of clinical learning environment and mentoring of culturally and linguistically diverse nursing students. J Clin Nurs. 2020;29(3–4):653–61. https://doi.org/10.1111/jocn.15112.

Moscato SR, Miller J, Logsdon K, Weinberg S, Chorpenning L. Dedicated education unit: an innovative clinical partner education model. Nurs Outlook. 2007;55(1):31–7. https://doi.org/10.1016/j.outlook.2006.11.001.

National Institute for Health and Care Excellence: Patient and public involvement. https://www.nice.org.uk/about/nice-communities/nice-and-the-public/public-involvement/public-involvement-programme/patient-public-involvement-policy (2013). Accessed 16 Feb 2020.

Needham J, McMurray A, Shaban RZ. Best practice in clinical facilitation of undergraduate nursing students. Nurse Educ Pract. 2016;20:131–8. https://doi.org/10.1016/j.nepr.2016.08.003.

Nestel D, Bearman M, editors. Simulated patient methodology: theory, evidence and practice. Chichester: Wiley Blackwell; 2015.

Nestel D, Kelly M, Jolly B, Watson M, editors. Healthcare simulation education: evidence, theory and practice. West Sussex: John Wiley & Sons; 2018.

Newton JM, Billett S, Ockerby CM. Journeying through clinical placements – an examination of six student cases. Nurse Educ Today. 2009a;29(6):630–4. https://doi.org/10.1016/j.nedt.2009.01.009.

Newton JM, Billett S, Jolly B, Ockerby CM. Lost in translation: barriers to learning in health professional clinical education. Learn Health Soc Care. 2009b;8(4):315–27. https://doi.org/10.1111/j.1473-6861.2009.00229.x.

Newton JM, Henderson A, Jolly B, Greaves J. A contemporary examination of workplace learning culture: an ethnomethodology study. Nurse Educ Today. 2015;35(1):91–6. https://doi.org/10.1016/j.nedt.2014.07.001.

Nursing and Midwifery Council: Standards for student supervision and assessment. https://www.nmc.org.uk/standards-for-education-and-training/standards-for-student-supervision-and-assessment/. (2018). Accessed 2020.

Nursing Council of New Zealand: Requirements for registration as a registered nurse. https://www.nursingcouncil.org.nz/Public/Nursing/How_to_become_a_nurse/NCNZ/nursing-section/How_to_become_a_nurse.aspx (2017). Accessed 5 March 2021.

Papastavrou E, Dimitriadou M, Tsangari H, Andreou C. Nursing students' satisfaction of the clinical learning environment: a research study. BMC Nurs. 2016;15(44):1–10.

Perry C, Henderson A, Grealish L. The behaviours of nurses that increase student accountability for learning in clinical practice: an integrative review. Nurse Educ Today. 2018;65:177–86. https://doi.org/10.1016/j.nedt.2018.02.029.

Philibert I, Elsey E, Fleming S, Razack S. Learning and professional acculturation through work: examining the clinical learning environment through the sociocultural lens. Med Teach. 2019;41(4):398–402. https://doi.org/10.1080/0142159X.2019.1567912.

Ratta C. The art of balance: preceptors' experiences of caring for deteriorating patients. J Clin Nurs. 2018;27:3497–509. https://doi.org/10.1111/jocn.14579.

Roxburgh M, Conlon M, Banks D. Evaluating hub and spoke models of practice learning in Scotland, UK: a multiple case study approach. Nurse Educ Today. 2012;32(7):782–9. https://doi.org/10.1016/j.nedt.2012.05.004.

Saarikoskia M, Leino-Kilpib H. The clinical learning environment and supervision by staff nurses: developing the instrument. Int J Nurs Stud. 2002;39:259–67.

Salamonson Y, Ramjan L, Lombardo L, Lanser L, Fernandez R, Griffiths R. Diversity and demographic heterogeneity of Australian nursing students: a closer look. Int Nurs Rev. 2012;59:59–65.

Seidlein A-H, Salloch S. Who cares about care? Family members as moral actors in treatment decision making. Am J Bioeth. 2020;20(6):80–2. https://doi.org/10.1080/15265161.2020.1754506.

Smith JH, Sweet L. Becoming a nurse preceptor, the challenges and rewards of novice registered nurses in high acuity hospital environments. Nurse Educ Pract. 2019;36:101–7. https://doi.org/10.1016/j.nepr.2019.03.001.

Smith MR, Grealish L, Henderson S. Shaping a valued learning journey: student satisfaction with learning in undergraduate nursing programs, a grounded theory study. Nurse Educ Today. 2018;64:175–9. https://doi.org/10.1016/j.nedt.2018.02.020.

Spence D, Zambas S, Mannix J, Jackson D, Neville S. Challenges to the provision of clinical education in nursing. Contemp Nurse. 2019;55(4–5):458–67. https://doi.org/10.1080/10376178.2019.1606722.

Stockhausen LJ. The patient as experience broker in clinical learning. Nurse Educ Pract. 2009;9(3):184–9. https://doi.org/10.1016/j.nepr.2008.06.006.

Suikkala A, Koskinen S, Leino-Kilpi H. Patients' involvement in nursing students' clinical education: a scoping review. Int J Nurs Stud. 2018;84:40–51. https://doi.org/10.1016/j.ijnurstu.2018.04.010.

Tanner C. Thinking like a nurse: a research-based model of clinical judgment in nursing. J Nurs Educ. 2006;45(6):204–21.

Tzouvara V, Papadopoulos C, Randhawa G. Systematic review of the prevalence of mental illness stigma within the Greek culture. Int J Soc Psychiatry. 2016;62(3):292–305. https://doi.org/10.1177/0020764016629699.

Vygotsky L. Mind and society: the development of higher mental processes. Cambridge: Cambridge University Press; 1978.

Wenger E. Communities of practice: learning, meaning and identity. Leaning in doing: social, cognitive, and computational perspectives. Cambridge: Cambridge University Press; 1998.

Williamson GR, Plowright H, Kane A, Bunce J, Clarke D, Jamison C. Collaborative learning in practice: a systematic review and narrative synthesis of the research evidence in nurse education. Nurse Educ Pract. 2020;43:102706. https://doi.org/10.1016/j.nepr.2020.102706.

Wong KK, Velasquez A, Powe NR, Tuot DS. Association between health literacy and self-care behaviors among patients with chronic kidney disease. BMC Nephrol. 2018;19:Article 196. https://doi.org/10.1186/s12882-018-0988-0.

World Health Organization: Europe: European Union Standards for Nursing and Midwifery: Information for Accession Countries https://www.euro.who.int/__data/assets/pdf_file/0005/102200/E92852.pdf (2009). Accessed.

Zolezzi M, Alamri M, Shaar S, Rainkie D. Stigma associated with mental illness and its treatment in the Arab culture: a systematic review. Int J Soc Psychiatry. 2018;64(6):597–609. https://doi.org/10.1177/0020764018789200.

Learning and Teaching in Clinical Settings: Expert Commentary from a Midwifery Perspective

47

Linda Sweet and Deborah Davis

Contents

Introduction	892
Midwifery	892
The Midwifery Philosophy	893
The Midwifery Scope of Practice	894
Models of Maternity Care	895
Evidence for Midwifery Care	895
Midwifery Education Governance	896
Models of Clinical Learning	900
Supporting Clinical Learning	900
Conclusion	905
Cross-References	906
References	906

Abstract

A midwife works in partnership with childbearing women to give the necessary support, care, and advice during pregnancy, labor, and the postpartum period. Midwifery is a regulated and licensed profession, and educational programs leading to registration as a midwife are required to meet minimum standards. Midwifery care is provided in a variety of contexts with a broad range of models of care. There is extensive evidence that midwives are crucial to improving the health and well-being of women and their babies globally, not only in low- and middle-income countries, and that continuity of midwifery care is the optimal means to achieve this. Teaching and learning in clinical settings may occur in hospitals, health centers, or women's own homes. This may occur in block

L. Sweet (✉)
Deakin University and Western Health Partnership, Melbourne, VIC, Australia
e-mail: l.sweet@deakin.edu.au

D. Davis
University of Canberra and Canberra Hospital and Health Services, Canberra, ACT, Australia
e-mail: Deborah.Davis@canberra.edu.au

© Springer Nature Singapore Pte Ltd. 2023
D. Nestel et al. (eds.), *Clinical Education for the Health Professions*,
https://doi.org/10.1007/978-981-15-3344-0_120

placements, regular weekly placement, or through continuity of care experience models. Midwifery education can be enhanced through learner activities, such as participatory practices and enacting learner agency. Teaching considerations include the practice curricula and practice pedagogies. Timing, sequencing, and affordance to learning opportunities that enhance the capacity for continuity of education are paramount. Teaching practices that are beneficial include positive role models, awareness of cognitive overload and teaching tasks in parts where necessary, using strategies that build clinical reasoning capacity such as think aloud technique, and providing regular and supportive feedback and effective assessments. All of these are strategies to support learning and teaching in midwifery clinical settings.

Keywords

Midwife · Midwifery education · Continuity of care · Woman-centered care · Continuity of education · Affordances · Teaching practices

Introduction

This chapter explores teaching and learning for midwifery. While we initially position midwifery in Australia, many of the issues raised will be applicable globally. Midwifery education in Australia has undergone significant changes of the last 20 years and continues to evolve and improve. To enable the reader insight into midwifery and the uniqueness of midwifery education, we start with describing what midwives do, the midwifery care philosophy, and a midwife's scope of practice. While there are international definitions, each country is likely to have slightly different scopes of practice for midwives. It is important to understand the midwifery philosophy and scope of practice, as these guide teaching and learning in clinical settings. There is substantial evidence of the value of continuity of midwifery care, and education providers should find ways to enhance continuity of care opportunities in curriculum. Following an overview of models of maternity care and models of clinical learning, we then explore learner-driven and teacher-driven actions that can be implemented to enhance clinical learning. Many of these are explained in detail throughout this book and we encourage you to read further on the concepts presented.

Midwifery

In many countries, the title "midwife" is protected and brings with it a variety of professional and legal responsibilities and accountabilities. The definition of the midwife according to the International Confederation of Midwives (ICM) (2017) is:

> ...a person who has successfully completed a midwifery education programme that is duly recognized in the country where it is located and that is based on the ICM Essential

Competencies for Basic Midwifery Practice and the framework of the ICM Global Standards for Midwifery Education; who has acquired the requisite qualifications to be registered and/or legally licensed to practice midwifery and use the title 'midwife'; and who demonstrates competency in the practice of midwifery.

The educational pathway to midwifery across the world is varied, although midwives must meet the standards for practice and attain/maintain registration as a midwife with the regulatory body in their respective country. In Australia, this is the Nursing and Midwifery Board of Australia. While education programs vary, they all incorporate the key element of providing learning opportunities in clinical settings. Many countries have mandated educational standards. In addition to any legislative requirements, education programs are shaped by professional and social forces. These include philosophical underpinnings of the profession, discourses on scope of practice, the maternity care system, and evidence for practice. The next paragraphs provide an outline of these factors to allow the reader to appreciate the broader context in which learning and teaching in clinical settings occurs for midwifery.

The Midwifery Philosophy

Becoming a health professional involves much more than acquiring the knowledge and skills that will be used in the practice of the profession. An important part of any professional education includes the process of socialization and the formation of a professional identity (Wald 2015). The philosophical underpinnings of a profession are central to a profession's identity.

The word "midwife" derives from the Old and Middle English terms for "with" (mid) and "woman" (wife) (Pelvin and Thompson 2015). Thus, the literal translation of midwife is "with woman." This concept forms the philosophical basis of the profession today. Various organizations from the Australian College of Midwives (2019) to the International Confederation of Midwives (2014) espouse a midwifery philosophy that is underpinned by a "with woman" approach. This approach recognizes the woman as an equal partner in her care, who has a right to bodily autonomy and to make informed decisions that are right for her own individual circumstances. The role of the midwife then, is to walk with the woman through her pregnancy, birth, and parenting journey providing professional advice, care, and support, and advocating for her when necessary. This approach is often also termed "woman-centered," recognizing the central role of the woman in her care and is akin to "person-centered" care often discussed in other healthcare contexts (Bhattacharyya et al. 2019). In a woman-centered approach, the woman and her needs take precedence over the needs of the clinician or organization (Fahy 2012). Ideally, all aspects of care will be tailored to the individual woman's needs, though this can be challenging within the context of large institutional settings. This approach does not exclude partners, family, or others who might be important to the woman. It is for each woman to decide who is important to her and who should be included. A "with woman" or "woman-centered" philosophy is implicitly feminist (Leap 2009) though this association is not always explicitly made in midwifery philosophy statements or education curricula. This is evident in the profession's focus on the empowerment of childbearing women and support of their right to self-determination and bodily autonomy.

Another important element of the midwifery philosophy is the belief that childbirth for most women is a normal physiological process (International Confederation of Midwives 2014); one for which a woman's body is well designed. This philosophical positioning contrasts with biomedical approaches to childbirth, which often focus on the potential for pathology and therefore risk. Midwifery education programs therefore need to thoroughly prepare the midwife for understanding and supporting the physiology of childbearing processes along with recognizing and managing deviations from these normal processes.

The Midwifery Scope of Practice

Midwifery is essentially a primary healthcare practice, and midwives have an autonomous role in the care of women who are well and for whom we expect a straightforward pregnancy, labor and birth, uncomplicated by medical or obstetric complexities. The International Confederation of Midwives' statement on the scope of midwifery practice (International Confederation of Midwives 2017) is worth repeating here:

> The midwife is recognised as a responsible and accountable professional who works in partnership with women to give the necessary support, care and advice during pregnancy, labour and the postpartum period, to conduct births on the midwife's own responsibility and to provide care for the newborn and the infant. This care includes preventative measures, the promotion of normal birth, the detection of complications in mother and child, the accessing of medical care or other appropriate assistance and the carrying out of emergency measures. The midwife has an important task in health counselling and education, not only for the woman, but also within the family and the community. This work should involve antenatal education and preparation for parenthood and may extend to women's health, sexual or reproductive health and childcare. A midwife may practise in any setting including the home, community, hospitals, clinics or health units.

The midwifery scope of practice varies from country to country and even state to state in some countries (such as in the United States of America) depending on legislation. Not all countries permit midwives to practice in accordance with the full scope of midwifery as described by the International Confederation of Midwives. Midwives can work anywhere along the spectrum from low to high risk though whatever the scope of practice, they form part of a maternity care system in which midwives and other health professionals including obstetricians, collaborate to ensure that women receive the care they need to optimize their experience and childbirth outcomes.

Aligning with the belief that childbirth is a normal, physiological process for most women and in recognizing that unnecessary intervention is associated with the potential for concomitant morbidities, the role of midwives is often constructed as "guardians of normal." Broadly, this can be understood as meaning that midwives draw on a range of skills and expertise to promote, protect, and support the physiology of childbirth. They work with women and their individual circumstances to provide them with the best possible experience and outcome, with the least possible interruption to physiological processes.

Models of Maternity Care

Midwifery students may find themselves in a variety of settings, experiencing a variety of models of maternity care. Maternity care can be delivered in many ways and the term "models of maternity care" is often used to represent this variety (Donnolley et al. 2016). Models of maternity care can range from private obstetric practice, to public hospital maternity care, shared care, midwifery group practice, through to private midwifery practice. The role of midwives and the scope of midwifery practice in each of these models vary significantly. The expected birth setting is another factor interacting with models of maternity care and these may include hospitals, birth centers, or home. Midwifery-led care usually refers to models of care in which midwives are practicing to their full scope; often but not always caring for well women at low risk of developing obstetric complications. Continuity of carer refers to a model of care in which the childbearing woman receives care from a known primary carer (and their backup person) throughout the spectrum of childbirth, from pregnancy, labor, and birth, to the postpartum period.

Models of maternity care in which midwives may be practicing to their full scope and across the spectrum of childbirth include private midwifery, team midwifery, and caseload midwifery group practice. Midwives also have a critical role to play in all other models of maternity care, and some have very specialized skill in caring for women with high levels of medical or social complexity. As Sandall (2012), p. 323) reminds us, "Every woman needs a midwife, and some women need a doctor too." Midwives, as critical members of the maternity care workforce, are usually found, wherever and in whatever model of maternity care a woman is experiencing.

Evidence for Midwifery Care

It is no exaggeration to refer to midwives as critical members of the maternity care workforce. The Lancet Global Series on Midwifery published a series of four studies focusing on maternity services globally (The Lancet 2014). They identified that midwives are crucial to improving the health and well-being of women and their babies globally, not only in low- and middle-income countries. The health and well-being of mothers and babies can be negatively impacted by "too much, too soon" referring to the over use of obstetric interventions in childbirth and also "too little, too late" (referring to a lack of access to or availability of appropriate obstetric interventions) (McDougall et al. 2016). Modelling focusing on the scaling up of midwifery in 78 countries found that midwifery (with family planning and interventions for maternal and newborn health) could avert a total of 83% of all maternal deaths, stillbirths, and neonatal deaths (Homer et al. 2014). As one commentator noted, "Midwifery therefore has a pivotal, yet widely neglected part to play in accelerating progress to end preventable mortality of women and children" (Horton and Astudillo 2014, p. 1075).

The availability of midwifery-led, continuity models of maternity care (such as midwifery group practices or caseload midwifery practices) has increased, especially in the public sector over the last decades. This has been driven in part by demand from women, and by the evidence supporting this model of maternity care. A systematic review and meta-analysis of data from 15 studies comparing midwife-led continuity to other models of maternity care (Sandall et al. 2016) found that midwife-led models produced superior outcomes to other models without any adverse effects. Women experiencing midwife-led, continuity models were less likely to experience obstetric intervention in childbirth and were more likely to be satisfied with their care. Importantly, women in this model of care were less likely to have a preterm birth or experience fetal loss.

Given the strong evidence for the impact of good quality midwifery care and midwifery-led, continuity models in particular, it is important that midwifery students are well-prepared to exercise their important and unique role in the maternity care system. Some countries, such as New Zealand and Australia, have mandated the inclusion of Continuity of Care Experiences, whereby students follow a woman through pregnancy, labor, birth, and 6 weeks postpartum. However, this is not consistent in midwifery education standards across countries.

Midwifery Education Governance

The past 10 years have seen significant change in the Australian regulatory environment for registration and education of health professionals including midwifery (Tierney et al. 2018; Australian Nursing and Midwifery Accreditation Council 2014). Higher education regulation and quality assurance have also undergone major transformation (Australian Nursing and Midwifery Accreditation Council 2014). To register as a midwife in Australia, individuals must first have completed a program of study accredited by the Australian Nursing and Midwifery Accreditation Council (ANMAC) and approved by the Nursing and Midwifery Board of Australia (NMBA) (Australian Nursing and Midwifery Accreditation Council 2014). Educational pathways to midwifery in Australia include "direct entry" undergraduate midwifery degrees, "double degree" undergraduate degrees in midwifery and nursing, and post basic programs for nurses; diploma or masters of midwifery programs where the student may be supernumerary or in the paid workforce as a nurse in maternity settings. Such programs may be as short as 1 year full time or up to 4 years full time, dependant on the curriculum and students' prior learning. This variation in program structure and content is not limited to Australia. Indonesia, for example, has entry to midwifery programs at Diploma Three Level through to

Bachelor Level, and vary from 3–5 years in duration. However, while regardless of the program all graduates can use the title "midwife," but only bachelor degree graduates are able to legally practice independently. In addition to the level of qualification and its duration, there are variations in content requirements across countries. Table 1 highlights some key similarities and differences across five countries/regions.

The current education standards for midwifery programs require that they be developed in collaboration with key stakeholders to reflect contemporary trends in midwifery practice, that theory and practice are integrated throughout the program in equal proportions, and that students are afforded a variety of supervised midwifery practice experiences in environments that provide suitable opportunities and conditions for students to meet the Midwife Standards for Practice (Australian Nursing and Midwifery Accreditation Council 2014). Furthermore, clinical learning is included as soon as possible in the first year of study to facilitate early engagement with the professional context of midwifery. In addition, formative and summative assessments exist across all midwifery practice experiences, with a summative assessment to evaluate students' abilities to meet the Midwife Standards for Practice (Nursing and Midwifery Board of Australia 2018) be undertaken by a midwife in an Australian midwifery setting before program completion (Australian Nursing and Midwifery Accreditation Council 2014). Given the scope of midwifery practice, the varied models of care in which midwives practice, and the overwhelming evidence of the benefit of continuity of carer for women, the education standards also require students to undertake a minimum number of continuity of care experiences as a component of their supervised midwifery practice experiences (Australian Nursing and Midwifery Accreditation Council 2014).

The continuity of care experience (CCE) in midwifery education requires students to follow women through their childbearing experience commencing during pregnancy, and concluding in the postnatal period, being a known carer in the woman's experience regardless of the model of maternity care she is receiving (Tierney et al. 2018). Such a model of clinical learning is not unique to Australia, similar models have been adopted in countries including New Zealand, the United Kingdom, the Netherlands, and Indonesia (Tierney et al. 2018). For CCE, students are expected to meet and care for a woman on a number of occasions during her pregnancy, be on-call to support and care for her during labor and birth, and to follow-up with her during the early postnatal period (Tierney et al. 2018). The CCE occurs separately to rostered clinical placement hours and always occurs under the supervision of a registered health professional (Tierney et al. 2018). Midwifery students commence CCE in the first year of study and continue undertaking them throughout their degree.

As shown above, the current education standards are a mix of minimum number of experiences and evidence of competence. This has the potential to create a dichotomy of number-focused learning within a competence-driven curriculum. Such an approach recognizes individual differences in learning experiences, progression, and time required to develop competence (ten Cate 2015). While ensuring a volume of practice experiences, competency-based education should acknowledge

Table 1 Comparison of education standards

Experiences	Australia (Australian Nursing and Midwifery Accreditation Council 2014)	New Zealand (Midwifery Council of New Zealand 2019)	Europe (Timmermans 2017)	United Kingdom (Nursing and Midwifery Council 2019a, b)	Indonesia (Association of Indonesian Midwife Education (AIPKIND) 2018a, b)
Antenatal care episode	100	100	100	100	100
Care of women in labor	10 in addition to 30 normal births	40	40	40	Not stated
Normal vaginal births	30	40	40 (or min 30 if participates in at least 20 further births)	40 (or min 30 if participates in at least 20 further births)	50
Breech births	Not stated	Included under complex birth	Active participation or simulation	Active participation or simulation	Included under complex birth
Episiotomy and suturing	Not stated	Not specified	Active participation or simulated	Active participation or simulated	Not stated
Care of women with complex needs	40 (pregnancy, labor and birth or postnatal)	40 complex birth	40 (pregnancy, labor and birth or postnatal)	40 (pregnancy, labor and birth or postnatal)	Not stated nationally
Postnatal care	100	100	100	100	100

Healthy newborn care and assessment	20		100	100	50
Continuity of care experiences	10		25	Not stated	5
Additional				Care of women with pathological conditions in the fields of obstetrics and gynecology. Initiation into care in the field of medicine and surgery.	Care of women with pathological conditions in the fields of obstetrics and gynecology. Initiation into care in the field of medicine and surgery.	Premarital and preconception care: 12 Family planning and contraception: 25 Baby, toddler, and preschool care: 100 Teenager: 10 Perimenopause care: 10
Ratio of theory to practice	50:50		50:50	50:50	Not stated
Minimum course duration and/or hours	Not specified		4800 h	Not stated	3 years and 4600 h or if RN 2 years and 3600 h or if RN 18 months and 3000 h +12 months professional practice	Diploma 3: 3 years Diploma 4: 4 years Bachelor of Midwifery: 5 years

individuals may require more or less experiences or practice than their peers (ten Cate 2015). What becomes important in such an approach is the provision of feedback for learning and quality assessment based on competence development.

Models of Clinical Learning

Midwifery education programs are required to provide a variety of midwifery practice experiences, over a range of practice contexts. These may include acute care public and private hospitals, community health services, and women's own homes. The way in which students are exposed to these practice-based experiences varies across programs, with some maintaining a traditional block placement model, some using a variant of the Dedicated Education Unit (whereby students attend 2–3 days per week at the same venue for a long period of time), and others prioritizing learning through the CCE (McKellar et al. 2018; McKellar and Graham 2017; Carter et al. 2015; Jayasekara et al. 2018). Much of the recent literature on clinical education in both nursing and midwifery has espoused a focus on models of placement, when actually they focus on the supervision or facilitation embedded within models (McKellar et al. 2018; McKellar and Graham 2017; Jayasekara et al. 2018; Hall-Lord et al. 2013). The concept of the structure of practice-based experiences, their regularity, frequency, and location are a different concern to the way in which these experiences are supported and facilitated. The educational outcomes of small regular experiences in a known venue, such as with the DEU model have been shown in nursing to be beneficial to student learning (Jayasekara et al. 2018). However, the more common model is a model of block placements in the same or varying clinical venues for 2–6 weeks. In some programs, students are supernumerary for their practice-based experiences, while for some registered nurse (RN) entry programs, the student may be employed as an RN undertaking a midwifery education program whereby, they receive their practice-based experiences during their paid employment. This wide variation brings educational challenges for learning and teaching in clinical settings. Regardless of the model of practice-based experiences and the subsequent facilitation, it is important that learning opportunities are optimized while on clinical placement, so that students can competently translate theory to practice (McKellar et al. 2018).

Supporting Clinical Learning

Teaching and learning in clinical settings has many stakeholders (Sweet and Glover 2013). We know that a student's involvement with authentic clinical practice is variable depending on their prior knowledge and experience, their progression level in an educational program, their personal agency, the health care providers, institutional expectations, and women's preferences (Sweet and Glover 2011). For the purpose of this chapter, we will first present ways in which learning can be enhanced through student actions, and then present ways in which teaching can enhance student learning.

Learner Actions for Enhancing Learning

No matter how much or the way teaching occurs, learning is the responsibility of the individual student. Learning occurs all the time, so it is the type and quality of everyday work experiences and individuals' responses to those experiences that shape what is learned (Billett 2016). As such, to maximize learning in clinical settings, it is important that students embrace learning opportunities, by being prepared for the experience, being motivated to learn, and engage in learning affordances. This is explained as participatory practices (Billett and Sweet 2019). Participatory practices are those that comprise a duality between what is afforded by the clinical setting on the one hand, and how the individual student elects to engage in and learn through those practices, on the other (Billett and Sweet 2019). No learning opportunity will necessarily produce the same learning for different learners, as how individuals come to experience, construe, and construct knowledge from the same experience will vary (Billett 2016; Billett and Sweet 2019). Therefore, it is important that students have clear learning goals prior to entering the clinical venue. This may be governed largely by the program of study but needs to be individualized to the learner's own needs. In order to identify meaningful goals, it is important that students learn what they need to know, do, and value to develop their midwifery practice (Billett 2016). Students may negotiate their learning goals with the academic staff, a clinical facilitator, or midwifery clinician with whom they are working. The key point is they have an intention for what they wish to learn every time they step into a clinical setting.

To meet individual learning goals, students need to enact their personal agency (Richards et al. 2013). Research with medical students has identified five salient factors that are central to developing and enacting learner agency during clinical education (Richards et al. 2013). These include (International Confederation of Midwives 2017) personal epistemologies, which are an individuals' beliefs about what knowledge is and its influence on their actions; (Wald 2015) maximizing opportunities in the self-directed learning environment, proactively seeking opportunities and guidance; (Pelvin and Thompson 2015) developing a positive sense of self, recognize learnings and personal growth; (Australian College of Midwives 2019) using assertive communication, to express opinions and needs, and minimize conflict; and (International Confederation of Midwives 2014) building resilience, through peer collaborations (Richards et al. 2013). These five factors would certainly assist midwifery students' learning in clinical settings. Therefore, to enhance learning in clinical settings, it is recommended that midwifery students reflect on and develop their own personal epistemology. That is, to understand what constitutes midwifery knowledge, what they value, and how they can learn from varied experiences. Midwifery students should seek advice and clarification from more experienced people to provide access to knowledge that is difficult to learn (Billett 2016). This requires declaration of learning goals, taking advice, and learning from colleagues. Through observation and listening to others' explanations and reasoning, learning occurs (Billett 2016). Active participation in routine practices, such as handover, and attending meetings, such as morbidity and mortality meeting, are invaluable for learning (Billett et al. 2018). Clinical education is in the most part a supernumerary workplace activity, and as such, students have the capacity to undertake different learning experiences. It is important that midwifery students declare their learning goals throughout placements and actively seek new and novel opportunities to develop their occupational capacities. This may involve focused activities such as deliberate practice (Clapper and Kardong-Edgren 2012), reflection and reflective writing (Sweet et al. 2019), and participating in interprofessional activities (Lapkin et al. 2013).

Moreover, clinical settings afford opportunities for practice, so students can hone their abilities to perform tasks effectively and build causal and propositional links among concepts for developing their clinical reasoning (Billett 2016). Building personal and professional resilience is an important component of professional development. The need for resilience is often triggered by exposure to an adverse event (Clohessy et al. 2019) and having self-confidence, optimism, and using reflection are ways to build resilience (Clohessy et al. 2019). Maximizing opportunities is about being an active participant in goal-directed, authentic work (Billett 2016).

While learning in the clinical setting is critically important, these environments present a variety of challenges including the need to prioritize the provision of healthcare in often busy environments over student learning, lack of knowledge, skill, or motivation in health professionals to precept students and in some settings, competition for clinical experiences among students in the health professions (medical and midwifery for example). Globally, the World Health Organization recognizes economic and political restrictions to exercise the full scope of midwifery practice, as one of the barriers to high quality midwifery education since students will have few opportunities if any, to experience the full scope of midwifery work in the clinical setting (World Health Organization 2019).

Teaching Actions for Enhancing Learning

Teaching in clinical settings occurs from many different people including midwives, doctors, allied health practitioners, other students and women. Much "teaching" is not necessarily intentional, as students learn from participating in everyday workplace activities. There are, however, a range of intentional teacherly activities that will enhance learning. It is of little importance as to who provides these activities, but that they are provided effectively for learning. For teaching in clinical settings, there are two key considerations: (i) the practice curricula – the types and sequencing of experiences and (ii) the practice pedagogies – the activities and interactions that augment learning (Billett 2016).

The practice curricula for midwifery in Australia is somewhat protected by the mandated education standards; however, these state minimum number of experiences, so the types, sequencing, and overall volume of experiences vary among programs. Placing students in clinical settings assumes they will be afforded appropriate learning opportunities. However, research has shown that there may be a lack of access to required activities, and insufficient guidance needed for learning in some settings (Sweet and Glover 2011; Billett 2016). It is important that supervisors/facilitators ensure students are afforded appropriate authentic learning opportunities for their level to promote continued learning. While it is up to students to also seek learning experiences, no amount of learner agency can compensate for the denial of access to requisite learning experiences (Richards et al. 2013). Moreover, learning activities beyond the scope of one's existing competence or skill level can lead to negative outcomes (Billett 2016), so it is important to consider the relevance of activities for individual learners. At times, there may be new or novel experiences which offer the potential for appropriate new learning; however, in such situations, and particularly if beyond the learners' current scope, there is a need for guidance by a more experienced clinician to ensure appropriate meaning making and clinical development (Billett 2016). New or novel experiences require carefully considered facilitation and may even require debriefing after the experience. Further to the type, sequencing, and volume of learning affordances is the increasing role of the student in active participation. Novice students may start with observation of practice and performing low risk skills, while over time, and by developing clinical capacities, will build up to practice without assistance. It is important that the oversight of student performance is scaffolded in a manner that allows increasing independence.

One aspect of the practice curricula that may be overlooked is continuity of education (Hirsh et al. 2007). Midwives are familiar with the value of continuity of care and carer, similarly continuity of education is valuable for learning. Educational continuity is said to include continuity of care, curriculum, and supervision (Hirsh et al. 2007). The CCE program in midwifery goes some way to provide educational continuity through continuity of care. This, however, is often the minority of clinical hours, with non-continuity models making up the bulk of clinical learning. Finding ways to increase the continuity of care in the curricula is one approach to improving midwifery education. Continuity of curriculum requires horizontal and vertical integration, that promotes learner centeredness education and assessment (Hirsh et al. 2007). Midwifery portfolios inclusive of evidence of performance, goal setting, reflection, and formative and summative authentic assessment is one way of integrating clinical learning across curriculum (Embo and Valcke 2016; Gray et al. 2019). A well-designed portfolio can evidence progressive development and positively contribute to students' self-esteem and is a useful tool for student advocacy for learning. Continuity of supervision is one way in which to monitor student progress, minimize a need for constant reorientating to new students, and promotes a sense of belonging. One Australian study found that midwifery preceptors have an important part to play in facilitating student learning and making students feel they belong in the clinical setting (McKenna et al. 2013). The sense of belonging encompassed feelings of acceptance by colleagues and of being valued. When they felt they belonged, students were comfortable asking for advice and assistance and could more actively engage with learning opportunities (McKenna et al. 2013).

Continuity of supervision may occur by allocation of a clinical mentor, preceptor, or facilitator, or a faculty staff member, and is more easily achieved if there is consistency in the venue in which clinical learning occurs. However, where students are required to attend multiple clinical venues, a named mentor is one approach to ensure some consistent professional advice and performance monitoring.

Strong collaborations between clinical venues and education providers are required for the practice curricula to be enacted well. However, these collaborations have been described as problematic (McKellar et al. 2018; Hall-Lord et al. 2013). The model of facilitation, the connection, and collaboration between staff across both institutions and mutual goals are important for success (McKellar et al. 2018; Hall-Lord et al. 2013; Sweet and Glover 2013).

There are numerous practice pedagogies known to benefit learning when done well. Ensuring the right learning opportunities for individual students based on their personal need is utmost important. In the midwifery setting, this can be complicated by the intimate nature of midwifery care, and it is vital that the woman's consent is obtained when engaging students in learning opportunities. Some countries such as New Zealand have an explicit code of rights for consumers of health care which include rights in respect of teaching or research (Health and Disability Commissioner 1996). This includes the right to uncoerced, informed choice and consent to be involved in teaching or research. Regardless of the existence of legislation to protect consumer rights, involvement in teaching must always be a choice and great care must be taken to elicit consent before involving a student in a woman's care.

Next is the power of role models – both positive and negative – which cannot be under estimated. Excellent role models demonstrate high standards of clinical competence, excellence in clinical teaching skills and humanistic personal qualities (Passi et al. 2013). However, students observe the practice of all clinicians and ascertain the practices they like and those they dislike. This has the potential to influence the workplace culture, the students' sense of belonging and their willingness to return to the clinical venue. Research has shown that it is often those who have no official teaching role, who are profoundly influential to learners' professional development (Osterberg et al. 2015). Whether formal or informal, role models play an important part in learning (Power and Wilson 2019) which often involves mimetic learning (Billett 2014), whereby learning is through observation and imitation of others.

When midwifery students enter clinical settings, they are expected to have the knowledge and skills relevant to their year level. This should include clinical skills for which they have learnt the theoretical background and then practiced in simulation settings. However, it is common for additional direct instruction and hands-on assistance by an experienced practitioner to be required. When teaching clinical skills, there is the potential for cognitive overload. For learners to understand the task, it is important they see the whole task or process from start to finish and in real-time performance, to provide a mental map on which to master the sub-tasks (Billett 2016; Nicholls et al. 2016). Learners may then be exposed to sub-tasks until mastery occurs and eventually build up to complete performance. Too often in practice clinicians expect learners to know how to complete whole tasks, and making use of skill teaching models is one way to enhance skills development, confidence, and retention (Nicholls et al. 2016). A useful bedside approach to assist learners to make meaning of theory and practice is the "think aloud" technique. The think aloud method requires individuals to verbalize their thoughts as they problem solve a case study or interpret a statement (Banning 2008). The think aloud method may be used by clinicians to make their thinking and acting more accessible to learners, or by students to allow the "teacher" to assess understanding and problem solving skills (Banning 2008; Carter et al. 2016). The think aloud approach promotes clinical reasoning, by bridging gaps in experience making use of multiple cue connections, hypothesis formation, and the use of meaningful and evidence-based information to predict health care outcomes (Banning 2008).

One of the most effective practice pedagogies for learning is feedback and assessment. No clinical experiences should occur without feedback for learning. Feedback is a process whereby learners obtain information about their performance in order to improve performance (Boud and Molloy 2013; Boud 2015). In order for feedback to be effective, it needs to be expected and valued, be generated through dialogue between the learner and the other, be based on performance standards of expectations, and be given at a time that allows for improved performance (Boud 2015). Ideally feedback that generates self-regulation is optimal, whereby learners are not dependent on others to ascertain performance (Boud 2015). Beyond feedback, the importance of effective assessment is required. A well-designed assessment tool, based on national standards, can facilitate learning and teaching in clinical practice, and enable monitoring of standards (Sweet and Henderson 2019; Sweet et al. 2020). Quality assessment processes should be valid, reliable, transparent, have educational effect, be acceptable and feasible, and where appropriate, provide effective feedback for learning (Norcini et al. 2011). Therefore, assessment of midwifery student competence should be based on the observation of routine authentic encounters and rated by assessors using reliable and valid tools (Sweet et al. 2020).

Often students are partnered with midwives who may be expert clinicians but are insufficiently prepared for the teaching role and may be unaware of the students' learning goals (Hall-Lord et al. 2013). It is important that staff development for practice pedagogies be provided for clinical staff supervising and assessing students (Wu et al. 2015).

Conclusion

Learning in clinical settings is a vital component of midwifery curriculum. So much so it is afforded approximately 50% of time in midwifery programs in Australia and elsewhere. We have shown how the midwifery philosophy, scope of practice, and model of maternity care influence learning in clinical settings. Ensuring midwifery curriculum incorporate educational continuity, through continuity of care, continuity of supervision, and continuity of curriculum will enhance midwifery student learning. Ensuring students learn through continuity is vital to progress the midwifery profession to meet the strong global evidence of midwifery-led continuity of care providing the best outcomes for women. We have presented the case for learning and teaching to be a shared responsibility, and shown how both learners and those they engage with in clinical settings can enhance learning outcomes.

Cross-References

▶ Focus on Selection Methods: Evidence and Practice
▶ Focus on Theory: Emotions and Learning
▶ Nursing and Midwifery Education: Historical Perspectives
▶ Obstetric and Midwifery Education: Context and Trends
▶ Optimizing the Role of Clinical Educators in Health Professional Education
▶ Teaching Simple and Complex Psychomotor Skills

References

Association of Indonesian Midwife Education (AIPKIND). Book 1: Curriculum Education of Midwife Professionals (Academic graduation and profession). Under consideration by the Indonesian Government. Jakarta Indonesia 2018a.

Association of Indonesian Midwife Education (AIPKIND). Book 2: Curriculum Guide Book, Education of Midwife Professionals (Academic graduation and profession). Under consideration by the Indonesian Government. Jakarta Indonesia 2018b.

Australian College of Midwives. Midwifery philosophy and values Canberra, Australia. 2019. https://www.midwives.org.au/midwifery-philosophy-values

Australian Nursing and Midwifery Accreditation Council. Midwife accreditation standards 2014 Canberra. 2014. www.anmac.org.au

Banning M. The think aloud approach as an educational tool to develop and assess clinical reasoning in undergraduate students. Nurse Educ Today. 2008;28(1):8–14.

Bhattacharyya O, Blumenthal D, Stoddard R, Mansell L, Mossman K, Schneider EC. Redesigning care: adapting new improvement methods to achieve person-centred care. BMJ Qual Saf. 2019;28(3):242.

Billett S. Mimetic learning at work: learning in the circumstances of practice. Cham: Springer International Publishing; 2014.

Billett S. Learning through health care work: premises, contributions and practices. Med Educ. 2016;50(1):124–31.

Billett S, Sweet L. Understanding and appraising medical students' learning through clinical experiences: participatory practices. In: Loo S, editor. Teaching and learning for occupational practice: a multi-disciplinary and multi-level perspective. Abingdon: Routledge; 2019.

Billett S, Noble C, Sweet L. Pedagogically-rich activities in hospital work: handovers, ward rounds and team meetings. In: Delany C, Molloy E, editors. Learning and teaching in clinical contexts: a practical guide. 1st ed. Sydney: Elsevier; 2018.

Boud D. Feedback: ensuring that it leads to enhanced learning. Clin Teach. 2015;12(1):3–7.

Boud D, Molloy E. Rethinking models of feedback for learning: the challenge of design. Assess Eval High Educ. 2013;38(6):698–712.

Carter AG, Wilkes E, Gamble J, Sidebotham M, Creedy DK. Midwifery students' experiences of an innovative clinical placement model embedded within midwifery continuity of care in Australia. Midwifery. 2015;31(8):765–71.

Carter AG, Creedy DK, Sidebotham M. Development and psychometric testing of the Carter assessment of critical thinking in midwifery (preceptor/mentor version). Midwifery. 2016;34:141–9.

Clapper TC, Kardong-Edgren S. Using deliberate practice and simulation to improve nursing skills. Clin Simul Nurs. 2012;8(3):e109–e13.

Clohessy N, McKellar L, Fleet J. Bounce back- bounce forward: midwifery students experience of resilience. Nurse Educ Pract. 2019;37:22–8.

Donnolley N, Butler-Henderson K, Chapman M, Sullivan E. The development of a classification system for maternity models of care. Health Inf Manage J. 2016;45(2):64–70.

Embo M, Valcke M. Workplace learning in midwifery education in Flanders (Belgium). Midwifery. 2016;33:24–7.

Fahy K. What is woman-centred care and why does it matter? Women Birth. 2012;25(4):149–51.

Gray M, Downer T, Capper T. Australian midwifery student's perceptions of the benefits and challenges associated with completing a portfolio of evidence for initial registration: paper based and ePortfolios. Nurse Educ Pract. 2019;39:37–44.

Hall-Lord ML, Theander K, Athlin E. A clinical supervision model in bachelor nursing education – purpose, content and evaluation. Nurse Educ Pract. 2013;13(6):506–11.

Health & Disability Commissioner. Code of health and disability services consumers' rights. 1996. [22/4/2020]. https://www.hdc.org.nz/your-rights/about-the-code/code-of-health-and-disability-services-consumers-rights/

Hirsh DA, Ogur B, Thibault GE, Cox M. "Continuity" as an organizing principle for clinical education reform. N Engl J Med. 2007;356(8):858.

Homer CSE, Friberg IK, Dias MAB, ten Hoope-Bender P, Sandall J, Speciale AM, et al. The projected effect of scaling up midwifery. Lancet. 2014;384(9948):1146–57.

Horton R, Astudillo O. The power of midwifery. Lancet. 2014;384(9948):1075–6.

International Confederation of Midwives. Philosophy and model of midwifery care. The Hague: International Confederation of Midwives; 2014. https://www.internationalmidwives.org/assets/files/definitions-files/2018/06/eng-philosophy-and-model-of-midwifery-care.pdf

International Confederation of Midwives. ICM international definition of the midwife. 2017. https://www.internationalmidwives.org/our-work/policy-and-practice/icm-definitions.html

Jayasekara R, Smith C, Hall C, Rankin E, Smith M, Visvanathan V, et al. The effectiveness of clinical education models for undergraduate nursing programs: a systematic review. Nurse Educ Pract. 2018;29:116–26.

Lapkin S, Levett-Jones T, Gilligan C. A systematic review of the effectiveness of interprofessional education in health professional programs. Nurse Educ Today. 2013;33(2):90–102.

Leap N. Woman-centred or women-centred care: does it matter? Br J Midwifery. 2009;17(1):12–6.

McDougall L, Campbell O, Graham W. Maternal Health. An executive summary for The Lancet's series. Lancet. 2016;388(10056)1–8.

McKellar L, Graham K. A review of the literature to inform a best-practice clinical supervision model for midwifery students in Australia. Nurse Educ Pract. 2017;24:92–8.

McKellar L, Fleet J, Vernon R, Graham K, Cooper M. Comparison of three clinical facilitation models for midwifery students undertaking clinical placement in South Australia. Nurse Educ Pract. 2018;32:64–71.

McKenna L, Gilmour C, Biro MA, McIntyre M, Bailey C, Jones J, et al. Undergraduate midwifery students' sense of belongingness in clinical practice. Nurse Educ Today. 2013;33(8):880–3.

Midwifery Council of New Zealand. Standards for approval of pre-registration midwifery education programmes and accreditation of tertiary education organisations, Midwifery Council of New Zealand 3rd ed. 2019.

Nicholls D, Sweet L, Muller A, Hyett J. Teaching psychomotor skills in the twenty-first century: revisiting and reviewing instructional approaches through the lens of contemporary literature. Med Teach. 2016;38(10):1056–63.

Norcini J, Anderson B, Bollela V, Burch V, Costa MJ, Duvivier R, et al. Criteria for good assessment: consensus statement and recommendations from the Ottawa 2010 conference. Med Teach. 2011;33(3):206–14.

Nursing & Midwifery Council. Realising professionalism: standards for education and training. Part 3: Standards for pre-registration midwifery programmes. 2019a.

Nursing & Midwifery Council. Standards of proficiency for midwives. 2019b.

Nursing and Midwifery Board of Australia. Midwife standards for practice. 2018. https://www.nursingmidwiferyboard.gov.au/Codes-Guidelines-Statements/Professional-standards.aspx

Osterberg L, Swigris R, Weil A, Branch WT Jr. The highly influential teacher: recognising our unsung heroes. Med Educ. 2015;49(11):1117–23.

Passi V, Johnson S, Peile E, Wright S, Hafferty F, Johnson N. Doctor role modelling in medical education: BEME guide no. 27. Med Teach. 2013;35(9):e1422–e36.

Pelvin B, Thompson T. Sustaining midwifery practice. In: Pairman S, Pincombe J, Thorogood C, Tracy S, editors. Midwifery, preparation for practice. 3rd ed. Sydney: Churchill Livingstone; 2015. p. 362–80.

Power A, Wilson A. Mentor, coach, teacher, role model: what's in a name? Br J Midwifery. 2019;27(3):184–7.

Richards J, Sweet L, Billett S. Preparing medical students as agentic learners through enhancing student engagement in clinical education. Asia-Pac J Coop Educ. 2013;14(4):251–63.

Sandall J. Every woman needs a midwife, and some women need a doctor too. Birth. 2012;39(4):323–6.

Sandall J, Soltani H, Gates S, Shennan A, Devane D. Midwife-led continuity models versus other models of care for childbearing women. Cochrane Database Syst Rev. 2016;4:1–118.

Sweet L, Glover P. Optimizing the follow through experience for midwifery learning. In: Billett S, Henderson A, editors. Developing learning professionals. Dordrecht: Springer; 2011. p. 83–100.

Sweet L, Glover P. An exploration of the midwifery continuity of care program at one Australian University as a symbiotic clinical education model. Nurse Educ Today. 2013;33(3):262–7.

Sweet L, Henderson A. Assessment of midwifery student practice: the value of a standardised assessment tool. Aust Midwifery News. 2019;19(9):24–5.

Sweet L, Bass J, Sidebotham M, Fenwick J, Graham K. Developing reflective capacities in midwifery students: enhancing learning through reflective writing. Women Birth. 2019;32(2):119–26.

Sweet L, Fleet J, Bull A, Downer T, Fox D, Bowman R, et al. Development and validation of the Australian Midwifery Standards Assessment Tool (AMSAT) to the Australian midwife standards for practice 2018. Women Birth. 2020;33(2):135–44.

ten Cate O. The false dichotomy of quality and quantity in the discourse around assessment in competency-based education. Theory Pract. 2015;20(3):835–8.

The Lancet. Midwifery: The Lancet; 2014. https://www.thelancet.com/series/midwifery

Tierney O, Sweet L, Houston D, Ebert L. A historical account of the governance of midwifery education in Australia and the evolution of the continuity of care experience. Women Birth. 2018;31(3):e210–e5.

Timmermans W. Workgroup training Flemish professional organization of midwives. Logbook for midwifery student. Directive 2013/55/EC of the European Parliament and the Council of 20 November 2013 on the recognition of professional qualifications 2017.

Wald HS. Professional identity (trans)formation in medical education. Acad Med. 2015;90(6):701–6.

World Health Organization. Strengthening quality midwifery education for universal health coverage 2030. 2019.

Wu XV, Enskär K, Lee CCS, Wang W. A systematic review of clinical assessment for undergraduate nursing students. Nurse Educ Today. 2015;35(2):347–59.

Learning and Teaching in the Operating Room: A Surgical Perspective

48

V. Chao, C. Ong, Debra Kiegaldie, and Debra Nestel

Contents

Introduction	910
Section 1: The Current State of Intraoperative Teacher and Learner Behaviors	913
Teacher Behaviors in the OR	913
Learner Behaviors in the OR	914
Section 2: Conditions Under Which Learning Takes Place and the Learning Process	915
What Affects Intraoperative Learning Opportunities?	915
What Can Affect the Learning Obtained from these Opportunities?	917
Section 3: Teaching Interventions and Models, Implications for Practice	920
Interventions: Description and Empirical Evidence	920
Models and Frameworks	924
Implications for Practice	924
Conclusions	926

V. Chao (✉)
National Heart Centre, Singapore, Singapore
e-mail: victor.chao.t.t@singhealth.com.sg

C. Ong
KK Women's and Children's Hospital, Singapore, Singapore
e-mail: caroline.ong.c.p@singhealth.com.sg

D. Kiegaldie
Faculty of Medicine, Nursing and Health Sciences, Monash University; Faculty of Health Sciences and Community Studies, Holmesglen Institute and Healthscope Hospitals, Melbourne, VIC, Australia
e-mail: debra.kiegaldie@holmesglen.edu.au

D. Nestel
Monash University Institute for Health & Clinical Education, Monash University, Clayton, VIC, Australia
Department of Surgery (Austin), University of Melbourne, Parkville, VIC, Australia
e-mail: debra.nestel@monash.edu

© Springer Nature Singapore Pte Ltd. 2023
D. Nestel et al. (eds.), *Clinical Education for the Health Professions*,
https://doi.org/10.1007/978-981-15-3344-0_64

Appendix I: Search Strategy Used in the Scoping Review 927
  Inclusion Criteria 927
  Exclusion Criteria 927
Cross-References 928
References 928

Abstract

The operating room (OR) is the main venue where trainee surgeons learn their craft. With educational challenges such as limited OR time and caseload, inconsistent faculty preparation and motivation, and the increasing complexity of cases, the case for efficient and structured intraoperative teaching in an environment optimized for learning is greater than ever.

A separate scoping review of literature of what is known about learner and teacher behaviors in the OR was undertaken and forms the basis of this chapter. We present a distillation of key features of this review. The intra-operative learning process and the factors which influence it are examined. The various interventions and models which may help in teaching and learning are summarized.

There are some findings that we intuitively know that enhance the learning experience, such as engaging learners and treating them well, giving learners consistent, constructive, and structured feedback, and allowing learners opportunities to operate with adequate supervision. What is less intuitive are findings on the use of humor, banter, and "war stories" to socialize trainees into the OR environment, the engagement of other stakeholders in the OR such as anesthesia and nursing colleagues to optimize learning, and the study of learning by motor and visual cues which has increasing relevance with the use of laparoscopic surgery where decisions are made on visual information alone.

The richness of the materials contributed by authors of the paper in this review provides a sound basis upon which to inform our practices, and to guide future research.

Keywords

Surgical skills training · Situated learning · Operating skills · Operating room · Operating theatre · Resident · Faculty · Postgraduate medical education

Introduction

There are concerns that graduates from surgical training programs are insufficiently prepared for independent practice (Klingensmith and Lewis 2013; Yeo et al. 2009). Contributory reasons for inadequate preparation include work-hour restrictions with consequent limited operating room (OR) time (Fairfax et al. 2010), insufficient caseload (Fairfax et al. 2010), and inadequate preparation of faculty for teaching (Gibson and Campbell 2000). Since many basic skills needed for surgery can be acquired outside the OR (Hamdorf and Hall 2000), this has resulted in a trend toward using wet labs (Bedetti et al. 2017), simulators, and task trainers (De Montbrun and Macrae 2012) to supplement traditional surgical training.

Nevertheless, the OR environment is "rich with complexity" (p.146, Glarner et al. 2017) and remains the primary teaching venue for surgeons in training (Kieu et al. 2015; Pernar et al. 2011; Scallon et al. 1992; Reznick 1993). The OR is where "a surgeon combines decision-making with technical" and many other aspects of professional surgical practice. Hence, optimal surgical training is required "both inside and outside the OR, creating a balance of practice and performance" (p.32, Levinson et al. 2010).

The complexity of surgical procedures has increased with advances in surgical science (Mateo Vallejo 2012), and these surgeries are being performed on sicker patients than before (Cooper and Gaba 2002). This imbalance between the increased scope of education and the reduced work-hours and clinical resources for training, highlights the need for more efficient and structured intra-operative teaching (Anderson et al. 2013).

While the OR has been the training ground where generations of surgeons have learned their craft, relatively little has been written about it. A 2017 systematic review described discordance between learners' and teachers' perceptions of quantity and quality of teaching in the OR, while suggesting that interventions could have a positive impact on learners' ratings of teaching performance (Timberlake et al. 2017). Another review on perioperative feedback highlighted the perceived need for more and better quality perioperative feedback (Mckendy et al. 2017). Both reviews focused mainly on teacher-learner interactions so did not include other aspects of intraoperative education, which will be made apparent later in this chapter.

This chapter reports what is known about intraoperative learning and teaching and is based on a scoping review of studies which were published prior to 31st Dec 2018. It also identifies research gaps for future investigation. Our preference was to present the chapter in a form meaningful to surgical teachers, trainees, and researchers rather than as a formal scoping review. However, Appendix I contains our search strategy and other relevant information to identifying papers for inclusion.

The chapter is divided into three sections that reflect the main themes identified during the scoping review. Box 1 summarizes our findings in analyzing the studies.

Box 1: Summary of Findings from Our Scoping Review

Section 1: The Current State of Intraoperative Teacher and Learner Behaviors
  Teacher behaviors in the OR

Ideal teacher characteristics and behavior
Actual teacher behavior from the perspectives of teachers, learners, and observers

(continued)

Box 1 (continued)
  Learner behaviors in the OR
  Section 2: Conditions Under Which Learning Takes Place and the Learning Process
  What affects intraoperative learning opportunities?

OR environment
Learner discrimination
Relationship between teacher and learner
Entrustment decisions
Participation and autonomy

  What can affect the learning obtained from these opportunities?

Goal setting
Concepts unique to psychomotor skills learning
Surgical skills learning during the operation is dynamic & influenced by multiple factors
Types of learning in the OR
Communication styles in OR culture
Teaching complex operations
Motivating Learners

  Section 3: Teaching Interventions and Models, Implications for Practice
  Interventions – description and empirical evidence

Enhancing learner preparation
Feedback interventions and structured briefing/debriefing tools
Use of video for demonstration
Coaching the teachers

  Models & frameworks
  Implications for practice

Curriculum design
Faculty development
Research opportunities

Section 1: The Current State of Intraoperative Teacher and Learner Behaviors

Teacher Behaviors in the OR

In this section, we explore the characteristics and behaviors of the ideal teacher from the perspectives of teachers and learners. This is then compared with actual teacher behaviors, as reported by teachers, learners, and observers.

Ideal Teacher Characteristics and Behavior

From the viewpoints of teachers and learners, the ideal teacher demonstrates confidence (Butvidas et al. 2011; Skoczylas et al. 2012; Iwaszkiewicz et al. 2008), patience, tolerance (Vollmer et al. 2011), and good communication skills (Butvidas et al. 2011; Vollmer et al. 2011). Before starting the case, s/he allows learners time to prepare (Butvidas et al. 2011) and discusses the case with them (Vollmer et al. 2011). During the operation, s/he gives learners autonomy (Butvidas et al. 2011, Vollmer et al. 2011) and constructive feedback (Jensen et al. 2012; Rose et al. 2011; Vollmer et al. 2011) as well as immediate feedback after the operation (Jensen et al. 2012; Kieu et al. 2015; Nathwani et al. 2017). Ideal feedback covers what went well and what did not go so well (Jensen et al. 2012), uses specific examples (Vollmer et al. 2011), covers technical skills and professional behaviors, and ends with an action plan for improvement. Ideal teachers ask learners for feedback on teaching skills (Vollmer et al. 2011).

Teacher and learner perspectives differ in that teachers believe the ideal teacher sets and communicates high standards, helps the learner avoid operative pitfalls, and demonstrates technical steps (Vollmer et al. 2011). While learners do value a competent teacher with technical expertise (Cox and Swanson 2002; Skoczylas et al. 2012), they prefer a calm and courteous teacher (Iwaszkiewicz et al. 2008; Skoczylas et al. 2012) with a positive attitude toward teaching (Iwaszkiewicz et al. 2008) who maintains a supportive learning climate of respect, support, and empathy (Cox and Swanson 2002; Vikis et al. 2008; Vollmer et al. 2011), and who has an explanatory or consultative leadership style (Kissane-Lee et al. 2016). The learners appreciate teachers who are sensitive to their needs (Cox and Swanson 2002), encourage learner participation and allow early surgical independence (Skoczylas et al. 2012; Vikis et al. 2008). Learners think that the ideal teacher provides "direct and ongoing feedback" regarding learner progress (p.253, Cox and Swanson 2002), and is willing to accept responsibility for mistakes and consequences (Skoczylas et al. 2012). Learners value an instructional plan (Vikis et al. 2008), emphasis on anatomical landmarks, and encouraging repetitive practice (Skoczylas et al. 2012).

Actual Teacher Behavior from the Perspectives of Teachers, Learners, and Observers

Both teachers and learners acknowledge that intraoperative education needs to be improved (Levinson et al. 2010; Rose et al. 2011). Teachers rarely asked for feedback on their own teaching skills or the trainee's learning objectives (Vollmer et al. 2011) and postoperative feedback was given far less often than it should (Kieu et al. 2015; Nathwani et al. 2017). Nevertheless, some teachers and learners agreed that procedures were discussed in advance (Levinson et al. 2010, Rose et al. 2011), that teachers demonstrated pertinent anatomy (Rose et al. 2011), asked relevant questions during the case (Levinson et al. 2010, Rose et al. 2011), gave learners constructive feedback (Levinson et al. 2010, Rose et al. 2011), and structured intraoperative teaching (Kieu et al. 2015).

In general, teachers' perceptions of the quality and/or quantity of their teaching were better than their learners' impressions (Butvidas et al. 2011; Claridge et al. 2003; Levinson et al. 2010; Rose et al. 2011; Vollmer et al. 2011). This included teaching about the steps of the procedure, surgical skills, instrument handling, and surgical technique (Rose et al. 2011). While teachers perceived that they gave frequent or adequate feedback, learners disagreed (Jensen et al. 2012; Levinson et al. 2010; Rose et al. 2011). A possible reason for the discrepancy could be because learners may not recognize teaching behaviors (Chen et al. 2014) during the flow of the operation (Ong et al. 2016). Learners reported that teachers did not routinely discuss their role in surgical procedures (Binsaleh et al. 2015; Mahoney et al. 2010), or help learners identify personal educational operative goals preoperatively (Snyder et al. 2012). Furthermore, teachers tended to have authoritative leadership styles, as opposed to the preferred explanatory or consultative styles (Kissane-Lee et al. 2016).

Independent observations of OR interactions corroborate learners' perspectives. Although teachers do make an effort to teach: in a study of the teaching of ACGME competencies in the OR, teachers spent an average of 34% of operative time instructing learners in patient care, with 22 teaching events per case (Greenberg et al. 2007); there are many areas for teaching improvement. Teacher-learner feedback occurred in less than half of all cases, with only about half of all teachable steps being taught (Pernar et al. 2016). Feedback when provided was done verbally and mostly unstructured, delivered in a corrective, unidirectional manner. Feedback on areas to improve was more common than affirmation of good performance; feedback as praise and affirmation when given was non-specific; and "action plans and strategies for improvement were rarely discussed." Feedback tended to be focused on technical skills (Pernar et al. 2016). Teaching–learning behaviors observed were "modeling," "coaching," and "scaffolding," while alternative cognitive apprenticeship methods of "exploration," "reflection," and "articulation" were less common (Ong et al. 2016). Teachers rarely capitalized on teaching opportunities toward the end of the operation during "closing" and in the recovery room (Scallon et al. 1992).

Learner Behaviors in the OR

There were fewer studies focused on learner behavior, as compared to teacher behavior. Both teachers and learners valued learner preparedness (Vollmer et al. 2011). In addition, learners recognized the importance of being receptive, prepared, and acknowledging their own limitations (Vikis et al. 2008). However, while learners believed they were adequately prepared for surgery by reading about procedures (Levinson et al. 2010, Rose et al. 2011) and by reviewing anatomy (Rose et al. 2011), this was not apparent to the teachers. Observers noted that learners occasionally did not register verbal feedback when they were concentrating on the operation (Ong et al. 2016).

Section 2: Conditions Under Which Learning Takes Place and the Learning Process

What Affects Intraoperative Learning Opportunities?

OR Environment
There is significant geographical variation in the perceived OR learning environment: Learners in Canada (Kanashiro et al. 2006), Australia/New Zealand (Mahoney et al. 2010), Nigeria (Ibrahim et al. 2013), and Pakistan (Soomro et al. 2017) found the OR learning environment to be satisfactory, while urology residents in Saudi Arabia "perceived the theater learning environment as less than ideal" (p.73, Binsaleh et al. 2015). The type of hospital also seemed to make a difference, where perceptions of learning at a tertiary referral hospital were lower when compared to community/regional hospitals (Diwadkar and Jelovsek 2010).

Several studies highlighted the fluid nature of the OR environment where time pressure and/or case scheduling affect learning opportunities (Chen et al. 2015; Kieu et al. 2015; Vollmer et al. 2011). Workflow disruptions – deviations from natural case progression – occur in up to 21% of operating time and may enable or hinder teaching. Some teachers used workflow disruptions to teach, though their teaching methods could shift from active to passive when they needed to take over surgery to ensure patient safety (Glarner et al. 2017). Distractions in the OR by pager interruptions had a mixed effect: a study where mostly non-urgent paging interrupted 55% of operations did not negatively impact learner's educational experience (Rose et al. 2012), while another study found learners who received pages in the OR were stressed and distracted (Binsaleh et al. 2015).

Learner Discrimination
Women learners reported reduced learning opportunities and support in multiple studies in the last decade from Canada, Nigeria, Pakistan, and the United States (Ibrahim et al. 2013; Kanashiro et al. 2006; Meyerson et al. 2017a; Soomro et al. 2017); however, a more recent study from the United States showed that faculty entrustment scores did not appear to differ for women and men learners in the OR (Thompson-Burdine et al. 2018).

Junior learners scored the OR lower in terms of learning environment, learning opportunities, workload, and support as compared to senior learners (Diwadkar and Jelovsek 2010; Kanashiro et al. 2006). This finding may be influenced by the factors described in the next few paragraphs.

The Relationship Between Teacher and Learner

Relationships between teachers and learners affect the learning environment since apprenticeship-style learning remains prominent in the OR (Kieu et al. 2015). The learners' relationships with their teachers "correlated most strongly with overall satisfaction" with the OR learning environment (p. 884, Mahoney et al. 2010), and increased familiarity and trust between teacher and learner allowed learners more access to operative opportunities (Torbeck et al. 2015). Early preoperative teacher-learner communication was also associated with learner participation (Bailey et al. 2018). On the other hand, poor teacher-learner rapport was perceived to reduce feedback. However, it has to be acknowledged that interactions between teachers and learners are "complicated by their shared responsibility towards the patient" (p. 91, Van Der Houwen et al. 2011).

Entrustment Decisions

Delegation of responsibility requires the teacher to manage the conflicting responsibilities of providing good care with the need to train (Reid et al. 2000). The entrustment process has been described as a "stepwise process" involving (1) "initial propensity to trust based on the perceived risk of the case and trustworthiness" of the learner; (2) deciding to trust the learner to begin the surgery; (3) "close observation of preliminary steps"; (4) "an evolving decision" based on the progress of the surgery;(5) intervention if the surgery goes "off-track" (withdrawal of trust); and (6) "re-evaluation of trust for future cases" (p.391, Salim et al. 2020).

Entrustment is influenced by several teacher factors: the teacher's ability to divide the operation into procedural segments to delegate some parts to the learner while remaining the principal operator for the rest; the teacher's "comfort level with their own technical skills in different procedures"; coping style with stress; level of interest in teaching, and supervising ability (p.308, Reid et al. 2000).

Important factors for entrustment in the OR are directly observed clinical skill, the confidence level of the teacher, and the ease of the operation (Teman et al. 2014). The teacher's confidence in the learner is enhanced by the learner's ability to do more in the OR (Park et al. 2017). The seniority of the learner was significantly correlated with teacher entrustment and learner entrustability behaviors (Sandhu et al. 2018). Recurring opportunities for learners to perform the same operation with the same teacher over an extended period of time (longitudinal contact) is important for progressive entrustment in the OR (Sandhu et al. 2017; Teman et al. 2014). Other systemic factors which may affect entrustment include hospital policies and duty-hour regulations (Sandhu et al. 2017).

The biggest barrier to entrustment in the OR is patient safety (Teman et al. 2014). The main reasons described for withdrawing trust are inability to follow instructions, failure to progress, and unsafe maneuvers (Salim et al. 2020). Teachers' focus on patient outcomes, a desire to increase efficiency and finish operations earlier, and expectations of attending surgeon involvement were barriers to entrustment (Teman et al. 2014).

Participation and Autonomy

While both teachers and learners had similar expectations of learner operative autonomy, actual levels achieved were significantly less than that expected (Meyerson et al. 2017b; Meyerson et al. 2014). Learner participation and autonomy in surgery are influenced by learner, teacher, and situational factors.

Learner factors include learner knowledge and preparation (Torbeck et al. 2015) and increased seniority (Bailey et al. 2018; Meyerson et al. 2017a, b), learner performance (Williams et al. 2017; Torbeck et al. 2015); learners who struggle or do not know their limitations tended to have their autonomy removed (Torbeck et al. 2015).

Teacher factors include teacher confidence in being able to "fix anything" (Torbeck et al. 2015), and teacher characteristics, habits, and beliefs (Williams et al. 2017); while teacher seniority has mixed effects. One study reported on low-rated teachers who seldom gave autonomy as being less mature surgeons (Torbeck et al. 2015), but others reported that junior teachers better understood learner's debriefing needs and were associated with increased learner involvement (Morgan et al. 2017a, b). Some teachers cite their moral responsibility for personally safely seeing the patient through the operation as a reason for limiting learner autonomy (Torbeck et al. 2015).

Situational factors limiting participation include operational complexity (Meyerson et al. 2017b; Morgan et al. 2017a, b; Williams et al. 2017), difficult anatomy, ill patients, and risky parts of the operation (Torbeck et al. 2015).

Factors which influence the teaching of surgical decision-making parallel those that influence participation and autonomy. Facilitators include reciprocal dialogue such as concept-driven feedback, safe struggle, and appreciation for retraction. Barriers include aberrant case characteristics, anatomic uncertainties, and time pressures (Hill et al. 2017). Learner seniority and case duration similarly affect learners' participation in intraoperative decision-making (Bezemer et al. 2016).

What Can Affect the Learning Obtained from these Opportunities?

Apart from the teacher-learner behaviors described above, other factors that may affect learning in the OR include goal setting, concepts unique to psychomotor skills learning, and the influence of situated learning (Brown et al. 1989) afforded by the cases, the OR team members, and the OR culture.

Goal Setting

Learners sometimes do not recognize intraoperative learning opportunities, as demonstrated by a study interviewing teacher-learner pairs that showed that teachers articulated more learning goals for learners than learners did for themselves (Pernar et al. 2011). Additionally, while teachers and learners both agreed on technical learning objectives, teachers identified the need to learn perioperative management, which was rarely identified by learners (Pernar et al. 2011).

Nebeker et al. found that gender differences may factor in the choice of learning objectives, with female learners tending to favor knowledge over technical skills. Learners who had female teachers were also more likely to select knowledge over skill, and attitude over skill than those with male teachers. Senior learners more frequently chose attitude-based learning objectives over their juniors (Nebeker et al. 2017).

Concepts Unique to Psychomotor Skills Learning

A qualitative study interviewing teachers and learners on what is learned in the OR identified sensory semiosis – learning to make sense of visual and haptic cues – as a key component of learning in the OR (Cope et al. 2015b; Skoczylas et al. 2012). Semiotics refers to the study of signs as elements that communicate meaning. For surgeons, making meaning was described as a way to translate what [surgeons] saw into "the 'known' abstract anatomy of the textbook" or "to recognize subtle changes in the tissues" visually or through touch (p.1127, Cope et al. 2015b). To develop sensory semiosis, teachers use verbal guidance to help learners to recognize visual cues of structures or pathology (Cope et al. 2015a; Feng et al. 2016). Compared to non-procedural specialties, physical guidance has increased importance for surgical teachers. Effective teachers often use perceptual-motor teaching that emphasizes the motor and tactile aspects of operating (Skoczylas et al. 2012).

Verbal and physical communications serve different but complementary functions during the surgery that allow the development of common ground, that is, a shared understanding about the operation including the maneuvers, timing, and coordination required. An analysis of teacher-learner interaction during laparoscopic cholecystectomy found that utterances or verbal communication provided detailed information for surgeons to develop "content common ground," whereas "actions contribute to process common ground development" (p.704, Feng and Mentis 2017). Verbal communication is required for introducing information (e.g., clarifying anatomy) while actions were used, not only for tacitly conveying information or guidance (e.g., the surgeon indicates a target area to dissect without speaking) (Feng and Mentis 2017; Sutkin et al. 2015b), but also to demonstrate understanding (e.g., the learner moves the instrument to the indicated target) (Feng and Mentis 2017).

Surgical Skills Learning During the Operation Is Dynamic and Influenced by Multiple Factors

During an operation, instances of teaching are interwoven within the procedure, and the operative team transitions between teaching moments and other activities required to advance the surgery (Svensson et al. 2009). This requires the teacher's and learner's cooperation and coordination (Sutkin et al. 2018), while the rest of the surgical and anesthetic team members need to adjust accordingly (Svensson et al. 2009). The progress of the procedure is valued both by teachers and learners. Learner hesitation impeding progress of the operation is interpreted negatively as a sign of incompetence (Ott et al. 2018) unlike expert "slowing down when you should" when recognizing uncertainty and difficulty (p.128, St-Martin et al. 2012).

Procedural variations due to teachers' individual preferences may also affect learning (Apramian et al. 2015; Hill et al. 2017). Apramiam et al. constructed the theory of "thresholds of principles and preference" where different teachers vary in which procedural variations they regard as negotiable (surgeon preference) vs. non-negotiable (surgical principle). Learners have to "spot" and "map" each teacher's thresholds as signposts to guide their behavior, and some learners eventually develop their own thresholds (Apramian et al. 2015).

Types of Learning in the OR

Some surgical competencies appear more difficult to learn and teach in the OR, with technical expertise most readily identified and learned, while health advocacy was least among the Royal Australasian College of Surgeons (RACS) competencies (Kieu et al. 2015). "Technical expertise was taught through watching, assisting with didactic instruction and demonstration," as compared with knowledge-based competencies which were taught by "active questioning and discussion," and behavioral competencies were taught by "observation and role-modeling" (p.27, Kieu et al. 2015). A case study of teacher-trainee pairs in observed operations found that teachers and trainees differed in their recall of the teaching and learning related to aspects of practice such as surgical reasoning and team management skills because of non-recognition of learning points and different learning goals (Ong et al. 2016).

Communication Styles in OR Culture

Observation in the OR has identified that verbal communication is used for teaching specific to the operation (findings, steps, tissue, and instrument handling) (Blom et al. 2007), teachings on clinical judgment, coaching for enhanced performance, and discussions on unrelated topics (Roberts et al. 2012). "Most teaching instances were prompted by errors in learner performance." "Instances of verbal teaching were numerous, arose opportunistically...and focused typically on multiple points" (p.643, Roberts et al. 2012).

Questions asked during the operation were mostly lower-level type questions (Barrett et al. 2017; Magas et al. 2017) focusing on recall/understanding, rather than analysis/evaluation (Magas et al. 2017). Teachers also did not wait long enough for learners to answer before intervening (Barrett et al. 2017). Learners often asked case-related questions focusing on operative techniques and logistics; these questions were mostly transactional rather than reflective (O'holleran et al. 2019). Teachers often "prefixed speech with polite terms and used terse language, colorful verbal analogies, and sometimes humor" (p.243, Sutkin et al. 2015a). Non-case-related discussion or "banter" was helpful to "humanize the participants" in the OR (p.647, Roberts et al. 2012). Several teachers used narrative stories from their personal experience to illustrate teaching points, which helped "socialize trainees in the culture of surgery" (p.63, Hu et al. 2012).

Teaching Complex Operations

Master surgeons employ many principles of learning theory when teaching uncommon and complex operations, including: graduated responsibility, development of a mental set, deliberate practice, deconstructing complex tasks, vertical transfer of information, and identifying principles to structure knowledge (Pernar et al. 2012).

Motivating Learners

Teachers often instinctively use techniques that motivate learners during intraoperative teaching, by activating both intrinsic and extrinsic learner motivation. They facilitate the learners' intrinsic motivation by facilitating learner autonomy, fostering responsible attitudes, modeling relational behavior, and encouraging learner self-motivation. Extrinsic motivation techniques include personal supervision, providing a "safe" learning environment with explicit instructions and motivating feedback (Dath et al. 2013). Others too have emphasized the motivational aspect of specific feedback, which "helped aid progression of learning" and "increased motivation and performance" of learners (p.1, Kamali and Illing 2018). In contrast, some forms of feedback – such as undermining or bullying – may have a detrimental effect on learner performance and well-being, and in some, may induce a "desire to pursue an alternative career" (p.1, Kamali and Illing 2018).

Section 3: Teaching Interventions and Models, Implications for Practice

In this section, we draw together several studies exploring structured teaching tools and models, and their implications for practice. While the level of evidence for the approaches is limited, they are underpinned by a range of educational theories (Table 1).

Interventions: Description and Empirical Evidence

The four interventions are enhancing learner preparation, feedback interventions and structured briefing/ debriefing tools, use of video for demonstration, and coaching the teachers.

Enhancing Learner Preparation

Strategies to enhance learner preparation include preoperative goal setting (Ahmed et al. 2013), encouraging patient familiarity through written scripts outlining patient-specific surgical management (Gas et al. 2017), and the institution of an "educational pause" in addition to the surgical time-out, which allows for discussion of learning objectives, in order to improve the learning experience (Clark Donat et al. 2016).

Feedback Interventions and Structured Briefing/ Debriefing Tools

Grantcharov et al. (2007) found that learners who received constructive feedback based on structured assessment made significantly greater improvement in their performance in the OR compared to those who did not receive feedback. Other educational interventions include the use of faculty development to improve the

Table 1 Interventions, models, and frameworks described for surgical education, which may be helpful in influencing practice

A.	Interventions – Description and empirical evidence
Enhancing learner preparation	*(a) Preoperative scripting* Prior to entering the OR, learners were asked to "script" a patient-centered surgical management plan that highlights specific patient information important for pre-, intra-, and post-operative surgical management. Learners who scripted randomized cases prior to entering the OR received higher performance scores (Gas et al. 2017). *(b) Discussing learning objectives pre-operatively (educational pause)* Learners who discussed their specific learning objectives with their teachers before beginning a surgical case were more likely to have surgical goals for the procedure, were better able to maximize learning opportunities, and were more satisfied with their participation in the case. Teachers were also more likely to be aware of learning objectives of learners (Clark Donat et al. 2016).
Feedback interventions and structured briefing/debriefing tools	*(a) Feedback improves performance* Learners who received detailed and constructive feedback after laparoscopic cholecystectomy showed significantly improved times to complete a second procedure and improved economy of movement scores as compared to controls (Grantcharov et al. 2007). *(b) 10 step pre- and post-operative briefing/debriefing structure* Introduction of a 10 step preoperative and postoperative briefing/debriefing structure not only reminded teachers that they needed to teach but also reminded learners what they needed to learn, resulted in more frequent and complete perioperative teaching, and perception of enhanced teaching by learners (Anderson et al. 2013). *(c) SHARP intervention* An educational intervention using a 5-in by 3-in card with 5 "prompts" – setting learning objectives, "how did it go," address concerns, review learning points, and actions to improve – resulted in improved objective scores of debriefing, as well as improvement in quality and style of debriefings, with user satisfaction in terms of usefulness, feasibility, and comprehensiveness of the tool (Ahmed et al. 2013). *(d) Surgical feedback cards* Surgical skills feedback (SurF) cards promoted "procedural 'key' step review" and immediate feedback, resulting in significantly more frequent and improved quality of feedback (Connolly et al. 2014). *(e) Structured teaching with BID model* Learners who underwent surgical training using a set format based on a surgical encounter template, including briefing, intraoperative teaching and debriefing (BID), reported satisfaction with the intervention, noting

(continued)

Table 1 (continued)

	improved feedback clarity, and increased opportunity to complete a procedure independently (Leung et al. 2015). *(f) Faculty members can improve their postoperative debriefing* Teachers were educated to initiate debriefing immediately after the procedure, ideally in the OR, addressing the overall flow of the case, what the learner performed well and what could be improved. Post-intervention, learners felt the teacher identified aspects of the case that they performed competently, they were more aware of the teacher's impression of their performance, and nearly all learners planned on making postoperative debriefing a routine part of self-assessment (Francis et al. 2016). *(g) Procedure feedback form* A flexible formative feedback process whereby learners initiated a postoperative feedback discussion and completed a feedback form with their teachers, supported learner self-reflection and was easily adaptable to a wide variety of clinical settings (Cook et al. 2015). *(h) QR code for portable electronic evaluation* Used immediately following surgical procedures, this streamlined portable electronic evaluation allows for direct, formative feedback for learners, and creates a longitudinal record of learner progress (Reynolds et al. 2014).
Use of video for demonstration	*Intraoperative video-enhanced surgical training* Use of on-demand video clips demonstrating anatomical landmarks, key elements, and operative techniques for each stage of the procedure in the OR, allowing playback before the learner attempts each stage, frees the teacher from having to take over to demonstrate how its done on the patient, allowing the learner more opportunity to operate on patients. Learners demonstrated improved technical and procedural skill improvement as compared to controls (Van Det et al. 2011). Learners who underwent this training method were subsequently able to perform more steps without needing supervisor intervention, with no increase in procedure time (Van Det et al. 2013).
Coaching the teachers	*Coaching teachers using a surgical encounter template* Teachers who underwent coaching via a surgical encounter template felt the program improved their confidence, technical, and teaching skills. Surgeons who previously did not have a structured approach to their surgical teaching adopted the BID structure when teaching (Leung et al. 2013).
B.	**Models and frameworks**
Teaching models	The **four-step** method (Demonstration, Deconstruction, Comprehension, Performance) and the "**stop and swap**," whereby the teacher takes-over part of surgery where the

(continued)

Table 1 (continued)

	learner has difficulty then swaps back for the learner to continue; rather than taking-over completely to finish the procedure (Haward and Webster 2016)
Zwisch model	The **Zwisch** model is a simple 4-stage model proposed to guide teacher-learners for entrustment decisions in the OR by designating the learner's level of earned autonomy for a given procedure. It comprises (1) Show and Tell; (2) Smart Help; (3) Dumb Help; and (4) No Help (Darosa et al. 2013). This framework translates the general concept of ACGME physician supervisory framework (direct supervision/ indirect supervision/ oversight) into a more practical approach for use in the OR.
BID model	The **briefing, intraoperative teaching, debriefing (BID)** model focuses both teacher and learner on shared learning objectives to guide intraoperative teaching. Teaching consists of immediate feedback and guidance directed by specific learning objectives and the teacher's existing teaching scripts. The debriefing aims to solidify the learning that occurred in the operation by enhancing learner reflection (Roberts et al. 2009).
Teaching operative judgment	**St-Martin** et al. propose a framework for teaching the "slowing-down moments of operative judgment" (St-Martin et al. 2012). Preoperative planning helps "identify both procedural-specific and patient-specific slowing-down moments, which ensures that intraoperative surprises are minimized and attention is directed appropriately on the critical moments, facilitating safe and mindful surgery." Unplanned or situationally responsive slowing-down moments are also valuable teaching opportunities, but if cognitive demands on the teacher are high, "the teaching moment can be delayed until the situation is controlled, but should not be lost completely" (St-Martin et al. 2012).

feedback skills of teachers (Francis et al. 2016), as well as the use of structured briefing/debriefing tools that aim to improve pre and postoperative briefing (Ahmed et al. 2013; Anderson et al. 2013; Connolly et al. 2014; Cook et al. 2015; Leung et al. 2015). Technology such as QR readers has also been shown to help create longitudinal records of resident progress (Reynolds et al. 2014).

Use of Video for Demonstration

Providing resources such as on-demand video clips that remove the need for demonstration upon the patient allowed the learner the opportunity to operate on the patient. This has resulted in reported improvement in technical skills with objective testing (van Det et al. 2011), with learners performing more steps without the need for the help of trainers within the same time period as controls (Van Det et al. 2013).

Coaching the Teachers (Professional Development)

A structured surgical coaching program for teachers resulted in participants gaining confidence in surgery, and reporting improvement in surgical skills; participating teachers expressed their intention to be more structured in their teaching (Leung et al. 2013).

Models and Frameworks

Models for teaching operative technique in the OR include the four-step method (Demonstration, Deconstruction, Comprehension, Performance) and the "stop and swap," whereby the teacher takes-over part of surgery where the learner has difficulty, then swaps back for the learner to continue; rather than taking-over completely to finish the procedure (Haward and Webster 2016). Other frameworks include the four-stage Zwisch model – Show and Tell, Smart Help, Dumb Help, No Help – which helps to guide entrustment decisions (Darosa et al. 2013), and the BID or Briefing, Intraoperative Teaching, Debriefing model which focuses both the teacher and learner on shared learning objectives (Roberts et al. 2009). Finally, the theoretical framework for understanding how surgeons think in practice as described by St-Martin et al. – attention and effort, situation awareness, and automaticity – helps the teacher understand learner behavior and cognition in the development of expertise, and to tailor their teaching in a more explicit and structured way (St-Martin et al. 2012).

Implications for Practice

The OR context adds unique teaching-learning elements – psychomotor skills development, operative entrustment decisions, and the presence of the OR team. These additional aspects need to be considered when designing curriculum and/or faculty development for intraoperative surgical skills development.

Curriculum Design

Curriculum design for surgical training should recognize the contribution of intraoperative teaching to the development of surgical skills in a trainee. Presently, intraoperative learning remains unstructured and opportunistic, being influenced by multiple factors related to the OR environment, the situational factors and the relational issues. Programs could restructure intraoperative teaching-learning practices based on the available evidence – as summarized above – in order to create better learning opportunities.

For example, junior learners find the OR less conducive to learning (Diwadkar and Jelovsek 2010), facing reduced entrustment and learner autonomy (Bailey et al. 2018; Meyerson et al. 2017a), which could possibly be a result of their lack of experience and confidence, relative lack of rapport with teachers, and their inability to navigate the procedural variations of their various teachers. Interventions that target junior learners could ease their transition into training by including OR team orientation, faculty mentor-matching, setting clear expectations regarding adequate preparation (Rose et al. 2011), and standardizing steps of common procedures to avoid confusion navigating procedural variation. Recurring opportunities for learners to perform the same operation with the same teacher over an extended period of time could improve entrustment in the OR (Sandhu et al. 2017; Teman et al. 2014). In addition, changing the focus from the number of operations performed, or the amount of time spent between learner and teacher, to a focus on achievement of proficiency in a series of entrustable tasks may help improve learning outcomes (Teman et al. 2014). The use of Entrustable Professional Activities (EPAs) would allow teachers to make competency-based decisions about the level of supervision required by learners for specific tasks, skills, and procedures (ten Cate 2005). Other systemic interventions to improve the OR learning environment include dedicated teaching lists with suitable cases, protected time for teachers, and learners including time for debriefing, reducing competing learners (Diwadkar and Jelovsek 2010), and the enlistment of the aid of other OR stakeholders such as anesthesia and the nursing team (Svensson et al. 2009).

Faculty Development

Surgical teachers who received faculty development on teaching practices contextualized to the OR have been found to have learner-perceived improvement in teaching behavior (Gardner et al. 2019). For instance, principles of effective feedback delivery are generic, but application in the OR may differ from the classroom/ward contexts in terms of timing (e.g., avoid concurrent feedback because the learner is fully occupied when performing surgery) or method (e.g., physical rather than verbal feedback). In addition, positive specific steps by faculty are more likely to be recognized and remembered, as compared to passive roles such as "assisting guidance" (Chen et al. 2014). By stating "I am giving you feedback," or words to that effect, a feedback session would not be misinterpreted as anything but exactly what it is (p.253, Jensen et al. 2012).

Training programs can provide teachers with resources such as structured tools to facilitate desired behaviors. For example, the SHARP intervention using a 5-in by 3-in card with 5 "prompts" – set learning objectives, "how did it go," address concerns, review learning points, and actions to improve (Ahmed et al. 2013) – reminds the teacher to set learning objectives before starting the procedure and to end with an action plan; steps that are often neglected during routine intraoperative teaching. Alternative frameworks like the BID model improve feedback clarity and increase learner participation (Leung et al. 2015). Even in the dynamic OR learning environment, it is possible to create more "teachable moments," as these unplanned learning opportunities can surface more often when teachers are primed to look for them. These include errors in learner performance (Roberts et al. 2012), workflow disruptions (Glarner et al. 2017), and hesitation (Ott et al. 2018). By setting a few specific learning goals at the outset of each case, these opportunities can be anchored to pre-determined objectives (Roberts et al. 2012),

The OR environment is often stressful, which impairs learning (Ng et al. 2019), thus efforts at communication by teachers can only help. The sharing of personal teacher stories is a form of role modeling, which informally "showcase core values in surgery" (p.66, Hu et al. 2012), and in doing so, "they teach the 'hidden curriculum'" (p.67, Hu et al. 2012), while humor and banter help to set a positive tone for the operation (Glarner et al. 2017; Roberts et al. 2012). In addition, communication by the teacher when reclaiming operating control in a case may "foster greater understanding" and empower learners "to maintain more ownership of the decision-making" (p.587, Hill et al. 2017).

Research Opportunities

The review that underpins this chapter also highlighted some gaps in current knowledge that can inform future research. While teacher behavior and the OR learning environment have been well-described in the literature, there has been less of an investigative focus on learners, particularly from an observer perspective. Understanding actual learner behavior as opposed to what they report, is valuable since learners sometimes have minimal insight into their lack of preparation (Levinson et al. 2010; Rose et al. 2011), and may not recognize when they are actually being taught (Chen et al. 2014; Ong et al. 2016). Another potential area of research is on the influence of learner agency on entrustment within the OR culture that expects learner preparation in order to "earn" the right to participate.

Learning by motor and visual cues is a new exciting area of study (Cope et al. 2015b; Skoczylas et al. 2012) as increasingly, in this age of video-assisted minimally invasive surgeries without haptic feedback, intraoperative judgment must be based on visual information alone (Cope et al. 2015a). Further research is needed on factors affecting sensory semiosis and effective strategies to facilitate this learning.

The relational elements of learning also require further investigation with few empirical studies considering both learner and teacher. Additionally, the influence of other healthcare professionals in the operating theater has been given limited consideration. As many operative procedures are undertaken on conscious patients, we need to better understand how to optimize learning under this condition.

In general, there is a lack of evidence for most educational interventions on sustainability in routine surgical practice, translation to the actual performance of learners, and ultimately patient care.

Conclusions

Teaching and learning intraoperative surgical skills follows general educational principles; however, pedagogical modifications are needed for the special requirements of psychomotor skills development, operative entrustment concerns, and the

OR environment. Surgical teachers who understand these contextual requirements are able to provide relevant education to enhance intraoperative skills learning.

Acknowledgments The authors would like to thank Ms. Anne Young (Monash University Library, Monash University, Melbourne), Mr. Patrick Condron (Brownless Biomedical Library, University of Melbourne), and Ms. Kim Kee Toh (Medical Library, National University of Singapore) for their assistance in the article search.

Appendix I: Search Strategy Used in the Scoping Review

VC performed a scoping review as part of a Master of Surgical Education thesis with the University of Melbourne, Australia. Scoping review methodology was chosen given the topic breadth, complexity, and heterogenous evidence, as it allows "a map of what evidence has been produced as opposed to seeking only the best available evidence to answer a particular question" (Arksey and O'Malley 2005). There were 94 out of 6383 English language suitable studies identified in online databases Ovid Medline, ERIC, and Embase published from the date of inception to 31 December 2018 using the following inclusion and exclusion criteria:

Inclusion Criteria

The Population (teachers and learners) was searched using text words: trainee, resident or residents, registrar, fellow or fellows, medical officer, consultant, attending, faculty, supervisor, mentor or mentors, coach or coaches, trainer or trainers, educator or educators, teacher or teachers, peer or peers, intern or interns.

The Context or setting was searched using text words: operating room, operating theatre, operating theater, intra-operative or intraoperative, peri-operative or perioperative, post-operative or postoperative, pre-operative or preoperative.

The Concept of learning and teaching was searched using text words: learn*, educat*, teach or teaching, instruct*, communicat*, train or training or trained or trains, debrief*, feedback.

Exclusion Criteria

Studies that were not in English, which studied the development of assessment tools, simulation including transfer from simulation to the OR, medical students, outcomes between trainees and consultants, tele-mentoring, patient safety, anesthesia, nursing, and non-technical skills, were excluded, as were opinion pieces and reviews of training programs/curricula. Studies on post-hoc teaching and/or coaching outside of the OR were also excluded.

Cross-References

▶ Coaching in Health Professions Education: The Case of Surgery
▶ Focus on Theory: Emotions and Learning
▶ Hidden, Informal, and Formal Curricula in Health Professions Education
▶ Surgical Education and Training: Historical Perspectives
▶ Surgical Education: Context and Trends
▶ Technology Considerations in Health Professions and Clinical Education

References

Ahmed M, Arora S, Russ S, Darzi A, Vincent C, Sevdalis N. Operation debrief: a SHARP improvement in performance feedback in the operating room. Ann Surg. 2013;258:958–63.
Anderson CI, Gupta RN, Larson JR, Abubars OI, Kwiecien AJ, Lake AD, Hozain AE, Tanious A, O'brien, T. & Basson, M. D. Impact of objectively assessing surgeons' teaching on effective perioperative instructional behaviors. JAMA Surg. 2013;148:915–22.
Apramian T, Cristancho S, Watling C, Ott M, Lingard L. Thresholds of principle and preference: exploring procedural variation in postgraduate surgical education. Acad Med. 2015;90:S70–6.
Arksey, O'Malley. Int J Soc Res Methodology. 2005;8(1):19–32
Bailey EA, Johnson AP, Leeds IL, Medbery RL, Ahuja V, Vandermeer T, Wick EC, Irojah B, Kelz RR. Quantification of resident work in colorectal surgery. J Surg Educ. 2018;75:564–72.
Barrett M, Magas CP, Gruppen LD, Dedhia PH, Sandhu G. It's worth the wait: optimizing questioning methods for effective intraoperative teaching. ANZ J Surg. 2017;87:541–6.
Bedetti B, Schnorr P, Schmidt J, Scarci M. The role of wet lab in thoracic surgery. J Vis Surg. 2017;3:61.
Bezemer J, Murtagh G, Cope A, Kneebone R. Surgical decision making in a teaching hospital: a linguistic analysis. ANZ J Surg. 2016;86:751–5.
Binsaleh S, Babaeer A, Rabah D, Madbouly K. Evaluation of urology residents' perception of surgical theater educational environment. J Surg Educ. 2015;72:73–9.
Blom EM, Verdaasdonk EG, Stassen LP, Stassen HG, Wieringa PA, Dankelman J. Analysis of verbal communication during teaching in the operating room and the potentials for surgical training. Surg Endosc. 2007;21:1560–6.
Brown JS, Collins A, Duguid P. Situated cognition and the culture of learning. Educ Res. 1989;18: 32–42.
Butvidas LD, Anderson CI, Balogh D, Basson MD. Disparities between resident and attending surgeon perceptions of intraoperative teaching. Am J Surg. 2011;201:385–9. discussion 389
Chen XP, Williams RG, Smink DS. Do residents receive the same OR guidance as surgeons report? Difference between residents' and surgeons' perceptions of OR guidance. J Surg Educ. 2014;71: e79–82.
Chen XP, Williams RG, Smink DS. Dissecting attending surgeons' operating room guidance: factors that affect guidance decision making. J Surg Educ. 2015;72:e137–44.
Claridge JA, Calland JF, Chandrasekhara V, Young JS, Sanfey H, Schirmer BD. Comparing resident measurements to attending surgeon self-perceptions of surgical educators. Am J Surg. 2003;185:323–7.
Clark Donat LE, Klatsky PC, Frishman GN. "Pause" for resident education in the operating room. J Reprod Med. 2016;61:534–40.
Connolly A, Hansen D, Schuler K, Galvin SL, Wolfe H. Immediate surgical skills feedback in the operating room using "SurF" cards. J Grad Med Educ. 2014;6:774–8.

Cook MR, Watters JM, Barton JS, Kamin C, Brown SN, Deveney KE, Kiraly LN. A flexible postoperative debriefing process can effectively provide formative resident feedback. J Am Coll Surg. 2015;220:959–67.

Cooper JB, Gaba D. No myth: anesthesia is a model for addressing patient safety. Anesthesiology. 2002;97:1335–7.

Cope AC, Bezemer J, Kneebone R, Lingard L. 'You see?' Teaching and learning how to interpret visual cues during surgery. Med Educ. 2015a;49:1103–16.

Cope AC, Mavroveli S, Bezemer J, Hanna GB, Kneebone R. Making meaning from sensory cues: a qualitative investigation of postgraduate learning in the operating room. Acad Med. 2015b;90:1125–31.

Cox SS, Swanson MS. Identification of teaching excellence in operating room and clinic settings. Am J Surg. 2002;183:251–5.

Darosa DA, Zwischenberger JB, Meyerson SL, George BC, Teitelbaum EN, Soper NJ, Fryer JP. A theory-based model for teaching and assessing residents in the operating room. J Surg Educ. 2013;70:24–30.

Dath D, Hoogenes J, Matsumoto ED, Szalay DA. Exploring how surgeon teachers motivate residents in the operating room. Am J Surg. 2013;205:151–5.

De Montbrun SL, Macrae H. Simulation in surgical education. Clin Colon Rectal Surg. 2012;25:156–65.

Diwadkar GB, Jelovsek JE. Measuring surgical trainee perceptions to assess the operating room educational environment. J Surg Educ. 2010;67:210–6.

Fairfax LM, Christmas AB, Green JM, Miles WS, Sing RF. Operative experience in the era of duty hour restrictions: is broad-based general surgery training coming to an end? Am Surg. 2010;76:578–82.

Feng Y, Mentis HM. Improving common ground development in surgical training through talk and action. AMIA Annu Symp Proc. 2017;2017:696–705.

Feng Y, Wong C, Park A, Mentis H. Taxonomy of instructions given to residents in laparoscopic cholecystectomy. Surg Endosc. 2016;30:1073–7.

Francis DO, Eavey RD, Wright HV, Sinard RJ. Incorporating postoperative debriefing into surgical education. J Surg Educ. 2016;73:448–52.

Gardner AK, Timberlake MD, Dunkin BJ. Faculty development for the operating room: an examination of the effectiveness of an intraoperative teaching course for surgeons. Ann Surg. 2019 Jan;269(1):184–90.

Gas BL, Mohan M, Jyot A, Buckarma EH, Farley DR. Does scripting operative plans in advance lead to better preparedness of trainees? A pilot study. Am J Surg. 2017;213:526–9.

Gibson DR, Campbell RM. Promoting effective teaching and learning: hospital consultants identify their needs. Med Educ. 2000;34:126–30.

Glarner CE, Law KE, Zelenski AB, Mcdonald RJ, Greenberg JA, Foley EF, Wiegmann DA, Greenberg CC. Resident training in a teaching hospital: how do attendings teach in the real operative environment? Am J Surg. 2017;214:141–6.

Grantcharov TP, Schulze S, Kristiansen VB. The impact of objective assessment and constructive feedback on improvement of laparoscopic performance in the operating room. Surg Endosc. 2007;21:2240–3.

Greenberg JA, Irani JL, Greenberg CC, Blanco MA, Lipsitz S, Ashley SW, Breen EM, Hafler JP. The ACGME competencies in the operating room. Surgery. 2007;142:180–4.

Hamdorf JM, Hall JC. Acquiring surgical skills. Br J Surg. 2000;87:28–37.

Haward RN, Webster DL. Teaching cataract surgery to trainees in the operating theatre. Clin Exp Ophthalmol. 2016;44:222–3.

Hill KA, Dasari M, Littleton EB, Hamad GG. How can surgeons facilitate resident intraoperative decision-making? Am J Surg. 2017;214:583–8.

Hu YY, Peyre SE, Arriaga AF, Roth EM, Corso KA, Greenberg CC. War stories: a qualitative analysis of narrative teaching strategies in the operating room. Am J Surg. 2012;203:63–8.

Ibrahim A, Delia IZ, Edaigbini SA, Abubakar A, Dahiru IL, Lawal ZY. Teaching the surgical craft: surgery residents perception of the operating theater educational environment in a tertiary institution in Nigeria. Niger J Surg. 2013;19:61–7.

Iwaszkiewicz M, Darosa DA, Risucci DA. Efforts to enhance operating room teaching. J Surg Educ. 2008;65:436–40.

Jensen AR, Wright AS, Kim S, Horvath KD, Calhoun KE. Educational feedback in the operating room: a gap between resident and faculty perceptions. Am J Surg. 2012;204:248–55.

Kamali D, Illing J. How can positive and negative trainer feedback in the operating theatre impact a surgical trainee's confidence and well-being: a qualitative study in the north of England. BMJ Open. 2018;8:e017935.

Kanashiro J, Mcaleer S, Roff S. Assessing the educational environment in the operating room-a measure of resident perception at one Canadian institution. Surgery. 2006;139:150–8.

Kieu V, Stroud L, Huang P, Smith M, Spychal R, Hunter-Smith D, Nestel D. The operating theatre as classroom: a qualitative study of learning and teaching surgical competencies. Educ Health (Abingdon). 2015;28:22–8.

Kissane-Lee NA, Yule S, Pozner CN, Smink DS. Attending surgeons' leadership style in the operating room: comparing junior residents' experiences and preferences. J Surg Educ. 2016;73:40–4.

Klingensmith ME, Lewis FR. General surgery residency training issues. Adv Surg. 2013;47:251–70.

Leung Y, Salfinger S, Tan JJ, Frazer A. The introduction and the validation of a surgical encounter template to facilitate surgical coaching of gynaecologists at a metropolitan tertiary obstetrics and gynaecology hospital. Aust N Z J Obstet Gynaecol. 2013;53:477–83.

Leung Y, Salfinger S, Mercer A. The positive impact of structured teaching in the operating room. Aust N Z J Obstet Gynaecol. 2015;55:601–5.

Levinson KL, Barlin JN, Altman K, Satin AJ. Disparity between resident and attending physician perceptions of intraoperative supervision and education. J Grad Med Educ. 2010;2:31–6.

Magas CP, Gruppen LD, Barrett M, Dedhia PH, Sandhu G. Intraoperative questioning to advance higher-order thinking. Am J Surg. 2017;213:222–6.

Mahoney A, Crowe PJ, Harris P. Exploring Australasian surgical trainees' satisfaction with operating theatre learning using the 'surgical theatre educational environment measure'. ANZ J Surg. 2010;80:884–9.

Mateo Vallejo F. General surgery: present and future. Int J Surg. 2012;10:176–7.

Mckendy KM, Watanabe Y, Lee L, Bilgic E, Enani G, Feldman LS, Fried GM, Vassiliou MC. Perioperative feedback in surgical training: a systematic review. Am J Surg. 2017;214:117–26.

Meyerson SL, Teitelbaum EN, George BC, Schuller MC, Darosa DA, Fryer JP. Defining the autonomy gap: when expectations do not meet reality in the operating room. J Surg Educ. 2014;71:e64–72.

Meyerson SL, Sternbach JM, Zwischenberger JB, Bender EM. The effect of gender on resident autonomy in the operating room. J Surg Educ. 2017a;74:e111–8.

Meyerson SL, Sternbach JM, Zwischenberger JB, Bender EM. Resident autonomy in the operating room: expectations versus reality. Ann Thorac Surg. 2017b;104:1062–8.

Morgan R, Kauffman DF, Doherty G, Sachs T. Resident and attending assessments of operative involvement: do we agree? Am J Surg. 2017a;213:1178–1185.e1.

Morgan R, Kauffman DF, Doherty G, Sachs T. Resident and attending perceptions of resident involvement: an analysis of ACGME reporting guidelines. J Surg Educ. 2017b;74:415–22.

Nathwani JN, Glarner CE, Law KE, Mcdonald RJ, Zelenski AB, Greenberg JA, Foley EF. Integrating postoperative feedback into workflow: perceived practices and barriers. J Surg Educ. 2017;74:406–14.

Nebeker CA, Basson MD, Haan PS, Davis AT, Ali M, Gupta RN, Osmer RL, Hardaway JC, Peshkepija AN, Mcleod MK, Anderson CI. Do female surgeons learn or teach differently? Am J Surg. 2017;213:282–7.

Ng R, Chahine S, Lanting B, Howard J. Unpacking the literature on stress and resiliency: a narrative review focused on learners in the operating room. J Surg Educ. 2019;76(2):343–53.

O'holleran B, Barlow J, Ford C, Cochran A. Questions posed by residents in the operating room: a thematic analysis. J Surg Educ. 2019;76:315–20.

Ong CC, Dodds A, Nestel D. Beliefs and values about intra-operative teaching and learning: a case study of surgical teachers and trainees. Adv Health Sci Educ Theory Pract. 2016;21:587–607.

Ott M, Schwartz A, Goldszmidt M, Bordage G, Lingard L. Resident hesitation in the operating room: does uncertainty equal incompetence? Med Educ. 2018;52:851–60.

Park J, Parker SH, Safford S. Surgical trainees' confidence in the operating room improves over time with a corresponding increase in responsibility. Am Surg. 2017;83:E421–3.

Pernar LI, Breen E, Ashley SW, Peyre SE. Preoperative learning goals set by surgical residents and faculty. J Surg Res. 2011;170:1–5.

Pernar LI, Ashley SW, Smink DS, Zinner MJ, Peyre SE. Master surgeons' operative teaching philosophies: a qualitative analysis of parallels to learning theory. J Surg Educ. 2012;69:493–8.

Pernar LI, Peyre SE, Hasson RM, Lipsitz S, Corso K, Ashley SW, Breen EM. Exploring the content of intraoperative teaching. J Surg Educ. 2016;73:79–84.

Reid M, Ker JS, Dunkley MP, Williams B, Steele RJ. Training specialist registrars in general surgery: a qualitative study in Tayside. J R Coll Surg Edinb. 2000;45:304–10.

Reynolds K, Barnhill D, Sias J, Young A, Polite FG. Use of the QR reader to provide real-time evaluation of residents' skills following surgical procedures. J Grad Med Educ. 2014;6:738–41.

Reznick RK. Teaching and testing technical skills. Am J Surg. 1993;165:358–61.

Roberts NK, Williams RG, Kim MJ, Dunnington GL. The briefing, intraoperative teaching, debriefing model for teaching in the operating room. J Am Coll Surg. 2009;208:299–303.

Roberts NK, Brenner MJ, Williams RG, Kim MJ, Dunnington GL. Capturing the teachable moment: a grounded theory study of verbal teaching interactions in the operating room. Surgery. 2012;151:643–50.

Rose JS, Waibel BH, Schenarts PJ. Disparity between resident and faculty surgeons' perceptions of preoperative preparation, intraoperative teaching, and postoperative feedback. J Surg Educ. 2011;68:459–64.

Rose JS, Waibel BH, Schenarts PJ. Resident perceptions of the impact of paging on intraoperative education. Am Surg. 2012;78:642–6.

Salim SY, Govaerts M, White J. The construction of surgical trust: how surgeons judge residents' readiness for operative independence. Ann Surg. 2020;271:391–8.

Sandhu G, Magas CP, Robinson AB, Scally CP, Minter RM. Progressive entrustment to achieve resident autonomy in the operating room: a national qualitative study with general surgery faculty and residents. Ann Surg. 2017;265:1134–40.

Sandhu G, Thompson-Burdine J, Nikolian VC, Sutzko DC, Prabhu KA, Matusko N, Minter RM. Association of faculty entrustment with resident autonomy in the operating room. JAMA Surg. 2018;153:518–24.

Scallon SE, Fairholm DJ, Cochrane DD, Taylor DC. Evaluation of the operating room as a surgical teaching venue. Can J Surg. 1992;35:173–6.

Skoczylas LC, Littleton EB, Kanter SL, Sutkin G. Teaching techniques in the operating room: the importance of perceptual motor teaching. Acad Med. 2012;87:364–71.

Snyder RA, Tarpley MJ, Tarpley JL, Davidson M, Brophy C, Dattilo JB. Teaching in the operating room: results of a national survey. J Surg Educ. 2012;69:643–9.

Soomro SH, Ur Rehman SS, Hussain F. Perception of educational environment in the operating theatre by surgical residents, a single-centre prospective study. J Pak Med Assoc. 2017;67:1864–79.

St-Martin L, Patel P, Gallinger J, Moulton CA. Teaching the slowing-down moments of operative judgment. Surg Clin North Am. 2012;92:125–35.

Sutkin G, Littleton EB, Kanter SL. How surgical mentors teach: a classification of in vivo teaching behaviors part 1: verbal teaching guidance. J Surg Educ. 2015a;72:243–50.

Sutkin G, Littleton EB, Kanter SL. How surgical mentors teach: a classification of in vivo teaching behaviors part 2: physical teaching guidance. J Surg Educ. 2015b;72:251–7.

Sutkin G, Littleton EB, Kanter SL. Intelligent cooperation: a framework of pedagogic practice in the operating room. Am J Surg. 2018;215:535–41.

Svensson MS, Luff P, Heath C. Embedding instruction in practice: contingency and collaboration during surgical training. Sociol Health Illn. 2009;31:889–906.

Teman NR, Gauger PG, Mullan PB, Tarpley JL, Minter RM. Entrustment of general surgery residents in the operating room: factors contributing to provision of resident autonomy. J Am Coll Surg. 2014;219:778–87.

ten Cate O. Entrustability of professional activities and competency-based training. Med Educ. 2005;39(12):1176–7.

Thompson-Burdine J, Sutzko DC, Nikolian VC, Boniakowski A, Georgoff PE, Prabhu KA, Matusko N, Minter RM, Sandhu G. Impact of a resident's sex on intraoperative entrustment of surgery trainees. Surgery. 2018;164:583–8.

Timberlake MD, Mayo HG, Scott L, Weis J, Gardner AK. What do we know about intraoperative teaching?: a systematic review. Ann Surg. 2017;266:251–9.

Torbeck L, Wilson A, Choi J, Dunnington GL. Identification of behaviors and techniques for promoting autonomy in the operating room. Surgery. 2015;158:1102–10. discussion 1110-2

Van Der Houwen C, Boor K, Essed GG, Boendermaker PM, Scherpbier AA, Scheele F. Gynaecological surgical training in the operating room: an exploratory study. Eur J Obstet Gynecol Reprod Biol. 2011;154:90–5.

Van Det MJ, Meijerink WJ, Hoff C, Middel LJ, Koopal SA, Pierie JP. The learning effect of intraoperative video-enhanced surgical procedure training. Surg Endosc. 2011;25:2261–7.

Van Det MJ, Meijerink WJ, Hoff C, Middel B, Pierie JP. Effective and efficient learning in the operating theater with intraoperative video-enhanced surgical procedure training. Surg Endosc. 2013;27:2947–54.

Vikis EA, Mihalynuk TV, Pratt DD, Sidhu RS. Teaching and learning in the operating room is a two-way street: resident perceptions. Am J Surg. 2008;195:594–8. discussion 598

Vollmer CM Jr, Newman LR, Huang G, Irish J, Hurst J, Horvath K. Perspectives on intraoperative teaching: divergence and convergence between learner and teacher. J Surg Educ. 2011;68:485–94.

Williams RG, George BC, Meyerson SL, Bohnen JD, Dunnington GL, Schuller MC, Torbeck L, Mullen JT, Auyang E, Chipman JG, Choi J, Choti M, Endean E, Foley EF, Mandell S, Meier A, Smink DS, Terhune KP, Wise P, Darosa D, Soper N, Zwischenberger JB, Lillemoe KD, Fryer JP. What factors influence attending surgeon decisions about resident autonomy in the operating room? Surgery. 2017;162:1314–9.

Yeo H, Viola K, Berg D, Lin Z, Nunez-Smith M, Cammann C, Bell RH Jr, Sosa JA, Krumholz HM, Curry LA. Attitudes, training experiences, and professional expectations of US general surgery residents: a national survey. JAMA. 2009;302:1301–8.

Learning and Teaching in the Operating Theatre: Expert Commentary from the Nursing Perspective

49

Rachel Cardwell, Emmalee Weston, and Jenny Davis

Contents

Introduction	934
History of Nurses in the Operative Environment	935
Roles in the Operating Theatre	936
Principal Surgical Team Members	936
Anesthetic Team	936
Transitional Surgical Staff	937
Management and Administration Staff	938
Nursing Roles Within the Perioperative Environment	938
Anesthesia Nursing	939
Intraoperative Environment – Perioperative Nursing	939
Recovery Nursing	942
Nontechnical Skills Within the Operating Theatre	943
Communication	944
Human Factors	944
Teamwork	945
Nursing Education – Operating Theatre	945
Perioperative Exposure at Undergraduate Level	945
Specialist Education	946
Continuing Professional Development (CPD)	946
Future Challenges for Learning and Teaching in the OT. Where Are We Headed?	947
Population	947
Workforce	947
Technology	947

R. Cardwell (✉)
Austin Health, La Trobe University, Melbourne, VIC, Australia
e-mail: r.cardwell@latrobe.edu.au

E. Weston
Austin Health, Melbourne, VIC, Australia
e-mail: Emmalee.WESTON@austin.org.au

J. Davis
School of Nursing and Midwifery, La Trobe University, Melbourne, VIC, Australia
e-mail: j.davis@latrobe.edu.au

© Springer Nature Singapore Pte Ltd. 2023
D. Nestel et al. (eds.), *Clinical Education for the Health Professions*,
https://doi.org/10.1007/978-981-15-3344-0_66

Strategies for Learning and Teaching in the Operating Theatre	947
Beginning a Career in the Operative Environment	948
Creating Positive Learning Experiences	948
Support for Learning and Teaching (Preceptor, Mentor)	949
Simulation	949
Safety in the Operating Theatre	950
The Safety of New Learners	950
Patient Safety	950
Biomedical Safety	951
Conclusion	952
References	952

Abstract

The operating theatre environment is dynamic, fast-paced, and challenging. Increasing complexity in modern surgical techniques and advancing technology means that patients require more intensive nursing care and interventions. Safe and effective surgical care relies heavily on the highly specialized skills and experience of operating theatre nurses who function as part of multidisciplinary teams. Nursing roles in the perioperative environment are diverse and highly specialized and continue to expand. This nursing workforce is however challenged by shortages and recruitment impacted by declining exposure of undergraduate nurses to this specialty area of practice. This chapter discusses learning and teaching in this unique clinical environment and begins with an introduction to the setting and roles of the operative team. It then discusses the challenges and approaches to learning and teaching in this specialist area of nursing practice.

Keywords

Education · Nurse · Operating theatre · Postoperative care · Patient safety · Surgical care

Introduction

Operative care is divided into three phases: the preoperative (preparation and management of a patient prior to surgery), intraoperative (the time the patient is admitted to the operating theatre until they are transported to the recovery room, or postanesthesia care unit (PACU)), and postoperative (immediate postanesthetic care) stages of surgery. Each phase of surgery requires a specific set of skills. Nurses may specialize to work within the anesthesia, intraoperative, or postoperative care teams. Nurses working in the operating theatre (OT) may also be referred to as "surgical" or "perioperative" nurses. OT nurses work as part of a multidisciplinary healthcare team. They facilitate timely assessment, care, treatment, education, discharge, and follow-up nursing care within a surgical setting. OT nurse responsibilities include planning, executing, directing, and evaluating nursing care of the surgical patient throughout preoperative, intraoperative, and postoperative phases.

Teamwork is imperative in OT. The value of teamwork, effective communication, standardized practices, and protocols all work together to provide safe patient care (CAN 2015). The workload can be unpredictable, physically and emotionally demanding. It can be noisy, busy, tense, confronting, and overwhelming. The impact of human factors on patient safety makes it a challenge to use this high-risk environment for learning and teaching purposes (Oeppen et al. 2019). Creating a positive learning environment in the OT is fundamental to attracting nurses and developing nursing roles within this setting.

History of Nurses in the Operative Environment

The development of surgery and surgical methods happened across the world at different times, first in China, India, South America, Mesopotamia, Persia, Arabia, and finally Europe (OPTIMUS 2019). The earliest documented "surgeons" were physicians, priests, or magicians who understood anatomy and who were experienced in the practices of amputation and trephination (drilling or cutting a hole in the skull to relieve pressure from head injuries, psychosis, or seizures). These skills were mostly used on the battlefield and are recorded as far back as 2,000 BC (South America), 5,100 BC (France), and 8,000 BC (Egypt) (OPTIMUS 2019).

Until the early 1800s, the most common surgeon was the battlefield surgeon who travelled around setting up a tent on the battlefield to remove foreign objects, apply bandages, undertake amputations, and give hope to the wounded and dying (OPTIMUS 2019). Between 1800 and 1900, Germany, France, Austria, England, and America began to build hospitals with spaces specifically dedicated to operating and teaching. Until the late 1900s, surgery was predominately a male-dominated profession. In the second half of that century, female surgeons began working in operating theatres, and doctors began accepting nurses as assisting practitioners with specific expertise and essential members of the surgical team (Schlich and Hasegawa 2017). Towards the twentieth century, the introduction of anesthesia transformed working conditions in the operating theatre and distinct areas of peri- and postoperative nursing care, antisepsis, and asepsis began to emerge.

By World War I, antisepsis was widely adopted to prevent infection. The wearing of gloves, gowns, masks and use of antiseptics for wash handing were well practiced in army surgical teams. During World War II, Korea expanded the hospital tent system to include operating theatres that allowed multiple surgery's to be done at the same time with the development of the mobile army surgical hospital (MASH) concept. This format became the foundation for modern operating theatre design and the development of individual nursing roles in anesthesia and perioperative. Surgery became known as a form of teamwork with each nurse having specific and central roles within the surgical team. Advances in surgical techniques and medical technology have seen expansion of professional roles and complexity of patient care in this practice environment, now recognized as a speciality area.

Roles in the Operating Theatre

Surgery involves a team of trained staff to assist with operating and will vary depending on the type of procedure being undertaken. Usually, a principal team of surgeons, anesthetists, and nurses work together throughout the entire operation. They are predominately responsible for the care, safety, and outcomes for patients before, during, and after surgery. Transitional staff also work in the OT, these members move in and out of the theatre at differing times through the operation, each having specialized skills to support patient care, procedures and achieve best possible outcomes.

Principal Surgical Team Members

Surgeons
The surgeon is responsible for assessment and diagnosis of the patient preoperatively. The surgeon is considered the leader of the surgical team, performs the surgery, and provides postoperative surgical orders, care, and treatment (Kaye et al. 2018).

Perioperative Nurses (Scrub/Instrument and Scout/Circulating)
Perioperative nurses provide care for patients in the period prior to and during surgery. They assume different roles within the operating theatre from scrubbing into a surgical procedure and assisting the surgical team with instrumentation, to scouting/circulating within the operating theatre to assist the scrub/instrument nurse and surgical team with any requirements they may have throughout the procedure (ACORN 2018). For further discussion, see Nursing roles within the perioperative environment.

Day Surgery Nurses
Day surgery nurses provide care for patients schedule to have same-day surgery. They provide care before and after surgery and assess the patient's condition for safe discharge home (Kaye et al. 2018).

Endoscopy Nurses
Endoscopy nurses work with physicians to assist with endoscopic-specific procedures. The role includes preparing equipment and assisting with procedures. They assist with patient sedation, monitoring, and providing postprocedure education (Kaye et al. 2018).

Anesthetic Team

Anesthetists
Anesthetists are responsible for preparing patients for administration of anesthesia during surgery. They assess patients for possible risks and side effects of anesthetic

medications, administer anesthesia, and monitor patients throughout surgery. They lead the operative team in resuscitating and stabilizing patients and managing postoperative pain (Kaye et al. 2018).

Anesthesia Nurses
Anesthesia nurses provide anesthetic nursing care under the guidance of the Anaesthetist (ACORN 2018). For further discussion, see Nursing roles within the perioperative environment.

Recovery Nurses
Recovery nurses assume responsibility for the care of the patient directly upon leaving the operating room. Their role is to monitor and assess a patient's condition postsurgical procedure (ACORN 2018). For further discussion, see Nursing roles within the perioperative environment.

Transitional Surgical Staff

Theatre Technicians
Theatre technicians are responsible for the movement of patients and equipment to and from and within the OT. They assist in the set-up and preparation of the operating theatres for surgery, including patient positioning. Their responsibilities include the setting up and checking of surgical equipment and providing technical assistance to surgeons, anesthetists, and nurses within the operating team (Kaye et al. 2018).

Pharmacists
The pharmacist role in operating theatres is to represent pharmacy services relating to patient care. They are available to contact before, during, and after surgery. They provide advice in relation to prescribing, efficacy, side effects, and safety of medications used before, during, and after surgery (Kaye et al. 2018).

Radiographers
The role of the radiographer in theatre is to use the imaging modalities to help diagnose and treat patient conditions during surgical procedures (Phillips 2016).

Biomedical Engineers
Biomedical engineers working within the operating theatre will have responsibilities involving medical systems and products specific to individual surgical procedures or patients. They install, maintain, and repair biomedical equipment used within the operating theatre (Phillips 2016).

Patient Service Attendants
Patient service attendants (PSAs) are responsible for the transport of patients to theatre and from the recovery room back to a ward or place for discharge (Kaye et al. 2018).

Medical Device Company Representative

Medical device company representatives work with the surgical team to support and train staff with the use of newly introduced products specific to a surgical procedure or operation (Kaye et al. 2018).

Central Sterilizing Services Department (CSSD) Staff

CSSD staff can be situated within the operative department or located nearby. They work to store and process instruments for sterilization and can source and provide instruments quickly when required (Phillips 2016).

Management and Administration Staff

Nurse Unit Managers

The nurse manager (NUM) role in perioperative settings leads the unit at operational and strategic levels. The NUM is defined as a person who is responsible for coordinating and managing an operating department or a day surgery unit (Siirala et al. 2019).

Associate Nurse Unit Managers

Associate Nurse Unit Managers (ANUM) support the NUM in management of the operating theatres. They are clinical and professional role models for all staff within the operating department and assume the NUM role in their absence (Kaye et al. 2018).

Clerical Staff

Clerical staff working in the operative environment provide administrative support and reception duties to all theatres (Phillips 2016).

Education Staff

Education staff create and support various models for learning and teaching across all multidisciplinary OT practice areas. Clinical support models often involved work integrated learning, mentors or preceptors, overseen by OT educational specialists from the different disciplines (Phillips 2016; Russell and Coventry 2019).

Nursing Roles Within the Perioperative Environment

Nurses working in the OT are commonly registered or certified nurses who have completed a bachelor's degree in nursing. In some settings, other levels of nurses including Enrolled Nurses (ENs) (or second level nurses) and Licenced Practice Nurses (LPN) can pursue formal education and experience in the following specialized areas of nursing.

Anesthesia Nursing

The word "anesthesia" comes from two Greek words: "an," meaning "without" and "aesthesis," which means "sensation" (ANZCA 2019). Anesthesia includes administering anesthetizing medications by inhalation or injection to block sensations of pain. The role of the anesthetic nurse (or Registered Nurse Anaesthetist [RNA]) is to assist the anesthetist in providing anesthesia to individual patient's requirements. Anesthesia nurses are required to have extensive knowledge of anesthetic agents (Table 1) and the procedures involved in their administration. The anesthetic nurse is expected to be able to care for patients requiring critical airway management, regional anesthesia (including nerve block/spinal/epidural), invasive, therapeutic, and monitoring procedures (Table 2) (ACORN 2018; Ireland and Osborne 2016).

Intraoperative Environment – Perioperative Nursing

Within the perioperative environment, there are two distinct nursing roles directly associated with assisting the surgeon. These roles include the circulating (scout) nurse and the instrument (scrub) nurse. These roles are either performed exclusively or the nurse will rotate between roles, depending on the country of training (ACORN 2018; Dunne 2019). The competence of the circulating and instrument nurse will directly influence the patient's surgical outcome (ACORN 2018). Planning patient care and identifying what nursing interventions will be required specific to the intraoperative environment are skills developed with experience. Understanding basic surgical techniques, such as the correct instruments and consumables required to address a bleeding vessel, is part of an intraoperative nurses' role. Knowing when and how to apply these techniques to different scenarios, while always maintaining the highest standard of asepsis, calls for both the instrument and circulating nurse to remain attentive, adaptable, responsive, and calm during surgical procedures. Operative nurses are governed by professional competency standards and practice guidelines for perioperative nursing in their global setting (ACORN 2018; AORN 2019; ORNAC 2017). The benefit of standardized practices in operating theatres is that common language and consistencies in roles and workflow are maintained for purposes of improving the quality and outcomes of surgical care.

Role of the Circulating Nurse

The role of the circulating nurse is to ensure optimal patient outcomes are reached. This is done by functioning and communicating effectively with all members of the healthcare team before during and after procedures. The circulating nurse participates in risk management activities including the World Health Organisation (WHO) Surgical Safety Checklist (Fig. 1) (O'Brien et al. 2017), double checking valid consent is present, assessing patient health and fasting status, and potential allergies. Core skills (Table 3) and responsibilities of the circulating nurse include: ensuring all

Table 1 Common medications used in anesthesia/recovery

Anesthetic agents	Emergency medications	Reversal agents	Other medications

Induction agents
  Propofol (Diprivan)
  Thiopental (Trapanal)
Opioids
  Alfentanil (Alfenta, Rapifen in Australia)
  Fentanyl
  Ketamine
  Morphine
  Oxycodone (Percodan, Endodan, Roxiprin, Percocet, Endocet, Roxicet, OxyContin)
  Remifentanil
Inhalation agents
  Desflurane
  Isoflurane
  Sevoflurane
Muscle relaxants
  Atracurium
  Cisatracurium (Nimbex)
  Pancuronium (Pavulon)
  Suxamethonium (succinylcholine)
  Rocuronium (Zemuron, Esmeron)
	Adrenaline (epinephrine)
	Amiodarone (Pacerone)
	Atropine
	Ephedrine (Akovaz, Corphedra)
	Glyceryl Tri Nitrate (Nitroglycerin)
	Metaraminol (Aramine, Metaramin, and Pressonex)
	Noradrenaline (Norepinephrine)
	Salbutamol (Ventolin)
		Flumazanil (flumazepil)
		Glycopyrolate (Cuvposa, glycopyrronium)
		Naloxone (Narcan)
		Neostigmine (Prostigmin)
		Sugammadex (Bridion)
			Calcium
			Clonidine (Catapres)
			Dexamethasone (dexasone, diodex, or hexadrol)
			Dexmedetomidine (Precedex)
			Droperidol (Inapsine)
			Esmolol (Brevibloc)
			Hydralazine (Apresoline)
			Insulin
			Ketorolac (Toradol)
			Magnesium
			Mannitol (Osmitrol)
			Metoprolol (Lopressor, Toprol XL)
			Ondansetron (Zofran)
			Paracetamol (acetaminophen, N-acetyl-para-aminophenol (APAP))
			Phentolamine (Regitine)
			Potassium
			Promethazine (Phenergan)
			Tramadol (Ultram, Conzip, Rybix ODT, Ultram ER)
			Tropisetron (Navoban)

Adapted from: Scarth and Smith 2017; Philip 2019

equipment and instruments required for the procedures are sterile, functioning, and available; performing and documenting surgical counts; and being present in the OR throughout the surgical procedure. These activities aim to recognize and respond to any changes in the patient's condition as well as monitoring for and acting on potential breaches in aseptic technique. For example, in the instance where a surgeon requests a specific item that is not already on the sterile field, it is the circulating nurse responsibility to source it and safely pass it to the instrument nurse for the surgeon to use. An important aspect of the circulating nurses' role is to act as patient advocate, respecting the patient's right to privacy, and preserving patient dignity pre-/post- and intraoperatively.

Table 2 Core anesthesia nurse clinical skills

Core anesthesia nursing skills
Completes anesthetic machine checking process
Meets with anesthetist and participates in discussion of plan for patient care
Preparation of IV fluid administration equipment
Preparation of patient and equipment for IV cannulation
Participation in the preoperative anesthetic surgery checklist
Provides validation for each component of the preanesthetic checklist
Assists with the setting up of the patient intubation airway trolley
Assists with connection of patient monitoring in the perioperative/operative environment
Assists in preparation for airway management/intubation of patient
Assists in preparation for extubating of patient postsurgery
Understands indications, action, and adverse reactions of anesthetic medications
Communicates issues that may delay surgery or cause surgery to be cancelled with surgical team

Source: ACORN (2016)

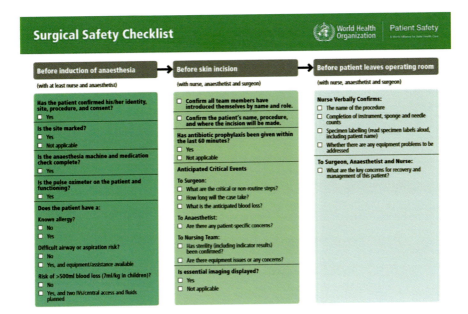

Fig. 1 WHO Surgical Safety Checklist (WHO 2016)

Role of the Instrument Nurse

The demands of an instrument nurse are complex due to the number of areas the role encompasses. Understanding the steps of the surgical procedure and how each patient's condition may impact on the intricacy of the surgery is part of the instrument nurses' role. Ensuring that correct equipment is available, functional, and safely prepared according to standards adds to the multifaceted nature of the instrument nurse' duties. While technical skills consume much of an instrument

Table 3 Core circulating nurse clinical skills

Core circulating nursing skills
Being aware of the hazards for both patients and staff within the physical environment. This including all persons entering the OT
Initiating and documenting the completion of the WHO Surgical Safety Checklist for every surgical procedure
Anticipate and identify the needs of the surgical team before and during surgery. Including opening the packaging of sterile items required during surgery
Maintain aseptic technique both before and during surgery while observing for any breach and initiate corrective action
Complete and document the surgical count with the instrument nurse to assist with the management of all equipment and consumables used during surgery
Correctly label and safely handle human tissue and explanted items that has been removed surgically
Complete the required documentation of intraoperative nursing care

Adapted from: ACORN (2016); IFPN (2019)

nurses' attention, it is paramount that the primary focus of their role is not distracted by these and continues to care for the patient.

The instrument nurse has a duty of care to assess the operating theatre environment and ensure that it is not only ready for the surgical procedure, but free from patient and staff risks (ACORN 2018; AORN 2019; ORNAC 2017). Confirming and communicating with all team members that documented and booked procedures have not been altered or updated will reduce potential theatre list errors and delays or patient complications – additionally part of the duties of an instrument nurse. The instrument nurse needs to adhere to the highest of standards of aseptic technique in line with following a unidirectional surgical flow (Standards Australia & Standards New Zealand 2018). Core skills (Table 4) include correctly performing a surgical scrub and safely glove and gowning – a fundamental feature of the instrument nurse role. Ensuring that asepsis is not compromised during set-up of the procedure is maintained throughout the surgical case, while also attending to surgeon requests provides an example of the situational awareness requirements of this nursing role.

Recovery Nursing

The principal role of the recovery room nurse (or postanesthesia care unit [PACU]) nurse is to monitor, critically evaluate, and clinically stabilize postoperative patients. The recovery room nurse anticipates and prevents the deterioration of patient complications as a direct result of the administered anesthesia and/or surgical procedure. Recovery room nurses undertake comprehensive systematic assessments of individuals immediately following transfer from the operating theatre. Assessment includes airway patency, levels of consciousness, sedation levels, and vital sign observations 10 minutely (ACORN 2018; AORN 2019; ORNAC 2017). The recovery room nurse core skills (Table 5) and considerations include direct patient observation, the anesthetic clinical handover, and the patients' medical history.

Table 4 Core instrument nurse clinical skills

Core instrument nursing skills
Prepare, check, and set up the required instruments and equipment needed for surgery
Observe the surgical case progression and identify the needs of the surgical team during surgery, including the passing of surgical instruments intraoperatively
Maintain aseptic technique both before and during surgery while observing for any breach and initiate corrective action
Initiate and complete the surgical count with the circulating nurse to assist with the management of all equipment and consumables used during surgery
Complete the required documentation of intraoperative nursing care

Adapted from: ACORN (2016); IFPN (2019)

Table 5 Core recovery nursing skills

Core recovery nursing skills
Completes a safety check of the recovery room bays
Identifies patient airway situation on arrival to recovery – has the pt. got an artificial airway in situ?
Identifies patient's level of consciousness
Participates in the handover process from anesthetist
Connects patient to vital sign monitoring equipment
Commences patient vital signs and interpretation
Documents patient vital signs and care delivered
Reviews patient's surgical procedure and medical history to direct nursing care
Reviews patient positioning postsurgery
Assess and manages patient pain
Assess and manages patient nausea
Completes a comprehensive patient handover from recovery to ward nurse

Source: ACORN (2016)

Recovery nursing is a specialty discipline that requires critical care nursing expertise.

The role, functions, and scope of practice of the operative nurse evolves through continuing education, time, and experience. Clinical skills and knowledge associated with each perioperative nursing role are continually developing as surgical procedures advance and patient care complexity increases. This leads to advanced skill development, more demanding tasks, and greater responsibility for the perioperative nurse.

Nontechnical Skills Within the Operating Theatre

Nontechnical skills (knowledge) within the OT are equally as important as having the technical ability to perform clinical skills. Professionally appropriate and effective communication between staff, patients, and family/ visitors is an imperative. Failure to effectively communicate, having an awareness of human factors and working as a team within the operating theatre are reasons frequently cited within the literature for surgical errors (Armour et al. 2019).

Communication

Effective interprofessional communication skills are essential when working in this specialized setting. Listening is an important aspect of interprofessional communication within the operating theatre. Since operating staff are wearing personal protective equipment (PPE) including masks during surgery, listening and understanding communication can be difficult. Speaking clearly and adopting a cooperative approach to understanding what has been communicated and ensuring it has been interpreted and understood correctly is important. Introductions of each member of the surgical team and their role help to identify individuals within the team. Eye contact is an essential part of communication within the operative setting; this ensures information is being communicated to the correct person, in a timely manner, helping to reduce errors (Colman et al. 2019). Working in the OT can be demanding and stressful, demonstrating respect and the use of common courtesy is essential to a calm environment (Weldon et al. 2013). Written and nonverbal communication are both key elements of effective communication within OT settings. Maintaining accurate clear documentation, on paper and/or electronic, allows others to easily and correctly interpret and follow instructions. This is crucial for continuing flow of safe patient care, from admission through to discharge of that same patient from the recovery room (Weldon et al. 2013).

Nonverbal communication in the OT is a special skill that is learnt with time and experience. When a new learner can focus learning in a specific surgical specialty, it helps to develop effective nonverbal communication and builds rapport and trust within the team. Focused learning allows individuals to develop a thorough understanding of procedures, skills required, possible complications, and equipment that is or may be required, during surgery. The constancy of working within specific surgical teams builds confidence and competence in individuals to work more efficiently and become effective confident team members (Sandelin et al. 2019; Weldon et al. 2013).

Human Factors

Human factors examine the relationships between human beings and their interactions with systems in the environment (WHO 2016). Surgical teams need to have a basic understanding of how human factor principles may affect the work environment during procedures. The OT is a high-pressure environment where errors can have momentous consequences. Stress (when perceived demands outweigh the perceived resources causing anxiety, irritability, or lack of concentration), fatigue, and interruptions (including noise) are all human factors that need to be recognized as important influences on performance and patient safety in the operative environment (Ng et al. 2019). Awareness of these factors and measures to counteract them and improve individual/team performance include staff introductions at the beginning of surgical lists, using WHO Surgical Safety Checklists, reducing foot traffic in/out of OT, double checking medications, and noise reduction can all improve patient outcomes.

Teamwork

To achieve optimal patient care, a clear understanding of team dynamics, how operating teams perform, and factors that facilitate or hinder teamwork is critical when working in the OT. Surgical teamwork involves complex interactions between all team members allocated to the surgical lists. To work together effectively as a team, each team member needs to understand their respective roles, responsibilities, and objectives throughout the surgical process. This helps to identify possible problems that may occur during surgery and any team dynamics that may negatively affect team performance, patient safety, and outcomes (Sandelin et al. 2019).

Teams working in the operating theatre need a heightened sense of situational awareness. Situational awareness is an awareness of the elements of the environment, taking into consideration three things:

1. What has just happened?
2. What is happening right now?
3. What is about to happen? (Oeppen et al. 2019)

Each member of the team in their professional capacity will frequently scan the environment taking into consideration these three questions and adjust their actions in response to the patient's condition. For nurses, the operative environment is different to other clinical settings they may have worked in. There are numerous different procedures/surgeries undertaken in 1 day, the workload requires high precision and quick actions, there is rapid turnover of patients, and an unpredictability with cases that may lead to acute and severe emergency situations at any time. New learners must adapt to caring for one patient as part of a team and in the OT the teams focus is exclusively on one patient, as opposed to one nurse having responsibility for four/five patients in other settings.

Nursing Education – Operating Theatre

Perioperative Exposure at Undergraduate Level

Globally not all undergraduate nursing programs offer the opportunity to undertake clinical placements in the operative environment (Foran 2016). Minimal exposure to the OT prior to registration could lead to fewer nurses choosing to work in the specialty (ACORN 2018). To continue to attract nurses to this specialty, mandatory perioperative placements during undergraduate education should be undertaken (ACORN 2018; AORN 2019; ORNAC 2017). Exposure to the operative environment at undergraduate level can be instrumental in inspiring people to pursue a career in this nursing specialty. It may increase students' knowledge and skills in the areas of anatomy/physiology, surgical procedures, patient condition/comorbidities and complexity of illness, patient assessment, and interdisciplinary communication (Foran 2016).

Specialist Education

Patient safety has been linked to increased knowledge and competence (Falk-Brynhildsen et al. 2019). Requirements for working as an OT nurse differ between countries. Sweden requires all operative nurses to be a registered nurse and to have completed a 3-year undergraduate degree and 1 year of postgraduate education specializing in either anesthesia or perioperative nursing. This is then followed by a 1-year advanced level postgraduate Master's in science (Falk-Brynhildsen et al. 2019). Further study to increase academic learning and clinical skills in the perioperative environment is encouraged in Australia (ACORN 2018). As patient safety is paramount in the operative environment, the promotion of an in-depth understanding of complex perioperative issues and increased knowledge and surgical skills is shown to improve patient outcomes (Russell and Coventry 2019).

Advanced practice and specialist postgraduate study options for OT nurses include hospital or university-based courses and online studies.

Continuing Professional Development (CPD)

Continuing professional development (also known as continual professional education, in-service, continuing education, life learning, and professional development) is any learning that helps maintain and improve current practice in an area of work. Its value and requirements vary between countries. For registered nurses in Australia working in any setting, including the operative environment, it is a requirement that a minimum of 20 h per year of CPD be completed (AHPRA 2019). CPD in the operative environment can include a range of learning activities, however, can be challenged by lack of organizational support and limited time during work hours to keep up with new knowledge (Sandelin et al. 2019). CPD can include meetings/conference attendance or other activities organized by national or international accredited perioperative bodies, joining specialist societies specific to an area of OT practice, internal learning activities such as teaching programs, clinical governance committee meetings, or personal study (Falk-Brynhildsen et al. 2019).

Future Challenges for Learning and Teaching in the OT. Where Are We Headed?

Population

The world's populations are aging and living longer, and with this comes increased demand on healthcare systems. Currently Australia and the United States have the greatest number of people aged above 65 years than in any other time in history (ACL 2019; ABS 2018). With continuing advances in medicine, people are not only living longer, they are also living longer with chronic diseases. As a result, the profile of patients requiring surgery is increasingly more complex due to multimorbid conditions and acuity, compounding critical care requirements (Haddad and Toney-Butler 2019). This places additional pressure on existing healthcare systems, including operating theatres.

Workforce

The healthcare workforce demographic is changing. Registered nurse populations globally are aging, one third (approximately one million) of registered nurses in Australia and the United States currently aged over 50 years and eligible for retirement in the next 10–15 years (Haddad and Toney-Butler 2019; AIHW 2016). Included in this number are OT nurse educators. While workforce demands have contributed to increased task shifting and role substitution in some settings, it has also influenced the introduction of dynamic and changing (global) roles for operative nurses including, surgical first assistant, nurse anesthetists, nurse endoscopists, and operating department practitioners (Royal College of Surgeons 2016).

Technology

Medical and digital technology integration into operating theatres has increased exponentially over the years (Blomberg et al. 2019). From the introduction of electronic medical records through to robotic-assisted surgery (e.g., prostate), the roles and demands of the operative nurse are continually expanding. The increasing use of technology also means change is ongoing for nursing workloads, roles, skills, and sense of value within delivery of patient care (McBride et al. 2019).

Strategies for Learning and Teaching in the Operating Theatre

The nature of perioperative nursing is challenging for all new learners. There is a need for nurses to have a high level of established and complex practical skills. Providing new learner perioperative nurses with supported and appropriate learning opportunities in high acuity clinical settings is a challenge many operating departments face (Hemingway et al. 2018; Ball et al. 2015; Freeling et al. 2017).

Operating theatres commonly experience a high volume of cases and are a fast-paced working environment. Nurses working in operative environments have a heightened awareness of time pressures. Becoming confident in their respective role takes time and practice. New learners must master technical (discussed previously) and nontechnical skills and must understand the why and not simply how to perform their duties (Wilson 2012).

Beginning a Career in the Operative Environment

Essentially all nurses who begin work in the operative environment for the first time are considered new learners. There are a limited number of acute nursing skills that are readily transferrable into the operating theatre. The physical learning environment of the OT is also unlike other clinical settings within healthcare. New learners must learn to navigate the physicality of the operating theatres, familiarize themselves with the culture and flow of surgery, and learn to adapt to the emotional effects of surgery on patients and the teams that work in this environment.

The operative environment is quite unique, enabling learners to create a clinical memory by combining real life pathology with tactile, visual, and verbal learning (Croghan et al. 2019). Learning within the operative setting is also very public. New learners predominately do their training within the OT during surgery and this is not simply a matter of "see one then do one" (Wilson 2012). After a comprehensive orientation, they are introduced as part of the team and begin work in appropriate surgical procedures, having a legitimate place within the team. This helps establish the new learner within the operative team, builds trust, and encourages the new learner to actively engage in their learning (Croghan et al. 2019).

New learners need clear learning objectives and to be guided to perform formal assessment requirements, at regular intervals to progress their learning. Having a clear understanding of what is required gives the new learner a sense of security that the objectives for working in theatre are clearly outlined. This enables the new learner to be able to retain knowledge and can reduce the stress of learning in the "real" environment, as opposed to the classroom (Croghan et al. 2019).

Allowing preparation time for new learners by preallocating surgical lists gives the learner the opportunity to preread, research, and revise specific surgical procedures, anatomy and physiology, medications, and possible complications. This can have a positive impact on the level of confidence and knowledge in the operating theatre (Croghan et al. 2019).

Creating Positive Learning Experiences

There are different approaches that support learning and teaching in OT. Students that feel welcomed into the operative clinical learning environment and who are encouraged to participate and contribute in their respective roles are more likely to pursue a future career in the OT (Ravindra et al. 2013). Creating an environment that is friendly and inclusive and where staff are approachable assists with learning. The current perioperative nursing workforce has a wealth of operative clinical experience, skills, and knowledge, however, is aging. Utilizing the clinical excellence of these experienced nurses to mentor and inspire others in the field before they retire is vital in developing new learners (Foran 2016). The future shortfall of clinical skills and knowledge in high acuity perioperative areas resulting from an aging workforce is a concern for many healthcare organizations (Freeling et al. 2017; Foran 2016). As a result, adequate planning is needed to identify opportunities to up-skill current new learner perioperative nurses. The benefit in encouraging career progression for new learners is parallel to the strength of care provided by healthcare organizations (Ball et al. 2015). In other words, by supporting novice nurses to develop their skills and knowledge, the efficacy of a department is also improved. This is advantageous in strengthening the clinical excellence of departments and has been argued as a factor that improves staff retention (Ball et al. 2015). Having a workforce plan that includes continual professional development for experienced mid-career nurses and career progression options may enhance the recruitment of additional staff into the perioperative field.

Support for Learning and Teaching (Preceptor, Mentor)

Preceptors or mentors (also known as peer/clinical instructors, clinical supervisors/facilitators) support, teach, and assess learners in clinical practice (Tuomikoski et al. 2019). Most learning and teaching in perioperative environments is facilitated by preceptors or mentors. In certain countries, it is a requirement for all registered nurses to participate in the education of new learners (O'Brien et al. 2014). However, successful transition from clinical nurse to a mentoring role is reliant on formal preparation. Mentors that work in the OT have a clear understanding of the pressures and realities of surgery. In order to be able to navigate new learners to the environment, qualities such as kindness, motivation, patience, and the ability to communicate clearly under pressure are required. Mentors need to be supported through education to develop strategies around providing and receiving feedback, handling challenging situations, adapting to differing learning styles as well as continually building their own skills (Tuomikoski et al. 2019). This can be achieved by encouraging mentors to develop a clinical portfolio within education. By doing so the competence and quality of mentoring will continue to improve, through the provision of regular feedback to the mentors themselves. The notion of mentoring mentors is one approach that can be utilized in the OT.

Simulation

The use of simulated learning in the OT can enhance interprofessional learning and communication together with theoretical knowledge and clinical skills relevant to specific surgical procedures. Its use in education can build confidence and competence among not only new learners but existing staff in the OT in a nonthreatening and safe environment (Blomberg et al. 2019; Hemingway et al. 2018). Using simulation to emulate surgical procedures for training purposes can progressively improve the skills of operative nurses through practical experience, repetition, constructive feedback, and critical thinking (Hemingway et al. 2018). The use of simulation to enhance learning in the OT can reduce the amount of time new learners require preceptor support, improve critical thinking, improve confidence and clinical judgment, and develop self-efficacy. This can strengthen the likelihood of new learners maintaining positions in the perioperative setting (Hemingway et al. 2018; Ball et al. 2015).

Safety in the Operating Theatre

The Safety of New Learners

Allowing new learners nurses to develop experience without compromising patient safety is a challenging scenario to balance. Without adequate support, new learners may be deterred from high acuity OT settings, heightening the issue of nursing shortages in these areas (Freeling et al. 2017).

A safe environment can be perceived from both patient and nursing perspective. The need to fulfill patient expectations by providing capable and confident staff contributes to a safe environment. In OT, the ability to provide safe learning opportunities for new learners to gain clinical experience may be a challenge (Hemingway et al. 2018). During surgery, the focus of experienced nursing staff may be entirely devoted to the needs of the patient, leaving minimal time available for new learners requiring support in these areas (Hemingway et al. 2018). Perceptions of heightened stress and fear related to the fast pace of surgery and not knowing what surgical stage the surgeon is up to can be barriers to learning, discouraging new learners from expanding their knowledge, and moving into higher acuity operating environments (Hemingway et al. 2018; Roberts and Greene 2011). Promoting the growth of new learners in a controlled environment is beneficial for healthcare organizations particularly when trying to address the shortage of nurses (Ball et al. 2015). Supporting new learners and retaining them into the future will enable high quality, patient-centered, evidenced-based care to be maintained in perioperative settings.

Patient Safety

Perioperative nurses face challenges in maintaining patient safety. An estimated 313 million surgical procedures occur globally each year and 4.2 million people die within 30 days of their surgery (Meara et al. 2019). In the perioperative environment, human error can contribute to morbidity and mortality. Reducing errors and improving patient safety is achieved by eliminating or reducing risks within the operative environment. Increasing complexity of surgery, heavy workloads, acute stress, and environmental risks from equipment, hazards, lasers, and instruments can all impact patient safety (AORN 2019). Clear communication between all staff and fostering a culture of risk awareness can improve patient outcomes (Lee et al. 2019).

Patient safety in the OT is guided by the World Health Organisation safety guidelines. This includes the continual assessment of patients in the preoperative, interoperative, and postoperative phases of surgery. The WHO Surgical Safety Checklist (SSC) was introduced into surgical settings in 2008. This 19-item checklist aims to increase communication and teamwork during surgery, can be modified for individual surgery centers, and used around the world to reduce patient morbidity and mortality (WHO 2019) (Fig. 1).

Checklists aid in the safe delivery of care to patients in the OT; however, if not implemented effectively and staff trained to use them properly, the potential for a positive patient outcome will be limited.

Biomedical Safety

Specimens

A common goal of performing surgery is often to obtain adequate pathology in order to diagnose, plan, or treat patients and their medical condition (Berryman 2009). In order to adequately obtain and preserve this pathology, it is necessary for healthcare professionals to safely and correctly follow guiding procedures.

From the initial stage of specimen collection during surgery, it is paramount that double checking of specimen details occurs. Errors relating to the inadequate identification, labeling, and handling of relevant pathology may result in detrimental outcomes for patients (ACORN 2018). Misdiagnosis or unnecessary follow-up treatment and surgery are avoidable adverse outcomes through correct and safe handling of specimens. For this reason, specimen labeling is included in the WHO Surgical Safety Checklist (WHO 2019) (Fig. 1).

Handling of biological specimens is also a potential hazard to staff safety. Chemicals, such as formaldehyde, are commonly used to preserve tissue specimens obtained during surgery. Formaldehyde is a toxic chemical and diligent education and training of staff is necessary to reduce the risk of hazardous exposures (ACORN 2018). Wearing appropriate personal protective equipment (PPE) and following safety procedures relating to the handling of specimens requiring formaldehyde is paramount.

Personal Protective Equipment (PPE)

The use of PPE in the OT is considered a standard infection control measure (ACORN 2018; AORN 2019; ORNAC 2017). All staff within the OT are required to wear perioperative attire, commonly known as surgical scrubs, to avoid compromise to any sterile fields. This is achieved by replacing outer garments of clothing with scrubs provided by the healthcare setting. Covered shoes that are cleanable provide staff with full protection from dropped items or splashes. Depending on local requirements, shoes may also need to be covered by the wearing specific outer covers that maintain the clean environment with the OT (ACORN 2018). Changing of perioperative attire is required daily or if the attire becomes wet or soiled.

All hair, including facial hair, must be covered by a disposable clean hat or balaclava (ACORN 2018; AORN 2019; ORNAC 2017). The wearing of cloth hats may be permitted provided they are replaced daily and adequately laundered. All OT staff are required to wear a surgical face mask which covers the nose and mouth, primarily to aid in protecting the wearer's face. Eye protection in the form of visors or goggles should be worn when there is any risk of splash to the wearer's eyes. This includes during intubation and extubation, when handling fluids, and always when scrubbed.

Gloves must be worn when handling chemicals, contaminants, blood, or other bodily fluids. Double gloving (wearing of two pairs of gloves at the same time) is widely promoted as the gold standard for surgical gloving (ACORN 2018; AORN 2019; ORNAC 2017). This practice reduces the risk to the wearer if there is a breach in the outer glove, such as a needle-stick or sharps injury. Double gloving reduces the risk of an acquired infection by up to 87% (ICT 2019). Lead gowns or use of protective screens are required to protect staff when X-Ray is being used in the OT (ACORN 2018; AORN 2019; ORNAC 2017) and should cover the torso, reproductive organs, and thyroid.

Conclusion

Learning and teaching in the OT setting is challenging because it is fast-paced, specialized and contains multiple distractions and heightened risks to patient safety. Appreciating these challenges is crucial in the development and implementation of learning and teaching strategies to support new and existing learners.

Safe and effective surgical care is dependent on team members having a range of well-developed interpersonal, communication, technical, and nontechnical skills. OT nurses with such specialized skills and experience are central to effective multidisciplinary surgical teams and patient outcomes. Growing and retaining these specialist nurses is important for safe patient-centered surgical care into the future.

References

Administration for Community Living (ACL). Aging and disability in America. 2019. Retrieved from https://acl.gov/aging-and-disability-in-america/data-and-research/minority-aging

Armour T, Ford R, Rasmussen B. Anaesthetic nurses' perceptions of learning during interprofessional simulation education. Clin Simul Nurs. 2019;35:5–9.

Association of periOperative Registered Nurses (AORN). AORN Standards 2019. Retrieved from https://www.aorn.org/guidelines/clinical-resources/aorn-standards

Australian and New Zealand College of Anaesthetist (ANZCA). What is anaesthesia? 2019. Retrieved from http://www.anzca.edu.au/patients/what-is-anaesthesia

Australian Bureau of Statistics (ABS) 3101.0 Australia Demographics Statistics, June 2018. Retrieved from https://www.abs.gov.au/ausstats/abs@.nsf/0/1CD2B1952AFC5E7ACA257298000F2E76?OpenDocument

Australian College of Operating Room Nurses, editor. ACORN standards for perioperative nursing including nursing roles, guidelines, position statements. 15th ed. Australian College of Operating Room Nurses; 2018.

Australian College of Operating Room Nurses. ACORN 2016. ACORN standards for perioperative nursing in Australia. 14th ed. Australian College of Operating Room Nurses.

Australian Health Practitioner Regulation Agency (AHPRA). Australia nursing and midwifery board. Continuing professional development. 2019. Retrieved from https://www.nursingmidwiferyboard.gov.au/codes-guidelines-statements/faq/cpd-faq-for-nurses-and-midwives.aspx.

Australian Institute of Health and Welfare (AIHW). Nursing and Midwifery workforce. 2016. Retrieved from https://www.aihw.gov.au/reports/workforce/nursing-and-midwifery-workforce-2015/contents/who-are-nurses-and-midwives

Ball K, Doyle D, Oocumma N. Nursing shortages in the OR: solutions for new models of education. AORN J. 2015;101(1):115–36.

Berryman R. The importance of specimens. ACORN J. 2009;22(3):16–7.

Blomberg AC, Lindwall L, Bisholt B. Operating theatre nurses' self-reported clinical competence in perioperative nursing: a mixed method study. Nurs Open. 2019;6(4):1–9.

Canadian Nurses Association (CAN). Framework for the practice of registered nursed in Canada. 2015. Retrieved from https://cna-aiic.ca/-/media/cna/page-content/pdf-en/framework-for-the-pracice-of-registered-nurses-in-canada.pdf?la=en&hash=55716DC66A8C15D13972F9E45BE4AC7AE0461620

Colman N, Figueroa J, McCracken C, Hebbar K. Simulation-based team training improves team performance among pediatric intensive care unit staff. J Pediatr Intensive Care. 2019;8(02):083–91.

Croghan SM, Phillips C, Howson W. The operating theatre as a classroom: a literature review of medical student learning in the theatre environment. Int J Med Educ. 2019;10:75–87.

Dunne N. Acorn international volunteering and teaching grant report: volunteering on board mercy ships, West Africa. J Perioper Nurs. 2019;32(3):43–4.

Falk-Brynhildsen K, Jaensson M, Gillespie BM, Nilsson U. Swedish operating room nurses and nurse anesthetists' perceptions of competence and self-efficacy. J Perianesth Nurs. 2019;34(4):842–50.

Foran P. The value of guided operating theatre experience for undergraduate nurses. ACORN J. 2016;29(1):10–8.

Freeling M, Parker S, Breaden K. Exploring experienced nurse's views, attitudes and expectations of graduate nurses in the operating theatre. ACORN J. 2017;30(1):23–8.

Haddad LM, Toney-Butler TJ. Nursing shortage. InStatPearls [Internet] 2019 Jan 19. StatPearls Publishing. Retrieved from https://www.ncbi.nlm.nih.gov/books/NBK493175/

Hemingway MW, Osgood P, Mannion M. Implementing a cardiac skills orientation and simulation program. AORN J. 2018;107(2):215–23.

Infection Control Today (ICT). Double gloving myth versus fact. 2019. Retrieved from https://www.infectioncontroltoday.com/personal-protective-equipment/double-gloving-myth-versus-fact

International Federation of Perioperative Nurses (IFPN). EORNA framework for perioperative nurse competencies. 2019. Retrieved from https://www.ifpn.world/application/files/8115/5480/6534/EORNA_Competencies_for_perioperative_nurses.pdf

Ireland S, Osborne S. Reviewing ACORN nursing role 'anaesthetic nurse'. ACORN: J Perioper Nurs Aust. 2016;29(4):54–7. [Online].

Kaye AD, Urman RD, Fox CJ III, editors. Operating room leadership and perioperative practice management. 2nd ed. Cambridge: Cambridge University Press; 2018.

Lee HF, Chiang HY, Kuo HT. Relationship between authentic leadership and nurses' intent to leave: the mediating role of work environment and burnout. J Nurs Manag. 2019;27(1):52–65.

McBride KE, Steffens D, Duncan K, Bannon PG, Solomon MJ. Knowledge and attitudes of theatre staff prior to the implementation of robotic-assisted surgery in the public sector. PLoS One. 2019;14(3):e0213840.

Meara JG, Leather AJ, Farmer PE. Making all deaths after surgery count. Lancet. 2019;393(10191):2587.

Ng R, Chahine S, Lanting B, Howard J. Unpacking the literature on stress and resiliency: a narrative review focused on learners in the operating room. J Surg Educ. 2019;76(2):343–53.

O'Brien A, Giles M, Dempsey S, Lynne S, McGregor ME, Kable A, Parmenter G, Parker V. Evaluating the preceptor role for pre-registration nursing and midwifery student clinical education. Nurse Educ Today. 2014;34(1):19–24.

O'Brien B, Graham MM, Kelly SM. Exploring nurses' use of the WHO safety checklist in the perioperative setting. J Nurs Manag. 2017;25(6):468–76.

Oeppen RS, Davidson M, Scrimgeour DS, Rahimi S, Brennan PA. Human factors awareness and recognition during multidisciplinary team meetings. J Oral Pathol Med. 2019;48(8).

Operating Room Nurses Association of Canada (ORNAC). ORNAC standards. 13th ed. 2017. Retrieved from https://www.ornac.ca/en/standards

OPTIMUS Integrated surgical environment. History of the operating room. 2019. Retrieved from https://www.optimus-ise.com/historical/history-of-the-operating-room/

Philip BK. Fast track recovery. In: Anesthesia in day care surgery. Singapore: Springer; 2019. p. 1–5.

Phillips N. Berry & Kohn's operating room technique. 13th ed. St Louis: Elsevier; 2016.

Ravindra P, Fitzgerald JE, Bhangu A, Maxwell-Armstrong CA. Quantifying factors influencing operating theater teaching, participation, and learning opportunities for medical students in surgery. J Surg Educ. 2013;70:495–501.

Roberts D, Greene L. The theatre of high-fidelity simulation education. Nurse Educ Today. 2011;31(7):694–8.

Royal College of Surgeons. A question of balance. The extended surgical team. 2016. Retrieved from https://doi.org/10.1308/rcsbull.2017.264

Russell KP, Coventry T. Innovations in postgraduate work integrated learning within the perioperative nursing environment: a mixed method. J Perioper Nurs. 2019;32(1):27–31.

Sandelin A, Kalman S, Gustafsson BÅ. Prerequisites for safe intraoperative nursing care and teamwork – operating theatre nurses' perspectives: a qualitative interview study. J Clin Nurs. 2019;28(13–14):2635–43.

Scarth E, Smith S. Drugs in anaesthesia and intensive care. 5th ed. New York: Oxford University Press; 2017.

Schlich T, Hasegawa A. Order and cleanliness: the gendered role of operating room nurses in the United States (1870s–1930s). Soc Hist Med. 2017;31(1):106–21.

Siirala E, Suhonen H, Salanterä S, Junttila K. The nurse manager's role in perioperative settings: an integrative literature review. J Nurs Manag. 2019;27(5):918–29.

Standards Australia Limited/Standards New Zealand (AS/NZS). Reprocessing of reusable medical devices in health service organizations (AS/NZS 4187:2014). 2018. Retrieved from SAI Global database.

Tuomikoski AM, Ruotsalainen H, Mikkonen K, Miettunen J, Juvonen S, Sivonen P, Kääriäinen M. How mentoring education affects nurse mentors' competence in mentoring students during clinical practice–a quasi-experimental study'. Scand J Caring Sci. 2019; https://doi.org/10.1111/scs.12728. Early View

Weldon SM, Korkiakangas T, Bezemer J, Kneebone R. Communication in the operating theatre. Br J Surg. 2013;100(13):1677–88.

Wilson M. Redesigning orientation. Assoc Oper Nurs J. 2012;95(4):453–62.

World Health Organisation (WHO). Human factors, Technical series on safer primary care. 2016. Retrieved from https://apps.who.int/iris/bitstream/handle/10665/252273/9789241511612-eng.pdf?sequence=1

World Health Organisation (WHO). WHO surgical safety checklist. 2019. Retrieved from https://www.who.int/patientsafety/safesurgery/checklist/en/

Learning and Teaching in Pediatrics

50

Ramesh Mark Nataraja, Simon C. Blackburn, and Robert Roseby

Contents

Introduction	956
Defining Pediatrics	957
Specialist College Frameworks	959
Key Qualities in a Successful Pediatric Healthcare Professional	961
General Versus Subspecialty Pediatrics	962
Educational Theory Applied to Pediatrics	963
Mastery Learning	963
Deliberate Practice	964
Feedback	964
Assessment	965
Experiential Learning	967
Reflective Practice	967
Communities of Practice	968
Simulation-Based Education	969
Types of Bench Trainer Simulators	970
Fidelity, Realism, and Educational Engagement	971
Scenario-Based Simulation	972
Simulated Patients and Roleplay	972
Integration of SBE into a Curriculum	973
Supported Returns to Training	973
Ethics in Pediatrics	975
Clinical Ethics Committees	975
Best Interests	975

R. M. Nataraja (✉) · R. Roseby
Monash Children's Hospital, Clayton, VIC, Australia

Department of Paediatrics, School of Clinical Sciences, Faculty of Medicine, Nursing and Health Sciences, Monash University, Clayton, VIC, Australia
e-mail: ram.nataraja@monashhealth.org; robert.roseby@monashhealth.org

S. C. Blackburn
The Learning Academy, Great Ormond Street Hospital for Children, London, UK
e-mail: simon.blackburn@gosh.nhs.uk

© Springer Nature Singapore Pte Ltd. 2023
D. Nestel et al. (eds.), *Clinical Education for the Health Professions*,
https://doi.org/10.1007/978-981-15-3344-0_68

Capacity and Consent 975
Consent, Assent, and Disclosure to Children 976
Child Protection 977
Interactions with Parents 978
Conclusion 979
Cross-References 979
References 979

Abstract

Pediatrics is unique in its scope and variability of clinical presentations. These range from an adolescent to a patient who has not yet been born, but has been diagnosed with an antenatal congenital abnormality. In this chapter, we discuss the various aspects of learning and teaching in pediatrics to allow readers to gain some insights into this complex, diverse, specialty. We describe the definition and scope of pediatrics itself, international training programs and curricula, general versus subspecialty pediatrics, and the specialist college frameworks. We also give an overview on the educational theories that underpin learning and teaching in pediatrics including mastery learning, deliberate practice, feedback, experiential learning, reflective practice, communities of practice, and the various types of simulators used in simulation-based medical education. Additionally, potentially controversial topics such as supported returns to practice are explored as this is especially relevant to pediatrics. Various ethical issues with relevance to pediatrics are also discussed. These include capacity and consent, disclosure to children, and child protection. The key differences in interactions with the pediatric patients are also discussed. Pediatrics as a speciality is a complex area to work, learn, and teach, but as for other disciplines, there are a few frameworks and theories that can help provide the structure. This chapter has been written within the frameworks of the authors' experiences and so is not intended to be a comprehensive resource for those aspects of pediatrics relating to non-medical healthcare professions, but it does identify the core essential characteristics for any healthcare professional working with children.

Keywords

Pediatrics education · Simulation-based medical education · Pediatric simulation · Educational theory · Pediatrics training · Ethics · Pediatrics training programs

Introduction

Clinicians are rightly proud of the history of medicine, reaching back to ancient civilizations, yet the treatment of pediatrics as a separate specialty is quite recent. It took almost 2000 years from the first recognition by the ancient Greek and Roman physicians that children were different from adults, to the introduction of the first formal academic course in pediatrics, in America at the Yale College of Medicine in

1813. The first children's hospital, The Hospital for Sick Children on Great Ormond Street in London, was built in 1852 (Rangroo 1992). It can be argued that the care of children occupies a status commensurate with the importance society places on children and childhood. In 1911, "recognition of the world as being the foremost civilized nation" was the target for the United States of America (USA) by recognizing their responsibilities toward children (Brosco 1999). This was in a call to reduce its infant mortality rate (IMR), which at that time was 135 per 1000, the 18th among 30 industrialized countries.

The training of specialists with expertise in the care of children, child development, and childhood diseases further developed over the course of the twentieth century. Today, teaching and learning in pediatrics are integral to present-day health systems, with medical schools and colleges training healthcare professionals in this field. This is becoming more relevant as "about half of the world's population is now younger than 25 years." (Resnick et al. 2012) This shift is accompanied by an increasing degree of subspecialization toward pediatrics within other healthcare professional domains such as nursing and allied health, with an increasing role for advanced practice in the care of children.

Defining Pediatrics

The lower limit of pediatric care appears initially easy to define, the birth of the patient. Although this may become less clear for example, pediatric subspecialists are requested to discuss potential diagnoses antenatally with pregnant women, participate in the emerging field of fetal cardiac imaging (Oepkes and Haak 2014) or are involved with fetal surgery (Deprest and Coppi 2012) and ex utero intrapartum treatment (EXIT) procedures. Although the start of pediatric care may extend antenatally, the upper limit of pediatric care is even harder to define. Pediatric centers may have different definitions of the age at which pediatric care ends, even within the same jurisdiction. When clustered, the somewhat arbitrary nature of the end of pediatric care and the start of adult care looks somewhat chaotic. Various studies have seen pediatric care end at any point between 12 and 19 years old, and even informally at the appearance of pubic hair. The US-based Society for Adolescent Health and Medicine recognizes the difficulty of using an age cut-off for definitions. They define young adulthood beginning at the age of 18 years based on evidence that the age group 18–25 years has higher mortality and risk factors different from the age groups below or above (Society for Adolescent Health and Medicine 2017). Our pediatric tertiary centers have a functional endpoint to pediatrics, whereby new patients after the age of 18 years are directed to adult health services, and the existing patients make the transition to adult healthcare by the first year after completing secondary school, between 18 and 19 years of age. It is increasingly recognized that transition to adult care should be a gradual and purposeful process (Blum et al. 1993). In the UK, for example, the current guidelines suggest that this should commence around the age of 14 years (National Institute for Health and Care Excellence (NICE) 2019). There are some conditions that necessitate earlier adult physician engagement, such as pregnancy in the context of chronic diseases, where adult specialists have more specific experience and expertise. There are also several areas where knowledge of pediatric diagnoses is required in looking after adult patients; the care of those young people who have complex congenital heart disease being one example. It can be seen, therefore, that precisely defining the beginning, and especially the end, of pediatric care is not as simple as it may initially seem. There are many barriers to this transition from pediatric to adult care, and this is an evolving area of medicine (Gray et al. 2017).

As pediatrics has evolved the specialty of adolescent medicine is emerging, as are the learning requirements for health professionals working with patients in this age group. Adolescence is defined by the World Health Organization as aged 10–19 years (Welfare AI of H 2017) and is recognized as a period of profound biological, social, and psychological change. While chronic disease survivors, ex-premature infants and those with congenital conditions are surviving into adolescence at rates higher than ever before (Myrhaug et al. 2019), diseases, disorders, and problems also emerge in this age group. These include eating disorders and other mental health diseases, risk taking behaviors, and their consequences such as sexually transmitted diseases including HIV, accidents, violence, drugs, tobacco, and the underage use of alcohol (Sawyer et al. 2012). All of these provide challenges to the learner. The first adolescent medicine-specific curriculum from the Society for Adolescent Health and Medicine (Table 1) (Coles and Greenberg 2017) has emerged in recognition of the unique needs of this group of patients.

The developmental focus of pediatric training fits well with the challenges of adolescent healthcare. Rapid developmental change, the impact of development on disease, and the impact of disease on development are common aspects of pediatric practice and sit well with the existing pediatric education models. Similarly, healthcare professionals dealing with chronic disease in young adults need to understand the impact of disease on the aspects of development such as relationships, career choice, reproductive decisions, and child rearing. We remain agnostic about whether training in adolescent health sits better with adult or pediatric programs.

Table 1 Curriculum domains for adolescent medicine (Coles and Greenberg 2017)

Adolescent medicine curriculum domains
1. Routine adolescent healthcare
2. Consent and confidentiality
3. Growth and development
4. Sexual and reproductive health
5. Psychological and behavioral health
6. Substance use and abuse
7. Safety and violence
8. Disordered eating
9. Sports medicine
10. Transition to adult care

The varied population from an antenatally diagnosed infant to an adolescent with a previous adult-based clinical diagnosis requires an extremely broad curriculum compared to other specialties. There is also the added complexity of approaching the complex emotional responses of a parent with an unwell child and the communication skills required to address them, as well as the more limited scope for hands-on experience while on the learning curve with pediatric patients, where the performance of practical procedures by relative novices is often felt to be unacceptable. Compared to the variability of conditions, treatments, and presentations in pediatrics, there is limited subspecialization compared to adult medical disciplines.

Specialist College Frameworks

The United Kingdom (UK), the United States of America (USA), Canada, Australia, and New Zealand frameworks for the qualities of specialists providing care for children are remarkably similar. However, the systems in which we work differ so specialist practice differs in different continents. For example, in the UK and Ireland, Australia and New Zealand pediatricians see only referred patients, whereas in the USA it may be a primary care specialty with subspecialist practice. There are different training programs to meet these differing workforce requirements, but the fundamental qualities of pediatric specialists remain similar (Fig. 1).

The Royal Australasian College of Physicians (Australia and New Zealand) framework describes ten domains of physician practice. This RACP framework has many similarities with other medical disciplines including pediatrics and surgery, Fig. 2.

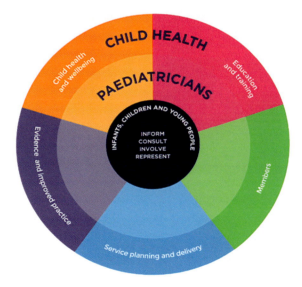

Fig. 1 RCPCH (the United Kingdom) framework (Royal College of Paediatrics and Child Health 2018)

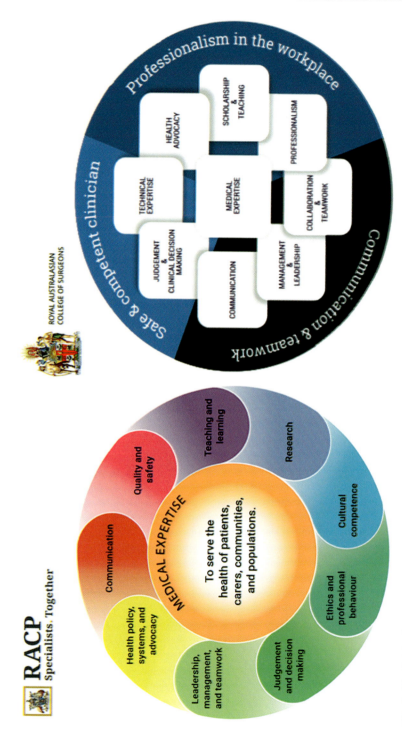

Fig. 2 The RACP framework for professional practice and Royal Australasian College of Surgeons (Royal Australasian College of Physicians Professional Practice Framework 2017)

Two decades ago, the purpose of a training program was seen as binary to prepare a trainee for their future practice or to lay a foundation for further training (Macnab et al. 1998). Educational theorists would view it more broadly than this now, and the emphasis on "life-long learning" in many aspects of training programs is related to this (Royal College of Paediatrics and Child Health 2018; Royal Australian College of Physicians Professional Practice Framework 2017).

As with the medical colleges, the nursing and midwifery pediatric frameworks are also well established internationally with generalized similarities. These include the Hong Kong College of Paediatric Nursing, which was established in 2012 and includes the subspecialities of Child & Adolescent Health, Paediatric Intensive Care, Neonatal Intensive Care, and School & Public Health Nursing. This curriculum involves three main core domains for pediatrics: generic, advanced practice, and specialty cores over 500 hours (Hong Kong College of Paediatric Nursing 2021). The Australian College of Nursing also has a dedicated pediatric stream, which offers a graduate certificate in pediatric nursing studies (Australian College of Nursing 2021). This graduate certificate qualification is commonly utilized by nursing staff as an entry level option for postgraduate education. The Royal College of Nursing in the UK has membership of 450,000 nurses, midwives, nursing support workers, and students with most established frameworks for the development of pediatric-specific skills (Royal College of Nursing (United Kingdom) 2020). These frameworks also have adapted to support the increased requirements for both Clinical Nurse Specialists and Advance Nurse Practitioners within the healthcare institutions especially in neonatology, emergency medicine, and pediatric oncology (Cooper et al. 2019; Mitchell et al. 2017). There has been an increase in the focus on specialist care and on the articulation of the role of the children's nurse and determinants of the quality of care they deliver (Brenner and Begley 2019). There is also an increased awareness for promoting other components of nursing practice such as research engagement in recent times (Newall and Khair 2020).

Key Qualities in a Successful Pediatric Healthcare Professional

Somewhat remarkably, there is a very limited evidence base in the published literature describing the influences on medical students and early career doctors on their choice to pursue pediatrics. In general terms, we know these include university admission policies, influence of individual educators, presence of mentoring, and the curriculum itself (Newton et al. 2010). Personal experiences in their non-professional lives are often cited by candidates in interviews for training positions. One of the limited studies to investigate this issue used survey data collected from graduating medical students from two medical schools in New York and North Carolina, USA, over an 11-year period (Newton et al. 2010). Of these, 337 intended to pursue careers in pediatrics, 175 in general, and 166 in subspecialty pediatrics. Common to both the groups were the highest ranked items on a 4-point scale of "helping others" followed by highly valuing "comprehensive patient care," with more generalist than subspecialist interested students indicating this second item. There were other differences between the groups also, with highly ranked items including lifestyle, working with the poor, income, prestige, and opportunity to participate in research (Newton et al. 2010).

This contrasts with other pediatric healthcare professionals such as nursing, as many nursing students enter the undergraduate training programs with preconceived ideas about their future career paths, which predominantly include pediatrics and midwifery (McKenna et al. 2010). These are often not based on the actual clinical exposure but rather an association with a "happy" area (Happell 2000). Although this will benefit pediatric nursing, it can have a negative influence on other domains such as geriatrics or other nonacute specialities (McKenna et al. 2010).

Regardless of the individual healthcare professionals' motivations for pursuing a career in either general or subspecialty pediatrics, there are essential qualities required for a successful practitioner. These include communication, empathy, adaptability, and the ability to reassure both the child and the parents in challenging situations. The practitioner needs to learn how to communicate with children, as a means of engagement, to gather information but also to explain things to a child. The experienced clinician will use play to understand and communicate with children. "A child's use of playthings such as dolls' houses, families of small animals or artworks can communicate all manner of issues which a child may otherwise not be able to articulate due to poor verbal skills or other reasons" (Roseby 2018).

General Versus Subspecialty Pediatrics

"Workforce planning in medicine is at best an inexact science and at worst a dark art" (Goddard 2010). In the United Kingdom (UK), the Shape of Training review (Klaber et al. 2015) mapped a future in which postgraduate training is shortened and aims to produce doctors who have a level of generic competence at the end of training, which can then be added with specialist "credentialing." The Royal College of Paediatrics and Child Health has argued that individual pediatric subspecialties are not special interests within a specialty but represent territories of knowledge that are the equivalent of their adult counterparts. For example, it could be argued that a pediatric neurologist requires as much specialist knowledge and skill as their adult counterpart. In the UK context, it has also been argued that "general pediatrics" is a specialty within its own right, rather than simply providing a building block for later subspecialist training. Regardless of the political context, it is clearly the case that pediatric practice requires the assimilation of skills in a variety of clinical areas, ranging from participating in antenatal care and learning the techniques needed to care for extremely small babies, to dealing with young adults making the transition into adult services. These skills must be acquired in the context of a training program that can deliver both the focus needed by future subspecialists and the breadth needed by those with a more general focus.

As for the medical training schemes, there is an increased subspecialization in pediatric-based nursing and midwifery practice. An example of this is the National Specialisation Framework for Nursing and Midwifery, which was developed in

Australia in 2006, (The National Nursing and Nursing Education Taskforce 2006). This occurred in response to the increasing healthcare specialization within the nursing workforce potentially leading to the fragmentation of care and inefficiency. Pediatric nursing was identified in the National Specialty Framework as one of the 18 areas of practice (The National Nursing and Nursing Education Taskforce 2006). Within pediatric nursing itself, there are many different subspecializations, for example, oncology, intensive care, emergency medicine, neonatology, gastroenterology, or pediatric urology. There is also a requirement for training subspecialty nurses in low- and middle-income countries as there has been a gradual improvement in the mortality associated with infectious diseases and hence a shift of focus to childhood cancers (Wilimas et al. 2003).

Educational Theory Applied to Pediatrics

There are many educational theories that underpin learning and teaching in pediatrics, and although there are many common themes with other specialties, we will discuss these theories within this context.

Mastery Learning

The concept of mastery learning is a key educational theory that underpins many competency-based training programs including pediatrics. In mastery learning, a complex task is divided into individual steps, which the learner must become competent to perform before proceeding to learn the next step (Mcgaghie et al. 2011). Therefore, there is a progressive cycle of achievement and performance competency demonstration, into which simulation-based learning can easily be implemented. This may include core pediatric skills such as establishing intravenous access with sequentially peripherally inserted intravenous cannulas, peripherally inserted central catheters, central venous catheters, and then intra-osseous access. While this scaffolding may exist informally in more traditional apprenticeship models, decreasing work hours and trainee case load demand greater structure and efficiency of skill learning. Simulation-based education can provide opportunities for practice when they do not exist clinically or where the skill is a rare clinical event. In pediatrics, there are many mastery domains including clinical, procedural, patient interaction, clinical decision-making, teamwork, collaboration, and professionalism.

One of the important aspects of mastery learning is that time is not a consideration, acknowledging that individual learners progress at a differing pace in different tasks. Therefore, the endpoint is the demonstration of competence, rather than other parameters. This does not mean that the mastery learning model finishes when competency has been obtained. Maintenance of optimal performance is essential and clinical practice, reflection, innovation, and successful adoption of new techniques can also be viewed through this framework. In pediatrics, the learning opportunities should be carefully considered for the trainee to discover their level of ability and then achieve mastery through focused effort with the application of constructive feedback. These should relate to both the cognitive and psychomotor domains. With more complex tasks, these should be subdivided into smaller individual steps for the learner to progress through, with their combination in the final step to achieve mastery (Block and Airasian 1971).

Deliberate Practice

Deliberate practice originated in the observation of the behaviors of elite performers in other nonclinical domains including elite musicians, professional athletes, typing experts, and chess grandmasters (Ericsson 2004). A minimum period of 10 years of sustained deliberate practice was required even with the most talented performers before they reached an established international level (Ericsson 2008). Deliberate practice describes the planned, purposeful repetition of all the aspects of a task to improve the individual's performance beyond their current level. Several elements are required to uniformly improve performance including a well-defined goal, the motivation to improve, provision of constructive feedback, and the opportunity for repetition resulting in gradual refinements of performance (Ericsson 2008). As the principles of deliberate practice are closely aligned to those of mastery learning, both can be applied to task components in pursuit of competency of a clinical skill. The combination of simulation-based medical education (SBE) with deliberate practice has been shown to be superior to more traditional clinical medical educational methods in achieving specific clinical skill competency (Mcgaghie et al. 2011).

Feedback

Effective learning will not occur without the integration of constructive feedback into every educational activity (Issenberg et al. 2005). Although feedback may be defined in many ways, one that resonates with clinical education is "specific information about the comparison between a trainee's observed performance and a standard, given with the intent to improve the trainee's performance" (Ridder et al. 2008). If there is no effective feedback, therefore, the learners are not able to place themselves according to their peers nor improve their performance having been given the means to do so. It should also be remembered that there may be a mismatch between the clinical educator's and trainees' perceptions of the quality of the feedback, including both its quantity and effectiveness. Although many clinical educators believe that they provide honest feedback, trainees themselves describe this as a rare event (Ridder et al. 2008). Although there are many described different techniques for the delivery of feedback in a clinical setting, the most applied technique is the Pendleton model (Pendleton 1984) (Table 2).

Feedback is more effective when it is provided as close in time to a learning experience as possible, although it should be delayed in high-tension environments. It should also be conducted in a neutral setting, away from peers and patients, with sufficient time and minimal chance of interruption. The time that is devoted to giving feedback is dependent on the individual learner, the points that need to be discussed and the current educational relationship. In the pediatric setting, the R2C2 model for effective feedback and coaching is highly effective and may supplement enhance the process (Sargeant et al. 2015; Atkinson et al. 2021) (Table 3).

Assessment

> *The candidate shall appear in the morning at the Royal Infirmary, and shall have a case submitted to him, for the examination of which one hour will be allowed....*
> *At four o'clock of the same day he shall appear for oral examination, which will last one hour, and shall be conducted by two examiners ...*
> *Royal College of Physicians Edinburgh, 1881 (*Royal College of Physicians of Edinburgh 2021*)*

Many training programs internationally are moving to workplace-based assessments.

Clinical examinations for doctors in specialist training have a long tradition. Today's specialist trainee "long case" examination, whereby a candidate sees a patient unknown to them for a clinical assessment and subsequently presents and discusses the case with examiners, is recognizable in the 1881 Royal College of Physicians of Edinburgh's exams (Royal College of Physicians of Edinburgh 2021), subsequently adopted by Glasgow and London counterparts (Fleming et al. 1974). From 1894 passing one of these examinations gave candidates a shared certificate of completion from the Royal Colleges of Physicians (UK). This clinical examination format and structure have evolved only a little over time and is found internationally in many specialties.

Table 2 Pendleton's framework for feedback (Pendleton 1984)

Pendleton's framework for feedback [Pendleton]
1. The learner describes what they think went well in the activity
2. The supervisor adds their observations of the positive aspects of performance and reinforces those already identified by the learner
3. The learner describes what could be improved next time and how this might be achieved
4. The supervisor adds recommendations for improvement and helps the learner identify learning opportunities

Table 3 The R2C2 model of effective feedback and coaching (Sargeant et al. 2015)

The R2C2 model for effective feedback and coaching
R: Build rapport with the trainee
R: Explore reactions to feedback
C: Explore the content of feedback by discussing what went well and what can be improved
C: Coach for change: Discuss how the learner can grow in skills and competence

With reference to Miller's classic pyramid, the clinical examination tests candidates' ability to "show how" they perform in clinical scenarios (Miller 1990).

Clinical examinations using real patients carry high face validity. Many of the domains within the specialist college frameworks can be encountered within such clinical examinations; however, clearly central to this modality of examination are domains such as medical expertise (i.e., history and examination, synthesis, judgment), communication, quality and safety, cultural competence, ethics and professional behavior, judgment, and decision-making.

Clinical examinations have a clear educational effect, whereby assessment drives learning. They require candidates to spend enormous time in preparation, which is almost certainly of greater value to individual learning compared to feedback regarding their performance on the day.

Clinical examinations have challenges, however, perhaps especially in pediatrics, as it is difficult to ensure standardization. When testing candidates using real cases, children with even relatively common syndromes present differently, and when factoring in different ages and stages of development as well as evolution of clinical features, candidates are often tested on quite different cases. Furthermore, when organizing children for clinical examinations, cases of particular ages or with particular conditions need to be excluded as they cannot be relied upon to behave as desired to allow the candidates to demonstrate their clinical skills.

The discipline of child health is well suited to workplace-based assessments (WBAs), which are growing in prominence internationally as formative assessment tools (Norcini et al. 2011), assessing on Miller's pyramid what a candidate "does" in their clinical work (Miller 1990). If a child's mood or behavior precludes assessment, an alternative case or different time for the consultation is generally able to be found. These also have high face validity because they are generally real patient encounters.

Modalities of assessment particularly suited to pediatrics include (Norcini and McKinley 2007):

Mini-Clinical Evaluation Exercise (mini-CEX): a specific clinical skill is demonstrated, such as history taking, physical examination, or patient counselling/explanation.
Direct Observation of Procedural Skills (DOPS): a specific procedure is demonstrated, such as intravenous canulation, application of plaster
Case-Based Discussion: a case being cared for by the doctor is discussed to test their understanding of nuances of history, examination, synthesis, investigations, and treatment
Entrustable Professional Activities: a clinical supervisor makes a judgment about trainee performance and the degree of supervision they require for a given activity

These WBAs are all designed for formative assessment, but many programs are now applying them as summative tools.

Experiential Learning

Experiential learning is the acquisition of novel skills by direct encounter and experiences. The learning cycle described by Kolb includes the four phases of experience, reflection, conceptualization, and experimentation (Kolb 2014). Feedback is an essential part of this process and helps to shape the cognitive modification of performance (abstract conceptualization) before this is applied to practice. Within this framework, the trainee is required to actively engage with the clinical environment with direct observation by the supervisor. Thus, active participation is required rather than direct observation of a senior clinician's performance. This approach enhances skill acquisition, which is particularly valuable in pediatrics as child health can be a relatively minor part of undergraduate learning, and thus, clinical exposure and resultant skill development opportunities may be reduced.

Such experiences could involve:

- Learning of pediatric-specific communication (Howells et al. 2006) and assessment (Schreiber et al. 2015) skills in general as well as skills around specific scenarios such as simulations of breaking bad news with parents (Gough et al. 2009).
- Maintaining the currency of rarely performed critical care skills (Craig et al. 2019).
- Learning about newly available investigations, especially those that may be important but used rarely (McClaren et al. 2020).

Reflective Practice

Reflective practice is the process of learning from past experiences, considering and evaluating previous knowledge regarding these experiences, and then incorporating this new knowledge considering these experiences (Jasper et al. 2013). In SBE activities debriefing is designed to promote reflection and is a crucial educational aspect. Although there is an evolving evidence base for the use of reflective practice, Gibbs's reflective cycle is an important aspect (Gibbs 1988) (Fig. 3).

These six stages are very closely linked to Kolb's learning cycle with the addition of the emotional dimension. The concept of reflective practice has also been incorporated into competency-based educational pediatric programs. Trainees are recommended to keep a reflective diary, which is confidential, and recommended to discuss this with their assigned educational supervisor as appropriate (Royal College of Paediatrics and Child Health 2018). Working with children with severe illness is emotionally difficult, especially for inexperienced learners. For example, reflective practice has been demonstrated to be useful for nursing students in the field of pediatric cancer care where their recorded experiences and emotions in a journal were discussed weekly with a mentor, enhancing learning and adjustment to the demands of the challenging field of practice (Mirlashari et al. 2017).

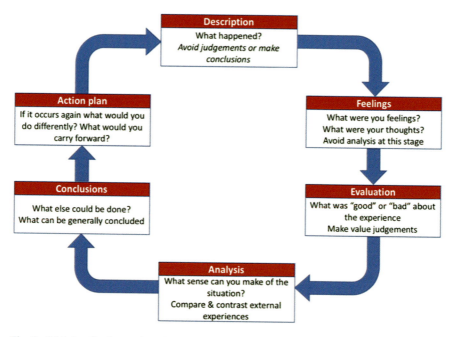

Fig. 3 Gibbs's reflective cycle (Gibb 1988)

Communities of Practice

The key basis of Communities of Practice (CoP) is that learning is a social activity, and interactions between individuals are crucial for engagement and learning. CoPs were originally described as a central element to the theory of "situated learning" (Lave and Wenger 1991). This was based on the observation that learning was more than simply acquiring knowledge as it involved a complex relationship between the novice and expert, peripheral participation in practice, becoming socialized into the practice and developing an identity within the community (Ranmuthugala et al. 2011). There are three domains that define a CoP:

1. Joint enterprise as there is a shared domain of interest and competency acquisition.
2. Mutual engagement as the activities enables collaborative learning and the development of learning partnerships.
3. A shared repertoire with the promotion of shared language, concepts, experiences, processes, practice, resources, and other educational tools.

CoPs can be important for learning in any discipline, but particularly in pediatrics where practice requires specific learning elements as well as enculturation into a style of practice. Special societies within nursing, allied health, and medical fields

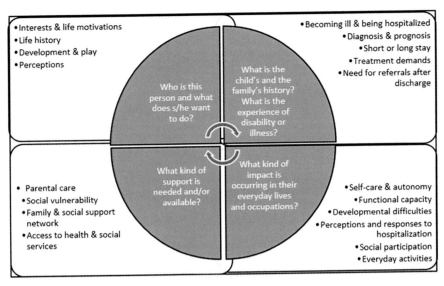

Fig. 4 A model of pediatric occupational practice derived from a community of pediatric occupational therapy in Brazil (from Galheigo et al. 2017)

pertaining to child health are important, as well as others that incorporate membership from all health disciplines, such as the Australasian Academy of Child and Adolescent Health.

Figure 4 demonstrates learning from research, which explicitly tapped into a community of practice within a pediatric occupational therapy community in Brazil (Galheigo et al. 2017). Such interesting methods can make visible and explicit practice-based knowledge, which can then become accessible to others in similar work environments.

Simulation-Based Education

The rapid evolution in healthcare education in the last few decades has been driven by changes such as the reduction in working hours, introduction of competency-based training programs and an increasing awareness of patient safety (Nataraja et al. 2018a). Simulation is one educational modality that has been incorporated into many training programs to improve their effectiveness within these constraints. Simulation-based education (SBE) as defined by Gaba is a "technique, not a technology, to replace or amplify real experiences with guided experiences that evoke or replicate substantial aspects of the real world in a fully interactive manner" (Issenberg et al. 2005). SBE allows the learner to acquire new skills, utilize techniques such as deliberate practice, and develop non-technical skills in an environment which is safe with its inherent patient safety implications. SBE incorporates many different educational modalities including part task trainers, bench trainers, mannequins with scenario-based simulation, virtual reality trainers, simulated patients, roleplay, hybrid simulation, and virtual or online simulation (Nataraja et al. 2018b). Simulation can be used to teach cognitive, psychomotor, and affective skills to either an individual or a team (Motola et al. 2013a). One of the most established simulation-based educational courses, Advanced Paediatric Life Support (APLS)™ is a requirement of many pediatric training programs. In Australia and the UK, all trainees must complete this at the commencement of the training program and ensure they hold current accreditation. Many of the other forms of SBE will be familiar to established educators such as the use of simulated patients for teaching complex communication skills, such as breaking bad news and issues surrounding obtaining consent, which are discussed in the relevant sections below. The terms technical and non-technical skills (NTS) are often used in simulation although in practice these skills are often fully integrated in delivering optimal clinical care. Most critical adverse events in a clinical setting occur after a failing of an NTS such as communication, situation awareness, or leadership. The terminology of NTS has also been challenged recently, and many medical educationalists prefer the term clinical cognitive skills.

Types of Bench Trainer Simulators

Simulation applied to teach psychomotor skills is one of its most recognizable educational forms and usually takes the form of a part-task, task, or bench trainer. These simulators are defined as whether the whole psychomotor skill or part of it can be taught. Examples include mannequins for basic or advanced pediatric life support, intubation simulators with increasing levels of complexity, lumbar puncture simulators, and stoma care with umbilical vascular access (Fig. 5). Some of these such as the Gaumard Advanced Newborn Care Simulator (Fig. 5A) have multiple functions depending on the educational requirements of the SBE session. These include training arm for intravenous access, external stoma sites, umbilical catheterization, temporal venous access, and male or female urinary catheterization. Many of these also have replaceable components after repeated use (Fig. 5B).

These simulators allow deliberate practice of a skill in a controlled safe environment until competency is achieved, which is dependent on regular constructive feedback. This can also occur in an environment without other potential external stressors to the learner such as the patient's parents. The use of deliberate practice in an SBE environment is highly applicable to pediatrics as this minimizes the patient's exposure to part of the trainee's learning curve. Although patient safety is at the core of this practice, there are also other considerations with children a decreased margin for error. An example of this is the placement of an ultrasound-guided percutaneous central line into the internal jugular vein. If performed incorrectly, the resultant hematoma can render subsequent venous access on that site impossible.

The SBE environment also enables the learner to experiment in technique without any direct patient safety implementations. Often there are different technique

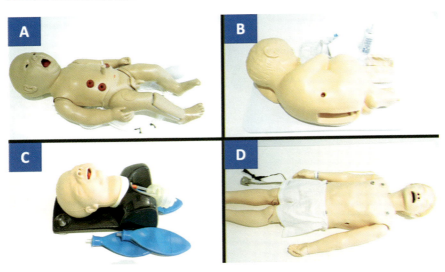

Fig. 5 Examples of pediatric simulators: (**a**) Newborn Advanced Care (Gaumard®, United States), (**b**) Paediatric Lumbar Puncture Simulator (Life/Form®, United States), (**c**) Pierre Robin AirSim Head (TruCorp®, Ireland), (**d**) Sim Junior (Laerdal®, Norway)

variations, all of which achieve a good clinical result, and this controlled safe environment allows the learner to ascertain which resonates with them the most.

Fidelity, Realism, and Educational Engagement

Traditionally, there has been a focus on the visual realism of simulators and a perception that if it does not appear exactly as the intended clinical situation, it is not educationally worthwhile. With a greater acceptance of the value of SBE, there has, however, been a shift in assessing simulators according to their fidelity and whether they confer the intended skills (Dieckmann et al. 2007). The question of the educational purpose of the SBE activity is crucial, so the conceptual and experiential fidelity is much more important than the physical fidelity. Traditionally, "high fidelity" mannequins included those with high technology, and although these often do translate into an effective activity, their presence does not guarantee it. When a simulator is chosen for an educational activity, the learning outcomes should determine which one is used rather than the physical appearance or the level of technology. Often this educational process is reversed in training programs with the acquisition of a high-technology simulator such as Sim Junior (Laerdal®, Norway), and then the activities are chosen according to its capabilities. This does not decrease the educational value of these high-technology simulators, but their use should be aligned with the individualized intended learning objectives of the session. This has also been highlighted by the shift in the perception of fidelity with simulators now being assessed with the lens of their functional task alignment rather than their conceptual, experiential, or physical fidelity (Hamstra et al. 2014).

Scenario-Based Simulation

Scenario-based simulation is one of the most recognizable forms of SBE as it forms the core the Advanced Paediatric Life Support (APLS©) course. In the APLS course, varying degrees of complexity emergency resuscitation scenarios are used both in the education and in the assessment of the participants. Although these are used for the acquisition of primarily psychomotor skills, it can be used for the development of non-procedural skills such as communication skills, situational awareness, expert judgment, decision-making skills, and cognitive task analysis (Dieckmann et al. 2007). Scenarios should be carefully designed; their timeline of crucial steps and clinical observation variations should be valid and believable for the participants. Scenario-based learning is also frequently combined with video debriefing, and this should be conducted by adequately trained facilitators to ensure effective and safe outcomes (Rudolph et al. 2014). The integration of feedback to promote reflection is vital as with any SBE activity. Although many of these learning activities occur in a purpose-built simulation center, they may also occur in situ within the pediatric clinical ward environment. These can involve pediatric mock codes and allow enriched learning activities in the trainee's own work environments. The acquisition of non-technical skills in SBE team-based training can potentially improve patient outcome, although the evidence base for this is still being established.

Simulated Patients and Roleplay

Simulated patients (SPs) are becoming an integral part of many aspects of medical education (Cleland et al. 2009; Nestel and Bearman 2014). This has been driven by the need to enhance non-technical skills such as communication and patient-contact skills. The most significant application of SPs has been in summative assessments such as OSCEs (Objective Standardized Clinical Examinations). This role was often performed by a relative or another facilitator on the course, but SPs are highly trained to represent patients or their relatives in SBE. This involves detailed role descriptions, ensuring that "patient" responses are standardized (Cleland et al. 2009). In pediatrics, they are often utilized as the parents of a child rather than a pediatric SP themselves being used, as there are various ethical concerns over their direct use in SBE (Nestel et al. 2020), including the limitations to differentiation between reality and play, emotional responses, reproducibility of reactions, and their psychological safety (Nestel et al. 2020). These concerns may also be countered with the use of emerging technologies such as virtual reality (VR). Virtual patients would allow the standardization of the interaction with a pediatric patient while ensuring the psychological safety of the child (Quail and Boyle 2019). VR has been successfully applied in pediatrics for venous canulation as a distraction technique (Goldman and Behboudi 2021; Caruso et al. 2020), and so these emerging technologies should be harnessed to enhance both clinical care and education.

Integration of SBE into a Curriculum

From a perspective of a training program, the effectiveness of SBE is the result of three interlinked components: training resources, trained educators, and curricular institutionalization (Issenberg 2006). This has occurred in many training programs including pediatrics regarding the availability of simulators, task trainers, simulated patients, and trained educators. However, the integration of SBE in the formal curriculum is still ongoing in various international pediatric training programs. Often when this does occur, it complements an existing program or curriculum rather than being fully integrated. The ideal framework for the integration of simulation involves a redesign of the curriculum with its expected outcomes, identification of outcomes better addressed with simulation, and then content development for the SBE activities, faculty training, and support mechanisms (Motola et al. 2013b). This involves constant evaluation and revision. SBE is not just an additional aspect of the curriculum as it becomes it wherever it is appropriate. The integration of SBE into training programs early will allow practitioners to continue to use it as an integral part of their careers moving forward. This is essential in a discipline such as pediatrics with the unique challenges as discussed above.

Supported Returns to Training

There are many reasons why there may be a prolonged absence from work in the pediatric setting including carer responsibilities, research time, long-term illness, or time spent abroad with an out-of-program experience. A significant proportion of pediatric trainees taking time out of postgraduate training will want to return on a less than full-time basis, lengthening training, although formal support for this is variable (Gordon et al. 2008). Career breaks and interruptions are circumstances in which trainees may either exit the training or hold its progress. In an ideal world, a trainee would re-join training and continue to make progress without a delay to their training or other adverse consequences. These training gaps are, however, combined with external pressures, which also reduce clinical environment exposure, such as the new Junior Doctors contract (2016) in the United Kingdom, which further limited working hours for trainees. A recent survey has shown that 96% of trainees experience an initial lack of confidence on returning to clinical practice (van Boxel et al. 2020). In the UK, Health Education England has reviewed and released guidelines on trainees' reintegration into the workplace after a prolonged absence (Health Education England (NHS) 2017) following an increased recognition that support is required for trainees returning to training (UK General Medical Council 2015). Postgraduate training is time constrained and demanding, with compulsory assessments or competencies (Royal College of Anaesthetists 2018). As trainees return to a time limited period, some of this time may be lost reintegrating and thus have an impact on their eventual ability to progress to the end of their training successfully. It is also the case that some key skills might have suffered from "fade" meaning that trainees are re-joining clinical practice with some loss of skills because of time away from clinical work (UK General Medical Council 2015). In the UK, the impact of such absences and the need for supportive reintegration strategies were highlighted in a high-profile case, in which a child died in the care of a doctor who had recently returned from 13 months parental leave (Royal Courts of Justice 2013).

This is not only limited to the medical workforce as gender imbalances in the wider healthcare professional workforce has also significantly changed in the last few decades (ALobaid AM, Gosling C, Khasawneh E, McKenna L, Williams B. 2020). A recent scoping review findings confirm that women healthcare professionals face circumstances that may affect their family lives, as well as factors relating to the workplace environment and stereotypes (ALobaid AM, Gosling C, Khasawneh E, McKenna L, Williams B. 2020). Implementing strategies such as reduced work hours, flexible timing, and part-time work can support women in the workplace, which then enhances and supports gender equality in healthcare organizations.

Prior to the Academy of Medical Royal Colleges (AoMRC) publication in 2012 (Academy of Medical Royal Colleges 2017), there was minimal literature on returning to clinical training after an absence. This AoMRC publication occurred as during the development of revalidation for doctors in the United Kingdom, significant concerns regarding the lack of guidance for doctor's returning to practice after a period of absence were revealed. Fears of returning to work have previously been voiced, and the expectation to return at the same level, as if the absence had not occurred, is known (Brightwell et al. 2013). The actual experience of returning to clinical work in pediatrics after a prolonged absence remains undocumented in published literature, although there has been some research in the context of pediatric surgery (Nash et al. 2018). In this context, there are increasing efforts to design and implement structures to facilitate a smooth transition back into the clinical environment. An example being the London School of Paediatrics offering a targeted course to help returning trainees reintegrate into the acute clinical environment (London School of Paediatrics 2019). This course offers pediatric SBE activities, key updates in pediatrics, as well as workshops addressing issues around flexible training, completing workplace-based assessments and the curriculum. This course also offers a resilience workshop supported by psychology and the opportunity to develop networks with other trainees who are in similar situations. Coaching sessions are also available. These are supported by Health Education England, which has appointed a Training Program Director for returns to practice. Resources are also increasingly being made available for educational supervisors to support trainees in this transitional phase. With an increasing demand for flexible working arrangements within Child Health, the ability of the educational system to support different models and durations of training will be key to the future health of pediatrics as a specialty.

Ethics in Pediatrics

Provision of clinical care for children raises unique ethical issues. There is usually a third party involved – the parent or the guardian (hereafter the term "parent" is taken to incorporate a second parent or non-parental guardian). With decreasing age, the parent is increasingly responsible for decision-making on behalf of the child. Parents are generally but not always in the best position to act in the best interests of the child.

Clinical Ethics Committees

A clinical ethics committee (CEC) is a reference group of clinicians trained in ethical decision-making, best constituted by a broad range of disciplines and seniorities. It is generally advisory rather than determinative. The authors' experience is that junior practitioners even as students have much to contribute as well as learn from participation. Seeking the views of CECs is increasingly common, especially around provision of pediatric care.

Most cases referred to CECs are around decision-making about appropriate care, where parents disagree with clinician views about appropriate care or where parents disagree with each other (i.e., best interests, benefits versus harms) (McDougall and Notini 2016; Nathanson et al. 2020). Other prominent issues include withdrawal or refusal of life-sustaining treatments including blood products and the use of complementary and alternative therapies (i.e., autonomy and decision-making) (McDougall and Notini 2014).

Best Interests

Consideration of a child's best interests limits the autonomy and authority of parents to make decisions on behalf of their child. It is a contested ethico-legal standard, which goes beyond a paternalistic approach of determining the best possible objective medical decision for a child. Rather, it incorporates shared decision-making, including views of parent and child, in addition to the usual ethical decision-making concepts (Streuli et al. 2021).

Capacity and Consent

One of the challenges for a clinician who looks after children is the movement of the patients through distinct stages during which their capacity to make decisions about their own lives and clinical care develop. Kenny and Grub described child development in terms of capacity in three distinct stages (Grubb et al. 2010). The first is that of a young child, who is completely reliant on an adult for consent. A young person of 16–17 years of age, by contrast, would normally be regarded as being able to consent as if there were an adult. Between these two stages is that of a competent child under the age of 16 years. UK case law has been accepted internationally as defining the standard for capacity of a child under 16 years to consent to medical treatment. The landmark decision coined the term "Gillick Competence" based on a 1986 case in which Mrs. Gillick contested the right of her General Practitioner to offer contraceptive advice to her daughter without her express knowledge or consent (Griffith 2016). The judgment in this case held that the child could consent for her own medical treatment if she had sufficient maturity and understanding to be able to weigh the risks and benefits of the treatment and to consider the longer-term effects of the treatment such as those on family life. It should be noted that Gillick competence is situation specific, and it requires significantly more decision-making maturity to consider a significant intervention such as a bone marrow transplant than it would to consent to the placement of a dressing on a minor wound. Before obtaining consent from a child on this basis, therefore, the treating clinicians must be satisfied that they meet the threshold of competence outlined in Gillick in the given clinical situation. While the Law in different countries treats the emerging competence of a child in slightly different ways, it remains an important principle, enshrined in the United Nations Convention on the Rights of the Child, that the evolving capacity of children must be respected by those involved in their healthcare (United Nations 2009).

There are other important case law decisions regarding consent and decision-making. These include Marion's case, whereby in 1993 a parent's request for a hysterectomy of their child with an intellectual disability was refused, as it was held that the child still had some decision-making capacity, which needed to be respected (McSherry and Waddington 2017).

There are numerous examples of cases where courts have denied permission for Jehovah's Witness parents to refuse blood transfusions for their children in many countries (Sagy et al. 2017). In Australia, in 2013, a court denied permission for a 17-year-old Jehovah's Witness to refuse lifesaving treatment for himself (Appeals Court of New South Wales 2013). The interesting thing about this case is that the 17-year old would have been able to consent to treatment but was not allowed to refuse it.

These examples demonstrate that the pediatric workforce faces ethical challenges and has learning needs not faced by practitioners dealing with adult patients.

Consent, Assent, and Disclosure to Children

Learners new to the field of child and adolescent health will find the concept of consent even more complex than just knowing who can and cannot give informed consent. Ability to consent is not a binary distinction, in which children either do or do not have capacity to consent, and is generally considered a spectrum, moving from limited to full capacity to agree to treatments at any age. This becomes particularly difficult when parents and treating clinicians have differing views about what constitutes a reasonable level of disclosure to a child about their illness and treatment. An American Academy of Pediatrics (AAP) position paper of 1995 and its revision in 2016 describe that "patients should participate in decision-making commensurate with their development; they should provide assent to care whenever reasonable" (Katz et al. 2016).

The AAP position is helpful. Disclosure respects and promotes involvement in decision making (Bartholome 1995), giving the child or young person a voice in their care. Disclosure also promotes involvement in the therapeutic relationship by the child and, as such, is likely to avoid restriction of future autonomy (Herbert and Dahlquist 2008), in that the child or young person will develop a voice within decisions about their care as they develop capacity. It is also the case that involvement of the child in discussions about their care demonstrates respect for them as a person (Bartholome 1995), as well as respecting the principles of truthfulness and fidelity. Finally, disclosure improves well-being (Dalton et al. 2019), so has a direct therapeutic implication for the child or young person. Conversely, avoidance of disclosure may lead to negative feelings of abandonment/unlovedness even in very young children.

Child Protection

Children are sometimes harmed by their carers or other adults. It is only since the 1960s that the child protection agenda has been a part of the pediatric health professional landscape (Fegert and Stötzel 2016).

Child abuse is an action by another person which causes significant harm to a child. This may take the form of active physical, sexual, or emotional harm but can also take the form of neglect or the withholding of love, care, and attention. In some jurisdictions, health professionals may be mandated to report reasonable suspicions of child abuse to responsible authorities such as the police or a child protection agency; in other jurisdictions, such a mandate falls on others such as education professionals or even any adult (Bath et al. 2010).

The threshold for state intervention to override parent rights as decision-makers for their child is generally around imminence and severity of harm. This dates to early publications in this field, which took the view that parents' rights to make decisions would be overturned only if it can be shown that no responsible mode of thinking warrants such treatment of a child (Schoeman 1985). With a high threshold for state intervention, it can be challenging for health professionals when they believe parent decision-making or behaviors with respect to a child are significantly suboptimal but are below the seriousness and imminence of harm threshold (McDougall and Notini 2014).

Pediatric education must equip learners to recognize acts of commission and neglect, and to know their reporting obligations. Such training is a requirement for healthcare professionals involved in caring for children and young people in many jurisdictions.

Interactions with Parents

Looking after children means that healthcare professionals are often faced with a child accompanied by an adult decision-maker. Medical care of the child therefore also demands care of their care givers and the ability to liaise with them in a way that leads to effective and collaborative decision-making. Unlike in adult practice, even children managed in intensive care environments have a cognitively able decision-maker acting as that advocate.

The ability of parents to make decisions on behalf of a child is restricted. For example, in the UK context, it is illegal for anyone under the age of 18 years to have a tattoo whether their parents consent to it or not (Government of the United Kingdom 1969). In most cases, skilled clinical teams can come to a consensus with a child's parents about the best way forward for their care. There are occasions, however, where the parent's views and those of the treating clinical team are different and not reconcilable. This may require these differences of opinion to be resolved in court. There have been recent legal cases in the United Kingdom where dispute has arisen around the issue of end-of-life decision-making, which have prominently shown difficulties associated with these situations (Royal Courts of Justice 2021).

In the educational context, it is important to remember that demands placed upon healthcare professionals dealing with children and families in situations in which the best course of action is disputed. Effective care for a child and family where such complex decisions are being made requires different both a high level of clinical knowledge and skill, and the ability to understand the issues, and argue from, an ethical and moral perspective. There is an increasing recognition of the demands placed on healthcare staff who are faced with delivering treatment for children where they do not feel this is in their best interests, or where there is parental refusal of this treatment (Kälvemark et al. 2004; Wocial and Weaver 2013). The difficulty caused by these situations is sometimes characterized as moral distress, which may be said to be the experience of "believing one knows the ethically correct thing to do, but something or someone prevents the individual from acting." This may occur when a person perceives the right course of action cannot be implemented because of institutional constraints. The ability to manage children in the context of moral uncertainty is part of being a professional (Huffman and Rittenmeyer 2012). It is arguable, however, that these situations occur frequently enough in pediatrics that staff need a framework of moral reasoning and ethical principles, as well as the ability to apply them to clinical situations such that they can make and understand the decisions pertaining to the care of the children for whom they have responsibility.

Part of the education of professionals in pediatric healthcare must, therefore, allow the discussion and education about these issues. In areas where these difficulties are common, the involvement of clinical ethicists has been shown to directly affect patient outcome by reducing length of PICU stay and by reducing moral distress in staff (Wocial and Weaver 2013).

Conclusion

In this chapter we have described some of the issues and challenges in learning and teaching in pediatrics. As for any postgraduate specialty, all the educational activities should be prepared with the learning objectives of the learner in mind and using the established educational theories behind them. Simulation is a technique, not a technology, and as for any other educational tool, should be used appropriately. The training programs differ internationally, but many of the key principles are the same as the characteristics of the trainees that they attract. Return to practice is an area that should be further refined in pediatrics as it has more of an impact than in many other specialties. There are also complex ethical issues that are unique to pediatrics, and the emergence of novel techniques, such as virtual reality, should be embraced in the education of this difficult area. First and foremost, the rights and optimal clinical outcomes of pediatric patients and their caregivers should be the primary driver in the design of educational programs.

Cross-References

▶ Focus on Selection Methods: Evidence and Practice
▶ Focus on Theory: Emotions and Learning

References

Academy of Medical Royal Colleges. Return to Practice Guidance 2017 Revision. 2017. published online June 15. http://www.aomrc.org.uk/wp-content/uploads/2017/06/Return_to_Practice_guidance_2017_Revison_0617-2.pdf.

Alobaid AM, Gosling C, Khasawneh E, McKenna L, Williams B. Challenges faced by female healthcare professionals in the workforce: a scoping review. J Multidiscip Healthc. 2020;13: 681–91.

Appeals Court of New South Wales. X v The Sydney Children's Hospitals Network. 2013. https://jwleaks.files.wordpress.com/2012/07/x-jehovahs-witness-child-v-the-sydney-childrens-hospitals-network-2013-nswca-320-27-september-2013.pdf.

Atkinson A, Watling CJ, Brand PLP. Feedback and coaching. Eur J Pediatr. 2021;2021:1–6.

Australian College of Nursing. Graduate Certificate in Child and Family Health Nursing. 2021. published online June 3. https://www.acn.edu.au/education/postgraduate-course/child-and-family-health-nursing#structure-fees. Accessed 3 June 2021.

Australian Institute of Health & Welfare. Aboriginal and Torres Strait Islander Health Performance Framework 2017 report: Northern Territory (Full Publication 13 nov 2017 edition) (AIHW). 2017; published online Nov 13. https://www.aihw.gov.au/getmedia/0e60dc3c-a582-4b7f-a4d1-1e623a91745e/aihw-ihw-186-2017-hpf-nt.pdf.aspx?inline=true. Accessed 2AD.

Bartholome WG. Informed consent, parental permission, and assent in pediatric practice. Pediatrics. 1995;96:981–2.

Bath H, Bamblett M, Roseby R. Growing them Strong, Together: Promoting the safety and wellbeing of the Northern Territory's children. 2010, Report of the board of inquiry into the

Child Protection System in the Northern Territory 2010. Darwin, 2010. https://digitallibrary.health.nt.gov.au/prodjspui/bitstream/10137/459/1/CPS%20Report%202010.pdf.

Block JH, Airasian PW. Mastery learning: theory and practice. New York: Holt Rinehart & Winston; 1971.

Blum RWM, Garell D, Hodgman CH, et al. Transition from child-centered to adult health-care systems for adolescents with chronic conditions A position paper of the Society for Adolescent Medicine. J Adolescent Health. 1993;14:570–6.

van Boxel E, Mawson I, Dawkins S, Duncan S, van Boxel G. Predicting risk of underconfidence following maternity leave. Arch Dis Child. 2020;105:1108–10.

Brenner M, Begley T. Children's nursing in Ireland: opportunities and challenges. Compr Child Adolesc Nurs. 2019;42:90–1.

Brightwell A, Minson S, Ward A, Fertleman C. Returning to clinical training after maternity leave. BMJ (Clinical research ed). 2013;347:f5965.

Brosco JP. The early history of the infant mortality rate in America: "A reflection upon the past and a prophecy of the future"1. Pediatrics. 1999;103:478–85.

Caruso TJ, George A, Menendez M, et al. Virtual reality during pediatric vascular access: A pragmatic, prospective randomized, controlled trial. Pediatr Anesth. 2020;30:116–23.

Cleland JA, Abe K, Rethans J-J. The use of simulated patients in medical education: AMEE guide no 42. Med Teach. 2009;31:477–86.

Coles MS, Greenberg KB. The time is here: A comprehensive curriculum for adolescent health teaching and learning from the Society for Adolescent Health and Medicine. J Adolesc Health. 2017;61:129–30.

Cooper MA, McDowell J, Raeside L, ANP-CNS Group. The similarities and differences between advanced nurse practitioners and clinical nurse specialists. Br J Nurs. 2019;28:1308–14.

Craig SS, Auerbach M, Cheek JA, et al. Preferred learning modalities and practice for critical skills: a global survey of paediatric emergency medicine clinicians. Emerg Med J. 2019;36:273.

Dalton L, Rapa E, Ziebland S, et al. Communication with children and adolescents about the diagnosis of a life-threatening condition in their parent. Lancet. 2019;393:1164–76.

Deprest J, Coppi PD. Antenatal management of isolated congenital diaphragmatic hernia today and tomorrow: ongoing collaborative research and development. Journal of Pediatric Surgery Lecture Journal of Pediatric Surgery Lecture. 2012;47:282–90.

Dieckmann P, Gaba D, Rall M. Deepening the theoretical foundations of patient simulation as social practice. Simul Healthc J Soc Simul Healthc. 2007;2:183–93.

Ericsson KA. Deliberate practice and the acquisition and maintenance of expert performance in medicine and related domains. Acad Med. 2004;79:S70.

Ericsson KA. Deliberate practice and acquisition of expert performance: a general overview. Acad Emerg Med Off J Soc Acad Emerg Med. 2008;15:988–94.

Fegert JM, Stötzel M. Child protection: a universal concern and a permanent challenge in the field of child and adolescent mental health. Child Adol Psych Men. 2016;10:18.

Fleming PR, Manderson WG, Matthews MB, Sanderson PH, Stokes JF. Evolution of an examination: M.R.C.P. Brit Med J. 1974;2:99.

Galheigo SM, Braga CP, Mieto FSR, et al. Exchanging knowledge within a community of practice: toward an epistemology of practice in occupational therapy paediatric hospital care. Cadernos Brasileiros De Terapia Ocupacional. 2017;25:449–59.

Gibb G. Learning by doing: A guide to teaching and learning methods Oxford. Further Education Unit; 1988.

Gibbs G. Learning by doing. Further Education Unit; 1988.

Goddard AF. Consultant physicians for the future: report from a working party of the Royal College of Physicians and the medical specialties. Clin Med. 2010;10:548–54.

Goldman RD, Behboudi A. Virtual reality for intravenous placement in the emergency department—a randomized controlled trial. Eur J Pediatr. 2021;180:725–31.

Gordon MB, McGuinness GA, Stanton BF, et al. Part-time training in pediatric residency programs: principles and practices. Pediatrics. 2008;122:e938–44.

Gough JK, Frydenberg AR, Donath SK, Marks MM. Simulated parents: developing paediatric trainees' skills in giving bad news. J Paediatr Child H. 2009;45:133–8.

Government of the United Kingdom. Tattooing of Minors Act 1969, c24. Tattooing of Minors Act 1969. n.d.. https://www.legislation.gov.uk/ukpga/1969/24/contents. Accessed 3 June 2021.

Gray WN, Schaefer MR, Resmini-Rawlinson A, Wagoner ST. Barriers to transition from pediatric to adult care: A systematic review. J Pediatr Psychol. 2017;43:488–502.

Griffith R. What is Gillick competence? Hum Vacc Immunother. 2016;12:244–7.

Grubb A, Laing J, McHale J, Kennedy I. Principles of medical law. Oxford: Oxford University Press; 2010.

Hamstra SJ, Brydges R, Hatala R, Zendejas B, Cook DA. Reconsidering Fidelity in simulation-based training. Acad Med. 2014;89:387–92.

Happell BM. "Love is all you need"? Student nurses' interest in working with children. J Spec Pediatr Nurs. 2000;5:167–73.

Health Education England (NHS). Supported Return to Training. 2017. published online Dec 7. https://www.hee.nhs.uk/sites/default/files/documents/Supported%20Return%20to%20Training.pdf. Accessed 2AD.

Herbert LJ, Dahlquist LM. Perceived history of anaphylaxis and parental overprotection, autonomy, anxiety, and depression in food allergic young adults. J Clin Psychol Med Settings. 2008;15:261–9.

Hong Kong College of Paediatric Nursing. 2021; published online June 3. http://hkcpn.com/training_curriculum.asp. Accessed 3 June 2021.

Howells RJ, Davies HA, Silverman JD. Teaching and learning consultation skills for paediatric practice. Arch Dis Child. 2006;91:367.

Huffman DM, Rittenmeyer L. How professional nurses working in hospital environments experience moral distress: A systematic review. Crit Care Nurs Clin North Am. 2012;24:91–100.

Issenberg SB. The scope of simulation-based healthcare education. Simulation in Healthcare: The Journal of the Society for Simulation in Healthcare. 2006;1:203–8.

Issenberg SB, Mcgaghie WC, Petrusa ER, Gordon DL, Scalese RJ. Features and uses of high-fidelity medical simulations that lead to effective learning: a BEME systematic review*. Med Teach. 2005;27:10–28.

Jasper M, Rosser M, Mooney G. Professional development, reflection and decision-making in nursing and healthcare. Chichester: John Wiley & Sons; 2013.

Kälvemark S, Höglund AT, Hansson MG, Westerholm P, Arnetz B. Living with conflicts-ethical dilemmas and moral distress in the health care system. Soc Sci Med. 2004;58:1075–84.

Katz AL, Webb SA, BIOETHICS CO. Informed consent in decision-making in pediatric practice. Pediatrics. 2016;138:e20161485.

Klaber RE, Lumsden DE, Kingdon C. Shape of training: the right people with the right skills in the right place. Arch Dis Child. 2015;100:119–20.

Kolb DA. Experiential learning. San Francisco: FT Press; 2014.

Lave J, Wenger E. Situated learning. Cambridge University Press; 1991.

London School of Paediatrics. Returning to clinical practice. 2019; published online July 29. https://londonpaediatrics.co.uk/current-trainees/returning-to-clinical-practice/. Accessed 2AD.

Macnab A, Martin J, Duffy D, Murray G. Measurement of how well a paediatric training programme prepares graduates for their chosen career paths. Med Educ. 1998;32:362–6.

McClaren BJ, Crellin E, Janinski M, et al. Preparing medical specialists for genomic medicine: continuing education should include opportunities for experiential learning. Frontiers Genetics. 2020;11:151.

McDougall RJ, Notini L. Overriding parents' medical decisions for their children: a systematic review of normative literature. J Med Ethics. 2014;40:448.

McDougall RJ, Notini L. What kinds of cases do paediatricians refer to clinical ethics? Insights from 184 case referrals at an Australian paediatric hospital. J Med Ethics. 2016;42:586.

Mcgaghie WC, Issenberg SB, Cohen ER, Barsuk JH, Wayne DB. Does simulation-based medical education with deliberate practice yield better results than traditional clinical education? A meta-analytic comparative review of the evidence. Academic Medicine: Journal of the Association of American Medical Colleges. 2011;86:706–11.

McKenna L, McCall L, Wray N. Clinical placements and nursing students' career planning: A qualitative exploration. Int J Nurs Pract. 2010;16:176–82.

McSherry B, Waddington L. Treat with care: the right to informed consent for medical treatment of persons with mental impairments in Australia. Australian J Hum Rights. 2017;23:109–29.

Miller GE. The assessment of clinical skills/competence/performance. Acad Med. 1990;65:S63–7.

Mirlashari J, Warnock F, Jahanbani J. The experiences of undergraduate nursing students and self-reflective accounts of first clinical rotation in pediatric oncology. Nurse Educ Pract. 2017;25: 22–8.

Mitchell L, Stuart-McEwan T, Panet H, Gupta A. Adolescents and young adults: addressing needs and optimizing care with a clinical nurse specialist. Clin J Oncol Nurs. 2017;21:123–6.

Motola I, Devine LA, Chung HS, Sullivan JE, Issenberg SB. Simulation in healthcare education: A best evidence practical guide. AMEE guide no. 82. Med Teach. 2013a;35:e1511–30.

Motola I, Devine LA, Chung HS, Sullivan JE, Issenberg SB. Simulation in healthcare education: A best evidence practical guide. AMEE guide no. 82. Med Teach. 2013b;35:e1511–30.

Myrhaug HT, Brurberg KG, Hov L, Markestad T. Survival and impairment of extremely premature infants: A meta-analysis. Pediatrics. 2019;143:e20180933.

Nash E, Curry J, Blackburn S. Returning to the theatre after an interval. Bulletin Royal Coll Surg Engl. 2018;100:277–81.

Nataraja RM, Webb N, Lopez PJ. Simulation in paediatric urology and surgery, part 2: an overview of simulation modalities and their applications. J Pediatr Urol. 2018b;14:125–31.

Nataraja RM, Webb N, Lopez P-J. Simulation in paediatric urology and surgery. Part 1: an overview of educational theory. J Pediatr Urol. 2018a;14:120–4.

Nathanson PG, Walter JK, McKlindon DD, Feudtner C. Relational, emotional, and pragmatic attributes of ethics consultations at a Children's hospital. Pediatrics. 2020;147:e20201087.

National Institute for Health and Care Excellence (NICE). Transition from children's to adults' services for young people using health or social care services. 2019; published online July 29. https://www.nice.org.uk/guidance/ng43. Accessed 2AD.

Nestel D, Bearman M. Simulated patient methodology. Chichester: John Wiley & Sons; 2014. https://doi.org/10.1002/9781118760673.

Nestel D, Ljuhar D, A G. Simulated participant methodology in paediatric surgical training: exploring contemporary practices. Semin Pediatr Surg. 2020;29:150907.

Newall F, Khair K. Research engagement in pediatric nursing practice: career pathways are the biggest barrier. J Pediatr. 2020;221:S62–3.

Newton DA, Grayson MS, Thompson LF. Money, lifestyle, or values? Why medical students choose subspecialty versus general pediatric careers. Clin Pediatr. 2010;49:116–22.

Norcini J, Anderson B, Bollela V, et al. Criteria for good assessment: consensus statement and recommendations from the Ottawa 2010 conference. Med Teach. 2011;33:206–14.

Norcini JJ, McKinley DW. Assessment methods in medical education. Teach Teach Educ. 2007;23: 239–50.

Oepkes D, Haak M. Extracardiac malformations: associations and importance: consequences for perinatal management of foetal cardiac patients. Cardiol Young. 2014;24:55–9.

Pendleton D. The consultation: an approach to learning and teaching. Oxford: Oxford University Press; 1984. https://books.google.com.au/books?id=njRrAAAAMAAJ

Quail NPA, Boyle JG. Virtual patients in health professions education. Adv Exp Med Biol. 2019;1171:25–35.

Rangroo V. The evolution of paediatrics from archaeological times to the mid-nineteenth century and the historical influence on present day practice. Acta paediatr. 1992;2008(97):677–83.

Ranmuthugala G, Plumb JJ, Cunningham FC, Georgiou A, Westbrook JI, Braithwaite J. How and why are communities of practice established in the healthcare sector? A systematic review of the literature. BMC Health Serv Res. 2011;11:273.

Resnick MD, Catalano RF, Sawyer SM, Viner R, Patton GC. Seizing the opportunities of adolescent health. Lancet. 2012;379:1564–7.

Ridder JMMVD, Stokking KM, Mcgaghie WC, Cate OTJT. What is feedback in clinical education? Med Educ. 2008;42:189–97.

Roseby R. Communication: as easy as child's play. J Paediatr Child Health. 2018;54:939–40.

Royal Australian College of Physicians Professional Practice Framework. 2017; published online July 25. https://www.racp.edu.au/fellows/professional-practice-framework.

Royal College of Anaesthetists. Returning to work after a period of absence. 2018; published online April 3. https://www.rcoa.ac.uk/system/files/ReturnToWork2015.pdf (accessed 2AD).

Royal College of Nursing (United Kingdom). Children and young people's nursing. 2020. https://www.rcn.org.uk/clinical-topics/children-and-young-people. Accessed 3 June 2021.

Royal College of Paediatrics and Child Health. 2018–2021 Strategy and 2018–2019 Council Identified Priorities. 2018; published online June 29. www.rcpch.ac.uk/about-us/aims-college.

Royal College of Physicians of Edinburgh. Membership Examinations. Methods of assessment. 2021; published online June 3. http://www.rcpe.ac.uk/sites/default/files/library_papers/history-of-membership-examinations/overview/index.php (accessed June 3, 2021).

Royal Courts of Justice. General Medical Council v. Dr Bawa-Garba Approved Judgement 2018. 2013. https://www.judiciary.uk/wp-content/uploads/2018/08/bawa-garba-v-gmc-final-judgment.pdf.

Royal Courts of Justice. Approved Judgment: Great Ormond Street Hospital vs. Guardian. 2021. https://www.judiciary.uk/wp-content/uploads/2017/07/gosh-v-gard-24072017.pdf.

Rudolph JW, Raemer DB, Simon R. Establishing a safe container for learning in simulation. Simulation in Healthcare: The Journal of the Society for Simulation in Healthcare. 2014;9:339–49.

Sagy I, Jotkowitz A, Barski L. Reflections on cultural preferences and internal medicine: the case of Jehovah's witnesses and the changing thresholds for blood transfusions. J Religion Heal. 2017;56:732–8.

Sargeant J, Lockyer J, Mann K, et al. Facilitated reflective performance feedback. Acad Med. 2015;90:1698–706.

Sawyer SM, Afifi RA, Bearinger LH, et al. Adolescent health 1 adolescence: a foundation for future health. Lancet. 2012;379:1630–40.

Schoeman F. Parental discretion and Children's rights: background and implications for medical decision-making. J Med Philos. 1985;10:45–62.

Schreiber J, Moerchen VA, Rapport MJ, et al. Experiential learning with children. Pediatr Phys Ther. 2015;27:356–67.

Society for Adolescent Health and Medicine. Young adult health and Well-being: A position statement of the Society for Adolescent Health and Medicine. J Adolesc Health. 2017;60:758–9.

Streuli JC, Anderson J, Alef-Defoe S, et al. Combining the best interest standard with shared decision-making in paediatrics—introducing the shared optimum approach based on a qualitative study. Eur J Pediatr. 2021;180:759–66.

The National Nursing and Nursing Education Taskforce. A National Specialisation Framework for Nursing and Midwifery. Australian Health Ministers' Advisory Council, 2006.

UK General Medical Council. Skills Fade: A Review of the Evidence That Clinical and Professional Skills Fade During Time Out of Practice, and of How Skills Fade May Be Measured or Remediated. 2015; published online May 16. https://www.gmc-uk.org/-/media/about/skills-fade-literature-review-full-report.pdf?la=en&hash=8B32071AF03167EE588EE574F6DCC4C85B1FEF0B. Accessed 2AD.

United Nations. United Nations Convention on the Rights of the Child. 2009; published online July10. https://www.unicef.org.au/Upload/UNICEF/Media/Our%20work/childfriendlycrc.pdf (accessed 2AD).

Wilimas JA, Donahue N, Chammas G, Fouladi M, Bowers LJ, Ribeiro RC. Training subspecialty nurses in developing countries: methods, outcome, and cost. Med Pediatr Oncol. 2003;41:136–40.

Wocial LD, Weaver MT. Development and psychometric testing of a new tool for detecting moral distress: the moral distress thermometer. J Adv Nurs. 2013;69:167–74.

Optimizing the Role of Clinical Educators in Health Professional Education

51

Simone Gibson and Claire Palermo

Contents

Introduction	986
Codeveloped Preclinical Learning	987
Enhancing the Skills and Qualities of Effective Clinical Educators	988
Creating a Positive Learning Culture in the Work Integrated Learning Setting	992
Conclusion	995
Index to Terms	995
References	996

Abstract

Clinical educators have a unique teaching role in that they need to support student learning while ensuring patient safety and service delivery. This chapter discusses the role of the clinical educator in preparing students for work integrated learning, and how they support students' learning trajectories during their practical placements. The skills and qualities of effective clinical educators are outlined including the intrinsic attributes that facilitate student learning, and other teaching skills such as organizational, assessment, and feedback skills. Methods for professional development for this group are proposed to assist in improving engagement and

S. Gibson (✉)
Department of Nutrition, Dietetics and Food, Medicine, Nursing and Health Sciences, Monash University, Clayton, VIC, Australia

School of Clinical Sciences, Medicine, Nursing and Health Sciences, Monash University, Clayton, VIC, Australia
e-mail: simone.gibson@monash.edu

C. Palermo
Department of Nutrition, Dietetics and Food, Medicine, Nursing and Health Sciences, Monash University, Clayton, VIC, Australia

Monash Centre for Scholarship in Health Education, Medicine, Nursing and Health Sciences, Monash University, Clayton, VIC, Australia
e-mail: claire.palermo@monash.edu

© Springer Nature Singapore Pte Ltd. 2023
D. Nestel et al. (eds.), *Clinical Education for the Health Professions*,
https://doi.org/10.1007/978-981-15-3344-0_125

both the student and clinical educator experience. This chapter also explores the role of the university in helping develop clinical educators and the importance of building productive relationships between academic and work integrated learning settings. Evidence from a range of health professions are used including allied health, medicine, and nursing.

Keywords

Clinical educator · Health professions · Student preparedness · Supervision · Teaching skills · Work integrated learning

Introduction

Clinical education aims to support health professions students achieve competence for entry-level practice across a range of practice areas and contexts. Experiential learning theory is one theory that assists understanding of the learning trajectory of students on practical placements, where students continually integrate their experiences with reflection and conceptualization to improve and practice future performance (Kolb et al. 2001). Upon entry to the workforce, students must be adept at one-on-one patient care, be able to work within individual systems such as wards or clinics, as well as the wider health system, and address the socio-ecological determinants of health (Sharma et al. 2018). This requires an appropriate and prepared workforce of educators within these settings to support student learning and competence development. In addition, the workplaces accepting students need to be adequately prepared to take on this important role in developing the future health care workforce.

Integral to student learning is the role of the clinical educator. Clinical educators work in complex environments and need to be proficient clinicians and competent teachers (Higgs and McAllister 2007). As clinical educators, their role encompasses that of being a mentor, role model, counselor, learning facilitator, evaluator, and supervisor to students on work integrated learning placement experiences (Higgs and McAllister 2007). Supervisory models vary across the health professions, work integrated learning (WIL) settings, funding models, and student year levels. While these differences need to be appreciated when examining and applying best evidence, it seems clinical educator roles have these common elements. Students on placement need to adapt to the busy, challenging, and complex health system. These sociocultural transitions can influence their development (Gibson et al. 2019). Sadly, bullying (Hakojärvi et al. 2014), violations of dignity (Davis et al. 2019), and unreliable assessment (Gibson et al. 2015) all can negatively impact learning on a placement. Enhancing the roles of clinical educators is essential in order to improve health workforce outcomes.

The aptitude of clinical educators in student supervision is key to the success of students participating in WIL (Kilminster and Jolly 2000). Clinical educators strongly influence student learning and satisfaction (Brown et al. 2013). High quality supervision can improve patient outcomes; however, inadequate supervision processes can compromise patient safety (Kilminster and Jolly 2000). Clinical educators may have specialist knowledge in their clinical areas, yet frequently lack sufficient training and support for their supervisory and assessment roles (Cleland et al. 2008, McClure and Black 2013). Universities play a role in equipping clinical educators for their educational responsibilities. Likewise, workplaces supporting student development need to embrace their role in developing the future health workforce.

In order to ensure effective learning experiences, a multifaceted, integrated approach is required to ensure the preparedness of all stakeholders for student placements. These include clinical educators, students, and the workplaces in which they will be based. The following chapter proposes that this requires: (i) a codeveloped learning curriculum focused on skill development, to optimize preparedness for work integrated learning (WIL); (ii) support and training of clinical educators to enthusiastically, proficiently, and efficiently support student learning; and (iii) creation of a positive culture toward student education in the workplace, by approaching clinical education as a clinician-student-academic team effort, with united goals. These will now be individually explored.

Codeveloped Preclinical Learning

Placement shortages, increasing patient complexity, rapidly evolving technology, and shorter patient lengths of stay create increasing challenges for clinical educators supporting students in the WIL environment (Sevenhuysen and Haines 2011). Ensuring students are adequately prepared to enter these complex environments is a priority for the safety and well-being of students, clinical educators, and the communities they serve. Clinical educator time and teaching intensity varies across students' learning trajectories, with students at the novice stage typically requiring more attention and resources (Hughes and Desbrow 2010, Sturman et al. 2011). Ensuring as much teaching, learning, and assessment as possible is achieved in the academic setting will assist in reducing the burden on the WIL environment.

In order to maximize expensive WIL time, students need solid foundation skills in professionalism prior to embarking upon placement and these include being able to effectively communicate, take initiative, and be flexible, resilient, and enthusiastic. (Chipchase et al. 2012, Gibson et al. 2015). It is on placement where they will encounter situations to build upon and develop these skills to be work-ready. National health professional registration bodies have developed competencies revised to reflect the diverse nature of health professionals' work, and there is a greater focus on professional skill competence (Frank and Danoff 2007, Scott 2008, Knox et al. 2016, Dart et al. 2019). Clinical educators supervising students support this emphasis (Gibson et al. 2015) but professional skill gaps including teamwork, communication and reflection skills, flexibility, and coping with uncertainty have been found in health professional graduates internationally (Gibson and Molloy 2012). Medical programs are increasingly training and assessing students in the areas such as emotional intelligence with positive results; however there is a lack of consensus with regard to definitions, training, and evaluation methods for this broad field (Satterfield and Hughes 2007, Arora et al. 2010).

Classroom-based activities may assist in students' feelings of confidence and preparedness for WIL. Translating theoretical lessons to clinical practice, where students perform authentic workplace activities, shows promise in addressing some of these parameters (Gibson et al. 2016, Palermo et al. 2019). Simulated activities have a wide range of applications ranging from teaching communication skills (Gibson and Davidson 2016, Kaplonyi et al. 2017), clinical and surgical skills (Theodoulou et al. 2018), to interprofessional practice (Bandali et al. 2008). Apart from simulation training, the evidence is still emerging regarding how to ensure students are truly placement-ready. Online training modules and clear and collaborative orientation processes for WIL appear to have benefit for health professional students starting placement (Robinson et al. 2008, Grace and O'Neil 2014).

To ensure that the classroom-based activities are relevant for WIL preparation, involving clinical educators in their development can assist with ensuring they are authentic. In addition, this also serves to promote a team-based approach to student training and ensures students are prepared for current and emerging issues in the workplace. Involving clinical educators in curriculum development can expose the informal and hidden curriculum that exists in health practice (Paul et al. 2014) while ensuring student training is relevant for WIL (McCluskey 2000). Examples include contributing to case-based learning development, helping to design and assess simulated learning activities, and being involved in health professional education research. Demonstrating that teaching is responsive to, and values, clinical educator inputs also supports a positive partnership between the university and workplace.

> **Key Points**
> - Optimally preparing students for placement is essential for the well-being of students, clinical educators, their patients, families, and communities.
> - Classroom-based activities that replicate real life workplace scenarios assist in preparedness.
> - Ensuring classroom-based learning has the ongoing input of clinical educators is essential to ensure they remain relevant to current workplace requirements and support the partnership between universities and workplaces.

Enhancing the Skills and Qualities of Effective Clinical Educators

Clinical educators are key to facilitating student progression in WIL and effecting student satisfaction (Brown et al. 2013), while carrying their role to ensure patient safety (Kilminster and Jolly 2000). Curriculum developers need to understand the skills required to inform development and support structures to create effective clinical educators and a sustainable system for delivering professional development and ongoing support of clinical educators in the area of education.

Identifying skills that make clinical educators effective is necessary to target training. These skills and qualities relate to all stages students experience during the experiential learning cycle, including having concrete experiences, reflection and observation, conceptualization, and active experimentation (Kolb et al. 2001). Clinical educator skills and qualities have been synthesized in the medical and allied health literature (Gibson et al. 2019, Sutkin et al. 2008) and include a range of personal attributes and interpersonal skills; high quality teaching and feedback skills; ability to promote collaborative learning between students and CEs; organization and planning skills; clinical educators having an integrated role in student assessment; and being excellent professional role models (Gibson et al. 2019).

Personal Attributes and Interpersonal Skills

The intrinsic traits of clinical educators have profound effects on student satisfaction and confidence (Gibson et al. 2019, Sutkin et al. 2008). Attributes such as kindness, patience, honesty, trust, and approachability foster a sense of students' belief in their own abilities. Students who feel valued as a future colleague develop a stronger sense of professional identity and feel supported to practice independently (Gibson et al. 2019). Clinical educators who are genuinely interested in their students are also more likely to identify and acknowledge external factors affecting student learning.

Creating a Collaborative Learning Culture

Self-aware clinical educators who demonstrate they are on a continuous learning journey along with their students have collective outcomes for both students and educators. Students feel more valued when they are treated as part of the team, and they appreciate clinical educators facilitating a positive attitude to clinical education. The collaborative environment is created by clinical educators taking the time to get to know students at placement commencement, being curious about students' viewpoints and experiences and sharing stories, as well as simple collegial activities such as staff having lunch with students. This collaboration extends to ensuring university-based academics, clinical educators and students have mutual understanding of expectations regarding the activities and tasks students undertake in the clinical setting as well as the standard at which they are expected to perform (Gibson et al. 2019).

High Quality Teaching and Feedback Skills

The principles of good teaching and learning that are promoted in academic settings hold true for clinical education as well. Clinicians may not necessarily see themselves as teachers, but strengthening their own identity around this role can enhance their confidence and ability, which translates to student learning. Teaching skills include adequately orientating students to tasks, clearly demonstrating and explaining techniques, linking theory to practice, allowing mistakes, and providing students opportunities to practice and demonstrate their learning. Clinical educators need to scaffold and tailor learning to student ability by building on students' previously acquired knowledge and skills. These evolving challenges need to be designed to meet the developing needs of students. Inextricably linked to this is the provision (and reception) of quality feedback. Feedback needs to be timely, useful, detailed, and directly related to individual student performance and needs (Dawson et al. 2019). To optimize student learning, clinical educators must allow students time to reflect and process feedback, which can be challenging in busy clinical environments with competing patient priorities. Encouraging student-led learning and feedback promotes student skill development, and is the beginning of lifelong learning.

Organization and Planning Skills

Students new to particular clinical settings value organized information ahead of time, so they can prepare themselves before they enter unfamiliar and often stressful environments. Clinical educators can provide policies, procedures, and manuals, as well as defined rotations, alleviating some of the uncertainty that comes with new placement appointments (Gibson et al. 2019).

The Clinical Educator's Role in Assessment

Clinical educators are required to not only observe and provide feedback to students, but to also monitor, assess, and report on student progress. To do this effectively, expectations of standards need to be shared among clinical educators, students, and the university. Programmatic approaches to assessment have been proposed as best practice in terms of work-based assessment (Dijkstra et al. 2010). Programmatic approaches involve a series of interdependent elements of learning and assessment methods that are connected to and dependent on each other. In this approach, assessment is viewed as *for* learning, rather than *of* learning. Instead of focusing on an individual assessment of isolated skills, it encompasses assessment of competence as a whole – whereby a range of skills, attitudes, and knowledge are integrated into performance of health care. Programmatic assessment also emphasizes the role of feedback, and as such, assessment occurs continuously through a range of learning activities (Schuwirth and Van der Vleuten 2011). Clinical educators play a vital role in work-based assessment and as such contribute vital information in the collection of evidence in a program of assessment. This may include the completion of assessment instruments on student performance or the provision of continuous feedback.

Providing feedback to underperforming students is highlighted as an area requiring attention in the literature (Cleland et al. 2008, Bearman et al. 2012). Clinical educators have multifaceted roles. They have competing priorities related to caring for their patients and providing education. Underperforming students add time and energy demands and clinical educators have reported a lack of support from universities and their employing health organizations, insufficient skills for managing this group, and that they devote significant emotional investment to help students pass and reach competency (Bearman et al. 2012). Australian physiotherapy clinical educators' strategies, when working with underperforming students, included providing more supervision and feedback, but they had limited alternative approaches to facilitate learning other than providing "more of the same" (Bearman et al. 2012).

Shifting the responsibility of competency achievement to students requires clinical educator skill development, support, and training (Bearman et al. 2012). University support for clinical educators to make clear and just assessment decisions is imperative. Taking a programmatic approach such that multiple pieces of evidence support students' understanding of their development will also support the provision of developmental feedback for the struggling student.

Be Role Models

Ultimately, clinical educators are performing roles that students aspire to, so they have a significant function as role models. Students value clinical educators who sincerely care about their patients and demonstrate leadership, both in their clinical and educational capacities. Students learn by watching, and seeing their clinical educators advocate for patients and their profession can instil the same in themselves. Clinical educators participating in research highlights the importance of lifelong learning. Educators working interprofessionally can provide students with the means to emulate this necessary practice to enhance current and future patient outcomes (Oandasan and Reeves 2005).

Training and Professional Development of Clinical Educators

Clinicians are often allocated students, yet receive little or no training in education or supervision. The literature consistently reports that clinical educators often feel undervalued and unsupported in their educational role with evidence from dietetics, medicine and general practice, and physiotherapy (Seabrook 2003, Gibson et al. 2015, Cleland et al. 2008, Barber et al. 2019). Studies of clinical educators in physiotherapy and nursing report feelings of isolation, particularly in making stressful competency assessment decisions (Bearman et al. 2012, McClure and Black 2013).

In supporting clinical educators to take on this role, training interventions involving active and experiential learning, social learning, and protected time have been found as mechanisms facilitating multiple improved positive supervisor outcomes (Rees et al. 2020). Both short and longer duration training appear to have similar effects (Rees et al. 2020). Training clinical educators for this role is essential to enhance their skills, and the literature suggests only modest investment, such as a once off workshop, may be required to build supervisory capability (Rees et al. 2019).

Provision of training and professional development for clinical educators needs to be accessible and targeted to their needs. Training programs should encompass the range of effective supervisory skills outlined above and involve active or experiential learning approaches that facilitate reflection. Kilminster et al. (2002) suggest a framework that incorporates learning about experiential learning and the skill development continuum; teaching, assessment and appraisal; interpersonal and counseling skills; and teaching and feedback skills. They also suggest that such training is credentialed to ensure clinical educators who supervise students are equipped and motivated to do so (Kilminster et al. 2002).

Clinical educators in primary care, and in isolated and rural settings, have unique challenges related to distance and the varied type of work they do (Gibson 2019, Barber et al. 2019). Their access to supervisor training is often limited, but these settings can provide rich opportunities for student learning, as well as meeting community needs and potentially addressing workforce shortages (Larsen and Perkins 2006). To facilitate clinical educator professional development, training must be made accessible. Strategies may include video conferencing, holding workshops at work-based locations, and creating webinars. Facilitating discussion between clinical educators and the university regarding individual student progress, and fostering discourse between clinical educators, may also assist to involve primary care educators. Communities of practice enable groups of professionals with similar interests to come together to achieve common goals (Barbour et al. 2018). Supporting the development of these communities of practice with a focus on education has been proposed as a mechanism to achieve this (Barber et al. 2019, Gibson 2019) and could also enhance health outcomes (Barbour et al. 2018).

> **Key Points**
> - Clinical educators require a set of knowledge, skills, personal attributes, and interpersonal skills to successfully complete their role
> - Creating a collaborative learning culture, having organization and planning skills, supporting assessment, providing feedback, and being role models are essential to clinical educator role and function.
> - Training and ongoing professional development of clinical educators is essential.

Creating a Positive Learning Culture in the Work Integrated Learning Setting

The relationship between academic and clinical settings is paramount to ensure the student experience is optimal (Kilminster and Jolly 2000). Improving perceptions and attitudes toward engagement in student learning is essential for moving WIL programs forward. Clinical educators derive much satisfaction and report improved clinical skills as a result of teaching students (Waters et al. 2018). There are clearly benefits to improving engagement between health focused organizations and universities. Tensions between clinical educators, WIL sites, and universities may exist, and although patient safety is considered to be fundamental, the focus on student learning can be of lower priority in WIL sites. Other sources of friction include financial restrictions on universities and health organizations alike, and differing expectations regarding student and graduate preparedness (Murray et al. 2010). Fostering relationships between organizations can assist in aligning these expectations. The following concepts may assist support the development of positive learning cultures in workplace learning settings.

University curriculum developers need to ensure curricula meet the needs of the community in terms of demand for qualified clinicians, limited placement numbers (Maillet et al. 2012), and patients. University-based curriculum designers and teachers need to consult with current practicing clinicians across diverse settings to develop appropriate preplacement training to be ready to learn in the constantly evolving clinical setting. Failure to do so results in emotional as well as monetary costs. For example, the cost of Australian physiotherapy students failing clinical placements accounting for university, health service, and government-related costs, has been estimated at nearly US$10,000 per failing student (Foo et al. 2017). Ensuring students are set up for success has significance for all stakeholders.

Understanding what roles and responsibilities clinical educators are expected to perform is the first step in improving culture and performance. Being cognisant of clinical educators' many roles beyond student supervision is important (Milosavljevic et al. 2014, McClure and Black 2013, Waters et al. 2018), and the body of published research is growing regarding health professionals and burnout (Milosavljevic and Noble 2015, Kreitzer and Klatt 2017). Increasing student supervision responsibilities need to be balanced with the often seemingly insurmountable workloads that clinicians already manage. However, society requires a sustainable skilled workforce to meet the demand, and with that comes work-based training which adds to clinicians' workloads.

Educational practice and supervisory expectations of clinical educators are variable (Kilminster and Jolly 2000, Kilminster et al. 2002), creating confusion around roles and responsibilities (McClure and Black 2013). Systemized training of clinical educators will assist in establishing understanding; however formal agreements and clear job descriptions are required. As described above, short duration, one-off training can support and develop clinical educators' confidence, knowledge, and skills in their supervisory practice (Rees et al. 2020). Furthermore, competencies related to student supervision have variable definitions in health profession competency standards. Accreditation standards and policies may be an avenue to ensure those involved in student training and development have been trained and have the required skills and attributes as clinical educators through prescription of accreditation standards related to WIL and assessment. In addition, competency descriptions specifically related to the student training aspect of clinical practice may be a way forward to value the implicit role of all health professionals in student training. A credentialing system for clinical educators may support this career trajectory and shared expectations of clinical education practice. This may serve to clarify supervisory roles and assist in gaining recognition and excellence of practice for clinical educators in both health organizations and within and across the health professions. When clinical educators are underperforming in their role, opportunities and mechanisms are usually lacking to provide support or feedback (Kilminster and Jolly 2000), so clear standards and policy will assist in performance management.

Shared expectations include acknowledging gender bias in some of the health professions. Experienced clinical educators in the female-dominated health professions may work part-time creating disjointed supervision, and the complex workloads of experienced clinicians (Milosavljevic and Noble 2015) may be challenging for novice students. These challenges must be factored for when designing the clinical education workforce.

Health professional education is commonly evaluated by student satisfaction and pass rates, which hold little value to the needs of health organizations. Health professional education has endeavored to discuss outcomes in terms of patients, which serves to add value for health care organizations (Dauphinee 2012). "Service learning partnerships" have been proposed as a work-based learning model that provide benefit to student learning and patient care, as the student learning programs are focused on patient care–related goals (Murray et al. 2010). These experiences have primarily been conducted in community-based organizations or in developing countries that generally require some baseline student skill proficiency; however they are highly evaluated by both students and the organizations in which they are based (Loewenson and Hunt 2011, Crawford et al. 2017). Other models of students adding benefit to organizations include students performing patient risk screening tasks, which have shown to enhance student learning, placement preparedness, and confidence (Gibson et al. 2016). In addition, medical students have been shown to add benefit to patient care the more years they are into their training (Molloy et al. 2018). Such experiences have the potential to translate to patient benefits while saving staff time (Gibson et al. 2016).

A challenge encountered when developing partnerships for clinical placements is the perception that students reduce productivity, however the evidence is unclear. Evidence indicates that productivity can increase while students are on placement (Rodger et al. 2012), however students, particularly novice students, can have negative impacts on clinical educators related to stress and work burden (Hughes and Desbrow 2010). Addressing these areas of concern, particularly balancing the support required for novice students with the benefits related to experienced students producing tangible outcomes in WIL can inform cost-benefit conversations that may assist in building a united approach for student placement training. Discovering other clinically relevant activities to assist in clinical educator workload management, as well as examining the mechanisms that make service learning partnerships valuable to all parties, is needed.

Nurturing interinstitutional relationships and determining effective strategies for changing culture is needed. Identifying placement-based clinical educator "champions," acknowledging excellence in clinical education practice, and providing assistance to organizations which host students to develop approaches to overcome barriers may cultivate improved engagement and attitudes to student education.

Encouraging clinical education as a career path for clinicians involved in education and assisting the development of an educational specialty related to their professional identity may strengthen their role and job satisfaction (Higgs and McAllister 2007, Barber et al. 2019). Acknowledging clinical educator excellence with awards and public recognition may assist in improving the profile of their essential role. Including them in educational and clinical research activities may also add value and prestige. Supporting clinical educators to join professional associations focused on health professional education may also promote continued professional development and a sense of professional identity in this area.

The engagement between universities and WIL sites is key to creating effective teaching and learning in clinical education. Curriculum designers need to consider the needs of students, clinical educators, and health services when creating learning activities to directly benefit all stakeholders. Conversations should occur at senior levels within health services with clearly articulated clinical educator and health service benefits. This may help ensure that clinical education holds value throughout health organizations from the executive level to the coalface of student learning with clinicians.

> **Key Points**
> - The relationship between academic and WIL settings is paramount to ensure successful outcomes for students, the organization, and patients. This relationship should be fostered through:
> - Shared understanding of roles and responsibilities between academic and clinical settings
> - Policies to support quality education practice (including, training, accreditation, and recognition systems)
> - Recognize the value students bring to organizations rather than emphasizing the burden

Conclusion

Optimally preparing students for clinical placements and supporting their competency development requires a unified and synergistic approach from all stakeholders including those from university, health care, and professional accreditation bodies. Involving clinical educators in the codesign of preplacement education, supporting the development and recognition of the unique set of skills required of clinical educators and creating a positive work integrated learning environment have been proposed as mechanisms to enhance both student and health outcomes. There is a need to embrace new ways of measuring the impact of clinical education away from perceptions and satisfaction to develop understanding of how these factors together influence student learning and ultimately improve health.

Index to Terms

Clinical Educator – individual health professional responsible for supporting health profession students achieve competence for entry-level practice across a range of practice areas and contexts (Gibson et al. 2019).

Work Integrated Learning – also known as placement, or fieldwork – are authentic work settings providing trainees with opportunities to practice and apply theoretical knowledge to practice (Gibson et al. 2015).

References

Arora S, Ashrafian H, Davis R, Athanasiou T, Darzi A, Sevdalis N. Emotional intelligence in medicine: a systematic review through the context of the ACGME competencies. Med Educ. 2010;44:749–64.

Bandali K, Parker K, Mummery M, Preece M. Skills integration in a simulated and interprofessional environment: an innovative undergraduate applied health curriculum. J Interprof Care. 2008;22:179–89.

Barber JRG, Park SE, Jensen K, Marshall H, Mcdonald P, Mckinley RK, Randles H, Alberti H. Facilitators and barriers to teaching undergraduate medical students in general practice. Med Educ. 2019;53:778–87.

Barbour L, Armstrong R, Condron P, Palermo C. Communities of practice to improve public health outcomes: a systematic review. J Knowl Manag. 2018;22:326–43.

Bearman M, Molloy E, Ajjawi R, Keating J. Is there a plan B?': Clinical educators supporting underperforming students in practice settings. Teach High Educ. 2012:1–14.

Brown T, Williams B, Lynch M. Relationship between clinical fieldwork educator performance and health professional students' perceptions of their practice education learning environments. Nurs Health Sc. 2013;15:510–7.

Chipchase LS, Buttrum PJ, Dunwoodie R, Hill AE, Mandrusiak A, Moran M. Characteristics of student preparedness for clinical learning: clinical educator perspectives using the Delphi approach. BMC Med Educ. 2012;12:112.

Cleland JA, Knight LV, Rees CE, Tracey S, Bond CM. Is it me or is it them? Factors that influence the passing of underperforming students. Med Educ. 2008;42:800–9.

Crawford E, Caine A-M, Hunter L, Hill AE, Mandrusiak A, Anemaat L, Dunwoodie R, Fagan A, Quinlan T. Service learning in developing countries: student outcomes including personal successes, seeing the world in new ways, and developing as health professionals. J Interprof Educ Pract. 2017;9:74–81.

Dart J, Mccall L, Ash S, Blair M, Twohig C, Palermo C. Toward a global definition of professionalism for nutrition and dietetics education: a systematic review of the literature. J Acad Nutr Diet. 2019;119:957–71.

Dauphinee WD. Educators must consider patient outcomes when assessing the impact of clinical training. Med Educ. 2012;46:13–20.

Davis C, King O, Clemans A, Coles J, Crampton P, Jacobs N, Mckeown T, Morphet J, Seear K, Rees C. Students' experiences of workplace dignity during work-integrated learning: a qualitative study exploring student and workplace supervisors' perspectives. Canberra: Australia & New Zealand Association for Health Professions Educaition; 2019.

Dawson P, Henderson M, Mahoney P, Phillips M, Ryan T, Boud D, Molloy E. What makes for effective feedback: staff and student perspectives. Assess Eval High Educ. 2019;44:25–36.

Dijkstra J, Van Der Vleuten C, Schuwirth LA. New framework for designing programmes of assessment. Adv Health Sci Educ. 2010;15:379–93.

Foo J, Rivers G, Ilic D, Evans DJR, Walsh K, Haines T, Paynter S, Morgan P, Lincke K, Lambrou H, Nethercote A, Maloney S. The economic cost of failure in clinical education: a multi-perspective analysis. Med Educ. 2017;51:740–54.

Frank JR, Danoff D. The CanMEDS initiative: implementing an outcomes-based framework of physician competencies. Med Teach. 2007;29:642–7.

Gibson SJ. Addressing the unique needs of training primary care-based educators. Med Educ. 2019;53:754–6.
Gibson SJ, Davidson ZE. An observational study investigating the impact of simulated patients in teaching communication skills in preclinical dietetic students. J Hum Nutr Diet. 2016;29:529–36.
Gibson S, Molloy E. Professional skill development needs of newly graduated health professionals: a systematic literature review. Foc Health Prof Educ. 2012;13:71–83.
Gibson S, Dart J, Bone C, Palermo C. Dietetic student preparedness and performance on clinical placements: perspectives of clinical educators. J Allied Health. 2015;44:101–7.
Gibson SJ, Golder J, Cant RP, Davidson ZE. An Australian mixed methods pilot study exploring students performing patient risk screening. Nurs Health Sci. 2016;18:203–9.
Gibson SJ, Porter J, Anderson A, Bryce A, Dart J, Kellow N, Meiklejohn S, Volders E, Young A, Palermo C. Clinical educators' skills and qualities in allied health: a systematic review. Med Educ. 2019;53:432–42.
Grace S, O'Neil R. Better prepared, better placement: an online resource for health students. Asia Pacific J Coop Educ. 2014;15:291–304.
Hakojärvi H-R, Salminen L, Suhonen R. Health care students' personal experiences and coping with bullying in clinical training. Nurs Educ Today. 2014;34:138–44.
Higgs J, Mcallister L. Being a clinical educator. Adv Health Sci Educ. 2007;12:187–200.
Hughes R, Desbrow B. An evaluation of clinical dietetic student placement case-mix exposure, service delivery and supervisory burden. Nutr Diet. 2010;67:287–93.
Kaplonyi J, Bowles KA, Nestel D, Kiegaldie D, Maloney S, Haines T, Williams C. Understanding the impact of simulated patients on health care learners' communication skills: a systematic review. Med Educ. 2017;51:1209–19.
Kilminster S, Jolly B. Effective supervision in clinical practice settings: a literature review. Med Educ. 2000;34:827–40.
Kilminster S, Jolly B, Vleuten C. A framework for effective training for supervisors. Med Teach. 2002;24:385–9.
Knox S, Dunne SS, Hughes M, Cheeseman S, Dunne CP. Regulation and registration as drivers of continuous professional competence for Irish pre-hospital practitioners: a discussion paper. Irish J Med Sci. 2016;185:327–33.
Kolb DA, Boyatzis RE, Mainemelis C. Experiential learning theory: previous research and new directions. In: Perspect think learn Cognit styles, vol. 1; 2001. p. 227–47.
Kreitzer MJ, Klatt M. Educational innovations to foster resilience in the health professions. Med Teach. 2017;39:153–9.
Larsen K, Perkins D. Training doctors in general practices: a review of the literature. Austr J Rural Health. 2006;14:173–7.
Loewenson KM, Hunt RJ. Transforming attitudes of nursing students: evaluating a service-learning experience. J Nurs Educ. 2011;50:345–9.
Maillet JOS, Brody RA, Skipper A, Pavlinac JM. Framework for analyzing supply and demand for specialist and advanced practice registered dietitians. J Acad Nutr Diet. 2012;112:S47–55.
Mcclure E, Black L. The role of the clinical preceptor: an integrative literature review. J Nurs Educ. 2013;52:335–41.
Mccluskey A. Collaborative curriculum development: clinicians' views on the neurology content of a new occupational therapy course. Austr Occup Ther J. 2000;47:1–10.
Milosavljevic M, Noble G. Burnout levels among dietitians working in the New South Wales public hospital system: a cross-sectional statewide survey. Nutr Diet. 2015;72:101–6.
Milosavljevic M, Noble G, Zaremba C. Day-to-day activities of clinical dietitians working in the inpatient and outpatient settings in a group of New South Wales public hospitals: the results of a direct observational study. Nutr Diet. 2014;71:10–5.
Molloy E, Lew S, Woodward-Kron R, Delany C, Dodds A, Lavercombe M, Hughson J. Medical student clinical placements as sites of learning and contribution. Melbourne: University of Melbourne; 2018.

Murray TA, Crain C, Meyer GA, Mcdonough ME, Schweiss DM. Building bridges: an innovative academic-service partnership. Nurs Outlook. 2010;58:252–60.

Oandasan I, Reeves S. Key elements for interprofessional education. Part 1: the learner, the educator and the learning context. J Interprof Care. 2005;19:21–38.

Palermo C, Kleve S, Mccartan J, Brimblecombe J, Ferguson M. Using unfolding case studies to better prepare the public health nutrition workforce to address the social determinants of health. Pub Health Nutr. 2019;22:180–3.

Paul D, Ewen SC, Jones R. Cultural competence in medical education: aligning the formal, informal and hidden curricula. Adv Health Sci Educ. 2014;19:751–8.

Rees CLS, Huang E, Denniston C, Edouard V, Pope K, Sutton K, Waller S, Ward B, Palermo C. Supervision training in healthcare: A realist synthesis. Adv Health Sci Educ. 2019. In press

Rees CE, Lee SL, Huang E, Denniston C, Edouard V, Pope K, Sutton K, Waller S, Ward B, Palermo C. Supervision training in healthcare: a realist synthesis. Adv Health Sci Educ Theory Pract. 2020;25:523–561.

Robinson A, Andrews-Hall S, Cubit K, Fassett M, Venter L, Menzies B, Jongeling L. Attracting students to aged care: the impact of a supportive orientation. Nurs Educ Today. 2008;28:354–62.

Rodger S, Stephens E, Clark M, Ash S, Hurst C, Graves N. Productivity and time use during occupational therapy and nutrition/dietetics clinical education: a cohort study. PLoS One. 2012;7:e44356.

Satterfield JM, Hughes E. Emotion skills training for medical students: a systematic review. Med Educ. 2007;41:935–41.

Schuwirth LW, Van Der Vleuten CP. Programmatic assessment: from assessment of learning to assessment for learning. Med Teach. 2011;33:478–85.

Scott SD. 'New professionalism'–shifting relationships between nursing education and nursing practice. Nurs Educ Today. 2008;28:240–5.

Seabrook MA. Medical teachers' concerns about the clinical teaching context. Med Educ. 2003;37:213–22.

Sevenhuysen SL, Haines T. The slave of duty: why clinical educators across the continuum of care provide clinical education in physiotherapy. Hong Kong Physiother J. 2011;29:64–70.

Sharma M, Pinto AD, Kumagai AK. Teaching the social determinants of health: a path to equity or a road to nowhere? Acad Med. 2018;93:25–30.

Sturman N, Régo P, Dick ML. Rewards, costs and challenges: the general practitioner's experience of teaching medical students. Med Educ. 2011;45:722–30.

Sutkin G, Wagner E, Harris I, Schiffer R. What makes a good clinical teacher in medicine? A review of the literature. Acad Med. 2008;83:452–66.

Theodoulou I, Nicolaides M, Athanasiou T, Papalois A, Sideris M. Simulation-based learning strategies to teach undergraduate students basic surgical skills: a systematic review. J Surg Educ. 2018;75:1374–88.

Waters L, Lo K, Maloney S. What impact do students have on clinical educators and the way they practise? Adv Health Sci Educ. 2018;23:611–31.

Well-Being in Health Profession Training

Andrew Grant

Contents

Introduction	1000
Mental Health in Students and Trainees in Healthcare Professions	1000
Well-Being	1000
Prevalence	1000
Stigma	1001
Risks	1002
Prevention/Well-Being Initiatives	1006
Recommendations	1012
Conclusion	1013
Cross-References	1013
References	1013

Abstract

In this chapter, the evidence in relation to the well-being of healthcare students is examined. In particular, the prevalence of mental health problems in this group is explored along with probable underlying causes. The stigma associated with mental illness is responsible for students and qualified practitioners seeking to conceal such illness when they occur. The use of drugs and alcohol by students and practitioners is also explored.

Interventions that have been shown to be beneficial to healthcare practitioners and students include support groups initiated by the institution including Schwarz rounds and Balint groups. A background to mindfulness-based stress reduction (MBSR) and mindfulness-based interventions (MBIs) is given along with evidence of their value when offered to healthcare professionals and students. While MSBR was initially introduced as a way of helping patients with physical health problems, particularly chronic pain, it is now also being used in a supportive and preventative

A. Grant (✉)
Emeritus Professor Swansea University, Swansea, UK
e-mail: a.j.grant@swansea.ac.uk

© Springer Nature Singapore Pte Ltd. 2023
D. Nestel et al. (eds.), *Clinical Education for the Health Professions*,
https://doi.org/10.1007/978-981-15-3344-0_136

way. Other interventions, including mental health first aid (MHFA), are presented as ways of ensuring that many people, staff and students, are aware of ways to help students or colleagues to access support or medical care when they need it. Finally, recommendations are made about provision of a tailor-made clinical service for healthcare practitioners and students based on the Practitioner Health Programme in London, and specific needs of practitioners working in rural areas are also explored.

Keywords

Student · Healthcare · Mental illness · Mindfulness · Stigma · Presenteeism

Introduction

Many students, when embarking on a career in one of the healthcare professions, will need to perform well academically and to demonstrate ability on other areas such as music and sport. Once they commence their training, they will, once again, need to work hard and may find themselves in a competitive environment. Their behavior will be monitored as if they were, already, members of the regulated profession which they aspire to join. It is not surprising, therefore, that healthcare professions students demonstrate higher levels of mental ill health than the general population. Healthcare students find themselves exposed to a double whammy. Prevalence of mental illness is raised but many are worried that to disclose their illness and to seek help may have a deleterious effect on their future healthcare career. Therefore, we examine ways of reducing the stigma attached to mental illness, ways of helping students maintain their well-being, and the provision of support for students which they find accessible.

Mental Health in Students and Trainees in Healthcare Professions

Well-Being

A variety of definitions of well-being exist. For the purposes of this chapter, the working definition has been adopted as a state that goes beyond absence of disease or pathology. Well-being refers to a state of positive good health, one of "thriving, not just surviving." For example, anticipatory support can be provided in a focused manner at stress points such as times of transition (school to university, first clinical placements, university to professional practice, etc.) (Drolet and Rodgers 2010).

Prevalence

Like most undergraduate or graduate entry university students, those studying to enter the healthcare professions are at a stage of their lives in early adulthood where mental illness is more likely to reveal itself for the first time. Research studies have indeed shown repeatedly, that healthcare students are more likely to experience mental illness than age-matched controls (Dahlin et al. 2005, 2007; Dyrbye et al. 2006; Compton et al. 2008; Jadoon et al. 2010; Aboshaiqah and Preposi Cruz 2018; Syed et al. 2018). The evidence which compares healthcare students with those in other university programs is less conclusive. A survey involving 376 first year medical students discovered that their initial scores for mental health were good but that these deteriorated during the course of their first year of study (Grant et al. 2013; Koter et al. 2016). A study carried out in Brazil found that 33% of dental, nursing, and medical students scored above the cut score for mental ill-health. There were strong correlations with female gender, lack of optimism for the future, feeling emotionally tense and finding the course to not be a source of pleasure (Fontes de Oliva Costa et al. 2014).

Effects of Applicant Population/Selection

It is worth examining the population who enter healthcare profession education and, subsequently, professional practice. In order to be admitted to vocational university programs, students need to perform to a very high academic standard. Many also show evidence of attainment in other areas of their lives including sport, music, and community work. In addition to their own ambition, applicants often carry the ambitions of their families, peer groups, and schools with them (Winter et al. 2017). Having obtained a place in a healthcare vocational program and, in many cases, having already graduated in a related subject, the stakes are very high for these students/professionals-to-be. Understandably, the atmosphere within classes is highly competitive. It is not surprising then that students in this competitive milieu are very reluctant to disclose a mental illness which, they perceive, will reduce their standing in comparison to their peers (Winter et al. 2017).

Stigma

Stigma, in relation to mental illness, is common within society. However, stigma has a particularly pernicious effect among current and future members of the health professions. There are prevailing views that are transmitted to medical students and trainees that "doctors don't get ill" (Grant et al. 2019a). While there is a clear understanding that mental illness among patients is a fact of life, the possibility of doctors being affected by a diagnosis of a mental illness is treated with a degree of denial. The tacit messages that students and doctors in training pick up are that for them to suffer a mental illness will make them appear weak among their peers and senior members of the profession who may have some say over their career progression in the future (Grant et al. 2019a). Stigmatization of mental illness is also recognized within the nursing profession. Nurses with mental illness report being the object of discrimination, and some even report negative perceptions of themselves as professionals in light of their illness (Ross and Goldner 2009).

Medical students often express a fear that disclosing a mental illness will result in them being referred for a fitness to practice investigation (Grant et al. 2013). There are then some commonly held and overvalued ideas that are frequently expressed by trainee doctors and medical students about the effect that disclosure of a mental illness might have on their future career. In fact, evidence shows that very few medical students are referred for fitness to practice procedures on health grounds alone. A small number may be referred where health problems have affected their behavior, but even these numbers are small.

There is a real danger, therefore, that health profession students may not seek the support and medical help they need if they experience mental illness. The threat that this poses, that of students and qualified professionals working in the clinical environment when they are unwell, is very real. A biographical narrative interview study was carried out with doctors in training who had personal experience of mental illness in England and Wales. They described being at work when they were unable to concentrate, communicate with patients, or make decisions.

There is a major need, therefore, to carry out myth-busting activities among health profession students and professionals (at all grades of seniority). This can take the form of poster campaigns (possibly giving the testimonies of famous people who have survived mental illness). A very powerful message can be given by respected senior members of health professions speaking about their own experiences of mental illness and showing that they have successfully continued in their careers. Information from peers is sometimes more approachable than information from the university, medical school, or employer. Students are able to make mental illness something more easily talked about among their peer group than staff from their educational institution (Grant et al. 2013).

Risks

In a recent study in the United Kingdom, focus groups were held with doctors in training examining their attitudes toward mental illness within the medical profession. The participants did not have personal histories of mental illness and said that they would turn up for work when they were ill. This was based on a sense of the need to do their job and not to place extra burden on their peers (Grant et al. 2019a). In a biographical narrative study (Wengraf 2008) carried out in England and Wales, doctors in training talked about practicing when mentally ill. This placed constraints on their ability to communicate with patients, concentrate, and be able to make clinical decisions. A junior doctor went into work for further 2 days after being given a medical certificate by their general practitioner (Grant et al. 2019b). They said that they did this because there was no chance that a locum could be found at such short notice. For some, presenteeism took the form of turning up, getting through the day as best they could, and carrying out their clinical commitments but with very little learning and no preparation for their future career, for example, for postgraduate exams.

Starkly put, as a consequence of being a doctor in training, some do not access mental healthcare when they need it. Similar prejudicial views toward colleagues with mental illness have been shown to exist in nursing (Ross and Goldner 2009). This must change as currently, because of their job, some health professionals will not receive the mental healthcare that they need but will continue to care for patients when their ability to do this may be impaired.

The Use of Alcohol and Recreational Drugs

The use of recreational drugs and hazardous use of alcohol are prevalent among health professional students. A study involving 855 medical students from 14 US medical schools showed that non-Caucasian students were likely to have consumed less alcohol than Caucasian students and to have consumed it less frequently (Eyala et al. 2017). Consumption of excessive amounts of alcohol was associated with loss of memory, risky sexual behavior, suicidal thoughts, and driving under the influence. A significant number of students smoked tobacco with smaller numbers of students using amphetamines, sedatives, and cocaine. The most common substances that respondents took were alcohol and cannabis. The authors point out the increasing severity of cannabis use and that in the last two decades the potency of street cannabis has increased significantly (Eyala et al. 2017). A study of risk-taking among healthcare students, medical students, and medical residents found that being male, slim, a habitual coffee drinker, a regular smoker, a medical student, or a resident physician correlated to regular alcohol use (Lamberti et al. 2017).

University Alcohol/Drug Policies

Although most higher education establishments have alcohol and drug policies, many students may not be aware of their existence. In a study in the United States that recruited 855 medical students, 40% of the students were not aware of its existence of their school's drug and alcohol policy (Eyala et al. 2017). Many higher education establishments around the world have clubs and traditions that involve consumption of excessive amounts of alcohol and some which involve initiation rituals, although attitudes toward these organizations may be less tolerated than they once were (Batty, 2018). It is essential that all Higher Education Institutions (HEIs) make clear that they do not condone or support such behavior. It is, therefore, regrettable that more students are not aware of their school's/college's alcohol policy which is one way of making clear to students that behavior involving excessive amounts of alcohol is completely unacceptable as is the coercion of other (possibly younger) students to drink more than they wish to or than is safe for them to do so.

A survey of medical students in Wales showed that out of 266 students who responded (12% of a population of 2,150), 65 reached the score for hazardous drinking on the CAGE questionnaire. Of the respondents, 23% had taken cannabis in the preceding year, 8% had taken ecstasy, 6% had taken cocaine, and 5% had taken ketamine (Farrell et al. 2019). A systematic review of problem drinking among nurses concluded that prevalence continued to be a problem (Kenna and Woo 2004). A cross-sectional survey of French medical, nursing, and physiotherapy students examined their risk-taking behavior over an 8-year period. Nursing students had higher risk-taking behavior than other students. Cannabis-taking dropped between the two time points (2007 and 2015). Binge drinking and exercise-taking increased (Tavolacci et al. 2018).

Disclosure

Fitness to practice procedures, or the fear of them and their consequences, are frequently cited by medical students and doctors in training as the reason for not disclosing any information about their mental illness to their clinical/educational supervisor or to their medical school (Grant et al. 2013; Winter et al. 2017). A systematic review of attitudes toward psychiatric illness and psychiatric services within the nursing profession also found that nurses with mental illness experienced negative attitudes toward mental illness from their colleagues (Ross and Goldner 2009).

For those students whose illness makes disclosure essential (for instance, where they have to take time out of scheduled activities for appointments with a therapist or doctor), they have no choice, and disclosure is unavoidable. There is no evidence that students who do disclose a mental illness to their medical school are, in any way, disadvantaged. However, the overvalued idea of the potential harm thrives regardless in the absence of evidence (Grant et al. 2013).

Barriers to Accessing Medical Care and Support

Many undergraduate medical students and junior (qualified) doctors will, if they can, conceal any problems with their mental health from their supervisors and fellow students. The strongly held view that exists among medical students that to reveal a mental illness can make them at risk of being seen as weak fuels the fear that being known to have a mental illness will have a damaging effect on students' future career and may even bring it to an end. This belief is, at least in part, responsible for the barrier that prevents many medical students and doctors in training from accessing medical or other support when they experience mental health problems (Grant et al. 2013; Grant et al. 2014; Grant et al. 2019b).

It is the combination of the prevalence of mental illness and fear of the consequences of disclosure that sets medical students apart from others in their age range, whether they are university students or not. There is debate about whether healthcare students and professionals in training have a sufficiently different set of demands that they need to be treated differently from other university students. It is often said that, unlike other students, medical students have to cope with life and death matters during the course of their training (Grant et al. 2013). The same can certainly, of course, be said of students in nursing and other healthcare professions (Ross and Goldner 2009). Health profession students' behavior falls under the jurisdiction of their regulatory body from the first day of their undergraduate training, not the day they graduate and begin practice. The code of practice of the professional bodies demands a far higher standard of behavior than the disciplinary code to which their contemporary university students are expected to conform. Students, particularly during the latter part of their training, when they are based in the clinical environment are usually expected to do a 9 to 5 working day, with additional time out of hours unlike most university students. This can make normal activities, such as keeping an appointment with their own doctor, more difficult.

Illness Behavior

What *is* different within medicine, and the evidence is that medical students pick this behavior up early in their training, is the access to qualified professionals' expertise about their personal health problems (Roberts 2000). These so-called corridor consultations involve the doctor or student self-referring in a place where there is no privacy and where a full history and examination is not possible. The consulting doctor may feel pressured into seeing the doctor or student in less than ideal conditions and concerned at being coerced into giving a consultation that has limited possibilities. In addition to self-referring for their own health problems, doctors are known to prescribe for themselves and to coerce colleagues into carrying out investigations without these being requested by a clinician (other than the student/doctor themselves). A commonly said expression about a lawyer who represents himself is that he "has a fool for a client." This situation of a doctor asking for a medical opinion is not dissimilar. In other words, a health professional or a student of a health profession needs the same professional relationship with any doctor who is treating them as any other patient. If, as many professionals do, they seek to bypass normal procedures, they will deprive themselves of an objective clinical opinion of their condition where the treating doctor has, at their disposal, all the usual diagnostic and therapeutic tools.

It is very unlikely that significant advances will be made in the way in which students and trainees in healthcare professions access support for mental health problems without the current levels of perceived stigma which students consistently appear to pick up once they begin their training being addressed (Ross and Goldner 2009). This requires direct and repeated delivery of information about dealing with mental illness to students starting as they at the university. It should include the following:

1. Mental illness is a common occurrence in the population, and in the healthcare professions, and is an expected event.
2. Almost everyone who experiences mental illness within the healthcare professions will make a full recovery and goes onto a happy, healthy career.
3. If students experience a mental health problem, it is perfectly acceptable for them to seek medical care away from the university or medical school. (By saying this, it is accepted that some students will, despite the best efforts of their school, still be very reluctant to disclose their illness and that it is far better that they seek medical help away from the institution than not feeling able to seek it at all).
4. Readily available accessible information on sources of medical care and support (see section "Sources of Support").
5. Information on how to support a friend/peer with a mental illness. (This may seem less personal or confrontational if it is couched in terms of "this is how to support a friend with a mental health problem" instead of "what to do if you experience mental health problems yourself") (see Mental Health First Aid, page 12).

Prevention/Well-Being Initiatives

It is not surprising that evidence shows that students who can be encouraged to take better care of their physical and emotional health enjoy a better sense of well-being. Regular exercise, healthy eating, and adequate sleep are all linked with improved mental health. Clearly, we can expect students who take no alcohol or a moderate amount to enjoy a better quality of life.

Pass/Fail Grading: Reducing Competitiveness

Reducing the burden on students to perform to an unnecessarily high level has been shown to improve well-being (Enns et al. 2001; Rohe et al. 2006; Bloodgood et al. 2009). Grades for written assignments can be replaced with a simple binary pass/fail system, thereby removing the incentive to strive for high marks/grades and to outperform peers. Student well-being is improved by the introduction of pass/fail grading without any determent to students' grades. A systematic review of the literature relating to pass/fail assessment of medical students identified four studies that included both student welfare and academic performance. They showed that pass/fail grading improved student well-being while making no difference to academic performance (Spring et al. 2011). Reducing competitiveness through the introduction of pass/fail assessment is recommended by Slavin and colleagues (Slavin et al. 2011) as one of the five ways of "helping students flourish." They also recommend promoting positive emotions, engagement with activities outside the classroom, development and maintenance of strong relationships, and encouraging students to celebrate achievement (Slavin et al. 2011).

Mindfulness

Mindfulness meditation in the form of mindfulness-based stress reduction (MSBR) is a format by which Buddhist-style meditation has been used with secular western audiences. Mindfulness-based stress reduction and other mindfulness-based interventions (MBIs) help the user to train their attention to stay in the present moment without judgment. MSBR was first introduced as a way of helping patients with chronic pain (Kabat-Zinn 1982). Both MSBR and MBIs have been used widely to help professionals across a broad spectrum of healthcare disciplines (Lomas et al. 2018). Initial training in MBSR, typically, consists of attendance at eight weekly classes of 2.5 hours each and one all-day weekend retreat. Participants are expected to practice medication daily during the 8-week period (Kabat-Zinn 1982).

A systematic review was carried out examining the effects of MBSR and MBIs on healthcare workers across a number of professional backgrounds. In total, 81 studies were included in the review although a significant proportion of these did not include a control group. The authors conclude that MBSR and MBI have a positive effect on stress, depression, and anxiety with medium or low to medium effect sizes. Results regarding effects of MBSR and MBI and stress were equivocal. The authors comment that many of the studies involved in their review involved small numbers but that they did not see any difference in results between participants from different healthcare professional groups (Lomas et al. 2018). Rosenzweig and colleagues carried out a controlled study measuring the effect of mindfulness-based stress reduction on medical students in Philadelphia, Pennsylvania (Rosenzweig et al. 2003). They used the Profile of Mood States (PoMS) to measure differences in mood states before and after the intervention in the active intervention and control groups. The PoMS has six subscales: tension-anxiety, depression-dejection, anger-hostility, vigor-activity, fatigue-inertia, and confusion-bewilderment. In addition, there was a holistic total mood disturbance (TMD) (Rosenzweig et al. 2003). The researchers found that the treatment (MSBR) group showed a statistically significant reduction in total mood disturbance, while the control group showed a rise. The MSBR group also showed a significant decrease in score for the tension/anxiety and confusion/bewilderment subscales.

Each medical school provides support for their students in different ways. Since September 2018, Swansea University Medical School has appointed a student representative elected by their peers as "welfare officer" with a brief for campaigning for better student support and signposting medical students in need of help. This post was created by the Medical Society and provides support only for medical students. The campus-based Welfare Office can see students within a day of making contact and will direct students to the right source of support (which will include financial advice, academic support, delays in submitting written work, etc.). The well-being service offers students one-to-one and group psychological support. Every cohort in the Graduate Entry Medicine (GEM) program at Swansea is allocated a cohort support tutor. This person provides support to the cohort throughout their 4 years on the GEM program. This is in addition to the personal tutor/academic mentor allocated to every student.

Cardiff University also has measures in place for their medical students; Medic Support has been running since 2001 and provides support and mentoring for students with all types of health concerns and long-term conditions.

The Vanderbilt Medical School in Nashville, Tennessee, has a major coordinated program of support for its students (Drolet and Rodgers 2010). The program is well resourced and able to pay salaries for key members of the program which was divided into three overlapping components:

1. *The Advisory College* which provided a structure for support and advice for students throughout the program but particularly on entry to medical school and at times of transition. Support was provided by faculty members but also by the students' peers.
2. *The Student Wellness Committee*. This committee supported by members of staff organized a major selection of healthy living activities including sport and yoga but also team-based activities including quizzes. There was an annual cup competition. This involved students from the four advisory committees competing. Student wellness committee activities came under five headings: mentoring, body, mind, social, and community.
3. *Vanderbilt Medical School Live*. This is a program of personal development which maximizes students' personal development as they progress through

medical school with the aim of helping them prepare for the role of practitioner which they are preparing to take on (Drolet and Rodgers 2010).

Sources of Support

It is not surprising that when students are reluctant to seek help from their educational institution, they turn, initially, to friends and family for support and advice (Winter et al. 2017). It behooves us, therefore, to ensure that university staff and a proportion of the student population (at least) have the knowledge and skills required to direct students who request help for a mental health concern to appropriate sources of help. Staff and peers should not enter into any clinical or therapeutic interaction with students who have a mental illness. However, they need to be well enough informed to recognize when their peers/students have a problem that may need professional intervention and how to enable the unwell, distressed student to access this help as soon as possible.

Mental Health First Aid (MHFA) consists of a brief training (typically 2 days) in which adults are prepared to be able to give initial support to their peers and colleagues when they experience mental health problems. There are 500,000 trained mental health first aiders in England, currently, and a number of providers offering the training (Hazards 2018). Mental Health First Aiders are given training in recognizing when a friend and/or colleague may be experiencing mental health problems, listening to them and helping identify appropriate sources of medical care and support. Mental Health First Aiders do not (must not) attempt to offer any kind of medical care or professional support (such as counseling). Some universities are seeking to provide networks of Mental Health First Aiders across the campus. Many nominate a second year or more senior student, not necesarily with mental health first aid or other training, to offer advice and support to new recruits. These students are often referred to as the "mums and dads" of new first year students (Grant et al. 2013). In some cases, relationships are built up over the years, and "families" containing students from all years are formed providing rich networks of support.

First Points of Contact

Most university students will be allocated a personal tutor or academic mentor. People in this role will have different titles in different establishments, but the role, that of a member of academic staff accessible and available to give support, exists in most universities. Unfortunately, there is not always one person who fulfills this or a similar role for professionals once qualified and practicing. Although there is some overlap between the undergraduate personal tutor role and that of educational supervisor for doctors in training, there is a difference in the way the role is perceived. For example, doctors in training do not see their educational supervisor as someone to whom they would disclose a mental illness and seek help and support (Grant et al. 2019a). The brief for the personal tutor role is broad and includes helping students access help with personal, academic, social, and health problems. The tutor is not expected to provide solutions to all the problems presented to them, but they need to be able to refer students on to appropriate sources of support. For this reason, personal tutors need to be given training in the role and the facilities that are available to students in need. Specifically, for students with mental health problems, personal tutors are not expected to provide counseling or therapy but should have an up-to-date knowledge of appropriate services on or off campus. Training in Mental Health First Aid may help tutors and other frontline university staff to provide an appropriate level of support and to direct students to sources of professional help.

Suicide Prevention

Moutier and colleagues offered mental health screening to 2,680 physicians, trainee doctors, and medical students. The program was set up with the specific aim of reducing suicide and mental ill health at a California medical school. They carried out a two-pronged attack which comprised a screening program and an educational campaign (Moutier et al. 2012). The screening was carried out using an online confidential screening tool, and the educational campaign was carried out in a number of formats including grand rounds for senior staff and similar formats for junior staff and students. From a population of 2,860, 374 people took up the offer of screening, and of these, 101 were found to meet the criteria for significant depression or suicide risk. Forty-eight were referred for psychiatric treatment (Moutier et al. 2012).

School Versus University Services (Relative Merits)

All medical students in the United Kingdom are able to access support for health, social, or personal problems from two sources. These are support from within the medical school itself and from university-wide, campus-based services. Although students do not criticize either source of support, the support offered by them differs significantly (see Fig. 1) (Grant et al. 2013). Support offered by the medical school is

	Support services	**Medical school**
Model	Social model of disadvantage	Medical model of incapacity
Services	Integrated, triage to specialists, holistic	Restricted to performance and pastoral
Resources	Large, breadth, depth	Small, focused
Transparency	Advertised widely, menu/portfolio	Formal system transparent, informal hidden
Confidentiality	Absolute except when danger to self or others	Conditional on circumstances
Options	Anything the student thinks is a good outcome	Course completion/becoming a doctor
Expectations	Flexibility	Compliance

Fig. 1 Comparison of campus-based and medical school sources of support (Grant et al. 2013). (Reproduced by kind permission of the General Medical Council (UK) and my co-authors)

likely to be delivered by members of academic staff whom students may encounter in other circumstances, for instance, in assessments and in making progression decisions about them. Conversely, university on-campus services are independent of schools and colleges and have no contact with students other than to provide support. They have an expressed confidentiality policy which will be broken only in very exceptional circumstances (e.g., where patient safety is in danger of being compromised or where a crime has been committed). Because of the dual roles that many medical school staff may have, it is more difficult, therefore, for them to have a clear, unequivocal, confidentiality policy to cover their supportive interactions with their students. As the same prejudices exist toward mental illness among practitioners and students in other healthcare professions, it is very likely that students will use sources of support strategically (Ross and Goldner 2009). In particular, they will avoid disclosure of any mental health problems to their teachers and the faculty members who will be making progression decisions about them.

Communicating Sources of Support

For healthcare practitioners and students, it is important:

(a) To communicate the presence of sources of support and how these might be accessed
(b) To communicate this information via multiple media (e.g., virtual learning environment, email, at inductions and via handbooks and other written media, such as posters)
(c) To communicate this information repeatedly

This information should be made available in several formats and on a "just in time" rather than a "just in case" basis. Students are less likely to assimilate where and when support is to be found when they don't need it. Conversely when they are unwell and in need of support, they will have strong motivation to find this information. As all students will be accessing the university's virtual learning environment on a regular basis, this is an obvious place to set up a well-being page with all relevant information about accessing support and healthcare. A named person needs to take responsibility for keeping this information up to date. It is also useful to include information about sources of support with the package of information that is given out at induction (often on a USB stick) and for the really key messages to be given face to face during induction week. Personal tutors should arrange to meet their students during the first week of term so that students have been introduced before they have to meet them to ask for support.

Preparation for Clinical Practice (PCP) at Swansea University Medical School

Preparation for clinical practice is a noncredit-bearing module which provides a framework to help students at Swansea University Medical School learn to develop healthy ways to cope with stress and challenges (i.e., to develop resilience), to ensure a good work-life balance, to deal with doubt and uncertainty, and to prioritize time well. Each session relies on facilitation by clinicians who have had personal experience of the challenges faced by medical students and doctors. Having the opportunity to have sessions at regular intervals is important – not only to develop learning but also to allow students to appreciate that fostering a healthy approach to work as a doctor needs frequent contemplation and reflection. To optimize student participation, it is important that the sessions are perceived as nonthreatening and conducted in a nonjudgmental manner, including using humor as a strategy for introducing difficult issues. The need for confidentiality is stressed at the outset. Tutors will broadly discuss the topic of the day, and an appropriate video (e.g., a TED Talk) may be used to elaborate on specific points. External speakers will visit and recount their personal experience of a time they encountered adversity and how they managed to cope along the way. The tutors guide this description if necessary, in order to highlight or clarify specific and important details. After this, students separate into smaller groups, are given prompting questions to consider between them (e.g., how would you act in a similar situation? where would you turn to for help?), and discuss the cases. The important focus points to consider include how individuals might cope/react if they were in a similar situation and what they might do to help prepare for this. At the end of the session, all students and tutors regather as a plenary, share their thoughts, and ask questions to tutors and speakers in an open forum. Care is taken to stress the most important points for the students to consider in their future careers.

The "topics" or "themes" covered include:

- Self-care – work and life
- Personal/professional difficulties (relationships, financial, etc.)
- Dealing with uncertainty, risk management
- "Mistakes" (regulator investigation, Coroner's Court attendance, etc.)
- Need for peer/mentor support for illness (physical/mental)
- Professional development and competence
- Failure to progress (exams, workplace-based assessments, etc.)
- Bullying

Schwarz Rounds and Balint Groups

Schwarz rounds are multi-professional, facilitated meetings in which any staff member can attend and can discuss the personal and emotional aspects of caring for patients (Point of Care Foundation). Meetings begin with presentations from three people presenting either different aspects of the same case or different cases with a common theme. Strict confidentiality is observed. Balint groups, which were originally created for general practitioners (family physicians) to discuss the psychological aspects of their work with patients, also involve the presentation and discussion of clinical cases presented by group members. While Balint groups are limited to certain groups of clinicians, Schwarz rounds are open to all staff, clinical and nonclinical (Salinsky 2013).

Recommendations

Bespoke Service

In the geographical area enclosed by the London Orbital Motorway, the M25, there is a health service which is exclusively for doctors and dentists, the Practitioner Health Programme (PHP). This is a service which doctors and dentists can access by self-referral. Users of the service are usually seen within a few days for an initial assessment, and the program has access to therapists from a variety of backgrounds (e.g., cognitive behavior therapy) as well as qualified psychiatrists (Practitioner Health).

What this service offers is:

(a) A route by which healthcare professionals who are worried about the effects of disclosing their illness somewhere where they can unburden themselves in an environment far enough away from their place of work. This makes it possible to allay their fears about the possible consequences of disclosure however unrealistic these may be.
(b) A service where medical attention and other therapeutic input are more readily, and more quickly available via the National Health Service.

Through economies of scale, it is, clearly, easier to provide a bespoke, dedicated health service for doctors and dentists in highly populated areas. The National Health Service England GP Health Service commits itself to putting a GP who is in need of help in touch with a practitioner within 1–2 h travelling time of their home.

Rural Areas

A problem that arises in rural areas is that there may be only one medical or specialist psychiatric team and the doctor in need of support may have past or present professional associations with that team or may be referring patients to them on a regular basis (Grant et al. 2019b). Referral to specialists outside the area requires an agreement for funding from the local trust or health board which in many cases will be the practitioner's employer. It is not reasonable to expect a health professional who is unwell to have to negotiate with senior staff in their own health board or trust for payment to be released for their treatment in a place where confidentiality and their feeling of safety are not compromised.

As a frequent and predictable event (a medical or dental practitioner having a mental health problem and needing professional help), there needs to be a protocol in place before it is needed by a practitioner with a health problem that they do not feel comfortable discussing with work colleagues.

- Work with the professional bodies across the healthcare professions to reverse current attitudes to mental health from within the professions.
- Recognize the particular needs of practitioners in rural areas.

Conclusion

Within this chapter, there are a number of recommendations to improve the support for students and professionals with mental health problems and the fears around disclosure. These include:

Ensuring that a significant proportion of students and faculty have training in mental health first aid
Awareness-raising initiatives to bring discussion about mental health out into the open
A recognition of the pernicious effect of fears that disclosure of a mental illness will damage students' and practitioners' careers and that this may act as a barrier to healthcare and support
Creating pathways to medical care that take account of students' and practitioners worries about the effect of disclosure of a mental illness on their career
Creating opportunities for staff to talk about the emotional aspects of their work in a safe environment, e.g., in Balint groups and Schwarz rounds

Cross-References

- Coaching in Health Professions Education: The Case of Surgery
- Conversational Learning in Health Professions Education: Learning Through Talk
- Developing Care and Compassion in Health Professional Students and Clinicians
- Developing Professional Identity in Health Professional Students

References

Alcohol Policy.
Aboshaiqah AE, Preposi Cruz J. Quality of life and its predictors among nursing students in Saudi Arabia. J Holist Nurs. 2018;37:200–8.
Batty, D. Cambridge drinking societies under threat as students reveal darkest secrets. The Guardian. London, Guardian Newspapers. (2018).
Bloodgood R, Short J, Jackson J, Martindale J. A change to pass/fail grading in the first two years at one medical school results in improved psychological well-being. Acad Med. 2009;84:655–62.
Compton MT, Carrera J, Frank E. Stress and depressive symptoms/dysphoria among US medical students: results from a large, nationally representative survey. J Nerv Ment Dis. 2008;196(12): 891–7.
Dahlin M, Joneborg N, Runeson B. Stress and depression among medical students: a cross-sectional study. Med Educ. 2005;39(6):594–604.
Dahlin M, Joneborg N, Runeson B. Performance-based self-esteem and burnout in a cross-sectional study of medical students. Med Teacher. 2007;29, 43(1):–48. Retrieved 7909593, mf9, 29, from http://ovidsp.ovid.com/ovidweb.cgi?T=JS&PAGE=reference&D=med4&NEWS=N&AN=17538833

Drolet BC, Rodgers S. A comprehensive medical student wellness program-design and implementation at Vanderbilt School of Medicine. Acad Med. 2010;85(1):103–10.

Dyrbye LN, Thomas MR, Huschka MM, Lawson KL, Novotny PJ, Sloan JA, Shanafelt TD. A multicenter study of burnout, depression, and quality of life in minority and nonminority US medical students. Mayo Clin Proc. 2006;81(11):1435–42. Retrieved 0405543, lly, 81, from http://ovidsp.ovid.com/ovidweb.cgi?T=JS&PAGE=reference&D=med4&NEWS=N&AN=17120398

Enns M, Cox B, Sareen J, Freeman P. Adaptive and maladaptive perfectionism in medical students: a longitudinal investigation. Med Educ. 2001;35:1034–42.

Eyala E, Roseman D, Winseman J, Mason H. Prevalence, perceptions, and consequences of substance use in medical students. Med Educ Online. 2017;22(1):1392824.

Farrell S, Molodynski A, Cohen D, Grant A, Rees S, Wullshleger A, Lewis T, Kadhum M. Wellbeing and burnout among medical students in Wales. Int Rev Psych. 2019;31:613–8.

Fontes de Oliva Costa E, Rocha EMV, de Abreu Santos AR, de Melo EV, Nogueira Martins LA, Andrade TM. Common mental disorders and associated factors among final-year healthcare students. Rev Assoc Med Bras. 2014;60(6):525–30.

Grant A, Kowalczuk J, Marrin K, Porter A, Rix A. Trainee doctors' views on mental illness among their peers and access to support services. Int Rev Psychiatry. 2019a; https://doi.org/10.1080/09540261.2019.1616893.

Grant A, Rix A, Mattick K, Winter P, Jones D. Identifying good practice among medical schools in the support of medical students with mental health concerns: a report prepared for the General Medical Council. Cardiff: Cardiff University; 2013.

Grant A, Rix A, Shrewsbury D. If you're crying this much you shouldn't be a consultant': the lived experience of UK doctors in training with mental illness*. Int Rev Psychiatry. 2019b; https://doi.org/10.1080/09540261.2019.1586326.

Grant A, Rix A, Winter P, Mattick K, Jones D. Support for medical students with mental health problems: a conceptual model. Acad Psychiatry. 2014;39:16–21.

Hazards. Is mental health first aid the answer? Hazards magazine, 141, (2018). From http://www.hazards.org/stress/mentalhealth.htm

Jadoon N, Yaqoob R, Raza A, Shehzad M, Zeshan SC. Anxiety and depression among medical students: a cross-sectional study. JPMA J Pakistan Med Assoc. 2010;60(8):699–702.

Kabat-Zinn J. An outpatient programme in behavioural medicine for chronic pain patients based on the practice of mindfulness meditation: theoretical considerations and preliminary results. Gen Hosp Psychiatry. 1982;4:33–47.

Kenna GA, Woo M. Substance use by pharmacy and nursing practitioners and students in a northeastern state. Am J Health Syst Pharm. 2004;61(9):921–30.

Koter T, Yanick T, Obst K, Voltmer E, Scherer M. Health-promoting factors in the freshman year of medical school: a longitudinal study. Med Educ. 2016;50(6):646–56.

Lamberti M, Napolitano F, Napolitano P, Arnese A, Crispino C, Panariello G, Di Giuseppe G. Prevalence of alcohol use disorders among under- and post-graduate healthcare students in Italy. PLoS One. 2017;12(4):e0175719.

Lomas T, Medina JC, Ivtzan I, Rupprecht S, Eiroa-Orosa FJ. A systematic review of the impact of mindfulness on the well-being of healthcare professionals. J Clin Psychol. 2018;74:319–55.

Moutier C, Norcross W, Jong P, Norman M, Kirby B, McGuire T, Zisook S. The suicide prevention and depression awareness program at the University of California, San Diego School of Medicine. Acad Med. 2012;87(3):320–6.

Point of Care Foundation. Schwarz rounds. Retrieved 05/05/2020, 2020., from https://www.pointofcarefoundation.org.uk/our-work/schwartz-rounds/

Practitioner Health, N. About Practitioner Health. Retrieved 05/05/2020, 2020., from https://www.practitionerhealth.nhs.uk/about-practitioner-health

Roberts LW. Caring for medical students as patients: access to services and care-seeking practices of 1,027 students at nine medical schools. Acad Med. 2000;75(3):272–7.

Rohe D, Barrier P, Clark M, Cook D, Vickers K, Decker P. The benefits of pass–fail grading on stress, mood, and group cohesion in medical students. Mayo Clin Proc. 2006;81:1443–8.

Rosenzweig S, Reibel D, Greeson J, Brainard G, Hojat M. Mindfulness based stress reduction lowers psychological distress in medical students. Teach Learn Med. 2003;15:88–92.

Ross C, Goldner E. Stigma, negative attitudes and discrimination towards mental illness within the nursing profession: a review of the literature. J Psychiatr Ment Health Nurs. 2009;16:558–67.

Salinsky, J. Balint groups and the Balint method. (2013). Retrieved 05/05/2020, 2020, from https://balint.co.uk/about/the-balint-method/

Slavin SJ, Hatchett L, Chibnall JT, Schindler D, Fendell G. Helping medical students and residents flourish: a path to transform medical education. Acad Med. 2011;86:e15.

Spring L, Robillard D, Gehlbach L, Simas TAM. Impact of pass/fail grading on medical students' well-being and academic outcomes. Med Educ. 2011;45(9):867–77.

Swansea University and Students' Union, Swansea University.

Syed A, Ali S, Khan M. Frequency of depression, anxiety and stress among the undergraduate physiotherapy students. Pak J Med Sci. 2018;34(2):468–71.

Tavolacci M, Delay J, Grigioni S, Déchelotte P, Ladner J. Changes and specificities in health behaviors among healthcare students over an 8-year period. PLoS One. 2018;13(3):e0194188.

Wengraf T. Life-histories, lived situations and ongoing personal experiencing: the biographic-narrative interpretive method (BNIM). Guide to BNIM interviewing and interpretation. London: London East Research Institute, University of East London, UK; 2008.

Winter P, Rix A, Grant A. Medical student beliefs about disclosure of mental health issues: a qualitative study. J Vet Med Educ. 2017;44(1):147–56.

Embedding a Simulation-Based Education Program in a Teaching Hospital

53

Rebecca A. Szabo and Kirsty Forrest

Contents

Introduction	1018
Embedding a Simulation Program in a Teaching Hospital	1019
Why the Term "Embed"?	1019
A Starting Guide to the Implementation Phase	1019
Implementation of SBE	1019
Understand Your Environment and Uncertainty	1020
Understand the 3Cs: Culture, Context, and Complexity	1020
Know How to Implement and/or Improve Something in that Environment and Culture	1021
Working with the Barriers and Enablers	1021
Barriers, Enablers and, What to Do with them	1023
Using Translational Simulation to Solve a hospital's Problem	1030
Know the External Landscape	1032
Understand Leadership and Change Management	1032
Leadership Versus Management	1033
The Power of the Narrative	1035
Conclusion	1036
References	1037

Abstract

This chapter provides an impression of why simulation and simulation-based education (SBE) in teaching hospitals are not yet as prevalent as they should be despite decades of experience and research. An overview of how someone might start and/or sustain an SBE program in a teaching hospital is provided with the

R. A. Szabo (✉)
Department of Obstetrics & Gynaecology and Department of Medical Education, Gandel Simulation Service The Royal Women's Hospital, University of Melbourne, Melbourne, VIC, Australia
e-mail: rebecca.szabo@unimelb.edu.au

K. Forrest
Faculty of Health Sciences and Medicine, Bond University, Gold Coast, QLD, Australia
e-mail: kiforres@bond.edu.au

© Springer Nature Singapore Pte Ltd. 2023
D. Nestel et al. (eds.), *Clinical Education for the Health Professions*,
https://doi.org/10.1007/978-981-15-3344-0_69

intention of embedding a program. Barriers and enablers to introducing and embedding an SBE program are intimately intertwined. Knowledge of barriers and enablers of SBE is important, as these will always exist particularly in complex organizations with uncertainty. While it would be nice to provide a practical step-by-step model of how to embed an SBE program in a teaching hospital, each hospital has its own culture, context, and complexity so any individual or team looking to embed SBE needs to appreciate these elements. Anyone directing SBE needs to understand change management, organizational complexity, and leadership for successful implementation of sustainable SBE in teaching hospitals such that they are embedded and treated as any other operational service a hospital cannot do without.

Keywords

Simulation · Simulation-Based Education (SBE) · Implementation · Barriers · Enablers · Leadership · Change Management · Uncertainty

Introduction

This chapter will:

1. Describe why simulation and SBE in hospitals are not yet as prevalent as it should be
2. Describe how you can start and/or sustain an SBE program in a teaching hospital
3. Explain how SBE can be embedded in a teaching hospital

There have been many decades of experience and evidence for simulation-based education (SBE) in healthcare, but SBE programs in teaching hospitals are still not seen as business as usual. Those hospitals that do have simulation centers often struggle as funding is in competition with healthcare service provision. For many organizations, it has been easier to stick with business as usual and maintain traditional healthcare education practices with either none or a little SBE.

Healthcare has changed significantly in the time that SBE has matured. There have been significant healthcare advancements, new medications, treatments, and an exponential growth of knowledge. In 1950, the doubling time of medical knowledge was 50 years, in 2020 it will be 73 days (Densen 2011). The impact is that people are living longer, often with more medical problems increasing the complexity and acuity seen in hospitals. All of this means more money is spent in healthcare and by hospitals than ever before. That is almost always without a similar increase in hospital budgets to allow for both service and education. Given this reality, if someone wants to either maintain or start an SBE program in a teaching hospital, what do they do?

This chapter is written as a guide. There is no easy recipe or checklist to follow. Just like most education and clinical encounters, every SBE program will need to be tailored to its local context. This is because primarily establishing and sustaining an SBE program is more about implementation science, change management, and leadership than it is about SBE specifically. The following provides an overview of these concepts and how they relate to establishing and sustaining or *embedding* SBE programs in a teaching hospital.

Embedding a Simulation Program in a Teaching Hospital

Why the Term "Embed"?

The definition of embed is for something to be fixed firmly and deeply. There are ongoing challenges for many SBE programs, even those at established centers worldwide. In 2004, Gaba stated that "The future of simulation in health care depends on the commitment and ingenuity of the healthcare simulation community to see that improved patient safety using this tool becomes a reality" (Gaba 2004). Over a decade later in 2015, Stefanidis et al. noted that "despite the scientific advances and strong evidence to support SBE, actual implementation remains variable and lagging substantially" (Stefanidis et al. 2015). Practically, how do we not just start an SBE program but embed it, so it is seen as much as core business as any other department in a hospital and not just that "training thing"?

A Starting Guide to the Implementation Phase

Implementation of SBE

> Good ideas with no ideas on how to implement them are wasted ideas. (Fullan 2001)

What Do We Do to Actually Implement, Sustain, and Embed SBE?

In education and training, before we introduce or substantially change a curriculum, we first take a step back and perform a "needs analysis." This is to identify the needs or gaps of learners to ensure the curriculum meets the users' needs. This is not dissimilar to the diagnostic phase of any clinical encounter. A similar approach is required to implement any new program particularly in something as complex as a hospital. Just saying so we need SBE because it's good or done at X hospital will set you up for failure.

Rostering interprofessional staff, funding, resources, and so on, are all challenges to implementing SBE. Additionally, hospitals are complex adaptive systems and any program implemented and sustained within such a system must coexist with the clinical service load. Therefore, a deep understanding of not only SBE pedagogy is needed, but the complex environment of a hospital, particularly the hospital in which you are trying to embed the program.

> *"So, you want to lead a SBE program in a teaching hospital...."*

Understand Your Environment and Uncertainty

Hospital are complex adaptive systems. Hospital and health service uncertainty is a reality of modern times, politics, and influences funding as well as healthcare and education making everything dynamic. Most people who implement any change management program in a hospital experience the realities of inherent uncertainty due to changes in leadership, government, and funding. This particularly impacts all education in hospitals, including SBE, as service understandably takes priority.

Fiscal challenges for SBE are not merely around finding money, but around showing worth and "return on investment" both initially and ongoing. This presents a very real challenge to all SBE experts regardless of geographical location. As described in the health policy literature, *"policy makers, hospital administrators and scholars of health policy are all interested to promote "value for money" technology adoptions at a hospital level. In particular, it is critical to avoid that technology that has been adopted with great fanfare and promise will become quickly a failure and abandoned"* (Lettieri 2009). This applies to SBE whereby decades of application and evidence is often viewed as an expensive innovation.

Those who have been successful in embedding SBE programs are acutely aware of this uncertainty. Anyone endeavoring to take on such a challenge needs to be equally aware and equipped to deal with this uncertainty which primarily means being flexible and able to lead regardless of any barriers or enablers and not just manage or deliver SBE. Some of the leadership qualities needed beyond a good understanding of SBE include persistence, dependability, sociability, creativity, and open-mindedness. Leaders over time, and often by necessity, develop skills to overcome uncertainty and challenges and should be supported in this by their organizations.

Understand the 3Cs: Culture, Context, and Complexity

> Culture in anthropology is the sum total of what any group, organization, or nation has learned throughout its history in coping with survival and managing its internal relationships. (Darling 2017)

Every organization will have its own culture and any strategy or change must occur within this cultural context (Szabo et al. 2017). Local context, culture, and politics of a hospital play a significant role and are likely more important than whether a hospital is within a public or private health service or its geographical location for successful outcome for change.

Teaching hospitals and healthcare systems have *"enormous complexity—both in lay terms by its complicated design and in scientific terms by its nonlinear, dynamic, and unpredictable nature"* (Lipsitz 2012). The leader understanding this complexity and unpredictability in the context of local culture and politics, and using this as a lever, is vital to being able to both implement and sustain SBE. This is key across financial challenges, engagement, and executive buy-in. Thus, leadership within the hospital cultural context is an important foundational concept. As Schein describes in "Organizational Culture and Leadership" – *"leadership and culture are fundamentally intertwined"* (Schein 1997).

Know How to Implement and/or Improve Something in that Environment and Culture

Two relatively new areas of scientific research can guide us in the implementation phase, **implementation science**, and **improvement science**. Implementation science and improvement science are distinct fields that share characteristics so there is significant overlap. The conceptual frame of reference for improvement science allows a broad scope of scientific study about which improvement strategies work best in a complex hospital system (Bauer et al. 2015). Implementation science scholars argue that the introduction of novel practices into established healthcare organizations requires much effort and needs to be "informed by an assessment of the likely barriers and enablers" (Braithwaite et al. 2014). Further reading and understanding of both these emerging sciences is useful for anyone leading an SBE program in a teaching hospital (Fig. 1).

Working with the Barriers and Enablers

Implementation scientists, Gardner and Lazzara, have previously explored implementation of SBE in hospitals. Lazzara et al., in 2014, described the eight success factors and tips for incorporating them into simulation programs (Lazzara et al. 2014). These eight "S" factors – science, staff, supplies, space, support, systems, success, and sustainability represent their synthesis of the most critical elements

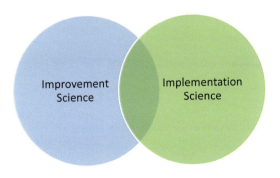

Fig. 1 Intersection of improvement and implementation science

necessary for successful simulation programs (Lazzara et al. 2014). Gardner et al. (2015) endeavored to outline a blueprint to success through identifying five domains – (1) Obtaining buy-in, (2) Funding, (3) Governance, (4) Space and equipment, and (5) Faculty development (Gardner et al. 2015). These constructs by Lazzara et al. and Gardner et al. provide guides and theoretical frameworks to what is needed. These themes are similar to each other and those outlined below demonstrating which is useful to understand. However, the fundamental key to bringing all this together is *leadership*.

Barriers and enablers to implementation of SBE in healthcare are often from similar categories such that they are enmeshed and interlinked (Stefanidis et al. 2015). Much of the guide and quotes below originate from research undertaken by Dr. Rebecca Szabo with Professor Margaret Bearman and Robert O'Brien looking at how to embed an SBE program or center in a teaching hospital (Szabo et al. 2017; Selected abstracts 2018). Six interlinked themes encompassing both barriers and enablers were identified. These themes are engagement of people, funding challenges, executive "buy-in," context playing a key role, research, and natural evolution of a program. Faculty development and promotion of SBE are the most important enablers and funding challenges particularly demonstrating "worth" and "return on investment" are the most significant barriers. Knowing the barriers and enablers is a useful starting point but it's important to remember there will always be barriers and enablers. The key is leadership, and an ability to adapt and be flexible to overcome and foresee barriers ahead, while also maximizeing enablers (Fig. 2).

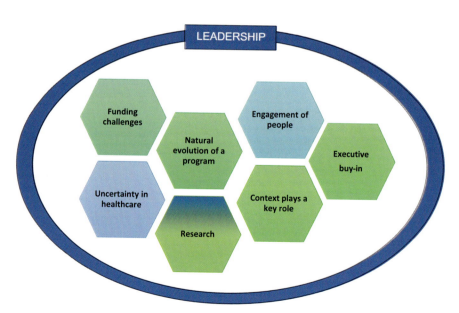

Fig. 2 Barriers and enablers to embed a sustainable SBE program in a teaching hospital (Szabo et al. 2017; Selected abstracts 2018)

Barriers, Enablers and, What to Do with them

Knowing the barriers and enablers is important to understand the landscape but perhaps matter less than the leadership attributes of SBE directors. Barriers will always exist given the complexity of hospitals and the inherent uncertainty in healthcare funding and of funding of education, particularly SBE (Szabo et al. 2017). What is paramount are the qualities and skills of the person implementing and running an SBE program to lead and transform culture to overcome whatever barriers exist and amplify any accessible enablers. The qualities and skills of the "leader" are as vital to successful implementation and sustainability. Without an understanding of leadership and uncertainty, there is a risk programs may have a false start and not be sustainable (Szabo et al. 2017).

Funding Challenges and Becoming Operational

Funding challenges in SBE are complex and can refer to the difficulty in both obtaining and maintaining funding. This can include the difficulties in implementing and sustaining an SBE program without a reliable and operational budget. This barrier is at times very significant and often emphasized by leaders in the field because it highlights the inherent uncertainty faced by SBE programs due to the intrinsic lack of reliable funding.

> I mean, if you don't have money, no money, no mission. (Expert2, USA)

Any SBE program or center requires initial funding for infrastructure, staff, and faculty hours and training, expensive simulation equipment, maintenance and audio-visual support. Funding, financial support or lack of it, fiscal drivers, and return on investment are interwoven acting as both barriers and enablers. Simplistically, if funding is available, a program can start. If further funding is obtained, the program can continue, and once the program has demonstrated its worth, it is more likely to obtain an operational budget. "Value" and showing "worth" were seen as important to demonstrate to hospital executives and staff.

> A very rigorous, well thought out realistic business plan that said to the organisation it's not always about money, that it will be a large investment and you may not recoup your investment in terms of monetary value, in allowing them to understand that you will recoup it in other ways, in terms of staff training and development, mitigating risk, research, promoting a culture of safety, all of those things, ticking all those boxes. (Expert1, Aus.)

We live in a world of ever-increasing healthcare costs compounded by reducing health budgets. It is a reality that in austere times hospitals will first cut money from education to ensure patient care is not compromised (Szabo et al. 2017). SBE programs need to get to a point of proving their "worth" and return on investment to overcome a lack of reliable funding and reliance on other mechanisms to ensure "survival."

In order to embed an SBE program, a leader needs to leverage any initial funding to ensure an operational budget is achieved by proving "worth." Often, seed funding has come from small grants or philanthropy. Finances required have often been minimized by staff volunteering and programs *"making do."* For a program to innovate and grow, as well as be sustainable within a teaching hospital, funding needs to be operationalized.

> In principle, they give us the best part of $1 million every year and I think that is now written into the hospital budget, it's an operating budget for us, so it's seen as just part of the norm… (Expert1, Aus.)

SBE program directors can secure and maintain an operational budget by knowing the barriers and removing or minimizing them. For example, paying a technician to set up and clean up reduced the amount required to pay senior medical specialists who then only needed to attend to teach.

> Your job as an operations person is to lower the barriers. Lower the barriers to simulation. (Expert3, Can)

Return on investment is part of ensuring ongoing funding and vital to demonstrating value and impact to senior management and any outside funders whether philanthropy or other grant bodies. Effective SBE experts recognize a need to demonstrate impact and value.

> "Someone has got to pay for it…they've got to recognise return on investment, or they've got to be visionary. Not many people are visionary, especially when it comes to money."
> "The people in the 'C' suite……they care about – if I put my money into this, am I going to get a return on investment?" (Expert2, USA)

Effectively demonstrating impact and value is an enabler for a program to both obtain and maintain funding. The ongoing challenge for SBE sustainability is the difficulty in evaluating and demonstrating return on investment and value to an organization particularly for rare emergencies and in countries with already low morbidity and/or mortality. SBE experts who have been able to successfully embed their programs have been able to convince their organizations of their worth. However, it is still seen as precarious and needing to be constantly proven. Knowing how to prove value relates to culture and context, as described earlier.

> Sustainability in terms of not just the dollar, sustainability to me means the value add. (Expert1, Aus.)

Having a business "strategy" is important. Understanding targets, managing the budget, and being able to justify SBE as a "business" are all important. These skills may be challenging to healthcare and education professionals not necessarily trained in business. Understanding the language of business and how to speak with the executives and donors is an essential enabler going forward, particularly in times of austerity.

> We need to speak the language of the CEOs and the CFOs. If we don't, we're going to be out of business. (Expert2, USA)

Additionally, the role of external revenue raising is important as both a potential barrier and enabler. The constant challenge of balancing external and internal business with one team of staff was deemed a significant barrier to sustainability and delivery of curriculum internally.

> External business and that's probably one of the constraints to us, is that at the end of the month, we are expected to get a certain amount of revenue but at the same time what counteracts that is they want to know what we've done internally and there is only a bucket of staff to go so far so that's probably our hardest thing at this point in time. (Expert1, Aus.)

Beyond this tension of "balance" is a need to think strategically, like a "businessperson," and be a step ahead of the perceived inevitable cost cutting because it is inevitable that education and SBE will be impacted early. Various strategies include diversifying to provide hospital design and testing, partnering with industry, use of a center or program by other industries including television, film, and sporting teams and international consulting. Significantly these challenges are independent of the type of health service, that is, public models in Australia and Canada versus private in the USA. Thus, the uncertainty and difficulty obtaining and maintaining funding may be an independent feature of SBE in healthcare.

National Evolution of a Program

Most SBE hospital programs tend to naturally evolve from a single course or simulation. They start small and build up from there. Most SBE hospital programs start with a single person or small group of people with more enthusiasm for SBE, rather than SBE leadership experience. This is also often true of funding, physical space, faculty, and equipment. The phrases "make-do" and "over time" are commonly heard from SBE experts.

You're working with a shoestring budget and you've just got to make do. Then gradually over time things evolve and people see value.... (Expert2, USA)

Traditionally in SBE programs much of this evolution has come about by persistence, perseverance, and experience. SBE experts describe successes and failures along the way leading to overall triumph of embedding SBE with time.

Start small. Get really good at it and then expand it. (Expert2, USA)

Purpose

Purpose and shared purpose can be a sometimes hidden but vital enabler. Making this shared purpose explicit to all those involved in an SBE program, as well as a hospital, can make a big difference in success or failure. Purpose or mission is important to aid program directors creating and adhering to strategic goals and objectives for themselves and the organization. If there is change in focus to external revenue raising or diversification, there is a risk of losing sight of the original purpose and not fulfilling the intended mission, thus alienating those who were engaged and had buy-in.

Innovation and Research

Innovation in SBE programs applies to both implementation and sustainability. It refers to both innovation of a program and having innovative ideas or solutions to move forward. SBE itself can still be viewed as an innovation and SBE experts as pioneers of this innovative pedagogy. While a physical center for SBE may not necessarily be needed, particularly with in situ simulation, a shared space may facilitate engagement and communication within the team and act as a catalyst for growth and innovation.

Research and data are important for funding, promotion, and integrity of SBE. Research as an enabler and barrier is a relatively new concept being introduced here. This can be represented by the challenge of conducting research in an educational setting and the need for research to further SBE. The reality is that research and evaluation are necessary to promote and publicize the efforts of any SBE program as well as to contribute evidence to the wider SBE and healthcare communities. Challenges faced by many programs to conduct research in SBE include not having the time or resources, partly due to a focus on "doing" and providing education.

We did a study and that proved that sim [simulation]-based training was more effective than traditional discharge teaching. (Expert3, Can)

Research has become an increasingly important feature of SBE for several reasons: (1) Potential grant funding and funding for research assistants, (2) Publications in high impact journals, and (3) Focus of hospital boards and executives on research and evidence-based medicine and education.

Several programs have overcome challenges to incorporate research by employing research assistants with education backgrounds who could contribute to both the education and research outputs of the SBE program and/or center. Going forward in increasingly austere times, opportunities to obtain research funding will be essential to sustainability of any SBE program. This can also help demonstrate influence of SBE to executives, universities, and healthcare professionals affiliated with hospitals.

Context Plays a Key Role: Politics and Culture

It is vital that you know your organization and identify both the things and people that will get in your way, and the things and people that will help you succeed. Context plays a key role and is specific to the actual institution and its own microcosm of politics and culture. This is an important notion impacting on sustainability of SBE and important for anyone leading an SBE program. As a leader of an SBE program it is important to understand your organization as a whole and what will assist with growth and what will hinder.

> The hard part is operationalising it, developing a strategy in your culture, in your political environment, in your financial environment that will allow you to grow simulation. (Expert2, USA)

Hospital politics is an unfortunate reality and understanding the "politics" is key to overcoming barriers. If we can understand "politics," we may be able to embed SBE in a hospital far earlier and far more effectively.

> It's all about politics. It's about understanding who your friends are, understanding who your enemies are, understanding who your champions are. (Expert2, USA)

The concept of "culture" encapsulates two aspects: (1) The culture, defined as values or beliefs, of the hospital acts to enable or hinder SBE implementation and sustainability; and (2) SBE has the ability to impact hospital culture particularly by encouraging a "culture of safety."

Engagement of People, Faculty Development, and Champions

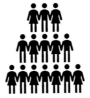

> Engagement of people and faculty development are probably the most important of the enablers and if this is not done effectively the most significant barrier.

Understanding of people to ensure engagement through a willingness to be inclusive and develop and promote others forms an important foundation to embed an SBE program in a teaching hospital. This requires transformational leadership by those directors and managers running SBE programs and clear modeling of leadership qualities.

> You've got to walk the walk and talk the talk. You can't just talk the talk. (Expert2, USA)

Part of this strategic leadership approach includes ensuring all departments and staff feel the SBE program is "theirs," that they have some level of ownership and entitlement to use it. There are different methods to achieve this result. At its core this is around collaboration, champions, and inclusiveness. Mostly, this requires the SBE director to have "leadership" qualities – to be someone who is well liked, well known to others, and someone who has a deep understanding of the hospital environment, culture, politics, and people to be able to influence those they did not necessarily have authority over.

As described, SBE program directors need to have a collaborative and inclusive approach to working with others including healthcare professionals, educators, and executives. This willingness to listen and ability to have others trust both you as the director and then by extension the pedagogy of SBE can enable and enhance engagement. This is key to sustaining SBE and being able to truly embed an SBE program in a teaching hospital.

Faculty development with some kind of formal training in SBE is vital for SBE programs. This ensures that faculty are well trained in simulation and as educators, thus able to provide best practice SBE.

> You've got to do faculty development. You've got to help people learn how to do this. (Expert2, USA)

This interlinks with collaboration, inclusion, and champions. Once trained, faculty from wide-ranging areas of the hospital may feel greater sense of ownership which strengthens collaboration, participation, and buy-in.

Champions and Promotion of SBE

A "champion" is defined as "a person who vigorously supports or defends a person or cause" (Oxford English Dictionary 2017). Champions can and will advocate for SBE and promote it further within the organization and elsewhere. Champions are people to be identified, developed, and mentored to act as exemplars of SBE faculty and can then assist both actively and passively by engaging others in SBE.

This is one form of "marketing" which can be a significant enabler to get the message out there to show worth to the executive and others. Having champions is one way to get the message of SBE and the specific program and/or center out, effectively, and with no advertising money required.

Champions. You need champions. You need to market every chance you get. You need to talk about it. I have a hotline to the public relations people. You've got to be self-promoting in that way. (Expert2, USA)

The reason such "self-promotion" is necessary alongside humbleness, collaboration, and inclusivity is to get the message out there and stay continually relevant. Engagement with patients, families, and the broader community is also important. Methods of promotion include tours of an SBE center by executive, patients and families, the local community, staff and media. Another key method of promotion in today's world is the use of social media particularly Twitter, Instagram, FaceBook, and LinkedIn.

Promotion of SBE by those outside the hospital to the executive can also be seen as making a substantial impact, particularly related to patient safety.

Other industries promoting simulation for us is a great thing, so it more or less helps validate us. If someone comes in who's a huge safety expert that says to every public hospital, every teaching hospital in Australia should have one of these.... that's one of the things that has helped promote simulation, that's one of the things that has made a difference, you know that helped embed simulation at the XX Hospital. (Expert1, Aus.)

Executive Buy-in and Visionary Leadership

Executive support is significant for embedding SBE in a hospital and may be too as "top-down," "buy-in," and executive leadership or engagement. Engagement by senior executives, including CEO, CFO, COO, and hospital board as well as any affiliated hospital foundations and donors, is vital to embed an SBE program. If there is no "buy-in" or worse, opposition from executives, this can be a significant barrier to SBE.

It is critical for success to have "buy-in" and support from above. This is in part to ensure the barriers to obtaining funds, resources, and space are not obstructed by leaders who do not believe in or support SBE in an already underfunded healthcare system. Different approaches to getting this "buy-in" can be taken, but any SBE leader must be acutely aware of this issue.

Those leading SBE also need to be aware this can change with any new executive member or change in board focus. This reinforces the underlying theme of inherent uncertainty for SBE that has been described above. If there is insufficient "buy-in" from CEO or other executive members, or the "buy-in" changes, funding, and resources for SBE may be removed. This particularly overlaps with the concepts of "champions and promotion" and "return on investment" to highlight how fundamental it is to ensure executives and donors, in particular, are aware of what the SBE program is achieving.

Simulation experts can be viewed as "pioneers and innovators" given the relatively young age of SBE. Visionary leadership, particularly in the 1990s and early 2000s, was seen as indispensable to enable SBE to be embedded and will be beneficial ongoing. Visionary leadership also applies to a hospital CEO who is able to greatly influence from the top-down. Being visionary means being prepared to take risks, being imaginative, resourceful, and inspired. These are all qualities that would assist in support of SBE even during especially austere times.

"Solve Someone's Problem"

To obtain support is one thing that is key in knowing how to "solve someone's problem" or "diagnosing the pain" and "fixing it." This can be very persuasive and useful to engage executives and hospital directors. Relating back always to quality and safety is key. This can also be used to demonstrate impact either on a large scale or by saving the hospital money or demonstrably mitigating significant risk particularly if related to recent incidents that is "problems." It can help get "traction" around SBE, "buy-in," and consequently funding and support.

> You've got to solve someone's problem. In order to get traction, you've got to solve a problem....Again top down. (Expert2, USA)

> Not only turned the execs head, turned the boards head and that's what they want us to do, turn the boards head. (Expert1, Aus.)

Solving someone's problem can also include using simulation to identify and solve problems for an organization. This is best described by the concept of translational simulation as first described by Professor Victoria Brazil (2017).

Using Translational Simulation to Solve a hospital's Problem

The term "translational simulation" is a more functional term for how simulation may be connected directly with health service priorities and patient outcomes, through interventional and diagnostic functions (Brazil 2017). Using in situ simulation, or in the clinical space simulation, new systems can be developed and implemented, such as introduction of new equipment or an Electronic Medical Record (EMR) to test how they would perform in real life and iron out any issues before actual implementation. In situ simulation is more than just a teaching tool because it can be used to test systems and improve the quality and delivery of healthcare in the actual clinical space. This can appeal significantly to hospital executives, quality and safety units and boards who need these "problems solved."

Keeping in mind some of the barriers above, including funding, the advantage of in situ simulation over a simulation center or "laboratory" includes reduced need for a physical center and associated resources. Translational simulation provides improved transfer of knowledge and skills into real-world practice, as well as opportunities to identify latent safety threats and other workplace-specific issues. In this way translational simulation can and has been used to test systems, demonstrate, and improve efficiency and usability (Petrosoniak et al. 2018), all things that address a hospital's problems (Fig. 3).

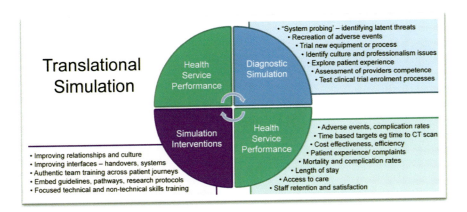

Fig. 3 Translational Simulation (Brazil 2017)

Potential applications of translational simulation to "solve problems," include:

- Examine workflow
- Improve culture
- Practice teamwork and communication
- Orient staff to new policies, procedures, and equipment
- Assess the efficacy of a system and identify gaps
- Practice rare events

Case Example: Implementation of an Electronic Medical Record (EMR)

The widespread implementation of EMRs globally has resulted in both benefits and unintended consequences, with the latter linked to the potential of causing significant adverse outcomes and patient harm, in part due to poor implementation strategies and EMR customization as well as lack of user training (Sittig et al. 2006; Mohan et al. 2016).

The Institute of Medicine (IOM) and American Medical Informatics Association (AMIA) have identified EMR development, implementation, and training as key areas for new research to improve healthcare quality and safety. The Institute of Medicine (IOM) and the National Institute of Standards and Technology (NIST) recommend the use of simulation to aid in EMR education (Stephenson et al. 2014). Simulation provides a tool to both identify these gaps and foster EMR-specific training at the same time as simulating clinical scenarios and applying evidence-based guidelines (Milano et al. 2014; March et al. 2013).

Simulation activities, particularly high-fidelity EMR-specific simulation training, afford an attractive potential solution that directly addresses some

(continued)

of these issues due to the fact that they can create realistic, reproducible environments without any chance of patient risk (Mohan et al. 2016; Rosen 2008). Simulation has also been used to reorient clinicians to ensure that negative EMR-related behaviors such as poor eye contact and prolonged screen gazing do not undermine patient-centerd communication (Lee et al. 2017).

Know the External Landscape

There are many factors driving the need to increase reliability within healthcare organizations to mitigate unwanted variability in the care we provide to patients. Several standards to drive the implementation of safety and quality systems and to improve quality care in hospitals have been published. Various government body safety reports have also been released to work to eliminate avoidable harm and strengthen quality of care. Additionally, globally several public and private hospital insurance underwriters have supported simulation as a risk management strategy. A model is used in Boston for the Harvard University affiliated group of hospitals and elsewhere.

An Australian Case Study: Understanding the Role of Insurance

The state-wide public hospital insurance body in Victoria, Australia, the Victorian Managed Insurance Authority (VMIA), has recognized the importance of team-based interprofessional simulation-based education for maternity and newborn emergencies by introducing an incentivization program "striving for better outcomes and encourage participation in best practice training, which has been demonstrated to improve care and outcomes for women and babies (VMIA 2018)."

VMIA introduced the Incentivising Better Patient Safety (IBSP) Guide. This program, focused on multi-professional simulation, means that "public maternity services that provide maternity training according to certain criteria will receive a refund of 5% on the obstetrics component of their medical indemnity premiums (VMIA 2018)."

Understand Leadership and Change Management

"The most dangerous phrase in the English language is, *'we've always done it that way'.*" [Rear Admiral Grace Hopper 1906–1992].

(continued)

> There's a commitment to start a simulation program. There's some money, some time, some equipment. How do you ensure it is not just started but also successful and lasting? People, invest in people and culture and the rest will follow.

> Successful leaders, whatever the organisation will listen, link and lead. In so doing, they bring about change not by implementing given visions from their powerbase but by reconciling factors and divisions to achieve reform that motivates groups to unify their change efforts. (Fullan and Scott 2009)

Knowing the barriers and enablers is useful but there will always be barriers and enablers. These may stay the same or change with changing culture, staff, and internal and external influences. In order to maximize enablers and overcome barriers, as well as have the foresight to predict what is ahead, it is vital to understand leadership and change management as essential elements to embedding an SBE program.

To embed an SBE program, directors need to be leaders and agents of change, not merely managers to overcome both the uncertainty and complexity inherent in hospitals and healthcare. Leadership models that best align for this type of change include *transformational leadership*, *dialogic change*, and *influence without authority* theories. An extensive list of ideal leadership traits has been described in business, change management, and healthcare literature (Northouse 2009). Some of these are diligence, trustworthiness, dependability, sociability, open-mindedness, intelligence, self-awareness, conscientiousness, and self-assurance (Northouse 2009). Many of these overlap with our views of ideal traits of educators and clinicians.

In embedding an SBE program experts' communication, networking and other interpersonal skills are encompassed by sociability and demonstration of ideal leadership traits.

Leadership Versus Management

Kotter defined "leadership" as separate to management (Kotter 2013). Leadership is about vision, about people buying-in, about empowerment, and most of all, about producing useful change. It is about innovation and vision but also enacting these (Kotter 2013). Management is a set of well-known processes, like planning, budgeting, structuring jobs, staffing jobs, measuring performance and problem-solving, which help an organization to predictably do what it knows how to do well (Kotter 2013). Good management is a necessity but understanding the value, importance, and distinction of good leadership is vital to embed and sustain SBE.

Transformational Leadership

Transformational leaders appeal to higher ideals and moral values and empower followers to produce profound and fundamental change (Yahaya and Ebrahim 2016). Burns, a political scientist, first delineated the notion of transformational leadership in 1978 (Sinclair 2007). He also advocated a values-based approach to leadership (Couto 2010). Beyond transactions that always occur between leaders and members of organizations, he advised leaders to develop their followers to be leaders themselves, thus being transformational and emphasizing growth of those being led as well as other outcomes (Couto 2010). This aligns with the concept of champions.

Bass and subsequent advocates have argued that such leadership raises followers to higher levels of consciousness independently of its context, task, or purpose (Sinclair 2007). True transformational leadership requires a toolbox of skills with different leadership styles depending on the context, time, project, and people. Leaders, especially transformational leaders, create visions and inspire followers toward new meanings and reinvigorated purpose (Sinclair 2007). This aligns with focusing on engagement of people and faculty development and less on equipment and space. Additionally, a focus of mentoring, promotion, and cultivation of others to further SBE and enact change wholly embraces this concept. The focus for SBE experts as leaders may be around transforming people and culture to both embed SBE and what it can achieve by creating a "culture of safety."

Influence Without Authority

Although a leader needs a toolbox of different skills and attributes, the Cohen and Bradford's Influence Without Authority (IWA) Model (Cohen and Bradford 2005a) corresponds to how many SBE experts create influence in their organizations (Fig. 4).

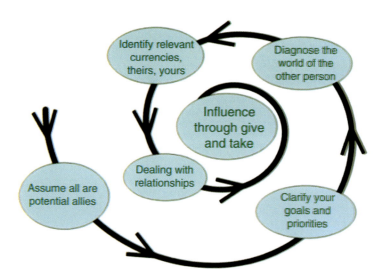

Fig. 4 The Cohen and Bradford Influence Without Authority Model (Cohen and Bradford 2005a)

The IWA model (Cohen and Bradford 2005a) describes one leadership approach taken and perhaps provides the best leadership theory for this complex situation where SBE experts often have no "authority" over the many people involved in hospitals and healthcare education. SBE directors must engage not only with those working directly in SBE programs but also with faculty who are in large part trained but not formally employed by most SBE programs, hospital staff from the varied healthcare professions including physicians, nurses, allied health, pharmacy, and support staff. There may or may not be external partners including universities, other hospitals or medical colleges, and external participants to liaise with. Moreover, they need to interact and engage with both middle management and executive level to ensure top-down support and buy-in. They are often also interacting with communications, media, industry, and philanthropy for funding and other opportunities.

Generally, the SBE director would only have direct authority over a handful of these many people and needs to capably and diplomatically engage and influence all other parties without any actual authority.

Cohen and Bradford's Influence Without Authority (IWA) Model (Cohen and Bradford 2005a) focuses on give and take where the leader needs to identify what others need and influence in this way (Cohen and Bradford 2005b). Communication, reciprocity, and exchange are vital to success. The IWA Model (Cohen and Bradford 2005b) also describes diagnosing the world of the other person which corresponds to the concept of "solve someone's problem" in order to influence and obtain "buy-in." Simulation educators and educators in general should be equipped with understanding their audience and use of debriefing skills to assist learners in transformational learning. Thus, these traits and skills may already be present and merely need reframing to a change management perspective and amplifying.

The Power of the Narrative

> Change your story and you can change your organisation. (Hilton and Anderson 2018)

The key to being heard as a leader is in delivering the message. Just as we need to know our audience as educators, we need to know our audience when first implementing such a program. We also need to be agile enough to change if the message is not being heard. Knowledge of the evidence is important but it's how we deliver this evidence to connect with people that is key.

> ***The message and the narrative are often more powerful than the actual evidence.***

To deliver that message with integrity the first thing you need will either to already be an expert in SBE and/or surround yourself with experts. Being able to provide a case for any program including SBE includes having legitimacy as an educator and simulation expert as well as knowing your organization's culture including the realities and pitfalls. To convince anyone, particularly those at executive levels, to take on something new, something different and something expensive means the person building and representing the business case needs to be both credible and knowledgeable.

A deep understanding of both the research and pedagogy is needed, but what is most vital is being able to be heard. The intended audience whether executive, finance, heads of units, philanthropy, university, and so on, needs to listen and connect with this information. For each group that may mean a different angle. For example, finance will be more interested in actual numbers and budget, while quality and safety will want to know the impact on patient care and outcomes, and education will want to know about training and so on.

Conclusion

Barriers and enablers to introducing and embedding an SBE program are intimately intertwined. Engagement of people through faculty development, champions, and promotion of SBE are important enablers. Funding challenges, particularly demonstrating "worth" and "return on investment," are significant barriers. While knowledge of barriers and enablers of SBE is important these will always exist particularly in complex organizations with uncertainty.

While it would be nice to provide a practical step-by-step model of how to embed an SBE program in a teaching hospital, based on identifying the barriers and enablers this is clearly not possible, different in every place and change over time. Each hospital has its own culture, context, and complexity so any individual or team looking to embed SBE needs to appreciate these elements. Anyone directing SBE needs to understand change management, organizational complexity, and leadership for successful implementation of sustainable SBE in teaching hospitals such that they are embedded and treated as any other operational service a hospital cannot do without.

> Developing this deeper feel for the change process by accumulating insights and wisdom across situations and time may turn out to be the most practical thing we can do—more practical than the best step-by-step models. (Fullan 2001)

> **Key Messages**
> - Simulation and SBE in hospitals are not yet even in well-established centers.
> - We know that enablers and barriers for SBE are intertwined and will always be present due to the inherent uncertainty and complexity of healthcare and healthcare education.

(continued)

- Good leadership is vital and will amplify enablers and overcomes barriers.
- Understanding of leadership and change management along with agility is essential to ensure sustainable embedded programs.

References

Bauer MS, Damschroder L, Hagedorn H, Smith J, Kilbourne AM. An introduction to implementation science for the non-specialist. BMC Psychol. 2015;3(1):32.

Braithwaite J, Marks D, Taylor N. Harnessing implementation science to improve care quality and patient safety: a systematic review of targeted literature. Int J Qual Health Care. 2014;26(3):321–9.

Brazil V. Translational simulation: not 'where?' but 'why?' A functional view of in situ simulation. Adv Simul. 2017;2(1):20.

Cohen AR, Bradford DL. The influence model: using reciprocity and exchange to get what you need. J Organ Excell. 2005a;1:57.

Cohen AR, Bradford DL. Influence without authority. 2nd ed. Hoboken: Wiley; 2005b.

Couto RA. Political and civic leadership. [electronic resource]: a reference handbook. Los Angeles/London: Sage; 2010.

Darling J. A conversation with Edgar Schein: aligning strategy, culture, and leadership. People & Strategy. 2017;40(2):64.

Densen P. Challenges and opportunities facing medical education. Trans Am Clin Climatol Assoc. 2011;122:48–58.

Fullan M. Leading in a culture of change. San Francisco: Jossey-Bass; 2001.

Fullan M, Scott G. Turnaround leadership for higher education. 1st ed. San Francisco: Jossey-Bass; 2009.

Gaba DM. The future vision of simulation in healthcare. Simul Healthc. 2004;13:127–129.

Gardner AK, Lachapelle K, Pozner CN, Sullivan ME, Sutherland D, Scott DJ, et al. Expanding simulation-based education through institution-wide initiatives: a blueprint for success. Surgery. 2015;158(5):1403–7.

Hilton K, Anderson A. IHI psychology of change framework to advance and sustain improvement. IHI white paper. Boston: Institute for Healthcare Improvement; 2018.

Kotter J. Management is (still) not leadership. Harv Bus Rev [Internet]. 2013 [cited 2017].

Lazzara EH, Benishek LE, Dietz AS, Salas E, Adriansen DJ. Eight critical factors in creating and implementing a successful simulation program. Jt Comm J Qual Patient Saf. 2014;40(1):21–9.

Lee WW, Alkureishi ML, Wroblewski KE, Farnan JM, Arora VM. Incorporating the human touch: piloting a curriculum for patient-centered electronic health record use. Med Educ Online. 2017;22(1):1396171.

Lettieri E. Uncertainty inclusion in budgeting technology adoption at a hospital level: evidence from a multiple case study. Health Policy. 2009;93(2/3):128–36.

Lipsitz LA. Understanding health care as a complex system: the foundation for unintended consequences. JAMA. 2012;308(3):243–4.

March CA, Steiger D, Scholl G, Mohan V, Hersh WR, Gold JA. Use of simulation to assess electronic health record safety in the intensive care unit: a pilot study. BMJ Open. 2013;3(4):e002549.

Milano CE, Hardman JA, Plesiu A, Rdesinski RE, Biagioli FE. Simulated electronic health record (Sim-EHR) curriculum: teaching EHR skills and use of the EHR for disease management and prevention. Acad Med. 2014;89(3):399–403.

Mohan V, Woodcock D, McGrath K, Scholl G, Pranaat R, Doberne JW, et al. Using simulations to improve electronic health record use, clinician training and patient safety: recommendations from a consensus conference. AMIA Annu Symp Proc. 2016;2016:904–13.

Northouse PG. Introduction to leadership: concepts and practice. Los Angeles: Sage; 2009.

Oxford English Dictionary. Oxford University Press; 2017. https://en.oxforddictionaries.com/definition/champion

Petrosoniak A, Brydges R, Nemoy L, Campbell DM. Adapting form to function: can simulation serve our healthcare system and educational needs? Adv Simul. 2018;3(1):8.

Rosen KR. The history of medical simulation. J Crit Care. 2008;23(2):157–66.

Schein EH. Organizational culture and leadership. 2nd ed. San Francisco: Jossey-Bass; 1997.

Szabo R. Selected abstracts from the 24th Annual Meeting of the Society in Europe for the Simulation Applied to Medicine. Adv Simul. 2018;3(2):1–11.

Sinclair A. Leadership for the disillusioned: moving beyond myths and heroes to leading that liberates. St Leonards: Allen & Unwin; 2007.

Sittig DF, Ash JS, Zhang J, Osheroff JA, Shabot MM. Lessons from "Unexpected increased mortality after implementation of a commercially sold computerized physician order entry system". Pediatrics. 2006;118(2):797–801.

Stefanidis D, Sevdalis N, Paige J, Zevin B, Aggarwal R, Grantcharov T, et al. Simulation in surgery: what's needed next? Ann Surg. 2015;261(5):846–53.

Stephenson LS, Gorsuch A, Hersh WR, Mohan V, Gold JA. Participation in EHR based simulation improves recognition of patient safety issues. BMC Med Educ. 2014;14(1):224.

Szabo R, Bearman M, O'Brien R. An exploratory study of experts' experiences of how to embed a sustainable simulation-based education program and/or centre in a teaching hospital. Melbourne: University of Melbourne; 2017.

VMIA. Incentivising better patient safety. Melbourne: VMIA; 2018.

Yahaya R, Ebrahim F. Leadership styles and organizational commitment: literature review. J Manag Dev. 2016;35:190.

Targeting Organizational Needs Through the Development of a Simulation-Based Communication Education Program

54

J. Sokol and M. Heywood

Contents

Introduction	1040
The Imperative to Address Organizational Needs Through Education	1040
Communication Training to Address Organizational Needs	1041
Simulation-Based Education Training as a Vehicle for Communication Training	1041
Development and Implementation of a Communication Simulation-Based Education Program	1043
Defining the Content of the Program	1043
Defining the Structure of the Program	1044
The Communication Framework	1046
Embedding Communication and Immersive Simulation Models	1048
Communication Models	1048
Evaluation of the Program	1049
Conclusion	1051
Cross-References	1052
References	1052

Abstract

Communication is challenging and complex but integral to patient and staff safety and well-being in health care. After review of our hospital critical incidents and staff feedback, we recognized a need to improve in the many facets of communication across the hospital. As a result, a simulation-based communication

---

J. Sokol (✉)
The Royal Children's Hospital Simulation Program, Department of Medical Education, The Royal Children's Hospital, Melbourne, VIC, Australia

University of Melbourne Department of Paediatrics, Melbourne, VIC, Australia
e-mail: jenni.sokol@rch.org.au

M. Heywood
The Royal Children's Hospital Simulation Program, Department of Medical Education, The Royal Children's Hospital, Melbourne, VIC, Australia
e-mail: melissa.heywood@rch.org.au

© Crown 2023
D. Nestel et al. (eds.), *Clinical Education for the Health Professions*,
https://doi.org/10.1007/978-981-15-3344-0_126

program was developed and implemented utilizing a framework that could be generalized across many aspects of health care. We discuss this program and how addressing organizational needs became the prime driver of this simulation program.

Keywords

Communication framework · Simulation · Education · Organizational needs · Communication skills training · Evaluation

Introduction

The Imperative to Address Organizational Needs Through Education

Kohn et al. (1999) targeted medical error in health care and highlighted the need to focus on team training of health care staff in order to mitigate the impact of human error on clinical outcomes and ultimately improving health care. Organizational and system factors have been increasingly recognized to contribute to health care outcomes (Reason 2000). Effective communication, in particular, can impact on patient and staff safety, experiences and satisfaction, and has become increasingly recognized to be a key factor in health care organizational structure and function (West 2000; Wilson et al. 1995). "High reliability organizations" (HRO) in health care focus on excellent patient outcomes emphasizing patient and employee safety, effective and open communication between all tiers of staff, acknowledgement and open discussion addressing the root cause(s) behind mistakes, consideration and respect of all staff and their expertise, and interprofessional collaboration between teams and professions (Weick and Sutcliffe 2007). Effective communication, despite being complex and challenging, has been recognized as an important factor to improving teamwork, patient, and staff safety and satisfaction in health care institutions (West 2000; Brock et al. 2013; Salas and Rosen 2013; Pronovost et al. 2006; Brindley and Reynolds 2011; Weller et al. 2014; Leonard 2004), and hence is crucial to HRO functioning at a high standard.

On review of our hospital critical incidents, adverse events, and staff surveys, we noted a need for improved communication between staff and with patients, across a broad range of areas. These included failure of staff to escalate concerns in various clinical and nonclinical situations, "everyday" and challenging communication interactions within and between clinical teams, providing information to families and their children about diagnoses, communicating with families when a procedure or clinical management does not go as planned, management of aggression in the workplace, giving feedback between staff, challenging conversations either face to face or over the phone with patients and families, and supporting staff after critical events.

This discussion explores how we addressed these organizational concerns. We review the current literature to identify the key elements required to deliver a robust simulation-based communication program to postgraduate clinicians and highlights how the structure and content of the communication framework can be developed to address these concerns. We discuss the educational tools utilized to deliver this knowledge through a simulation-based education program. Lastly, we will describe the impact of this interprofessional simulation-based education program on postgraduate clinicians through qualitative evaluation of our program, in order to provide some direction for others who may wish to embark on this type of program.

Communication Training to Address Organizational Needs

There is little doubt that effective communication is one of the most important skills that a health care professional can possess. Over the past decade there has been a growing body of evidence demonstrating the benefits to patients when clear, empathic communication skills are utilized. Evidence suggests skilled communication interactions may enhance information recall, provide greater satisfaction with care, and improved adherence to treatment (Armas et al. 2018; Gordon et al. 2015), in addition to purported improved patient outcomes through enhanced patient safety (Brock et al. 2013; Halverson et al. 2011; Lingard 2004). Communication plays a key role in building relationships, information gathering, information provision, making decisions, responding to emotions, managing uncertainty, and enabling patient and family self-management. Sensitive and caring communication is an important source of emotional support for patients and families. In addition, effective communication between clinicians and within clinical teams plays an important role in staff and patient satisfaction (Street and De Haes 2013; de Haes and Bensing 2009). Conversely, poor communication between clinicians and families, and within health care teams can add significantly to the distress associated with illness and hospitalization, and can ultimately lead to loss of trust, in addition to contributing to increased rates of patient safety incidents (Leonard 2004; Lingard 2004; Murphy and Dunn 2010; Kennedy et al. 2014). The latter is demonstrated in two reviews. Lingard's observational study concluded that 30% of team interactions in the operating room resulted in communication failure, with a third of those contributing to patient safety incidents during operating procedures (Lingard 2004). In addition, Leonard (2004) reviewed sentinel events in their institution and found 70% of critical incidents were related to poor communication. Our own institutional experience is not dissimilar. When we reviewed hospital incidents over the 2 years prior to commencement of this communication program, human factors were thought to contribute in 76% of incidents, with 47% of these attributed to poor communication.

Simulation-Based Education Training as a Vehicle for Communication Training

Communication skills training with health care professionals is thought to improve the patient experience, through improving patient-centered care, perception of communication, confidence, and empathy with patients, in addition to communication within teams (Wouda and Hulsman 2013; Maatouk-Burmann et al. 2016; Pehrson et al. 2016; Awad et al. 2005; Ammentorp and Kofoed 2011). While communication challenges have been addressed through the introduction of improved checklists, particularly in the operating room (Leonard 2004), we examine the utility of simulation-based education for postgraduate clinicians in this setting. Utilizing simulation-based education for communication training is not new. Fossili Jensen et al. (2011) and Maatouk-Burmann et al. (2016) utilized simulation methodology to explore the efficacy of communication skills training with randomized controlled trials. They found an improvement in patient-centered behavior during the physician–patient interaction (assessed by patient feedback and rating of video recordings). Learning was thought to improve due to the opportunity for repetitive practice (Maatouk-Burmann et al. 2016). Simulation-based communication training has been utilized for training physicians and/or nurses to enhance communication interactions with patients (Kennedy et al. 2014; Maatouk-Burmann et al. 2016; Pehrson et al. 2016; Fossili Jensen et al. 2011; Gabrielson and Karlsen 2016; Subramanian and Sathanandan 2016) and to strengthen team communication (Awad et al. 2005) in a variety of clinical settings with varied methodology. A number of communication skills training programs sessions have been reported that are similar to our communication program (Kennedy et al. 2014; Pehrson et al. 2016; Gabrielson and Karlsen 2016; Subramanian and Sathanandan 2016). Self-reported pre- and postevaluations suggested didactic sessions followed by role-plays (Pehrson et al. 2016) and simulations (Gabrielson and Karlsen 2016; Subramanian and Sathanandan 2016) were perceived to be a feasible and acceptable means of teaching communication skills to improve confidence with communication during patient interactions. Kennedy (Kennedy et al. 2014) assessed year-to-year patient feedback following physician communication training. They found statistically significant improvements in many important facets of patient communication including listening, involvement of patients in decision-making, courteousness, provision of clear instruction, and explanation of the medical condition, knowing the patient as a person, patient perception of the quality of the doctor, and overall quality of care. Awad et al. (Awad et al. 2005) employed didactic discussion and simulated role-play methodology with the aim of improving communication teamwork skills in the operating room. They reassessed a communication score 4 months after training, finding the communication score to improve among anesthetists and surgeons but not nursing staff. They attributed this result to the fact that fewer nurses had received the training. They did not, however, consider that these results may have been impacted by the content, training method, and application of training packages for nurses, nor whether the learning styles of the nurses might be different to that of the surgeons and anesthetists; all of which may influence the impact of communication training.

The evidence for the efficacy of communication skills training, however, is not yet established. Blackmore et al. (2018) and Selman et al. (2017) completed independent meta-analyses of general and palliative care communication training research, respectively. Neither found conclusive evidence that communication training was of definite benefit, with both demonstrating included studies to be limited by their methodology. They did suggest that communication training with simulation may improve the ability of staff to demonstrate empathy. Recommendations to achieve higher level of evaluation outcomes include improving methodology to consider repetitive practice through multiple training sessions (Maatouk-Burmann et al. 2016; Blackmore et al. 2018), facilitating in situ simulation sessions (Blackmore et al. 2018) and employing video feedback for participants (Selman et al. 2017).

Development and Implementation of a Communication Simulation-Based Education Program

In order to improve the consistency of communication and enhance recognition of the phases in which to base communication between staff, and staff and families, we developed a common communication framework that would lend itself to broad range of communication topics, building on the concept of deliberate repetitive practice, developed by Ericsson (2004), and the communication model described by de Haes and Bensing (2009). Our intention was to develop a communication framework that could be utilized consistently across diverse communication situations and practiced within these communication training sessions, providing staff with the tools (words, approach, and communication framework) to address challenging situations. We define the content and development of the communication programs, and structure of the framework below. Following each session participants were asked to complete a questionnaire which included with both quantitative (Likert scales) and qualitative inquiry (free text), enquiring about perceptions of learning outcomes, confidence in achieving behavioral learning objectives, facilitation of the program, and suggestions for program improvement. Completion of the evaluation surveys was voluntary, and completion was considered as consent to utilize data for quality assurance purposes. The evaluation surveys informed iterative review of the programs over time. The project was approved as a quality assurance project by the hospital research and ethics committee (HREC QA/65619/RCHM-2020).

Defining the Content of the Program

Program content (Table 1) was mapped to the Australian National Safety and Quality Health Service Standards (Australian Commission on Safety and Quality in HealthCare 2017) and developed as a result of feedback from organizational surveys in addition to direct staff feedback and critical incident review. Interprofessional participation was encouraged to create realistic scenarios. A consistent communication framework was utilized to consolidate the framework concept across the different communication programs. These included "graded assertiveness training" (later renamed as "speaking up for safety"), "giving feedback," "breaking bad

Table 1 Communication programs

Communication program	Content
Communication 101	General communication principles
Giving and receiving feedback	Providing feedback to colleagues
Graded assertiveness	Speaking up for patient and staff safety
Clinical handover	Effective delivery of handover for patient safety
The impact of human factors on patient safety	The interaction of human factors with team communication
Supportive leadership following critical events	Training clinical and nonclinical staff to delivery of psychological first aid to colleagues
Building trust in teams	Emotional intelligence, giving feedback, and communicating with colleagues
Breaking bad news	Empathy, active listening, verbal, and nonverbal communication techniques
Difficult conversations	Empathy, active listening, verbal, and nonverbal communication techniques
Open disclosure	Hospital-wide organizational strategy, dedicated to improving open disclosure
Management of clinical aggression	Simulation-based session added to the "management of clinical aggression" study day
End of life conversations	Empathy, listening, verbal, and nonverbal communication techniques
Advanced care planning	Empathy, listening, verbal, and nonverbal communication techniques, specific guidelines

news," "difficult conversations," "psychological first aid" (supporting staff after a challenging clinical or nonclinical event), "advanced care planning," and "end of life care." In addition, an interprofessional hospital-wide committee developed guidelines for providing information on how to disclose clinical error and patient harm to families, known in Australia as "Open Disclosure." Other programs utilizing a predefined communication strategy rather than our communication framework were included. These programs encompass "management of clinical aggression" (de-escalation of aggressive behavior) and "clinical handover" which utilized the ISBAR (Marshall et al. 2009) (or SBAR), (Leonard 2004; Dingley et al. 2008) format. ISBAR is an acronym for introduction, situation, background, assessment, and review/recommendations. This communication strategy is a recognized and well-established communication strategy for handing over patients between health care workers or teams has been documented to improve clinical handover between teams (Leonard 2004; Marshall et al. 2009; Dingley et al. 2008).

Defining the Structure of the Program

The program structure utilizes a scaffolded educational approach and is based on Miller's theory of assessment (Miller 1990). Learning is based on providing background knowledge, followed by opportunity to observe and then practice skills, followed by consolidation of concepts through demonstration of what they have learned. The latter aims to facilitate behavioral change. We adapted Miller's pyramid (Miller 1990) to our communication simulation education program strategy by developing interactive program-specific workshops to learn theory (with pre-reading and/or completion of e-Learn modules prior to the workshop), role-plays for skills training to practice the communication framework, and simulated scenarios to enable behavioral change for particular situations (Fig. 1). Ideally, participants would attend all three components, but this is not always possible.

The communication workshops commence with different "ice-breakers" to emphasize specific aspects of communication. Theories pertinent to the communication topic are discussed where needed, in addition to the general principles of communication, with interactive activities. We utilize video clips (either downloaded from the Internet or developed by the RCH simulation team) to emphasize relevant theory and behavior, in addition to group discussion with brainstorming, to debrief the videos. Communication principles and strategies are discussed within the communication framework, particularly exploring the concept of "empathy" and its role in these conversations. Discussion also includes the importance of ascertaining "frames" of colleagues or families involved in the conversation, as described in "Debriefing with Good Judgment" (Rudolph et al. 2007). A simple communication framework that can be utilized across a broad range of communication discussions is then discussed, before putting this into practice with simulated role-plays and immersive simulation with an actor.

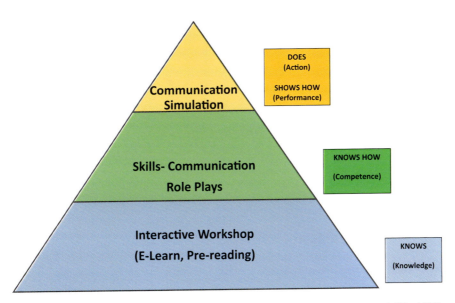

Fig. 1 Communication workshop structure, based on Miller's pyramid of assessment (Miller 1990)

The Communication Framework

This communication framework (Fig. 2) is modified from some aspects of Rudolph's "Debriefing with Good Judgment" (35)and the "Program to Enhance Relational and Communication Skills" (PERCS) model (Browning et al. 2007). The communication framework includes a "pre-huddle," "conversation," and "post-huddle," and is repeated with the various communication programs. This enables familiarity, enhancing recognition and thus facilitation of a simple communication strategy.

The "pre-huddle" is emphasized to ensure the clinicians discuss how they will prepare to facilitate the conversation with the family, prior to entering the room: which staff will be present for the conversation, what questions will they ask, who will ask them, and how might the staff support each other and the family members.

The "conversation" incorporates specific content relevant to the communication topic in addition to general communication strategies. For instance, we utilize a recognized model for training staff to speak up when they have a concern (PACE: probe, alert, challenge, and escalate) and for supporting staff after challenging events (the "look," "listen," and "link" model for "Psychological First Aid" (WHO WTF, and World Vision 2011)) within the "conversation" section of the communication framework. Likewise, concepts of the "Open Disclosure" guideline are included

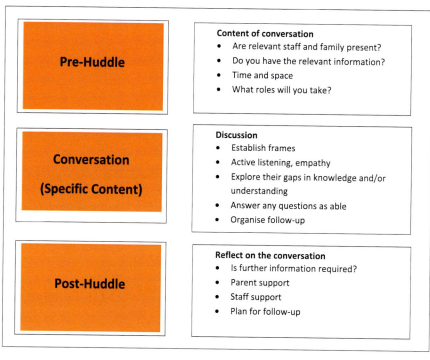

Fig. 2 The Royal Children's Hospital communication framework. Framework adapted from Browning et al. (2007) and Rudolph et al. (2007)

within the conversation, providing staff with appropriate words, phrases, and a consistent approach to supporting families, when faced with this situation. In addition to content-specific strategies, approaches discussed and practiced include active listening and acknowledgment of emotions, recognition of verbal and nonverbal cues, and recognition for the importance of enabling and empowering questions and allowing time for patients and families to absorb the conversation. The strategy to "close the gap" of knowledge or learning (Rudolph et al. 2007), relevant to the conversation, then follows. This training allows staff to recognize that families must have the opportunity to ask and have questions answered. They learn to disclose that not all questions can be answered immediately, but follow-up will be provided. Provision for planning a follow-up family meeting, in addition to time for families to grieve if required, is imperative, and brings closure of the conversation component of the framework.

A "post-huddle" is a reinforcement to staff that the "conversation" with the family is not the end of the discussion. The "post-huddle" allows time for teams to reflect on and document the conversation, consider and conduct any research that is required for previously unanswered patient or family questions, and then organize the follow-up conversation with families. This time is also used to "check in" on staff after what are often challenging conversations.

Following the workshop, participants practice the communication framework in a structured, safe, educational environment through simulated role-plays. In the more extensive training sessions, simulation sessions with an actor follow. Bell et al. (2014) documented perceived additional educational value when an actor was involved with the communication education session. As not all participants can participate directly in a simulation, we utilize role-plays to enable all participants the opportunity to practice using the framework. The role-plays are developed by the simulation team in conjunction with clinicians and are specific to departments to accurately portray specific communication issues within their department that are realistic to their situation. At the end of the role-play, participants are invited to provide feedback to each other. Additional group discussion enables sharing of challenges when utilizing the communication framework and an opportunity for questions, to promote learning.

The communication simulation session with an actor enables full immersion, practice of the framework, and discussion of the challenges pertaining to providing effective communication in each domain. We aim for the simulation component to be interprofessional, with the team participating in the conversation to reflect the true clinical team who may attend a family meeting. In addition, both the "pre-" and "post-huddle" are streamed to the observers and debriefers, so the debriefing can include discussion around all components of the framework.

A facilitated debriefing follows the simulation scenario. The actor participates in the debriefing to provide direct feedback to participants, particularly around some of the verbal and nonverbal cues. They also facilitate the participants to consider the family's emotions, rather than focusing solely on facts. Bell et al. (2014) documented the value of actor participation in simulations and the debriefings that followed and found similar themes arose from participant learners, faculty, and actors alike. Themes included bringing realism to the scenarios, providing feedback particularly the "lay person" perspective, the ability to change the depth of emotions depending on how participants interacted with them, and bringing another layer of education to the discussion. The facilitated debriefing sessions include all learners (participants and observers of the simulation) to enable reflective discussion of the relevant framework and how to adapt newly found skills to the specific situations, as the simulation component does not sometimes enable all attending staff to participate in the simulated exercise. Observers have attended the workshop and practiced the framework in the role-plays, and so after observing the simulation are able to actively participate in, and learn from, the debriefing. The learning benefits for observers of simulation sessions were reinforced by O'Regan et al. (2016). Data from this meta-analysis suggested observed simulation sessions are an effective means of learning in simulation-based education as long as the observers are provided with a tool to reflect upon during the simulation and are included in the debriefing.

Embedding Communication and Immersive Simulation Models

To reinforce learning, we combined deteriorating patient and communication simulation scenarios following some communication-based workshops. This involved particularly "Breaking Bad News" communication workshops simulation and sessions for the critical care areas (Paediatric Intensive Care, Neonatal Intensive Care, Neonatal and Paediatric Retrieval, and the Emergency Departments). This involves staff participating in a deteriorating patient simulation and debriefing, followed by a communication simulation with an actor as the "parent" in which they are required to deliver the "bad news" to the family, utilizing the communication framework. This training has been extremely well received, being perceived to provide a realistic situation of having to break bad news to parents following a devastating event. These combined scenarios enable participants to incorporate learned communication skills from the workshop into the simulated situation. We believe participation in an initial deteriorating patient simulation has improved "buy-in" for the communication simulation as emphasized in this reflection:

> One of the best SIM scenarios I have seen. Thought the clinical communication mix (although painful) was excellent, made communication much more real.
> I feel more confident in delivering bad news to parent following a critical event.

Communication Models

The structured communication framework aims to assist clinicians when undertaking these conversations. The framework should provide the necessary components to ensure the clinician is addressing all aspects of communication. A variety of communication models have emerged over the past decades, each containing similar facets of communication strategies (Kennedy et al. 2014; Kurtz et al. 2003; Baile et al. 2000;

Makoul 2001; Milan et al. 2010; Frankel and Stein 1999; Peterson et al. 2014). The Calgary Cambridge framework (Kurtz et al. 2003) highlights information gathering during the medical interview in addition to facets of communication techniques. SPIKES, a six-point protocol for communicating bad news, focuses on factors to consider prior to the communication interaction, the conversation including patient perceptions and empathy, and then a summary phase (Baile et al. 2000). The SEGUE (Makoul 2001) and the Kalamazoo (Peterson et al. 2014) communication frameworks are checklists, used for assessment of communication interactions. They include items such as establishing relationships during medical information gathering, active listening, building empathy, providing time for patients to ask questions, as well as other facets of communication. The PEARLS framework is based on six aspects of communication: partnership, empathy, apology, respect, legitimization, and support, and has been utilized in varied aspects of communication training such as giving feedback (Milan et al. 2010) and improving the patient–physician interaction (Kennedy et al. 2014). The Four Habits four habits communication framework (Frankel and Stein 1999) is based on four facets of communication: beginning the conversation (setting up rapport and creating relationships), understanding patient perspectives, demonstrating empathy, and a conclusion involving information delivery, education, patient decision-making, and follow-up. de Haes and Bensing (2009) base their communication model on Rogerian theory, which espouses a person-centred approach to the communication interaction. The model focuses on six principles including establishing and fostering the patient–clinician relationship, gathering, and providing information, demonstrating empathy, allowing patient decision-making, and responding to emotions by providing communication that influences change behavior. This framework shares similar principles to the SPIKE (Baile et al. 2000), and Four Habits (Frankel and Stein 1999) frameworks, and our own framework. We address the first five of these components within the "pre-huddle" and "conversation." The sixth principle is addressed in the "post-huddle" or follow-up phase of our framework and involves enabling a change in behavior.

Evaluation of the Program

Over 3,500 participants have attended 244 communication education sessions across 5 years of the program. An education program should not be static: this communication simulation program has had ongoing development through an iterative process. This was enabled through qualitative (free text) and quantitative confidential evaluations (Likert scales) focusing on specific communication learning objectives across the varied communication themes.

Both quantitative and qualitative data were positive for content reinforcement, delivery of the program, and confidence for utilizing the framework in varied situations:

> I liked the spectrum of approaches and importance of the fact there are no right answers but some good guiding principles.

The importance of self and team preparation and using a brief huddle prior to approaching family.

Participant learning outcomes about communication strategies focused on benefits of the scaffolded learning approach, interprofessional nature of the sessions, and benefits of a communication program:

I was quite nervous, but it was really great. Was good having mixture of team and personalities to de-stress with.
Appropriate content and structure of information, practical framework, role play and feedback supported my learning.

Participants also reflected on the importance of learning communication through role-plays or simulation scenarios:

Communication is crucial and affects the performance of all other technical and personal skills.
Continue to include scenarios where treatment does not resuscitate effectively as is invaluable to practice the dying situation.

Learning the significance of effective communication within their teams was also highlighted:

Communication is a team thing, and we can all contribute to improving the end result.
Learning factors that influenced the successful functioning of a team during a (communication) scenario.

In addition, the realization of the need for empathy and active listening was emphasized:

I learned to be mindful that everyone has their very own story which we forgot all too often.
Be straight forward and clear but also gentle and empathic in delivering bad news. Also, that listening is VERY important in all clinical situations.
I learned the importance of validating and exploring a parent's care of their child.

Reflections from utilizing the communication model to give feedback emphasized respect, the importance of providing feedback, and trying to understand different perspectives:

To consider the other persons frame and be respectful when giving feedback also to be understanding when receiving feedback.
Positive and negative feedback are both equally as important to improve practice.

Learning to speak up when concerned about safety frequently highlighted uncomfortable emotions when dealing with hierarchy. Reflections suggested the training sessions were perceived to assist in overcoming these fears:

> Learning to be assertive and explain if I feel uncomfortable and ask for help
> Patient safety is key- don't be afraid to speak with consultants.

The learning outcomes from "open disclosure" sessions highlighted the need to provide guidance to staff to communicate clinical error to families:

> Use the structure to provide guidance for open disclosure.
> Wording is important, and every person reacts different - stay flexible
> It's ok to apologise.

Training to provide "psychological first aid" highlighted the desire to support colleagues, but recognized challenging content:

> Look-be aware of those around us and learn the signs of emotional stress.
> I like the simulation and putting the framework into practise. I found the first 1 1/2 hours of input a lot to take in.

Despite the positive evaluations, at this stage we have evaluated our communication program only to Kirkpatrick level 2 (Kirkpatrick and Kirkpatrick 2006). Evaluation of the effectiveness of this communication program to atleast Kilpatrick level 3 is essential, as emphasized in the two meta-analyses (Blackmore et al. 2018; Selman et al. 2017), and others (Kiessling et al. 2017). Kiessling et al. (2017) describe the key facets to enable evaluation of communication programs, including which aspects of a program to assess, choosing the appropriate educational tool and level of outcome, and how to construct the research. Patient feedback was considered as one of the constructs used to evaluate at a higher level of outcome. As there were several communication training strategies and programs being facilitated across our hospital concurrently, it was challenging to assess any measure of changes in care delivered through family feedback, or any cost-effectiveness of our program. In addition, measured improvement within departments has not been possible as the communication sessions sometimes included staff from varied departments rather than a single department. Utilizing a common communication framework across several communication programs has, however, anecdotally enabled our staff to deal with common communication situations with greater empathy, clarity, and confidence.

Conclusion

With the aim of addressing organizational concerns, this scaffolded simulation-based education approach enabled participants to practice various communication discussions for diverse clinical and interpersonal situations, utilizing a shared communication framework. The purpose was to enable repetitive practice of a common framework across a broad range of communication situations. Role-play and simulation were utilized to provide opportunity to reinforce behavioral learning and implement a change in behavior through repetitive practice and reflection. Staff participating in multiple communication programs have become familiar with the framework and have highlighted the usefulness of this in their evaluations. We have found this approach to communication education to be increasingly requested by departments and individuals alike, throughout the hospital.

Our communication simulation program delivered a broad range of communication-based education sessions that were identified by the organization and by staff themselves. The enablers of this communication program have arisen from not only organizational leaders, but also health care workers themselves, through recognition for the need, and desire, to improve. There have been challenges facilitating the program. The main challenge is sustainability, as the cost of educators and actors, along with the increasing popularity of the program, result in the need for more trained staff to deliver the sessions. Attributing any direct positive impact on patient interactions may be difficult; however it is imperative that future directions include exploring the effectiveness of this program. The common communication framework, role-plays, and simulation sessions with an actor have anecdotally been successful, with evaluations demonstrating a high regard for the realism of the simulated situation, and the embedding of the framework. We intend to review the hospital incident reporting and patient complaint systems after 5 years, in order to review whether implementation of this communication program has had an impact on patient or staff complaints, or on the many varied aspects of communication that we are faced with every day that contribute to our critical incidents.

Cross-References

▶ Conversational Learning in Health Professions Education: Learning Through Talk
▶ Developing Patient Safety Through Education
▶ Embedding a Simulation-Based Education Program in a Teaching Hospital
▶ Focus on Theory: Emotions and Learning
▶ Simulation for Clinical Skills in Healthcare Education
▶ Supporting the Development of Patient-Centred Communication Skills
▶ Team-Based Learning (TBL): Theory, Planning, Practice, and Implementation

References

Ammentorp J, Kofoed PE. Research in communication skills training translated into practice in a large organization: a proactive use of the RE-AIM framework. Patient Educ Couns. 2011;82(3):482–7.

Armas A, Meyer SB, Corbett KK, Pearce AR. Face-to-face communication between patients and family physicians in Canada: a scoping review. Patient Educ Couns. 2018;101(5):789–803.

Australian Commission on Safety and Quality in HealthCare. National safety and quality health service standards. 2nd ed. Sydney: ACSQHC; 2017.

Awad SS, Fagan SP, Bellows C, Albo D, Green-Rashad B, De la Garza M, et al. Bridging the communication gap in the operating room with medical team training. Am J Surg. 2005;190 (5):770–4.

Baile W, Buckman R, Lenzi R, Glober G, Beale E, Kudelka A. SPIKES-A six-step protocol for delivering bad news: application to the patient with cancer. Oncologist. 2000;5:302–11.

Bell SK, Pascucci R, Fancy K, Coleman K, Zurakowski D, Meyer EC. The educational value of improvisational actors to teach communication and relational skills: perspective of interprofessional learners, faculty, and actors. Patient Educ Couns. 2014;96:381–8.

Blackmore A, Kasfiki EV, Purva M. Simulation-based education to improve communication skills: a systematic review and identification of current best practice. BMJ Simul Technol Enhance Learn. 2018;4(4):159–64.

Brindley P, Reynolds S. Improving verbal communication in critical care medicine. J Crit Care. 2011;26:155–9.

Brock D, Abu-Rish E, Chiu CR, Hammer D, Wilson S, Vorvick L, et al. Interprofessional education in team communication: working together to improve patient safety. Postgrad Med J. 2013;89 (1057):642–51.

Browning D, Meyer E, Truog R, Solomon M. Difficult conversations in health care: cultivating relational learning to address the hidden curriculum. Med Educ. 2007;82:905–13.

de Haes H, Bensing J. Endpoints in medical communication research, proposing a framework of functions and outcomes. Patient Educ Couns. 2009;74(3):287–94.

Dingley CD, Daugherty K, Derieg MK, Persing R. Improving patient safety through provider communication strategy enhancements. In: Henriksen K, Battles J, Keyes MA, et al., editors. Advances in patient safety: new directions and alternative approaches. 3: Performance and tools. Rockville: Agency for Healthcare Research and Quality (US); 2008.

Ericsson KA. Deliberate practice and the acquisition and maintenance of expert performance in medicine and related domains. Acad Med. 2004;79(10):S70–81.

Fossili Jensen B, Gulbrandsen P, Dahl FA, Krupa tE, Frankel RM, Arnstein F. Effectiveness of a short course in clinical communication skills for hospital doctors: results of a crossover randomized controlled trial. Patient Educ Couns. 2011;84:163–9.

Frankel RM, Stein T. Getting the most out of the clinical encounter: the four habits model. Permanente. 1999;3(3):79–88.

Gabrielson AK, Karlsen M-MW, Falch AL, Stubberud D-G. Communication training course with simulation. Opphavsrett Sykepleien.no/Forskning 10.4220. Sykpleienf.2016.57832

Gordon J, Deland E, Kelly R. Let's talk about improving communication in healthcare. Columbia Med Rev. 2015;1(1):23–7.

Halverson AL, Casey JT, Andersson J, Anderson K, Park C, Rademaker AW, et al. Communication failure in the operating room. Surgery. 2011;149(3):305–10.

Kennedy DM, Fasolino JP, Gullen DJ. Improving the patient experience through provider communication. Patient Exp J. 2014;1(1):56–60.

Kiessling C, Tsimtsiou Z, Essers G, van Nuland M, Anvik T, Bujnowska-Fedak MM, et al. General principles to consider when designing a clinical communication assessment program. Patient Educ Couns. 2017;100(9):1762–8.

Kirkpatrick D, Kirkpatrick J. Evaluating training programs: the four levels. 3rd ed. San Francisco: Berrett-Koehler Publishers; 2006.

Kohn LT, Corrigan JM, M D. To err is human: building a safer health system. Washington, DC: Institute of Medicine; 1999.

Kurtz S, Silverman J, Benson J, Draper J. Marrying content and process in clinical method teaching: enhancing the Calgary-Cambridge guides. Acad Med. 2003;78:802–9.

Leonard M. The human factor: the critical importance of effective teamwork and communication in providing safe care. Qual Saf Health Care. 2004;13(Suppl 1):i85–90.

Lingard L. Communication failures in the operating room: an observational classification of recurrent types and effects. Qual Saf Health Care. 2004;13(5):330–4.

Maatouk-Burmann B, Ringel N, Spang J, Weiss C, Moltner A, Riemann U, et al. Improving patient-centered communication: results of a randomized controlled trial. Patient Educ Couns. 2016;99(1):117–24.

Makoul G. The SEGUE framework for teaching and assessing communication skills. Patient Educ Couns. 2001;45:23–34.

Marshall S, Harrison J, Flanagan B. The teaching of a structured tool improves the clarity and content of interprofessional clinical communication. Qual Saf Health Care. 2009;18:137–40.

Milan FB, Parish SJ, Reichgott MJ. A model for educational feedback based on clinical communication skills strategies: beyond the "Feedbacl Sandwich". Teach Learn Med. 2010;18(1):42.

Miller G. The assessment of clinical skills/competence/performance. Acad Med. 1990;65(9):63–7.

Murphy JG, Dunn WF. Medical errors and poor communication. Chest. 2010;138(6):1292–3.

O'Regan S, Molloy E, Watterson L, Nestel D. Observer roles that optimise learning in healthcare simulation education: a systematic review. Adv Simul. 2016;1:4.

Pehrson C, Banerjee SC, Manna R, Shen MJ, Hammonds S, Coyle N, et al. Responding empathically to patients: development, implementation, and evaluation of a communication skills training module for oncology nurses. Patient Educ Couns. 2016;99(4):610–6.

Peterson EB, Calhoun AW, Rider EA. The reliability of a modified Kalamazoo consensus statement checklist for assessing the communication skills of multidisciplinary clinicians in the simulated environment. Patient Educ Couns. 2014;96(3):411–8.

Pronovost PJ, Thompson DA, Holzmueller CG, Lubomski LH, Dorman T, Dickman F, et al. Toward learning from patient safety reporting systems. J Crit Care. 2006;21(4):305–15.

Reason J. Human error: models and management. BMJ. 2000;320:768–70.

Rudolph J, Simon R, Rivard P, Dufresne R, Raemer D. Debriefing with good judgment: combining rigorous feedback with genuine inquiry. Anesthesiol Clin. 2007;25:361–76.

Salas E, Rosen M. Building high reliability teams: progress and some reflections on teamwork trainng. BMJ Qual Saf. 2013;22:369–73.

Selman LE, Brighton LJ, Hawkins A, McDonald C, O'Brien S, Robinson V, et al. The effect of communication skills training for generalist palliative care providers on patient-reported outcomes and clinician behaviors: a systematic review and meta-analysis. J Pain Symptom Manag. 2017;54(3):404–16 e5.

Street RL Jr, De Haes HC. Designing a curriculum for communication skills training from a theory and evidence-based perspective. Patient Educ Couns. 2013;93(1):27–33.

Subramanian P, Sathanandan K. Improving communication skills using simulation training. BJMP. 2016;9(2):911–3.

Weick K, Sutcliffe K. Managing the unexpected: resilient performance in an age of uncertainty. 3rd ed. Jossey Bass: San Francisco; 2007, 2015.

Weller J, Boyd M, Cumin D. Teams, tribes and patient safety: overcoming barriers to effective teamwork in healthcare. Postgrad Med J. 2014;90(1061):149–54.

West E. Organisational sources of safety and danger: sociological contributions to the study of diverse events. Qual Health Care. 2000;9:120–6.

WHO WTF, and World Vision. Psychological first aid: guide for field workers. Geneva: WHO; 2011.

Wilson R, Runciman W, Gibberd R, Harrison BT, Newby L, Hamilton J. The quality in Australian health care study. Med J Aust. 1995;163:458–71.

Wouda JC, Hulsman RL. Pathways towards designing effective medical communication curricula. Patient Educ Couns. 2013;93(1):1–2.

Effective Feedback Conversations in Clinical Practice

55

C. E. Johnson, C. J. Watling, J. L. Keating, and E. K. Molloy

Contents

Introduction	1056
The Role of Feedback	1056
Problems with Feedback in Clinical Practice	1057
Learner-Centered Feedback	1058
Who, When, and Where	1058
The Feedback Quality Instrument (FQI): A Learner-Centered Framework to Guide Practice	1059
Components in Formal Feedback Discussions	1060
Set the Scene	1060
Analyse Performance	1060
Plan for Improvement	1064
Foster a Psychologically Safe Learning Environment	1065
Foster Learner Understanding and Learner Agency	1067
Summary and Conclusion	1068

C. E. Johnson (✉)
Monash Doctors Education, Monash Health and Faculty of Medicine, Nursing and Health Sciences, Monash University, Melbourne, VIC, Australia
e-mail: Christina.johnson@monashhealth.org

C. J. Watling
Centre for Education Research and Innovation, Schulich School of Medicine and Dentistry, Western University, London, ON, Canada
e-mail: chris.watling@schulich.uwo.ca

J. L. Keating
Department of Physiotherapy, School of Primary and Allied Health Care, Faculty of Medicine Nursing and Health Science, Monash University, Melbourne, VIC, Australia
e-mail: jenny.keating@monash.edu

E. K. Molloy
Department of Medical Education, Melbourne Medical School, University of Melbourne, Melbourne, VIC, Australia
e-mail: elizabeth.molloy@unimelb.edu.au

© Springer Nature Singapore Pte Ltd. 2023
D. Nestel et al. (eds.), *Clinical Education for the Health Professions*,
https://doi.org/10.1007/978-981-15-3344-0_53

Cross-References 1068
References 1069

Abstract

Feedback plays a crucial role in health professionals' training in clinical practice. The aim of feedback is to help learners improve their performance using an interactive learning conversation. This offers learners the opportunity to understand more about the desired standard and the standard of their own work, and to problem solve difficulties with an expert (or another collaborator). In this chapter, we discuss the core components of effective feedback and the key literature that supports it. As our objective is to assist health professionals to make the most of feedback opportunities, the chapter focuses on practical strategies with multiple illustrative examples of dialogue.

Keywords

Effective feedback · Formative feedback · Health professions education · Workplace learning · Performance improvement · Performance enhancement · Performance analysis

Introduction

In this chapter we present educators and learners with our thoughts on how to make the most of feedback interactions. To be effective, feedback interactions demand care and skill, to engage learners and educators in an authentic learning dialogue that leads to improvements. Feedback in clinical practice occurs in a variety of ways but we focus on face-to-face feedback, as might occur at scheduled meetings to review a specific task performance or a more cumulative performance discussion at the end of a day or mid/end of a clinical attachment. We describe the different components of verbal feedback and their importance in optimizing benefits for learners. These suggestions for quality feedback practice are supported by research findings and brief explanations of important underlying theory. As our focus is on practical skills, examples of best practice are presented throughout. Many of these are derived from real encounters, stemming from an in-depth study on authentic verbal feedback encounters in routine clinical practice (Johnson et al. 2019, 2020a; Johnson and Molloy 2018). We have used the generic terms "learner" and "educator," to indicate the person whose performance is being reviewed and the other person, respectively. Often the learner is a student or junior clinician and the educator is their supervisor but alternatively could be a peer, another health professional, a clinical educator, or a patient.

The Role of Feedback

Feedback is a process whereby learners use performance information to generate improvements (Molloy and Boud 2013; Carless and Boud 2018). Feedback can have a major impact on improving performance (Hattie and Timperley 2007; Ericsson

2015; Ende 1983; Johnson et al. 2020b). A useful feedback conversation helps learners to understand how their skills are progressing (which aspects meet the expected standard and which do not, yet) and then to take action to develop their skills further (Sadler 1989; Boud and Molloy 2013; Dweck and Yeager 2019). Thus feedback involves performance information with *purpose*, offering direction and motivation for learning (Watling and Ginsburg 2019). Furthermore, feedback should make a difference. When feedback is viewed as a system designed to optimise performance, its value depends on the outcome, as the indicator of success (Molloy and Boud 2013).

An educator can assist with this process of performance improvement by helping learners to take advantage of learning experiences available in clinical practice and utilize multiple sources of performance guidance such as role models, interactions with other health professionals or patients, and educational resources (van der Leeuw et al. 2018). Subsequent to a feedback session, a learner needs opportunities to practice so they can implement planned changes. This allows the learner and educator to test whether the strategies developed during the feedback discussion were successful, in which case they can turn their attention to the next steps in skill development. However, if the learner runs into unexpected difficulties, they can develop potential ways to overcome them. This emphasizes the value of designing training to include (or identify) incrementally difficult tasks that are spaced across time, to enable learners to implement action plans and demonstrate progression in learning (Molloy and Boud 2013).

During feedback conversations, an educator can help the learner to reflect on their performance, consider what would be most useful to improve next and how they could do it effectively (Sargeant et al. 2005; Johnson et al. 2016). An educator's expert understanding of what characterizes quality performance and their ideas on how to nurture it can be highly valuable in guiding next steps (Ende et al. 1995) and in helping learners calibrate their own judgement (Johnson and Molloy 2018). Providing opportunities for learners to reflect on their performance and propose improvement strategies, may mean that an additional function of feedback (beyond improvement of the next iteration of work) is to build clinicians' self-regulated learning strategies, including evaluative judgement (Nicol and Macfarlane-Dick 2006; Butler and Winne 1995). In addition, interactive dialogue fosters co-construction of new insights and improvement strategies tailored for the learner, as educator and learner perspectives mingle and evolve (Telio et al. 2015, 2016).

Problems with Feedback in Clinical Practice

Despite consensus that feedback is important for learner development, feedback practice seems to be fraught with problems that may threaten its effectiveness (Kluger and DeNisi 1996; Bangert-Drowns et al. 1991). Learners often report that when they do get feedback, it can be hard to makes sense of what the educator is trying to say or make use of the information to improve (Sargeant et al. 2005, 2008; Bing-You et al. 1997). Further, even when plans are made, learners may not have the opportunity to test improvement strategies because of the busy and unpredictable nature of clinical practice (Noble et al. 2020; Watling et al. 2016). In addition, feedback is an emotional business (Molloy et al. 2013). This may be particularly true for health professionals, as they highly value their professional identity (Ende 1983; Butler and Winne 1995; Kluger and DeNisi 1996; Sargeant et al. 2008). In particular, when feedback conversations broach substandard performance, even when carefully done, it may be an uncomfortable experience for learners. Negative emotional reactions such as disappointment, anxiety, shame, and demotivation are particularly likely when the learner did not foresee any performance concerns and these feelings can persist over extended periods of time (Sargeant et al. 2008). Strong emotions may interfere with a learner's ability to process, integrate and use feedback information, even if it is valid. Hence an important role for educators during feedback conversations is to help learners to consider the performance analysis and explore their reactions to it, to reduce the risk of initial emotions overwhelming productive use of the information (Sargeant et al. 2015, 2018; Pelgrim et al. 2012).

On the other hand, many educators say they do not feel skilled in feedback. They find it stressful as they do not wish to damage their collegial relationship with the learner or cause the learner to feel embarrassed, upset or demotivated (Ende et al. 1995; Hewson and Little 1998). In addition, educators may struggle with the pressure to make credible evaluative judgements and highlight what is important. Considering these findings, there appear to be opportunities to positively evolve feedback experiences for both educators and learners.

Learner-Centered Feedback

Traditionally, feedback was characterized as an educator telling a learner what they did right or wrong, and how to fix it. Recent research indicates that this scenario is still common (Johnson et al. 2019). It may be driven by an educator's wish to help the learner by delivering as much knowledge as possible in a limited amount of time. This behavior is influenced, in part at least, by the demands and pressures of clinical work (Molloy 2009). However, despite good intentions, such a monologue contains information that may not be useful if the educator has not tapped into the needs, concerns or goals of the learner (Sadler 1989). In contrast, contemporary concepts of feedback are learner-centered and focus on learners proactively driving the process. As such, feedback can be described as a process in which learners gather information about the quality of their work, use it to generate plans for improvements, analyze the effect of implementing those plans, and then start a new improvement cycle (Carless and Boud 2018; Boud and Molloy 2013; Ramani et al. 2019). Importantly, *the effect* of feedback becomes the focus in these learner-centred notions of feedback. That is, it is not just about *what is said* but rather, *what students do* with the information.

Who, When, and Where

When designing an effective feedback process, in addition to the core conversation which this chapter focuses on, other aspects that need to be considered include *who*, *when*, and *where*. Starting with *who*, some assume that senior clinicians are always the most useful partner in a feedback discussion. However, if the learner wants to find out whether their explanation of discharge medications was clear, or the way they repositioned a patient caused discomfort, it is the patient who is in the best position to provide this information. Peer feedback interactions offer some advantages too. Conversations involving peers (or near peers) may be less anxiety-provoking and hence more candid. Peers may be more available than senior clinicians and they may be better at explaining concepts using simple language (Tai et al. 2016a). The peer acting in the educator role is likely to gain too because analyzing performance, explaining concepts, and debating ideas are valuable learning activities (Tai et al. 2016b). Even though this chapter is focused on the learner-educator interaction, the supervising educator can play an important role in helping learners to make the most of this "feedback rich environment."

When to have a feedback discussion is another factor affecting learner outcomes. Often learners are interested in performance information as soon as they have completed a task because they are motivated to solve any difficulties or dilemmas they have just experienced. For example, in studies in surgical environments, feedback conversations are often held during wound closure, when surgeons do not need to devote all their attention to this comparatively simple task (Molloy and Denniston 2018). However, delaying a feedback discussion is likely to be better if the learner is exhausted, upset, or distracted due to a catastrophe or if they urgently need to be elsewhere, for example, to pick-up a child from day care. Taking a broader perspective, the way training programs are designed can greatly influence feedback. Potential strategies to promote meaningful conversations include integrating opportunities for observation, finding ways to create longer educator-learner relationships so trust can build and creating a culture focused on continuing development (Watling and Ginsburg 2019). In addition, feedback at the midpoint of an attachment is likely to be more valuable than at the end; feedback is only useful if a learner can apply it and this gives a learner the chance to make changes during the remaining time in the same context.

Considering *where* to have feedback discussions, typically it is recommended that they occur in private as performance evaluations pose risks to professional and social standing, which is magnified when others are present (this is further discussed in the section on psychological safety). On the other hand, if respectful and valuable feedback is routinely embedded into clinical practice, observers may also benefit and it provides the advantage of addressing performance promptly.

The Feedback Quality Instrument (FQI): A Learner-Centered Framework to Guide Practice

The Feedback Quality Instrument (FQI) describes key components of high quality formal face-to-face feedback interactions. It was developed through a research process including an extensive literature review, expert analysis, and psychometric tests (explained in detail elsewhere), involving three of us (CJ, JK, EM) (Johnson et al. 2016, 2019). It describes what educators can do to engage, motivate, and enable a learner to improve. As part of the FQI development 36 authentic feedback interactions between educators and learners during routine clinical practice were analysed; reflection on this analysis in the context of the broader field of feedback research led us to construct a framework for impactful feedback conversations, which we describe in detail below.

Components in Formal Feedback Discussions

Formal feedback discussions can be characterized by five core components. Three components occur more or less sequentially: set the scene, analyse performance, and plan improvements. The other two components occur throughout a feedback exchange: foster psychological safety, and foster learner agency and understanding.

Set the Scene

Educators rarely set the scene at the beginning of feedback conversations (Johnson et al. 2019), and so the opportunity to lay the groundwork for optimizing the interaction is missed. This introduction is similar to a "prebrief" or "brief" in simulation education (Kolbe et al. 2019; Rudolph et al. 2014). By explicitly highlighting the purpose, discussing expectations for the process and each person's role in the interaction, and clarifying the time available, the feedback arrangements become more transparent and predictable. If the learner knows what to expect and has some control over it, anxiety related to these uncertainties can be reduced. Anxiety impairs complex thinking and memory, which are key capabilities underpinning learning. Involving the learner in negotiating expectations for the feedback process sets a tone of equity and collaboration for the whole session. It might sound something like this:

> Educator: Today we have about 20 minutes to discuss the urinary catheter insertion you did for Mr P this morning. The aim of this is to help you get a step closer to passing your competency assessment next month. You and I haven't had a feedback discussion before, so I'd like to describe what I think works well and then I'm keen to hear what you think would be most useful. I usually like to start by asking you to compare what you did, with what you saw me do when I demonstrated the procedure. Then we can clarify which aspects hit the mark and do not, yet. Let me know what you were unsure of and ask any questions you like as we go because I am keen to help you. Together we can decide exactly what will be most useful for you to work on next, to continue your progress. What would you like to add to or modify about this plan?

Analyse Performance

Evaluation involves the educator and learner comparing the learner's performance with the expected standards (the target "quality performance"), to identify both similarities and differences. This is a collaborative process with the aim of developing a shared understanding of the learner's capabilities and identifying which aspect to refine next.

It is important for a learner to develop skills in identifying quality work, and to make judgements about how their own work, or the work of others, compares to this standard. This capacity is known as "evaluative judgment" (Tai et al. 2016b; Dawson et al. 2018). It facilitates a learner's ability to independently monitor and improve their performance, including whenever educators are not available (Johnson and Molloy 2018; Tai et al. 2017). Once a learner has a strong vision of the key characteristics of a "good performance," any differences in their own performance become more apparent. So, one of the most useful things an educator can do is to help the learner to develop a clear vision of "what it should look like" and understand why these features are important. This can be done through educator modelling of clinical practice (ideally accompanied by an explanation), or through description of good practice.

Often evaluation looks like this:

Educator: So why don't you start off by telling me how you went?
Learner: I thought it was okay.
Educator: So I thought.....

Here, when the educator asks the learner for their self-assessment, the learner just makes a vague and superficial comment and then the educator starts to explain their own assessment. This suggests that neither believe that a learner's self-assessment is worthwhile. However, a learner's self-assessment plays an important role in feedback. It allows the learner to practice evaluating their own work by comparing it with the target performance, and to raise key issues they would like to focus on. This process is thought to develop a learner's evaluative judgement (Johnson and Molloy 2018; Tai et al. 2016b). From the educator's perspective, it often reveals gaps or inaccuracies in the learner's understanding of the target performance (and hence in the judgment of their own work), which the educator can address. It helps calibrate the learner's judgment if the educator explains why they agree or disagree with the learner's analysis. In addition, when a learner reveals they are having difficulties with one aspect of the performance and asks for help, this invitation for assistance indicates that the learner is open to advice and motivated to work on this area.

Here's what a collaborative evaluation could look like:

Educator: So, tell me how did things go during the session with Mrs J this afternoon?
Learner: Yeah, it went pretty well. I asked how she found the exercises I gave her last week and if she had any difficulties . . . I checked if she'd done any walking and if that caused any pain. I think I addressed her concerns well, because she was a bit worried about doing the more difficult squats, so I talked about how she could modify the exercises. It's hard to know if she is doing the other exercises properly but I had given her the handouts.
Educator: I agree, you've built up a good rapport with Mrs J. Your review was well structured - you covered all the important points and you modified the squats appropriately. I might have missed this but did you ask her to show you how she's been doing each exercise?
Learner: Now I remember that you did that last week when we worked together but I did not think of it at the time. That would have helped me sort out whether or not she was correctly interpreting the exercise handout.

Educator: Yes, I find that it can be revealing when you check exactly what people are doing. Did you think that her English was good enough to understand the instructions?
Learner: She seemed to speak English fairly well… I guess her first language is Greek. I could have checked if she preferred the handout in Greek.

The language of feedback matters; it should set the tone for a collaborative and supportive discussion with a focus on the learner's continuing development (Johnson et al. 2020a). A candid interaction, as illustrated here, suggests the learner feels psychologically safe, as they honestly reflect on their work, raise difficulties and propose improvements. Within this excerpt, the educator responds to the learner's comments and uses questions to encourage further reflection and suggest ideas. These strategies show the educator values the learner's perspective and is keen to assist, thereby fostering psychological safety (see the section on psychological safety for more details).

A learner needs to understand three pieces of information to help them navigate their path to improvement: (i) the key features of the target "quality performance" (ii) similarities and differences between their own performance and the target performance, and (iii) what they can do to get closer to the target performance (Hattie and Timperley 2007; Sadler 1989). The last one equates to the action plan, which is discussed later.

If the educator selects a suitable example in the learner's practice and describes the learner's actions and their consequences, this creates a foundation for an open discussion covering the learner's version of the event, their intentions, and reasoning behind their actions (Silverman and Kurtz 1997; Rudolph et al. 2016). It is essential for learners and educators to work together to identify the underlying reasons for observed behaviors. For example, a learner could make a wrong diagnosis for a patient's wrist pain for a number of reasons. Possibilities include that the learner had never been taught about common wrist conditions; they did not know how to correctly examine the wrist or interpret the clinical findings; they only examined the patient's wrist briefly because it was so painful; or they could not recall the name of the correct condition under the stress of presenting to an intimidating professor and so, called it something else. Different reasons for an error could need different solutions. This illustrates the benefits of an educator directly observing a learner undertaking a task as it gives an educator first-hand information, which provides a better basis for discussion. Nevertheless, an educator's memory and interpretation of what happened presents only one viewpoint, so educators should check these with learners' own accounts. In addition, learners may alter what they do when they are being observed, so what is observed may not represent a learner's "normal practice" (Watling et al. 2016; Pelgrim et al. 2012). When feedback does rely on reports from other clinicians, descriptions of specific instances provide a better starting point for feedback discussions than observers' inferences.

Identifying aspects that met expected standards, and those that did not, serve different purposes. When educators describe which aspects learners did correctly (or have improved), especially those skills that learners have been working on, it highlights progress and achievement. This engenders feelings of competence and satisfaction, that "I can do this" and "the hard work is worth it." This motivates learners to continue applying effort and effective strategies into the next phase of development (Locke and Latham 2002; Ten Cate et al. 2011). In addition, it helps to calibrate learners' evaluative judgement. Alternatively, when educators clarify aspects of performance that still need improvement, this focuses learners' attention on the performance gap, and what they could do differently to continue improving. Here is an example of an educator giving clear, specific and actionable information. The educator describes key features of "quality," compares it with the learner's performance and then suggests one way to do it more effectively:

> Educator: I thought you answered the question for him when you said, "How are you going at home? You're obviously doing pretty well: you told me you cook and look after yourself without any help". He's an elderly gentleman and sometimes people aren't doing as well as it initially seems. If you had asked 'How are you managing at home?' and included the daughter in that conversation, I think you might have got more accurate information about how he was really coping alone at home since his wife died.

Educator Reticence to Broach Substandard Performance

Typically, educators are reluctant to raise performance concerns, even though this offers the best chance for learners to improve their practice (Johnson and Molloy 2018; Ende et al. 1995; Ramani et al. 2017). Educators report they fear it will elicit negative emotional responses or a loss of self-esteem in learners, and damage their collegial relationship. This manifests in educators trying to "soften the blow." At times, educators attempt to raise issues indirectly by making vague, ambiguous or camouflaged comments. Another common technique used is to attempt to "sweeten" comments by "sandwiching" them between praise delivered before and afterwards (Molloy et al. 2019).

On the other hand when an educator directly discusses substandard performance in an open-minded and collaborative way, it gives the best opportunity for a learner to clearly understand "what the problem is" and focus on "how to fix it," or to consider how the performance might have been impacted by context or circumstance. In addition, it helps to create a "continuing improvement" atmosphere where skill gaps or mistakes are expected and characterized as useful learning opportunities (Dweck and Yeager 2019).

Experts recommend the following strategy to honestly and openly discuss aspects of substandard performance (Silverman and Kurtz 1997; Rudolph et al. 2007). The educator starts by describing the specific actions observed (what was done, said or decided), as this helps the learner to focus on the particular event under review. Actions are best described as effective (or not) for achieving the desired objective, instead of "good" or "bad." The educator clearly explains their provisional concern or opinion, keeping in mind that their subjective interpretation of events may be incorrect. Some examples of language that invite the learner to offer a different perspective include "I am wondering if...but I may have misunderstood so I am interested to hear your view" or "I am beginning to think...can you help me understand what I am missing?" An educator can only know *what* happened, not *why*. Importantly, the educator invites the learner to share their own perspective. This is crucial, as there are frequently alternative reasons for specific behaviors. For example, if a learner is seen arriving late to an interprofessional team meeting, it could be because they preferred to stay longer at a colleague's farewell morning tea; the wrong meeting room was listed on the meeting invitation; they were delayed because they helped a visitor to find the outpatient clinic; or took an urgent phone call about their child. All of these explanations warrant different interventions. Often a learner is reluctant to contest an educator's comments, so it is up to the educator to encourage a learner to voice their thoughts by emphasizing the educator's intention to help the learner, their desire to understand the real reason for what happened and tailor an effective solution. Exploring the learner's reasoning, including aims, options, priorities or assumptions, helps identify underlying learning needs.

> Educator: I notice that you didn't check Mr L's reflexes. What was your reasoning there?
> Learner: Yes, I know I should have done that but he was getting agitated so I figured he'd had enough. I thought I would come back to do it later.
> Educator: Assessing reflexes is an important part of the neurological examination because it is a key sign for differentiating upper and lower motor neurone disorders. Delaying it causes problems because further investigations need to be arranged, based on the examination. Plus testing reflexes is fairly quick to complete but it does need patient cooperation. How else could you have helped his agitation?
> Learner: I really didn't know what to do. I just tried to finish my examination as quickly as possible.
> Educator: You could have asked him why he seemed restless. There may have been something simple you could have done for him, to settle him down. For example, he might have needed to use the bathroom. Let's go back in and see if we can complete the examination together.

Describing actions and decisions focuses learners' attention on actions that can be corrected (Ende 1983). In contrast, comments regarding inherent personal attributes focuses attention directly at a person's "self," which tends to evoke strong negative emotions as a protective response (Kluger and DeNisi 1996). Once aspects for improvement have been agreed on, the pair can turn their attention to developing plans for improvements.

Plan for Improvement

Action plans involve specifying the practical steps a learner can take to improve their performance. This may include developing task performance, learning strategies or professional identity. It is frequently missing in feedback conversations in the clinical environment (Johnson et al. 2019; Fernando et al. 2008). Action plans may involve simple educator tips or more extensive strategies for improvement, for example, practicing a psychomotor task, like tying surgical knots; making a stroke rehabilitation program more patient centered, by starting with identifying what the patient would like to achieve; trying a new strategy to be more organized, such as by getting to work 15 minutes before the shift starts so there is time to prepare the day's task list; or watching a YouTube video on how to screen for delirium in hospitalized patients. The best action plans – those which are most likely to be successfully implemented by the learner – are developed by the learner and educator working together (Sargeant et al. 2015). People like to learn in different ways depending on their preferences and circumstances, so it is a good idea to design the action plan to match these preferences whenever possible. For example, one learner might prefer more "hands on" practice with a colleague, while another may prefer listening to podcasts during a long commute. Using a coaching approach, it is useful to consider various options including any expected difficulties, in order to refine strategies to overcome them (Sargeant et al. 2015, 2018).

People are more likely to achieve goals that are specific (so they know when you have achieved it), measurable (so they can monitor progress), achievable (so there is a high likelihood that putting in the effort will lead to success), relevant (pertinent to their objective) and time based (has defined timelines). This is known as developing SMART goals (Locke and Latham 2002).

Plan a Review

Another important aspect of effective feedback is to plan a review, after the learner has implemented the action plan, to see whether the strategies were effective:

> Educator: How do you feel like you've gone with your patient this week?
> Learner: I feel that my management has been getting a bit better. After we discussed creating a problem list last week, I found it was helpful to identify what her main problems are. Do you want to take a look at my notes and see if I got them correct? Also, I found it hard to specify a problem in a short phrase, so I think they are a bit long winded.

This demonstrates how feedback is best handled as an ongoing conversation, rather than a one-off, as this enables "closing of the loop" and setting new goals to continue advancing practice. In addition, this example shows a learner practicing their evaluative judgement by outlining their evaluation of their work and seeking to calibrate this against the educator's perspective.

Modern clinical education environments are often characterized by fragmented supervision. This can make it difficult for educators to trace the effect of their feedback conversation on the learner's performance (Watling and Ginsburg 2019). Without "seeing the effect" of feedback, it is harder for educators to calibrate and refine their own feedback approaches. Learners can proactively create links between separate educator's sessions and drive ongoing improvements themselves by relaying a previous educator's comments in a subsequent session and asking the educator to analyze their progress in that specific area. At the organizational level, it could be useful to consider how longitudinal teacher-learner relationships can be promoted when creating work and learning schedules (Molloy et al. 2019).

Foster a Psychologically Safe Learning Environment

The most useful outcomes from feedback discussions are likely to arise when a learner and educator engage in an interactive discussion, incorporating both their perspectives, to co-construct new insights and plans. A learner is more likely to fully engage in a feedback discussion about their learning needs if they feel psychologically safe (Carless 2013). Psychological safety is defined as "a shared belief that the team is safe for interpersonal risk taking" which gives rise "to a sense of confidence that the team will not embarrass, reject or punish someone…due to mutual respect and trust" (Edmondson 1999). Typical learning behaviors such as asking questions, trialling a new technique, proposing a solution, making mistakes or asking for help, all reveal learners' limitations. In addition, there is often a substantial power imbalance between the learner and educator, especially if the educator is responsible for assessing the learner at the end of their clinical attachment or could be a potential referee. Therefore, a learner may not want to reveal their difficulties, in case it negatively influences the educator's opinion of the learner's professional credibility. A learner's dilemma could be summarized as "what is the likelihood of a beneficial outcome including valuable help and support, compared to a detrimental outcome such as experiencing embarrassment or humiliation, or having my progress impeded" (Cook and Artino Jr 2016)? Hence, achieving psychological safety is a tricky enterprise, for all the reasons outlined here.

Psychological safety can be enhanced by an educator demonstrating respect, support and assistance, and focusing on continuing improvement (Johnson et al. 2020a). Learners gauge the safety of a learning interaction based on a number of factors: their past experience with an educator, their observations of that educator interacting with others, and the stories they hear from their peers. (Edmondson 1996, 1999). Herein lies the potential value of longitudinal relationships between educators and learners, so they can get to know each other and establish a safe learning environment (Voyer et al. 2016). Nevertheless, it seems likely that educators can develop skills in fostering psychological safety with learners in once-off interactions, just as they need to do with patients (Silverman et al. 2013).

Educators can demonstrate respect for learners in many ways. This includes being courteous, valuing learners' views, recognizing learners' autonomy and appreciating learners' current expertise and future potential. Educators can use inclusive language, such as "we," to show they include the learner in the health professional community (Johnson et al. 2020a). For example, an educator might say, "It is important that we discuss treatment options with patients." If educators convey that mistakes and difficulties are valuable opportunities for learning and that any skill can be improved by applying effective learning strategies, effort and persistence, this is likely to convey a "growth mindset" (Dweck 1986). Educators can show they value learners' contributions to feedback discussions by exploring learners' perspective, listening attentively, taking their ideas into account and responding thoughtfully. These are crucial activities in creating a shared understanding, and a springboard for innovative ideas. Educators can assist learners by collaborating with them to develop effective strategies to enhance performance. Learners' confidence can be strengthened when educators indicate they want to work alongside the learner and believe the learner can succeed. Educators can communicate compassion by empathizing with difficulties that learners experience during clinical practice. The power differential can be reduced by an educator showing their own vulnerability. They might do this, for example, by openly stating that they do not know everything or that they remember when they had a similar struggle at a comparable stage in their own training (Molloy and Bearman 2019; Bynum and Artin 2019).

Foster Learner Understanding and Learner Agency

Learning can be viewed as a process of interpreting and building on experiences, by creating mental schemas that encompass key information about concepts and that link to related mental schemas (Wadsworth 1996). A learner draws on the relevant schema to make sense of what is going on around them and to solve problems. Whenever a learner's mental schema is insufficient or clashes with an experience, attempting to solve this problem stimulates correcting, extending or adding further detail to the schema, to make it more useful. Learning can be promoted by discussing the topic with others, including reflecting, reasoning and making decisions (Epstein et al. 2008; Kaufman 2010). It drives the brain to review an idea from different perspectives, and to compare and connect it with (or divide it from) other concepts. Educators can promote these active learning strategies by encouraging a learner to explain their thinking, consider alternatives, ask questions and try to problem-solve.

When educators are conveying information, they can make it easier to understand by explaining it simply and clearly, describing specific examples, clarifying the meaning of technical terms, explaining the rationale and encouraging questions. It is useful if an educator starts with basic information and avoids unnecessary details that do not contribute to helping a learner understand core concepts. Learning involves processing information via the working memory, to build mental schemas. This requires sustained attention and mental energy, which limits the rate of processing, particularly for novel or complex information. Processing of valuable information can be impeded by extraneous information, tiredness or distractions (Fraser et al. 2015; Van Merrienboer and Sweller 2010). As a learner is only going to be able to process limited information at one time, an educator can help by focusing discussions on just one or two aspects of the performance, instead of trying to address a long list. An educator can find out which aspects might be the "most useful to focus on next" by asking what the learner found difficult or wants to learn.

In wrapping up a feedback session, it can be useful to check the learner's understanding of the goals and action plan. One useful tactic is to ask the learner to explain it to you in their own words:

> Educator: What do you think are the key things to take out of today that you need to use in the future?

Learner agency refers to a learner's capacity to achieve goals by utilizing available resources, such as their time, effort, intellect, access to educational information or personal advice (Molloy and Boud 2013; Nicol and Macfarlane-Dick 2006).

During feedback exchanges, educators can facilitate learners' development in various ways. They may use their expertise to demonstrate a new technique to improve an examination, advocate for a learner to prioritize improving one particular aspect of a performance or assist learners to develop their learning strategies, such as making learning goals "SMART." As the effect of feedback depends on the learner, the learner could be described as "the enactor" of feedback and the educator as "the enabler" (Johnson et al. 2016). In addition, educators can support learners' intrinsic motivation by fostering learners' feelings of competence, connection and autonomy (Ten Cate et al. 2011; Deci and Ryan 2000). A learner is more likely to be successful when they have a clear understanding of exactly what they need to do to improve and why this will help them to achieve their goals, so they feel motivated to work at it.

Individuals prize autonomy. They resist being controlled but will happily devote considerable time and effort to pursuits that interest them. In clinical practice, learners have their own goals and are motivated to achieve them (Deci and Ryan 2000). Hence, they prioritize activities that will move them closer to achieving them. So, if an educator offers assistance that will help them reach their goals faster, it is more likely to be used. On the other hand, if an educator talks about a topic that holds no interest or relevance for the learner, a learner may tend to ignore the educator or only reluctantly comply. However, there are times that learners need to master skills that may not particularly interest them. In this setting, an educator needs to find ways to promote autonomy and ensure learners develop their competence across required domains. A potentially useful approach involves the educator explaining why the skill is important for the learner while explicitly acknowledging their lack of interest and collaborating with them to develop efficient strategies that suit them by seeking the learner's ideas first and then the learner's opinions on the educator's suggestions.

Summary and Conclusion

Experts agree that feedback is crucial for optimizing performance, although it is rarely done well in practice. In this chapter we have shared our reflections on the key components of effective feedback conversations, accompanied by practical examples based on observational research focussing on clinical interactions. We propose using the Feedback Quality Instrument to reinforce the key elements of effective feedback: psychologically safe, collaborative conversation about performance that inspires continuous improvement. We hope that educators and learners will find our reflections useful in thinking about their own practice, and unlock more of the potential power in their feedback.

Cross-References

- ▶ Coaching in Health Professions Education: The Case of Surgery
- ▶ Conversational Learning in Health Professions Education: Learning Through Talk

► Debriefing Practices in Simulation-Based Education
► Written Feedback in Health Sciences Education: "What You Write May Be Perceived as Banal"

References

Bangert-Drowns RL, Kulik C-LC, Kulik JA, Morgan M. The instructional effect of feedback in test-like events. Rev Educ Res. 1991;61(2):213–38.

Bing-You RG, Paterson J, Levine MA. Feedback falling on deaf ears: residents' receptivity to feedback tempered by sender credibility. Med Teach. 1997;19(1):40–4.

Boud D, Molloy E. What is the problem with feedback? In: Boud D, Molloy E, editors. Feedback in higher and professional education. London: Routledge; 2013. p. 1–10.

Butler DL, Winne PH. Feedback and self-regulated learning: a theoretical synthesis. Rev Educ Res. 1995;65(3):245–81.

Bynum WE, Artin AR. Why we should strive for emotional candour in medical education, too. Med Educ. 2019;53(7):745–6.

Carless D. Trust and its role in facilitating dialogic feedback. In: Boud D, Molloy E, editors. Feedback in higher and professional education. London: Routledge; 2013. p. 90–103.

Carless D, Boud D. The development of student feedback literacy: enabling uptake of feedback. Assess Eval High Educ. 2018;43(8):1315–25.

Cook DA, Artino AR Jr. Motivation to learn: an overview of contemporary theories. Med Educ. 2016;50(10):997–1014.

Dawson P, Ajjawi R, Boud D, Tai J. Introduction: what is evaluative judgement? In: Boud D, Ajjawi R, Dawson P, Tai J, editors. Developing evaluative judgement in higher education assessment for knowing and producing quality work. London: Routledge; 2018. p. 1–4.

Deci EL, Ryan RM. The 'what' and 'why' of goal pursuits: human needs and the self-determination of behavior. Psychol Inq. 2000;11:227–68.

Dweck CS. Motivational processes affecting learning. Am Psychol. 1986;41:1040.

Dweck CS, Yeager DS. Mindsets: a view from two eras. Perspect Psychol Sci. 2019;14(3):481–96.

Edmondson AC. Learning from mistakes is easier said than done: group and organizational influences on the detection and correction of human error. J Appl Behav Sci. 1996;32(1):5–28.

Edmondson AC. Psychological safety and learning behavior in work teams. Adm Sci Q. 1999;44(2):350–83.

Ende J. Feedback in clinical medical education. J Am Med Assoc. 1983;250(6):777–81.

Ende J, Pomerantz A, Erickson F. Preceptors' strategies for correcting residents in an ambulatory care medicine setting: a qualitative analysis. Acad Med. 1995;70(3):224–9.

Ericsson KA. Acquisition and maintenance of medical expertise: a perspective from the expert-performance approach with deliberate practice. Acad Med. 2015;90(11):1471–86.

Epstein RM, Siegel DJ, Silberman J. Self-Monitoring in Clinical Practice: A Challenge for Medical Educators J Contin Educ Health Prof 2008;28(1):5–13

Fernando N, Cleland J, McKenzie H, Cassar K. Identifying the factors that determine feedback given to undergraduate medical students following formative mini-CEX assessments. Med Educ. 2008;42(1):89–95.

Fraser KL, Ayres P, Sweller J. Cognitive load theory for the design of medical simulations. Simulation in Healthcare. 2015;10(5):295–307.

Hattie J, Timperley H. The power of feedback. Rev Educ Res. 2007;77(1):81–112.

Hewson MG, Little ML. Giving feedback in medical education: verification of recommended techniques. J Gen Intern Med. 1998;13(2):111–6.

Johnson CE, Molloy EK. Building evaluative judgement through the process of feedback. In: Boud D, Ajjawi R, Dawson P, Tai J, editors. Developing evaluative judgement in higher education assessment for knowing and producing quality work. London: Routledge; 2018. p. 166–75.

Johnson CE, Keating JL, Boud DJ, Dalton M, Kiegaldie D, Hay M, et al. Identifying educator behaviours for high quality verbal feedback in health professions education: literature review and expert refinement. BMC Med Educ. 2016;16(1):96.

Johnson CE, Keating JL, Farlie MK, Kent F, Leech M, Molloy EK. Educators' behaviours during feedback in authentic clinical practice settings: an observational study and systematic analysis. BMC Med Educ. 2019;19(1):129.

Johnson CE, Keating JL, Molloy EK. Psychological safety in feedback: what does it look like and how can educators work with learners to foster it? Med Educ. 2020a;54(6):559–70.

Johnson CE, Weerasuria MP, Keating JL. Effect of face-to-face verbal feedback compared with no or alternative feedback on the objective workplace task performance of health professionals: a systematic review and meta-analysis. BMJ Open. 2020b;10(3):e030672.

Kaufman DM. Applying educational theory in practice. In: Cantillon P, Wood D, editors. ABC of learning and teaching in medicine. Oxford: Blackwell Publishing; 2010.

Kluger AN, DeNisi A. The effects of feedback interventions on performance: a historical review, a meta-analysis, and a preliminary feedback intervention theory. Psychol Bull. 1996;119(2):254–84.

Kolbe M, Eppich W, Rudolph J, Meguerdichian M, Catena H, Cripps A, et al. Managing psychological safety in debriefings: a dynamic balancing act. BMJ Simul Technol Enhanc Learn. 2019. https://doi.org/10.1136/bmjstel-2019-000470.

Locke EA, Latham GP. Building a practically useful theory of goal setting and task motivation. A 35-year odyssey. Am Psychol. 2002;57(9):705–17.

Molloy E. Time to pause: feedback in clinical education. In: Delany C, Molloy E, editors. Clinical education in the health professions. Sydney: Elsevier; 2009. p. 128–46.

Molloy E, Bearman M. Embracing the tension between vulnerability and credibility: 'intellectual candour' in health professions education. Med Educ. 2019;53(1):32–41.

Molloy E, Boud D. Changing conceptions of feedback. In: B D, Molloy E, editors. Feedback in higher and professional education. London: Routledge; 2013. p. 11–33.

Molloy E, Denniston C. The role of feedback in surgical education. In: Nestel D, Dalrymple K, Paige P, Aggarwha R, editors. Advancing surgical education: theory, evidence and practice. New York: Springer; 2018.

Molloy E, Borrell-Carrio F, Epstein R. The impact of emotions in feedback. In: Boud D, Molloy E, editors. Feedback in higher and professional education. London: Routledge; 2013. p. 50–71.

Molloy E, Ajjawi R, Bearman M, Noble C, Rudland J, Ryan A. Challenging feedback myths: values, learner involvement and promoting effects beyond the immediate task. Med Educ. 2019;54(1):33–9.

Nicol DJ, Macfarlane-Dick D. Formative assessment and self-regulated learning: a model and seven principles of good feedback practice. Stud High Educ. 2006;31(2):199–218.

Noble C, Billett S, Armit L, Collier L, Hilder J, Sly C, et al. "It's yours to take": generating learner feedback literacy in the workplace. Adv in Health Sci Educ 2020;25:55–74. https://doi.org/10.1007/s10459-019-09905-5

Pelgrim EA, Kramer AW, Mokkink HG, van der Vleuten CP. The process of feedback in workplace-based assessment: organisation, delivery, continuity. Med Educ. 2012;46(6):604–12.

Ramani S, Post SE, Könings K, Mann K, Katz JT, van der Vleuten C. "It's just not the culture": a qualitative study exploring residents' perceptions of the impact of institutional culture on feedback. Teach Learn Med. 2017;29(2):153–61.

Ramani S, Konings KD, Ginsburg S, van der Vleuten CPM. Twelve tips to promote a feedback culture with a growth mindset: Swinging the feedback pendulum from recipes to relationships, Medical Teacher, 2019;41(6)625–631. https://doi.org/10.1080/0142159X.2018.1432850

Rudolph JW, Simon R, Rivard P, Dufresne RL, Raemer DB. Debriefing with good judgment: combining rigorous feedback with genuine inquiry. Anesthesiol Clin. 2007;25:361.

Rudolph JW, Raemer DB, Simon R. Establishing a safe container for learning in simulation: the role of the presimulation briefing. Simul Healthc. 2014;9(6):339–49.

Rudolph JW, Simon R, Dufresne RL, Raemer DB. There's no such thing as "nonjudgmental" debriefing: a theory and method for debriefing with good judgment. Simul Healthc. 2016;1(1):49–55.

Sadler DR. Formative assessment and the design of instructional systems. Instr Sci. 1989;18(2):119–44.

Sargeant J, Mann K, Ferrier S. Exploring family physicians' reactions to multisource feedback: perceptions of credibility and usefulness. Med Educ. 2005;39(5):497–504.

Sargeant J, Mann K, Sinclair D, Van der Vleuten C, Metsemakers J. Understanding the influence of emotions and reflection upon multi-source feedback acceptance and use. Adv Health Sci Educ. 2008;13(3):275–88.

Sargeant J, Lockyer J, Mann K, Holmboe E, Silver I, Armson H, et al. Facilitated reflective performance feedback: developing an evidence- and theory-based model that builds relationship, explores reactions and content, and coaches for performance change (R2C2). Acad Med. 2015;90(12):1698–706.

Sargeant J, Lockyer JM, Mann K, Armson H, Warren A, Zetkulic M, et al. The R2C2 model in residency education: how does it Foster coaching and promote feedback use? Acad Med. 2018;93(7):1055–63.

Silverman J, Kurtz S. The Calgary-Cambridge approach to communication skills teaching II: the set-go method of descriptive feedback. Educ Gen Pract. 1997;8(7):288–99.

Silverman J, Kurtz S, Draper J. Building the relationship. Skills for communicating with patients. 3rd ed. London: Radcliffe Publishing; 2013. p. 118–48.

Tai J, Molloy E, Haines T, Canny B. Same-level peer-assisted learning in medical clinical placements: a narrative systematic review. Med Educ. 2016a;50(4):469–84.

Tai JH, Canny BJ, Haines TP, Molloy EK. The role of peer-assisted learning in building evaluative judgement: opportunities in clinical medical education. Adv Health Sci Educ. 2016b;21(3):659–76.

Tai JH, Ajjawi R, Boud D, Dawson P, Panadero E. Developing evaluative judgement: enabling students to make decisions about the quality of work. High Educ. 2017;76:467. https://doi.org/10.1007/s10734-017-0220-3.

Telio S, Ajjawi R, Regehr G. The "educational alliance" as a framework for reconceptualizing feedback in medical education. Acad Med. 2015;90(5):609–14.

Telio S, Regehr G, Ajjawi R. Feedback and the educational alliance: examining credibility judgements and their consequences. Med Educ. 2016;50(9):933–42.

Ten Cate TJ, Kusurkar RA, Williams GC. How self-determination theory can assist our understanding of the teaching and learning processes in medical education. AMEE guide no. 59. Med Teach. 2011;33(12):961–73.

van der Leeuw RM, Teunissen PW, van der Vleuten CPM. Broadening the scope of feedback to promote its relevance to workplace learning. Acad Med. 2018;93(4):556–9.

Van Merrienboer JJG, Sweller J. Cognitive load theory in health professional education: design principles and strategies. Medical Education. 2010;44(44):85–93

Voyer S, Cuncic C, Butler DL, MacNeil K, Watling C, Hatala R. Investigating conditions for meaningful feedback in the context of an evidence-based feedback programme. Med Educ. 2016;50(9):943–54.

Wadsworth BJ. Piaget's theory of cognitive and affective development: foundations of constructivism. 5th ed. White Plains: Longman Publishing; 1996.

Watling C, Ginsburg S. Assessment, feedback and the alchemy of learning. Med Educ. 2019;53(1):76–85.

Watling C, LaDonna KA, Lingard L, Voyer S, Hatala R. 'Sometimes the work just needs to be done': socio-cultural influences on direct observation in medical training. Med Educ. 2016;50(10):1054–64.

Supervision in General Practice Settings

James Brown and Susan M. Wearne

Contents

Introduction	1074
GP as a Training Environment, Trainee Progression and Theoretical Models	1076
Three Theoretical Perspectives on GP Work-Based Learning	1076
Trainee Trajectories and Supervision in GP	1078
The Tasks of Supervision in GP	1080
Engaging the Trainee in the Working Community	1080
Conducting the Ad Hoc Supervisory Call-In	1082
Teaching	1084
Mentorship and Role Modelling	1086
Monitoring and Feedback	1087
Assessment	1089
Facilitating an Understanding of Good Practice	1090
Shared Supervision	1091
Supervisor Recruitment	1092
Inducting the New Supervisor to the Role	1093
Supporting the Supervisor	1093
Facilitating Supervisor Peer Networks	1094
Supervisor Professional Development	1094
Engaging the Supervisor in Program Development and Delivery	1094
Conclusion	1095
Cross-References	1095
References	1095

J. Brown (✉)
Royal Australian College of General Practice, East Melbourne, VIC, Australia

Gippsland Medical School, Monash University, Churchill, VIC, Australia
e-mail: jamesboyerbrown@gmail.com

S. M. Wearne
Health Workforce Division, Commonwealth Department of Health, Canberra, ACT, Australia

Academic Unit of General Practice, Australian National University, Canberra, ACT, Australia
e-mail: susan.wearne@health.gov.au

© Springer Nature Singapore Pte Ltd. 2023
D. Nestel et al. (eds.), *Clinical Education for the Health Professions*,
https://doi.org/10.1007/978-981-15-3344-0_54

Abstract

Supervision in the general practice (GP) setting is work-based education. This chapter draws on three social theories of work-based education to provide a focus for exploring the tasks of GP supervised practice. Based on this, we consider the roles and needs of the trainee, the supervisor, and the training practice. We also consider how training organizations that oversee the whole of GP training delivery might support the GP supervisor. We view the trainee as on a trajectory towards becoming a fully credentialed clinician with the associated responsibilities. This requires a change over time in the way that the trainee is identified and identifies themselves. The way that the trainee engages with the work-based training environment is crucial for how this happens. We view the supervisor as a key facilitator for enabling the trainee to effectively and safely engage with the training practice working community and its work. The supervisor also has an important role in scaffolding the trainee's development. The attitude of the supervisor and the nature of the supervisory relationship are key for these activities. The culture of the training practice and the way that the training practice engages with the trainee also matter. Functioning well, training practices can benefit from the trainee as both a contributor to the work and as a resource for keeping the training practice up to date. Finally, the support provided to supervisors by the broader training organization is a significant determinant for the way the supervisor engages with their supervisory role.

Keywords

General practice · Work-based learning · Supervision · Training · Theory and practice

Introduction

This chapter is about clinical education in the context of supervision in general practice (GP). It is intended as a resource for trainees, supervisors, and faculty who are teaching and learning in this context. The content draws on relevant theoretical models, research, scholarly opinion, and the authors' practical experience.

By "general practice" we refer to the delivery of primary medical care overseen by a primary care physician in the community context (Greenhalgh 2007). In some contexts, this is referred to as "family medicine." By "supervision," we draw on Wearne et al.'s definition of the GP supervisor:

> A GP supervisor is a general practitioner who establishes and maintains an educational alliance that supports the clinical, educational and personal development of a resident. (Wearne et al. 2012)

Both authors are general practitioner supervisors and educational researchers in Australia. James Brown also oversees the professional development program for supervisors under a GP training organization. Susan M. Wearne also works as a senior medical adviser for the Australian Department of Health.

In Australia, GP is mostly delivered by medically trained generalists working in private group practices that provide GP medical consultations together with a range of nursing and allied health services. These practices receive funding to host medical students and GP trainees. Senior medical students and GP trainees learn as they contribute to the work of patient care by attending patients themselves under varying levels of supervision. A nomenclature of levels of supervision is provided in Table 1 (Medical Board of Australia 2017). This supervision is provided by a fully qualified general practitioner who is usually on-site attending to their own patients.

In Australia, universities oversee the placement and training of medical students and GP regional training organizations oversee the placement and training of postgraduate GP trainees. GP trainees have educational and supervision requirements based on their stage of training. Qualification (fellowship) as a general practitioner requires at least 4 years of postgraduate experience. For postgraduate training, practices and supervisors are accredited by one or both of the two GP professional colleges, Australian College of Rural and Remote Medicine and Royal Australian College of General Practice. Training standards are set by those colleges. Training and support is also provided for supervisors by regional training organizations. In other countries, universities, professional colleges, or training organizations may oversee postgraduate training and between 2 and 6 years postgraduate experience is required (Gupta and Hays 2016).

In the GP context, supervision is principally about patient safety and enabling the trainee to contribute to the work of patient care (Morrison et al. 2015). Education for the student and trainee is an important secondary agenda and provides the means for both trainee development and for work-place maintenance and evolution. Learning within supervision in GP is work-based education. In most settings, the supervisory relationship is over an extended period of time.

This chapter is divided into three sections. The first introduces three applicable work-based learning theoretical frameworks and describes a conceptualization of the learning trajectory of supervised trainees in GP. The second section examines seven core supervisory activities and draws on the theoretical frameworks, relevant research, and the experience of the authors to recommend initiatives that supervisors, trainees, and the GP practice community might take to support learning. The third

Table 1 Levels of supervision

Level 1	(a) Supervisor is present as the trainee consults overseeing all consultations
	(b) Supervisor joins all trainee consultations for the consultation conclusion
Level 2	Supervisor is called in as required and all consultations are reviewed at the end of each clinical session
Level 3	(a) Supervisor is available to attend as required by the trainee and monitors trainee practice
	(b) Supervisor is available for advice by phone
Level 4	Mentorship and loose oversight

section examines the role of training organizations for supporting supervisors in their work of trainee education.

GP as a Training Environment, Trainee Progression and Theoretical Models

Work-based learning in GP under supervision is the main learning context for becoming a general practitioner (Gupta and Hays 2016). In this setting, trainees from medical student through to senior pre-fellowship trainee, learn as they contribute to the work of GP patient care.

In this section, first we consider three social learning theories that give different useful viewpoints for understanding work-place learning in GP; then we draw on these for the concept of a trajectory taken by the trainee towards becoming a fully credentialed general practitioner. We also look at the changing place of supervision depending on where the trainee is on the trajectory.

Three Theoretical Perspectives on GP Work-Based Learning

Theories of work-based learning are helpful for understanding supervision in general practice. While a detailed exploration of these theories is beyond the scope of this chapter, we introduce three prominent theories of work-based learning to inform the discussion. These theories are: Engestrom's Activity Theory (Engeström et al. 1999), Wenger's Communities of Practice (Wenger 1998), and Billett's theory of work-place pedagogy (Billett 2002) and personal epistemologies (Billett 2009). These theories view work-place learning as a social activity framed around four things: the work that is done; the community of workers who undertake the work; the learner; and, the resources and rules that the work-place uses to achieve its work.

Engestrom's Activity Theory takes the shared work object as its starting point. The concept is that work activities are defined by a common object and motive shared by a work team. In GP, this common object and motive is to create a plan for the patient (Brown et al. 2018). An activity system is a set of linked actions in a particular context bounded by a set of rules to achieve the object. Important in achieving the object is the use of artifacts which are resources that are both physical, such as a computer, and nonphysical, such as knowledge. Learning in an activity system is at two levels. The first is learning by the participants in the activity system in gaining access to the tools to achieve the object, particularly the tools of knowing. The second is learning by the system as a whole as it addresses the need to change over time so that it continues to achieve its object. This change may involve changing the conception of the object or be driven by the object itself, that is, the plan for the patient and the patient themself. For a trainee coming into the system of a GP clinic, they will need to re-learn the object of the clinical practice, gain access to new tools, and learn new knowledge including an understanding of the rules that govern the clinic and GP more broadly. The community itself will also need to change in order to effectively incorporate the trainee as a contributor to achieving the object.

Wenger's Community of Practice theory starts with the community of practice engaged in a common endeavor. Learning is principally about the longevity of the community of practice through inducting and enabling the development of newcomers and with this, adapting the community itself so that it remains relevant to a changing task. Learning in a GP from this perspective is about bringing newcomers into the clinic community to be members of that community and to be part of ensuring that the clinic community remains current and has longevity. A newcomer engages on a trajectory which moves them from the periphery of the community towards becoming an integral part of that community. This trajectory of changing identity is determined by their engagement with the community of practice and the meaning that they come to own in this. This means that the trainee in GP develops an identity that is defined by their participation and mutual engagement with the practice community within which they are working and training, and the meaning that the trainee and the practice community make of the trainee's participation.

Billett's work-place pedagogy and personal epistemologies foregrounds the interface between the work-place and its trainee. On the one side, the work-place is characterized by the affordances or resources and privileges it does or doesn't offer the trainee including the degree and manner of invitation to the trainee. On the other side, the trainee engages with and embraces whatever it is that the work-place offers depending on the trainee's personal characteristics, motives, and the meaning that the work has for them. Learning for the trainee in GP then is about the trainee gaining whatever they need to contribute to the work of the practice which depends on what they offered and on their personal orientation.

All three theoretical frameworks view the trainee and supervisor as culturally bound in the education that they engage in. The trainee and supervisor, however, within the bounds of their cultural context, have agency. That is, they have the capacity to be purposeful in their choices and this has an impact on learning and development.

Bringing these three theoretical perspectives together offers important concepts for framing supervision in GP (Table 2). These theories also point to imperatives for: the object of the work – patient care; the community of practice – maintaining its capacity to get the work done and enabling the trainee to be an effective contributor to the work; and the trainee – their engagement and development.

From this, we can generate an overarching list of seven imperatives for supervision of trainees in GP:

1. Ensuring patient safety
2. Enabling the practice to get the work done
3. Keeping work practices up to date
4. Enabling the trainee to contribute effectively to the work of the practice
5. Engaging the trainee effectively
6. Keeping the trainee safe
7. Scaffolding the trainee's development

Table 2 Selected theoretical concepts from work-based learning theories

Concept	Concept in the context of GP training
Object (of an activity) (Engeström et al. 1999)	The purpose of an activity. In GP patient care, this is usually to craft a plan with the patient. In trainee education, this is usually to enable them to contribute to care
Artifacts (Engeström et al. 1999)	The tools to achieve an object. In GP these are things such as an ECG, clinical software, and clinical knowledge used to achieve a plan for the patient
Rules (Engeström et al. 1999)	The explicit and implicit procedures and ways of doing things that the GP clinic working community works within
Community of practice (Wenger 1998)	The group of individuals within the GP clinic working to provide GP clinical care for the clinic's patients
Participation and mutual engagement	The engagement of the trainee and the GP clinic's working community in providing patient care
Trajectory of identity (Wenger 1998)	Over time, moving on a trajectory from the position of newcomer to the position of an experienced contributing member of the clinic community. There is also the trajectory from medical student to senior clinician
Affordances (Billett 2002)	Privileged access given to the trainee by the clinic working community to the resources it uses to achieve patient care
Personal epistemology (Billett 2009)	A trainee's specific stance towards learning and engaging with the work of the clinic based on their individual history and beliefs

Trainee Trajectories and Supervision in GP

All three theoretical models identify learning as a process of change for the learner, the working community, and the working community's systems.

Wenger's theory describes the change for the learner as a trajectory (Wenger 1998). This is a trajectory of increasing engagement in a working community and has three components: (1) a developing repertoire of competencies; (2) increasing ownership of meaning; and, (3) increasing privilege and accountability. For the trainee in GP, this equates to: (1) increasing GP relevant knowledge and skills; (2) developing disposition and identity (Cruess et al. 2016) of a general practitioner; and (3) increasing independence with decreasing level of supervision (Yardley et al. 2012).

To explore this trainee trajectory in GP, we examine three levels of trainee and their typical development with regards to: knowledge and skills, disposition and identity as a GP, and their required level of supervision.

The Senior Medical Student in GP

Senior medical students will typically enter the GP environment equipped with: basic clinical information knowledge; the skills to undertake a history and examination; and, the ability to present their findings to others. Their clinical reasoning skills are usually not well developed. The senior medical student's identity is still that of a student but also as a nascent clinician.

There are many areas of informational knowledge these students won't know that are needed in GP contexts. This may be new information particular to the GP context; or, it may be new application of information learned elsewhere. The student's lack of rational clinical thinking skills and credentialing limits their clinical engagement to doing things on the supervisor's behalf such as collecting information, writing notes, and organizing investigations and treatment. Level-1 supervision is required. At this stage of their trajectory, the learning tasks are to: gain the necessary informational knowledge; understand its application; and, to develop the clinical reasoning skills to be able to craft credible differential diagnoses and management options. The knowledge demands of the work drive student information learning as gaps in their knowledge are made apparent. Recognizing the need for clinical reasoning skills and the means of gaining these depends on a supervisor engaging the student in the process of making diagnostic and management conclusions and showing them how to derive these from the patient clinical information the student gathers. Being enabled to contribute to clinical decisions is important for the student to begin to conceive of themselves as a clinician.

The Postgraduate Junior GP Trainee

The junior postgraduate trainee typically will have accumulated sufficient clinical knowledge to function as a junior doctor in the hospital setting. The junior trainee will usually have developed the core clinical reasoning skills required to build basic diagnostic assessments and management plans (Bearman et al. 2011). The junior GP trainee can be expected to have the identity of junior clinician and perhaps also that of nascent general practitioner. Not long after commencing a placement in the GP work place, they will be expected to be attending patients themselves under level 2 or level 3 supervision (Ingham et al. 2019). They too will be confronted by an information knowledge deficit. GP has its own spectrum of clinical presentations and issues; and, in community based medicine, appropriate management for a given condition can be different to best-practice in a hospital setting. There are clinical skills that the junior trainee will need to build in order to address patient needs in the GP setting. These include: learning to establish rapport and common agendas with patients; dealing with the undiagnosable; and navigating complex problems at the interface of the biological, psychological, and social (Greenhalgh 2007). They also need to learn the disposition of the general practitioner; particularly that of a patient-centered approach (McWhinney and Freeman 2009). This stage of the trainee's trajectory in GP can be highly stressful as they find themselves in a position of responsibility for which they are inadequately equipped (Morrison et al. 2015).

For the junior postgraduate trainee, the supervisor is required: for ensuring the trainee is allocated clinical responsibility that is commensurate with their ability; to be a resource for addressing gaps in the trainee's knowledge and skills; for clinical back up and oversight to ensure trainee and patient safety (Morrison et al. 2015); and, for being a senior mentor for supporting the trainee identity formation.

The Pre-fellowship GP Trainee

The pre-fellowship GP trainee conducts most of their consultations independently. Their knowledge and skill sets are sufficient for most circumstances. Their learning is a refining of these and preparing for practice following full credentialing as a general practitioner. This requires assuming the identity of general practitioner where they project themselves confidently in the role of general practitioner and receive recognition as such by both the patient and professional communities. They need to learn how to practice without supervision. This means learning to evaluate and develop their own clinical practice, developing referral networks and practices, and developing professional support networks. For the senior postgraduate trainee, the supervisor's role becomes primarily a mentoring one.

The Tasks of Supervision in GP

In this section, we build on the theoretical principles of learning under supervision and the concept of the trainee trajectory in general practice to examine the activities of the GP supervision. We identify these activities as:

1. Engaging the trainee in the working community
2. Conducting the ad hoc supervisory call-in
3. Teaching
4. Mentorship
5. Monitoring and feedback
6. Assessment
7. Facilitating an understanding of good practice

We draw on relevant research and the experience of the authors to provide recommended initiatives that supervisors, trainees, and the GP practice community might take support learning.

Engaging the Trainee in the Working Community

Consistent with the theoretical frameworks for work-place learning, engagement of the trainee in the GP work community is fundamental to achieving the imperatives of GP trainee supervision. The objective is for the trainee to be engaged and participating in the work-place in a way that contributes to the work while protecting patient and trainee safety and for the trainee to find meaning in being part of the working community. Key determinants of how this happens are the overall culture of the work-place (Wiener-Ogilvie et al. 2014), the attitude of the supervisor (Pront et al. 2016), and the response of the trainee (Billett 2009). A recent review of GP supervision literature identified key elements of the culture of the GP work-place for enabling trainee engagement as inclusivity and a flat hierarchy (Jackson et al. 2019). Cottrell et al. identified availability and approachability as being key supervisor attributes (Cottrell et al. 2002). In achieving engagement of the trainee in the GP work community, there are important practical tasks for each of the supervisor, trainee, and the work-place community; and important resources to achieve these.

Orientation of the new trainee to the environment is foundational to engaging the trainee in the clinic working community and introducing them to the procedures and the resources it uses for providing patient care. This warrants significant investment of time and effort as so much of what follows depends on this. Ideally orientation should involve a staged engagement of the trainee with the work; as it is by engaging in the work, that meaning can be made of the work environment. In the GP setting, there are four discrete physical work areas to become familiar with. These are: the consulting room, the treatment area, the reception area, and the community external to the clinic premises including patients' homes, residential care, and GP-based hospital care. The trainee needs time of orientation in each of these work areas where they are introduced to the tasks, procedures, and resources as they guided in contributing to the activity. In the consulting room they might sit in with the supervisor and take the clinical notes; in the treatment area there will be patient treatments that they can contribute to as they are shown the procedures and facilities; in the reception area they can receive patients under the oversight of a receptionist.

There needs to be physical resources and set procedures to support the orientation itself. We recommend two physical resources. The first is an orientation checklist; Table 3 provides an example of areas of orientation that such a checklist might be organized around. The second is a summary of organizational procedures and frameworks that can be used by the trainee for making sense of the environment during orientation and later as a reference.

Table 3 Important areas of orientation

Physical facilities
  Within the clinic
  External to the clinic

Social connections
  Who's who
  Informal social activities and places – e.g., lunches and tea room
  Formal social events

Clinical consultation resources
  Within the consulting room
  External to the consulting room

Policies and procedures
  Routine activities and processes
  Policy manuals
  Employment terms

Communication
  Internal
  External

Safety
  Patient safety
  Trainee safety
  Accessing support
  Emergency procedures

Education
  Reference resources
  Areas of expertise held by members of the team
  Scheduled educational activities

Table 4 Summarises the key actions for the supervisor, the trainee, and the practice community in supporting the trainee's engagement in the working community

For the supervisor
Be available and approachable
Prioritize developing a relationship with the trainee
Schedule time with the trainee
Provide clear guidelines on when and how to call for assistance
For the trainee
Engage with the people within the practice community and their work
Respond positively to efforts by the practice community to engage with you
For the practice community
Orientate of the trainee to the procedures and resources of the work through guided engagement of the trainee in tasks with others in each work area
Provide
An orientation checklist
A reference manual of organizational procedures
A trainee designated work space, signage, and information fliers
Actively invite and include the trainee into both the practice work social environments

Material recognition of the trainee in the work environment enhances a sense of place and engagement for the trainee. These might include a designated consulting room or computer station. Signage and information fliers, that include the trainee, add to the sense of welcome and belonging.

The supervisor needs allocated time to develop a common vision with the trainee on the objectives and planned activities of the placement, ensuring that the aspirations and requirements of the trainee, the work-place, and the overseeing educational institution are addressed. This discussion needs to include clear delineation of the safety structures in place for when the trainee finds themselves in a situation beyond their capacity to manage on their own.

Engaging the trainee on a social level is important. This includes introducing and inviting them to the social component of the work-place including informal tea-room gatherings and organized social events. It is also valuable for the supervisor and trainee to spend time outside of the work-place for acquainting each with the other in a more informal way.

The trainee themselves is a key player in engaging with the working community. This means responding positively to invitations of inclusion by the practice community and the supervisor and reciprocating this with an interest in the people within the practice and the work that they do.

Key actions for engaging the trainee in the working community are summarised in Table 4.

Conducting the Ad Hoc Supervisory Call-In

The trainee in GP will be attending patients under a level of supervision that should match their competency and experience (Table 1). Fundamental to working under supervision is for the trainee to be able to call on their supervisor for immediate help with the patient that they are attending at the time. We call this the "ad hoc supervisory call-in." We have conducted two in depth investigations into "ad hoc supervisory call-ins" in GP and identified the importance of this occurrence for: enabling the trainee to complete the consultation; protection of patient and trainee safety; learning; and, for trainee identity formation (Morrison et al. 2015; Brown et al. 2018; Clement et al. 2016).

There are several determinants that need to be in place to ensure that the "ad hoc supervisory call-in" occurs when it is needed. The first is that the trainee needs to know that they need help. The second is that the trainee needs to feel safe in calling in the supervisor; this requires addressing fears of inconveniencing the supervisor and of loosing of credibility with the patient or the supervisor (Stewart 2008). The third is ease of access to the supervisor (Kilminster et al. 2007). Therefore, in order to ensure that supervisory call-ins occur when required, the following need to be addressed. The trainee needs guidance on when they need to call the supervisor in. Building a checklist of presentations that require an automatic call in is valuable. The second is that the supervisor needs to be both approachable and accessible (Cottrell et al. 2002). This means a clearly articulated line of easy access to the supervisor by the trainee and for the trainee to be given a clear message from the supervisor that the interruption is welcome. This clearly depends on the attitude of the supervisor and the degree to which they feel inconvenienced. Allocating time within the supervisor's consulting session to accommodate "ad-hoc supervisor call-ins" is therefore essential. The third is that the call is conducted in a way that meets the trainee's needs and does not undermine the trainee in the patient's eyes.

There are several suggested formats for how the call in might be conducted to enhance the educational value of the supervisory call-in (Ingham 2012; Irby and Wilkerson 2008). Important for the identity of the trainee is how the supervisor and trainee position themselves during the supervisory call-in. In broad terms: the supervisor can take over; the supervisor can coach the trainee to a conclusion using prompts and leading questions; or, the supervisor can be a resource for the trainee to use to complete the consultation themselves with the supervisor providing an opinion, a piece of information, or an affirmation. Each of these three modes of engagement is indicated in different circumstances depending on the trainee capability and the patient need. An important consideration is the hierarchy between the supervisor and trainee expressed in this positioning as a pronounced hierarchical positioning of the supervisor over the trainee, which can undermine the trainee with the patient and therefore undermine the trainee's identity as a clinician in their own right. In order to avoid the trainee being undermined, the trainee needs to retain overall control of the call-in. For this, the trainee needs to be clear about what it is that they want and need from the supervisor to complete the consultation and then to make this clear to both the patient and the supervisor. In this way, even when the supervisor takes over, having the supervisor comply with an explicit request by the trainee keeps the trainee as the overarching arbiter of the outcome. This is a complex skill and the trainee is likely to need coaching to be able to do this. The supervisor

Table 5 Summarises the key actions for the supervisor, the trainee, and the practice community in supporting the supervisory call-in

For the supervisor
Guide the trainee on when and how to call for assistance when attending patients
Be available and accessible
Avoid undermining the trainee with their patient
Use a model for conducting a call-in
Make a deliberate choice on whether to take over, coach, or be a resource
For the trainee
Be clear what is wanted of the supervisor and articulate this to the patient and supervisor
For the practice community
Have the systems in place to ensure that there is always an accessible supervisor and that this is clear to both the trainee and supervisor

also needs to be aware of the way they position themselves when with the trainee and the trainee's patient and to be willing to allow the trainee to take the lead.

Key actions that support the supervisory call-in are summarised in Table 5.

Teaching

Teaching is a means of facilitating the trainee to gain the resources of knowledge, understanding, skills, and disposition to undertake the work of patient care. Teaching is also an important medium for the supervisor to engage with the trainee. Teaching in GP is both formal and informal. Work tasks are the main context and frame for teaching with the primary driver being to enable the work to be done.

The supervisor call-ins, as described above, have been identified as powerful informal learning experiences (Morrison et al. 2015). The other main venue for informal teaching is the so-called "corridor conversation" (Long et al. 2007). These are when the trainee and supervisor engage in unscheduled conversations in the absence of the patient to talk about the trainee's clinical work. These "corridor conversations" are not dissimilar to the supervisory call-in in that the main focus is to enable the trainee to complete immediate tasks of patient care. However, with the patient absent, "doctor-talk" can be used more freely; and, the trainee's learning needs can be explored more explicitly without the risk of undermining the credibility of the trainee with their patient (Kennedy et al. 2009).

Most GP training programs also cater for formal teaching with time scheduled specifically for education, usually when patients are not being attended. There are two approaches to using formal teaching time. The first is reactive, and the second is proactive. Both are important.

Reactive teaching is teaching based on the current challenges the trainee is dealing with in attending specific patients. This teaching ideally happens soon after the trainee has attended their patient. A regular formal end of session debrief can provide effectively for this.

Proactive learning is learning in anticipation of what the trainee is likely to be faced with and challenged by. Proactive learning requires identification of trainee learning needs and planning a means to address these (Garth et al. 2016). Areas of "learning need" can be categorized as information knowledge, skills knowledge, and dispositional knowledge (Billett 1993). Information knowledge includes both clinical and bureaucratic information. Skills knowledge includes managing the GP consultation in all its challenging variations (Neighbour 2019), integration of the psychosocial, biomedical, and procedural skills and how to access resources to support clinical care. Dispositional knowledge is attitudinal and an important component of identity formation.

Identification of educational learning needs is supported by a structured and revisited dialogue between the trainee and the supervisor about the trainee's learning needs, and by specific activities to identify needs that might not be obvious to the trainee. Trainees identify learning needs as they are confronted with clinical issues in their work; experienced supervisors identify learning needs drawing on their own experiences particularly with previous trainees; and, the literature contains guidance on areas of likely learning needs (Neighbour 2019; Morgan et al. 2014).

Two educational activities that are particularly useful for identifying trainee learning needs that may not be otherwise obvious are trainee consultation observation (Kogan et al. 2017) and post consultation clinical note review (Morgan and Ingham 2013). Consultation observation may be by video or in person. Clinical note review is a review of the trainee's clinical notes by the supervisor and the trainee together to reflect on the consultation outcomes and the clinical thinking behind these. These activities can also serve as an assessment and monitoring purpose.

Having identified a learning need, a decision needs to be made on how to best address the need. This depends on the type of knowledge and being aware of where expertise is likely to lie.

For clinical information, authoritative references are likely to be the most reliable source of information. It can be unhelpful to view the supervisor as necessarily the authority on clinical information as while the supervisor's clinical knowledge should be adequate for the task, it is not necessarily up to date. The supervisor can provide advice on what references might be used for clinical information and how to access them.

While not necessarily being the best source of clinical information, the supervisor does know how to apply that clinical information to the contexts at hand (Cantillon and de Grave 2012). Therefore, if teaching is to focus on a particular topic area, the supervisor's skills are most applicable to contextualizing content knowledge that the trainee themself has sourced in preparation for the teaching session.

Skills knowledge and dispositional knowledge are best learned by a combination of observation, doing, and feedback on doing. This can be done by mutual consultation observation and role play. When the trainee observes the supervisor, it is valuable for them to have a framework of analyzing the supervisor's consultation with particular events and maneuvers within the consultation to identify. This is then used to frame a discussion afterwards to explore the process of the consultation and the supervisor's thinking within the consultation. When the supervisor observes the trainee's consultation, a framework of consultation debrief is helpful. Table 6 details

Table 6 Domains of consultation assessment identified by Govaerts et al. (2013)

1. Doctor Patient relationship
Rapport
Appropriate confidence and authority
Facilitating common ground
In the consultation agenda
In the management plan
2. Structuring the consultation
Establishing the full agenda early
Signposting
Clean sequencing of the components of the consultation
3. Clinical knowledge

Table 7 Summarises the key actions for the supervisor, the trainee, the supervisor and trainee together, and the practice community in supporting teaching of the trainee

For the supervisor
Be available and approachable
Use corridor conversations for giving advice to trainees that might undermine the trainee if given in front of the patient
Have a bank of scripted role plays for challenging consultations
For the trainee
Use corridor/tea room conversations for seeking advice that require "doctor talk"
Source best practice protocols and factual clinical information from reliable evidence-based references
For the supervisor and trainee together
Schedule end of clinical session debriefs
Engage in regular learning/teaching planning dialogues
Utilize the supervisors' expertise in contextualizing the application of clinical knowledge rather than as an authoritative source of factual knowledge
Engage in mutual consultation observation and debrief
Engage in formal trainee clinical note review
For the practice community
Schedule time for formal teaching
Allow time buffers for informal teaching

the domains of assessment used by supervisors in consultation observation that Govaerts et al. identified in their research (Govaerts et al. 2013).

Role plays also provide a powerful means for trainees to develop consultation schemas for difficult consultations. Pre-prepared role play formats can be a useful resource for this activity.

Key actions that support teaching are summarised in Table 7.

Mentorship and Role Modelling

Wenger's theorizing positions the "old-timer" as instrumental in enabling the newcomer to join a community of practice and embark on a trajectory of identity from being an outsider to becoming an integral part of the working community (Wenger

Table 8 Summarises the key actions for the supervisor and the trainee community in establishing an effective mentor relationship

For the supervisor
Generate a genuine concern for, and an investment in, the trainee's professional journey
Be willing to share your own professional journey and challenges particularly in balancing multiple roles
Articulate the rationale behind what you do

For the trainee
Be proactive in engaging with your supervisor reciprocating their interest
Be willing to share personal challenges in engaging with the work

1998). An important part of what the "old-timer" gives to the newcomer is a vision of what it is to be an "old-timer" and how the new-comer might become an "old-timer" themselves. They do this through both talk and through example. The GP supervisor occupies the position of the "old-timer" for the GP trainee. In this position, they offer the GP trainee a model and vision for becoming a GP clinician both in their clinic community and in the community of medicine more broadly. They do this through role modelling and mentorship.

Role modelling can be by happenstance and can be deliberate. Deliberate role modelling and mentorship go together. Deliberate role modelling and mentorship depend on an investment by the supervisor in the trainee and their journey in becoming a clinician. This requires time, genuine interest, and a willingness to expose their thinking and to share their dilemmas and stories. Exposure of thinking is articulating to the trainee the rationale behind what they do either in the course of undertaking tasks or in purposeful reflection within a scheduled time together. Sharing dilemmas and personal stories are acts of vulnerability (Bearman and Molloy 2017). Exposure of thinking and story sharing can provide powerful exemplars for the trainee in developing their own practice and perceptions of what it is to be a GP. It can also give them a frame for developing strategies for managing the role of clinician within the context of multiple other life roles – what Wenger calls the "nexus of multi-membership" (Wenger 1998).

Role modelling and mentorship are important for the trainee in developing internal models of good practice (Tai et al. 2018) against which to judge their own practice. This is discussed further later.

As with all relationships, effective mentorship relationships are two way. Just as it is important for the supervisor to invest in the relationship, so too, it is important for the trainee to invest in the relationship. Identity formation is also two way. Research has indicated that the supervisor's identity as a supervisor is impacted on significantly by the degree to which the trainee places trust in the supervisor and is willing to be vulnerable with the supervisor (Garth et al. 2019).

Key actions that support a mentor relationship are summarised in Table 8.

Monitoring and Feedback

From a work-based theory perspective, trainee monitoring and feedback has three purposes. The first is to achieve conformity by the trainee to the norms of the workplace, the second is to determine trainee privileging, and the third is to provide guidance for the trainee in building the knowledge required for the work-place (Billett 2009). The norms of a GP work-place are strongly framed by the more global norms of the profession and by the expectations and requirements of the society at large (Wenger 1998).

Feedback from the trainee to the practice is also important for ensuring the GP work-place remains current with its own practices.

Trainee monitoring and feedback require the supervisor to know how the trainee is performing. Some information about trainee performance will be gained by happenstance through their interactions as they work and learn together and through incidental feedback from patients and other staff. However, in GP, particularly for trainees working under level 2 supervision or higher, the trainee will be attending patients largely on their own with the supervisor having little direct view of the trainee's actual clinical work. This can be hazardous for patient care (Ingham et al. 2019; Byrnes et al. 2012). It is therefore essential for the supervisor to be proactive in gaining a view on the trainee's clinical practice. Regular consultation observation is the cornerstone for this and can be done by sitting in on trainee consultations, viewing videotaped trainee consultations and joint consultations. Important information on trainee performance can also be gained from reviewing the trainee's clinical notes (Morgan and Ingham 2013). Third party impressions of trainee performance are also valuable and can be sourced by actively seeking feedback from other team members or undertaking formal patient and colleague surveys (Wright et al. 2012).

There has been considerable focus recently on feedback in the medical education literature (Ramani et al. 2019). Feedback is understood as a core educational activity, as without knowing how we are performing, we don't know what we need to change and learn (Cantillon and Sargeant 2008). Feedback can be affirming, directive, or corrective. The academic conversation on feedback has moved from understanding feedback as something that is dispensed to the trainee to viewing feedback as a relational process. It has been described as a dialogue (Askew and Lodge 2004), an alliance (Telio et al. 2015), and a dance (Bing-You et al. 2017).

The measure of the value of feedback is its impact. The impact of feedback depends on: the way it is given; the receptiveness of the receiver; the nature of the relationship that frames the feedback; and, the cultural context that the feedback sits with in (Lefroy et al. 2015). There are well-used frameworks for engaging in feedback such as the Pendleton model, Calgary Cambridge approach, and the Reflective Feedback Conversation (Cantillon and Sargeant 2008). The receptiveness of the trainee to feedback depends on their readiness for feedback. This means that it is important for the trainee to have a voice in what they will receive feedback on. Receptiveness of the trainee to feedback also depends on the credibility that the supervisor has in the eyes of the trainee for both their clinical expertise and educational expertise (Telio et al. 2016). Telio et al.'s educational alliance model gives guidance on the features of a supervisory relationship that support effective feedback (Telio et al. 2015). These are a shared understanding of the trainee's

Table 9 Summarises the key actions for the supervisor, the trainee and the practice community in supporting monitoring and feedback

For the supervisor
Proactively collect data relating to the trainee's performance
Have a framework for giving and receiving feedback
Develop a shared educational agenda with the trainee
Normalize feedback exchanges by having these frequently including at scheduled times
Ask the trainee what they would like feedback on
Ask for feedback on yourself – both as a clinician and as an educator
For the trainee
Share your educational goals with your supervisor
Determine what you seek feedback on and ask for this
Give feedback to your supervisor
For the practice community
Normalize feedback across the whole practice
Promote a culture of professional integrity and "no blame"

educational goals and activities; a joint commitment to these; and, for the trainee to believe that the supervisor is invested in the trainee's well-being.

A culture within the practice that normalizes feedback is important for feedback to occur and to be effective (Ramani et al. 2019; Denny et al. 2019). When feedback is normalized, it becomes a frequent event that occurs both formally and informally across the whole practice. Trainee orientation needs to include an overview of feedback events and processes. It is also important for the supervisor to actively seek feedback from the trainee and to use this to demonstrably adapt their own practice. As well as normalizing feedback, this: increases the credibility of the supervisor with the trainee; models the use of feedback; and provides a means for developing the supervisor's clinical and educational practice. It is problematic if feedback only occurs in the context of a critical incident as this invites negative reactions of blame, guilt, and defensiveness.

Giving corrective feedback is often inhibited by its perceived risks (Denny et al. 2019). These relate to the potential reaction by the recipient of the corrective feedback who may find the experience destabilizing and respond with withdrawal or retaliation. This is particularly an issue for the trainee giving corrective feedback to the supervisor or the practice as they are dependent on their goodwill. These risks need to be addressed to enable frank feedback. Bing-You's metaphor of feedback as a tango is helpful (Bing-You et al. 2017). Drawing on this metaphor, feedback is a shared two-way endeavor where each is attuned and in step with each other.

Key actions that support monitoring and feedback are summarised in Table 9.

Assessment

Assessment sits alongside monitoring and feedback. Trainee assessment in the GP work-place concerns making judgments about the trainee for three areas of decision-making: (1) the level of supervision required by the trainee; (2) trainee learning needs that require addressing; and (3) trainee readiness for progression to the next stage of training (Wearne and Brown 2014).

Judgment of the level of supervision required is a process of entrustment of responsibility to the trainee. Because of the implications this has for patient and trainee, it is important for there to be a rigor behind this judgment. We suggest that these decisions be based on repeated observation of the trainee at work and that initial impression be tested with other information such as team review of the trainee and review of clinical notes (Wearne and Brown 2014). Ten Cate et al., have developed the concept of "Entrustable Professional Activities (EPAs)" as units of practice that can be used as signposts of developing competency (Ten Cate et al. 2015). An example of such an activity in GP might be managing a request for a termination of pregnancy. EPAs are a useful framework for developing a folio of clinical activities that require deliberate entrustment decisions before the registrar can determine themselves that they don't require supervision for the activity. Such clinical activities are those with higher stakes such as managing a sick child.

Supervisors can be in a position to make well-informed assessments of trainee performance and competence because they work closely with the trainee. However, using supervisor assessments for high-stake decisions on progress of training can be problematic for the supervisory relationship. Depending on supervisors for high-stakes trainee progress judgments adds to the supervisor/trainee power differential which can compromise the trainee's willingness to be frank with the supervisor and therefore compromise educational agendas (Garth et al. 2016). We recommend that supervisor assessments of trainees should be part of programmatic assessment but not be used as a stand-alone high-stakes assessment unless the trainee is engaging in reprehensible behavior. We suggest that high-stakes work-based assessments be undertaken by external experts such is currently done in New Zealand.

Trainee assessment of training placements is an important source of feedback for the supervisor, the training placement, and faculty. It is important to protect trainee safety in seeking trainee assessments of their training practices and supervisors. Strategies to do this are: building a culture of feedback; systematically collating and anonymizing trainee feedback for each site; and obtaining feedback from graduating trainees who have completed their fellowship requirements when their level of risk in giving a negative assessment is less.

Key actions that support assessment are summarised in Table 10.

Facilitating an Understanding of Good Practice

An important challenge for trainees is to develop a concept of good practice as conceived by and judged by the community within which they work (Wenger 1998). The GP supervisor is a key conduit for the GP trainee to learn this. Likewise, it is important for local working communities to bench mark their practice against external concepts of good practice as judged by the more global communities. The GP trainee has the potential to be a significant conduit for bringing concepts of good

Table 10 Summarises the key actions for the supervisor and the practice community in supporting assessment

For the supervisor
Be deliberate in assessing the trainee for decisions on the level of supervision required
Observe your trainee at work
Add rigor to level of supervision-related assessments by collecting information from multiple sources
Advise trainees early in the placement how they will be assessed
Assess your trainee for competency in high-stake presentations before entrusting them with the decision whether or not to call for assistance

For the practice community
Use external assessors for high-stake trainee progress assessments
Protect trainee safety if seeking trainee assessments of placements

practice from the broader medical community to their local GP training practice (Engeström et al. 1999). Trainees will have recently worked in hospitals and they are exposed to global ideas of good practice through out-of-practice education.

For the trainee to learn good practice from their supervisor, they need to know what their supervisor does in particular situations and to understand the rationale behind this. Good practice in the local context may differ from good practice as conceived by the more global medical community. If the reasons for this are unavailable to the trainee, there is the risk that the trainee mistakenly judges the supervisor's practice as poor and thus, the supervisor's credibility is undermined (Denny et al. 2019).

For the training practice and the supervisor to learn good practice from their trainee, they need a nonhierarchical attitude to the ownership of knowledge (Jackson et al. 2019). This provides an environment that is safe for trainees to share what they know, particularly if it is at odds with the supervisor's practice.

Development of a mutual understanding of good practice requires two-way dialogue about clinical practice. It requires opportunities for the trainee to observe the supervisor's practice, to be privy to the thinking behind this practice, and to be invited by the supervisor to critique the supervisor's practice.

Experiences of the supervisor changing their practice based on information from the trainee can be key moments for building the supervisory relationship and for trainee development. These events build trust and a sense of safety for the trainee within the supervisory relationship; they build credibility for the supervisor; they provide a model for lifelong learning; and, they support the trainee's trajectory towards identifying themselves as a full member of the GP clinical community.

Key actions that support the trainee to develop a model of good practice are summarised in Table 11.

Shared Supervision

Supervision of a trainee in GP is increasingly shared between several general practitioners (Thomson et al. 2011). This arrangement has potential value and potential compromises. The value is trainee access to different clinical and

Table 11 Summarises the key actions for the supervisor, the trainee and the practice community to support the trainee to develop a model of good practice

For the supervisor
Articulate the rationale behind clinical decisions
Invite critique of own clinical practice by the trainee
Modify clinical practice when indicated by new knowledge brought by the trainee
For the trainee
Observe your supervisor at work
Recognize that context may alter best-practice
For the practice community
Build a culture of democratic rather than hierarchical ownership of knowledge

supervisory approaches and expertise. The compromise is a dilution in the contact with any one supervisor for the purpose of forming a supervisory relationship. This can be addressed by having an identified primary supervisor for mentorship and support. If there are multiple supervisors for a trainee, it is important that they function as a team with the shared objective of supporting the trainee's learning.

Building and Sustaining GP Supervisory Capacity

Organizations that oversee the whole of GP training delivery have an important role in building and sustaining supervisory capacity (Garth et al. 2019). Just as the trainee and the supervisor can be usefully viewed as participants in a clinical community of practice, so too, the supervisor can be usefully viewed as a participant in an educational community of practice. This educational community of practice overlaps with the clinical community of practice with the supervisor being a member of both. In this section, we take a summary overview of how an organization overseeing training might provide a community of practice in which the supervisor participates where the shared enterprise is the education of trainees. We look at six core training organization activities that engage the supervisor with the object of enabling the supervisor in their work of trainee education. These activities are:

1. Supervisor recruitment
2. Inducting the new supervisor to the role
3. Supporting the supervisor
4. Facilitating supervisor peer networks.
5. Supervisor professional development
6. Engaging the supervisor in program development and delivery

In exploring these things, we again draw on the theoretical and research literatures on work-based learning.

Supervisor Recruitment

The motivation to supervise is important. For a prospective supervisor to desire the role of supervisor, the activity of supervision needs to fit with the general practitioner's narrative about themselves (Billett 2009; Garth et al. 2019). Our personal narratives are built on: past experience, trajectories that we can imagine for ourselves, and desired cultural rewards (Holland 2001). Therefore, it is important for training providers to: consider and foster trainees as future supervisors; have a clear trajectory for development as a supervisor; and, ensure that being a supervisor is rewarding (Garth et al. 2019; Ingham et al. 2015).

The roles and requirements of supervision need to be clearly articulated and documented. Credentials, sufficient remuneration, and privileging also need to be attached to the role of supervisor.

Inducting the New Supervisor to the Role

As with inducting the new trainee, the new supervisor will make meaning of the supervisor's role if their induction is done alongside an initial engagement in the work of supervision and scaffolding of this is supported by someone who is already an experience member of the supervisory community. Ideally, induction provides a staged increase in supervisory responsibility with expert oversight and support which decreases as the new supervisor becomes more experienced. A designated, experienced supervisor or educator is an obvious candidate to provide this. In doing so, they need to engage with the new supervisor proactively and to be reliably available for guidance, mentorship, and information as required. The training organization also needs to provide easy and reliable access to training-related information and advice that can be accessed by the new supervisor at short notice as needed. Ideally the administrator is a known contact for the supervisor. On-line reference resources can be useful for immediate access as needed. Many training organizations also provide orientation workshops that have the added value of enabling new supervisors to connect with each other. The standards and requirements of supervision need to be clearly articulated and documented for reference as required.

Supporting the Supervisor

Training organizations are important for supporting supervisors through: compensation for the impost of supervision; support for the work of supervision; and, social recognition to underline the importance of supervision (Brown et al. 2019).

Compensation for the impost of supervision includes adequate financial recompense and provision of relief from consulting responsibilities. Support for the work of supervision includes educational resources, supervisor professional development, and provision of structures to support supervisor peer networking. Social recognition includes certification and positions of status such as university appointments.

Supervisors require easy access to immediate advice for providing supervision and for meeting bureaucratic requirements. This can be provided through online references and expertise accessible by the phone.

There will also be times when training organization expertise is required for addressing problematic supervisory relationships.

Facilitating Supervisor Peer Networks

Supervisors being connected with other supervisors is important for: identifying as a supervisor; building supervisory skills; and for developing an understanding of good supervisory practice (Garth et al. 2019). This connection can be supported by program facilitation of in-practice supervisor mentorship, facilitated small group networks and small group interactions at workshops.

Supervisor Professional Development

Supervision is a complex task that justifies a defined professional development curriculum and syllabus (Morgan et al. 2015). In section "The Tasks of Supervision in GP" of this chapter, we identified and explored seven areas of activity required of supervision. These provide a framework for a supervisor professional development syllabus:

1. Engagement of the trainee in the working community
2. The supervisory clinical encounter
3. Teaching
4. Mentorship
5. Monitoring and feedback
6. Assessment
7. Understanding good practice

We also add:

8. Supervisor well being
9. Critical thinking

This syllabus can be delivered: online, through educational activity; on-site at the training practice; in small groups and in large workshops. In deciding what mode of delivery, it is worth considering the type of learning that is being supported. Online delivery for factual learning has the advantage of efficiency and convenience. In-practice, delivery enables direct connection with the actual work of supervision. Small group delivery enables peer-benchmarking, and large group enables connection with the broader community of supervisory practice (Garth et al. 2019).

Engaging the Supervisor in Program Development and Delivery

Engaging supervisors in program development and program delivery outside of their own practice is important for supervisor engagement and identification as an educator. It also provides a means for recruiting supervisors into medical education work beyond supervision and ensures education is based on their real-world expertise. Engaging supervisors in this way facilitates what Wenger calls "ownership of meaning" (Wenger 1998). Formal engagement of supervisors in program development also ensures that program development aligns with the realities of the work-based training that occurs within training practices.

Conclusion

Supervision in the GP settings is at its core, work-based learning. The supervisor's role therefore sits at the interfaces of trainee development, the work that needs to done, and maintenance of the training practice's capacity to do that work. In this setting, building trainee competencies is a part of a much bigger whole. This bigger whole includes the endeavors of: engagement and relationship building; making and owning meaning in the work; supervisor and trainee identity development; and the maintenance and development of the work-place. The ways that the supervisor, the trainee, and the training organization engage in these activities are key determinants of learning outcomes.

Cross-References

▶ General Practice Education: Context and Trends

References

Askew S, Lodge C. Gifts, ping-pong and loops–linking feedback and learning. In: Feedback for learning. Abingdon: Routledge; 2004. p. 13–30.
Bearman M, Molloy E. Intellectual streaking: the value of teachers exposing minds (and hearts). Med Teach. 2017;39(12):1284–5.
Bearman M, Lawson M, Jones A. Participation and progression: new medical graduates entering professional practice. Adv Health Sci Educ. 2011;16(5):627–42.
Billett S. Authenticity and a culture of practice within modes of skill development. Aust NZ J Vocat Educ Res. 1993;2(1):1–29.
Billett S. Toward a workplace pedagogy: guidance, participation, and engagement. Adult Educ Q. 2002;53(1):27–43.
Billett S. Personal epistemologies, work and learning. Educ Res Rev. 2009;4(3):210–9.
Bing-You R, Hayes V, Varaklis K, Trowbridge R, Kemp H, McKelvy D. Feedback for learners in medical education: what is known? A scoping review. Acad Med. 2017;92(9):1346–54.
Brown J, Nestel D, Clement T, Goldszmidt M. The supervisory encounter and the senior GP trainee: managing for, through and with. Med Educ. 2018;52(2):192–205.
Brown J, Kirby C, Wearne S, Snadden D. Remodelling general practice training: tension and innovation. Aust J Gen Pract. 2019;48(11):6.
Byrnes PD, Crawford M, Wong B. Are they safe in there?: patient safety and trainees in the practice. Aust Fam Physician. 2012;41(1/2):26.
Cantillon P, de Grave W. Conceptualising GP teachers' knowledge: a pedagogical content knowledge perspective. Educ Prim Care. 2012;23(3):178–85.
Cantillon P, Sargeant J. Giving feedback in clinical settings. Br Med J. 2008;337:a1961.

Clement T, Brown J, Morrison J, Nestel D. Ad hoc supervision of general practice registrars as a "community of practice": analysis, interpretation and re-presentation. Adv Health Sci Educ. 2016;21(2):415–37.

Cottrell D, Kilminster S, Jolly B, Grant J. What is effective supervision and how does it happen? A critical incident study. Med Educ. 2002;36(11):1042–9.

Cruess RL, Cruess SR, Steinert Y. Amending Miller's pyramid to include professional identity formation. Acad Med. 2016;91(2):180–5.

Denny B, Brown J, Kirby C, Garth B, Chesters J, Nestel D. 'I'm never going to change unless someone tells me I need to': fostering feedback dialogue between general practice supervisors and registrars. Aust J Prim Health. 2019;25(4):374–9.

Engeström Y, Miettinen R, Punamäki R-L. Perspectives on activity theory. Cambridge: Cambridge University Press; 1999.

Garth B, Kirby C, Silberberg P, Brown J. Utility of learning plans in general practice vocational training: a mixed-methods national study of registrar, supervisor, and educator perspectives. BMC Med Educ. 2016;16(1):211.

Garth B, Kirby C, Nestel D, Brown J. 'Your head can literally be spinning': a qualitative study of general practice supervisors' professional identity. Aust J Gen Pract. 2019;48(5):315–20.

Govaerts JM, Van de Wiel WM, Schuwirth WL, Van der Vleuten PC, Muijtjens MA. Workplace-based assessment: raters' performance theories and constructs. Adv Health Sci Educ. 2013; 18(3):375–96.

Greenhalgh T. Primary health care: theory and practice. Oxford, UK: Blackwell Publishing; 2007.

Gupta TS, Hays R. Training for general practice: how Australia's programs compare to other countries. Aust Fam Physician. 2016;45(1/2):18.

Holland D. Identity and agency in cultural worlds. Cambridge, MA: Harvard University Press; 2001.

Ingham G. Avoiding 'consultation interruptus': a model for the daily supervision and teaching of general practice registrars. Aust Fam Physician. 2012;41(8):627.

Ingham G, Fry J, O'Meara P, Tourle V. Why and how do general practitioners teach? An exploration of the motivations and experiences of rural Australian general practitioner supervisors. BMC Med Educ. 2015;15:190.

Ingham G, Plastow K, Kippen R, White N. Tell me if there is a problem: safety in early general practice training. Educ Prim Care. 2019;30:212.

Irby DM, Wilkerson L. Teaching when time is limited. Br Med J. 2008;336(7640):384–7.

Jackson D, Davison I, Adams R, Edordu A, Picton A. A systematic review of supervisory relationships in general practitioner training. Med Educ. 2019;53:874.

Kennedy TJ, Regehr G, Baker GR, Lingard L. Preserving professional credibility: grounded theory study of medical trainees' requests for clinical support. Br Med J. 2009;338:b128.

Kilminster S, Cottrell D, Grant J, Jolly B. AMEE guide no. 27: effective educational and clinical supervision. Med Teach. 2007;29(1):2–19.

Kogan JR, Hatala R, Hauer KE, Holmboe E. Guidelines: the do's, don'ts and don't knows of direct observation of clinical skills in medical education. Perspect Med Educ. 2017;6(5):286–305.

Lefroy J, Watling C, Teunissen P, Brand P. Guidelines: the do's, don'ts and don't knows of feedback for clinical education. Perspect Med Educ. 2015;4(6):284–99.

Long D, Iedema R, Lee BB. Corridor conversations: clinical communication in casual spaces. In: The discourse of hospital communication. Abingdon: Routledge; 2007. p. 182–200.

McWhinney IR, Freeman T. Textbook of family medicine. 3rd ed. Oxford/New York: Oxford University Press; 2009. xii, 460 p.

Medical Board of Australia. Supervised practice for international medical graduates guidelines. Medical Board of Australia; 2017 [updated 24 Aug 2019]. Available from: https://www.medicalboard.gov.au/Codes-Guidelines-Policies/Supervised-practice-guidelines.aspx

Morgan S, Ingham G. Random case analysis: a new framework for Australian general practice training. Aust Fam Physician. 2013;42(1/2):69.

Morgan S, Henderson K, Tapley A, Scott J, Thomson A, Spike N, et al. Problems managed by Australian general practice trainees: results from the ReCEnT (Registrar Clinical Encounters in Training) study. Educ Prim Care. 2014;25(3):140–8.

Morgan S, Ingham G, Wearne S, Canalese R, Saltis T, McArthur L. Towards an educational continuing professional development (EdCPD) curriculum for Australian GP supervisors. Aust Fam Physician. 2015;44(11):854–8.

Morrison J, Clement T, Nestel D, Brown J. Perceptions of ad hoc supervision encounters in general practice training: a qualitative interview-based study. Aust Fam Physician. 2015;44(12):926–32.

Neighbour R. Challenging consultations. InnovAiT. 2019;12(1):24–9.

Pront L, Gillham D, Schuwirth LW. Competencies to enable learning-focused clinical supervision: a thematic analysis of the literature. Med Educ. 2016;50(4):485–95.

Ramani S, Könings KD, Ginsburg S, van der Vleuten CP. Twelve tips to promote a feedback culture with a growth mind-set: swinging the feedback pendulum from recipes to relationships. Med Teach. 2019;41(6):625–31.

Stewart J. To call or not to call: a judgement of risk by pre-registration house officers. Med Educ. 2008;42(9):938–44.

Tai J, Ajjawi R, Boud D, Dawson P, Panadero E. Developing evaluative judgement: enabling students to make decisions about the quality of work. High Educ. 2018;76(3):467–81.

Telio S, Ajjawi R, Regehr G. The "educational alliance" as a framework for reconceptualizing feedback in medical education. Acad Med. 2015;90(5):609–14.

Telio S, Regehr G, Ajjawi R. Feedback and the educational alliance: examining credibility judgements and their consequences. Med Educ. 2016;50(9):933–42.

Ten Cate O, Chen HC, Hoff RG, Peters H, Bok H, van der Schaaf M. Curriculum development for the workplace using entrustable professional activities (EPAs): AMEE guide no. 99. Med Teach. 2015;37(11):983–1002.

Thomson JS, Anderson KJ, Mara PR, Stevenson AD. Supervision – growing and building a sustainable general practice supervisor system. Med J Aust. 2011;194(11):S101.

Wearne S, Brown J. GP supervisors assessing GP registrars-theory and practice. Aust Fam Physician. 2014;43(12):887.

Wearne S, Dornan T, Teunissen PW, Skinner T. General practitioners as supervisors in postgraduate clinical education: an integrative review. Med Educ. 2012;46(12):1161–73.

Wenger E. Communities of practice: learning, meaning, and identity. Cambridge: Cambridge University Press; 1998.

Wiener-Ogilvie S, Bennison J, Smith V. General practice training environment and its impact on preparedness. Educ Prim Care. 2014;25(1):8–17.

Wright C, Richards SH, Hill JJ, Roberts MJ, Norman GR, Greco M, et al. Multisource feedback in evaluating the performance of doctors: the example of the UK General Medical Council Patient and Colleague Questionnaires. Acad Med. 2012;87(12):1668–78.

Yardley S, Teunissen PW, Dornan T. Experiential learning: AMEE guide no. 63. Med Teach. 2012;34(2):e102–15.

Further Reading

Engeström Y, Miettinen R, Punamäki R-L. Perspectives on activity theory. Cambridge: Cambridge University Press; 1999.

Greenhalgh T. Primary health care: theory and practice. Oxford, UK: Blackwell Publishing; 2007.

Neighbour R. The inner apprentice: an awareness-centred approach to vocational training for general practice. Abingdon: Routledge; 2018.

Wenger E. Communities of practice: learning, meaning, and identity. Cambridge: Cambridge University Press; 1998.

Conversational Learning in Health Professions Education: Learning Through Talk

57

Walter J. Eppich, Jan Schmutz, and Pim Teunissen

Contents

Introduction	1100
The Problem	1100
Purpose of This Chapter	1101
Chapter Overview	1101
What Is "Talk" and Why It Matters	1102
Talk in Main Scholarly Perspectives of Learning	1103
Talk and Learning from Clinical Work	1104
Talk and Explicit Learning Conversations	1108
Talk and Tensions	1110
Talk and Psychological Safety	1111
Conclusion	1114
Cross-References	1114
References	1114

Abstract

Health professions educators have increasingly focused on communication as a key skill to be mastered, which has had implications for curriculum development. However, communication in modern team-based healthcare also has explicit and intrinsic learning potential. Communication – or "talk" – can be viewed as the

W. J. Eppich (✉)
RCSI SIM Centre for Simulation Education and Research, RCSI University of Medicine and Health Sciences, Dublin, Ireland
e-mail: weppich@rcsi.ie

J. Schmutz
Department of Psychology, University of Zurich, Zurich, Switzerland
e-mail: jsschmutz@ethz.ch

P. Teunissen
Faculty of Health Medicine and Life Sciences (FHML), School of Health Professions Education (SHE), Maastricht University, Maastricht, The Netherlands
e-mail: p.teunissen@maastrichtuniversity.nl

© Springer Nature Singapore Pte Ltd. 2023
D. Nestel et al. (eds.), *Clinical Education for the Health Professions*,
https://doi.org/10.1007/978-981-15-3344-0_48

verbal content of speech and its associated "paralanguage" along with their social implications. Viewed in this light, talk is not only a skill that enables patient care but also represents a social medium of learning. This chapter explores the role of talk in the main scholarly perspectives of learning and examines conversational learning in both clinical workplaces and in explicit learning conversations in a variety of settings. Finally, the authors explore how conversational tensions influence learning and how psychological safety promotes productive conversational activities such as speaking up.

Keywords

Learning conversations · Talk · Debriefing · Simulation · Workplace learning · Team reflection

Introduction

In modern healthcare, individual clinicians from various professions work in highly interdependent team-based settings (Edmondson 2012), and communication breakdowns threaten patient safety (Sutcliffe et al. 2004). The "work" in clinical practice includes two important components (Bowers et al. 1997): (a) taskwork, which involves what needs to happen for patient care in terms of assessment and management, and (b) teamwork, which denotes how team members work together to achieve patient care, including communication, coordination, etc. Therefore, teamwork serves to support completion of taskwork. This realization has placed increasing emphasis on "communicative competence" (Hymes 1972) to enable interprofessional collaboration (Hammick et al. 2009) and teamwork (Schmutz et al. 2019).

This trend has wide-reaching impacts for clinical education. For example, "communication skills" comprise several core competencies in postgraduate clinical education, as evidenced by the CanMeds roles of "Collaborator" and "Communicator" from the Royal College of Physicians and Surgeons of Canada (CanMeds). The Accreditation Council on Graduate Medical Education from the United States also provides developmental milestones as assessment guidelines for many medical specialties (ACGME). For example, general pediatric trainees in the United States must achieve milestones in several domains for which "communicative competence" is reflected wholly or in part by core competencies related to managing interpersonal communications (Benson 2014) and interprofessional teamworking (Guralnick et al. 2014).

The Problem

This emphasis on "communicative competency," with communication as a skill to be mastered, has become a dominant discourse in health professions education (HPE) and led to widespread adoption of "team and communication skills training." This focus on communication as a learning outcome, however, deemphasizes another fundamental contribution of "communication" in HPE: communication represents a primary medium of our learning. Broadly, we can view "communication" as "talk," which we define as joint social activity between conversation partners (Clark 1996; Garrod and Pickering 2004) comprised by the verbal content of speech and its associated "paralanguage" (Abercrombie 1968; Zant and Berger 2020; Wouters et al. 2020). These paralinguistic cues, or not-worded elements, include acoustic properties of speech, such as tone of voice, volume, and pitch that accompany verbal behavior (Wouters et al. 2020). A broader yet controversial perspective also includes nonvocal phenomena such as body gestures or facial expressions that convey emotion and meaning (Abercrombie 1968).

Thus, "talk" not only contributes to team processes that enable the work required for safe patient care but also mediates the learning required to engage in that work in team settings. Psychological and sociocultural theorists support this view (Hicks 1995; Vygotsky 1978, 1986; Wells and Wells 1984; Wells 1999). This fundamental role of talk in healthcare makes learning inseparable from patient care. The dominant focus on communicative competence as a learning outcome draws attention to skills in talking and shifts attention away from talk as an essential learning process in HPE. In this regard, Wells (1999) highlights "the role of language in knowing and coming to know" (p. 140). By viewing talk primarily as an individual outcome of learning (i.e., communicative competency), health professions educators may overlook talk itself as an important social medium of learning in clinical education. Therefore, we may be losing opportunities to augment and accelerate learning since related theory and conceptual frameworks of healthcare talk remain underdeveloped.

Purpose of This Chapter

Talk plays a prominent role in both clinical workplaces and in formal curricular elements such as healthcare simulation across the spectrum of HPE from undergraduate and postgraduate training to continuing professional development. Therefore, we explore talk from two vantage points: learning through talk *from* practice in clinical workplaces and learning through talk *for* practice in formal educational settings. Readers will be able to clarify how talk contributes to learning in these two settings by: (a) identifying key similarities and differences as well as potential synergies and (b) applying practical strategies to steer healthcare talk to promote in the service of both learning and patient care.

Chapter Overview

This chapter has seven sections, many of which draw substantially from unpublished content in the primary author's doctoral thesis entitled "Learning through talk: The role of discourse in medical education."

1. What Is Talk and Why It Matters
2. Talk in the Main Scholarly Perspectives of Learning
3. Talk and Learning from Clinical Work
4. Talk and Learning from Explicit Learning Conversations
5. Talk and Tensions
6. Talk and Psychological Safety
7. Conclusions

What Is "Talk" and Why It Matters

Viewed broadly, talk encompasses the terms "discourse," "dialogue," "communication," and "conversation" depending on the field of literature. Given the ubiquitous nature of talk in settings inside and outside of work, health professions educators can lose sight of its integral role in a variety of processes beyond "communication."

While healthcare simulation and workplace learning research has focused primarily on how students and residents learn from "doing" (Dornan et al. 2007; Yardley et al. 2012; Teunissen et al. 2007; Teunissen 2015), much of their clinical practice involves "talking" not only with patients but with other clinicians as part of interprofessional, multidisciplinary teams. Therefore, "learning by doing" often refers to "learning by talking." As in other occupations (Iedema and Scheeres 2003; Scheeres 2003), talk comprises an integral aspect of clinical work for doctors-in-training. In teaching hospitals, Atkinson (1995) noted that "spoken performances are constitutive of the work" (p. 5). Examples of "talk as work" include giving oral patient presentations in a variety of contexts, handing off patients to other providers, talking with subspecialists on the telephone to seek patient care advice, or communicating with team members while caring for deteriorating patients. Talk not only reflects the discursive work of patient care, talk contributes to the learning process of becoming a healthcare provider, exemplified by research on how medical students learn to perform case presentations (Lingard et al. 2003a, b; Lingard and Haber 1999; Haber and Lingard 2001).

Medical discourse has garnered attention both as an essential vehicle for socialization in medicine and a means of socially constructing medical knowledge (Arluke 1977; Anspach 1988; Hunter 1991; Atkinson 1995). For example, young doctors gain competence while also learning to don a "cloak of competence" as part of their professionalization (Haas and Shaffir 1977, 1982). Further, Haas and Shaffir (1977) noted that early year medical students confront difficulties when beginning "to communicate in the symbolic system that defines medical work and workers" (p. 73, emphasis added). They must manipulate "the symbols of the profession," including language, to create "an imagery of authoritativeness and competence" (pp. 85–86). In Medical Talk and Medical Work, Atkinson (1995) refers to "discursive acts" (p. 39) and socially organized practices around talk in medicine, which comprise the work of medical knowledge production within clinician teams. Hunter (1991) viewed ritualistic case presentations as "central to the discourse of medicine" and "the medium of clinical thought and communication" (p. 56) since medical knowledge achieves structure through narratives. Further, Erickson (1999) explored the tensions junior doctors face when learning to present patients – and thus one's self – competently to their clinical supervisors. Junior doctors must put aside the rigid presentation style of the medical student and present one's self as "both tough and casual in the face of difficult circumstances of professional work" (p. 123) by balancing the use of formal and informal language. These uses of language and ways of talking both contribute to and reflect the hidden curriculum in medical training (Haas and Shaffir 1982).

In summary, talk reflects discursive work that shapes socialization in healthcare; talk contributes fundamentally to patient care; and talk as "communication" can be viewed both as an interactional and relational process as well as a learning outcome related to communication skills to be mastered. Finally, talk is inseparable from the process of learning and patient care. We now explore the place of talk in main scholarly perspectives of learning.

Talk in Main Scholarly Perspectives of Learning

Sfard (1998) articulated two metaphors of learning representing opposite ends of a spectrum that provide a valuable lens to view the roles of talk in learning, namely "learning as acquisition" and "learning as participation." The acquisition metaphor foregrounds cognitive processes that lead to knowing and personal enrichment. Thus, talk serves to convey knowledge to be processed and acquired by learners. Reddy (1979) referred to a conduit metaphor that captured a now outdated conception that language simply transmits thought. Other expressions of "learning as acquisition" from experiential learning (Kolb 1984) and reflective practice (Schon 1983) highlight the supportive role educators can play in the reflective dialogue of both "in" and "on" action. Swanwick (2005) pointed out that these cognitive perspectives view the functioning of the mind as independent from social contexts.

At the other end of the spectrum, "learning as participation" views knowing as a process of "belonging, participating, communicating" (p. 7) (Sfard 1998). Participatory forms of learning in workplaces exemplify sociocultural theories, foregrounding the role of discourse within specific social contexts to construct knowledge (Brown et al. 1989; Lave and Wenger 1991; Wenger 1998). Thought and the symbols used to mediate that thought interrelate during goal-oriented joint activity (Vygotsky 1978, 1986; Wells 1999). Language represents a highly versatile system of symbols that significantly influences this process referred to as "semiotic mediation" (Wells 1999). Talk as joint social action manifests within specific contexts, making learning a highly situated and social process (Brown et al. 1989; Lave and Wenger 1991). Further, three dimensions contribute to learning within communities of practice (Wenger 1998): mutual engagement in the work, joint enterprise borne of shared purpose, and a shared repertoire. Importantly, this shared repertoire includes customary ways of talking within communities. As Lave and Wenger (1991) described, newcomers gain access to the community through participation in legitimate activities commensurate with their newcomer status. For example, junior doctors often call subspecialists on the telephone to seek advice, which represents a prime example of this legitimate peripheral participation in authentic clinical workplace activities since the most junior doctors often take on this work. In these participation frameworks (Wenger 1998), "learning to talk" plays a vital role as both social and cultural practice that provides access to the community and allows newcomers to move from peripheral to central members. As a result, talk and the use of jargon drive socialization in medicine. Further, ways of talking become reified or formalized as "the way things are done around here"; these reifications (Wenger 1998) capture cultural practices within a community. Highly contextualized and reified ways of talking shape culture, thinking, and knowing in various settings with powerful influences on clinical education (Teunissen 2015).

Talk and Learning from Clinical Work

Talk represents discursive work and contributes significantly to both patient care and learning from patient care activities in modern team-based healthcare. Physicians-in-training spend a vast majority of their time engaged in authentic patient care experiences. Several key considerations about workplace-based learning touch on aspects of learning "by acquisition" and "by participation." Clinical education encompasses both formal and informal aspects, requiring clear distinction between each. Formal learning takes place in institutions and classrooms; since educators direct the learning, high degrees of structure characterize it (Marsick and Watkins 1990). Examples during clinical education include lunch-hour teaching conferences or simulation-based training sessions in which learners "acquire" specific medical knowledge and skills articulated by objectives to be achieved.

Informal learning, on the other hand, is highly context-specific and takes various forms. Learning can be "incidental" or a by-product of other activities (Marsick and Watkins 1990), as in learning about power and hierarchy in healthcare during resuscitations of critically ill patients. If this learning fails to reach awareness, it remains implicit and taken for granted (Eraut 2000, 2004). Such tacit learning abounds in healthcare, part of which contributes to the "hidden curriculum" in medical training (Haas and Shaffir 1982). Alternately, informal learning can have intentional elements, either reactively in response to emergent learning opportunities or deliberately in learning for future patient care episodes (Eraut 2000).

Since participation in patient care activities comprises most of the workplace curriculum (Billett 1996, 2000), sociocultural perspectives have great relevance for learning from clinical work since learning is embedded within social relationships (Vygotsky 1978; Swanwick 2005; Wenger 1998). Wenger (1998) noted that talk represents a means of acting in the world, thus comprising participatory skills that enable access to social interactions in communities of practice. A valuable example to illustrate intrinsic learning potential of workplace conversations, telephone talk represents a significant social activity during the workday of trainee physicians.

Using constructivist grounded theory methodology, Eppich et al. (2019) studied work-related telephone talk as a social phenomenon to explore how workplace talk influenced physicians' clinical education. "Work-related telephone talk" referred to those conversations between doctors-in-training and other clinicians to achieve patient care goals. During in-depth individual interviews, 17 doctors-in-training from various specialties and training years described their telephone interactions with healthcare team members such as their clinical supervisors, fellow doctors-in-training, subspecialists, nurses, and other allied health professionals. Through a sociocultural analytic lens, the authors highlighted conversational tensions that appeared to influence learning positively: (a) dealing with power differentials, (b) dealing with pushback, and (c) expressing uncertainty while embodying trustworthiness. In contrast to prior work that framed tensions negatively, the authors identified productive components to conversational tensions. These unpleasant yet "productive conversational tensions" served as potent motivators to change future behavior, namely their telephone talk, in ways to prevent or mitigate these tensions by modifying what they said and how they said it (see Fig. 1). For example, doctors reported the unpleasantness of dealing with subspecialists who initially pushed back over the telephone, such as questioning or even denying legitimate requests or bluntly disagreeing with proposed courses of action. Many doctors-in-training highlighted the added difficulty of communicating over the phone, especially when pushback arose. They lamented being unable to see facial expressions or body language to offset quite negative paralinguistic cues such as a harsh tone of voice. Early experiences of pushback led to concrete changes in their telephone talk:

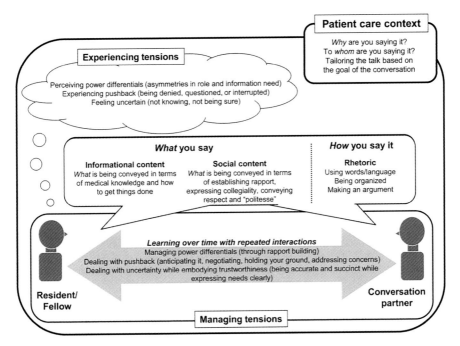

Fig. 1 How tension during telephone talk can promote learning for doctors-in-training. (With permission from Eppich et al. (2019))

- Anticipating their conversations partner's needs
- Framing clinical questions clearly at the outset of the call
- Conveying relevant information concisely and persuasively using words that grabbed the listener's attention
- Modulating the conversation to provide a sense of urgency when required
- Recognizing the limits of telephone communication and, when necessary, seeking an in-person conversation at the patient's bedside

The paralanguage that accompanies vocal speech also contributes to perceptions of urgency and persuasiveness. Wouters et al. (2020) examined working strategies of telephone triage nurses and highlighted the important role that paralinguistic cues play in helping these nurses accurately assess the urgency of a patient's condition. Depending on the situation, cues such as tone of voice or shortness of breath supplemented more objective information. At times, these global assessments of illness severity then led telephone triage nurses to override computer decision support systems, justified by their judgments of paralanguage to create a more robust mental image of the patient's condition. Further illustrating the contribution of paralanguage in communication, Zant and Berger (2020) demonstrated the impact paralinguistic cues on persuasiveness. They found that people not only speak louder and vary their speech volume when seeking to persuade, these same modulations in paralanguage also signaled confidence. Although Eppich et al. (2019) did not specifically examine how doctors-in-training learn to modulate their paralanguage, this aspect of their learning through telephone talk came through in "learning to sound confident" when conveying trustworthiness.

In a related study, Eppich et al. (2018) used qualitative thematic analysis to identify both formal and informal aspects of workplace telephone talk that contributed to learning. Formal educational practices such as teaching and explicit feedback provide a target for faculty development strategies. The main findings, however, related to informal aspects of these conversations. Specifically, conversational questions and interruptions served as "disguised feedback" for doctors-in-training. For example, when junior doctors did not anticipate information needs for respective conversation partners, conversation partners (such as subspecialists or supervising doctors) posed information-seeking questions to aid clinical decision-making. Based on these questions, junior doctors identified which information to include proactively in future telephone case presentations. Using van der Leeuw et al.'s (2017) notion of "performance relevant information" as a lens, Eppich et al. (2018) surmised that sensitizing doctors-in-training to disguised feedback had potential to impact their future workplace learning. Thus, the authors proposed several potential educational strategies to enhance telephone talk: (a) embedding telephone communication skills in existing simulation activities and (b) developing stand-alone curricular elements to sensitize junior doctors to "disguised" feedback during telephone talk as a mechanism to augment future workplace learning. Rather than a traditional view of "simulation as learning to perform" for future clinical work, Eppich and colleagues suggested a complementary and novel approach to simulation, namely "simulation as learning how to learn" from future clinical work.

As a further example of workplace conversational learning, Schmutz and Eppich (2017) delineated the potential influences of team interactions on both performance and learning. The authors used a theoretical construct from the psychology and management literature called team reflexivity (TR). TR describes "the extent to which team members collectively reflect on the team's objectives, strategies, and processes, as well as their wider organizations and environments, and adapt accordingly" (West and Sacramento 2009, p. 907). Since TR captures a team-level phenomenon, shared reflection necessarily requires talk among team members. Traditional views of TR captured only reflection after events occurred, akin to post-event debriefings (Schippers 2012). Schmutz and Eppich (2017) extended this view through a novel conceptual framework for TR in healthcare that encompasses three phases during which TR may occur: pre-action TR (reflection before patient care, e.g., during a briefing), in-action TR (deliberations during active patient care), and post-action TR (reflection after patient care, e.g., during a debriefing). Accordingly, TR addresses goals, taskwork, teamwork, or resources with various outcomes depending on the phase. These main outcomes include: optimal preparation (before), adaptation to dynamic situations (during), or learning (after). Schmutz and Eppich (2017) conceptualized how teams create shared understanding before, during, and after active joint clinical care through the talk of TR – including among clinical supervisors and doctor-in-training. These embedded conversations may contribute to highly situated forms of clinical workplace learning and enable collective competence. These team reflexive moments are characterized by discursive team behaviors, including:

- Recapping and summarizing (either initiated by team leaders or requested by team member)
  - "Let's review what we have done so far" or "Can we review what we have done so far?"
  - "Let's recap to make sure we are on the same page" or "Can we recap to make sure we are on the same page"
- Inviting input from team about clinical decision-making, prioritizing, and planning future actions
  - "What do you think?"
  - "What are we missing?"
  - "What else could be going on?"
  - "Any other ideas or suggestions?"
  - "What are our next steps?"

Further, empiric evidence from analysis of simulated emergency situations revealed that reflection in the heat of the moment during patient care episodes improved team performance especially for larger teams (Schmutz et al. 2018). Further, these team reflexive behaviors that characterize this form of workplace talk can now be measured with the Team Reflection Behavioral Observation System (TuRBO) for Acute Care Teams (Schmutz et al. 2021). This observation system may facilitate team training and future work on the impacts of TR on both team performance and learning in various settings.

Building on these ideas, Eppich and Schmutz (2019) described concrete strategies to foster "team inclusiveness" to begin overcoming a workplace mentality characterized by "tribalism" and uniprofessional learning. In addition to team reflexive behaviors previously outlined, team inclusiveness also encompasses key behaviors shown to enhance critical team dialogue, such as:

- Inclusive leadership: explicitly inviting and appreciating input (Nembhard and Edmondson 2006).
- Inclusive leader language: implicit use of first-person plural pronouns such as "we," "us," and "our"; rather than, "What are *you* going to do about it? instead, "What are *we* going to do about it?" (Weiss et al. 2018).
- Speaking up by team members with questions, concerns, or suggestions (Eppich 2015; Edmondson and Besieux 2021).

In summary, multiple empiric studies have addressed the contribution of learning through clinical workplace talk. Here we have illustrated the intrinsic learning potential of workplace interactions using two specific instances: work-related telephone conversations and team reflection during various timepoints in relation to patient care episodes. This work highlights four main areas: (a) sociocultural aspects related to power and pushback and how they serve to promote learning due to productive conversational tensions, (b) formal aspects of talk related to process and content in the workplace, (c) informal conversational elements as "disguised feedback," and (d) team interactions as a mechanism that drives learning. These informal opportunities to learn through talk supplement more obviously deliberate conversations with learning as an explicit goal.

Talk and Explicit Learning Conversations

Some conversations occur to promote learning explicitly. Both feedback and debriefing conversations both fall into this category. Tavares et al. (2020) traced the origins of the originally distinct terms "feedback" and "debriefing." In their conceptual analysis, the authors identified distinct theoretical roots of these terms in how they have been studied and used in practice. More recently, similar theories advance the study and enactments of feedback and debriefing as explicit experiential learning conversations. These commonalities relate to the varied types of experiential events or performances that form the substance of these learning conversations in which learners participate and educators may observe. Educators who facilitate these learning conversations promote reflection. As Fig. 2 illustrates, several contextual factors shape these learning conversations, including educator and learner characteristics, their preexisting relationship, social norms, and learning goals to name a few. These additional factors influence how educators, whether in clinical workplaces or in simulation, engage with learners and what conversations strategies and models inform the approach to the conversation.

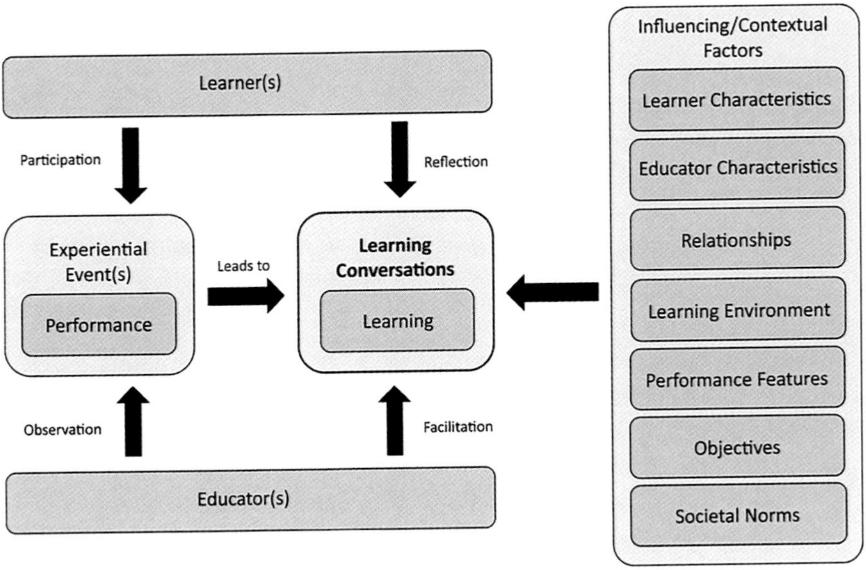

Fig. 2 A conceptualization of how learning conversations between a learner and an educator share common antecedents and how influencing/contextual features may need to be aligned with and/or shape conversational choices. An *experiential event* in a simulation or clinical context begins the process where a learner participates by responding to clinical stimuli and an educator(s) observes the performance. The learner and educator then engage in a unique pattern of dialogue, or *learning conversation*, shaped by conversational choices suited to a number of influencing/contextual factors. The list of *influencing/contextual* factors shown in the figure represents those commonly included in theoretical orientations and is not intended to be comprehensive. (With permission from Tavares et al. (2020))

While this model of experiential learning conversations denotes similarities between practice-based learning and simulation, important differences exist which emphasize the need for authenticity in the learning activities in simulation settings. Specifically, Bligh and Bleakley (2006) offered a critique of simulation-based education in healthcare, however, questioning whether "learning by simulation can become a simulation of learning" (p. 606). They observed that simulation may in some instances no longer accurately reflect actual clinical practice. The authors called for greater dialogue between work-based learning and simulation-based learning, pointing out that the "work-based learning movement can benefit from studying how the simulation culture structures the learning environment, where scaffolding and feedback are regularly employed" (p. 607). The learning conversations model by Tavares et al. (2020) represents one unifying mechanism that plays an integral role in learning from both workplaces and simulation. See additional chapters in this volume for more detail on feedback ("Feedback and supervision in health professions education") and debriefing (▶ Chap. 38, "Debriefing Practices in Simulation-Based Education").

We should also highlight that Tavares et al. (2020) explored debriefings as a learning conversation, not debriefing with a therapeutic aim such as "psychological debriefing." Kolbe et al. (2021) added granularity to our understanding of the term "debriefing" related to team debriefings that might arise in clinical settings after stressful or highly consequential clinical events, such as a resuscitation, unanticipated deterioration of an otherwise stable patient, or an unexpected poor clinical outcome. As Kolbe et al. (2021) outline, intention and potential impacts should be aligned for debriefings. The authors differentiate between two common approaches to debriefing: "debriefing-to-learn" and "debriefing-to-treat." When debriefing-to-learn, facilitators explore events in detail using structured approaches and strive to maximize group participation in order to identify areas of learning and improvement and promote future performance. The value of debriefing-to-learn has been demonstrated for simulation debriefing (Cheng et al. 2013) and workplace after-action reviews (Allen et al. 2018). However, debriefings-to-treat intended to support clinical staff after extremely stressful clinical events require unique training and expertise to avoid potential harm. When debriefing-to-treat, trained facilitators strive to minimize psychological morbidity and structure these therapeutic conversations quite differently with different aims in mind. Kolbe et al. (2021) propose a third debriefing intention, namely debriefing-to-manage, to offer guidance when a learning-oriented debriefing unexpectedly elicits strong emotional reactions that veers into a potentially therapeutic space. When debriefing-to-manage, facilitators should avoid exploring events in detail, providing participants control and space and respecting individual preferences about whether to contribute or to remain silent in the group setting. Importantly, facilitators should offer additional supports after the debriefing. We offer this nuanced discussion about alignments between debriefing intentions and impacts to raise awareness about required skill sets and approaches as the use of clinical debriefing expands.

Talk and Tensions

While healthcare simulation values supportive learning environments, unfortunately the situation in clinical workplaces varies greatly. Empiric work has consistently demonstrated the detrimental impact of rudeness on cognition and performance (Flin 2010; Porath et al. 2007; Porath and Pearson 2010; Riskin et al. 2015). Although the term "tension" generally invokes negative connotations (Lingard et al. 2002; Wadhwa and Lingard 2006; Chan et al. 2014), the notion of "productive conversational tension" Eppich et al. (2019) highlighted earlier adds a more nuanced view to our understanding of workplace talk since some tensions appeared to motivate junior doctors to change future behavior and craft their telephone talk in ways to minimize tensions while achieving patient care goals. Eppich et al. (2019), however, warned against creating intentional tensions given the risks of disruptive behavior and incivility. Olmos-Vega et al. (2017) also identified potentially beneficial tensions in clinical supervisor-supervisee dyads if safe learning environments allowed for productive negotiation. While team conflict is generally viewed negatively and something teams should avoid (Chan et al. 2014; Greer et al. 2012; Janss et al. 2012), certain collectivistic (rather than individualistic) conflict processes have benefits for team performance (DeChurch et al. 2013). These notions of productive tensions and constructive conflict processes have great relevance also for the discursive practice of TR. The extent to which TR surfaces tensions and promotes productive collectivistic processes in the service of learning and patient care requires further study.

A fine line exists between productive and highly unproductive conversational tensions. Incivility in the workplace threatens psychological safety and social relations (Flin 2010; Pearson and Porath 2005) and thus hinders the dialogue that promotes learning and patient care. The relationship between communication breakdowns and patient safety is well documented (Eppich 2015; Kohn et al. 2000). Even witnessing rudeness impairs cognitive functioning in onlookers (Porath and Erez 2009), even when they are not party to the rude interactions, a finding with relevance for healthcare (Flin 2010; Riskin et al. 2015). Issues of civility most certainly impact clinical practice, for example, during telephone conversations when clinical supervisors or subspecialists interrupt junior doctors abruptly or rudely question management decisions. Further, doctors-in-training face threats to supportive clinical learning environments from disjointed team interactions in traditional clinical rotational structures (Holmboe et al. 2011; Bernabeo et al. 2011). By rotating to different clinical services every few weeks, doctors-in-training fail to build meaningful collegial relationships that enable the conversations that promote their clinical and professional development in team-based healthcare settings (Pugh and Hatala 2016). Especially such variable learning conditions demand attention to psychological safety to tip the scale from unproductive to productive conversational tensions.

Talk and Psychological Safety

An extensive literature highlights the essential role of psychological safety for both learning and performance in workplace (Kessel et al. 2012; Ortega et al. 2014; O'Donovan et al. 2021) and simulation-based settings (Rudolph et al. 2014; Kolbe et al. 2020; Purdy et al. 2022). Psychological safety refers to a willingness to take interpersonal risks (Edmondson 1999) and a belief that one will not be punished, blamed, or humiliated when speaking up with questions, concerns, or mistakes (Edmondson and Lei 2014). In short, psychological safety can be viewed as "a sense of permission for candour" (p. 271) (Edmondson and Besieux 2021). Psychological safety contributes to mutual trust and fosters productive learning relationships. Indeed, supportive yet challenging learning environments are fundamental for all learning conversations, including effective post-simulation debriefings (Kolbe et al. 2020) and candid workplace talk (Edmondson and Lei 2014). Recommendations exist for strategies to establish a "safe container" in simulation settings (85), yet Purdy et al. (2022) recently added nuance to our understanding of psychological safety in an elegant qualitative study. The authors identified bidirectional impacts of psychological safety between team simulations in workplace settings such as emergency departments, showing that the "safe container" may actually be leaky. Team members bring their perceptions of workplace psychological safety into simulation activities, for good or for ill, which may influence interactions during simulation and debriefing. However, team simulations also had the potential to "incubate" psychological safety which increased team familiarity and shaped future real-world practice. As Purdy et al. (2022) recommend, these bidirectional impacts highlight the need to foreground psychological safety in all aspects of simulation: how we think about it, how we design it, how we implement it, and how we debrief it.

Along these lines, recent research highlighted the role of building and managing relationships and rapport in facilitator-guided post-event debriefings to create and maintain a productive space for learning. Loo et al. (2018) used a rapport management model to critique debriefing frameworks identified through a systematic literature search. In their critical review, the authors assessed the extent to which existing debriefing frameworks integrated formal language to address main aspects of rapport management, namely (a) face sensitivities that deal with personal/social values like respect, status, and competence, (b) sociality rights and obligations related to personal/social entitlements such as being treated fairly, and (c) interactional goals in terms of tasks and relationships. Of 34 debriefing frameworks identified in this review, 15 considered all three components of the rapport management model. The authors noted that debriefing scripts should incorporate "culture-specific linguistic conventions" (p. 58) and phrases to manage rapport. Needless to say, debriefing scripts are only words on a page; how they are enacted in practice may be another matter. Yet these findings underscore the potential for scripts to help manage key aspects of the talk, especially for novice educators, until these important elements become second nature. Sargeant et al. (2015) also highlighted relationship-building as a precursor to exploring reactions and content in their framework for facilitated feedback. Clinical event debriefings (Kessler et al. 2015), a form of post-action TR (Schmutz and Eppich 2017), also rely on rapport and relationships that promote psychological safety and open a safe space to discuss otherwise undiscussable topics (Argyris 1980).

As it relates to the influence of psychological safety and tensions on conversational learning, Edmondson and Besieux (2021) recently published a helpful conceptual matrix to outline productive workplace conversations. In outlining this framework, the authors highlight the respective contribution of voice behaviors versus silence related to overall productiveness of a conversation. While this important paper stems from the management literature, the principles are imminently applicable to healthcare sectors, in which voice behaviors are more commonly referred to as speaking up. Voice represents critical moments of agency related to conversational contributions since these moments reflect a conscious choice to engage in voice behaviors over silence (Eppich 2015). The productive conversation matrix elegantly positions voice behaviors to the type of contribution and also integrates silence – or the absence of talk – as a vital element of conversation. The four quadrants of the productive conversational matrix (see Fig. 3) include essential group conversational activities that contribute to goal attainment:

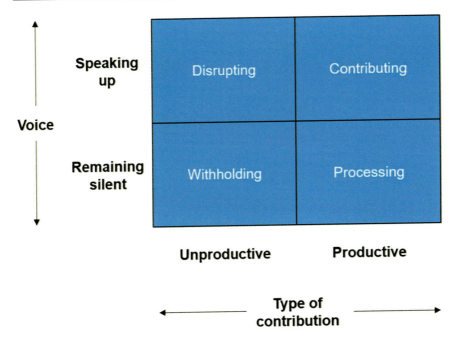

Fig. 3 The productive conversational matrix. (With permission from Edmondson and Besieux (2021))

1. Productive voice: speaking up with question, contributing ideas and opinions; psychological safety fosters candor.
2. Productive silence: taking time to process, thinking time; active listening – requires group norms that encourage processing.
3. Unproductive voice: disrupting the group, creating unhelpful tensions, being rude – threatens psychological safety.
4. Unproductive silence: keeping valuable suggestions or concerns to one's self; insufficient psychological safety limits candor.

When viewing the productive conversational matrix in HPE settings, we can recognize how these productive ebbs and flows of voice and silence contribute to debriefings or workplace conversations such as telephone talk or interdisciplinary rounds. In both contexts, posing questions freely and having time to process information contributes to learning. Of course, the contrary applies – in environments of poor psychological safety, disruptive behaviors potentiate suboptimal learning climates and foster withholding behaviors. In formal and informal learning contexts, health professions educators contribute to learning culture (Watling 2015) in ways that promote psychological safety. At a granular level, educators in a variety of settings can take explicit steps to create challenging yet supportive learning environment that promote productive and limit unproductive behaviors.

Conclusion

Rather than viewing talk as "communicative competency" and as a learning outcome, this chapter treats talk as joint social activity that contributes to both learning for practice as well as learning from practice. This chapter addresses the following overarching question: How does "talk" contribute to learning in clinical education? The aim was twofold: to identify lessons from these respective from formal and informal conversations settings that might inform each other, and to articulate practical strategies to steer healthcare talk and promote both meaningful learning and patient care.

We have integrated distinct literature streams in health professions education and workplace learning, psychology and team science, and healthcare debriefing to illustrate how talk contributes to clinical education. Lessons from explicit experiential learning conversations demonstrate the potential in deliberately steering the talk of practice by attending to both process and content elements. When viewed through a sociocultural lens, talk represents social activity that drives learning, highlighting the integral role of relationships and rapport. "Productive conversational tensions" add a more nuanced view to our understanding of workplace talk in recognizing that some tensions motivate junior doctors to adapt their talk in ways to minimize future tensions. The potential for unproductive tensions, disruptive voice, and withholding behaviors highlight the vital importance of psychological safety in a variety of learning contexts.

Cross-References

▶ Communities of Practice and Medical Education
▶ Debriefing Practices in Simulation-Based Education
▶ Effective Feedback Conversations in Clinical Practice
▶ Simulation for Clinical Skills in Healthcare Education

References

Abercrombie D. Paralanguage. Int J Lang Commun Disord. 1968;3(1):55–9.
ACGME Milestones by Specialty. Accreditation Council on Graduate Medical Education. http://www.acgme.org/What-We-Do/Accreditation/Milestones/Milestones-by-Specialty. Accessed on 5 September 2022.
Allen JA, Reiter-Palmon R, Crowe J, Scott C. Debriefs: teams learning from doing in context. Am Psychol. 2018;73(4):504–16.
Anspach RR. Notes on the sociology of medical discourse: the language of case presentation. J Health Soc Behav. 1988;29(4):357–75.
Argyris C. Making the undiscussable and its undiscussability discussable. Public Adm Rev. 1980;40(3):205–13.
Arluke A. Social control rituals in medicine: the case of death rounds. In: Dingwall R, Heath C, Reid M, Stacey M, editors. Health care and health knowledge. New York: Prodist; 1977.

Atkinson P. Medical work and medical talk: the liturgy of the clinic. London: Sage Publications; 1995.

Benson BJ. Domain of competence: interpersonal and communication skills. Acad Pediatr. 2014;14(2 Suppl):S55–65.

Bernabeo EC, Holtman MC, Ginsburg S, Rosenbaum JR, Holmboe ES. Lost in transition: the experience and impact of frequent changes in the inpatient learning environment. Acad Med. 2011;86(5):591–8.

Billett S. Towards a model of workplace learning: the learning curriculum. Stud Contin Educ. 1996;18(1):43–58.

Billett S. Guided learning at work. J Work Learn. 2000;12(7):272–85.

Bligh J, Bleakley A. Distributing menus to hungry learners: can learning by simulation become simulation of learning? Med Teach. 2006;28(7):606–13.

Bowers C, Braun CC, Morgan BB. Team workload: its meaning and measurement. In: Brannick MT, Salas E, Prince C, editors. Team performance assessment and measurement: theory, methods, and applications. Mahwah: Lawrence Erlbaum Associates; 1997. p. 85–108.

Brown JS, Collins A, Duguid P. Situated cognition and the culture of learning. Educ Res. 1989;18(1):32–42.

CanMeds Framework. Royal College of Physicians and Surgeons of Canada. http://www.royalcollege.ca/rcsite/canmeds/canmeds-framework-e. Accessed 5 September 2022.

Chan T, Bakewell F, Orlich D, Sherbino J. Conflict prevention, conflict mitigation, and manifestations of conflict during emergency department consultations. Acad Emerg Med. 2014;21(3):308–13.

Cheng A, Hunt EA, Donoghue A, Nelson-McMillan K, Nishisaki A, Leflore J, et al. Examining pediatric resuscitation education using simulation and scripted debriefing: a multicenter randomized trial. JAMA Pediatr. 2013;167(6):528–36.

Clark HH. Using language. Cambridge, UK: Cambridge University Press; 1996. p. 1–436.

DeChurch LA, Mesmer-Magnus JR, Doty D. Moving beyond relationship and task conflict: toward a process-state perspective. J Appl Psychol. 2013;98(4):559–78.

Dornan T, Boshuizen H, King N, Scherpbier A. Experience-based learning: a model linking the processes and outcomes of medical students' workplace learning. Med Educ. 2007;41(1):84–91.

Edmondson A. Psychological safety and learning behavior in work teams. Adm Sci Q. 1999;44:350–83.

Edmondson AC. Teaming: how organizations learn, innovate, and compete in the knowledge economy. San Francisco: Wiley; 2012.

Edmondson AC, Besieux T. Reflections: voice and silence in workplace conversations. J Chang Manag. 2021;21(3):269–86.

Edmondson AC, Lei Z. Psychological safety: the history, renaissance, and future of an interpersonal construct. Annu Rev Organ Psychol Organ Behav. 2014;1:23–43.

Eppich W. "Speaking up" for patient safety in the pediatric emergency department. Clin Pediatr Emerg Med. 2015;16(2):83–9.

Eppich WJ, Schmutz JB. From "them" to "us": bridging group boundaries through team inclusiveness. Med Educ [Internet]. 2019;53(8):756–8.

Eppich WJ, Rethans J-J, Dornan T, Teunissen PW. Learning how to learn using simulation: unpacking disguised feedback using a qualitative analysis of doctors' telephone talk. Med Teach. 2018;40(7):661–7.

Eppich WJ, Dornan T, Rethans J-J, Teunissen PW. "Learning the lingo": a grounded theory study of telephone talk in clinical education. Acad Med. 2019;94(7):1033–9.

Eraut M. Non-formal learning and tacit knowledge in professional work. Br J Educ Psychol. 2000;70(Pt 1):113–36.

Eraut M. Informal learning in the workplace. Stud Contin Educ. 2004;26(2):247–73.

Erickson F. Appropriation of voice and presentation of self as a fellow physician: aspects of a discourse of apprenticeship in medicine. In: Sarangi S, Roberts C, editors. Talk, work, and institutional order. New York: Mouton de Gruyter; 1999. p. 109–43.

Flin R. Rudeness at work. BMJ. 2010;340:c2480.

Garrod S, Pickering MJ. Why is conversation so easy? Trends Cogn Sci. 2004;8(1):8–11.

Greer LL, Saygi O, Aaldering H, Dreu CKWD. Conflict in medical teams: opportunity or danger? Med Educ. 2012;46(10):935–42.

Guralnick S, Ludwig S, Englander R. Domain of competence: systems-based practice. Acad Pediatr. 2014;14(2 Suppl):S70–9.

Haas J, Shaffir W. The professionalization of medical students: developing competence and a cloak of competence. Symb Interact [Internet]. 1977;1(1):71–88.

Haas J, Shaffir W. Ritual evaluation of competence: the hidden curriculum of professionalization in an innovative medical school program. Work Occup. 1982;9(2):131–54.

Haber RJ, Lingard LA. Learning oral presentation skills: a rhetorical analysis with pedagogical and professional implications. J Gen Intern Med. 2001;16(5):308–14.

Hammick M, Olckers L, Campion-Smith C. Learning in interprofessional teams: AMEE guide no. 38. Med Teach. 2009;31(1):1–12.

Hicks D. Discourse, learning, and teaching. Rev Res Educ. 1995;21(1):49–95.

Holmboe E, Ginsburg S, Bernabeo E. The rotational approach to medical education: time to confront our assumptions? Med Educ. 2011;45(1):69–80.

Hunter KM. Doctors' stories. Princeton: Princeton University Press; 1991.

Hymes DH. On communicative competence. In: Pride JB, Holmes J, editors. Sociolinguistics: selected readings. Harmondsworth: Penguin Books; 1972. p. 269–93.

Iedema R, Scheeres H. From doing work to talking work: renegotiating knowing, doing, and identity. Appl Linguis. 2003;24(3):316–37.

Janss R, Rispens S, Segers M, Jehn KA. What is happening under the surface? Power, conflict and the performance of medical teams. Med Educ. 2012;46(9):838–49.

Kessel M, Kratzer J, Schultz C. Psychological safety, knowledge sharing, and creative performance in healthcare teams. Creat Innov Manag. 2012;21(2):147–57.

Kessler DO, Cheng A, Mullan PC. Debriefing in the emergency department after clinical events: a practical guide. Ann Emerg Med. 2015;65(6):690–8.

Kohn SC, Corrigan J, Donaldson M. To err is human: building a safer health system. Washington, DC: National Academy Press; 2000.

Kolb D. Experiential learning: experience as the source of learning and development. Saddle River: Prentice Hall; 1984.

Kolbe M, Eppich W, Rudolph J, Meguerdichian M, Catena H, Cripps A, et al. Managing psychological safety in debriefings: a dynamic balancing act. BMJ Simul Technol Enhanc Learn. 2020;6(3):164.

Kolbe M, Schmutz S, Seelandt JC, Eppich WJ, Schmutz JB. Team debriefings in healthcare: aligning intention and impact. BMJ. 2021;374:n2042.

Lave J, Wenger E. Situated learning: legitimate peripheral participation. Cambridge, UK: Cambridge University Press; 1991.

Lingard L, Haber RJ. Teaching and learning communication in medicine. Acad Med. 1999;74(5):507–10.

Lingard L, Reznick R, Espin S, Regehr G, DeVito I. Team communications in the operating room: talk patterns, sites of tension, and implications for novices. Acad Med. 2002;77(3):232–7.

Lingard L, Garwood K, Schryer CF, Spafford MM. A certain art of uncertainty: case presentation and the development of professional identity. Soc Sci Med. 2003a;56(3):603–16.

Lingard L, Schryer C, Garwood K, Spafford M. "Talking the talk": school and workplace genre tension in clerkship case presentations. Med Educ. 2003b;37(7):612–20.

Loo ME, Krishnasamy C, Lim WS. Considering face, rights, and goals: a critical review of rapport management in facilitator-guided simulation debriefing approaches. Simul Healthc. 2018;13(1):52–60.

Marsick VJ, Watkins KE. Informal and incidental learning in the workplace. London: Routledge; 1990.

Nembhard IM, Edmondson AC. Making it safe: the effects of leader inclusiveness and professional status on psychological safety and improvement efforts in health care teams. J Organ Behav. 2006;27:941–66.

O'Donovan R, Brún AD, McAuliffe E. Healthcare professionals experience of psychological safety, voice, and silence. Front Psychol. 2021;12:626689.

Olmos-Vega FM, Dolmans DHJM, Vargas-Castro N, Stalmeijer RE. Dealing with the tension: how residents seek autonomy and participation in the workplace. Med Educ. 2017;51(7):699–707.

Ortega A, den Bossche PV, Sánchez-Manzanares M, Rico R, Gil F. The influence of change-oriented leadership and psychological safety on team learning in healthcare teams. J Bus Psychol. 2014;29(2):311–21.

Pearson CM, Porath CL. On the nature, consequences and remedies of workplace incivility: no time for "nice"? Think again. Acad Manag Exec. 2005;19(1):7–18.

Porath CL, Erez A. Overlooked but not untouched: how rudeness reduces onlookers' performance on routine and creative tasks. Organ Behav Hum Decis Process. 2009;109:29–44.

Porath CL, Pearson CM. The cost of bad behavior. Organ Dyn. 2010;39(1):64–71.

Porath C, Macinnis D, Folkes V. Witnessing incivility among employees: effects on consumer anger and negative inferences about companies. Acad Manag J. 2007;109(5):1181–97.

Pugh D, Hatala R. Being a good supervisor: it's all about the relationship. Med Educ. 2016;50(4): 395–7.

Purdy E, Borchert L, El-Bitar A, Isaacson W, Bills L, Brazil V. Taking simulation out of its "safe container" – exploring the bidirectional impacts of psychological safety and simulation in an emergency department. Adv Simul. 2022;7(1):5.

Reddy MJ. The conduit metaphor – a case for frame conflict in our language about language. In: Ortony A, editor. Metaphor and thought. Cambridge, UK: Cambridge University Press; 1979. p. 284–324.

Riskin A, Erez A, Foulk TA, Kugelman A, Gover A, Shoris I, et al. The impact of rudeness on medical team performance: a randomized trial. Pediatrics. 2015;136(3):487–95.

Rudolph JW, Raemer DB, Simon R. Establishing a safe container for learning in simulation: the role of the presimulation briefing. Simul Healthc. 2014;9(6):339–49.

Sargeant J, Lockyer J, Mann K, Holmboe E, Silver I, Armson H, et al. Facilitated reflective performance feedback: developing an evidence- and theory-based model that builds relationship, explores reactions and content, and coaches for performance change (R2C2). Acad Med. 2015;90(12):1698–706.

Scheeres H. Learning to talk: from manual work to discourse work as self-regulating practice. J Work Learn. 2003;15(7/8):332–7.

Schippers MC. Why team reflexivity works. RSM Insight. 2012;4:18–9.

Schmutz JB, Eppich WJ. Promoting learning and patient care through shared reflection: a conceptual Framework for team reflexivity in health care. Acad Med. 2017;92(11):1555–63.

Schmutz JB, Lei Z, Eppich WJ, Manser T. Reflection in the heat of the moment: the role of in-action team reflexivity in health care emergency teams. J Organ Behav. 2018;39(6):749–65.

Schmutz JB, Meier LL, Manser T. How effective is teamwork really? The relationship between teamwork and performance in healthcare teams: a systematic review and meta-analysis. BMJ Open. 2019;9(9):e028280.

Schmutz JB, Lei Z, Eppich WJ. Reflection on the fly: development of the Team Reflection Behavioral Observation (TuRBO) system for acute care teams. Acad Med. 2021;96(9):1337–45.

Schon DA. The reflective practitioner. New York: Harper & Collins; 1983.

Sfard A. On two metaphors for learning and the dangers of choosing just one. Educ Res. 1998;27(2):4–13.

Sutcliffe KM, Lewton E, Rosenthal MM. Communication failures: an insidious contributor to medical mishaps. Acad Med. 2004;79(2):186–94.

Swanwick T. Informal learning in postgraduate medical education: from cognitivism to "culturism". Med Educ. 2005;39(8):859–65.

Tavares W, Eppich W, Cheng A, Miller S, Teunissen PW, Watling CJ, et al. Learning conversations: an analysis of the theoretical roots and their manifestations of feedback and debriefing in medical education. Acad Med. 2020;95(7):1020–5.

Teunissen PW. Experience, trajectories, and reifications: an emerging framework of practice-based learning in healthcare workplaces. Adv Health Sci Educ. 2015;20(4):843–56.

Teunissen PW, Scheele F, Scherpbier AJJA, Vleuten CPMVD, Boor K, van Luijk SJ, et al. How residents learn: qualitative evidence for the pivotal role of clinical activities. Med Educ. 2007;41(8):763–70.

van der Leeuw RM, Teunissen PW, van der Vleuten CPM. Broadening the scope of feedback to promote its relevance to workplace learning. Acad Med. 2017;93(4):556–9.

Vygotsky LS. Mind in Society. Cambridge: Harvard University Press; 1978.

Vygotsky LS. Thought and language. Cambridge, MA: MIT Press; 1986.

Wadhwa A, Lingard L. A qualitative study examining tensions in interdoctor telephone consultations. Med Educ. 2006;40(8):759–67.

Watling C. When I say . . . learning culture. Med Educ. 2015;49(6):556–7.

Weiss M, Kolbe M, Grote G, Spahn DR, Grande B. We can do it! Inclusive leader language promotes voice behavior in multi-professional teams. Leadersh Q. 2018;29(3):389–402.

Wells G. Language and education: reconceptualizing education as dialogue. In: Language use in professional contexts, vol. 19. Cambridge, UK: Cambridge University Press; 1999. p. 135–55.

Wells G, Wells J. Learning to talk and talking to learn. Theory Pract. 1984;23(3):190–7.

Wenger E. Communities of practice: learning, meaning, and identity. New York: Cambridge University Press; 1998.

West MA, Sacramento C. Team reflexivity. In: Levine JM, Hogg MA, editors. Encyclopedia of group processes & intergroup relations, vol. 1. 1st ed. Thousand Oaks: Sage Publications; 2009. p. 907–9.

Wouters LT, Zwart DL, Erkelens DC, Huijsmans M, Hoes AW, Damoiseaux RA, et al. Tinkering and overruling the computer decision support system: working strategies of telephone triage nurses who assess the urgency of callers suspected of having an acute cardiac event. J Clin Nurs. 2020;29(7–8):1175–86.

Yardley S, Teunissen PW, Dornan T. Experiential learning: AMEE guide no. 63. Med Teach. 2012;34(2):e102–15.

Zant ABV, Berger J. How the voice persuades. J Pers Soc Psychol. 2020;118(4):661–82.

Underperformance in Clinical Education: Challenges and Possibilities

58

Margaret Bearman

Contents

Introduction	1120
Experiences of Underperformance, Remediation, and Failure	1121
Learners' Experiences of Underperformance in the Clinical Environment	1121
Clinical Educators' Experiences of Underperformance	1122
Strategies for Working with Underperformance: Recommendations from the Literature	1123
Five Program Level Strategies	1123
Five Educator-Level Recommendations	1125
Beyond the "Five Strategies Approach": Supporting Learner Autonomy, Competency, and Relatedness	1128
Building Autonomy: Feedback for Future Learning	1129
Conclusions	1130
References	1130

Abstract

This chapter outlines the challenges and possibilities for working with underperformance in clinical education, based on theory and evidence. It commences by describing the experiences of underperformance from both learner and educator perspectives. Two comprehensive literature reviews on remediation from 2019 and 2021 are synthesized into ten strategies: five at program level and five at educator level. Drawing from self-determination theory, the guiding principles of building learners' autonomy, competence, and relatedness are suggested as a useful frame for understanding how to frame any response to underperformance. Finally, feedback for future learning through building evaluative judgment is explored as a potential avenue for learners to build their capabilities beyond the area of immediate deficit. This chapter recognizes the complexity of working with underperformance, acknowledging there may be no

M. Bearman (✉)
Centre for Research in Assessment and Digital Education (CRADLE), Deakin University, Melbourne, VIC, Australia
e-mail: margaret.bearman@deakin.edu.au

© Springer Nature Singapore Pte Ltd. 2023
D. Nestel et al. (eds.), *Clinical Education for the Health Professions*,
https://doi.org/10.1007/978-981-15-3344-0_55

easy solutions for this inherently challenging situation but offering a variety of different means to approach this educational problem.

> **Keywords**
>
> Clinical education · Underperformance · Remediation · Feedback

Introduction

Clinical educators often struggle with managing underperformance. There is almost always some challenge in assisting learners who cannot do what is expected of them. This can compound in clinical environments, where a teaching and learning consideration becomes integrated with a workplace problem. Indeed, clinical educators identify underperformance as one of the most time-consuming and difficult aspects of their role (Bearman et al. 2013). Working with underperformance can be stressful and lead to very strong emotions, such as anger and guilt (Luhanga et al. 2008). Frequently, clinical educators simply do not know what to do about underperformance (Bearman et al. 2013). This leads, among other things, to an avoidance of providing necessary performance information to the learner, what is termed "vanishing feedback" (Ende 1983). At its most extreme, this can manifest as "failure to fail," where clinical educators pass students who they think are not meeting requirements (Dudek et al. 2005).

Underperformance is not just about the educator-learner relationship. Clinical contexts vary enormously while some offer wonderful learning opportunities, others may provide little support. Steinert (2013) suggests it is always worth asking where the "problem" lies. The issue at hand may indeed not be the student or the teacher but the clinical environment or the educational system. The significance of systemic issues is underlined by the persistent differential attainment between white and ethnic minority cohorts in the UK (Woolf 2020), which suggests that progression has less to do with capability and more to do with context. While much of the solution from a medical education perspective rests with program design and particularly the educator-student relationship, underperformance may also speak to broader problems with the clinical culture, the opportunities afforded by the particular environment, the curriculum itself, or even assessment processes. Kalet et al. (2017) make this point strongly with respect to societal, professional, and institutional dimensions surrounding underperformance, noting "remediation is socially constructed within educational ecosystems, and it sends messages about the nature of learning, support, assessment, regulation, process, identity..."

This chapter aims to provide those who work in health professional education insights regarding possible means of supporting underperformance, drawing from the extensive literature. First, it considers how various types of underperformance are experienced by educators and students. Next, it outlines strategies at program level and at individual educator level, synthesized from two recent literature reviews. The potential for self-determination theory to provide guiding principles is then explored, particularly with respect to the significant problem of boosting learner autonomy during underperformance. Finally, developing the learner's evaluative judgment is proposed as a means to counter the observation that for most, underperformance tends to remediate past deficits, not inform future successes.

Experiences of Underperformance, Remediation, and Failure

Ellaway et al. (2018) describe three "zones" in clinical education. The first zone is referred to as *success*, where learners are within the usual curriculum and the whole progressing appropriately; the second is *remediation*, where learners temporarily have to focus on specific areas of deficit; and the third is *formal failure*, where learners must redo or exit the program altogether. Underperformance cuts across all three zones. In the first instance, the underperformance can be managed within the usual curriculum, whether momentary or sustained. Less frequently, redressing underperformance requires separate and intensive attention alongside a formal label that progression is of concern. This is usually what is termed "remediation." Finally, the level of underperformance may mean that the learner will not meet the necessary standards and the implications of this for the progression pathway must be considered. Much of the underperformance literature focusses on remediation, but educational approaches and strategies should be coherent across the usual curriculum, remedial programs, and any re-exit or exit strategies. This does not mean that educational strategies should be the same at all points, but rather that managing underperformance is ideally aligned across the mainstream curriculum, remedial programs, and at the point of formal failure or beyond.

One thing that is consistent across all three zones is that underperformance is an emotional business. Teachers and learners alike can find underperformance distressing. The combination of the general emotionality associated with feedback (Ajjawi et al. 2021) as well as the need to ensure safe practitioners may be part of the reason that underperformance can be very difficult to manage. Understanding the experiences of learners and teachers provides context for any educational strategies.

Learners' Experiences of Underperformance in the Clinical Environment

For all the work on remediation and underperformance in the clinical environment, there is surprisingly little that investigates the perspective of the learner (Davenport et al. 2018). This may be a natural consequence of the difficulties in seeking data from participants who can be labeled "underperformers." However, there are some published studies. For example, experiences of failure from the nursing literature speak of surprise and distress: "I had a lot of anger and of course disappointment, devastation in myself" (Handwerker 2018). Bynum et al. (2021) describe how shameful medical students felt with respect to underperforming even momentarily or relative to others ("below average"). As McGregor (2007) notes, a student may try to be "a chameleon" in order to meet expectations.

McGregor's 2007 study of an academically capable student who fails in the clinical environment shows the significance of relationship: "... [the student] experienced disconnecting relations—she was not trusted or respected, and her voice was misunderstood and discounted" (McGregor 2007). However, others can also be blamed or included in the narrative of failure: LaDonna et al.'s (2018) study of academic physician's experiences noted that in recounting narratives of their underperformance, physicians tended to "deflect or share responsibility." The need to distribute responsibility may be a means of protecting the self from unpleasant emotions (LaDonna et al. 2018; McGregor 2007) associated with loss of future trajectory (Handwerker 2018; McGregor 2007). Experiencing underperformance may be so distressing that it results in behaviors that are counter to learning. This suggests the need for compassion with respect to underperformance, particularly when it leads to outright failure. Indeed, Bellini et al. (2019) describe "compassionate off-ramps" out of medical school as a moral imperative.

Clinical Educators' Experiences of Underperformance

Clinical educators describe working with underperformance as highly challenging: They use words like "stressful," "exhausting," and "struggle" (Bearman et al. 2013). A particular concern is trying to balance roles as a provider of safe patient care and as an educator (Bearman et al. 2013). There is significant literature investigating the "failure to fail" phenomenon, and the difficulties that clinical educators find in making a judgment that will result in "negative expected outcomes" for the student (Cleland et al. 2008). Yepes-Rios et al.'s (2016) systematic review around failure-to-fail describes the personal guilt experienced by many clinical educators. Some educators can feel positively about failing students (Luhanga et al. 2008); likely these will not be studied within the failure-to-fail literature.

A recurrent theme in the literature, and one that has significant implications for educational strategies, is educators and researchers' view that successful remediation is dependent on insight (Price et al. 2021). However, as LaDonna et al. (2018) point out, even when academic physicians require insight and taking of responsibility from their own learners, they seem unable to grapple with these same issues in their own narratives of underperformance. Indeed, insight itself may be a well-overstated notion. There may be a difference between the internal insights that lead to behavior change and the performative insights, which are contingent on the "chameleon" nature described by McGregor (2007). As one clinical supervisor described, learners will often: "...keep up the big fake bravado keep the blind down – 'I'm not going to let you know anything about me because that might expose some weakness that you might see in me'" (Bearman et al. 2018).

These types of emotional and relational tensions suggest the many reasons that underperformance feels intractable. It is easy to write that clinical educators should be compassionate and simultaneously not take responsibility for the negative outcomes of their students, but managing emotions is not readily dictated despite intentions. It is equally easy to suggest that students need insight, but promoting insights, when the student is trying to guess what the educators wants to hear, is inherently difficult. While the next section provides useful educational strategies for navigating these complex cross-currents, it is worth remembering that these represent aspiration rather than the messiness of educating within clinical environments. Working with underperformance in clinical education may always be complex and challenging. At the same time, working with a learner, to help them move from underperformance to excellence, can be highly fulfilling.

Strategies for Working with Underperformance: Recommendations from the Literature

Two recent comprehensive literature reviews provide valuable information around how to work with underperformance (Price et al. 2021; Chou et al. 2019). These are synthesized and reinterpreted here bringing together different elements from both reviews to create a series of recommended strategies. Readers are referred to the original publications for further details and reference to the original literature, particularly to explore the level of evidence (Chou et al. 2019), and the specific context-mechanism-outcomes patterns described within the realist review (Price et al. 2021).

Five Program Level Strategies

As mentioned, systems surrounding underperformance have a considerable impact on both clinical educators and learners' experiences. While issues such as difficult clinical environments are beyond the remit of most programs, there are some program design approaches that can help with remediation. The following are mostly synthesized from Chou et al. (2019), as noted below. Box 1 provides an illustrative example of these five strategies in practice.

Program strategy 1: Design robust selection and assessment processes with well-described standards of practice (Chou et al. 2019). While this may seem self-evident, it is necessary for much of the latter strategies: Working with underperformance is easiest with clear, appropriate, and accepted expectations.

Program strategy 2: Scaffold underperformance within the normal curriculum. One of the problems of underperformance is that being labeled as poorly performing may be a self-fulfilling prophecy. Therefore, it is recommended to manage underperformance within the overall curriculum to avoid formal remediation as far as possible (Chou et al. 2019). Ideally, every learner should experience good supports, frequent assessment opportunities, and clear expectation-setting; this means that the commencement of these activities is not regarded as a tacit marker for underperformance (Bearman et al. 2018).

Program strategy 3: Design any remediation program with reference to the current literature. This strategy takes account of shifting evidence as future studies may offer new insights. At present, as Chou et al. (2019) note, the current literature suggests programs frame remediation as routine and educative rather than exceptional and punitive; it suggests intervening early and proactively. Use of small groups with expert facilitators may also be helpful (Chou et al. 2019).

Program strategy 4: Consider the role of clinical educators and how they can be supported. Chou et al. (2019) suggest a number of guidelines regarding educators. These are grouped together here. First, any program should support frontline educators, who may be least equipped in terms of educational strategies to deal with underperformance. Next, within remediation programs ensure that assessors and educators/mentors are not the same person; Price et al. (2021)'s realist review also makes this recommendation. Finally, cautiously consider how information about underperformance is shared between educators. The purpose here must always be to develop the learner, and such information sharing should be with full knowledge by the student.

Program strategy 5: Design formal institutional processes around underperformance, remediation, and failure that are transparent, fair, and compassionate. This strategy summarizes Chou et al.'s (2019) guidelines for fair due processes, which take into account the individual learner and the responsibility to patient safety as well their suggested need for compassionate exit strategies. In addition, the need for documentation of all processes, concerns and agreements is key (Chou et al. 2019; Bearman et al. 2018). While Chou et al. (2019) suggest processes must balance the tension between the learner support and the need for communities to have competent care, Bearman et al. (2018) propose that it may not be in an individual's best interest for them to continue in a career when they are not competent.

Box 1: Illustrative Example of the Program Principles: An "At Risk" Program for Undergraduate Physiotherapy

A new physiotherapy program has been designed and implemented in the last three years. During this time, the curriculum committee has developed carefully considered selection processes and assessment practices; the program employs well-articulated competency-based standards aligned with professional standards (*Program Strategy 1*). Sam has been asked to develop a new program to support students who are "at risk" of failing while on clinical placement (*Program Strategy 2*). They consult widely in setting up processes and procedures, including with clinical educators, disability liaison officers, and student representatives. This is not a straightforward process and, after consultation with policy advisors, policies and procedures are refined. The policy advisors suggest that the procedures particularly will need some iterative refining, and Sam agrees to a review after twelve months (*Program strategy 5*).

(continued)

Box 1 (continued)

Sam is very keen to ensure that students who underperform or are at risk of failure can navigate their circumstances with the least distress possible. Therefore, Sam consults the literature and ensures that orientation processes to the clinical environment raise the possibility of underperformance and the possible need for remediation. In particular, students attend a half-day session focusing on transition to the clinical environment. As part of this, a student from previous years explains how, despite academic success, they struggled at first in the clinical environment. Educators then reinforce that it is normal for students to find the transition difficult and some may need extra support but they too can take responsibility by reaching out for help (*Program Strategy 3*).

Another feature is to establish a part-time academic clinical liaison to work with and support clinical educators around underperformance (*Program Strategy 4*); the budget expenditure is justified by the higher engagement with placement environments as a consequence of this type of support. This liaison officer therefore can act as a first port of call if there are early concerns, can help educators design activities to assist learners before they need any additional attention, and can work with students if necessary without taking an assessment responsibility. Additionally, they ensure that documentation standards are met for all students (*Program Strategy 5*).

While no program or bureaucracy is perfect, Sam is pleased to see that student experiences of remediation improve and clinical educators, when surveyed, rate the support they receive from the clinical liaison officer highly. The number of students requiring formal intervention reduces after the introduction of the "at-risk" program, and although a small number of students continue to fail, the number of complaints and appeals are almost a third of what they were prior to the program's commencement.

Sam, excited by opportunities for further innovation, starts to plan early intervention strategies including peer networks for students who are at risk of failure.

Five Educator-Level Recommendations

Both Chou et al. (2019) and Price et al. (2021) emphasize the need for effective feedback processes within remediation programs. Note the emphasis on term "feedback process," which reflects the contemporary view that feedback is relational and not just the positive and negative message (Molloy et al. 2020). By this definition, most recommendations from the literature revolve around feedback. Price et al. (2021) also suggest that educator activities should optimally build motivation and insight. As noted above, insight is a challenging concept, and motivation may be a more valuable goal for the educator (Bearman et al. 2018). Chou et al.'s (2019) and

Price et al.'s (2021) work are interpreted into the following five recommendations; Box 2 provides an illustrative example.

Educational strategy 1: Build trust. Trust is often in short supply at the point where learners are at risk of failing (McGregor 2007). The provision of environments where learners feel sufficiently comfortable to be vulnerable about their deficits ("psychologically safe") and where the educator is cast as an advocate for the learner ("on the same team") can build trust in both the educator and the overall remediation process. It is important for learners to experience empathy, positive regard, and to feel that discussions are confidential (Price et al. 2021). In this way, the learner can examine their own performance in order to improve rather than to make a definitive judgment about their competence.

Educational strategy 2: Create opportunities for learner autonomy. Chou et al. (2019) and Price et al. (2021) both underline the importance of involving the learner in planning and goal setting regarding any program to redress deficits. Further, as Price et al. (2021) outline, it is important for learners to identify for themselves where problems lie. Not only will they be more receptive, but through this process of identification, they may also come to start to manage their own concerns into the future. Another way of supporting learner autonomy is to focus learners on identifying the things that can be improved and to avoid any suggestion that the underperformance is due to an inherent deficit (Price et al. 2021).

Educational strategy 3: Reference standards and multisourced data. Performance is optimally judged relative to an expected standard. Framing learner perceptions of their underperformance, relative to these standards, can therefore assist in helping the learner understand why they may need to change what they are doing (Price et al. 2021). Often, learners find it easier to understand deficits against what they see as objective data, and so feedback processes are often helped by asking learners to focus on concrete data (not hearsay) from many triangulating sources (Chou et al. 2019; Price et al. 2021) and to therefore help identify areas for improvement.

Educational strategy 4: Situate learning in its broader contexts. As stated, one of the most significant influences upon underperformance can be situations outside of the workplace. For instance, caring responsibilities, financial problems, and illness can lead to learners not being at their best at particular moments in time. Recognizing these broader contextual issues can help educators work with underperformance. Indeed, most people underperform at least some of the time, and asking educators to frame underperformance and remediation as an often temporary state that is frequently part of clinical training (Price et al. 2021; Chou et al. 2019) can help increase motivation and reduce feelings of shame. Price et al. (2021) describe how affirming strengths can foster professional identity, which may in turn build the motivation for making changes.

Educational strategy 5: Developing sustained changes to practice. One of the most notable insights from Cleland et al.'s (2013) literature review on remediation was that the included studies focused on redressing underperformance by helping students scrape a pass within the particular instance at hand. Both Chou et al.

(2019) and Price et al. (2021) suggest strategies that build learners' capabilities look beyond the minimum pass. First, Price et al. (2021) suggest sustaining learning through repeated practice, mediated by feedback and guided reflection. These latter reflective processes, including reflective logs and coaching, may help the learner make sense of their experiences (Chou et al. 2019; Price et al. 2021). Chou et al. (2019) emphasize the need for learners to come to self-regulate.

The five educator recommendations, while targeting underperformance, are also ones that are generally good principles to undertake in any kind of learning. And to a certain extent, that is how it should be. Educators employ the same principles to work with learners at all levels, although clearly there are differences in focus, scaffolding, and sequencing. One thing that is not mentioned in these reviews, but has been noted elsewhere (Bearman et al. 2018), is clinical educators may very well need to acknowledge and address their own stresses and emotions that arise when working with underperformance. While educating is often a pleasure, there may be little delight found in negotiating between a busy clinical environment and a trainee who cannot take necessary responsibility or a learner who requires extra oversight. If reflective practice is necessary for learners to manage underperformance, it may be equally critical for educators as well. Being strategic about where energy is expended may also help ensure that one's own emotional load does not lead to provide inappropriate tacit or explicit feedback information.

> **Box 2: Illustration of the Educator Principles: Supervision Within a General Practice Training Rotation**
>
> Lee has commenced a second placement within general practice training, and Jo, their supervisor, notes that they are floundering with respect to consultation skills, particularly time management. Most trainees struggle at first, but Lee does not seem to be improving and is becoming overwhelmed by their clinical workload and heavily reliant on senior colleagues for guidance. And Lee seems to be avoiding Jo, despite Jo's "open door" efforts (*Educational Strategy 1*).
>
> Jo wants to intervene early before things get out of hand, so they arrange to meet after a shift. To make sure the conversation is not pressured, Jo speaks to the practice staff and makes sure that they both have fewer appointments that afternoon. Jo starts off the conversation by asking Lee how they are doing (*Educational Strategy 1*).
>
> Lee's response is surprising. Their mother is seriously unwell, and they have carer duties. They know that they are overwhelmed but cannot seem to do anything about it. When Jo reinforces that consultation skills often challenge most new general practitioners, Lee seems relieved (*Educational Strategy 4*). Lee also is pleased with the suggestion that they put together a plan. Together, they decide to focus on time-management skills, and they talk through some of

(continued)

> **Box 2** (continued)
>
> the ways time can be managed (*Educational Strategy 2*). Jo offers some useful heuristics on how to manage the patient interaction and offers to observe immediately, but Lee wants to hold off on the observation until they have had a chance to put the heuristics into practice. Jo respects this (*Educational Strategy 2*) but suggests buddying with another trainee at the practice to do some observation of each other, with particular focus on time management and standards of patient communication (*Educational Strategy 3*).
>
> By the time that Jo comes to observe Lee, they find enormous improvement, not only in the consultation skills but also in Lee's confidence. However, Jo asks Lee to arrange a schedule of regular meetings where Lee presents challenging consultations. This has the dual purpose of not only following up on changes to practice (*Educational Strategy 5*) but also ensuring that Lee can balance their carer responsibilities with their training.

Beyond the "Five Strategies Approach": Supporting Learner Autonomy, Competency, and Relatedness

The literature provides a range of strategies to help address underperformance, and as outlined above, this can usefully inform both how programs are designed and how educators teach. However, strategies run the risk of becoming too instrumental. For example, affirming strengths can easily become tokenistic while being transparent can easily tip into reductionism and may overlook the value of professional judgment. Educational theory serves as a counter to this potential instrumentalism by providing guiding principles.

Previous work has suggested Self-Determination Theory (SDT) provides a useful frame to help navigate the emotional and relational tensions within underperformance (Bearman et al. 2018). Certainly, SDT helps with understanding *why* some of the strategies outlined above may be successful. Additionally, SDT may also help in educators' decisions when contextualizing educational ideas into local contexts.

SDT is a theory of motivation (Deci et al. 2001). It therefore describes reasons that people choose to engage or disengage with their education. Ryan and Deci (2020) propose that in order to develop, people need to fulfill three foundational psychological needs: They must experience feelings of autonomy, competency, and relatedness. If these three states are undermined, motivation diminishes. SDT explains why working with underperformance causes challenges for clinical educators and learners. Underperformance generally suggests a lack of competence; educationally, it is significant for learners to recognize this in order to address this. However, feeling incompetent undermines the motivation to address any deficits. Moreover, in clinical education, if learners are not competent, their autonomy must be reduced in order to ensure patient safety. Finally, if learners feel like their professional identity is under attack, relatedness to clinical colleagues and educators may reduce.

If SDT provides an explanation for the challenges facing educators and learners, it also offers solutions. Many of the strategies listed above provide programs or suggest ways of interacting that boost these three needs. *Educational strategies 2 and 5* directly address the issue of supporting learner autonomy. Some of the proposed approaches within *Educational strategy 4* are about building feelings of competence by looking beyond the immediate deficit area. Building trust as outlined in *Educational strategy 1* likely builds relatedness.

In addition to providing support for the strategies listed above, SDT also provides insight into how to work with learners when implementing a strategy does not provide the desired result. This is the advantage of theory: While a strategy offers specific research-based approaches, they tend to be somewhat normative and presuppose ideal learning environments. In reality, standards are very difficult to articulate well, learners will not attend orientations, and clinical educators may be reluctant to engage with academic institutions. Therefore, in any particular situation, with all its attendant real-world messiness, it may be necessary to reflect on how to build motivation. By considering the domains of learner autonomy, competence, and relatedness, educators may gain insight into how to help a particular learner or how to troubleshoot a challenge in curriculum or remediation processes.

There is no ideal or single solution here: Autonomy and patient safety may be in tension; the learner may need to struggle with feelings of incompetence as a necessary part of learning; and not everyone needs to like each other. However, thinking with an SDT lens can help an educator reframe what they are doing and prevent them doing "more of the same" but look for good educational alternatives. For example, when planning any activity or sequence of activities designed to redress underperformance, a clinical educator can consider how the intended programs impact on the learner's feelings of competence, autonomy, and relatedness. This may include simulating tasks to build feelings of competence or allowing the learner to choose tasks to build autonomy or enhancing relatedness via extended debriefs that are high on interpersonal exchange and low on didactics.

Building Autonomy: Feedback for Future Learning

Consider SDT prompts examination of the gaps within the literature and hence with the strategies outlined above. One area which may deserve more attention is considering how to build autonomy into the future, so that the learner can continue to develop once the remediation and support processes have ended. Often, remedial processes leave the learner dependent on the educator telling them whether they are doing well or poorly. However, once in practice, the learner must assume this responsibility for themselves. SDT would suggest learners will be more likely to continue to be motivated and engaged in their learning, if autonomy can be extended beyond the "guided reflective practice" recommended by Chou et al. (2019) and Price et al. (2021).

One possible solution is to develop the learner's insight into the qualities of good performance, a capability often called evaluative judgment (Tai et al. 2018; Bearman et al. 2021; Fawns and O'Shea 2019). Tai et al. (2018) define evaluative judgment as the capability to: "judge the quality of work of self and others." By focusing on evaluative judgment, the learner can look beyond the particular deficit at hand, which can breed defensiveness and other unhelpful emotions, toward how the learner can assess whether a performance is good or bad. This helps build autonomy as the learner themselves can take responsibility for considering their performance against others' views or against data or against standards.

The idea of feedback for future learning is that learners can be supported in recognizing the features of good practice (Bearman et al. 2021). In current feedback approaches, learners are often asked: How do you think you are performing? In feedback for future learning, the emphasis is on asking the learners to point to examples of good or poor practice, so that they can then understand how they fit within these possibilities. This allows learners to see how often tacit standards play out in action and how types of data, including comments from colleagues or patient data, help construct notions of good practice.

A very useful way to develop evaluative judgment is association with colleagues or students at the same level. Peer learning, in particular peer feedback, can build evaluative judgment (Tai et al. 2016). While many people emphasize the problems with "receiving" peer feedback as dismissing it as inaccurate or unhelpful, the key value in peer feedback is making the judgments about other people's work. Often peers are overlooked to help with underperformance or remediation programs or are cast as slightly less threatening sources of information. The value of peers is that they provide many opportunities for learners who may be underperforming to observe and judge work, as well as providing an opportunity for relatedness. In this way, peer interactions can build a sense of what quality work looks like in a nonthreatening environment, building a sense of autonomy.

Conclusions

Underperformance in clinical environments challenges learners, educators, and systems. A significant body of literature provides helpful guidance on how to work with underperformance. However, program designers and educators still must translate these into practice, mindful that the goal of working with underperformance is not to "fix" the learner. Rather, it is to provide learners with the opportunities, activities, and frameworks that can help them develop, both with respect to the immediate deficit, and into their future training as a health professional.

References

Ajjawi R, Kent F, Broadbent J, Tai JH-M, Bearman M, Boud D. Feedback that works: a realist review of feedback interventions for written tasks. Stud High Educ. 2021:1–14. https://doi.org/10.1080/03075079.2021.1894115.

Bearman M, Molloy E, Ajjawi R, Keating J. 'Is there a Plan B?': clinical educators supporting underperforming students in practice settings. Teach High Educ. 2013;18(5):531–44. https://doi.org/10.1080/13562517.2012.752732.

Bearman M, Castanelli D, Denniston C. Identifying and working with underperformance. In: *Learning and teaching in clinical contexts: a practical guide*; 2018. p. 236–50.

Bearman M, Brown J, Kirby C, Ajjawi R. Feedback that helps trainees learn to practice without supervision. Acad Med. 2021;96(2):205–9. https://doi.org/10.1097/acm.0000000000003716.

Bellini LM, Kalet A, Englander R. Providing compassionate off-ramps for medical students is a moral imperative. Acad Med. 2019;94(5):656–8. https://doi.org/10.1097/acm.0000000000002568.

Bynum WE IV, Varpio L, Lagoo J, Teunissen PW. 'I'm unworthy of being in this space': the origins of shame in medical students. Med Educ. 2021;55(2):185–97. https://doi.org/10.1111/medu.14354.

Chou CL, Kalet A, Costa MJ, Cleland J, Winston K. Guidelines: the dos, don'ts and don't knows of remediation in medical education. Perspect Med Educ. 2019;8(6):322–38. https://doi.org/10.1007/s40037-019-00544-5.

Cleland J, Knight LV, Rees CE, Tracey S, Bond CM. Is it me or is it them? Factors that influence the passing of underperforming students. Med Educ. 2008;42(8):800–9. https://doi.org/10.1111/j.1365-2923.2008.03113.x.

Cleland J, Leggett H, Sandars J, Costa MJ, Patel R, Moffat M. The remediation challenge: theoretical and methodological insights from a systematic review. Med Educ. 2013;47(3):242–51. https://doi.org/10.1111/medu.12052.

Davenport R, Hewat S, Ferguson A, McAllister S, Lincoln M. Struggle and failure on clinical placement: a critical narrative review. Int J Lang Commun Disord. 2018;53(2):218–27. https://doi.org/10.1111/1460-6984.12356.

Deci EL, Koestner R, Ryan RM. Extrinsic rewards and intrinsic motivation in education: reconsidered once again. Rev Educ Res. 2001;71(1):1–27. https://doi.org/10.3102/00346543071001001.

Dudek NL, Marks MB, Regehr G. Failure to fail: the perspectives of clinical supervisors. Acad Med. 2005;80(10):S84–7.

Ellaway RH, Chou CL, Kalet AL. Situating remediation: accommodating success and failure in medical education systems. Acad Med. 2018;93(3). https://doi.org/10.1097/ACM.0000000000001855

Ende J. Feedback in clinical medical education. J Am Med Assoc. 1983;250(6):777–81.

Fawns T, O'Shea C. Evaluative judgement of working practices. Ital J Educ Technol. 2019;27(1):5–18.

Handwerker SM. Challenges experienced by nursing students overcoming one course failure: a phenomenological research study. Teach Learn Nurs. 2018;13(3):168–73. https://doi.org/10.1016/j.teln.2018.03.007.

Kalet A, Chou CL, Ellaway RH. To fail is human: remediating remediation in medical education. Perspect Med Educ. 2017;6(6):418–24. https://doi.org/10.1007/s40037-017-0385-6.

LaDonna KA, Ginsburg S, Watling C. Shifting and sharing: academic physicians' strategies for navigating underperformance and failure. Acad Med. 2018;93(11):1713–8. https://doi.org/10.1097/acm.0000000000002292.

Luhanga F, Yonge O, Myrick F. Precepting an unsafe student: the role of the faculty. Nurse Educ Today. 2008;28(2):227–31. https://doi.org/10.1016/j.nedt.2007.04.001.

McGregor A. Academic success, clinical failure: struggling practices of a failing student. J Nurs Educ. 2007;46(11):504–11.

Molloy E, Ajjawi R, Bearman M, Noble C, Rudland J, Ryan A. Challenging feedback myths: values, learner involvement and promoting effects beyond the immediate task. Med Educ. 2020;54(1):33–9. https://doi.org/10.1111/medu.13802.

Price T, Wong G, Withers L, Wanner A, Cleland J, Gale T, et al. Optimising the delivery of remediation programmes for doctors: a realist review. Med Educ. 2021; https://doi.org/10.1111/medu.14528.

Ryan RM, Deci EL. Intrinsic and extrinsic motivation from a self-determination theory perspective: definitions, theory, practices, and future directions. Contemp Educ Psychol. 2020;61:101860. https://doi.org/10.1016/j.cedpsych.2020.101860.

Steinert Y. The "problem" learner: whose problem is it? AMEE Guide No. 76. Med Teach. 2013;35 (4):e1035–45. https://doi.org/10.3109/0142159X.2013.774082.

Tai J, Canny BJ, Haines TP, Molloy EK. The role of peer-assisted learning in building evaluative judgement: opportunities in clinical medical education. Adv Health Sci Educ. 2016;21(3):659–76.

Tai J, Ajjawi R, Boud D, Dawson P, Panadero E. Developing evaluative judgement: enabling students to make decisions about the quality of work. High Educ. 2018;76(3):467–81.

Woolf K. Differential attainment in medical education and training. BMJ. 2020;368:m339.

Yepes-Rios M, Dudek N, Duboyce R, Curtis J, Allard RJ, Varpio L. The failure to fail underperforming trainees in health professions education: a BEME systematic review: BEME Guide No. 42. Med Teach. 2016;38(11):1092–9. https://doi.org/10.1080/0142159X.2016.1215414.

Part V

Assessment in Health Professions Education

Approaches to Assessment: A Perspective from Education

Phillip Dawson and Colin R. McHenry

Contents

Introduction	1136
Educational Assessment: Foundations and Emerging Big Ideas	1136
Foundational Ideas from Educational Assessment	1136
Big Ideas in Assessment	1140
Conclusion	1144
Cross-References	1144
References	1144

Abstract

There is a large body of research literature on assessment in health professions education. However, there is an even larger body of literature on assessment in the broader field of higher and professional education. This chapter investigates some foundational and emerging ideas in the education research literature on assessment that may be useful to health professions educators. It first covers basic ideas from educational assessment: standards-based approaches; the multiple roles of assessment; and the aligning of assessment with learning outcomes. It then addresses some new "big ideas" in assessment research: new perspectives on feedback; the development of students' capabilities in dealing with feedback; and the promotion of academic integrity. Throughout, links are made between those ideas and how they may work in health professions education. We hope it will provide both a useful foundation for investigating other chapters on assessment within this text, as well as a prompt to pursue some new concepts from the broader field of education.

P. Dawson (✉)
Centre for Research in Assessment and Digital Learning (CRADLE), Deakin University, Geelong, VIC, Australia
e-mail: p.dawson@deakin.edu.au

C. R. McHenry
School of Medicine and Public Health, University of Newcastle, Newcastle, NSW, Australia
e-mail: colin.mchenry@newcastle.edu.au

© Springer Nature Singapore Pte Ltd. 2023
D. Nestel et al. (eds.), *Clinical Education for the Health Professions*,
https://doi.org/10.1007/978-981-15-3344-0_74

Keywords

Assessment · Constructive alignment · Feedback · Feedback literacy · Academic integrity · Cheating

Introduction

To assess is to "make judgements about students' work, inferring from this what they have the capacity to do in the assessed domain, and thus what they know, value, or are capable of doing" (Joughin 2009, p. 16). But what does it mean to assess well? This chapter first covers some of the foundational ideas underpinning educational assessment, and then explores some of the emerging big ideas in educational assessment research. It aims to provide a grounding in the broader education literature that will support a reading of other more specialized chapters on assessment in this book.

Educational Assessment: Foundations and Emerging Big Ideas

Foundational Ideas from Educational Assessment

Standards-Based Assessment

We begin with what may be an obvious point: that assessment is performed with respect to clearly stated standards or criteria (i.e., "standards-based"), rather than assigning grades to predetermined proportions of a student cohort ("norm-referenced"). The logic behind this is explained in detail within the education literature (e.g., Biggs 1999; Boud 2000) and is uncontroversial within that discipline. The relevance of standards-based assessment to professional degrees such as medicine and allied health is clear: competent professionals are those who can practice at a specified standard, not simply the top 50% (for example) of a student intake. Despite the near-universal adoption of standards-based assessment in secondary education (Stiggins 2005), uptake of standards-based assessment can be patchy within the university system; academic culture in some disciplines can lag somewhat (Biggs 1999; Boud 2000; Elton and Johnston 2002). In our experience many university departments cling to the idea, even if not explicitly articulated, that for example only the top 20% of a class should be accorded the highest grade and that variations from that proportion indicate something amiss. Under standards-based assessment the proportion of students achieving a particular grade is irrelevant as long as they have demonstrated achievement to that standard, and that standard is authentically linked to professional practice (Ajjawi et al. 2021; Tabish 2008).

Three points of interest follow from this. Firstly, the language of grades should be free of holdovers from norm-referenced grading; "A," "B," etc. tend to communicate rank order and "Distinction" is explicitly norm-referencing, whereas terms such as "Pass," "Competent," and "Exceeds expectations" communicate achievement against a standard (Biggs 1999). Secondly, the curriculum should reflect the standards that the grades are based upon, and be aligned with those standards via assessment (Drake 2007, and see section "Alignment" below). Thirdly, those standards must be appropriate so that graduates are competent to progress to the next stage of practice without being a danger to themselves or others; this is especially relevant to health professions (Epstein 2007).

One of the obvious signs of a move toward standards-based assessment is the construction of marking guides and rubrics for assessment tasks. The writing of rubrics that help students understand what specific standards mean and look like is important and requires attention; exemplars of work at the different standards are also particularly useful (Hendry et al. 2012; Carless and Boud 2018).

The Multiple Roles of Assessment

Most involved with teaching are aware of summative assessment and formative assessment; the former is used to assign grades, while the latter is a means of providing feedback to students about the progress of their learning. This has been termed the "double duty" of assessment (Boud 2000). We will discuss feedback in more detail later; here, we explore some of the tensions between these two forms of assessment and introduce an additional aspect of assessment that has received attention more recently.

Summative assessment first; within professional contexts this is the assessment that provides the basis for certification, and although conceptually straightforward, there are some key points worth emphasizing. The first is that, as far as the students are concerned, these assessments define the curriculum (Biggs 1999). Irrespective of what is published in the course learning goals, or delivered in lectures and tutorials, the operational curriculum is driven by the summative assessment, and life is much easier for all concerned if the Intended Learning Outcomes (ILOs) and the delivery match the assessment (again, more on alignment of these below).

Secondly, summative assessment across a program such as medicine should "sum" to function as a meaningful assessment across the entire program (van der Vleuten et al. 2012). This programmatic role of assessment is particularly challenging, especially when certification is reduced to a single overall mark. What does an overall mark of, for example, 61% across the program mean in terms of a student's competence to progress to the next phase of the profession? In which aspects were they competent, and in which are they not? A single mark does not carry any of that information. The process of converting standards-based assessments against particular criteria for particular tasks into a single number leads to the loss of significant information.

Thirdly, summative assessment often operates to inhibit genuine learning (Boud 2000). In particular, "learning for assessment" (also known as "teaching to the test") is often accused of promoting superficial learning approaches (Blazer and Pollard 2017; Firestone et al. 2004; Popham 2001; Posner 2004). However, this problem with summative assessment is magnified by poor alignment between ILOs (or objectives as Biggs previously referred to them) and the assessments themselves;

hence explicit use of standards offers a solution as "the objectives are embedded in the assessment tasks" (Biggs 1999).

Finally, the results of summative assessment in themselves provide a basis for feedback and often function as a valid pedagogical approach – hence the growing literature on "learning by assessment" (also known as "assessment for learning" or "learning-oriented assessment") (Baird et al. 2017; Carless 2005, 2007, 2015; Hawe and Dixon 2017; Carless et al. 2006; Wiliam 2011; Panadero et al. 2018).

In a health professions education context, a particularly effective use of assessment for learning is problem-based learning (PBL) (Barrows and Tamblyn 1980; Savery 2006), which places the assessment task at the start of the learning activities rather than the end; the ILOs and curriculum are thus necessarily aligned with the summative assessment (Biggs 1999; Hmelo-Silver 2004), and as long as the assessment tasks are authentic (e.g., clinical cases), all of the learning activities can be well directed toward professional practice (Boud and Feletti 1997). Although the widespread use of PBL in medical schools has attracted some criticism (Bokey et al. 2014; Glew 2003), and its efficacy compared with other teaching and learning approaches has yet to be demonstrated at large scales (Polyzois et al. 2010; Hartling et al. 2010), it remains a key pedagogical approach in medical education. Assessment practices that work well with PBL are regular formative and summative tests rather than infrequent "high stakes" exams, and more recent developments include the integration of competency-based medical education (CBME) and programmatic assessment with PBL (van der Vleuten and Schuwirth 2019).

Formative assessment: This assessment type is designed to enable feedback for students with the aim of enhancing their learning (Boud 2000; Boud et al. 2010; Carless 2017). However, formative assessment is sometimes neglected compared with summative assessment; its role in connection with feedback should mean that is a central part of pedagogy, but often this is not the case. Providing an appropriate focus on formative assessment will thus require a change in approach for many teachers.

For any educators looking to improve formative assessment, an obvious initial step is to provide detailed and useful feedback information on summative assessment tasks; the task is then performing both duties. However, when feedback information is provided along with grades, the value of the feedback may be diminished (Black and Wiliam 1998; Harrison et al. 2016). Another issue is with combining the two forms: one of the strengths of formative assessment is that mistakes can be viewed as learning opportunities, rather than as failures as they appear under summative assessment (Boud 2000), and if the formative and summative assessment tasks are not separated then this strength of formative assessment is lost. Fortunately, an emphasis on low-stakes assessment can provide a useful formative component across multiple summative assessment tasks that can be integrated into programmatic approaches to assessment (Bok et al. 2013); note the synergies with the above discussion of PBL. Feedback is especially important with the context of professional learning (e.g., in clinical placements), but must have credibility and constructiveness in order to be effective (Watling et al. 2013). In clinical contexts, qualitative feedback ("comments") can be more effective than scores and can even serve as a programmatic assessment tool (Ginsburg et al. 2013, 2017). Clinical supervisors should be aware that enabling effective feedback in these professional learning contexts can be complex (Lefroy et al. 2015).

Increasing the emphasis on effective formative assessment does have significant logistical implications. One specific issue concerns the banks of questions used for summative assessment. In the context of the preclinical phase of medical education, summative tests often use question banks of, for example, MCQs that are reused from year to year; these banks are perceived as being difficult and time-consuming to construct. Generic feedback comments on test results is of little value to students, who need specific information about their own performance in order to learn from the assessment (Boud et al. 2010), but providing detailed formative comments on summative assessment tasks requires providing access to the questions used in the task, and as that access in turn creates obvious issues for academic integrity – specific questions become "public" and are thus seen as compromised and unavailable for future summative assessment – educators can be reluctant to provide that detailed feedback on tests. If summative tests are to be used as effective formative feedback, then those question banks will need to be updated regularly, which has important implications on the resources required to maintain them. These logistical demands need to be acknowledged as part of efforts to place formative assessment at the heart of pedagogy.

Sustainable assessment can be summarized as "life-long assessment" (Boud 2000; Boud and Falchikov 2006; Carless et al. 2011) and stems from the idea that the acquiring of a degree is an early stage in the development of professional competency and expertise (Berliner 1988; Epstein 2007), and that subsequent progress by the graduate should occur within the context of ongoing (hence "sustainable") assessment. Some of this assessment might be formal, and thus similar to the formats used during the degree program (examples include formal examinations run by professional bodies, observation by supervisors during clinical placement, or "360" assessments (Epstein 2007)). However, Boud and colleagues argue self-assessment is a particularly important feature of sustainable assessment, and so the development of the skills required for self-assessment should be a focus of education (Boud and Falchikov 2006; Boud and Molloy 2013). In this context, the foundation for sustainable assessment may be grown from the formative assessment practices used in the undergraduate program (Boud 2000). The development of lifelong learning and reflection within a professional context is linked to the emerging field of evaluative judgment, which is closely connected to the principles of sustainable assessment (Tai et al. 2018). In this view, one of the goals of assessment is that learners develop their capabilities to make decisions about the quality of their own work and the work of others.

Alignment

When Biggs (1999) outlined the principles of constructive alignment, he was formalizing what may appear to be common sense in curriculum design: (i) make sure that the official ILOs (which may be drawn from professional standards) detail what students need to learn from the course, (ii) ensure that the course's materials and activities develop learners to achieve these ILOs, and (iii) make especially sure that the assessment reflects these ILOs. Common sense this might seem, but as Biggs himself noted universities are notoriously poor at aligning their curricula, and in our experience his comments are as relevant today as they were 20 years ago.

Constructive alignment provides an approach for integrating standards, ILOs, delivery and assessment across a curriculum, and as such can be used to address many of the potential issues identified above (Kandlbinder 2014; Treleaven and Voola 2008). The process of constructive alignment is a particularly good tool for designing assessment that drives learning; by ensuring that the ILOs and content delivery are aligned with the assessment, it can thus turn "teaching to the test" from a weakness to a strength.

An important part of the process of constructive alignment is to ensure that the ILOs are (i) aligned, and (ii) useful. Their utility comes from being sufficiently detailed to inform and describe the delivered and assessed curriculum, and for this they need to be detailed and specific (fine-grained). However, when we think about ILOs, we tend to focus on the 7 to 10 generic (course-grained) bullet points learning outcomes ("learning goals" in the taxonomy of McMahon and Thakore 2006) that we are required to formulate for the course handbook; while these describe in general terms the content and assessment of the course, they are of limited help in the process of constructive alignment. Finer-grained learning objectives can provide a useful basis for mapping the teaching content delivered, and especially for aligning that content with assessment. That fine-grained mapping in turn can allow the standards in the assessments to be explicitly compared with professional requirements, and even tracked over the course of the entire program, thus addressing one of the significant challenges of programmatic assessment.

Of particular interest to health professions educators is Biggs' argument that problem-based learning and learning portfolios are inherently aligned (Biggs 1999); it is therefore likely that those programs that use PBL have already undergone the process of constructive alignment, even if they have not explicitly set out to do so.

Big Ideas in Assessment

Building on the fundamentals set out in the previous section, this section explores three advances that have happened in the education assessment literature that may be useful for health professions education: feedback as a process; feedback literacy; and academic integrity. While these ideas have been considered to some degree by health professions education researchers, we think there is benefit to be had from engaging in the broader education understandings of these ideas, which is what we present here.

Feedback as a Process

Traditionally in education, feedback has been thought of as information, usually provided by a teacher to a student. Prominent reviews and meta-analyses in education (Hattie and Timperley 2007; Shute 2008), as well as surveys of students (Winstone and Pitt 2017), tended to reinforce this idea of feedback-as-information. When feedback is viewed as information, its quality is judged on the quality of the information, rather than on the effects of that information (Boud and Molloy 2013). But for feedback to be a worthwhile process, surely it requires learners to actively engage with whatever feedback information is being provided?

Recently in the higher and professional education feedback literature there has been a shift from a focus on feedback as information to a focus on feedback as a process (Boud and Molloy 2013; Carless et al. 2011; Dawson et al. 2019; Winstone and Carless 2019). In this view, feedback is not the comments educators provide, but what learners do with those comments. Proponents of this view of feedback argue that this is not a new definition of feedback, but instead it is a return to feedback's roots in science and engineering, echoing arguments by Sadler (1989). Moves to define feedback as a process have also been made in medical education (Ajjawi and Regehr 2019).

Regardless of if one agrees with this (re-)definition, an explicit focus on feedback processes, rather than just feedback information, provides some new ways to think about what matters in feedback. In education, significant investments are often made into improving feedback that exclusively focuses on providing higher quality comments to learners. However, in many educational contexts, students do not routinely make use of feedback comments (Winstone et al. 2017). A process view of feedback leads us to view this problem as not just one of the quality of the comments, but on the systems, designs and scaffolds used to ensure learner engagement with feedback.

Substantial guidance is provided by Boud and Molloy (2013) on how to design feedback systems that will promote active engagement with feedback. Their "Feedback Mark 2" is distinguished from the dominant feedback approaches used in education by: learners being oriented to the purposes and expectations of feedback; active engagement with criteria and standards, perhaps through the use of exemplars or being required to provide peer feedback; learners being required to make feedback requests; learners being required to demonstrate how they have responded to previous feedback; among other factors. Underpinning Feedback Mark 2 is the view of learners as the active agents of feedback. Much like Biggs' mantra from his work on constructive alignment that learning is "what the student does" (Biggs 1999), learning from feedback is something that only learners can do, and it requires learners to be actively engaged. However, not all students (or educators) are fully equipped to participate in these feedback processes, as this is something that itself needs to be learned. The next section explores emerging research into feedback literacy, which is an attempt to capture the capabilities required to effectively engage in feedback.

Feedback Literacy

The shift toward viewing feedback as a process places extra requirements on learners. Rather than being passive recipients of feedback, learners now need to be able to seek out, understand and make use of feedback. They also need to make productive use of their emotions throughout this process. This set of capabilities has been labeled "feedback literacy" by Carless and Boud (2018), building on earlier work by Sutton (2012). Carless and Boud define feedback literacy as "the understandings, capacities and dispositions needed to make sense of information and use it to enhance work or learning strategies" (p. 1316).

Feedback literacy can be conceptualized as four interconnected components (Carless and Boud 2018). *Appreciating feedback* means not just understanding what feedback is and what it is for, but actively seeking out feedback and trying to make sense of it. *Making judgments* involves decisions about how useful any particular feedback information is, making evaluative judgments (Tai et al. 2018) about the quality of work, and making decisions about what to do with the information. *Taking action* involves using feedback to improve work, as well as taking other actions that might make the feedback interaction more useful, such as storing the information in a safe place for the future. *Managing affect* includes not just being resilient to critical feedback, but also not being overly swayed by praise, and productively using emotion to maximize the feedback process. The feedback literacy literature argues that if learners possess these capabilities they will be best able to participate in feedback processes.

As conceptualized by Carless and Boud (2018), feedback literacy is a set of capabilities for learning at university. However, it could fruitfully be reconceptualized as a set of capabilities for work and life in general. Workplaces can spend millions of hours per year on feedback processes (Buckingham and Goodall 2015), and equipping learners to engage with these processes could support their transition to graduate life. However, the degree to which feedback literacy is transferrable from context to context remains an open question. Rather than relying on transfer, there is emerging work in health professions education that suggests learners can develop feedback literacy directly within healthcare settings (Noble et al. 2020).

Cheating and Academic Integrity

Over the past few decades the higher education literature has seen an increasing focus on responses to cheating. These have shifted from an exclusive focus on the negative side of the problem, such as how to detect and punish cheating, to an additional focus on the positive side: the promotion of academic integrity. The International Centre for Academic Integrity defines academic integrity as "a commitment to five fundamental values: honesty, trust, fairness, respect, and responsibility" (Fishman 2014, p. 1). Academic integrity tends to be viewed as something that can be cultivated through teaching and learning, rather than being an innate, unchangeable part of students' character (Bretag 2019). The academic integrity community argues for a need to focus on promoting academic integrity, using a range of strategies, including incorporating academic integrity in the curriculum, working with student organizations, and the use of honor codes.

Much of the education research on academic integrity has focused on plagiarism (Bretag 2019). However, more recent research has also focused on seemingly newer threats to integrity, particularly "contract cheating" (Lancaster and Clarke 2007).

This form of cheating occurs when learners get a third party to undertake assessed work instead of doing it themselves. The "contract" part of the term comes from the term's originators' experiences observing computer science students contracting out their assessed work online; however the term has come to include both paid and nonpaid outsourcing of assessed work. Estimates for the prevalence of contract cheating range from 2% to 16% (Bretag et al. 2018; Newton 2018). While robust evidence is not available comparing the rates of contract cheating across the health professions, nursing has been the site of several contract cheating scandals and several research papers (see some studies cited in Newton 2018, for further information).

Contract cheating presents a great threat to both integrity and public safety. Unlike copy-paste plagiarism, which can be spotted through text-matching tools that compare student work against a database of sources, in some circumstances it can be very challenging to tell if a learner has completed their own work. Most contract cheating goes undetected, as when people are not specifically primed to detect it they tend not to (Lines 2016; Medway et al. 2018). However, when educators are alerted to the potential existence of contract cheating and asked to detect it, they can often detect a significant proportion of it (58% in Dawson and Sutherland-Smith 2019). Training programs and specialist software have also shown promise at significantly increasing contract cheating detection rates (Dawson and Sutherland-Smith 2019; Dawson et al. 2020). However, educators who suspect contract cheating often do not report it through their institutional disciplinary procedures, with many stating they felt it was too time consuming, or too hard to prove, in one large-scale Australian survey study (Harper et al. 2018).

Education regulators are increasingly taking an interest in the academic integrity of providers. In Australia, the Tertiary Education Quality and Standards Agency was recently provided with new criminal powers targeting businesses that help students cheat ("Tertiary Education Quality and Standards Agency Amendment (Prohibiting Academic Cheating Services) Bill 2019," 2020). There is limited evidence as to the effectiveness of these sorts of laws (Amigud and Dawson 2020); however, they possess some power symbolically as they show that cheating is not just ethically wrong, it is a matter society deems has a criminal element.

Beyond plagiarism and outsourcing, academic integrity also overlaps conceptually with professionalism and professional integrity (Guerrero-Dib et al. 2020; Kenny 2007). Lapses in academic integrity by health professions students are arguably also lapses in professionalism. Evidence of student embellishment in reflective tasks (Maloney et al. 2013) and admissions essays (Kumwenda et al. 2013) in health professions are therefore particularly concerning. Some health professions accrediting bodies now view academic integrity breaches as very significant problems; for example, the UK General Medical Council lists various academic integrity breaches such as cheating as unprofessional behavior that "could lead to fitness to practise proceedings" (General Medical Council and Medical Schools Council 2016, p. 48).

Conclusion

This chapter has drawn concepts from the education research literature on assessment, including both fundamental and emerging topics. To conclude, we would like to encourage educators to consult the other chapters in this text that cover assessment. But we do not want them to stop there. Beyond the world of health professions education there is a range of work on assessment that is directly relevant. The top journal for practitioners hoping to engage with this literature is *Assessment & Evaluation in Higher Education*, and the peak conference is Assessment in Higher Education, currently held biennially in Manchester, UK. Health professions educators and researchers are warmly welcomed in these communities. Many ideas now prominent in the broader education research literature, such as programmatic assessment and problem-based learning, first gained traction in medical education. It is our hope that stronger relationships between higher education and health professions education may lead to better assessment in both communities.

Cross-References

▸ Measuring Performance: Current Practices in Surgical Education
▸ Programmatic Assessment in Health Professions Education

References

Ajjawi R, Regehr G. When I say ... feedback. Med Educ. 2019;53(7):652–4. https://doi.org/10.1111/medu.13746.

Ajjawi R, Bearman M, Boud D. Performing standards: a critical perspective on the contemporary use of standards in assessment. Teach High Educ. 2021;26(5):728–741. https://doi.org/10.1080/13562517.2019.1678579.

Amigud A, Dawson P. The law and the outlaw: is legal prohibition a viable solution to the contract cheating problem? Assess Eval High Educ. 2020;45(1):98–108. https://doi.org/10.1080/02602938.2019.1612851.

Baird J, Andrich D, Hopfenbeck TN, Stobart G. Assessment and learning: fields apart? Assess Educ Princ Policy Pract. 2017;24(3):317–50. https://doi.org/10.1080/0969594X.2017.1319337.

Barrows HS, Tamblyn RM. Problem-based learning: an approach to medical education. New York: Springer; 1980. 201 pp

Berliner DC. The development of expertise in pedagogy. American Association of Colleges for Teacher Education Publications; 1988. p. 3–34.

Biggs J. What the student does: teaching for enhanced learning. High Educ Res Dev. 1999;18(1): 57–75. https://doi.org/10.1080/0729436990180105.

Black P, Wiliam D. Inside the black box: raising standards through classroom assessment. London: School of Education, King's College; 1998.

Blazer D, Pollard C. Does test preparation mean low-quality instruction? Educ Res. 2017;46(8): 420–33. https://doi.org/10.3102/0013189X17732753.

Bok HGJ, et al. Programmatic assessment of competency-based workplace learning: when theory meets practice. BMC Med Educ. 2013;13:123.

Bokey L, Chapuis PH, Dent OF. Problem-based learning in medical education: one of many learning paradigms. Med J Aust. 2014;201(3):134–6. https://doi.org/10.5694/mja13.00060.

Boud D. Sustainable assessment: rethinking assessment for the learning society. Stud Contin Educ. 2000;22(2):151–67. https://doi.org/10.1080/713695728.

Boud D, Falchikov N. Aligning assessment with long-term learning. Assess Eval High Educ. 2006;31(4):399–413. https://doi.org/10.1080/02602930600679050.

Boud D, Feletti G. The challenge of problem-based learning. London: Kogan-Page; 1997. 349 pp

Boud D, Molloy E. Rethinking models of feedback for learning: the challenge of design. Assess Eval High Educ. 2013;38(6):698–712. https://doi.org/10.1080/02602938.2012.691462.

Boud D, et al. Assessment 2020: seven propositions for assessment reform in higher education. Sydney: Australian Learning and Teaching Council; 2010.

Bretag T. From 'perplexities of plagiarism' to 'building cultures of integrity': a reflection on fifteen years of academic integrity research, 2003–2018. HERDSA Rev High Educ. 2019;6:5–35.

Bretag T, Harper R, Burton M, Ellis C, Newton P, Rozenberg P, ... van Haeringen K. Contract cheating: a survey of Australian university students. Stud High Educ. 2018;1–20. https://doi.org/10.1080/03075079.2018.1462788.

Buckingham M, Goodall A. Reinventing performance management. Harv Bus Rev. 2015;93:40–50.

Carless D. Prospects for the implementation of assessment for learning. Assess Educ Princ Policy Pract. 2005;12(1):39–54.

Carless D. Learning-oriented assessment: conceptual bases and practical implications. Innov Educ Teach Int. 2007;44(1):57–66.

Carless D. Excellence in university assessment: learning from award-winning practice. London: Routledge; 2015.

Carless D. Scaling up assessment for learning: progress and prospects. In: Carless D, Bridges SM, Chan CKY, Glofcheski R, editors. Scaling up assessment for learning in higher education. Singapore: Springer; 2017. p. 3–17. https://doi.org/10.1007/978-981-10-3045-1_1.

Carless D, Boud D. The development of student feedback literacy: enabling uptake of feedback. Assess Eval High Educ. 2018;43(8):1315–25. https://doi.org/10.1080/02602938.2018.1463354.

Carless D, Joughin G, Mok M. Learning-oriented assessment: principles and practice. Assess Eval High Educ. 2006;31(4):395–8.

Carless D, Salter D, Yang M, Lam J. Developing sustainable feedback practices. Stud High Educ. 2011;36(4):395–407. https://doi.org/10.1080/03075071003642449.

Dawson P, Sutherland-Smith W. Can training improve marker accuracy at detecting contract cheating? A multi-disciplinary pre-post study. Assess Eval High Educ. 2019;44(5):715–25. https://doi.org/10.1080/02602938.2018.1531109.

Dawson P, Henderson M, Mahoney P, Phillips M, Ryan T, Boud D, Molloy E. What makes for effective feedback: staff and student perspectives. Assess Eval High Educ. 2019;44(1):25–36. https://doi.org/10.1080/02602938.2018.1467877.

Dawson P, Sutherland-Smith W, Ricksen M. Can software improve marker accuracy at detecting contract cheating? A pilot study of the Turnitin Authorship Investigate alpha. Assess Eval High Educ. 2020;45(4):473–482. https://doi.org/10.1080/02602938.2019.1662884.

Drake SM. Creating standards-based integrated curriculum: aligned curriculum, content, assessment, and instruction. Thousand Oaks: Corwin Press; 2007. 240 pp

Elton L, Johnston B. Assessment in universities: a critical review of research. Learning and Teaching Support Network; 2002. 97 pp

Epstein RM. Assessment in medical education. N Engl J Med. 2007;356(4):387–96.

Firestone WA, Monfils LF, Schorr RY. The ambiguity of teaching to the test: standards, assessment, and educational reform. Mahwah: Lawrence Erlbaum Associates; 2004. 237 pp

Fishman T. The fundamental values of academic integrity. 2nd ed. International Center for Academic Integrity, Clemson University; 2014.

General Medical Council and Medical Schools Council. Achieving good medical practice: guidance for medical students. Manchester: General Medical Council; 2016.

Ginsburg S, Eva K, Regehr G. Do in-training evaluation reports deserve their bad reputations? A study of the reliability and predictive ability of ITER scores and narrative comments. Acad Med. 2013;88(10):1539–44. https://doi.org/10.1097/ACM.0b013e3182a36c3d.

Ginsburg S, van der Vleuten CPM, Eva KW. The hidden value of narrative comments for assessment: a quantitative reliability analysis of qualitative data. Acad Med. 2017;92(11):1617–21. https://doi.org/10.1097/ACM.0000000000001669.

Glew R. The problem with problem-based learning in medical education: promises not kept. Biochem Mol Biol Educ. 2003;31(1):52–6. https://doi.org/10.1002/bmb.2003.494031010158.

Guerrero-Dib JG, Portales L, Heredia-Escorza Y. Impact of academic integrity on workplace ethical behaviour. Int J Educ Integr. 2020;16(1):2. https://doi.org/10.1007/s40979-020-0051-3.

Harper R, Bretag T, Ellis C, Newton P, Rozenberg P, Saddiqui S, van Haeringen K. Contract cheating: a survey of Australian university staff. Stud High Educ. 2018;44:1–17. https://doi.org/10.1080/03075079.2018.1462789.

Harrison CJ, Könings KD, Dannefer EF, Schuwirth LWT, Wass V, van der Vleuten CPM. Factors influencing students' receptivity to formative feedback emerging from different assessment cultures. Persp Med Educ. 2016;5:276–84. https://doi.org/10.1007/s40037-016-0297-x.

Hartling L, Spooner C, Tjosvold L, Oswald A. Problem-based learning in pre-clinical medical education: 22 years of outcome research. Med Teach. 2010;32:28–35.

Hattie J, Timperley H. The power of feedback. Rev Educ Res. 2007;77(1):81–112. https://doi.org/10.3102/003465430298487.

Hawe E, Dixon H. Assessment for learning: a catalyst for student self-regulation. Assess Eval High Educ. 2017;42(8):1181–92. https://doi.org/10.1080/02602938.2016.1236360.

Hendry GD, Armstrong S, Bromberger N. Implementing standards-based assessment effectively: incorporating discussion of exemplars into classroom teaching. Assess Eval High Educ. 2012;37(2):149–61. https://doi.org/10.1080/02602938.2010.515014.

Hmelo-Silver CE. Problem-based learning: what and how do students learn? Educ Psychol Rev. 2004;16(3):235–66. https://doi.org/10.1177/003172170508700414.

Joughin G. Assessment, learning and judgement in higher education: a critical review. In: Joughin G, editor. Assessment, learning and judgement in higher education. Dordrecht: Springer; 2009. p. 13–27.

Kandlbinder P. Constructive alignment in university teaching. HERDSA News. 2014;36(3):5–6.

Kenny D. Student plagiarism and professional practice. Nurse Educ Today. 2007;27(1):14–8. https://doi.org/10.1016/j.nedt.2006.02.004.

Kumwenda B, Dowell J, Husbands A. Is embellishing UCAS personal statements accepted practice in applications to medicine and dentistry? Med Teach. 2013;35(7):599–603. https://doi.org/10.3109/0142159X.2013.798402.

Lancaster T, Clarke R. The phenomena of contract cheating. In: Roberts T, editor. Student plagiarism in an online world: problems and solutions. Hershey: Idea Group; 2007. p. 144–58.

Lefroy J, Watling C, Teunissen P, Klinieken I. Guidelines: the do's, don'ts and don't knows of feedback for clinical education. Persp Med Educ. 2015;4:284–99. https://doi.org/10.1007/s40037-015-0231-7.

Lines L. Ghostwriters guaranteeing grades? The quality of online ghostwriting services available to tertiary students in Australia. Teach High Educ. 2016;44:1–26. https://doi.org/10.1080/13562517.2016.1198759.

Maloney S, Tai JH-M, Lo K, Molloy E, Ilic D. Honesty in critically reflective essays: an analysis of student practice. Adv Health Sci Educ. 2013;18(4):617–26. https://doi.org/10.1007/s10459-012-9399-3.

McMahon T, Thakore H. Achieving constructive alignment: putting outcomes first. Qual High Educ. 2006;3:10–9.

Medway D, Roper S, Gillooly L. Contract cheating in UK higher education: a covert investigation of essay mills. Br Educ Res J. 2018;44(3):393–418. https://doi.org/10.1002/berj.3335.

Newton PM. How common is commercial contract cheating in higher education and is it increasing? A systematic review. Front Educ. 2018;3:67. https://doi.org/10.3389/feduc.2018.00067.

Noble C, Billett S, Armit L, Collier L, Hilder J, Sly C, Molloy E. "It's yours to take": generating learner feedback literacy in the workplace. Adv Health Sci Educ. 2020;25(1):55–74. https://doi.org/10.1007/s10459-019-09905-5.

Panadero E, Andrade H, Brookhart S. Fusing self-regulated learning and formative assessment: a roadmap of where we are, how we got here, and where we are going. Aust Educ Res. 2018;45:13–31.

Polyzois I, Claffey N, Matheos N. Problem-based learning in academic health education. A systematic literature review. Eur J Dent Educ. 2010;14:55–64.

Popham WJ. Teaching to the test. Educ Leadersh. 2001;58(6):16–20.

Posner D. What's wrong with teaching to the test? Phi Delta Kappan. 2004;85(10):749–51.

Sadler DR. Formative assessment and the design of instructional systems. Instr Sci. 1989;18(2):119–44. https://doi.org/10.1007/BF00117714.

Savery JR. Overview of problem-based learning: definitions and distinctions. Interdiscip J Prob Based Learn. 2006;1(1):9–20.

Shute VJ. Focus on formative feedback. Rev Educ Res. 2008;78(1):153–89. https://doi.org/10.3102/0034654307313795.

Stiggins R. From formative assessment to assessment for learning: a path to success in standards-based schools. Phi Delta Kappan. 2005;87(4):324–8.

Sutton P. Conceptualizing feedback literacy: knowing, being, and acting. Innov Educ Teach Int. 2012;49(1):31–40. https://doi.org/10.1080/14703297.2012.647781.

Tabish SA. Assessment methods in medical education. Int J Health Sci. 2008;2(2):3–7.

Tai J, Ajjawi R, Boud D, Dawson P, Panadero E. Developing evaluative judgement: enabling students to make decisions about the quality of work. High Educ. 2018;76(3):467–81. https://doi.org/10.1007/s10734-017-0220-3.

Tertiary Education Quality and Standards Agency Amendment (Prohibiting Academic Cheating Services) Bill 2019, Commonwealth of Australia. 2020.

Treleaven L, Voola R. Integrating the development of graduate attributes through constructive alignment. J Mark Educ. 2008;30(2):160–73. https://doi.org/10.1177/0273475308319352.

van der Vleuten CPM, Schuwirth LWT. Assessment in the context of problem-based learning. Adv Health Sci Educ. 2019;24:903–14. https://doi.org/10.1007/s10459-019-09909-1.

van der Vleuten CPM, Schuwirth LWT, Driessen EW, Dijkstra J, Tigelaar D, Baartman LKJ, van Tartwijk J. A model for programmatic assessment fit for purpose. Med Teach. 2012;34(3):205–14. https://doi.org/10.3109/0142159X.2012.652239.

Watling C, Driessen E, van der Vleuten CP, Vanstone M, Lingard L. Beyond individualism: professional culture and its influence on feedback. Med Educ. 2013;47(6):585–94. https://doi.org/10.1111/medu.12150.

Wiliam D. What is assessment for learning? Stud Educ Eval. 2011;37(1):2–14.

Winstone N, Carless D. Designing effective feedback processes in higher education: a learning-focused approach. Routledge; 2019.

Winstone N, Pitt E. Feedback is a two-way street. So why does the NSS only look one way? Times Higher Education. 2017, September 14. Retrieved from https://www.timeshighereducation.com/opinion/feedback-two-way-street-so-why-does-nss-only-look-one-way

Winstone N, Nash RA, Rowntree J, Parker M. 'It'd be useful, but I wouldn't use it': barriers to university students' feedback seeking and recipience. Stud High Educ. 2017;42(11):2026–41. https://doi.org/10.1080/03075079.2015.1130032.

Measuring Attitudes: Current Practices in Health Professional Education

60

Ted Brown, Stephen Isbel, Mong-Lin Yu, and Thomas Bevitt

Contents

Introduction	1150
What Are Attitudes?	1151
Why Are Attitudes Important?	1152
How Do Attitudes Develop?	1153
How Do Attitudes Change and Evolve?	1154
Approaches and Techniques to Gathering and Measuring Attitude Data	1154
Types of Attitude Measurement Scales	1156
Qualitative Approaches to Exploring Attitudes	1160
Features of Quality Attitude Measures to Consider	1162
Constructing Attitude Measurement Scales	1163
Relevance of Attitudes to Health Professional Clinical Education	1164
Traditional Methods Used to Develop Attitudes	1164
Simulation-Based Education	1165

T. Brown (✉)
Department of Occupational Therapy, School of Primary and Allied Health Care, Faculty of Medicine, Nursing and Health Sciences, Monash University – Peninsula Campus, Frankston, VIC, Australia
e-mail: ted.brown@monash.edu

S. Isbel
Faculty of Health, University of Canberra, Canberra, ACT, Australia
e-mail: Stephen.Isbel@canberra.edu.au

M.-L. Yu
Department of Occupational Therapy, School of Primary and Allied Health Care, Faculty of Medicine, Nursing and Health Sciences, Monash University, Frankston, VIC, Australia
e-mail: mong-lin.yu@monash.edu

T. Bevitt
Faculty of Health, The University of Canberra Hospital, Canberra, Bruce ACT, Australia
e-mail: Thomas.Bevitt@canberra.edu.au

© Springer Nature Singapore Pte Ltd. 2023
D. Nestel et al. (eds.), *Clinical Education for the Health Professions*,
https://doi.org/10.1007/978-981-15-3344-0_76

Practice-Based Education 1166
Types of Attitudes Relevant to Health Professional Education 1166
Conclusion 1168
References 1172

Abstract

Attitudes are an enduring set of beliefs, perceptions, and ideas. Students enrolled in health professional courses may have strong beliefs and opinions on certain topics related to professional education and their clinical practice. These attitudes may become more apparent while health professional students are completing clinical placements. This chapter provides an overview of definitions of what attitudes are; why attitudes are important; how attitudes develop, change, and evolve; approaches to the measurement of and gathering attitude-related data; types of quantitative attitude scales; qualitative approaches to gathering attitude data; the steps involved in constructing an attitude measurement scale; and the relevance of attitudes to health professional clinical education. Academic and clinical educators need to be conversant on the topic of students' attitudes and its relationship to clinical education.

Keywords

Attitudes · Beliefs · Measurement · Students · Health professional · Clinical education · Fieldwork · Internships

Introduction

Attitudes are part of us as human beings and an intrinsic aspect of health professional students' inner selves when completing clinical education placements, internships, or clerkships. Attitudes are an internal component of our psyche, are enduring, and influence our values, beliefs, and internal dialogue. As such, it is important for academic and clinical educators to be mindful of health professional students' attitudes. This is particularly relevant for the health care disciplines when providing care and services involves interacting with patients, families, and other health care team members. No doubt health professional students' attitudes towards certain cultural groups, social issues, diagnostic groups, and clinical decision making will be challenged when completing practicums, internships, and placements. Part of the role of academic and clinical educators is to respond to these 'attitude-challenge' or 'attitude-confrontation' incidences and provide 'just-right' learning experiences and feedback that will promote students' critical reflection, attitude refinement, and professional growth. This chapter will cover the topic of attitudes and their measurement. A definition of what attitudes are, how attitudes develop and evolve, why attitudes are important (including in relation to clinical education), approaches and techniques to gathering and measuring attitude data, and examples of attitude research applied to health professional students will be discussed.

What Are Attitudes?

Attitudes are numerous and varied, reflected in the range of definitions of what constitutes an attitude. Allport (1935, p. 810) defined an attitude as "a mental and neural state of readiness, organized through experience, exerting a directive or dynamic influence upon the individual's response to all objects and situations with which it is related." An object, event, location, or individual (including oneself) that is the focus of specific attitudes is referred to as an *attitude object* (Solomon 2017).

Attitudes that people possess can be permanent or transitory, basic or fleeting, complex or simple, and/or permanent or transient (Guyer and Fabrigar 2015). Anastasi (1988, p. 584) described an attitude as "a tendency to react favorably or unfavorably toward a designated class of stimuli, such as a national or ethnic group, a custom or an institution." Attitudes are learned, include features of personality (such as interests, values, motivations, views, and social beliefs), can fall anywhere along a continuum from acceptable/favorable to completely unacceptable/unfavorable, and can assume a number of aspects (including intensity, course, generality, and/or specificity) (Crano and Gardikiotis 2015). All people develop, hold, and express attitudes regardless of their gender, ethnicity, level of educational attainment, socioeconomic status, age, status, or intelligence (Reid 2006).

By and large, people from a country or political region hold similar attitudes on a range of issues. For example, values that Australian citizens espouse include freedom and dignity of the individual, freedom of religious beliefs, equality of men and women, a sense of egalitarianism, fair play, and tolerance, and care for those in need. Codes of conduct and ethical behavior for specific health care disciplines require health professionals to demonstrate specific types of attitudes. Examples of these attitudinal behaviors include altruism, respect, dignity, compassion, empathy, openness, cultural awareness, equality, accountability, honesty, autonomy, motivation, and social justice awareness. Conversely, attitudes considered undesirable in health professionals include being judgmental, dishonest, negative, intimidating, and self-centered. Therefore, health professional students completing practice education placements need to have appropriate attitudes modelled to them, and also be given constructive feedback on unacceptable attitudes they may express or behavior(s) they may demonstrate.

Rosenberg and Havland (1960, p. 3) described attitudes as "predispositions to respond in a particular way towards a specific class of objects." Since attitudes are predispositions, they are not measurable or visible, but in its place are delineated from the way individuals respond to specific stimuli. Attitudes can be implicit or explicit. Implicit attitudes operate at the conscious level with individuals being aware of them, whereas explicit attitudes impact behavior unconsciously with no recognition of them (Hahn et al. 2013). For this reason, even when attitudes are characterized, they cannot be clearly observed, but instead must be implied from observable verbal and nonverbal behavior(s). Students completing clinical placements may demonstrate implicit attitudes towards certain clients or approaches to professional practice, and it is the role of the fieldwork educator to provide feedback to the student if these attitudes are deemed to be inappropriate or unprofessional in nature.

There are different conceptualizations of attitudes. There is the 'single component model of attitudes' where attitudes represent a person's feelings, subjective reactions, and sentiments towards an attitude object. In sum, it is a unidimensional view of an attitude as the emotions and affect linked to the attitude object. On the other hand, the 'three components of attitudes' view takes a multidimensional perspective (Eagly and Chaiken 1993). The three components connected to the tripartite model are *affective* responses (such as moods, feelings, and emotions); *behavioral* responses (explicit actions that individuals demonstrate to the attitude object); and *cognitive* responses (such as thoughts, ideas, or beliefs based on information). In relation to the attitude object, the three responses are all observable, but the attitude is inferred from the overt reaction of the individual. This framework has also been referred to as the ABC model of attitudes since it "emphasizes the interrelationships among knowing, feeling, and doing" (Solomon 2017, p. 286).

Why Are Attitudes Important?

Attitudes are significant for a number of reasons, including the fact they are predictive of behavior towards attitude objects, they are prevalent, are a discriminating influence on perceptions and memories, and underpin several mental functions. Attitudes are accurate behavioral barometers if the attitudes themselves are consistent, strong, based on familiarity and experience, and connected to the actions being predicted. Katz (1960) proposed a functionalist theory of attitudes whereby attitudes are governed by the functions they provide. He identified four types of psychological functions that attitudes serve: (i) *adaptive-adjustment/utilitarian function* (e.g., when a person expresses socially acceptable attitudes and is then rewarded by others with approval and social acceptance; this relates to the principles of reward and punishment); (ii) *ego-defensive function* (e.g., attitudes that guard one's self-esteem from internal feelings and external threats or that rationalize actions that make one experience guilt); (iii) *value-expressive function* (e.g., attitudes a person articulates that are indicative of, or central to, who he/she is; and (iv) *knowledge function* (e.g., attitudes provide meaning, worth, order, structure, and knowledge for one's life).

Overall, knowing peoples' attitudes helps others in predicting their behavioral responses. For example, a person may like people who are quiet, engaging, sensitive, and gentle and be put off by individuals who are loud, boisterous, opinionated, and discourteous. It is likely the impact of a person's social-personal attitude in this instance is to stay away from people who are outspoken and sure of themselves and gravitate towards individuals who are a better social fit for them. It is interesting to note that some researchers now believe that there is little to no association between verbal assessments of attitude and explicit behaviors of individuals (Guyer and Fabrigar 2015).

How Do Attitudes Develop?

A number of factors have been found to impact how and why attitudes form in human beings. These can include the social environment, cultural context, religious beliefs, family and home environment, maturity level, educational attainment, socioeconomic status, existing prejudices, political environment, and personal life experiences in general. Attitudes can form directly as a consequence of direct personal experience or observation (Fabrigar et al. 2005).

Social norms and roles can have a powerful impact on a person's attitudes. *Social norms* comprise society's guidelines for what activities are viewed as appropriate, whereas *social roles* relate to how people are supposed to act in a specific environment or life role (Mackie et al. 2015). For example, international students from Asia-Pacific countries often see their placement supervisors as 'authority figures' and as 'superior' in social and workplace contexts and tend to 'listen' to their supervisors as opposed to being actively involved in discussions or asking questions. An additional attitudinal concept is *subjective norms* which refers to the influence of what a person believes others think or perceive what he/she should do. Subjective norms are composed of two factors: (i) the *intensity* of a normative belief and (ii) the *motivation* to comply with that belief (Solomon 2017).

According to the *Learning Theory of Attitude Change*, classical conditioning, operant conditioning, and observational learning can be applied to alter people's attitudes. Learning in the form of *classical conditioning* can be used to modify attitudes. People develop a favorable association with specific events, items, or individuals (e.g., association of stimuli and responses) and henceforward will have a positive attitude towards attitude objects. *Operant conditioning* can also be utilized to change people's behavior. For example, if a smoker receives enough negative feedback (in the form of negative reinforcement) about their habit, they might consider stopping smoking (Solomon 2017). Referred to as *observational learning*, individuals also learn attitudes by observing the people in their immediate environment (Fabrigar et al. 2005). For example, people may spend time watching their favorite news program, and this will influence their attitudes on specific news topics presented. Friends, peers, significant others, and family members may influence a person's attitudes through observational learning.

Another type of attitude model is the *Fishbein Expectation-Value Model* (Fishbein 1963), which is composed of three elements: (i) *salient beliefs* that people have about an attitude object; (ii) *objective-attribute linkages* which is the probability that a specific object has a significant trait or feature; and (iii) *evaluation* of each of the significant features.

Attitudes are typically integrated into a *cognitive structure* that is interconnected (Schwarz 2015). Altering one attitude will necessitate a change in other attitudes. Attitudes are linked horizontally and vertically. *Vertical attitude structure* refers to connections between fundamental core beliefs, whereas a *horizontal attitude configuration* occurs when two or more underlying beliefs are linked. Horizontally structured attitudes are much more enduring and difficult to modify (Crano and Gardikiotis 2015).

How Do Attitudes Change and Evolve?

Attitudes change and evolve over a person's life span. Some types of attitudes are deeply entrenched and are not readily open to influence or modification (Reid 2006). This could be referred to as 'attitude rigidity.' Other types of attitudes fluctuate or develop in response to a specific situation. Exhibiting 'attitude flexibility' implies that a person's attitude is adaptable and able to shift or evolve based on the environmental demands placed on it. There are several potential hurdles to attitude change including a desire for consistency with what is familiar and comfortable, not enough information, lack of an incentive to change, insufficient motivation, or lack of adequate resources needed to make a substantial change.

There are several ways that attitudes can be changed or modified even though they may be deeply entrenched. Attitudes will often change via direct experience in life situations. Since harmful attitudes may result due to insufficient information, the provision of new evidence will assist to change attitudes. Another useful means to change attitudes is to settle differences between attitudes and behaviors. Finally, a person's attitudes may change to better match his/her behavior. This occurs due to a person experiencing a state of *cognitive dissonance,* a behavioral concept connected to *Dissonance Theory of Attitude Change* (Reid 2006). It happens when a person experiences psychological distress due to incompatible thoughts or beliefs. To decrease this sense of stress, a person may modify his/her attitudes so that they are in better alignment with their other beliefs or actual behaviors. Individuals try to reduce dissonance by eliminating, adding, or changing components of their attitudes (Solomon 2017).

Students completing clinical education placements may experience episodes of cognitive dissonance related to their learning, experience, and constructive feedback they receive. For example, final year students completing their final placement may be expected to independently manage their own caseload to meet the specified learning goals to pass the placement, and they may feel distressed if they are not given 'enough' cases to be responsible for. Hence, it is important that clear expectations are negotiated and communicated between the supervisor and student so that the fieldwork educators set clear expectations at the start of the placement to reduce dissonance experienced by the student.

Approaches and Techniques to Gathering and Measuring Attitude Data

Typically, there are four primary approaches towards gathering and measuring attitude data: self-reports, reports of others, sociometrics, and records (Zikmund et al. 2013). *Self-reports* involve individuals reporting directly about their own attitudes, beliefs, feelings, and ideas about a specific topic. This type of self-report attitude information is generated in one of two formats, written or oral. Written attitude self-reports can take the form of questionnaires, quantitative rating scales, logs, blogs, reflective journals, online surveys, or diaries. Oral self-report of attitudes can take the form of focus groups, key informant interviews, surveys, or polls. *Reports of others* occur where a third person reports about the attitudes of a person, group, or organization. Often parents/caregivers are asked to report on behalf of their children by health care professionals. Structured interviews, standardized questionnaires, journals, reports, or direct observation techniques can be used to generate this type of attitude data.

Sociometric techniques are employed when members of a group, team, department, or organization describe their attitudes and beliefs about one another. This can supply an overview of the attitude patterns within a group, for example, a multidisciplinary treatment team on a rehabilitation unit or members of a nongovernmental organization. Finally, another approach to attitude measurement is through the use of *records*. Records are the systematic documentation of regular events. Records can take the format of inventories, class attendance reports, medical reports, written or audio recordings of minutes of meetings that take place, spread sheets with academic grades, or the ratings of students' fieldwork performance using a standardized tool (Desselle 2005).

Within the use of self-reports, reports of others, sociometrics, and records, attitude measurement is achieved via one of the following techniques: questionnaires, interviews, written accounts, and observational ratings (Boateng et al. 2018). *Questionnaires* present the respondent with a range of items that they are asked to answer. Questionnaires can be presented in hard-copy written format or as an online survey. One type of item often included as part of a questionnaire is a rating scale where respondents are asked to rate individual items. *Interviews* occur via person-to-person interactions, on the telephone, or via online videoconferences. Interviews are face-to-face meetings between two or more people in which the respondent answers questions and they often take the format of a highly structured interview.

Written accounts can take several different forms including journals, logs, blogs, online posts, and diaries. Written accounts can be formal or informal. *Observations* are usually based on formal observations of an individual or groups of participants and bring to the fore actions and attitudes that otherwise may be unnoticed (Fabrigar et al. 2005). Questionnaires, interviews, written accounts, and observational ratings are all types of attitudinal measurement approaches that could be used with students completing clinical education placements.

Although the emotional and belief constituents of an attitude are internal to a person, his/her attitudes can be viewed based on his or her resulting behavior. Since attitudes are not always overt, they are measured via inferences and observations. Currently, several indirect approaches are used to measure attitudes including *physiological* tests (such as blood pressure, facial electromyography, pupillary reflex, dilation or response measures, or galvanic skin responses [GSR]), *projective* or *implicit* assessments (such as the Implicit Association Test, House-Tree-Person drawing, Draw a Person Task, Thematic Apperception Test, Rotter Incomplete Sentence Blank, Implicit PsyCap Questionnaire, or Rorschach Inkblot Test), *behavioral* measures (where behavior is utilized as an index that represents a given attitude towards the target object) (see Fig. 1) and written or verbal *self-report questionnaires* (Schwarz 2015; Maitland 2011). The primary weakness of all indirect attitude

Please evaluate each attribute on how important it is to you when completing a fieldwork placement by placing an X at the position on the horizontal line that best describes your feeling

Supervisor communication   Not important _____ Very important

Supervisor approach   Not important _____ Very important

Workplace culture   Not important _____ Very important

Fig. 1 Example of a rating scale

measurement approaches is their lack of sensitivity and objectivity to different levels or gradations of an attitude; however, the one advantage is that they are less likely to generate socially desirable responses.

Written and verbal self-report attitude questionnaires require respondents to carry out one of four activities: rating, ranking, sorting, or making a choice (Zikmund et al. 2013). A *rating* task requires a respondent to appraise the size of some trait or factor. *Ranking* involves a respondent being asked to grade or rank order a number of attitude statements, feelings, or other traits of an attitude object. *Sorting* involves a respondent being given a number of response option cards, objects, pictures, or other relevant materials and then being asked to sort them into different piles or to categorize them. Respondents are then asked to verbally identify the piles or categories of the attitude objects. Finally, *making a choice* is a "measurement task that identifies preferences by requiring respondents to choose between two or more alternatives" (Zikmund et al. 2013, p. 313).

Types of Attitude Measurement Scales

Items on attitude questionnaires can take a variety of formats including *Thurstone scales, Likert scales,* s*emantic-differential scales, numerical rating scales, single-item direct measures, constant-sum scale, graphic rating scales,* and *Stapel scale* (DeCastellarnau 2017; Lovelace and Brickman 2013; Russell 2011). Thurstone scales include an assortment of statement items, and the respondent selects those he/she agrees with (Solomon 2017). The strengths of Thurstone scales are that the items express the direction and intensity of the attitude it is measuring, and there is an assumption of equal intervals between each rating point. These types of scales are time-consuming and expensive to construct, are less precise than Likert scales, and can possess value-laden biases (Maitland 2011).

Another common format for questionnaire items is the use of *Likert scales*. Likert scales need to have a minimum of three response options of either increasing or decreasing value and provide a method for summated ratings (see Fig. 2). The number of response options can be even or odd in number, but the most common number used is 5 (e.g., strongly disagree, disagree, no opinion, agree, strongly agree) or 7 (e.g., very unsatisfied, somewhat unsatisfied, unsatisfied, neither unsatisfied or

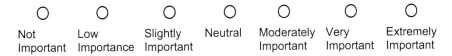

Fig. 2 Example of a seven-point Likert scale

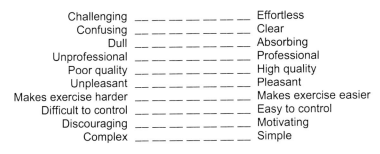

Fig. 3 Example of a semantic differential scale. (© D. Stevens, 2019)

unsatisfied, satisfied, somewhat satisfied, very satisfied). By their nature, Likert scales are relatively easy to design, inexpensive, and sensitive.

The responses to a number of Likert scale items may be added or averaged together to generate one or more composite scales. Each individual item is meant to represent a part or facet of the latent attitudinal construct that is being measured. The composite scales are intended to be a quantitative summation of the attitude domains being assessed. Only a group of items that are found to be reliable and valid should be added together or averaged to calculate a total score that represents a dimension, construct, or factor.

Next, *semantic-differential scales* utilize a list of contrasting bipolar adjectives with seven rating spaces between the two of them (Osgood et al. 1957). The respondent is asked to mark which end of the rating scale is most similar to their opinion, feeling, or view using the adjective pairs provided (see Fig. 3). Examples of the descriptive rating scale adjective pairs for a semantic-differential scale might include big–small, expensive–inexpensive, ugly–beautiful, happy–sad, curious–apathetic, personal–public, simple–complex, dull–exciting, or indispensable–unnecessary. For scoring purposes, a numerical rating is assigned to each of the spaces, with potential score ranges being 1, 2, 3, 4, 5, 6, 7 or −3, −2, −1, 0, +1, +2, +3.

The semantic-differential rating scale approach provides data about three components of attitudes, those being evaluation, potency (e.g., strength), and activity. *Evaluation* refers to whether a respondent views the attitude theme in a negative or positive light. *Potency* denotes how strongly a respondent feels about the attitude topic. Lastly, *activity* indicates whether the attitude topic is viewed as active or passive. Semantic-differential scales are relatively straightforward to complete but can be prone to positional response bias (Russell 2011).

A variation of a Likert scale and a semantic-differential scale is a *numerical rating scale*. A numerical rating scale provides numbers instead of a space/line or written descriptors as response options to indicate response positions (Desselle 2005). The numerical rating scale uses opposing adjectives in the same way as a semantic differential scale but swaps the empty spaces with numbers.

Single-item direct attitude scales are used by researchers to measure a targeted construct via a single targeted question. However, while there may be benefits in relation to brevity and reduced participant response burden, single-item attitude scales are problematic. For instance, *acquiescence bias* refers to the fact that when respondents read an item and then have to decide on the spot if they agree or disagree with it, this can cause an overestimation in the ratings (Fabrigar et al. 2005).

Another type of scale is the *constant-sum scale* where respondents are asked to divide a specified number up into smaller amounts to indicate the relative or degree of importance among a list of qualities or traits (Dudek and Baker 1956). The default for the specified number to be divided up is either 50 or 100 (see Fig. 4). The constant-sum approach can be used as a rating scale or as a sorting activity with cards. With this scaling approach, as the number of response categories increase, the technique becomes increasingly complex for the respondent to complete (Desarbo et al. 1995). One prerequisite skill that respondents need to complete attitude items that utilize the constant-sum scale approach is the mathematical ability to add and subtract.

Using a pictorial approach to attitude assessment, one can use a variety of *graphic rating scales*. This involves measuring attitudes where respondents rate a graphical picture of an object that may or may not contain a number that is along a continuum. When completing a graphic scale, participants are allowed to select any point along the rating range to signpost their attitude. Usually, a participant's score is calculated

---

A constant-sum scale requires participants to divide a fixed number of points among several attributes corresponding to their relative importance.

Divide 100 points among the following characteristics of fieldwork placement and how important they are to you.

_____ Location to your home

_____ Traveling time to placement

_____ Communication from supervisor

_____ Workplace culture

_____ Staff attitude toward placements

_____ **100 Points**

Fig. 4 Example of a constant-sum scale. (© D. Stevens, 2019)

by measuring the length of the rating scale line to the closest millimeter where he/she has placed a mark. Typically, the graphic continuum should be 100 mm in length so that a score out of 100 can be generated. These can also be referred to as a visual analogue scale. Picture or figurine response options are also available including a ladder scale (DeCastellarnau 2017), a thermometer scale (Wilcox et al. 1989) (see Fig. 5), LEGO Pictorial scale (Obaid et al. 2015), and a happy-face scale (Jackson et al. 2006; Hicks et al. 2001) (see Figs. 6 and 7).

Another version of a rating scale is the *Stapel scale* (Russell 2011) (see Fig. 8). It can be used as an alternative to a semantic-differential scale and involves the use of one single adjective. The stimulus adjective is placed in the center of an even number

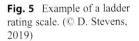

Fig. 5 Example of a ladder rating scale. (© D. Stevens, 2019)

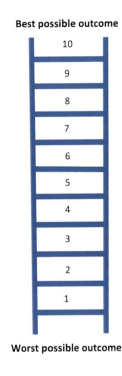

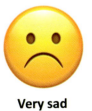

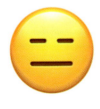

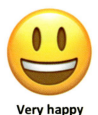

Fig. 6 Example of a simple facial rating scale. (© D. Stevens, 2019)

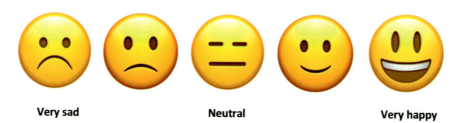

Fig. 7 Example of a more complex facial rating scale. (© D. Stevens, 2019)

Fig. 8 Two examples of a Stapel scale. (© D. Stevens, 2019)

	-5
	-4
-3	-3
-2	-2
-1	-1
Ease of accessibly	Quality of service
+1	+1
+2	+2
+3	+3
	+4
	+5

of numerical values, typically a range of −3 to +3 or −5 to +5. The rating scale gauges how close or far away from the target adjective an opinion or attitude is sensed or felt to be by the respondent. The one advantage of the Stapel scale is that it is easier to construct and administer.

Qualitative Approaches to Exploring Attitudes

Qualitative research approaches are useful for understanding attitudes by providing a means to study human experiences, feelings, emotions, perceptions, and the meanings a target audience may give to a behavior or a specific topic (Liamputtong 2013). Four commonly used methods to collect qualitative information include in-depth interviews, focus group discussions, observation, and record keeping (Liamputtong 2013; Silverman 2010). An in-depth interview is usually conducted face-to-face via one-on-one interactions between an interviewer and an interviewee where the perspectives and attitudes that an individual may have on a chosen topic are explored. A focus group typically involves a small group of six to ten people who usually have similar experiences, concerns, or cultural or social background participating in a planned discussion on a targeted topic. Observation refers to information that is gathered by observing people's behaviors within their natural environments of their daily life. Record keeping uses existing documentation, such as existing interview transcripts, diaries, journals, or newspapers to collect relevant data.

Of the many different methods available for analyzing qualitative information, content analysis, thematic analysis, narrative analysis, discourse analysis, and grounded theory are five of the most widely used techniques (Liamputtong 2009). *Content analysis* is used to organize, classify, or sort the qualitative information into categories to summarize and extract meaning from the information. *Thematic analysis* methods critically review the qualitative information and focuses on examining and identifying patterns or themes of meaning within collected information. *Narrative analysis* involves making sense of stories recounted by one or more respondents and considering individual respondent's background and experiences to find answers for a question. *Discourse analysis* is a method to analyze conversations (both written and spoken) between people in their social context. *Grounded theory* involves understanding a phenomenon through systematic data collection and data analysis to develop a new theory based on the data.

To ensure that qualitative information truly represents a picture of one's attitude(s), a rigorous research process is imperative. Rigor refers to the quality of being very thorough, careful, exact, and accurate, and trustworthiness is the model used to appraise the rigor of the qualitative research process (Carasco and Lucas 2015). Lincoln and Guba (1985) introduced four criteria to establish trustworthiness, including credibility, transferability, dependability, and confirmability. *Credibility* ensures that qualitative research findings are 'believable,' meaning the degree to which the researchers correctly represent the respondents' views. Many techniques can be used to address credibility, including prolonged engagement, persistent observations, data collection triangulation, researcher triangulation, peer debriefing, referential adequacy, and member checking. Among these techniques, triangulation and member checking are most commonly used.

Transferability is the generalization of the findings to another situation or context. This can be established by providing thorough descriptions of the study context so people can decide if the information is transferable. To achieve *dependability*, the qualitative process needs to be logical and documented with sufficient detail so that another researcher could easily replicate the process, understand and follow the decisions trail, and achieve the same or similar conclusions (Lincoln and Guba 1985). *Confirmability* critiques the level of confidence that the researchers' interpretations and conclusions are based on the information collected. An audit trail details the research process (such as rationale for the choice of theory, methodology, data analysis, and interpretations of the data) and is a popular method for establishing dependability and confirmability (Tobin and Begley 2004).

Qualitative approaches are useful when conceptualizing an attitude towards a specific issue and can be used to inform and improve the designs of quantitative attitude measurement scales such as those completed by health professional students. Qualitative information related to attitudes is able to provide in-depth understanding and interpretation of the results generated from attitude measurement scales. Therefore, both qualitative approaches and quantitative attitude measurement scales are indispensable and complement each other for measuring attitudes. A mixed-methods approach integrating both qualitative and quantitative attitude data provides an informed perspective for comprehensively measuring and understanding attitudes particularly in relation to the measurement of attitudes in clinical education contexts.

Features of Quality Attitude Measures to Consider

Reid (2006, p. 20) said that "absolute measures of attitudes are impossible. Only comparisons can be made." There are several general features of measurement that quality attitude scales should exhibit. Quantitative attitude measures need to be valid, reliable, replicable, responsive to change, and straightforward to complete, explain, and comprehend (Fabrigar et al. 2005). In measurement terms, establishing the validity of an attitude scale is the first thing that should be addressed before considering its other psychometric properties. The items that make up an attitude scale need to adequately represent the construct, trait, or feature it claims to measure; this is referred to as construct, factorial, or structural *validity*. If a scale claims to measure nursing students' attitudes to completing fieldwork placements in a mental health setting, then the items need to be reflective of that domain.

An attitude scale needs to generate consistent results, otherwise known as *reliability*. For example, if a group of medical students completed a measure of empathetic attitudes towards patients in palliative care settings on two occasions during the first and third week of a semester, then the results should be relatively consistent or repeatable. There are several types of reliability that are often reported about a scale including test-retest validity, internal consistency, and split-half reliability. The following strategies are recommended to ensure quality reliability results are obtained: using large samples, careful pretesting, ensuring the conditions of the scale completed are socially desirable and that a sufficient number of items are used to allow cross-check questions in the format of repeated questions and similar questions.

A good quality attitude scale should also be *replicable*. One fieldwork educator should be able to utilize an anxiety attitude scale with a group of nursing students commencing a placement at a children's hospital, and another educator should be able to administer the same attitude scale to a group of physiotherapy students at a subacute rehabilitation center. In other words, there should be no variation in how well the anxiety attitude scale measures its target factors with the two different student groups.

Another important feature of a quality attitude scale is that it should be sensitive to small gradations of change in the target variable being assessed. This is referred to as *responsiveness to change* (Zikmund et al. 2013). This is particularly relevant if an attitude scale is being used as an outcome measure or being used to measure change in a group of participants over time. Finally, an attitude scale should be *simple* to administer, understand, complete, and explain. If an attitude scale is going to be used by a variety of researchers, understood by a variety of clinical educators, and completed by a range of different respondent groups, then its *clinical utility* needs to be ensured (Zikmund et al. 2013).

Attitudinal scales can be susceptible to different types of response bias including: (i) *bias to middle responding* where participants avoid extreme responses on a rating scale; (ii) *halo effect* where a respondent allows prejudices and preconceptions to impact his/her answers; (iii) *Hawthorn effect* where respondents' answers are influenced based on positive encounters between the researchers and participants when conducting a study; (iv) *social desirability* effect where respondents want to appear capable, competent, worthy, unprejudiced, open-minded, democratic, or in a positive light based on their answers; or (v) *response set* which involves respondents' inclination to constantly agree or disagree to a set of items (Smith and Noble 2014). When selecting an existing attitude scale to use or designing a new attitude measure, it is essential to consider the types of biases it might be susceptible to (Pannucci and Wilkins 2010).

Constructing Attitude Measurement Scales

When considering the measurement of attitudes, it is suggested that researchers investigate whether a valid attitude scale that assesses the desired attitude construct is already available. In the event that the needed attitude scale does already not exist, then a valid, reliable, and responsive quantitative measure composed of items that are representative of the target attitude construct is required. The development of such a scale should follow a number of steps (Carpenter 2018; Streiner et al. 2015):

(a) Conceptualization: identifying and defining the attitude construct(s) to be measured.
(b) Operationalization: generate items for the attitude scale through a comprehensive review of the relevant cognate research and theoretical literature, conferring with known content experts, and reviewing existing measures; this provides a source of potential items and ensures the content validity of the scale is broad, inclusive, and comprehensive.
(c) Scaling: selection of the rating scale method that will be adopted, for example, will a Likert, Stapel or semantic-differential scale be selected?
(d) Formatting: working version of the attitude scale is reviewed by content experts and items are pretested on respondents with feedback sought; working version of the scale is revised based on feedback.
(e) Refinement: item reduction techniques are implemented and viable attitude factors are extracted using a Classical Test Theory approach such as exploratory factor analysis (Carpenter 2018; Streiner et al. 2015).
(f) Dimensionality investigation: evaluation of dimensionality and construct validity of attitude scale factors is completed using an Item Response Theory approach such as the Rasch Measurement Model (Carpenter 2018; Streiner et al. 2015).

(g) Validity enhancement: other aspects of validity can be examined such as convergent and divergent validity, concurrent validity, predictive validity, and discriminative validity.
(h) Reliability examination: evaluation of the attitude scale's reliability completed: test-retest reliability, internal consistency, split-half reliability, and alternate form reliability.
(i) Consideration of other psychometric properties: other aspects of the attitude scale are evaluated including responsiveness to change, clinical utility, and cross-cultural applicability.
(j) Presentation and ongoing fine-tuning: psychometric properties of the attitude scale need to be summarized, analyzed, and reported; this involves the ongoing revision and critique of the attitude scale to ensure currency, relevance, sensitivity, and accuracy.

The development, validation, and refinement of any attitude scale is an ongoing, dynamic process. In sum, it is a complex, time-consuming, and resource-intensive process. However, there is an ongoing need for high-quality attitude measures with accompanying evidence of validity, reliability, and clinical utility that academic and clinical educators can use with health professional students completing clinical education placements.

Relevance of Attitudes to Health Professional Clinical Education

Education methods that are used to promote, develop, inform, or modify health professional students' attitudes can broadly be categorized into three main areas: traditional education, simulation-based education, and practice-based education. Traditional methods of education include face-to-face lectures, tutorials, and workshops. Simulation-based education methods include but are not limited to the use of case studies, vignettes, role play, immersive scenarios, and actors, while practice-based education involves the use of real patients or consumers in context.

Traditional Methods Used to Develop Attitudes

Many universities incorporate content into their health professional courses aimed at developing attitudes that are critical in the delivery of health care. The incorporation of lectures, tutorials, and workshops have been used to develop positive attitudes around patient safety (Walpola et al. 2015), empathy (Miller 2013), sexual health (Gerbild et al. 2018), and communication (Lichtenstein et al. 2018). In a survey of 23 medical schools in the United Kingdom (Stephensen et al. 2006), the components of curricula that were seen as supporting attitudinal learning included:

- Involving students in setting objectives related to attitudes
- Being explicit about codes of behavior

- Student learning contracts
    Formal teaching of communication, ethics, and diversity
- Problem-based learning
- Reflective practice.

Walpola et al. (2015) describe the successful introduction of a program embedded into a pharmacy course aimed at developing positive attitudes towards patient safety. The program consisted of two lectures and a tutorial guided by the WHO Patient Safety Curriculum Guide (2011). Following the program, students' attitudes improved significantly around errors, questioning behavior, and open disclosure. Miller (2013) developed audiovisual material containing the narratives of people with disabilities which was presented to health care students who were asked to reflect on what they saw. Following the program, students reported a significantly more positive attitude towards people with disability. Gerbild et al. (2018) developed a two-week course for health professional students based on sexual health and rehabilitation, including the examination of norms, values, and attitudes towards sexuality and sexuality at different stages in life. These students reported a sustained change in attitude towards addressing sexual health in their future profession.

Simulation-Based Education

Simulation-based education has been described as an artificial representation of a real-world process to achieve educational goals through experiential learning (Al-Elq 2010). Simulation has been successfully used in many health professions, including medicine (Peltan et al. 2015), occupational therapy (Imms et al. 2018), and nursing (Wang et al. 2015) to teach clinical skills. Simulation offers students an opportunity to learn clinical skills in a way that encourages deep learning while eliminating associated risks to patients. Simulation has also been used to develop and modify health professional students' attitudes towards interprofessional learning (Yang et al. 2017; Lawlis et al. 2017), to promote empathy in specific clinical groups (Chen et al. 2015), and attitudes towards aging (Lucchetti et al. 2017).

For example, when a multidisciplinary simulated ward experience was conducted using Mask-Ed™ characters and simulated case conferences, improvements were seen in interprofessional collaboration including improved knowledge of and attitudes towards multidisciplinary roles in the care of patients (Lawlis et al. 2017). Chen et al. (2015) used a simulated game (referred to as the Geriatric Medication Game) to show improvement in empathy towards older people in pharmacy students, particularly when thinking about how disabilities can affect older people and how older people may be treated differently in the health care system. In the Geriatric Medication Game, students are required to role play being an older adult presenting with a physical, financial, or psychological problem who engages with the health care system and completes several tasks (Chen et al. 2015). At the end of the game, students are asked to reflect on any stereotypes or misperceptions they may have had about older adults. Lucchetti et al. (2017) used a game simulating some of the physiological changes in aging to improve attitudes and empathy towards older people. Attitude data was collected using self-report scales about their attitudes towards older adults, empathy, knowledge about aging, and overall cognitive knowledge (Lucchetti et al. 2017).

Practice-Based Education

Just as in real life, practice-based education is seen as important in developing and practicing clinical skills and the teaching of attitudes that are critical for safe and ethical practice in health care. Meeting, intervening, and generally being involved with patients' and consumers' care have been shown to improve attitudes around dementia (Roberts and Noble 2015), stigma (Patten et al. 2012), and attitudes towards home caring (Yamanaka et al. 2018).

Patten et al. (2012) invited people with lived experience of mental illness to share their experiences with pharmacy students in an interactive format, following which students reported a significant reduction in stigma towards people with mental illness. In another study, exposing medical students to home care interventions for 2 weeks significantly improved their attitude toward home care (Yamanaka et al. 2018), while Roberts and Noble (2015) demonstrated that medical students' attitudes towards people with dementia improved after engaging with dementia patients in a structured, museum-based arts program.

Exposure to people with a variety of clinical diagnoses and cultural backgrounds may improve attitudes in specific circumstances but the opposite may also occur. That is, continual exposure to the same groups without critical reflection of the attitudes that shape the therapeutic relationship may not be conducive to developing positive attitudes. For example, health professionals are expected to display compassion towards patients and consumers but continuous and intense exposure to patients has been shown to reduce the level of compassion in nursing (Zhang et al. 2018), medicine (Kleiner and Wallace 2017), and among other health care workers (Cocker and Joss 2016; Kopera et al. 2015). It is, therefore, important for students and clinicians to continually reflect on how attitudes shape and affect the therapeutic relationship with patients and consumers.

Types of Attitudes Relevant to Health Professional Education

All health care professions expect their members to treat each other and the people they treat in a way that is fair, empathic, and respectful. Most professions enshrine these expectations in a code of ethics that explicitly describes the behaviors and attitudes that are expected of their members. For example, doctors are expected to treat patients as individuals, and to do so with respect, dignity, and compassion (Australian Medical Association 2019). Occupational therapists need to ensure the privacy, dignity, and autonomy of the people they see (Occupational Therapy Australia 2019), while nurses are expected to treat all people with compassion and dignity regardless of their social, economic, or health status (American Nurses Association 2019). Inherent in the expected behaviors and attitudes described in professions' codes of ethics is the maxim that health care professionals should respect the diversity of the people they encounter. Health care professionals should treat all people respectfully regardless of race, gender, religion, age, sexual orientation, or any other factor that differs from their own culture.

Negative attitudes towards specific diagnostic groups also exist in the general community. For example, people with mental illness are often stigmatized as being violent, dangerous, and unpredictable (Hinshaw and Stier 2008); people with addictions are seen as unwilling and disinterested in ceasing their substance abuse (Sheals et al. 2016); older people are often regarded as frail, unfriendly, and a burden on society (Kusumastuti et al. 2017). Health care professionals are expected to engage with people presenting with a range of diagnoses and from different backgrounds in a nonjudgmental and caring way. However, the literature reports entrenched negative attitudes towards diagnostic groups among health care professionals and students. For example, Chapman et al. (2013) describe how doctors may unwittingly perpetuate health inequalities through implicit biases around race, age, and weight. Health care professionals and students are reported to stereotype, hold negatively implicit attitudes about, and stigmatize people with mental illness (Jacq et al. 2016; Murphy et al. 2016). Negative attitudes and/or implicit bias have also been reported in other diagnostic groups such as the elderly (Kusumastuti et al. 2017), obese people (Sabin et al. 2015a), people with substance abuse (Sheals et al. 2016), and people from marginalized groups such as those from the lesbian-gay-bisexual-transsexual-intersex (LGBTI) community (Sabin et al. 2015b).

Although entrenched negative attitudes have been reported in the health professions and among health care students, programs have been successful in changing attitudes. For example, a simulation game was used to improve pharmacy students' empathy for older people (Lucchetti et al. 2017), while another used educational films to improve trainee dietitians' and doctors' attitudes towards obese people (Swift et al. 2013). Other educational programs have reported success in changing attitudes towards people with mental illness (Ng et al. 2017), patients with pain (Puri Singh et al. 2015), and from the LGBTI community (Tsingos-Lucas et al. 2016; Sekoni et al. 2017).

As mentioned previously, some attitudes are deeply entrenched and are hard to modify (Reid 2006). When these attitudes adversely affect a student's performance or lead to poor patient outcomes, educators have a responsibility to address the underlying entrenched attitude. Students may not be aware of the effect their entrenched attitudes are having and may need strategies to identify and address any negative outcomes. A successful way of allowing students to identify how their own beliefs, values, and experiences positively and negatively affect interactions with patients is through reflective practice. Tsingos-Lucas et al. (2016) showed that the integration of reflective activities into a pharmacy curriculum increased the reflective capacity of students. Reflective learning activities such as reflective writing in portfolios and journals (Hogg et al. 2011) have been used to develop a range of professional attributes including clinical reasoning (Croke 2004) and communication skills (Lonie 2010). Inherent in reflecting on clinical reasoning and communication skills within a diverse population is examination of how and why decisions are made. Engaging in this sort of reflection can facilitate students to challenge and question how some of their entrenched attitudes may affect the therapeutic relationship and their interactions with patients.

Better patient outcomes have been identified when health care is delivered by competent interdisciplinary teams (Helitzer et al. 2011). One of the aims of interprofessional education is for students to develop an understanding of the roles and responsibilities of other health care disciplines. From this understanding, positive attitudes are developed regarding the roles and responsibilities of other disciplines which ultimately lead to improvements in patient care. Interdisciplinary teaching is carried out in several ways, including simulation (Brock et al. 2013), immersion or exposure to interprofessional teams (Jacobsen and Lindqvist 2009), teacher-facilitator reflection (Hylin et al. 2007), and shared learning where students share their interprofessional experiences with peers (Hutchings et al. 2013).

The following section highlights selected studies from the domain of attitude research in health care education. The list cited in Table 1 is not meant to be exhaustive but rather highlights the breadth and scope of the research in terms of the disciplines involved, the attitudes being researched, and novel methodologies used.

Conclusion

The role of attitudes in the clinical education of health professional students is clearly a relevant research topic. In their interactions with clients and families, students as well as other professional staff are required to demonstrate appropriate and professional attitudes. Students need to be self-aware and possess the ability to modify their attitudes when needed according to the environmental cues they receive. In this chapter, a number of relevant topics have been covered including how attitudes are defined; how attitudes develop and evolve; quantitative and qualitative data collection of attitudes; the steps to go through to construct a sound attitude scale; and, finally, the relevance of attitude measurement within health professional student education.

Table 1 Examples of attitude research completed with health professional students

Authors	Study location	Sample size and health professional student groups involved	Data gathering tools	Methodology	Implications for practice
Sullivan and Mendonca (2017)	United States of America	n = 32; first year occupational therapy students n = 30; second year occupational therapy students n = 6; first year public health students	Attitudes Toward Intellectual Disabilities (Morin et al. 2013)	Nonrandomized pretest posttest following lecture and fieldwork	Empirical work examining if a lecture or fieldwork impacts attitude change. Positive change in attitude towards people with an intellectual disability occurred following fieldwork only. There was no change following a disability awareness lecture
Patterson et al. (2018)	Australia	n = 23; nursing students who completed a nontraditional fieldwork placement n = 27; nursing students who completed a traditional placement	Mental Health Clinical Placement Survey for First Day of Placement (Hayman-White and Happell 2005)	Nonexperimental comparative approach	Paper explores the impact of diverse placement settings on attitude change within mental health settings for nursing students. Students who completed nontraditional placements self-reported more positive attitudes and better preparedness towards mental health nursing; decreased anxiety and negative stereotyping of mental illness; and the same level of desire to pursue future career in mental health nursing

(continued)

Table 1 (continued)

Authors	Study location	Sample size and health professional student groups involved	Data gathering tools	Methodology	Implications for practice
Oren et al. (2018)	Turkey	n = 650; midwifery students	Purpose developed questionnaire plus Sexuality Attitudes and Beliefs Survey (Reynolds and Magnan 2005)	Descriptive cross-sectional survey	Students were aware of the importance of sexual counselling and reported positive attitudes towards the taboo subject for the cohort. However, students felt that a lack of training prevented them from providing a service, particularly to minority groups
Sim and Mackenzie (2016)	Australia	n = 9; occupational therapy students	Semistructured interviews	Qualitative; grounded theory approach	This paper is an example of how a qualitative research approach can demonstrate sustained attitude change from a placement experience. It also presents a framework to assist students and professionals to prepare for placements in developing countries
Kritsotakis et al. (2017)	Greece	n = 1007; nursing, social work and medical students	Attitude Toward Disabled Persons Form B (Yuker and Block 1986) and Community Living Attitude Scale – Intellectual Disability (Henry et al. 1998)	Descriptive cross-sectional survey	A descriptive paper examining attitudes of nursing, social work, and medical students towards people with a disability. The paper provides a statistical summary of the results from all previous studies

				that used the data collection tools. The study found that students had poor overall attitudes towards people with a disability, prompting a recommendation for educational reform
Van de Pol et al. (2018)	Netherlands	n = 36; medical students	Essays and focus groups	Qualitative content analysis	Previous research of medical students' attitudes indicated a negative association with geriatric medicine and care for older persons. This study utilizes qualitative methods to understand the reasons for students' attitudes and perceptions. The paper identified that teaching the complexity of clinical practice and focusing on professional identity may develop positive attitudes towards geriatric medicine and encourage graduates to work within the area of elderly care

References

Al-Elq AH. Simulation-based medical teaching and learning. J Fam Community Med. 2010;17(1): 35–40. https://doi.org/10.4103/1319-1683.68787.

Allport GW. Attitudes. In: Murchison CM, editor. Handbook of social psychology. Winchester: Clark University Press; 1935. p. 798–844.

American Nurses Association. American Nurses Association code of ethics 2015. http://nursing.rutgers.edu/civility/ANA-Code-of-Ethics-for-Nurses.pdf. Accessed 10 Jan 2019.

Anastasi C. Psychological testing. 6th ed. New York: Macmillan; 1988.

Australian Medical Association. AMA code of ethics 2016. https://ama.com.au/articles/code-ethics-2004-editorially-revised-2006-revised-2016. Accessed 10 Jan 2019.

Boateng GO, Neilands TB, Frongillo EA, Melgar-Quiñonez HR, Young SL. Best practices for developing and validating scales for health, social, and behavioral research: a primer. Front Public Health. 2018;6:149. https://doi.org/10.3389/fpubh.2018.00149.

Brock D, Abu-Rish E, Chiu CR, Hammer D, Wilson S, Vorvick L, et al. Interprofessional education in team communication: working together to improve patient safety. BMJ Qual Saf. 2013;22(5): 414–23. https://doi.org/10.1136/postgradmedj-2012-000952rep.

Carasco JA, Lucas K. Workshop synthesis: measuring attitudes; quantitative and qualitative methods. Transp Res Procedia. 2015;11:165–71. https://doi.org/10.1016/j.trpro.2015.12.014.

Carpenter S. Ten steps in scale development and reporting: a guide for researchers. Commun Methods Meas. 2018;12(1):25–44. https://doi.org/10.1080/19312458.2017.1396583.

Chapman EN, Kaatz A, Carnes M. Physicians and implicit bias: how doctors may unwittingly perpetuate health care disparities. J Gen Intern Med. 2013;28(11):1504–10. https://doi.org/10.1007/s11606-013-2441-1.

Chen A, Yehle M, Plake K. Impact of aging simulation game on pharmacy students' empathy for older adults. Am J Pharm Educ. 2015;79(5):65. https://doi.org/10.5688/ajpe79565.

Cocker F, Joss N. Compassion fatigue among healthcare, emergency and community service workers: a systematic review. Int J Environ Res Public Health. 2016;13(6):618. https://doi.org/10.3390/ijerph13060618.

Crano WD, Gardikiotis A. Attitude formation and change. In: Wright J, editor. International encyclopedia of the social & behavioral sciences. 2nd ed. Amsterdam: Elsevier; 2015. p. 169–74.

Croke E. The use of structured reflective journal questions to promote fundamental development of clinical decision-making abilities of the first-semester nursing student. Contemp Nurse. 2004;17 (1–2):125–36.

DeCastellarnau A. A classification of response scale characteristics that affect data quality: a literature review. Qual Quant. 2017;52(4):1523–59. https://doi.org/10.1007/s11135-017-0533-4.

Desarbo W, Ramaswamy V, Chatterjee R. Analyzing constant-sum multiple criterion data: a segment-level approach. J Mark Res. 1995;32:222–32. https://doi.org/10.2307/3152050.

Desselle SP. Construction, implementation, and analysis of summated rating attitude scales. Am J Pharm Educ. 2005;69(5):Article 97. https://doi.org/10.5688/aj690597.

Dudek FJ, Baker KE. The constant-sum method applied to scaling subjective dimensions. Am J Psychol. 1956;69(4):616–24. https://doi.org/10.2307/1419084.

Eagly AH, Chaiken S. The psychology of attitudes. Orlando: Harcourt Brace Jovanovich College; 1993.

Fabrigar LR, Krosnick JA, MacDougall BL. Attitude measurement. In: Brock TC, Green MC, editors. Persuasion: psychological insights and perspectives. Thousand Oaks: Sage; 2005. p. 17–40.

Fishbein M. An investigation of the relationships between beliefs about an object and the attitude towards that object. Hum Relat. 1963;16(1):233–40. https://doi.org/10.1177/001872676301600302

Gerbild H, Larsen C, Rolander B, Areskoug-Josefsson K. Does a 2-week sexual health in rehabilitation course lead to sustained change in students' attitudes? A pilot study. Sex Disabil. 2018;36(4):417–35. https://doi.org/10.1007/s11195-018-9540-1.

Guyer JJ, Fabrigar LR. Attitudes and behavior. In: Wright J, editor. International encyclopedia of the social & behavioral sciences. 2nd ed. Amsterdam: Elsevier; 2015. p. 162–7.

Hahn A, Judd CM, Hirsh HK, Blair IV. Awareness of implicit attitudes. J Exp Psychol Gen. 2013;143(3):1369–92. https://doi.org/10.1037/a0035028.

Hayman-White K, Happell B. Nursing students' attitudes toward mental health nursing and consumers: psychometric properties of a self-report scale. Arch Psychiatr Nurs. 2005;19(4): 184–93. https://doi.org/10.1016/j.apnu.2005.05.004.

Helitzer DL, Lanoue M, Wilson B, Hernandez BUD, Warner T, Roter D. A randomized controlled trial of communication training with primary care providers to improve patient-centeredness and health risk communication. Patient Educ Couns. 2011;82(1):21–9. https://doi.org/10.1016/j.pec.2010.01.021.

Henry D, Keys C, Jopp D. The community living attitude scale – reference manual (Tech rep). Chicago: Department of Disability and Human Development, University of Illinois at Chicago; 1998.

Hicks CL, Baeyer CLV, Spafford PA, Korlaar IV, Goodenough B. The faces pain scale – revised: toward a common metric in pediatric pain measurement. Pain. 2001;93(2):173–83.

Hinshaw SP, Stier A. Stigma as related to mental disorders. Annu Rev Clin Psychol. 2008;4: 367–93. https://doi.org/10.1146/annurev.clinpsy.4.022007.141245.

Hogg G, Ker J, Stewart F. Over the counter clinical skills for pharmacists. Clin Teach. 2011;8(2): 109–13. https://doi.org/10.1111/j.1743-498X.2011.00437.x.

Hutchings M, Scammell J, Quinney A. Praxis and reflexivity for interprofessional education: towards an inclusive theoretical framework for learning. J Interprof Care. 2013;27(5):358–66. https://doi.org/10.3109/13561820.2013.784729.

Hylin U, Nyholm H, Mattiasson AC, Ponzer S. Interprofessional training in clinical practice on a training ward for healthcare students: a two-year follow-up. J Interprof Care. 2007;21(3): 277–88. https://doi.org/10.1080/13561820601095800.

Imms C, Froude E, Chu E, Sheppard L, Darzins S, Guinea S, et al. Simulated versus traditional occupational therapy placements: a randomised controlled trial. Aust Occup Ther J. 2018;65(6): 556–64. https://doi.org/10.1111/1440-1630.12513.

Jackson D, Horn S, Kersten P, Turner-Stokes L. Development of a pictorial scale of pain intensity for patients with communication impairments: initial validation in a general population. Clin Med (Lond). 2006;6(6):580–5. https://doi.org/10.7861/clinmedicine.6-6-580.

Jacobsen F, Lindqvist S. A two-week stay in an interprofessional training unit changes students attitudes to health professionals. J Interprof Care. 2009;23(3):242–50. https://doi.org/10.1080/13561820902739858.

Jacq KD, Norful AA, Larson E. The variability of nursing attitudes toward mental illness: an integrative review. Arch Psychiatr Nurs. 2016;30(6):788–96. https://doi.org/10.1016/j.apnu.2016.07.004.

Katz D. The functional approach to the study of attitudes. Public Opin Q. 1960;24(2):163–204. https://doi.org/10.1086/266945.

Kleiner S, Wallace JE. Oncologist burnout and compassion fatigue: investigating time pressure at work as a predictor and the mediating role of work-family conflict. BMC Health Serv Res. 2017;17(1):639. https://doi.org/10.1186/s12913-017-2581-9.

Kopera M, Suszek H, Bonar E, Myszka M, Gmaj B, Ilgen M, et al. Evaluating explicit and implicit stigma of mental illness in mental health professionals and medical students. Community Ment Health J. 2015;51(5):628–34. https://doi.org/10.1007/s10597-014-9796-6.

Kritsotakis G, Galanis P, Papastefanakis E, Meidani F, Philalithis AE, Kalokairino UA, et al. Attitudes towards people with physical or intellectual disabilities among nursing, social work and medical students. J Clin Nurs. 2017;26(23–24):4951–63. https://doi.org/10.1111/jocn.13988.

Kusumastuti S, van Fenema E, Polman-van Stratum E, Achterberg W, Lindenberg J, Westendorp R. When contact is not enough: affecting first year medical students' image towards older persons. PLoS One. 2017;12(1):e0169977. https://doi.org/10.1371/journal.pone.0169977.

Lawlis T, Frost J, Eckley D, Isbel S, Kellett J. Enhancing health care student inter-professional learning through a pilot simulation ward experience using Mask-Edtm (KRS Simulation). Aust J Clin Educ. 2017;2(1):Article 5. https://doi.org/10.1186/s12909-017-0872-9.

Liamputtong P. Qualitative data analysis: conceptual and practical considerations. Health Promot J Austr. 2009;20:133–9. https://doi.org/10.1071/HE09133.

Liamputtong P. Qualitative research methods. South Melbourne: Oxford University Press; 2013.

Lichtenstein NV, Haak R, Ensmann I, Hallal H, Huttenlau J, Krämer K, et al. Does teaching social and communicative competences influence dental students' attitudes towards learning communication skills? A comparison between two dental schools in Germany. GMS J Med Educ. 2018;35(2):Doc18. https://doi.org/10.3205/zma001165.

Lincoln Y, Guba EG. Naturalistic inquiry. Newbury Park: Sage; 1985.

Lonie JM. Learning through self-reflection: understanding communication barriers faced by a cross-cultural cohort of pharmacy students. Curr Pharm Teach Learn. 2010;2(1):12–9. https://doi.org/10.1016/j.cptl.2009.12.002.

Lovelace M, Brickman P. Best practices for measuring students' attitudes toward learning science. CBE Life Sci Educ. 2013;12(4):606–17. https://doi.org/10.1187/cbe.12-11-0197.

Lucchetti AL, Lucchetti G, de Oliveira IN, Moreira-Almeida A, da Silva Ezequiel O. Experiencing aging or demystifying myths? Impact of different "geriatrics and gerontology" teaching strategies in first year medical students. BMC Med Educ. 2017;17(1):35. https://doi.org/10.1186/s12909-017-0872-9.

Mackie G, Moneti F, Shakya H, Denny E. What are social norms? How are they measured? San Diego: Center on Global Justice, University of California/UNICEF; 2015.

Maitland A. Attitude measurement. In: Lavrakas PJ, editor. Encyclopedia of survey research methods. Thousand Oaks: Sage; 2011. p. 1–4. https://doi.org/10.4135/9781412963947.n25.

Miller SR. A curriculum focused on informed empathy improves attitudes toward persons with disabilities. Perspect Med Educ. 2013;2(3):114–25. https://doi.org/10.1007/s40037-013-0046-3.

Morin D, Crocker AG, Beaulieu-Bergeron R, Caron J. Validation of the attitudes toward intellectual disability – ATTID questionnaire. J Intellect Disabil Res. 2013;57(3):268–78. https://doi.org/10.1111/j.1365-2788.2012.01559.x.

Murphy AL, Phelan H, Haslam S, Martin-Misener R, Kutcher SP, Gardner DM. Community pharmacists' experiences in mental illness and addictions care: a qualitative study. Subst Abuse Treat Prev Policy. 2016;11:6. https://doi.org/10.1186/s13011-016-0050-9.

Ng YP, Rashid A, O'Brien F. Determining the effectiveness of a video-based contact intervention in improving attitudes of Penang primary care nurses towards people with mental illness. PLoS One. 2017;12(11):e0187861. https://doi.org/10.1371/journal.pone.0187861.

Obaid M, Dünser A, Moltchanova E, Cummings D, Wagner J, Bartneck C. LEGO pictorial scales for assessing affective response. In: Abascal J, Barbosa S, Fetter M, Gross T, Palanque P, Winckler M, editors. Human-Computer Interaction – INTERACT, vol. 9296; 2015. p. 263–80. https://doi.org/10.1007/978-3-319-22701-6_19.

Occupational Therapy Australia (Internet). Code of ethics 2014. https://www.otaus.com.au/sitebuilder/about/knowledge/asset/files/76/codeofethics%282014%29.pdf. Accessed 10 Jan 2019.

Ören B, Zengin N, Yazıcı S, Akıncı AÇ. Attitudes, beliefs and comfort levels of midwifery students regarding sexual counselling in Turkey. Midwifery. 2018;56:152–7. https://doi.org/10.1016/j.midw.2017.10.014.

Osgood CE, Suci G, Tannenbaum P. The measurement of meaning. Urbana: University of Illinois Press; 1957.

Pannucci CJ, Wilkins EG. Identifying and avoiding bias in research. Plast Reconstr Surg. 2010;126(2):619–25. https://doi.org/10.1097/PRS.0b013e3181de24bc.

Patten SB, Remillard A, Phillips L, Modgill G, Szeto AC, Kassam A, et al. Effectiveness of contact-based education for reducing mental illness-related stigma in pharmacy students. BMC Med Educ. 2012;12(1):120. https://doi.org/10.1186/1472-6920-12-120.

Patterson C, Perlman D, Taylor EK, Moxham L, Brighton R, Rath J. Mental health nursing placement: a comparative study of non-traditional and traditional placement. Nurse Educ Pract. 2018;33:4–9. https://doi.org/10.1016/j.nepr.2018.08.010.

Peltan ID, Shiga T, Gordon JA, Currier PF. Simulation improves procedural protocol adherence during central venous catheter placement: a randomized controlled trial. Simul Healthc. 2015;10(5):270–6. https://doi.org/10.1097/SIH.0000000000000096.

Puri Singh A, Haywood C, Beach MC, Guidera M, Lanzkron S, Valenzuela-Araujo D, et al. Improving emergency providers' attitudes toward sickle cell patients in pain. J Pain Symptom Manag. 2015;51(3):628–32. https://doi.org/10.1016/j.jpainsymman.2015.11.004.

Reid N. Thoughts on attitude measurement. Res Sci Technol Educ. 2006;24(1):3–27. https://doi.org/10.1080/02635140500485332.

Reynolds KE, Magnan MA. Nursing attitudes and beliefs toward human sexuality collaborative research promoting evidence-based practice. Clin Nurse Spec. 2005;19(5):255–9. https://insights.ovid.com/pubmed?pmid=16179857

Roberts H, Noble J. Changing medical student perceptions of dementia. Neurology. 2015;85(8):739–41. https://doi.org/10.1212/WNL.0000000000001867.

Rosenberg MJ, Havland CI. Attitude organization and change: an analysis of consistency among attitude components. New York: Yale University Press; 1960.

Russell GJ. Itemized rating scales (Likert, semantic differential, and Stapel). In: Kamakura W, editor. Wiley international encyclopedia of marketing volume 2: marketing research. Hoboken: Wiley; 2011. https://doi.org/10.1002/9781444316568.wiem02011.

Sabin JA, Moore K, Noonan C, Lallemand O, Buchwald D. Clinicians' implicit and explicit attitudes about weight and race and treatment approaches to overweight for American Indian children. Child Obes. 2015a;11(4):456–65. https://doi.org/10.1089/chi.2014.0125.

Sabin JA, Riskind R, Nosek B. Health care providers' implicit and explicit attitudes toward lesbian and gay men. Am J Public Health. 2015b;105(9):1831–41. https://doi.org/10.2105/AJPH.2015.302631.

Schwarz N. Attitude measurement. In: Wright J, editor. International encyclopedia of the social & behavioral sciences. 2nd ed. Amsterdam: Elsevier; 2015. p. 178–82.

Sekoni AO, Gale NK, Manga-Atangana B, Bhadhuri A, Jolly K. The effects of educational curricula and training on LGBT-specific health issues for healthcare students and professionals: a mixed-method systematic review. J Int AIDS Soc. 2017;20(1):216–24. https://doi.org/10.7448/IAS.20.1.21624.

Sheals K, Tombor I, McNeill A, Shahab L. A mixed-method systematic review and meta-analysis of mental health professionals' attitudes toward smoking and smoking cessation among people with mental illnesses. Addiction. 2016;111(9):1536–53. https://doi.org/10.1111/add.13387.

Silverman D. Doing qualitative research: a practical handbook. London: Sage; 2010.

Sim I, Mackenzie L. Graduate perspectives of fieldwork placements in developing countries: contributions to occupational therapy practice. Aust Occup Ther J. 2016;63(4):244–56. https://doi.org/10.1111/1440-1630.12282.

Smith J, Noble H. Bias in research. Evid Based Nurs. 2014;17:100–1. https://doi.org/10.1136/eb-2014-101946.

Solomon MR. Attitudes and persuasive communications. In: Solomon MR, editor. Consumer behavior: buying, having and being; global edition. Boston: Pearson; 2017. p. 284–333.

Stephensen A, Adshead L, Higgs R. The teaching of professional attitudes within UK medical schools: reported difficulties and good practice. Med Educ. 2006;40:1072–80. https://doi.org/10.1111/j.1365-2929.2006.02607.x.

Streiner DL, Norman GR, Cairney J. Health measurement scales: a practical guide to their development and use. Oxford, UK: Oxford University Press; 2015.

Sullivan A, Mendonca R. Impact of a fieldwork experience on attitudes toward people with intellectual disabilities. Am J Occup Ther. 2017;71(6):7106230010p1–8. https://doi.org/10.5014/ajot.2017.025460.

Swift JA, Tischler V, Markham S, Gunning I, Glazebrook C, Beer C, et al. Are anti-stigma films a useful strategy for reducing weight bias among trainee healthcare professionals? Results of a pilot randomized control trial. Obes Facts. 2013;6(1):91–102. https://doi.org/10.1159/000348714.

Tobin GA, Begley CM. Methodological rigour within a qualitative framework. J Adv Nurs. 2004;48:388–96. https://doi.org/10.1111/j.1365-2648.2004.03270.x.

Tsingos-Lucas C, Bosnic-Anticevich S, Schneider CR, Smith L. The effect of reflective activities on reflective thinking ability in an undergraduate pharmacy curriculum. Am J Pharm Educ. 2016;80(4):65. https://doi.org/10.5688/ajpe80465.

van de Pol MHJ, Lagro J, Koopman EL, Olde Rikkert MGM, Fluit CRMG, Lagro-Janssen ALM. Lessons learned from narrative feedback of students on a geriatric training program. Gerontol Geriatr Educ. 2018;39(1):21–34. https://doi.org/10.1080/02701960.2015.1127810.

Walpola RL, Fois RA, Carter SR, Mclachlan AJ, Chen TF. Validation of a survey tool to assess the patient safety attitudes of pharmacy students. BMJ Open. 2015;5(9):e008442. https://doi.org/10.1136/bmjopen-2015-008442.

Wang R, Shi N, Bai J, Zheng Y, Zhao Y. Implementation and evaluation of an interprofessional simulation-based education program for undergraduate nursing students in operating room nursing education: a randomized controlled trial. BMC Med Educ. 2015;15(1):115. https://doi.org/10.1186/s12909-015-0400-8.

Wilcox C, Sigelman L, Cook E. Some like it hot: individual differences in responses to group feeling thermometers. Public Opin Q. 1989;53(2):246–57. https://doi.org/10.1086/269505.

World Health Organization (Internet). Multi-professional patient safety curriculum guide 2011. Cited Feb 2019. Available from: https://www.who.int/patientsafety/education/mp_curriculum_guide/en/.

Yamanaka T, Hirota Y, Noguchi-Watanabe M, Tamai A, Eto M, Iijima K, et al. Changes in attitude of medical students toward home care during a required 2-week home care clinical clerkship program. Geriatr Gerontol Int. 2018;18(4):655–6. https://doi.org/10.1111/ggi.13268.

Yang L, Yang Y, Huang C, Liang J, Lee F, Cheng H, et al. Simulation-based inter-professional education to improve attitudes towards collaborative practice: a prospective comparative pilot study in a Chinese medical centre. BMJ Open. 2017;7(11):e015105. https://doi.org/10.1136/bmjopen-2016-015105.

Yuker H, Block J. Research with the attitude toward disabled persons scales (ATDP): 1960–1985. Hempstead: Hofstra University Center for the Study of Attitudes Toward Persons with Disabilities; 1986.

Zhang YY, Zhang C, Han XR, Li W, Wang YL. Determinants of compassion satisfaction, compassion fatigue and burn out in nursing: a correlative meta-analysis. Medicine (Baltimore). 2018;97(26):e11086. https://doi.org/10.1097/MD.0000000000011086.

Zikmund WG, Babin BJ, Carr JC, Griffin M. Attitude measurement. In: Zikmund WG, Babin BJ, Carr JC, Griffin M, editors. Business research methods. 9th ed. Boston: Cengage Learning US; 2013. p. 310–32.

Measuring Performance: Current Practices in Surgical Education

61

Pamela Andreatta, Brenton Franklin, Matthew Bradley, Christopher Renninger, and John Armstrong

Contents

Introduction	1178
Introduction to Assessment	1178
Surgical Competencies: Knowledge, Abilities, Perceptions	1180
Assessment in Surgery	1181
Cognitive (Knowledge) Assessment	1181
Motor Behavior (Abilities) Assessment	1186
Affective (Perceptions) Assessment	1190
Performance (Integrated Abilities) Assessment	1191
Synthesis and Best Practices	1193
Cross-References	1196
References	1196

Abstract

Assessment requirements within the domain of surgery are equal in complexity and scope to the performance domain itself. There are numerous performance requirements in each of the cognitive, motor, and affective dimensions, and equally complex requirements for integration across a broad spectrum of performance contexts. Current assessment practices largely focus on the cognitive dimensions; however, there are initiatives and developing trends that include assessment of motor and affective dimensions as training program components. Precision of measurement remains challenging in all performance dimensions, with concomitant constraints on the accuracy and justness of assessment outcomes as definitive confirmation of performance competency in the domain.

P. Andreatta (✉) · B. Franklin · M. Bradley · C. Renninger
The Norman M. Rich Department of Surgery, Uniformed Services University & the Walter Reed National Military Medical Center "America's Medical School", Bethesda, MD, USA
e-mail: pamela.andreatta@usuhs.edu; brenton.franklin@usuhs.edu; matthew.j.bradley22.mil@mail.mil

J. Armstrong
University of South Florida Morsani College of Medicine, Tampa, FL, USA

© Springer Nature Singapore Pte Ltd. 2023
D. Nestel et al. (eds.), *Clinical Education for the Health Professions*,
https://doi.org/10.1007/978-981-15-3344-0_77

Increasing the accuracy and precision of assessment instrumentation and defining explicit performance criteria within the domain will lead to improved assessment implementation and value to surgeons, patients, and other stakeholders.

Keywords

Assessment in surgery · Performance assessment in surgery · Competency assessment · Surgical assessment · Testing in surgery · Surgical performance assessment · Surgical skills assessment · Surgical performance dimensions

Introduction

Introduction to Assessment

Assessment is a process by which the acquisition of understanding, abilities, and perceptions is measured. It is frequently used during education and training to determine the extent to which instruction has successfully facilitated its aims in increasing one or more of those dimensions for learners. The results of formative assessment outcomes are used to provide information to learners about their progress in mastering what they are studying and where they need to focus additional effort to achieve mastery, as well as to inform those who facilitate instruction where to make adjustments to pedagogical processes to assure that learners achieve mastery. The results of summative assessment confirm to others that learners have achieved and continue to maintain mastery in their areas of study, and as such require more rigorous psychometric integrity (Harlen and James 1997; Messick 1989; Andreatta et al. 2011; Wiggins 1998). Conceptually, this is a straightforward construct: measure baseline understanding, ability, and perceptions of learners before and after instruction, and calculate the difference to determine if the instruction was successful. Practically, the construct is anything but straightforward. This is largely because measuring understanding, abilities, and perceptions often requires the measurement of covert processes and neurocognitive responses that take place in the brain and are therefore not easily measured directly. For complex domains where the seamless integration of knowledge (cognitive), physical abilities (motor behavior), and perceptions (affective) are essential to performance mastery, assessment requirements are concomitantly complex. To assure mastery in such a domain, it is necessary to complete assessment for each dimension (cognitive, motor behavior, affective), and their integration in practice (Bennett 2011; Bearman et al. 2013; Dougherty and Andreatta 2017; Andreatta and Dougherty 2019; Moss 1992; Miller 1990).

Cognitive assessment measures the understanding of facts, concepts, and content relationships in a domain, including the higher level cognitive and meta-cognitive processing abilities required for application, analysis, synthesis, and generation of new knowledge in a domain (Bloom et al. 1956; Anderson and Krathwohl 2001;

Krathwohl 2002). Because all cognitive activities occur in the brain, their acquisition and mastery are covert, and we must rely on overt indicator behaviors for assessment. An easy example of this is to confirm an understanding of the proximal and directional concepts of "left" and "right." To confirm proximal understanding, one could ask a learner to raise their right/left hand, which would provide an indicator that they understood the concept. To confirm directional understanding, one could ask to learner to move one step to the right/left, rotate 45 degrees to the right/left, toss a ball to the right/left, or any number of similar indicator behaviors. These example indicators include motor behaviors, which are overt actions that are more directly measurable than cognitive processes. The motor behavior dimension is more directly measurable because the associated motor behaviors are largely overt in nature. For example, it is possible to measure the ability to run a 10-minute mile using a stopwatch to capture the start and finish times of a runner. However, there are qualitative attributes to most ability dimensions that include both cognitive and affective components of refinement, both of which are covert (Clark and Fiske 1982; Krathwohl et al. 1964; Anderson and Bourke 2000). This is evidenced in sports domains like gymnastics, where assessment includes both technical scores (motor behavior) and artistic scores that are based on the qualitative perception of those behaviors (cognitive and affective).

The affective dimension is often the most challenging to measure because it is contextually dependent, covert, qualitatively dynamic, and depending on the instrumentation, subjectively unreliable (Clark and Fiske 1982; Krathwohl et al. 1964; Anderson and Bourke 2000). For example, assessing a learner's feelings about eating eggs for breakfast can be measured any number of ways, from a direct open-ended question about their like or dislike of eggs for breakfast to a complex rating scale encompassing various preparations of egg dishes. However, the individual's own interpretation of their feelings about eggs may not be clear, may change depending on how hungry they are or whether they have recently eaten a lot of eggs, or may be confounded by something that is unrelated to eggs themselves but favorably or unfavorably reminds them of eggs. The latter influence is extremely important when assessing perceptions because affect stimulated from contexts unrelated to the domain of interest can also positively or negatively impact performance of the other dimensions (cognitive, motor behavior) Harrow 1972; Clark and Fiske 1982). For example, anxious feelings can adversely impact both cognitive processes and motor behaviors.

How to assess the concept of right/left, running and gymnastics abilities, or preference for eggs at breakfast are simple examples of assessments in each of the three performance dimensions. Assessment of a gymnast performing a floor routine that included running flips and twisting layouts to the right and left while eating eggs would be an example of an integrated performance assessment that includes these three dimensions. This chapter examines something far more challenging: assessment in the domain of surgery.

Surgical Competencies: Knowledge, Abilities, Perceptions

To understand the complexity of assessment requirements in the domain of surgery, one needs to first understand the performance requirements for surgeons in day-to-day professional practice, and the trajectory by which they acquire professional proficiencies in the domain. On any given day, a surgeon may be required to coordinate with the clinical staff to schedule patients, meet with new patients, and enact the processes associated with diagnosing and determining treatment alternatives for their respective conditions, check-in with preoperative patients and the surgical team to assure all preoperative requirements are completed, perform a variety of operative procedures that may require several hours of precise execution of fine motor skills and unrelenting situational awareness of patient status and team coordination, coordinate postoperative patient requirements with the nursing team, discuss postoperative patient outcomes with families, examine and evaluate postoperative patients and patients who remain hospitalized, complete all documentation associated with all clinical and surgical activities, access and respond to dozens of email, phone, and text messages, consult with colleagues, contribute to quality and safety initiatives, attend hospital committee meetings, and review recent published findings in medicine and the surgical specialty. If surgeons are affiliated with academic medical institutions, they will be required to train medical students, residents and fellows, as well as secure funding and perform research, serve on institutional committees, provide peer-review service to professional journals and granting agencies, publish in scholarly journals, volunteer for activities associated with one or more professional societies, make presentations at professional conferences and short courses, provide topical opinions for media outlets, and assemble a portfolio for promotion. For military surgeons, there are the additional requirements for deployments and casualty care in high intensity environments (Andreatta et al. 2021; Tyler et al. 2012; Edwards et al. 2018).

Within each of these performance areas, there are numerous detailed competencies that span all three performance dimensions. These requirements begin during medical school, and continue unabated through residency, fellowship, and professional practice. Additionally, surgical culture prioritizes patient well-being over personal well-being, which frequently leads to challenges in sustaining personal health and family and social relationships. To perform well as a surgeon requires masterful integration of deep and complex knowledge sets, fine and gross motor controls sequenced through specific routines and intermittent exigent applications, and the ability to manage fatigue, stress, emotions, anxiety, and other affective perceptions effectively. Surgeons are required to perform in this capacity while limiting error, with its attendant risks for their patients, colleagues, and practice, as well as their professional status and personal well-being. Routine assessment within this performance construct would benefit surgeons by providing them with the information they need to minimize risk and maximize their abilities in the domain. That is, providing surgeons with evidence to help them perform as well as possible benefits all of the same stakeholders that are adversely affected when performance errors occur. This chapter will consider how this information is captured and provided to surgeons and other stakeholders at each phase of post-medical school professional development. The authors provide a detailed look at the assessment processes that are implemented in the USA, with the understanding that these practices vary between countries around the world and a thorough review of all of them could encompass a multi-volume book. Nonetheless, the foundational components of assessing knowledge, skills, interpersonal abilities, and implementation of professional strategies remain common even if some of the specifics vary by location.

Assessment in Surgery

Cognitive (Knowledge) Assessment

The cognitive (knowledge) dimension of performance involves the recall of specific facts, concepts, and associated interrelationships; and the identification and consolidation of procedural patterns are required to accurately interpret, differentiate, and render decisions in complex environments. It also includes the ability to implement metacognitive strategies and derive original solutions to novel situations in the domain of expertise (Bloom et al. 1956; Anderson and Krathwohl 2001; Krathwohl 2002). Over time, experts develop elaborate knowledge structures in long-term memory that allow them to use fewer cognitive resources and rapidly grasp the essence of complex situations by discerning information, disregarding less informative elements, and reducing complexities. This ability to recognize patterns enables experts to interpret situations inferentially, including other situational aspects that may or may not be obvious to non-experts. They are able to do this because they are able to automatically activate the domain-specific knowledge stored in long-term memory and compare the new situation with previously encountered situations. Fundamentally, the development of the cognitive dimensions of performance in surgery also establishes the core of performance in the motor and affective dimensions because of shared reliance on these same knowledge structures for pattern recognition and dimensional response. Not surprisingly, knowledge assessment is the primary method for measuring the competency of surgeons across the continuum of training and professional practice. It is also the performance dimension that has the greatest degree of precision and psychometric support for assessment instrumentation.

During residency, there are few formal knowledge assessments; however, there are options to engage with discretionary assessments made available through professional organizations. There are also assessment components embedded within specialty-specific instruction and certification requirements for patient care privileging.

Resident In-Training Examinations

Most postgraduate training programs have their residents and fellows take in-training examinations (ITE). ITEs are designed to assess the progress of residents during training and provide program directors with comparative knowledge assessment data to evaluate the progress and areas of deficiency for residents relative to others at the same training level. ITEs are the same for all residents, but they are scored according to training year. Both the American Board of Surgery (ABS) and the American College of Osteopathic Surgeons (ACOS) offer annual exams for general surgery residency programs that are comprised of multiple choice questions designed to measure knowledge of applied science and management of clinical problems related to surgery (ABS 2021; ACOS 2021). Some ITE questions include previous board exam questions. There are similar exams for Neurosurgery, Orthopedic Surgery, Otolaryngology, Plastic Surgery, and other surgical subspecialties (AOAN 2021; ABO 2021; AAOS 2021; ASPS 2021).

ITEs can be taken on a yearly basis. The intended purpose of ITEs is to identify residency program strengths and weaknesses, and scores are released to program directors to share discretely with individual trainees. In this regard, ITEs are useful for program evaluation but not for formative assessment, which requires that specific information be provided to each test taker about his/her performance on each test item (Sadler 1989). Missed items are cataloged by topic for presentation to the test taker. As such, individual assessment from these exams limits the information about where individuals are performing well and where they require additional work to increase their abilities.

This is further complicated by the misuse of ITE scores for high-stakes decisions, such as promotion, remediation, and retention, even though the ITE is designed as a low-stakes formative examination. Although there is evidence that ITE scores correlate with board qualifying exam (QE) scores, they do not predict passing the board certifying exam, which requires the ability to articulate decision-making and technical steps in surgical cases. These higher order thinking abilities are best supported by detailed assessment information from which the learner can modify understanding of complexity in the domain. Without providing the assessment details to the learner, the ITEs may serve less as formative assessments that develop deep knowledge structures and more as test preparation that helps residents learn how to take multiple choice exams covering content in the domain (Jones et al. 2014; de Virgilio et al. 2010; Nguyen et al. 2021).

Certification and Course Specific Knowledge Assessment

There are several training requirements and certifications that surgical trainees must complete in order to perform their work in clinical settings and be eligible for board certification. Each one includes an embedded knowledge assessment of some form. These include courses such as Advanced Cardiac Life Support (ACLS), Pediatric Advanced Life Support (PALS), Advanced Trauma Life Support (ATLS), Fundamentals of Laparoscopic Surgery (FLS), and Fundamentals of Endoscopic Surgery (FES) (AHA 2021; ATLS 2021; FLS 2021; FES 2021).

The Surgical Council on Resident Education (SCORE) provides a web-based portal for general and subspecialty surgical trainees that includes a wide variety of resources designed to support the curriculum requirements of a five-year general surgery residency program, including self-assessment. Each learning module includes multiple choice questions that assess understanding and acquired knowledge, and the portal features a new topic each week with related content and a 10-question quiz. Although the portal content focuses on all areas of a general surgery residency, there is also fellowship-level content and curricular content for pediatric surgery, surgical critical care, surgical oncology, and vascular surgery. Resident usage of the SCORE portal increases as annual ITEs approach, and there is evidence that completion of the learning modules increases ITE scores (SCORE 2021; Joshi et al. 2017; Winer et al. 2019).

Like the SCORE portal, Orthobullets provides educational content and knowledge assessment opportunities for orthopedic surgery residents and fellows, yet also for practicing orthopedic surgeons. The portal facilitates the development of personalized assessment for individuals, as well as groups. Individuals are able to create personalized tests from a library of several thousand multiple choice questions, many of which are from prior board exams. Personalized tests provide the test takers with immediate feedback to help guide their learning. The group test function allows residency program directors to create customized tests for residents and use test outcomes to track and identify any deficits that require improvement. However, residents are unable to view the results until the program director permits it. Orthobullets is a for-profit company, and users must subscribe to one of several pricing packages to access the various content areas (Al Farii 2020). As such, outcomes are restricted to subscribers and do not inform decisions by oversight and accrediting bodies. Likewise, there is no validation process in place for the content presented through the site. Nonetheless, there is evidence suggesting that access to Orthobullets is beneficial for exam preparation and acquisition of procedural knowledge for orthopedic surgeons (Rogers et al. 2019).

There are other commercially available web-portals that include both instructional content and assessment options for residents, fellows, and practicing surgeons across the spectrum of surgical specialties. Although providing easy access to content, these web-portals do not include external review processes and credentialing oversight, so the accuracy and validity of these resources must be considered with discretion.

Certifying Examinations

After completion of a postgraduate training program, whether residency or fellowship, surgical trainees take one or more board certifying examinations. These exams are considered pass/fail high-stakes summative assessments, and qualify and detailed score reports are not provided to examinees.

The American Board of Surgery requires completion of a qualifying exam (QE) and a certifying exam (CE). The QE consists of about 300 multiple choice questions that are designed to assess the examinee's knowledge of general surgical principles, applied science, and professional practice requirements. The exam questions align with the curriculum ascribed by the surgical council of resident education, which covers 27 organ-based categories of patient care that are further separated into associated diseases/conditions and operations/procedures. There are two levels of content stratification, with core content reflecting situations that would be frequently encountered by most general surgeons and for which they must be able to provide comprehensive care, including procedural competency. The advanced content stratification reflects diseases and procedures that are not consistently part of general surgery practice, but for which the examinee should be able to make a diagnosis and provide initial management. Additional content includes knowledge of applied science and clinical medicine, professionalism, interpersonal and communication skills, practice-based learning and improvement, and systems-based practice. The QE is subjected to conventional psychometric analysis to assure that validity and reliability standards for high stakes assessments are met (ABS 2021). The American Osteopathic Board of Surgeons (AOBS) administers a similar exam with equally rigorous psychometric standards (AOBS 2021).

Upon successful completion of the QE, surgical residents take the CE oral exam, which is the last step for board certification in general surgery. The CE is designed to assess the examinee's diagnostic aptitude, comprehension of therapeutic alternatives, surgical judgment, clinical reasoning abilities, problem-solving capabilities, technical operative and procedural acumen, and ethical and humanistic qualities. Board examiners place emphasis on examinees' ability to apply their knowledge to manage a broad range of clinical problems safely, effectively, and promptly.

The American Board of Orthopedic Surgeons (ABOS) implements a similar approach for board certifying examinations. The ABOS board certification process includes Level 1 and Level 2 exams; however, ABOS requires that examinees be in practice for 17 months at one location, association, and affiliation before qualifying for Level 2 examination. The ABOS obtains peer review feedback about examinees from their affiliated hospital chiefs of staff, chiefs of orthopedics, surgery, and anesthesia, and operating room nursing staff before determining eligibility for the Level 2 examination. Once admitted for the oral examination, examinees must provide an institutionally verified list of all cases performed during a specified six-month period. Twelve cases are selected for inquiry by the board examiners, who score the examinees responses to questions using an ordinal rating scale with categorical anchors (ABOS 2021).

In addition to board certifying examinations for general and orthopedic surgery, there are certifying examinations for otolaryngology, plastic surgery, thoracic surgery, neurological surgery, and associated sub-specialties (ABS 2021; AOBS 2021; ABOS 2021; ABMS2 2021; ABMS2 2021; ABIM 2021). These exams follow a similar two-level structure that includes both written and case-based oral examination. For vascular surgeons, there is an option to complete the Registered Physician Vascular Interpretation (RPVI) examination, which is a formal assessment of the knowledge, skills, and abilities deemed essential for physicians practicing vascular surgery and vascular medicine. In addition to multiple choice questions, the exam includes questions that require the application of interpretation and reasoning capabilities using a simulated workstation (APCA 2021).

Professional Practiced

After surgeons are certified for their primary practice areas, they must complete the recertification processes required by their specialty board(s) to maintain their certification. The goal of the recertification process is to ensure that all surgeons are both competent and current their respective practice areas. Historically, most recertification requirements included the completion of a high stakes knowledge test every 10 years, with similar content to the certification exams for residents and fellows. However, there has been a significant shift toward more frequent, practice-centered assessment in recent years, with most specialty boards now employing a multi-component assessment process for recertification every 2 years.

The ABS has shifted to recertification every 2 years through a Continuous Certification Assessment process for all surgical specialties and sub-specialties. In addition to information about ongoing surgical practice, surgeons complete a 40-question open book exam that includes both core surgical principles and practice-specific content. Depending on the discipline, examinees are provided with articles and references in advance of the exam to help with preparation. Examinees are given immediate feedback for each question, and they have two attempts to answer each question correctly. A final score of 80% is required to pass the exam (ABS 2021).

AOBS-certified specialty and subspecialty surgeons must also maintain specified requirements for ongoing surgical practice, as well as complete a practice-centered written examination. The Osteopathic Continuous Certification (OCC) exams follow a more traditional format, with a single 2.25-h time-delimited proctored administration. Each exam consists of 100 multiple choice questions designed to assess basic science and clinical knowledge, skills, and principles that are critical for each respective specialty area. As with other similar certifying examinations, AOBS continuous certification exams meet rigorous psychometric standards for validity and reliability (AOBS 2021).

The ABOS enacts a maintenance of certification (MOC) process as part of recertification in orthopedic surgery and associated subspecialties. ABOS also requires documented evidence of ongoing surgical practice and the completion of a practice-centered knowledge assessment. Examinees may choose to complete the knowledge assessment component through one of three formats (computer-based exam, oral exam, web-based longitudinal assessment). The computer-based exam is a proctored 3-h test comprised of 150 multiple choice questions either covering general and clinical content that all orthopedic surgeons are expected to know, or content that includes subspecialty-specific information. The oral examination alternative is similar in format to the oral component (Level 2) of initial certification and includes questioning on 12 cases submitted by the examinee for consideration. Examiners assess data gathering, diagnosis and interpretive skills, treatment plans, technical skills, patient outcomes, and applied knowledge using a similar ordinal rating scale to the Level 2 exam. The web-based longitudinal assessment option is a practice-centered approach that is conceptually similar to the ABS's continuous certification assessment. Exam content is identified by the American Academy of

Orthopaedic Surgeons (AAOS) and orthopedic subspecialty societies, and ABOS selects more than 200 of these knowledge sources to generate test questions. Examinees may review and select 15 practice-centered knowledge sources as the foundation for their 30-question, multiple choice exam (two questions per source). The knowledge source is identified before examinees view each question and the exam is open book; however, there is a 3-min time limit for each question (ABOS 2021).

Recertification in other surgical subspecialties follows one or more of these formats, depending on the specialty board. Most specialty and subspecialty boards require routine MOC; however, the intervals between assessment requirements for recertification vary from 2 to 10 years (ABMS2 2021; ABIM 2021).

Motor Behavior (Abilities) Assessment

Performance of clinical and surgical abilities is paramount for quality and safe patient care (Etchells et al. 2003). Clinical or surgical abilities refer to motor behaviors that involve the use and control of the body to complete an intended objective. The development of motor behaviors includes the ability persistently to control the force, speed, precision, and kinesthetic integration of the body to effect the desired outcome (Wulf et al. 2010; Newell and Ranganathan 2010; Bingham 1995). This kinematic information is stored in the brain as a motor program, where a series of individual complex movements have been grouped together as a unit, or chunk, to enable execution of domain specific actions (▶ Chap. 18, "Cognitive Neuroscience Foundations of Surgical and Procedural Expertise: Focus on Theory"). For surgeons, the habituated ability to control their fingers, hands, and arms deliberately and with bimanual dexterity, as well as proprioceptively control their bodies during operations, is consistent with the activation of these types of motor programs and establishes the foundation for performance mastery in this dimension (Kauffman et al. 1987; Wulf et al. 2010).

Abilities (skills) assessment refers to the process of measuring those actions and comparing the measured outcome to explicit criteria (Dave 1970; Harrow 1972). Assessment of surgical abilities typically includes measurement of accuracy, precision, efficiency, comprehensiveness, consistency, and safety (Kauffman et al. 1987). Motor programs are developed through the deliberate practice of focused actions that include timely and specific feedback (formative assessment) to assure accurate acquisition (Kauffman et al. 1987). The sequencing of activities designed to develop complex abilities is an integral component of deliberate practice and assures that necessary steps are not overlooked. Implementation of assessment is optimally structured to align strategically with progression from one ability level to the next (Dave 1970; Ericcson 1993; Gist et al. 1990). Motor programs require activation to assure retention over time, so it is important routinely to refresh surgical abilities that are infrequently used in practice (Fleishman and Parker 1962). Summative assessment confirms that these abilities have been acquired and once achieved, maintained over time (Kauffman et al. 1987). Additionally, these abilities are vulnerable to stress, fatigue, irritation, and other perception challenges associated with the affective dimension (Beilock and Gray 2012; Maurer and Munzert 2013; McCaskie et al. 2011).

Residency and Fellowship

Formal skills assessment is not generally required for residents and fellows, and they primarily rely on feedback given to them by their attending faculty during the provision of clinical and operative care. However, training programs have the discretion to implement various forms of formative and summative assessment mechanisms for progress tracking or patient care privileging. These types of assessments are often associated with corresponding instruction, but not always. For example, most residents are required to complete the AHA Advanced Cardiovascular Life Support (ACLS) course, which is designed for healthcare professionals who either direct or participate in the management of cardiopulmonary arrest or other cardiovascular emergencies (AHA 2021). ACLS uses patient manikin simulators to assess the ability of learners to perform the clinical and procedural skills required for treating pre-arrest, arrest, or post-arrest patients. For residents and fellows working with pediatric patients, AHA provides certification through Pediatric Advanced Life Support (PALS), which follows a similar structure and includes similar skills assessment requirements (AHA 2021).

Residents and fellows who are training in the various surgical specialties complete the American College of Surgeons (ACS) Advanced Trauma Life Support (ATLS) course, which focuses on patient assessment, implementation of resuscitation and stabilization strategies, determination of a facility's capacity to meet the patient needs, and facilitation of inter-hospital transfer (ATLS 2021). Although the ATLS course does not have a formal skills assessment component, learners are required to perform various procedures at skills stations and receive associated feedback from course faculty.

The ACS and the Society of American Gastrointestinal and Endoscopic Surgeons (SAGES) jointly offer two courses focusing on the acquisition of minimally invasive surgical skills. Successful completion of both courses is required to take the QE. The Fundamentals of Laparoscopic Surgery™ (FLS) course includes hands-on training and assessment of basic laparoscopic surgical abilities; the skills assessment component consists of five simulation exercises designed to quantify ambidexterity, depth perception, hand-eye coordination, controlled movement of instruments, and efficiency of movement. Although many surgical training programs require the use of FLS, there are many challenges to its validity for use as an assessment platform, especially for high stakes summative assessment. The simulation fidelity of several exercises is poorly defined and not reflective of an operative environment, which is a foundational requirement for assessment validity (Sroka et al. 2010; Scott et al. 2013). The scores for each exercise include efficiency (time) and precision (accuracy); however, the scoring formulas for each task are not clear, and more challenging skills are not appropriately weighted for their differential score contribution. Additionally, there are requirements for repetitive performance within each task that are not evidence-based. Although the psychometric evidence supporting these measures is minimal, there are several studies confirming the value of FLS for formative assessment, especially during the early phases of laparoscopic skill development. In addition to skills assessment, the course includes a test designed to measure understanding and application of the basic fundamentals of laparoscopy with emphasis on clinical judgment or intraoperative decision-making. A 10-year certificate is awarded upon successful completion of FLS; however, evidence suggests that laparoscopic skills degrade without use in a much shorter interval, as soon as 6 weeks (Andreatta et al. 2014; Brackmann et al. 2017).

The Fundamentals of Endoscopic Surgery™ (FES) is a correlate to FLS but focuses on the performance of basic gastrointestinal (GI) endoscopic surgery (endoscopy). The course includes assessment of the basic endoscopic skills required for the uses of flexible gastrointestinal (GI) endoscopy, including navigation, loop reduction, retroflexion, mucosal evaluation, and targeting (tool manipulation). Skills are assessed using proprietary simulators that include built-in scoring mechanisms. Like FLS, studies suggest that FES skills assessments meet the rigorous psychometric standards required for high-stakes examinations; however, there are significant weaknesses in the study designs supporting these conclusions (Vassiliou et al. 2014). Specifically, the methodologies rely on self-reported experience as the foundation for expertise; this is an imprecise measurement that neither provides accurate information about the capabilities of the sample nor performance consistency. As such, there is no reported evidence that demonstrates a relationship between performance on the simulator and performance in operative contexts. Additionally, there is a lack of transparency for the simulator's scoring algorithms, which is problematic for establishing an evidence base for asserting both validity and reliability. These elements are essential for high stakes summative assessment, which must be both accurate and fair. Although there is evidence that the training on a simulator using the FES tasks improves the ability to perform those tasks on the simulator, there is no evidence to confirm that these abilities transfer to the applied practice of endoscopic surgery (Ritter et al. 2018). The value of FES for formative assessment during the process of acquiring endoscopic skills is unclear.

The Accreditation Council for Graduate Medical Education (ACGME) indirectly captures information about various skills that are embedded within 18 competency areas, each of which includes performance milestones that describe the overall professional requirements for surgeons in that competency area (ACGME 2021). The achievement of each competency is biannually captured for every trainee using an ordinal scale with categorical anchors (Levels 1–5, 5 highest). The ordinal scale has nine options and assumes that progression is equivalent across the spectrum of performance (e.g., each level has the same implications for failure or achievement). Although these scales can provide a global view of a trainee's progress and identify areas for improvement, they do not meet the standards required for either formative or summative assessment purposes. They provide no explicit performance criteria or actionable information about the numerous skills that are required during the provision of patient care. Notwithstanding the uses of categorical anchors, the scales rely on a subjective view of trainees over an extended period of time (6 months) by a variable number of faculty with whom they have worked. Inconsistent training of faculty in the use of the scales, both within and across training programs, further diminishes the assessment value of the milestones.

The American Board of Surgery (ABS) requires periodic assessment of operative and clinical performance as part of an ongoing effort to standardize the knowledge and skills performance criteria for general surgery residents. Every trainee is required to obtain at least six operative performance assessments and six clinical performance assessments during their residency program. Although the ABS does not collect completed assessment forms, the program director must attest that the 12 assessments have been completed. The ABS provides assessment forms for 13 procedures, each of which is based on an ordinal scale with partial anchors provided for procedural steps, implementation of technique and instrumentation, and overall independent ability to perform procedure. The ABS also allows for discretionary use of other assessment instruments, such as the objective structured clinical examination (OSCE) and objective structured assessment of technical skills (OSAT); however, these forms have uncontrolled content and measurement structures and do not meet the requirements for summative assessment purposes (Hodges 2003; Regehr et al. 1998). Additionally, the unspecified content and periodicity requirements of the assessment framework render any resulting data less informative for formative or summative assessment purposes (Faulkner et al. 1996; Anderson et al. 2016; Darzi et al. 2001). Still, it is a step in the right direction, and the ABS is acknowledged for its shift toward competency-based training and credentialing, even if there is room for improvement in assessment rigor and value.

Professional Practice

After surgeons complete their training and associated requirements, there are few, if any, specifications for assessment of clinical and surgical skills to maintain professional licensure or certification. Depending on the specialty and practice privileges, most surgeons are required to maintain certifications acquired during residency (e.g., ACLS, ATLS). However, it is largely assumed that surgeons will maintain their acquired skills within the context of providing clinical and surgical care to patients. It is also assumed that surgeons will continue to acquire and hone their skills through relevant continuing medical education (CME) activities, such as professional courses, industry-specific training, and other opportunities for learning how to use new technologies, techniques, and resources. There are three well-established CME courses for trauma surgery: Advanced Trauma Life Support (ATLS), Advanced Surgical Skills for Exposure in Trauma (ASSET), and Advanced Trauma Operative Management (ATOM). Although these courses include skills assessment components, they are formative by design and intended to document successful completion of the instruction rather than demonstrated competence. For example, the ASSET course provides training for critical surgical exposures in key anatomical areas of the neck, chest, abdomen and pelvis, and upper and lower extremities, including hands-on implementation of procedural skills. Although learners receive feedback from their instructors, the course does not include concomitant skills assessment (Bowyer et al. 2013; Mackenzie et al. 2019). A revised version of the course (ASSET+) includes detailed performance assessment of surgical skills for every procedure, before and after training. These assessment data provide learners with explicit information about their baseline performance gaps and help them to focus their efforts to improve specific skills performance during the course, with significant gains over the prior course version (Elster et al. 2020, Bowyer et al. 2021). Rather than course completion, these assessment data document actual acquired abilities and associated competencies in performing the procedures.

There are numerous examples of continuing medical education and industry-supported skills training for surgical specialties. To the extent meaningful procedural skills assessment could be implemented during these activities, an evidence base of surgical skills competency would be rapidly realized. More importantly, identification of gap areas would facilitate focused skill development, leading to increased quality and safety of patient care.

Affective (Perceptions) Assessment

The affective (perceptions) dimensions of surgery include the values, attitudes, attributions, feelings and emotional control that influence motivation, self-efficacy, interpersonal associations, job satisfaction, leadership, and goal setting. Societal expectations associated with overt displays of perceptions are culturally dependent, and the uses and interpretation of affective assessments must accommodate those dependencies. Perceptions are characterized by three attributes: target, intensity, and direction. The target is the entity that stimulates the perception, the intensity is the strength of feeling associated with the perception, and the direction ascribes a feeling as positive, negative, or neutral (Anderson and Bourke 2000). There are significant positive and negative affective dimensions associated with surgery, which have historically been managed through various techniques designed to sublimate overt display or recognition within the contexts of professional interactions and patient care. Positive perceptions may be tempered to control expectations, and negative perceptions may be internalized to avoid the appearance of vulnerability or incompetence.

The positive value affective assessment and associated cultural change that it brings to workplaces is substantiated with theoretical and empirical support, including increased job satisfaction, productivity, quality, safety, achievement, attendance, retention, and profitability (Madlock and Booth-Butterfield 2012; Sardzoska and Tang 2012; Riketta 2008). The reason why even small changes in perception have such pronounced impacts on performance is because perceptions are designed to alert human beings to potential harm, and therefore, they assert themselves hierarchically over other performance dimensions. Perceptions are deeply enmeshed with cognitive processes and motor behaviors, and strongly negative perceptions can adversely impact performance across all three dimensions. For example, if a surgeon is experiencing significant stress, compensatory control mechanisms will recruit cognitive resources to manage that stress at the expense of increased effort and behavioral tradeoffs in the other performance dimensions (Hockey 1997; Kahneman

1973). Experts exhibit an economy of motor planning both at the level of central neural programming and subsequent motor unit activation that is not evident in novices. The experienced or expert surgeon is ergonomically more efficient than the novice, uses fewer, more efficient, and more precise movements, and demonstrates better instrument handling skills (Milton et al. 2007). As expertise and automaticity develop, knowledge processes and abilities require fewer cognitive resources, and the destructive impacts of negative perceptions are more readily accommodated and moderated. Individuals can also be taught to enact affective control in productive ways, such as deliberate attentional focus (Kenny 2009; Arora et al. 2011; Andreatta et al. 2010).

Despite its integral component to surgical performance, assessment in the affective dimension is rarely implemented during residency, fellowship, or professional practice, and there is minimal evidence of its inclusion during medical school (Cate and de Haes 2000; de Haes et al. 2005; Hodges et al. 2011). There are components within the ACGME milestones that include dimensionally relevant competencies, such as professionalism, interpersonal communication, and maintaining wellness. Likewise, many medical schools and residency programs are discussing the challenges associated with this performance dimension, and some include both instructional and community-building activities that are designed to raise awareness and address affective management. Nonetheless, perception-related challenges remain prevalent in health services care and training environments. The contextual and cultural antecedents for these challenges are beyond the scope of this chapter, but individuals can acquire expertise in the affective dimension of surgery in the same way that they can in cognitive and psychomotor abilities. Performance hindering perceptions can be identified through purposeful assessment and mitigated through focused training to develop affective control strategies, such as cognitive reappraisal and mindfulness techniques (Song 2009; Beilock and Gray 2012; Arora et al. 2011).

Performance (Integrated Abilities) Assessment

Proficient performance in surgery requires the seamless integration of the three performance dimensions described in the previous sections; however, these dimensions are not discretely separate and are interdependent in practice. Cognitive understanding influences affective perceptions and vice versa, and both dynamically influence psychomotor behaviors. To characterize and document surgical performance capabilities comprehensively, it is essential to assess the performance of individuals in the contextually relevant circumstances of patient care and its associated constituent parts. Performance assessment serves this purpose by measuring the ability to apply knowledge, motor behaviors, and perceptions in situationally appropriate ways, with the aim of achieving an intended outcome in the performance domain. If the assessment instrumentation has psychometric rigor, the outcomes have very high predictive validity because they measure performance in actual work environments. Therefore, performance assessment is considered a gold standard for complex domains with performance characteristics across the three dimensions, such as surgery.

Residency and Fellowship

Two clinical assessment forms are frequently used during post-graduate medical education, each of which relies on ordinal rating scales with partial categorical anchors for each assessed component. The Mini-Clinical Evaluation Exercise (Mini-CEX) includes global performance dimensions for patient encounters, including medical interviewing, physician examination, humanistic qualities/professionalism, clinical judgment, counseling skills, organization, efficiency, and overall clinical competence (ABIM 2021; Norcini et al. 2003). The Clinical Assessment and Management Exam-Outpatient (CAMEO) includes global performance dimensions for test ordering and understanding, diagnostic acumen, history taking, physical examination, communication skills, and overall performance, as well as a survey component for patients to rate their perceptions of the trainee (Wilson et al. 2015). As described in the skills section, the ABS requires six performance assessments in both clinical and operative care environments (ABS 2021). While there are clear validity advantages for implementing these assessments in the context of applied patient care, there are measurement limitations associated with the instrumentation for all of these exams. For example, although the score records facilitate recognition of case complexity, there are no concurrent scoping adjustments to account for the complexity. These scales also restrict the variance of data by limiting the scope of performance options and assume equivalent weight between each interval and the categorical anchors.

Professional Practice

Post-training performance assessment for surgeons is not widely implemented, although there have been some incremental advances in this area through initiatives from the Royal Colleges of Surgeons and Surgical Specialty Associations in the United Kingdom, Australia, and New Zealand (Beard et al. 2009). These initiatives are supported by workplace assessments (WPA) and procedural based assessments (PBA) of various performance dimensions using similar instrumentation to those described for surgical training programs, including the Mini-CEX, the Ottawa clinical assessment tool (OCAT), direct observation of procedural skills (DOPS), and procedural specific PBA forms. Other assessment mechanisms include chart-stimulated recall (CSR) and peer assessment using the Peer Assessment Tool (Mini-PAT), multi-sources feedback (MSF), and formal and informal letters, recommendations, and institutionally driven 360 performance evaluations (Norcini 2013). There remain significant challenges with the uses of these instruments in practice, as well as with the integrity of measurement and scoring validity for summative and other certification purposes. However, they are useful for formative assessment and provide information about potential performance gaps ahead of the realization of errors during patient care. Most health service institutions have both formal and informal processes for documenting and assessing performance errors, especially if they are associated with adverse or near miss events. Although these types of assessments are essential for assuring care quality and safety, optimal ongoing performance assessment would provide greater assurance that surgeons are maintaining accurate and current capabilities in their specialty practice while limiting the occurrence of adverse events.

Synthesis and Best Practices

This chapter provides a review of the foundational performance requirements for surgeons during residency, fellowship, and professional practice, and the various methods of assessment that are implemented to assure performance standards are realized. We examined each of the three primary performance dimensions (cognitive, motor, and affective), as well as their integration in applied clinical and surgical practice. Surgery is an extremely complex performance domain, with rigorous performance requirements for each dimension and numerous interrelationships between the three dimensions. As such, assessment requirements for the domain are equally complex and involve the specification and measurement of numerous details for each dimension, while at the same time accommodating the variability inherent in the environments within which surgeons work. It is not an ideal environment for capturing the types of accurate, precise, comprehensive, and fair assessment information that benefits surgeons and other stakeholders (e.g., hospitals, payers, patients, colleagues, and families). The intricacies of the environment are further complicated by the inherent challenges in measuring certain performance attributes in each dimension, especially the cognitive and affective dimensions where performance is largely covert in form. Nonetheless, there are established methods and mechanisms for measuring every attribute of each performance dimension, even if the value of doing so risks the possibility of over-assessing within the domain.

Historically and presently, abilities within the domain of surgery are primarily assessed in the cognitive dimension through examinations in written or verbal formats. These may be formative or summative in use, but most take the form of multiple choice questions that require the examinee to identify the best response to a question. Culminating oral examinations for credentialing purposes include higher order cognitive reasoning as well. The assessment of motor and affective abilities has largely been formative and subsumed within the context of providing surgical care. More recently, other forms of assessing motor abilities have evolved to include simulation-based methods and rating-scales that quantify performance of specific tasks. This is an important step toward implementing defensible assessment frameworks for measuring the spectrum of motor abilities required for surgery. However, these frameworks encompass substantial variance in both the contextual fidelity of the simulation and the uses of weakly defined assessment instrumentation. The inclusion of affective elements as specific competencies is also a step toward realizing deliberate assessment within this dimension. The emphasis on the cognitive dimension as the proxy indicator for surgical competency is evident when considering the incongruence of cognitive performance outcomes when compared with motor and affective performance outcomes (Shah et al. 2018). Especially during training, individuals will focus on what will be assessed, which will lead to an imbalance of capabilities in other performance dimensions.

Optimally, assessment would align with the trajectory of mastery learning, where incremental achievement of increasingly complex dimensional abilities is formatively assessed, and summative assessment confirms mastery. Once mastered, abilities would require periodic reassessment to assure retention. This minimizes the burden of assessment within training environments, while assuring that cross-dimensional competencies are attained and maintained in the domain. We propose a framework for leveraging the assessment processes that have demonstrated effective value for developing and confirming competencies across the performance dimensions while improving the overall assessment processes. This approach identifies and minimizes content and measurement gaps, aligns implementation with content sequencing and retention periodicity, and assures the accuracy, completeness, and justness of outcomes used for credentialing purposes. An overview of the types of assessment requirements that might be implemented across residency, fellowship, pre-certification and post-certification professional practice is delineated in Table 1. This overview incorporates the foundational taxonomies for each performance dimension, aligns with the principles of mastery learning for achievement of competencies, and follows best practices for authentic performance assessment in professional practice contexts. The information presented in Table 1 provides a foundation for determining comprehensive assessment that encompasses all performance dimensions in surgery; however, both formative and summative assessment requirements and associated instrumentation would need to be tied to specific competency objectives at each provider level. The descriptions for each level of the dimensional taxonomies included in the table are beyond the scope of this chapter, and we refer readers to the cited literature for further exploration.

Assessment requirements within the domain of surgery encompass a broad scope and include many details because the performance domain is complex and requires the integration of multifaceted knowledge structures, precise motor abilities, and affective control to achieve mastery. Current assessment practices largely focus on the cognitive dimensions, and these are well developed across the profession, from training through professional practice. There are initiatives and developing trends that include assessment of motor and affective dimensions as training program components, although these remain discretionary for practicing surgeons. Current assessment methods in motor and affective dimensions are challenged by measurement precision and concomitant constraints on the accuracy and justness of assessment outcomes as confirmation of competencies. Increasing the accuracy and precision of assessment instrumentation, as well as defining explicit performance criteria, will lead to improved assessment value to surgeons, patients, and other stakeholders.

Table 1 Comprehensive competency-based assessment plan for surgery

	Provider level			
	Residency	Fellowship	Pre-certified professional	Certified professional
Cognitive Dimension	Bloom Levels 1–4 for each program specific competencies	Bloom Levels 3–5 for each program specific competencies	Bloom Levels 3–5 in specialty domain	Bloom Levels 3–5 in specialty domain
Motor Dimension	Dave Levels 1–4 for each program specific competencies	Dave Levels 3–5 for each program specific competencies	Dave Levels 3–5 in specialty domain	Dave Levels 3–5 in specialty domain
Affective Dimension	Krathwohl Levels 1–5 for program specific competencies	Krathwohl Levels 3–5 for program specific competencies	Krathwohl Levels 3–5 in specialty domain	Krathwohl Levels 3–5 in specialty domain
Integrated Performance	Performance criteria specified for each of the following contexts: Clinical care Operative care Hospital care Care coordination Administrative Research Academic Service	Performance criteria specified for each of the following contexts: Clinical care Operative care Hospital care Care coordination Administrative Research Academic Service	Performance criteria specified for each of the following contexts: Clinical care Operative care Hospital care Care coordination Administrative Research Academic Service Teaching Leadership	Performance criteria specified for each of the following contexts: Clinical care Operative care Hospital care Care coordination Administrative Research Academic Service Teaching Leadership
Competency Documentation	*Formative Assessment:* Two assessments per month, including all dimensions *Summative Assessment:* One assessment per competency per year for all dimensions	*Formative Assessment:* Two assessments per month, including all dimensions *Summative Assessment:* One assessment per competency per year for all dimensions	*Formative Assessment:* Two peer-to-peer assessments per year for cognitive and motor dimensions Three 360-degree assessments per year for Integrated Performance *Summative*	*Formative Assessment:* Two peer-to-peer assessments per year for cognitive and motor dimensions Three 360-degree assessments per year for Integrated Performance *Summative*

(continued)

Table 1 (continued)

	Provider level			
	Residency	Fellowship	Pre-certified professional	Certified professional
	Portfolio: All formative assessments Summative assessment outcomes Credentialing requirements as specified by program	*Portfolio:* All formative assessments Summative assessment outcomes Credentialing requirements as specified by program	*Assessment:* 1 assessment per year for all dimensions Certification examinations/ requirements *Portfolio:* All formative assessments Summative assessment outcomes Credentialing requirements for specialty	*Assessment:* 1 assessment per year for all dimensions Re-certification examinations/ requirements Expansion of practice examinations/ requirements *Portfolio:* All formative assessments Summative assessment outcomes Credentialing requirements for specialty

Cross-References

▸ Entrustable Professional Activities: Focus on Assessment Methods
▸ Focus on Theory: Emotions and Learning
▸ Learning and Teaching in the Operating Theatre: Expert Commentary from the Nursing Perspective
▸ Supporting the Development of Professionalism in the Education of Health Professionals
▸ Surgical Education and Training: Historical Perspectives
▸ Surgical Education: Context and Trends

References

AAOS Orthopaedic In-Training Examination. American Academy of Orthopaedic Surgeons. 2021. https://www.aaos.org/education/about-aaos-products/orthopaedic-in-training-examination-oite/. Accessed 19 May 2021.

ABMS Guide to Medical Specialties. American Board of Medical Specialties. 2021. https://www.abms.org/wp-content/uploads/2020/11/ABMS-Guide-to-Medical-Specialties-2020.pdf. Accessed 19 May 2021.

Advanced Trauma Life Support. American College of Surgeons. 2021. https://www.facs.org/quality-programs/trauma/atls. Accessed 19 May 2021.

Al Farii H. The impact of the Orthobullets website as a learning tool among orthopaedic surgery residents in two different residency programmes. Orthopaedic Proceedings. 2020;102-B (SUPP_60).

Anderson LW, Bourke SF. Assessing affective characteristics in the schools. Mahwah: Lawrence Erlbaum Associates; 2000. p. 24–48.

Anderson LW, Krathwohl DR. A taxonomy for learning, teaching, and assessing: a revision of Bloom's taxonomy of educational objectives. New York: Longman; 2001.

Anderson DD, Long S, Thomas G, Putnam MD, Bechtold JE, Karam MD, et al. Objective structured assessment of technical skills does not assess the quality of the surgical result effectively. Clin Orthop Relat Res. 2016;478:874–81.

Andreatta P, Dougherty P. Supporting the development of psychomotor skills. In: Nestel D, Dalrymple K, Paige J, Aggarwal R, editors. Advancing surgical education: theory, evidence and practice. New York: Springer; 2019. p. 183–96.

Andreatta PB, Hillard ML, Krain LP. The impact of stress factors in simulation-based laparoscopic training. Surgery. 2010;147(5):631–9.

Andreatta PB, Marzano DA, Curran DS. Validity: what does it mean for assessment in obstetrics and gynecology? Am J Obstet Gynecol. 2011;204(5):384.e1–6.

Andreatta P, Marzano DA, Curran DS, Klotz JJ, Gamble CR, Reynolds RK, et al. Low-hanging fruit: a clementine as a simulation model for advanced laparoscopy. Simul Healthc. 2014;9(4):234–40.

Andreatta PB, Bowyer MW, Remick K, Knudson MM, Elster EA, et al. Evidence-based surgical competency outcomes from the clinical readiness program. Ann Surg. 2021; https://doi.org/10.1097/sla.0000000000005324.

Arora S, Aggarwal R, Moran A, Sirimanna P, Crochet P, Darzi A, Kneebone R, Sevdalis N, et al. Mental practice: effective stress management training for novice surgeons. J Am Coll Surg. 2011;212:225–33.

Beard J, Rowley D, Bussey M, Pitts D. Workplace-based assessment: assessing technical skill throughout the continuum of surgical training. ANZ J Surg. 2009;79(3):148–53.

Bearman M, Nestel D, Andreatta P. Simulation-based medical education. In: Walsh K, editor. Oxford textbook of medical education. Oxford: Oxford University Press; 2013. p. 186–200.

Beilock SL, Gray R. From attentional control to attentional spillover: a skill-level investigation of attention, movement, and performance outcomes. Hum Mov Sci. 2012;31(6):1473–99.

Bennett RE. Formative assessment: a critical review. Assess Educ: Princ Policy Pract. 2011;18(1):5–25.

Bingham GP. The role of perception in timing: feedback control in motor programming and task dynamics. In: Covey E, Hawkins HL, Port RF, editors. Neural representation of temporal patterns. Boston: Springer; 1995.

Bloom B, Englehart M, Furst E, Hill W, Krathwohl D, et al. Taxonomy of educational objectives: the classification of educational goals. Handbook I: cognitive domain. New York: Longmans, Green; 1956.

Bowyer MW, Kuhls DA, Haskin D, Sallee RA, Henry SM, Garcia GD, Luchette FA, et al. Advanced surgical skills for exposure in trauma (ASSET): the first 25 courses. J Surg Res. 2013;183(2):553–8.

Bowyer MW, Andreatta PB, Armstrong JH, Remick K, Elster EA, et al. A novel paradigm for surgical skills training and assessment of competency. JAMA Surg. 2021;156(12):1103–1109

Brackmann MW, Andreatta P, McLean K, Reynolds R. Teaching and assessing laparoscopic camera navigation: validation of a novel box-trainer simulator. Surg Endosc. 2017;31(7):3033–9.

Cate TJ, De Haes JCJM. Summative assessment of medical students in the affective domain. Med Teach. 2000;22(1):40–3.

Certification Examinations. American Board of Orthopaedic Surgery. 2021. https://www.abos.org/certification/. Accessed 19 May 2021.

Certifications & Examinations. Alliance for physician certification & advancement. 2021. https://www.apca.org/certifications-examinations/. Accessed 19 May 2021.

Clark MS, Fiske ST. Affect and cognition. Hillsdale: Lawrence Erlbaum Associates; 1982.

CPR & ECC. American Heart Association. 2021. https://cpr.heart.org/en. Accessed 19 May 2021.

Darzi A, Datta V, Mackay S. The challenge of objective assessment of surgical skill. Am J Surg. 2001;181:484.

Dave RH. Psychomotor levels. In: Armstrong RJ, editor. Developing and writing behavioral objectives. Tucson/Arizona: Educational Innovators Press; 1970.

de Haes JCJM, Oort FJ, Hulsman RL. Summative assessment of medical students' communication skills and professional attitudes through observation in clinical practice. Med Teach. 2005;27(7):583–9.

de Virgilio C, Yaghoubian A, Kaji A, Collins JC, Deveney K, Dolich M, Easter D, Hines OJ, Katz S, Liu T, Mahmoud A, Melcher ML, Parks S, Reeves, Salim A, Scherer L, Takanishi D, Waxman K, et al. Predicting performance on the American Board of Surgery Qualifying and Certifying Examinations: a multi-institutional study. Arch Surg. 2010;145(9):852–6.

Dougherty P, Andreatta P. Competency based education-how do we get there? Clin Orthop Relat Res. 2017;475(6):1557–60.

Edwards MJ, White CE, Remick KN, Edwards KD, Gross KR, et al. Army general surgery's crisis of conscience. J Am Coll Surg. 2018;226(6):1190–4.

Elster EA, Andreatta PB, Ritter EM, Galante J, Bowyer MW. et al. Preliminary clinical readiness outcomes from the KSA program for the advancement of forward surgical care. Military Health System Research Symposium (MHSRS). Bethesda, MD. August 2020.

Ericsson KA, Krampe R, Th., & Tesch-Roemer C. The role of deliberate practice in the acquisition of expert performance. Psychological Review, 1993;100, 363–406.

Etchells E, O'Neill C, Bernstein M. Patient safety in surgery: error detection and prevention. World J Surg. 2003;27:936–41.

Faulkner H, Regehr G, Martin J, Reznick R. Validation of an objective structured assessment of technical skill for surgical residents. Acad Med. 1996;71:1363.

Fleishman EA, Parker JF Jr. Factors in the retention and relearning of perceptual-motor skill. J Exp Psychol. 1962;64(3):215–26.

FLS Program Description. Fundamentals of laparoscopic surgery. 2021. https://www.flsprogram.org. Accessed 19 May 2021.

General Surgery In-Service Examination. American College of Osteopathic Surgeons. 2021. https://www.facos.org/OS/Navigation/Education/Residents/Inservice_Examination.aspx. Accessed 19 May 2021.

Gist ME, Bavetta AG, Stevens CK. Transfer training method: its influence on skill generalization, skill repetition, and performance level. Pers Psychol. 1990;43(3):501–23.

Harlen W, James M. Assessment and learning: differences and relationships between formative and summative assessment. Assess Educ: Princ Policy Pract. 1997;4(3):365–79.

Harrow AJ. A taxonomy of the psychomotor domain. New York: David McKay; 1972.

Hockey GRJ. Compensatory control in the regulation of human performance under stress and high workload: a cognitive-energetical framework. Biol Psychol. 1997;45(1–3):73–93.

Hodges B. Validity and the OSCE. Med Teach. 2003;25(3):250–4.

Hodges BD, Ginsburg S, Cruess R, Cruess S, Delport R, Hafferty F, Ho M-J, Holmboe E, Holtman M, Ohbu S, Rees C, Cate O, Tsugawa Y, Van Mook W, Wass V, Wilkinson T, Wade W, et al. Assessment of professionalism: recommendations from the Ottawa 2010 conference. Med Teach. 2011;33(5):354–63.

In-Service Exam. American Osteopathic Association Neurosurgery. 2021. http://aoaneurosurgery.org/in-service.html. Accessed 19 May 2021.

In-Service Exams for Residents. American Society of Plastic Surgeons. 2021. https://www.plasticsurgery.org/for-medical-professionals/education/events/in-service-exam-for-residents. Accessed 19 May 2021.

In-Training Examination. American Board of Surgery. 2021. https://www.absurgery.org/default.jsp?certabsite. Accessed 19 May 2021.

Jones AT, Biester TW, Buyske J, Lewis FR, Malangoni MA, et al. Using the American Board of Surgery In-Training Examination to predict board certification: a cautionary study. J Surg Educ. 2014;71(6):e144–8.

Joshi ART, Salami A, Hickey M, Barrett KB, Klingensmith ME, Malangoni MA, et al. What can SCORE web portal usage analytics tell us about how surgical residents learn? J Surg Educ. 2017;74(6):e133–7.

Kahneman D. Attention and effort. Englewood Cliffs: Prentice-Hall; 1973.

Kaufman H, Wiegand RL, Tunick RH. Teaching surgeons to operate – principles of psychomotor skills training. Acta Neurochir. 1987;87:1–7.

Kenny DT. The role of negative emotions in performance anxiety. In: Juslin P, Sloboda J, editors. Handbook of music and emotion: theory, research, applications. Oxford, UK: Oxford University Press; 2009.

Krathwohl D. A revision of Bloom's taxonomy: an overview. Theory Pract. 2002;41(4):212–8.

Krathwohl DR, Bloom BS, Masia BB. Taxonomy of educational objectives: handbook 2. Affective domain. New York: David McKay; 1964.

Mackenzie CF, Tisherman SA, Shackelford S, Sevdalis N, Elster E, Bowyer MW, et al. Efficacy of trauma surgery technical skills training courses. J Surg Educ. 2019;76(3):832–43.

Madlock PE, Booth-Butterfield M. The influence of relational maintenance strategies among coworkers. J Bus Commun. 2012;49(1):21–47.

Maintaining Certification (MOC) American Board of Internal Medicine. 2021. https://www.abim.org/maintenance-of-certification/. Accessed 19 May 2021.

Maurer H, Munzert J. Influence of attentional focus on skilled motor performance: performance decrement under unfamiliar focus conditions. Hum Mov Sci. 2013;32(4):730–40.

McCaskie AW, Kenny DT, Deshmukh S. How can surgical training benefit from theories of skilled motor development, musical skill acquisition and performance psychology? Med J Aust. 2011;194(9):463–5.

Messick S. Validity. In: Linn RL, editor. Educational measurement. 3rd ed. New York: American Council on Education and Macmillan; 1989. p. 13–103.

Miller GE. The assessment of clinical skills/competence/performance. Acad Med. 1990;65:S63–7.

Milton J, Solodkin A, Hlutík P, Small SL. The mind of expert motor performance is cool and focused. NeuroImage. 2007;35:804–13.

Mini-CEX: Mini-Clinical Evaluation Exercise. American Board of Internal Medicine. 2021. https://www.abim.org/Media/qlvp1fhb/mini-cex.pdf. Accessed 19 May 2021.

Moss PA. Shifting conceptions of validity in educational measurement: implications for performance assessment. Rev Educ Res. 1992;62(3):229–58.

Newell KM, Ranganathan R. Instructions as constraints in motor skill acquisition. In: Renshaw I, Davids K, Savelsbergh GJP, editors. Motor learning in practice: a constraints-led approach. London: Routledge; 2010. p. 17–32.

Nguyen J, Liu A, McKenney M, Elkbuli A. Predictive factors of first time pass rate on the American Board of Surgery Certification in general surgery exams: a systematic review. J Surg Educ. 2021; S1931–7204(21)00020–9.

Norcini J. Workplace assessment. In: Swanwick T, editor. Understanding medical education: evidence, theory and practice. 2nd ed. Hoboken: Wiley; 2013. p. 279–92.

Norcini JJ, Blank LL, Duffy FD, Fortna GS. The mini-CEX: a method for assessing clinical skills. Ann Intern Med. 2003;138(6):476–81.

Otolaryngology Training Examination (OTE). American Board of Otolaryngology- Head and Neck Surgery. 2021. https://www.aboto.org/ote.html. Accessed 19 May 2021.

Primary Certification in General Surgery. American Osteopathic Board of Surgery. Updated 2021. Accessed 19 May 2021. https://certification.osteopathic.org/surgery/certification-process-overview/general-surgery/.

Program Description. Fundamentals of endoscopic surgery. 2021. https://www.fesprogram.org/about/. Accessed 12 May 2021.

Regehr G, MacRae H, Reznick RK, Szalay D. Comparing the psychometrics properties of checklists and global rating scales for assessing performance on an OSCE-format examination. Acad Med. 1998;73(9):993–7.

Resident Performance Assessment. American Board of Surgery. 2021. https://www.absurgery.org/default.jsp?certgsqe_resassess. Accessed 12 May 2021.

Riketta M. The causal relation between job attitudes and performance: a meta-analysis of panel studies. J Appl Psychol. 2008;93(2):472–81.

Ritter EM, Taylor ZA, Wolf KR, Franklin BR, Placek SB, Korndorffer JR, Gardner AK. Simulation-based mastery learning for endoscopy using the endoscopy training system: a strategy to improve endoscopic skills and prepare for the fundamentals of endoscopic surgery (FES) manual skills exam. Surg Endosc. 2018;32:413–20.

Rogers MJ, Zeidan M, Flinders ZS, Presson AP, Burks R. Educational resource utilization by current orthopaedic surgical residents: a nation-wide survey. J Am Acad Orthop Surg Glob Res Rev. 2019;3(4):e041.

Sadler DR. Formative assessment and the design of instructional systems. Instr Sci. 1989;18:119–44.

Sardzoska EG, Tang TLP. Work-related behavioral intentions in Macedonia: coping strategies, work environment, love of money, job satisfaction, and demographic variables. J Bus Ethics. 2012;108:373–91.

SCORE Curriculum Outline for General Surgery. Surgical Council on Resident Education. 2020–2021. http://files.surgicalcore.org/2020-2021_GS_CO_Booklet_v3editsfinal.pdf. Accessed 19 May 2021.

Scott DJ, Hafford M, Willis RE, Gugliuzza K, Wilson TD, Brown KM, Vansickle KR. Ensuring competency: are fundamentals of laparoscopic surgery training and certification necessary for practicing surgeons and operating room personnel? Surg Endosc. 2013;27(1):118–26.

Shah D, Haisch CE, Noland SL. Case reporting, competence, and confidence: a discrepancy in the numbers. J Surg Educ. 2018;75(2):304–12.

Song S. Consciousness and the consolidation of motor learning. Behav Brain Res. 2009;196:180–6.

Specialty and Subspecialty Certificates. American Board of Medical Specialties. 2021. https://www.abms.org/member-boards/specialty-subspecialty-certificates/. Accessed 19 May 2021.

Sroka G, Feldman LS, Vassiliou MC, Kaneva PA, Fayez R, Fried G. Fundamentals of laparoscopic surgery simulator training to proficiency improves laparoscopic performance in the operating room – a randomized controlled trial. Am J Surg. 2010;199:115–20.

The Accreditation Council for Graduate Medical Education. Surgery Milestones. Second Revision: January 2019. https://www.acgme.org/Portals/0/PDFs/Milestones/SurgeryMilestones.pdf. Accessed 19 May 2021.

Training & Certification. The American Board of Surgery. 2021. https://www.absurgery.org/default.jsp?certcehome. Accessed 19 May 2021.

Tyler JA, Ritchie JD, Leas ML, Edwards KD, Eastridge BE, White CE, Knudson MM, Rasmussen TE, Martin RR, Blackbournes, et al. Combat readiness for the modern military surgeon: data from a decade of combat operations. J Trauma Acute Care Surg. 2012;73(2 Suppl 1):S64–70.

Vassiliou MC, Dunkin BJ, Fried GM, Mellinger JD, Trus T, Kaneva P, Lyons C, Korndorffer JR Jr, Ujiki M, Velanovich V, Kochman ML, Tsuda S, Martinez J, Scott DJ, Korus G, Park A, Marks JM, et al. Fundamentals of endoscopic surgery: creation and validation of the hands-on test. Surg Endosc. 2014;28(3):704–11.

Wiggins G. Educative assessment: designing assessments to inform and improve student performance. San Francisco: Jossey-Bass; 1998.

Wilson AB, Choi JN, Torbeck LJ, Mellinger JD, Dunnington GL, Williams RG, et al. Clinical Assessment and Management Examination – Outpatient (CAMEO): its validity and use in a surgical milestones paradigm. J Surg Educ. 2015;72(1):33–40.

Winer LK, Cortez AR, Kassam A, Quillin RC, Goodman MD, Makley AT, Sussman JJ, Kuethe JW, et al. The impact of a comprehensive resident curriculum and required participation in "this week in SCORE" on general surgery ABSITE performance and well-being. J Surg Educ. 2019;76(6):e102–9.

Wulf G, Shea C, Lewthwaite R. Motor skill learning and performance: a review of influential factors. Med Educ. 2010;44:75–84.

Programmatic Assessment in Health Professions Education

62

Iris Lindemann, Julie Ash, and Janice Orrell

Contents

Introduction	1204
Programmatic Assessment for Learning	1204
Assessment and Feedback are Aligned with Program-level Learning Outcomes and Longitudinal Development of Integrated Competencies	1206
Program Design and Educational Processes Focus on Accumulated Informational Assessments	1208
Feedback to Students on their Progress is a Pivotal Educational Process	1210
Students are Coached to be Effective Self-Regulated Learners	1211
Progress Decision-Making Moments are Fewer and not Bound to Single Assessment Activities	1215
Making PAL Work	1216
Conclusion	1218
Cross-References	1218
References	1218

Abstract

This chapter recounts the learning gained by a group of assessment developers in one Australian medical education program as they implemented a comprehensive approach to curriculum development supporting greater emphasis on assessment as, and for, learning. This was a major work that challenged the dominant culture of a psychometric approach to assessment *of* learning. This chapter describes programmatic assessment for learning (PAL) (not to be confused with peer-assisted learning) which is a curriculum approach that uses a diverse range of assessment tasks that, over time, generates comprehensive information to inform students and educators of students' progress towards achieving whole-of-program learning outcomes. This information assists students in developing and prioritizing their learning plans. The PAL curriculum approach constitutes a

---

I. Lindemann (✉) · J. Ash · J. Orrell
Prideaux Centre for Health Professions Education, Flinders University, Adelaide, SA, Australia
e-mail: iris.lindemann@gmail.com; julie.ash@flinders.edu.au; janice.orrell@flinders.edu.au

© Springer Nature Singapore Pte Ltd. 2023
D. Nestel et al. (eds.), *Clinical Education for the Health Professions*,
https://doi.org/10.1007/978-981-15-3344-0_79

significant cultural shift and requires a significant change in understanding the educational role of assessment for curriculum designers, academic teachers, university policy makers, and students alike. This chapter will describe the persuasive benefits for adopting a PAL curriculum and recount the challenges and barriers that were experienced by those involved in the process of implementation.

Keywords

Programmatic assessment · Programmatic assessment for learning · Assessment · Feedback · Learning coach

Introduction

This chapter provides a rich description of an emerging approach to curriculum design called programmatic assessment for learning (PAL). This approach to curriculum development utilizes end-of-program-level learning outcomes as its core element and assessment as an enabler rather than a measure of learning. In describing PAL, this chapter will identify the essential elements for adopting this curriculum approach and discuss the benefits and the challenges inherent in introducing PAL and in confronting the significant cultural shift required by all of its stakeholders.

Programmatic Assessment for Learning

Programmatic assessment for learning (PAL) is a curriculum concept that originated in medical education (Schuwirth and van der Vleuten 2011; van der Vleuten and Schuwirth 2005; van der Vleuten et al. 2012) and is increasingly being adopted and adapted in other professional education programs of study (Bacon et al. 2018; Jamieson et al. 2017; Bok et al. 2013; Gadbury-Amyot and Overman 2018). PAL is not a new concept but is now "coming of age" as experts in medical education and education assessment are coming to the same conclusions about ways for assessment to drive effective learning, particularly in professions-based education (Torre et al. 2019).

Recent advances in quality assessment in medical education support a focus away from atomistic progress decisions based on individual assessment tools towards programs of assessment where feedback information from diverse individual assessment activities inform student decision-making about their learning efforts to support their achievement of program-level learning outcomes. PAL assessment processes recognize the complex integration of competencies required for the preparation of health professionals for practice and the need to draw credible conclusions about students' performance achievements from a broad base of evidence (van der Vleuten and Schuwirth 2005; Schuwirth and van der Vleuten 2019). Traditionally, in medical education especially, assessment evidence has been mainly drawn from objective testing tools that can be psychometrically analyzed for reliability and statistical inferences (Dijkstra et al. 2010). Problematically, this highly objective information tends to be least representative of the complexity inherent in professional practice. In contrast, highly authentic assessment, while valid, is often judged to be too "subjective" and, therefore, not reliable. Validity is the most important feature of assessment and yet assessment programs often sacrifice validity in order to achieve high levels of reliability (Knight 2000). There is growing support for using comprehensive, highly authentic, and valid assessment, including subjective evidence, or judgments, by professional experts, that can be collected systematically and inform credible and trustworthy assessment decisions (Schuwirth and van der Vleuten 2019; Driessen et al. 2012). In PAL, student responses to assessment judgments and feedback are essential contributions to assessment information. Student responses are collated in a dossier or portfolio as evidence of students' regular reviews and reports on their progress, and contribute to summative evaluation and progress decision-making.

PAL curricula have core key features that address contemporary critical educational challenges and are summarized in Box 1 below.

> **Box 1 A Summary of Key Features of PAL**
> Key features of **PAL** include the following attributes (Torre et al. 2019; Pearce and Prideaux 2019).
>
> - *Assessment and feedback are aligned with program-level learning outcomes and longitudinal development of integrated competencies.*
> - *Program design and educational processes focus on accumulated informational assessments.*
> - *Feedback to students on their progress is a pivotal educational process.*
> - *Students are coached to be effective self-regulated learners.*
> - *Assessment decisions and progress decisions are separated.*
> - *Progress decision-making moments are fewer and draw from the triangulation of multiple assessment outcomes from multiple assessment tools over time.*

Building these key education features of PAL into the curriculum requires adjustments to resourcing, assessment policies, and infrastructure to make implementation possible while offering opportunities for significant improvements in assessment and its impact on student uptake of feedback on their learning (Heeneman et al. 2015). Implementing PAL will require significant organizational change, including improved staff development opportunities. It also provides fertile educational research opportunities to improve the education of the next generation of health professionals.

The key features of PAL provided in Box 1 are now elaborated in the following discussion, with a focus on the benefits of a PAL curriculum as well as some of the challenges faced in implementing PAL in higher education and some of the key tools which make implementation more effective.

Assessment and Feedback are Aligned with Program-level Learning Outcomes and Longitudinal Development of Integrated Competencies

PAL requires the design of all program assessment activities and feedback to align with the end-of-program outcomes. Typically, the number of integrated outcomes that define a program are limited. There are no guidelines for the number of program-level learning outcomes which can be defined; however, it is important in PAL to limit the number of outcomes so that they are manageable for students and staff to understand and report on. Too many outcomes can result in assessment tasks compartmentalized into competencies, with the effect of losing the holistic and integrated nature of practice competence (Schuwirth and van der Vleuten 2019).

Unlike conventional assessment, in PAL, students can legitimately draw evidence of their progress in a program-level outcome from any assessment activities occurring within a designated time frame, regardless of the location of the assessment activity within the curriculum. To illustrate this, students may demonstrate their progress in an outcome such as "leadership," with evidence of their leadership from their research experiences, as well as from their clinical experiences. Students may also include leadership evidence from their external activities. Additionally, students in clinical placements may demonstrate their progress for an outcome such as communication, from a range of clinical observational feedback forms plus from documented peer feedback provided during tutorials. Such diverse sources of assessment evidence allow the capture of a holistic view of students' competence and their development of competence over time, rather than relying on a mere single snapshot within a specific component of a program.

An important difference between conventional and PAL curricula is the need for students to be able to readily access assessment information from different areas of their curriculum over time in order to demonstrate their competency. Multiple small study units which are all assessed separately can be a limiting factor to such assessment (The term study unit is used to mean a unit of study within the curriculum which traditionally has defined credit units and assessment activities. Different terms are used in different institutions such as topic, subject, module, or course.). Curriculum design is more usable when smaller study units are integrated into a single overarching study unit which may extend over a whole semester or even a year. However, for programs where curricula are currently divided into smaller study units within semesters and year levels, transitioning to PAL does not necessarily require a change to curriculum content. Rather, the change involves integration of existing content into larger study units. A more integrated curriculum enables student development towards program-level outcomes to be expressed as development over time using data from all areas of the curriculum, rather than from a summation of separate assessments from discrete study units. A more integrated curriculum also enhances students' abilities to monitor their development over time in important skills such as professionalism, communication, and leadership. These important aspects of professional practice are difficult to assess in one-off events, because their development occurs over time and is often difficult to isolate, identify, and develop within a single study unit.

Designing an integrated curriculum also allows for the use of longitudinal assessment tools, such as progress tests and portfolios. In medical education, progress testing has been used extensively to provide students with regular feedback on how their knowledge building is developing and the knowledge gaps they should address (Freeman et al. 2010; Tio et al. 2016). The progress test is a longitudinal knowledge test which measures student development of knowledge over the duration of a complete program. Progress tests are designed to assess the end-of-program level of knowledge and capabilities and yet are held regularly throughout the program, enabling students to monitor their knowledge development against a long-term goal. Longitudinal testing promotes focused attention to knowledge gaps, improves learning, and encourages retention of knowledge (van der Vleuten et al. 2012; Albanese and Case 2015). Longitudinal testing principles have also been applied to OSCE (objective structured clinical examination) clinical assessments with some promising results (Pugh et al. 2014, 2016).

Changing the design of curricula does not occur without challenges. Creating larger study units from small ones requires negotiation with university policy makers and accreditation bodies. Small, discrete study units which are separately assessed are the norm in higher education and are used to offer students wider choices in study unit selection as well as assisting students to manage the financial commitments of their study. Creating larger, integrated study units limits flexibility and student choice. However, it is not uncommon for health professional programs to limit study unit selection choice due to stringent accreditation requirements. In our experience, our rationale for successful negotiations with university policy makers and accreditation boards to achieve this integration was based on enhancing students' use of feedback and enhanced learning attainment of the required program outcomes.

In our experience, a negative aspect of changing the design of curricula was that it disrupted the allocated roles and responsibilities of study unit and program coordinators. Some existing study unit coordinators lost their titles, but not their roles, because they remained responsible for content areas, but without clear recognition. Thus, those responsible for content areas within an integrated PAL study unit need to have their responsibilities made explicit so these are recognized for workload and career advancement purposes. These aspects of change need to be clearly documented and agreed on, in guidelines for coordination and teaching roles, as part of the process of planning to implement PAL.

A prerequisite for implementing PAL is to have well-defined, publicly explicit, end-of-program learning outcomes that are communicated and accepted by all students and educators, in order for student progress to be effectively evaluated across all program-level learning outcomes. Thus, the establishment of an online curriculum database will provide access to the curriculum for all students and their educators across all locations, mapping learning across the curriculum towards the program-level learning outcomes. The curriculum database outlines and aligns the educational content, the teaching, learning, and assessment activities. It also provides pathways to achieving competency in all learning outcomes. This clarity of learning outcomes provides a substantial basis for dialogue about the academic program between the professions, their practitioners, and students. This dialogue is especially important in the clinical years when most clinical supervisors are not employed within university boundaries. Easy access to curriculum information allows workplace supervisors to more readily gain insight into what is being taught in health professions programs, to provide better, more relevant, and consistent feedback when they interact with students in clinical settings.

Program Design and Educational Processes Focus on Accumulated Informational Assessments

In PAL, students are provided with the opportunity to view their development longitudinally across all program-level learning outcomes **in a centralized online assessment database**. The assessment database aligns with information in the curriculum database, with each assessment activity clearly linked to program-level learning outcomes. The information in the assessment database is derived from all assessment results and feedback of assessment activities for each student which are documented, collected, and collated across all years of their study program. The assessment database is an important tool, providing an ongoing record of students' learning, enabling students to reflect and report accurately on their progress and ensures that progress can be verified by their learning coach.

Students are required to utilize the data in the assessment database to reflect on their feedback from individual assessment activities, to make plans for future learning, and to chart their progress over time for each program-level learning outcome. Students' responses to the feedback they have received is an important aspect of their assessment and, as such, they are required to regularly document their reflections and planning as well as improvements in their learning in a portfolio (see "Learning Portfolio" below).

Assessment activities are staged so students can identify gaps or difficulties in learning with ample time to remediate issues as they arise. Students can also engage in additional learning and assessment activities as they see fit to generate evidence of remediation in their portfolio. Since PAL enables and requires students to respond rapidly to identified learning challenges and provide ongoing evidence of their progress, at the end of the study unit, a student should have a very clear idea of their progress status.

If a student has significant and persistent learning difficulties in any area, they will be expected to have made efforts to address these issues and thus they will know if difficulties require more time. This makes pass-fail decisions less of a surprise for students or their educators as a students' levels of competence is likely to have been on discussed multiple occasions with them by the end of a study unit. In our experience, this aspect of a PAL approach contrasts sharply with traditional assessment, where students often experience a lack of timely feedback, and no explicit expectation that they will be accountable for acting on the feedback they receive and subsequently, poor results are often unexpected.

PAL is designed so that the delineation between formative and summative assessments is removed. All assessment is designed to be "informative" both for students and their educators. In PAL curricula, all informative assessment contributes to a final progress decision, usually at key progress decision points when each student's progress is evaluated, summarized, and judged.

In contemporary clinical settings, there is evidence that students continue to describe feedback as inadequate and unhelpful (Al-Mously et al. 2014; Daelmans et al. 2004; Maher et al. 2015; Noble et al. 2019). Feedback is often viewed as "telling" the student, with an expectation they will follow through on responding to the feedback and with the role of the student in feedback neglected (Molloy and Boud 2013). In PAL, students self-evaluate their assessment feedback and use this to enable further learning. The PAL assessment database enables those "lost" aspects of the curriculum to be reclaimed explicitly, as all significant feedback is documented, collected, collated, and used for learning and provides a rich source of evidence of a student's competency on which to base a final progress decision.

The Learning Portfolio

The learning portfolio is key to decision-making about students' progression. Students regularly analyze, integrate, and interpret their assessment feedback and make entries into their portfolio. A portfolio report is submitted prior to each learning coach meeting which summarizes the resulting learning in terms of how students perceive they are achieving the program-level learning outcomes. The portfolio report is structured in alignment with the program-level learning outcomes and provides a trail of evidence on their progress in each program learning outcome. The evidence which informs the portfolio report is based primarily on information from the assessment database, and hence students' portfolio reports can be verified by learning coaches who also have access to students' assessment information in the portfolio. Areas of discrepancy or omissions between information in the assessment database and the students' portfolio report can be discussed at learning coach meetings, often leading to useful learning. An electronic portfolio format provides advantages of access for students and staff across diverse locations and readily enables information to be recorded in succinct formats and to link relevant information. For example, students are able to provide a portfolio report, which they can verify by linking to relevant portfolio entries or to feedback from a specific assessment activity, which are also situated within the portfolio.

The portfolio report is the students' contribution to evidence of learning and is a key document determining student progress. Engagement in the portfolio and portfolio report allows students to exercise some control of their assessment, promoting agency (Schut et al. 2018). In addition to the portfolio report, the student portfolio includes recommendations for progression from the students' learning coach and relevant educators who have worked with the students. Formal program assessment documentation, such as a "statement of assessment methods," positions the portfolio as the primary assessment. Thus, students who do not engage with and produce evidence in the portfolio are at risk of not progressing.

In health professional programs, it is important to discuss privacy issues with students. Students need to understand what they can document in their portfolio. A student reflecting on a failure of workplace practice in their portfolio as a relevant learning experience may have concerns that they or others could be reported for negligent practice. Thus, programs need clear policy as to who can access student portfolio information and how this information can be used.

Feedback to Students on their Progress is a Pivotal Educational Process

PAL encourages students to seek and value high quality feedback, including feedback on how they can improve to meet program-level learning outcomes. Without such feedback, students' engagement in self-regulated learning will be limited, and as a consequence, they will have difficulty generating evidence of learning development which is needed for progression decisions. Often conventional assessment practice provides limited feedback to students on their performance with little expectation that students will act on it or provide evidence of having done so. For example, if student assessment is scored, they may receive minimal or no information on the basis for the score and little information about their areas of strength and weakness. Feedback is an essential element for student learning, however, only when this feedback is meaningfully used by the student to direct future learning (Boud and Molloy 2013) has feedback truly occurred.

Failure to provide meaningful feedback can be a significant stumbling block when implementing PAL. Assessment activities in which the assessor function of the clinical educator dominates their role as facilitator of learning are seen by students as providing poor quality feedback (Bok et al. 2013). Conversely, assessment activities which are relevant and which promote student agency enhance students' acceptance of feedback and their aspiration to improve (Harrison et al. 2016). Within a clinical setting, students often work with numerous clinical educators who are variable in their experience of clinical assessment and knowledge of the curriculum. Without faculty development in assessment, some educators may construe PAL's informative ongoing assessment practice as "formative assessment," which can lead to a casual attitude to assessment with provision of minimal relevant feedback (Bok et al. 2013). Formative assessment is different to informative assessment as the latter requires students to make meaning from feedback to inform the development of personal learning goals (Schuwirth and van der Vleuten 2019). Personal beliefs of assessment are often aligned with a summative assessment culture and may be difficult to change towards an assessment for learning culture (Harrison et al. 2017). To ensure high quality feedback, clinical educators and students need systematic learning opportunities on understanding assessment culture and on the provision of meaningful and informative feedback that students can apply usefully.

Students are Coached to be Effective Self-Regulated Learners

Most clinical education programs have program-level outcomes relating to students being self-directed, independent, or self-regulated learners, and this expectation is especially evident in the clinical learning setting (Teunissen and Westerman 2011; White 2007). Being a self-regulated learner is especially important in the clinical setting where the learning structure is generally more flexible than in the more familiar classroom setting. During placements, students need to navigate their learning in an unfamiliar setting, where their learning and assessment often takes second place to patient care, which can be challenging (Cooper et al. 2010).

Programmatic assessment is designed to require students to take ownership and responsibility for learning and assessment and demonstrate how they have achieved this in their portfolio. In the clinical setting, as in conventional curricula, students are provided with an overall plan of assessment activities with the student being responsible for ensuring these are completed to an adequate standard. In PAL, there is an expectation that students will arrange learning in response to both the feedback they receive and to their self-evaluation of their performance in assessment activities and their overall progress, to identify strengths and deficits in learning, and to make plans for ongoing learnings (Schuwirth and van der Vleuten 2019). Students are also required to document this progress.

The difference in PAL to more traditional assessment is that student progression is based on the evidence in their assessment portfolio which shows that they are:

1. Self-regulated learners and progressing in their capabilities as self-regulated learners.
2. Achieving the standard of competence required by their program as explicitly demonstrated in relation to program-level learning outcomes.

PAL ensures that students have an accurate perception of their progress towards and performance in all program-level learning outcomes and that they remediate any poor performance in any learning outcomes. Inaction on poor performance in a single learning outcome can be the basis for deferring a decision regarding a student's progression. This process makes the requirement explicit that all learning outcomes are to be achieved and ensures that poor performance in one learning outcome is not masked or compensated by good performance in other learning outcomes, as might happen when assessment results are simply summed. This condition makes PAL different to conventional assessment and empowers students as agents of their own learning. It is also critical that curricula and educators support students' abilities to demonstrate learning across all outcomes through careful integration of learning across the curricula.

Students need support to develop their deliberate learning capabilities (Colthorpe et al. 2019; Rascón-Hernán et al. 2019). Students experience multiple barriers in higher education to using feedback and subsequently may not know how to use feedback effectively (Noble et al. 2019; Winstone et al. 2016). Even self-regulating students may find they are not provided with opportunity to be agentic learners despite this being an explicit program requirement. Thus, the continual self-evaluation work in PAL can be tiring and stressful for students within a demanding curriculum. This is especially the case when PAL principles are not followed within the PAL curriculum (Heeneman et al. 2015). Changing existing cultures of assessment away from existing teaching practices, which cultivate student overreliance on their educators for knowing what to learn and when, is difficult to change at both a personal and organizational level (Harrison et al. 2017). In cases where PAL principles are not upheld, students can misguidedly perceive all assessments as summative assessment rather than treating each informative assessment activity as a learning moment. If students perceive each assessment as high-stakes summative tasks, they are then inclined to "learn to pass" rather than "learn to learn" (Heeneman et al. 2015).

The Role of the Learning Coach

In a PAL curriculum, ongoing support is provided to help students to understand what is required of them, including how to use feedback effectively and to self-regulate learning. To this end, PAL includes the provision of learning coaches as an essential element in the assessment infrastructure.

The learning coach role "moves a step beyond providing feedback and focuses upon identifying performance goals in response to feedback and developing plans to address them" (Armson et al. 2019). The PAL learning coach role requires full access to students' assessment results so they can assist students to interpret results and other feedback so students can develop their own strategies for ongoing learning. The learning coach advises students, especially in the early years on how they might manage and draft their portfolio report to address all the program-level learning outcomes.

The role of the learning coach in PAL is relatively new, and ongoing research reveals that effective coaching methods afford long-term benefits for learning. A literature review of coaching in medical education found academic benefits for student learning; however, the definitions of coaching varied considerably (Lovell 2018). The terms coaching and mentoring are often used interchangeably despite key differences, with coaching being more performance and goal oriented (Irby 2012). An evaluation of a newly established PAL program in veterinary medicine revealed students identified this support for student learning as important. Students reported that they highly valued individual meetings with a "mentor" who provided personalized guidance to "scaffold self-directed learning" (Bok et al. 2013). Medical students, similarly, valued the safe and trusted relationship with the coach in dealing with academic issues (Wolff et al. 2019).

The ideal approach in PAL is for students to meet at regular intervals throughout their program with a dedicated learning coach. Sustaining this relationship over time is important for the student and the coach to establish trust in the working relationship. Mentoring relationships may not always be positive experiences, as preexisting cultural and gender barriers and unconscious bias can emerge (Han and Ju 2019). Thus faculty development for coaches is important to build the critical skill set required to be an effective learning coach (Armson et al. 2019; Wolff et al. 2019; Meeuwissen et al. 2019) as this role is a less didactic than other educational roles (Gordon and Brobeck 2010).

Learning coaches generally are recruited from the existing pool of educators working with students in the medical program. There is some debate regarding whether learning coaches should be people involved in student assessment or not, because the learning coach role may be seen to conflict with the assessment role (Wolff et al. 2019; Cavalcanti and Detsky 2011). It can also be counter argued that having the additional assessment role can draw on the coach's long-term rich understanding of a student's progress. In reality, available staff and resources will likely determine who is selected to be a learning coach.

Training for learning coaches on both the role of coach and assessment is important because coaches who hold authoritarian concepts of teaching tend to experience more role conflict than those whose approach supports student-directed development and achievement (Meeuwissen et al. 2019). To address these concerns, there are benefits in appointing a coordinator for learning coaches who can provide ongoing training and support for learning coaches and ensure consistency in the coaching process, and in the evaluation of portfolios and feedback to students. The coordinator can also be catalytic in developing the learning coach role by creating a learning coach community of practice so that the coaches can learn more about the role from each other. The coordinator can also act as a point of contact for dealing with any issues arising such as help with difficulties.

The following case study (Box 2) is an illustration of the role of the learning coach. Students are fictional and examples are drawn from a compilation of learning coaching experiences.

Box 2 Case Study: Reflections of a Learning Coach (Ashley)

The second round of learning coach sessions is completed and Ashley, the learning coach, reflects on the progress of two students seen that day.

Ashley reflects:

Micky is progressing well, consistently using the strategies identified in their previous meeting to resolve group learning problems that had affected Micky's early assessment results. Micky was quietly happy with the PAL process and stated that having a learning coach was pretty cool and something Micky had not experienced before. What a transformation from miserable to confident in just 8 weeks.

Ashley's thoughts turned to the next student.

Max has been very dismissive of the entire portfolio process and his second submitted portfolio summary report showed this attitude had not changed.

(continued)

Box 2 (continued)

Recent assessment feedback recorded in the assessment database indicated Max is performing poorly in a number of learning outcomes and is an "at-risk" student. Also, Max's portfolio report does not reflect these poor performances.

Ashley has reinforced the assessment-for-learning process, encouraging Max to reflect on his portfolio report and whether it considered all his assessment feedback. They then looked together at his assessment feedback and Ashley prompted Max to consider what strategies might address the concerns identified. Max agreed he needed to respond to his feedback and use his portfolio to reflect and work out better strategies for learning. But Max was also resentful. *"I've always gotten good marks in the past, medicine's a bit more intense, so really I just need to study harder and memorise the stuff."* Max also divulged that he was homesick and that this was affecting his study and possible strategies to address this were discussed. Ashley was still concerned, but thought there had been a step forward.

After the subsequent learning coach meeting, Ashley prepared a progression recommendation for each student to submit to the Progress Review Board. Micky was clearly ready to progress. Mickey's portfolio report accurately reflected on feedback received and demonstrated a capacity to learn from feedback. Mickey's feedback also indicated a satisfactory standard of competence had been met. These factors together represented an overall satisfactory performance and a recommendation to progress.

Max, however, had not followed through on plans made at the previous meetings. Max's portfolio report entries were sparse and shallow and continued to overlook feedback received. Max's report did not address all learning outcomes, and learning development was addressed only in one learning outcome related to knowledge building. This is despite Max's feedback on assessments in the assessment database continuing to reveal an unsatisfactory standard across a number of learning outcomes.

The learning coach process enables coaches to offer remediation and Ashley decide to meet with Max again to ensure he understood why he was at risk of not progressing. Ashley wanted to ensure Max understood that the progression decision was based on a holistic judgment of Max's progress and not only marks achieved in assessments. Max took the meeting seriously and undertook the agreed actions. Two weeks later, Max resubmitted a portfolio report which addressed the concerns discussed and included a realistic plan for future learning. Max was recommended to progress; however, he was flagged as an "at-risk" student which meant this decision was reviewed by a nominated academic, before formal submission to the Progress Review Board.

Progress Decision-Making Moments are Fewer and not Bound to Single Assessment Activities

In programmatic assessment, high-stakes decisions about student progression are not based on any single assessment outcome, rather they are based on an aggregation of:

- Information and outcomes from students' individual assessment activities collated in the assessment database (multiple assessment activities and multiple assessors) across a designated study unit.
- Student portfolio report which provides a summary of evidence from portfolio entries and assessment outcomes. It also includes students' reflective evaluation of their own achievement of required learning including their critique, analysis, planning, monitoring, adapting, and reflecting on learning.
- Students' evidence of outcomes of any additional learning and assessment undertaken, for example, after a poor assessment performance or after self-evaluating overall gaps and improvements needed from accumulated assessment evidence in the portfolio.
- Evaluations from significant educators who have worked with the student (including the learning coach).
- Other evidence of learning as applicable.

The portfolio provides the student with some choice as to what they include as evidence of learning and how they present this. The approach to assessment encourages students to engage in prescribed assessment, as it becomes clear to them that it is in their best interest to use assessment activities as learning experiences and to use their portfolio to demonstrate their developing competence and achievement of the program-level learning outcomes. Students successful navigation of this process is dependent on the clear alignment between the assessment activities and the articulation of the curriculum and program-level learning outcomes.

The Progress Review Board

In PAL, progression decisions are made by a Progress Review Board (PRB), comprising a team with expertise in programmatic assessment, the curriculum, assessment requirements, and the standards required for progression. The PRB requires clear policies and procedures which determine the decision-making processes and membership (Tweed and Wilkinson 2019). All information presented in the assessment database and in the student's portfolio is considered by the PRB, and this information is considered holistically in making a final decision as to whether a student is ready to progress to the next stage of their program. Given the large body of evidence available on each student, the progress decision can be considered to be valid, trustworthy, credible, and comprehensive. It can be argued that this is a fairer judgment process than in traditional assessment because the resulting progress decision is based on students' entire learning journey and does not hinge on single high-stakes assessments or exam results. The use of a wide variety of assessment information and use of an PRB, which is an expert panel, to make progress decision in PAL, might be criticized as an approach that is subjective in comparison to more objective methods, such as collation of marks, which are often perceived to be more reliable and defensible. It can be counter argued, however, that no assessment is ever truly objective because most rely on the expert judgment of a single assessor, who is asked to interpret performance into numeric scales or marks. Reliable assessment judgments can only be made if there is sufficient information upon which judgments are based and if the assessor has the appropriate expertise (Schuwirth et al. 2017). Both of these conditions are met through the use of the PRB and through the review of comprehensive assessment information for progression decisions, and thus PAL can be argued as reliable and defensible.

While it may seem an overwhelming amount of work for the PRB to fully review each student's portfolio, in practice, the decision for most students' progressions is clear, either to progress or not, requiring minimal deliberation by the panel. Few students' progression will be in doubt or contestable, and where doubt arises, time is required for the PRB to consider all the available evidence before coming to a final decision. Evidence from one school using programmatic assessment revealed assessment information contained in the portfolio enabled high consensus between assessors, adding support to the portfolio assessment process (de Jong et al. 2019).

Allowing assessment tasks and progress decisions to occur at separate times is a unique feature of PAL. This concept is challenging for some educators to accept as plausible, especially where there is a tradition of valuing one-off and high-stakes examinations as critical to assess end-point knowledge and skills building. Conventional assessment decisions rely on the collation of numbers to determine final progress decisions. In PAL, scores are still important; however, they are valuable information considered alongside narrative reports of a student's performance in making any high-stakes decisions. Rather than a process of weighting and adding scores, the PRB looks for evidence of students' engagement in achieving each program-level learning outcome. This of course is an important capability in a health professional career.

Making PAL Work

It is evident that implementing PAL requires a significant paradigm shift in understanding how curricula are designed and how assessments are structured and supported. The paradigm shift that PAL entails in assessment practice requires time and effort to communicate to students, educators, and administrators. It is critical to build a pervasive culture of assessment for learning in which emphasis on the learning function of assessment is placed in all aspects of the program. Without this emphasis, students will likely judge some assessments as more important than others for progression decisions and start behaving in ways which are undesirable for their learning. There is evidence from PAL programs that when the learning environment is not fully supportive of PAL, students can become confused about the purpose of assessment and can increasingly view informative assessments as summative (Bok et al. 2013; Heeneman et al. 2017). There is also evidence that in some cases, clinical supervisors become resistant to changing their approach to assessment to emphasize feedback, in contrast to their preference to give just a pass – fail grade. Some feel in doing so they are relinquishing their influence as assessors (Bok et al. 2013).

Developing a new culture of assessment which prioritizes learning requires clear articulation of the curriculum and alignment of the many players who design, influence, and engage in assessment with students. Recent studies in PAL emphasize that curriculum design needs to be true to the underlying principles of PAL for educational advantages to flow to students and that faculty development and student training, especially in the delivery and use of quality feedback are critical aspects of PAL implementation (Heeneman et al. 2015; Schut et al. 2018). Adaptation to this different assessment paradigm requires ensuring that clear assessment expectations are communicated and that a safe culture of assessment is fostered in which student agency in assessment is promoted and students and their educators are supported in the process of change.

A decision to implement PAL requires long-term vision and investment, since the changes will impact all aspects of an education program. Resources will need to be redistributed to provide the infrastructure PAL requires. Such infrastructure will include reliable methods for collecting and collating assessment feedback, personnel and systems for supporting student self-regulation, and a PRB for progression decision-making. Not all of these resources are specific to PAL as they are evident in a range of educational settings; however, in combination, they are integral to its functioning. An additional advantage of both the curriculum and assessment databases is that they constantly generate information that can be used for internal program review, evaluation, and for external accreditation. This results in an integration of quality improvement and quality assurance processes into ongoing program management, rather than as stand-alone data generation events.

A framework for the design of programmatic assessment curricula emphasizes the critical role of central governance (Timmerman and Dijkstra 2017). It is critical that program and institutional leaders act as advocates and enablers supporting the implementation of PAL. As discussed earlier, an institutional assessment policy needs to support the essential features of PAL. A major change of leadership and unexpected changes to educational policy during implementation can disrupt the implementation if these are not understood fully.

Reflecting on the costs of PAL, van der Vleuten and Heeneman (2016) conclude that all assessment is costly, including programmatic assessment; however, programmatic assessment is affordable if the focus remains on what matters most for learning, such as student feedback and support, and defensible assessment decisions. This may mean foregoing some assessment activities, such as expensive high-stakes end-of-year examinations, which have limited value for student learning and arguably limitations for decision-making about student progress.

Conclusion

Implementing PAL is a complex sociocultural process that requires vision and opportunities, for educators and students to critically reflect on the prevailing hidden curriculum, including examining conceptions of assessment and its fundamental purposes and opportunity to problematize the processes that tacitly support the status quo. Key stakeholders need to be provided with the means and time to acquire a deep understand of what PAL is, and what it is not, since it will affect every element of the educational program. The positive benefits of introducing PAL is that it promotes student agency in developing self-regulated learning and is the means for more comprehensive and integrated program enhancement and quality assurance.

PAL makes the fundamental role of feedback consequential in the teaching and learning process. Teachers must build meaningful feedback into everything they do as well as helping students to develop into active participants in the feedback process. This is commonly recognized by researchers and practitioners as desirable but is rare in practice. Trust is another important aspect of PAL. Teachers and practitioners must trust students to be actively engaged and to self-manage their learning; then they will learn. This capacity to take responsibility for being the agents of their own learning is a feature of being a professional and is a capability and a disposition for the future careers of health practitioners. PAL enables this feature to become an authentic aspect of the conversation between curriculum designers, curriculum enablers, and students.

Cross-References

- Approaches to Assessment: A Perspective from Education
- Coaching in Health Professions Education: The case of Surgery
- Future of Health Professions Education Curricula
- Self-Regulated Learning: Focus on Theory
- Written Feedback in Health Sciences Education: "What You Write May Be Perceived as Banal"

References

Albanese M, Case S. Progress testing: critical analysis and suggested practices. Adv Health Sci Educ. 2015;21(1):221–34.

Al-Mously N, Nabil N, Al-Babtain S, Fouad Abbas M. Undergraduate medical students' perceptions on the quality of feedback received during clinical rotations. Med Teach. 2014;36(supl): S17–23.

Armson H, Lockyer J, Zetkulic M, Könings K, Sargeant J. Identifying coaching skills to improve feedback use in postgraduate medical education. Med Educ. 2019;53(5):477–93.

Bacon R, Kellett J, Dart J, Knight-Agarwal C, Mete R, Ash S, et al. A consensus model: shifting assessment practices in dietetics tertiary education. Nutr Diet. 2018;75(4):418–30.

Bok H, Teunissen P, Favier R, Rietbroek N, Theyse L, Brommer H, et al. Programmatic assessment of competency-based workplace learning: when theory meets practice. BMC Med Educ. 2013;13(1):1–9.

Boud D, Molloy E. Rethinking models of feedback for learning: the challenge of design. Assess Eval High Educ. 2013;38(6):698–712.

Cavalcanti R, Detsky A. The education and training of future physicians. Why coaches Can't be judges. JAMA. 2011;306(9):933–4.

Colthorpe K, Ogiji J, Ainscough L, Zimbardi K, Anderson S. Effect of metacognitive prompts on undergraduate pharmacy students' self-regulated learning behavior. Am J Pharm Educ. 2019;83(4):526–36.

Cooper L, Orrell J, Bowden M. Work integrated learning. Abingdon: Routledge; 2010.

Daelmans HEM, Hoogenboom RJI, Donker AJM, Scherpbier AJJA, Stehouwer CDA, van der Vleuten CPM. Effectiveness of clinical rotations as a learning environment for achieving competences. Med Teach. 2004;26(4):305–12.

de Jong L, Bok H, Kremer W, van der Vleuten C. Programmatic assessment: can we provide evidence for saturation of information? Med Teach. 2019;41(6):678–82.

Dijkstra J, Van der Vleuten C, Schuwirth L. A new framework for designing programmes of assessment. Adv Health Sci Edu. 2010;15(3):379–93.

Driessen E, van Tartwijk J, Govaerts M, Teunissen P, van der Vleuten CPM. The use of programmatic assessment in the clinical workplace: a Maastricht case report. Med Teach. 2012;34(3):226–31.

Freeman A, Van Der Vleuten C, Nouns Z, Ricketts C. Progress testing internationally. Med Teach. 2010;32(6):451–5.

Gadbury-Amyot C, Overman P. Implementation of portfolios as a programmatic global assessment measure in dental education. J Dent Educ. 2018;82(6):557–64.

Gordon S, Brobeck S. Coaching the Mentor: facilitating reflection and change. Mentoring Tutoring. 2010;18(4):427–47.

Han H, Ju A. The complexity of mentoring observed through engagement with programmatic assessment. Med Educ. 2019;53(6):542–4.

Harrison C, Könings K, Dannefer E, Schuwirth LT, Wass V, van der Vleuten C. Factors influencing students' receptivity to formative feedback emerging from different assessment cultures. Perspect Med Educ. 2016;5(5):276–84.

Harrison C, Könings K, Schuwirth L, Wass V, van der Vleuten C. Changing the culture of assessment: the dominance of the summative assessment paradigm. BMC Med Educ. 2017;17(1):73–undefined.

Heeneman S, Oudkerk Pool A, Schuwirth L, van der Vleuten C, Driessen E. The impact of programmatic assessment on student learning: theory versus practice. Med Educ. 2015;49(5):487–98.

Heeneman S, Schut S, Donkers J, van der Vleuten C, Muijtjens A. Embedding of the progress test in an assessment program designed according to the principles of programmatic assessment. Med Teach. 2017;39(1):44–52.

Irby B. Editor's overview: mentoring, tutoring, and coaching. Mentoring Tutoring. 2012;20(3):297–301.

Jamieson J, Jenkins G, Beatty S, Palermo C. Designing programmes of assessment: a participatory approach. Med Teach. 2017;39(11):1182–8.

Knight P. The value of a Programme-wide approach to assessment. Assess Eval High Educ. 2000;25(3):237–51.

Lovell B. What do we know about coaching in medical education? A literature review. Med Educ. 2018;52(4):376–90.

Maher J, Pelly F, Swanepoel E, Sutakowsky L, Hughes R. The contribution of clinical placement to nutrition and dietetics competency development: a student-centred approach. Nutr Diet. 2015;72(2):156–62.

Meeuwissen S, Stalmeijer R, Govaerts M. Multiple-role mentoring: mentors' conceptualisations, enactments and role conflicts. Med Educ. 2019;53(6):605–15.

Molloy E, Boud D. Changing conceptions of feedback. In: Boud D, Molloy E, editors. Feedback in higher and professional education. Oxon: Routledge; 2013. p. 11–33.

Noble C, Billett S, Armit L, Collier L, Hilder J, Sly C, et al. "It's yours to take": generating learner feedback literacy in the workplace. Adv Health Sci Educ. 2019;25(1):55–74.

Pearce J, Prideaux D. When I say … programmatic assessment in postgraduate medical education. Med Educ. 2019;53(11):1074–6.

Pugh D, Touchie C, Wood T, Humphrey-Murto S. Progress testing: is there a role for the OSCE? Med Educ. 2014;48(6):623–31.

Pugh D, Bhanji F, Cole G, Dupre J, Hatala R, Humphrey-Murto S, et al. Do OSCE progress test scores predict performance in a national high-stakes examination? Med Educ. 2016;50:351–8.

Rascón-Hernán C, Fullana-Noell J, Fuentes-Pumarola C, Romero-Collado A, Vila-Vidal D, Ballester-Ferrando D. Measuring self-directed learning readiness in health science undergraduates: a cross-sectional study. Nurse Educ Today. 2019;83:104201.

Schut S, Driessen E, van Tartwijk J, van der Vleuten C, Heeneman S. Stakes in the eye of the beholder: an international study of learners' perceptions within programmatic assessment. Med Educ. 2018;52(6):654–63.

Schuwirth LWT, van der Vleuten CPM. Programmatic assessment: from assessment of learning to assessment for learning. Med Teach. 2011;33(6):478–85.

Schuwirth L, van der Vleuten CPM. How 'testing' has become 'programmatic assessment for learning'. Health Prof Educ. 2019;5(3):177–84.

Schuwirth L, van der Vleuten C, Durning SJ. What programmatic assessment in medical education can learn from healthcare. Perspect Med Educ. 2017;6(4):211–5.

Teunissen P, Westerman M. Opportunity or threat: the ambiguity of the consequences of transitions in medical education. Med Educ. 2011;45(1):51–9.

Timmerman A, Dijkstra J. A practical approach to programmatic assessment design. Adv Health Sci Educ. 2017;

Tio RA, Schutte B, Meiboom AA, Greidanus J, Dubois EA, Bremers AJA. The progress test of medicine: the Dutch experience. Perspect Med Educ. 2016;5(1):51–5.

Torre D, Schuwirth L, Van der Vleuten CPM. Theoretical considerations on programmatic assessment. Med Teach. 2019:1–8.

Tweed M, Wilkinson T. Student progress decision-making in programmatic assessment: can we extrapolate from clinical decision-making and jury decision-making? BMC Med Educ. 2019;19(1):176–undefined.

van der Vleuten C, Heeneman S. On the issue of costs in programmatic assessment. Perspect Med Educ. 2016;5(5):303–7.

van der Vleuten CPM, Schuwirth L. Assessing professional competence: from methods to programmes. Med Educ. 2005;39(3):309–17.

van der Vleuten CPM, Schuwirth L, Driessen E, Dijkstra J, Tigelaar D, Baartman LKJ, et al. A model for programmatic assessment fit for purpose. Med Teach. 2012;34(3):205–14.

White C. Smoothing out transitions: how pedagogy influences medical students' achievement of self-regulated learning goals. Adv Health Sci Educ. 2007;12(3):279–97.

Winstone N, Nash R, Rowntree J, Parker M. 'It'd be useful, but I wouldn't use it': barriers to university students' feedback seeking and recipience. Stud High Educ. 2016;42(11):2026–41.

Wolff M, Morgan H, Jackson J, Skye E, Hammoud M, Ross P. Academic coaching: insights from the medical student's perspective. Med Teach. 2019:1–6.

# Entrustable Professional Activities: Focus on Assessment Methods

63

Andrea Bramley and Lisa McKenna

Contents

Introduction	1222
What is an EPA?	1222
Evolution of EPAs in Health Care	1223
Application of EPAs in Health Professional Education	1224
EPAs and Training Improvement	1228
EPAs and the Clinical Education Relationship	1228
Case Study 1	1229
Case Study 2	1230
Conclusion	1230
Cross-References	1231
References	1231

Abstract

This chapter describes the evolution and application of Entrustable Professional Activities (EPAs) an emerging concept in healthcare professional education and clinical assessment. Entrustable Professional Activities are observable actions that define the work of a health care professional in a vocational context. They describe the duties or tasks that a competent health professional can do independently and are linked, usually in a matrix, to professional competency standards. As EPAs are defined and observable, they offer an additional and practical means of assessment of clinical skills in a workplace setting and are a valuable addition to other methods of clinical skill assessment such as Objective Structured Clinical Examinations (OSCEs) and simulations. EPAs have emerged from medicine and

A. Bramley (✉)
Department of Dietetics and Human Nutrition, La Trobe University, Melbourne, VIC, Australia
e-mail: a.bramley@latrobe.edu.au

L. McKenna
School of Nursing and Midwifery, La Trobe University, Melbourne, VIC, Australia
e-mail: l.mckenna@latrobe.edu.au

© Springer Nature Singapore Pte Ltd. 2023
D. Nestel et al. (eds.), *Clinical Education for the Health Professions*,
https://doi.org/10.1007/978-981-15-3344-0_82

their use is expanding to other disciplines such as nursing, medical specialties and allied health professions such as dietetics and pharmacy. In this chapter, strategies for defining, describing and assessing EPAs are presented. Inherent in EPAs is the concept of trust which can be used as a framework to develop an educational alliance between learner and supervisor. The degree of independence or the level of trust a supervisor might have in a trainee can fluctuate in a dynamic clinical environment with trust being inversely related to clinical risk. Furthermore, the level of trust given to a trainee will be influenced by the behavior of the trainee or the intrinsic propensity to trust present within a supervisor. Being a key concept in EPAs, this chapter concludes by exploring the concept of trust and how is this can enhance clinical supervision skills through exploring two case studies.

Keywords

Clinical assessment · Competency · Competency-based assessment · Entrustable professional activities · EPAs · Trust

Introduction

The use of competency-based education has been a predominant feature of health professional education for many decades. Many professions have mandated achievement of competency standards to regulate professional practice and as pre-requisite for initial registration in the specific field. While they have been a mainstay in health professions education, competency-based approaches have been critiqued as being difficult to measure and assess, having lack of shared understanding of performance expectations with focus on attributes, rather than technical skills performance (Pilj-Zieber et al. 2014; ten Cate 2013a). It is from this basis that the concept of entrustable professional activities (EPAs) emerged (ten Cate 2013a).

This chapter examines the rapidly evolving use of EPAs in health professional education. It outlines the evolution of EPAs and their relationship to competency development and examines how they have been used in health professions to the present time, including their application to clinical practice, learning and assessment. The chapter concludes with two case studies demonstrating how EPAs can be used in clinical practice contexts.

What is an EPA?

An EPA is essentially a professional task or responsibility entrusted to an individual to perform their role independently. In the case of the learner in a health profession, an EPA is entrusted to them by a clinical teacher or supervisor when they are deemed able to take on the associated responsibility (Ross 2015; Ten Cate and Scheele 2007). Hence, the concept of "trust" is inherent in EPAs and underpins their application in practice. Trust is a key component in the work of health professionals and underpins the delivery of safe, quality and effective care delivery. People receiving care must be able to trust the health professional, while health professionals must be able to trust each other, both inter- and intra-professionally in delivering effective, quality care (ten Cate 2013b). Hence, EPAs align well with health professional practice and responsibility and allow students in the disciplines to develop their associated necessary attributes.

It is necessary to explore how EPAs are different to competencies that have been previously used for many decades across health disciplines to assess professional practice. According to ten Cate (2013b), EPAs provide a mechanism by which competencies can be transferred into clinical practice. He views competencies as descriptors of the professional, while EPAs serve to describe the work performed by the professional. As a result, one EPA could incorporate a number of different competencies. For example, the EPA of "Developing and implementing a patient management plan" requires the performer to demonstrate performance in several CanMEDS roles; Medical expert, Communicator, Collaborator, Scholar and Health advocate (ten Cate et al. 2010, p. 672). Competencies, by their nature, encompass a broad scope of knowledge, skills and attitudes (Frank et al. 2010). On the other hand, EPAs constitute task lists required in particular contexts that can be readily observed. According to Moon et al. (2018), EPAs are developed for "tasks or responsibilities that are observable, executable, and measurable in process and outcome" (p. 1597a).

Evolution of EPAs in Health Care

Entrustable professional activities first emerged in 2005 (ten Cate 2005) in undergraduate medicine as a response to challenges encountered in implementing a competency framework into a curriculum (ten Cate and Scheele 2007). Prior to that time, education had been largely competency-based following broad introduction across many fields internationally in the 1990s. As introduced above, competency-based education focuses on individual elements of the health professional's knowledge, skills and attitudes. While important in development of the professional, competencies are general and do not describe the tasks that a particular professional needs to be able to do. Educational assessment strategies such as simulations and OSCEs are useful to assess clinical skills in an academic environment but may be resource intensive and pose logistical challenges (ten Cate and Scheele 2007). Hence, the gap between competencies and practice and the challenge of clinical skills assessment led to the development of EPAs (ten Cate 2018).

EPAs originally emerged from the United States where, in 2012, the Alliance for Academic Internal Medicine (AAIM) Educational Redesign Committee released a set of 16 proposed EPAs that all graduating internal medicine residents needed to be able to perform. In 2013, the Association of American Medical Colleges (AAMC) in the United States subsequently constituted a panel with a view to developing a set of fundamental behaviors that could be required of medical graduates, drive development of future medical curricula and guide the assessment of competence (Angus et al. 2017).

From our observations, EPAs are now being applied across a range of different health professions and are expanding from pockets of early adoption. There are now many increasing examples of the creation and use of EPAs outside of medicine including examples from pharmacy, dentistry, dietetics and nutrition and nursing. Wright and Capra (2017) describe the process of the development of EPAs in nutrition and dietetics education. In this example, academics and clinical educators used an iterative process to define 10 EPAs with each consisting of between 12 and 21 tasks or elements. Students reviewed the new methodology positively and reported a higher recognition of learning and skill development compared to previously used competency-based methods. An Australian national working party of dietetic academics and clinical educators has since been established to develop national consensus and further define milestones (Community of Practice for Dietetic Educators 2018). Beyond dietetics, Van Houwelingen et al. (2016) describe development of EPAs for the area of telehealth nursing, a specific area of nursing practice. Several authors also describe EPAs being developed for nurse practitioners (Foret Giddens et al. 2014; Bargagliotti and Davenport 2017; Hoyt et al. 2017). Significant work has also taken place in pharmacy practice in the USA, where Haines et al. (2017) describe the development of EPA for graduate pharmacists and suggest that there is potential for EPAs to be customized to different workplace settings or used to define and develop advanced practice roles (Pittenger et al. 2016).

EPAs can be used to describe entry level expectations, but they can also be layered to inform curricula for postgraduate specializations. Postgraduate training programs are time-based, and the development of EPAs can potentially inform the curriculum in different years of training programs. An example of this approach has been adopted by the Australian and New Zealand College of Psychiatry across each year of training in the psychiatry program (Boyce et al. 2011). The paper by Boyce et al. describes the approach of developing four EPAs for the first year of training with plans to develop specific EPAs for various rotations in subsequent years (Aimer et al. 2016). Other examples of EPAs in medical specialties include radiology (Ryan et al. 2017), gastroenterology (Rose et al. 2014), pathology (Powell and Wallschlaeger 2017), neonatology (Parker et al. 2017) and palliative medicine (Myers et al. 2015), just to name a few.

More recently, EPAs have been described as being developed for academic faculty development. Iqbal et al. (2018) conducted a review of EPA use in the education of health professional educators, finding only nine studies. Of these, only two demonstrated using EPAs in their training programs, one in a Master of Health Professions Education program in the United States, and the other in a Fundamental Teaching Activities program in Canada. Hence, while their use is not necessarily widespread as yet, it is expanding into new contexts.

Application of EPAs in Health Professional Education

EPAs present a practical and feasible method for providing assessment in a dynamic clinical environment by practicing clinicians who may not be educators or academics (Englander and Carraccio 2014). As EPAs describe the expected skills and work activities of the health professional, the development of a mutual understanding of expectations of the trainee/student and the assessor/supervisor is fostered. When an entrustment decision is made, the student is deemed able to perform the activity independently. The entrustment scale clearly describes student progress from dependence to independence promoting shared understandings of the expected level of performance. The learner is able to progress from observation to execution with decreasing levels of supervisor intervention until a level of mastery is reached where the learner then had the capacity to supervise more junior colleagues (ten Cate 2013b).

The Association of American Medical Colleges (AAMC) defined 13 essential EPAs that a graduate of a medical training program should be able to perform on the first day of their internship without supervision. This project was initially motivated by patient safety concerns, as it was known that the skills of new medical residents could be variable, and they were expected to perform a high range of tasks independently from the first day of their residency. The EPAs and an extensive toolkit with supporting materials are available online and the process of development has been published (Englander et al. 2016). The title of the EPAs, Core Entrustable Professional Activities for Entering Residency, is framed in a vocational manner and is relevant to undergraduate and graduate training pathways.

Several methods for developing EPAs and embedding them in curricula have been reported in the literature. A three-step process is described by Mulder et al. (2010) and is illustrated using an example from the Dietetic Program at La Trobe University Australia (Fig. 1):

Step 1 Select the EPAs
Step 2 Describe the EPAs
Step 3 Plan learning and assessment

Although this may seem quite straightforward, there are challenges associated with each step. The authors suggest starting from clinical practice and focusing on the desired outcomes of the health education training program (Mulder et al. 2010). Implicit in this step is that the profession is well defined with a clear scope of practice. Several methods have been described in the literature including the use of a working party consisting of clinicians, program directors, educators and health service researchers (Chang et al. 2013) or through the use of a Delphi approach (Hauer et al. 2013) sourcing input from educators and recent graduates. Although wide consultation is recommended, there may still be lack of buy-in by those who feel that EPA may not cover all aspects of the profession, or who feel that the EPAs reduce practice to a list of tasks. The number and range of EPAs may vary across disciplines and there is contention between EPAs being over-arching or specific to an area of practice (Chang et al. 2013). The range and number of EPAs varies, with Warm et al. (2014) noting that numbers of EPAs can range from five to 25, citing examples from internal medicine, psychiatry and pediatrics.

The second step of the process, describing the EPA is important to ensure clear links to competency frameworks and that there is sufficient information provided to

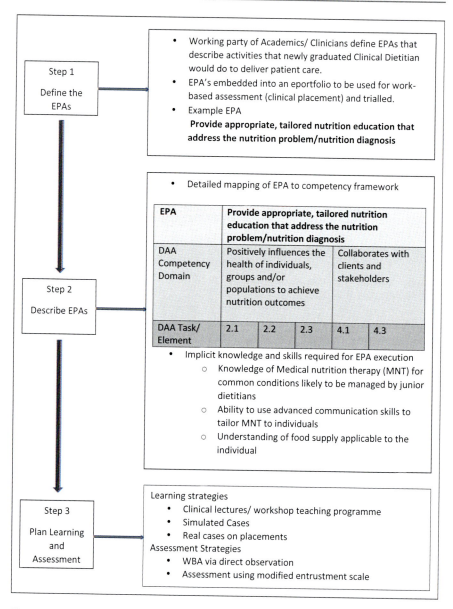

Fig. 1 Development and implementation of a Dietetics EPA using methodology described by Mulder et al. (2010)

students, academics and clinical educators or supervisors to be able to use them. It is also important that all domains of competence are covered by the developed EPAs. It may also be important to define those competencies that are essential to the individual EPA and those that would enhance proficiency or involve advanced practice. The use of milestones to describe behavioral performance of an EPA may also be advantageous with a clear description of a novice learner who would need a large amount of direct supervision and one of an independent learner who would not need the supervisor to be physically present in the room to perform the activity independently to the required standard (Englander et al. 2016; Haines et al. 2017). This is an important factor in building a shared vision of a work-ready professional between students, clinical supervisors and educators and communicates the desired learning outcomes.

The third step is not without challenge as well. Designing learning, such as providing opportunities to practice and develop skills, as well as the assessment of performance in the clinical setting, can be challenging and require careful planning and thought. In clinical placements or experiential learning, the types of learning opportunities or rotations need to be considered. Similarly, in the classroom, considered thought and planning are required to develop learning and assessment resources. Thompson et al. (2017) describe the process of developing five high fidelity case study simulations to inform assessment of the American Medical Colleges EPA 10, "Recognize a Patient Requiring Urgent or Emergent Care and Initiate Evaluation and Management" (Englander et al. 2014). Thompson et al. (2017) propose the simulation model to address concerns regarding patient safety and lack of real-world opportunity for students to practice and demonstrate this EPA which requires a deteriorating patient requiring emergency care.

An additional possible pitfall is the potential to formulate large lists of EPAs that may frustrate students and teachers, however if EPAs are too broad, they may lose their impact in assessment. Potential to mitigate these challenges may be through the use of the Observable Practice Activity (OPA), a smaller process or outcome-based examples of practice that can be viewed as a series of nesting dolls that fit into a bigger EPA (Warm et al. 2014). Warm et al. (2014, p. 1178) provide an example of an OPA, "minimize unfamiliar terms during patient encounters" that is mapped to the broader competency of communication skills. The specific description of the observable skill provides explicit instruction to both the learner and the teacher as to what is required in a specific work-based context.

As EPAs are vocationally oriented and immediately relatable in the workplace, inexperienced assessors are likely to be comfortable understanding and using them as they will be activities that they would perform as part of their current work. Peters et al. (2017) in describe their use of EPAs in medicine as a tool to develop learning goals that are explicit to students. As the concept of trust is central to EPAs, the use of student self-assessment regarding performance on an EPA can aid the supervisor to facilitate a conversation about why more supervision might be required in the case of an overconfident student and what might facilitate independence in an underconfident student. EPAs can be used for formative assessment, as well as summative assessment, and lend themselves to a longitudinal framework where, with continuing practice and feedback, the learner should progress up the scale of entrustment. O'Leary et al. (2016) describe a slightly different process with supervised learning events being used for formative assessment and EPAs for summative assessment in psychiatry. A challenge in using EPAs for assessment is that observation is required to inform entrustment but there may be little guidance as to how, when and who makes the observations and provides feedback (Tully et al. 2016). Similarly, Touchie et al. (2014) describe that differences in the level of supervision expected by subject matter experts was higher than that actually received by first year medical residents in their study. In addition to direct observation, feedback from other sources such as other health professionals or capturing the patient's perspective (Chang et al. 2013) should potentially be included when assessing an EPA.

EPAs and Training Improvement

There may be an important role for EPAs to drive improvements and inform the development of healthcare professional training programs in continual adaptation to meet ever-changing needs of the healthcare system. As Entrustable Professional Activities describe the work, an independent competent practitioner is expected to be able to do, any gaps in performance that students or recent graduates show can potentially be measured, analyzed and can help guide future curriculum and assessment design (Angus et al. 2017). EPAs also offer potential to guide expanding the professions and help with defining advanced practice roles, particularly in nursing and allied health.

EPAs and the Clinical Education Relationship

Intrinsic to the concept of EPAs is the concept of trust. Trust is important in healthcare and a key component of the relationship between patients and their clinicians, and between members of the multidisciplinary team. Patients "trust" that the person caring or treating them knows what they are doing, they can execute the clinical activity with competence and that the activity has a purpose or and desired effect. Healthcare workers understand the concept of trust, and this can be extended to enhance the relationship between the trainee and supervisor, potentially improving the learning environment (Damodaran et al. 2017).

As a result of the nature of the clinical learning environment, clinical education, supervision and assessment will always have an aspect of subjectivity, and therefore the potential for bias. Trust is separate to feelings of liking or disliking that may bias assessment and could be used to describe behaviors, rather than personal qualities, thereby decreasing some of the emotion that inevitably comes with being assessed or judged. The five-point entrustment scale rates students' performance on how much support is required by the supervisor to perform the task independently (ten Cate 2013b). Discussions around performance can be linked back to what is required to enable more trust and therefore, independence.

The use of EPAs can help students to identify areas of knowledge or skill deficiency and plan and develop targeted learning goals to increase independence. As EPAs are linked to multiple competencies, it is possible that a student may not yet possess one of the competencies that is required to perform the EPA independently. If a problem area can be identified and targeted, then detailed learning goals can be identified to bridge the gap. Furthermore, as EPAs are workplace specific, they can be useful for educators to provide orientation or training specific to that workplace context to enable autonomy (Carraccio et al. 2016).

How much autonomy or independence is granted to a learner is also dependent on the risk of the situation. Risk can be influenced by condition of the patient, nature of the clinical situation or factors in the clinical environment. These are extrinsic to the learner and can help learners to understand why they may be granted independence to perform an EPA in a certain situation, but not in another. It also important for supervisors to understand attainment of an EPA does not equal a fully developed health practitioner and that all students and graduates will continue to need feedback, particularly when starting a new practice area or in a healthcare setting that they are not experienced with (Haines et al. 2017). How much direct supervision a student receives depends of the amount of risk, the learning context and level of trust established in the relationship (Babbott 2010; Sterkenburg et al. 2010)

In addition to level of risk, the degree of trust in a learner can be influenced by the supervisor's style, with some people having a higher propensity to trust than others, a perceived or real gap in the knowledge or skill a student demonstrates or the professional behavior of the student (Damodaran et al. 2017). It is useful for supervisors to reflect on what student factors increase trust and to be able to explain these to students. For example, is it the ability of students to recall theory when questioned, is it the student using a standardized patient handover tool, or do they need to have a certain level of direct supervision or observation before they are sufficiently prepared to allow the student to be independent? The aim of clinical education is to progress the level of trust in the relationship to an agreed point, often to the point of post hoc or indirect supervision. Through a shared understanding of factors impacting trust, a space is created where students and educators can have meaningful conversation about how to increase trust and therefore achieve independence (Choo et al. 2014). From a student perspective, some students may thrive with close supervision and find this reassuring while others could find high levels of observation to undermine their confidence or increase anxiety. Discussing supervision and teaching styles can help students and supervisors connect and form an educational relationship with the objective of progressing the level of student independence. The following case studies examine how trust within the clinical education relationship might play out.

Case Study 1

A dietetics student is placed in a diabetes nutrition clinic with a new supervisor who has not supervised the student before. The handover from another supervisor is that this student has performed with autonomy all required aspects of a similar Type 2 diabetes focused nutrition clinic. A referral is received to see a 65-year-old gentleman with newly diagnosed Type 1 diabetes mellitus. The student has not assessed or provided education for a person with Type 1 DM before but feels confident to do so. Despite the slightly usual presentation of the referral, 65 years old is uncommon but not unheard of for a new diagnosis of Type 1 diabetes mellitus, the supervisor decides to allow the student to conduct the session and step in only as required.

During the appointment it becomes quickly apparent that the diabetes has been triggered by an immunotherapy regimen to treat cancer that was not apparent in the referral. In addition to the diabetes, the patient has underlying disease-related malnutrition and significant gastrointestinal side effects that will impact on nutrition management. The supervisor takes over and completes the consultation.

Following the consultation, the student expresses frustration and disappointment that they were not able to complete the consultation. Using the concepts of trust and clinical risk, the supervisor explains that the risks were much higher than initially assessed and that this reason (combined with the time pressures of an outpatient clinic) rather that the student's performance caused the decreased level of student autonomy. The supervisor reinforces that she would still trust the student to see less complex patients with post hoc supervision.

Case Study 2

A nursing student is deemed at risk of failing a clinical placement due to aspects of professional behavior. When observed with patients the student easily builds rapport, has excellent communication skills and implements appropriate interventions but often but not always rushes or skims over patient assessment and spends a lot of time talking to the multidisciplinary team socially.

During a formative assessment the clinical educator uses the framework of trust to provide feedback to the student. She explains that the student's inconsistency in approach to patient assessment decrease the trust that the supervisor has in the student's ability to correctly assess patients if presented with a new clinical condition or in a different healthcare setting. While the interventions have all been appropriate, the supervisor explains that if the clinical risk of the situation escalated, the supervisor would not have the confidence to trust the student to work independently in this situation. Similarly, conducting large amounts of social discussion with staff decreases the level of trust the supervisor has in the student coping with an increased workload. If the student had finished their work, then a behavior that would improve the trust between the student and supervisor would be for the student to contact the supervisor to provide handover and assign new work or learning activities.

Conclusion

The use of EPAs has potential to enhance practice-based education in all healthcare professions and is increasing. As they describe the work of professionals, EPAs help operationalize competency frameworks that may seem vague or abstract to clinicians responsible for providing clinical supervision and training. Although the process of creating, defining and assessing EPAs is not without challenges the potential benefits make them worth pursuing. A key reason why EPAs are worthwhile lies in the additional vocational assessment opportunities that will help inform programmatic assessment. EPAs and the trust framework create opportunities for feedback, and therefore improvement both for students individually and potentially for training programs. For students, using EPAs can help drive a targeted learning plan that is linked towards increasing independence. A trust framework can enhance the student/supervisor relationship and help move towards an environment of assessment for learning, as well as providing opportunities in assessment of learning. EPAs can help define professions and help build shared understandings of what entry level, and possibly graduate, practitioners should be able to do. For training programs, any performance gaps can be used to help improve student training and inform the curriculum to meet the workplace needs.

Cross-References

- Conversational Learning in Health Professions Education: Learning Through Talk
- Focus on Theory: Emotions and Learning
- Measuring Performance: Current Practices in Surgical Education
- Programmatic Assessment in Health Professions Education
- Supporting the Development of Professionalism in the Education of Health Professionals

References

Aimer M, de Beer W, Evans B, Halley E, Kealy-Bateman W, Lampe L, et al. Developing entrustable professional activities for the comptency-based fellowship program for psychiatry in Australia and New Zealand. Aust N Z J Psychiatry. 2016;50:39–40.

Angus SV, Vu TR, Willett LL, Call S, Halvorsen AJ, Chaudhry S. Internal medicine residency program directors' views of the core entrustable professional activities for entering residency: an opportunity to enhance communication of competency along the continuum. Accad Medica. 2017;92:785–91.

Babbott S. Commentary: watching closely at a distance: key tensions in supervising resident physicians. Acad Med J Assoc Am Med Coll. 2010;85(9):1399–400.

Bargagliotti LA, Davenport D. Entrustables and entrustment: through the looking glass at the clinical making of a nurse practitioner. J Nurs Pract. 2017;13(8):e367–e74.

Boyce P, Spratt C, Davies M, McEvoy P. Using entrustable professional activities to guide curriculum development in psychiatry training. BMC Med Educ. 2011;11:96.

Carraccio C, Englander R, Holmboe ES, Kogan JR. Driving care quality: aligning trainee assessment and supervision through practical application of entrustable professional activities, competencies, and milestones. Acad Med. 2016;91(2):199–203.

Chang A, Bowen JL, Buranosky RA, Frankel RM, Ghosh N, Rosenblum MJ, et al. Transforming primary care training – patient-centered medical home entrustable professional activities for internal medicine residents. J Gen Intern Med. 2013;28(6):801–9.

Choo KJ, Arora VM, Barach P, Johnson JK, Farnan JM. How do supervising physicians decide to entrust residents with unsupervised tasks? A qualitative analysis. J Hosp Med. 2014;9(3):169–75.

Community of Practice for Dietetic Educators. Entrustable professional activities (EPAs) and milestones for student dietitians. Version 1; 2018.

Damodaran A, Shulruf B, Jones P. Trust and risk: a model for medical education. Med Educ. 2017;51(9):892–902.

Englander R, Carraccio C. From theory to practice: making entrustable professional activities come to life in the context of milestones. Acad Med. 2014;89(10):1321–3.

Englander R, Flynn T, Call S, et al. Core entrustable professional activities for entering residency: curriculum developers guide. Washington DC: Association of American Medical Colleges MedEdPORTAL iCollaborative. 2014; Resource ID 887. Available at: https://www.mededportal.org/icollaborative/resource/887. Accessed 4 Aug 2019.

Englander R, Flynn T, Call S, Carraccio C, Cleary L, Fulton TB, et al. Toward defining the foundation of the MD degree: core entrustable professional activities for entering residency. Acad Med. 2016;91(10):1352–8.

Foret Giddens J, Lauzon-Clabo L, Gonce Morton P, Jeffries P, McQuade-Jones B, Ryan S. Re-envisioning clinical education for nurse practitioner programs: themes from a national leaders' dialogue. J Prof Nurs. 2014;30(3):273–8.

Frank JR, Mungroo R, Ahmad Y, Wang M, De Rossi S, Horsley T. Toward a definition of competency-based education in medicine: a systematic review of published definitions. Med Teach. 2010;32(8):631–7. https://doi.org/10.3109/0142159X.2010.500898.

Haines ST, Pittenger AL, Stolte SK, Plaza CM, Gleason BL, Kantorovich A, et al. Core entrustable professional activities for new pharmacy graduates. Am J Pharm Educ. 2017;81(1):S2.

Hauer KE, Kohlwes J, Cornett P, Hollander H, Ten Cate O, Ranji SR, et al. Identifying entrustable professional activities in internal medicine training. J Grad Med Educ. 2013;5(1):54–9.

Hoyt KS, Ramirez EG, Proehl JA. Making a case for entrustable professional activities for nurse practitioners in emergency care. Adv Dermatol. 2017;39(2):77–80.

Iqbal MZ, Al-Eraky MM, AlSheikh MH. Designing entrustable professional activities for training health professional educators: a review of current practices. Med Sci Educ. 2018;28:797–802.

Moon JY, Lounsbery JL, Schweiss S, Pittenger AL. Preceptor and resident perceptions of entrustable professional activities for postgraduate pharmacy training. Curr Pharm Teach Learn. 2018;10:1594–9.

Mulder H, Ten Cate O, Daalder R, Berkvens J. Building a competency-based workplace curriculum around entrustable professional activities: the case of physician assistant training. Med Teach. 2010;32(10):e453–9.

Myers J, Krueger P, Webster F, Downar J, Herx L, Jeney C, et al. Development and validation of a set of palliative medicine entrustable professional activities: findings from a mixed methods study. J Palliat Med. 2015;18(8):682–90.

O'Leary D, Al-Taiar H, Brown N, Bajorek T, Ghazirad M, Shaddel F. Workplace assessment in crisis? The way forward. BJPsych Bull. 2016;40(2):61–3.

Parker TA, Guiton G, Jones MD Jr. Choosing entrustable professional activities for neonatology: a Delphi study. J Perinatol. 2017;37(12):1335–40.

Peters H, Holzhausen Y, Boscardin C, Ten Cate O, Chen HC. Twelve tips for the implementation of EPAs for assessment and entrustment decisions. Med Teach. 2017;39(8):802–7.

Pilj-Zieber EM, Barton S, Konkin J, Awosoga O, Caine V. Competence and competency-based nursing education: finding our way through the issues. Nurs Educ Today. 2014;34:676–8.

Pittenger AL, Chapman SA, Frail CK, Moon JY, Undeberg MR, Orzoff JH. Entrustable professional activities for pharmacy practice. Am J Pharm Educ. 2016;80:57.

Powell DE, Wallschlaeger A. Making sense of the milestones: entrustable professional activities for pathology. Hum Pathol. 2017;62:8–12.

Rose S, Fix OK, Shah BJ, Jones TN, Szyjkowski RD. Entrustable professional activities for gastroenterology fellowship training. Neurogastroenterol Motil. 2014;26(8):1204–14.

Ross M. Entrustable professional activities. Clin Teach. 2015;12:223–5.

Ryan AG, Laurinkiene J, Hennebry J, Stroiescu A, Moriarty HK, Knox M, et al. Entrustable professional activities for interventional radiologist trainers. Cardiovasc Intervent Radiol. 2017;40(2 Supplement 1):S323.

Sterkenburg A, Barach P, Kalkman C, Gielen M, ten Cate O. When do supervising physicians decide to entrust residents with unsupervised tasks? Acad Med. 2010;85(9):1408–17.

Ten Cate O. Entrustability of professional activities and competency-bases training. Med Educ. 2005;39:1176–7.

Ten Cate O. Competency-based education, entrustable professional activities, and the power of language. J Grad Med Educ. 2013a;5:6–7.

Ten Cate O. Nuts and bolts of entrustable professional activities. J Grad Med Educ. 2013b;5:157–8.

Ten Cate O. A primer on entrustable professional activities. Korean J Med Educ. 2018;30:1–10.

Ten Cate O, Scheele F. Viewpoint: competency-based postgraduate training: can we bridge the gap between theory and clinical practice? Acad Med. 2007;82(6):542–7.

Ten Cate O, Snell L, Carraccio C. Medical competence: the interplay between individual ability and the health care environment. Med Teach. 2010;32(8):669–75.

Thompson LR, Leung CG, Green B, Lipps J, Schaffernocker T, Ledford C, et al. Development of an assessment for entrustable professional activity (EPA) 10: emergent patient management. West J Emerg Med. 2017;18(1):35–42.

Touchie C, De Champlain A, Pugh D, Downing S, Bordage G. Supervising incoming first-year residents: faculty expectations versus residents' experiences. Med Educ. 2014;48(9):921–9.

Tully K, Keller J, Blatt B, Greenberg L. Observing and giving feedback to novice PGY-1s. South Med J. 2016;109(5):320–5.

Van Houwelingen CTM, Moerman AH, Ettema RGA, Kort HSM, ten Cate O. Competencies required for nursing telehealth activities: a Delphi-study. Nurs Educ Today. 2016;39:50–62.

Warm EJ, Mathis BR, Held JD, Pai S, Tolentino J, Ashbrook L, et al. Entrustment and mapping of observable practice activities for resident assessment. J Gen Intern Med. 2014;29(8):1177–82.

Wright ORL, Capra SM. Entrustable professional activities for nutrition and dietetics practice: theoretical development. Focus Health Profess Educ. 2017;18:31–47.

Workplace-Based Assessment in Clinical Practice

64

Victor Lee and Andrea Gingerich

Contents

Introduction to Workplace-Based Assessments	1236
Case Vignette	1237
The Goals for WBAs	1237
Tracking	1239
Feedback	1239
Assessment Judgments	1240
What Are the Stakes?	1240
Reviewing WBA Forms	1241
The Implementation of WBAs	1243
Quality Improvement Issues for WBAs	1244
Differing Perspectives of WBAs	1245
Final Considerations	1246
Conclusion	1247
Cross-References	1247
References	1247

Abstract

In this chapter, we will provide an overview of the assessment modality referred to as workplace-based assessments. This newer assessment method has evolved over the last two to three decades and focuses on assessing performance in routine clinical practice. It can be easy to be confused by the multitude of workplace-based assessment tools out there and lose sight of the purpose and practice of this method of assessment. Using a case vignette as a practical example, we will

V. Lee (✉)
Centre for Integrated Critical Care, The University of Melbourne, Melbourne, VIC, Australia

Austin Health, Melbourne, VIC, Australia
e-mail: victor.lee@austin.org.au

A. Gingerich
Northern Medical Program, University of Northern British Columbia, Prince George, BC, Canada
e-mail: Andrea.Gingerich@unbc.ca

© Springer Nature Singapore Pte Ltd. 2023
D. Nestel et al. (eds.), *Clinical Education for the Health Professions*,
https://doi.org/10.1007/978-981-15-3344-0_83

explore the process of implementing workplace-based assessment into an educational program in the undergraduate or postgraduate setting. Our aim is to provide a systematic approach to navigating the various considerations and challenges in order to develop, implement, and maintain a quality workplace-based assessment program.

Keywords

Workplace-based assessment · Direct observation · Clinical competency · Feedback

Introduction to Workplace-Based Assessments

Workplace-based assessments (WBAs) are used to assess learners as they participate in routine clinical activities in the workplace. WBAs allow learners to be assessed while participating within different domains of professional health care practice and forms of patient care (Pangaro and ten Cate 2013). They are particularly useful because they are one of the few assessment modalities that assess the highest level of Miller's pyramid of clinical assessment known as the "Does" level that is the "*action* component of professional activity" in routine daily practice (Miller 1990). In summary, WBAs are authentic assessment modality that enables the assessment of performance in diverse real-world contexts while relying primarily on direct observation.

Workplace-based assessments are an assessment modality comprised of multiple tools too numerous to list individually, but a few common examples are the mini-clinical evaluation exercise (Mini-CEX), case-based discussion (CbD), and direct observation of procedural skills (DOPS). The Mini-CEX was one of the first WBA tools used in medicine and it can be used to assess a patient encounter, including history taking, physical examination, clinical judgement, professionalism, and overall clinical care (Norcini and Blank 1995). CbDs often focus on written communication, clinical synthesis or reasoning, and patient management based on the clinical records or notes (Al-Wassia et al. 2015). DOPS focuses on assessment of a procedural, technical, or operative skill (Khanghahi and Azar 2018). For each of these tools, there have been different versions developed by different institutions, postgraduate specialties, and professional bodies. They are most useful when they are linked to an underlying competency-based framework or curriculum.

WBA tools are diverse in terms of what they focus on, what data is recorded, and even who completes the assessment form. For example, clinical logbooks, sometimes also known as shift report cards or encounter cards, are used to document activities during a clinical shift (Schüttpelz-Brauns et al. 2016). They are completed by supervisors or learners. Multisource feedback (MSF) or 360 degree assessment are WBAs completed by supervisors, peers, allied health professionals, or patients the learner has interacted with to provide performance information from multiple unique perspectives (Donnon et al. 2014). Entrustable professional activities (EPAs)

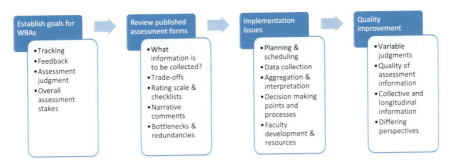

Fig. 1 Process for implementing WBAs

are a form of assessment that document which activities have been entrusted to learners or documents the level of supervision that was provided for the learner to safely and effectively participate in the clinical activity (ten Cate et al. 2016).

It could be easy to become overwhelmed by the variety of WBA tools available and for this reason we will use the following case vignette as the context for describing the suggested steps for implementing workplace-based assessments into an educational program. These steps involve establishing the goals for WBAs, reviewing published assessment forms, examining implementation issues, and, finally, ensuring quality improvement (Fig. 1).

Case Vignette

Kirsty is a program director and is keen to use more direct observation to assess learner performance. She has read that workplace-based assessments make use of direct observation to provide feedback and assessment for learners. This is important because she wants to better determine learner performance in actual clinical practice. Although she has read that individual workplace-based assessments may not be very reliable, when they are used collectively, they can provide a better picture of learner competence in the workplace. This collated information would enable her to determine that her learners are ready to progress to the next stage of training. And so, Kirsty would like to know more about workplace-based assessments in order to set up a more robust system of performance assessment in her training program.

The Goals for WBAs

To help Kirsty select the most appropriate tools for her program we would encourage her to specify her assessment goals. Workplace-based assessments can allow for learners to be assessed while they interact with real patients in authentic work environments, to have feedback about their performance in a clinical workplace recorded, and for some of their clinical experiences to be documented (Norcini and Burch 2007). It is not easy to make decisions about which tools to use and how to implement them. One of the key questions for Kirsty to ask is: What are the current gaps in assessing clinical performance for her learners? In other words, what information does she need for workplace-based assessments to provide that cannot be provided by other assessment modalities? This means surveying other forms of assessment that her program may already utilize to assess at the knows (e.g., multichoice or select-choice questions), knows how (e.g., extended matching questions or short answer questions), or shows how (e.g., objective structured clinical examinations) levels. For example, the latter (otherwise known as OSCEs) may be more suited to assessing performance in simulated contexts for high-stakes decision-making purposes whereas WBAs can be used to assess performance in actual clinical practice (Norcini et al. 2003). Our advice to program directors like Kirsty would be to specify her goals for workplace-based assessment.

In this section we will offer a framework to help Kirsty with identifying the differing goals of WBAs. It is our guess that if she was to ask her faculty why workplace-based assessment should be implemented at her institution, she would hear more than one goal described. Since WBA is assessment that is situated in the workplace, and this is where the bulk of clinical learning occurs, it is not surprising that workplace-based assessment has been closely tied to learning and feedback. WBAs have been used as a way to promote teaching and learning within the workplace (Lörwald et al. 2018). They can be used to emphasize what is important and prioritized in clinical learning. For example, WBAs can direct learners to the "must see" and "must do" clinical activities and record their participation in these activities. The timing of WBAs can help to reinforce the curriculum's content and timeline by acting as a reminder for learners and supervisors. The rating scales and checklists on assessment forms can include details about evidence-based best practices and clinical guidelines. When used to assess learners, they are also communicating information about the latest best practices to learners and faculty. Checklists and rating scales can also be used to frame feedback conversations, and learners can use them as learning aids to review the key steps. In this section we will tease apart three main goals from the varied practices used to implement workplace-based assessment (Table 1).

Table 1 Representative examples of workplace-based assessments with corresponding goals

Goals		Examples
Tracking	*Only*	Clinical logbooks
Tracking	*plus* feedback	Field notes
		Multisource feedback
		Surgical or procedural checklists
Tracking	*plus* assessment judgments and comments	360 degree assessment
		Mini-CEX
		Direct observation of procedures
		Case-based discussions
Tracking	*plus* level of supervision or entrustment	Entrustable professional activities
		Zwisch scale
Assessment judgments and comments *only*		In-training assessments or evaluation reports

Tracking

Much of the teaching and learning that will take place in the lecture halls, classrooms, laboratories, and simulation centers can be predicted. This allows for the curricula to be predetermined, designed, reviewed, and shown to others. Much of the learning that happens in the clinical workplace cannot be predicted and is not easily recorded in curricula documents. One of the goals of WBAs is to function as a record-keeping device to verify learners' clinical learning activities through documentation. Quite often the tracking information is included as the first portion of an assessment form. Location, setting, case type, patient demographics, and complexity of the case may be included as checkboxes to provide context for the subsequent assessment judgments and/or written comments.

Tracking is the primary goal for some workplace-based assessments and may be the only information required on the form. Clinical logbooks, for example, can act as passports that record where the learner was, who they interacted with, or what they experienced. This could be an appropriate technique for junior learners who are observing but not yet participating with patient care or for more senior learners when they are on rotation to other units or services. Encounter cards or logbooks can be used to monitor learners' activities and provide some evidence to administrators of learners' attendance, patient mix, and case mix at various clinical sites (Starmer et al. 2020). Recent research is working to leverage the documentation of electronic medical records to compile tracking information on learners (Sebok-Syer et al. 2019). It has the potential to be much more comprehensive in documenting patient mix and case type than learner-generated forms. Tracking information is volume of practice evidence for learners and their coaches or mentors to review for gaps in learning experiences to inform plans for upcoming learning activities. For example, it is possible for tracking to reveal limited exposure to a certain patient type and extensive observation of a particular surgical technique. Tracking tools document volume and breadth of experience that can be included in portfolios and can contribute to progression decisions. When aggregated, tracking information is evidence that can be used for program evaluation to inform changes to curricula such as length of exposure to specific disciplines or clinical rotations as well as for reporting for accreditation purposes.

Feedback

Feedback has been identified as an important aspect of workplace learning and is discussed in the chapter "Feedback and Supervision in Health Professions Education." Workplace-based assessments have been used in many ways to support feedback exchange in the workplace. The requirement to complete WBAs can initiate direct observation moments that may otherwise not take place. They can also be used to regulate a minimum number of feedback conversations during a specific period of time. Through the promotion of direct observation, learners may be able to receive more frequent and more specific feedback on their skills. Feedback and assessment are often intertwined. In differentiating the two, we see feedback as identifying what can be changed or improved and then discussing why and how to go about doing that. Multisource feedback and field notes are examples of WBAs where the primary purpose is to gather and document written feedback. Field notes are an assessment technique where brief feedback comments pertaining to specific skills are immediately recorded after directly observed events. They were originally employed as a feedback prescription utilizing the equivalent of a prescription pad where the bulk of the form was for recording feedback. Selection of "stop, important correction," "in progress," or "carry on, got it" quickly summarizes the nature of the feedback comments and helps with organizing the field notes (Donoff 2009). By having the feedback documented, the comments can be aggregated and reviewed to inform personal learning plans. The content of the feedback comments can also contribute to progression decisions both by serving as evidence of demonstrated skills and by capturing how the learner has responded to feedback in subsequent learning opportunities (Ross et al. 2011).

Assessment Judgments

Most often the goal of WBAs is to gather assessment judgments. Assessment judgments identify how well something has been done or how well someone is doing. For example, they may indicate an evaluative judgment of how well something has been done or if it has been performed in accordance with a stated criteria. Or they may indicate if someone is doing as well as others or as expected for their level of training. Assessment judgments tend to be documented using a score on a rating scale or ticking off a checkbox. They may be accompanied by written assessment comments that elaborate on or justify assessment judgments. Decision-makers tend to rely on the written comments to interpret the ratings, make sense of the learner's performance, and to help them make progression decisions. These comments may be combined with written feedback comments that specify how something can be improved.

Assessment judgments documented with rating scales can be analyzed to measure the amount of competence someone has. Assessment judgments can also be used to monitor the longitudinal development of competence. This analysis may involve psychometrics or Bayesian analysis such as plotting trajectories using rating scales, using the number of procedures performed (e.g., volume of practice), or displaying patterns of performance in large databases to reveal a typical patterns. Kirsty may want to consult with an assessment expert when designing scales and analysis procedures.

What Are the Stakes?

Now that Kirsty has considered the differences between collecting tracking, feedback, and assessment judgment data, she will need to determine what is ultimately done with the collected assessment information. There are different ways to think about it. The phrase "assessment for learning" has been used to describe assessment information that is collected for the benefit of the learner's own learning and not used to make assessment decisions (Schuwirth and van der Vleuten 2011). It tends to be a systematic process for collecting feedback information. It is related to the term "formative assessment" that also focuses on using assessment information as feedback to the learner. Both of these terms are connected to the concept of "stakes" or how much the assessment counts or impacts a learner's progression through the program. Formative assessment for learning tends to have no or low stakes attached to each assessment data point. This means that a single assessment form cannot stop a learner from progressing. Assessments with no stakes would be ones that are optional and have no influence on the learner's academic record. This may be the case when a new assessment form or process is first introduced and piloted.

There are two common ways for an assessment to be low stakes. One is a mandatory deliverable, such as an assessment that must be completed but it does not matter what is documented. Logbooks are an example because there is often a minimum number that must be completed. The other way an assessment can be low stakes is when the form's content matters but only when numerous completed assessments are reviewed together to reveal a pattern. Field notes are an example because numerous pieces of feedback are collected and a concerning pattern of feedback would be used to initiate additional learning opportunities and eventually formal remediation. The concept of stakes can be confusing because many low-stakes assessments can be used to make a high-stakes assessment decision. For example, many entrustable professional activities are reviewed to decide when a learner can progress to a reduced level of supervision and progress within the program.

The phrase "assessment of learning" captures the concept of collecting assessment information to determine how well the learner is performing and if they are competent enough to progress within the program (Schuwirth and van der Vleuten 2011). It tends to emphasize judgments and ratings of ability used to measure competence. It is related to the term "summative assessment" that is used to describe assessments that count and have impact on the learner's progression. The stakes may be low, such as when many Mini-CEX assessment forms are collected and analyzed to inform assessment decisions, or high as is the case with end of rotation assessments where a single failing rating can impede progression. The highest stake decision that programs must make is determining who has successfully completed the requirements of the program. A programmatic assessment approach purposefully combines various assessment modalities to inform assessment decisions and is further discussed in ▶ Chap. 62, "Programmatic Assessment in Health Professions Education."

Reviewing WBA Forms

After identifying the goal or goals for introducing WBAs into Kirsty's program, the next step is to review the available WBA tools. There are many published assessment forms and one or more might align with Kirsty's goals for tracking her learners' activities, documenting feedback comments, and/or capturing assessment judgments. As she critiques the forms she may see where trade-offs have been made in the design. Perhaps one form is specific to a single clinical activity (such as providing bad news or performing a lumbar puncture) and provides comprehensive relevant details to support faculty in making targeted assessment judgments and providing meaningful feedback. However, the trade-off for the comprehensiveness of the form is that a large set of forms would be needed if there were many learning activities to be assessed. It may be cumbersome for faculty to access the correct form quickly and easily and this may be a barrier to assessment completion.

There are other trade-offs to consider. A WBA form that includes tracking, feedback, and assessment judgments will take longer to complete than a form that addresses only one goal. If the form takes too much time to complete, while simultaneously observing the learner or immediately after having a feedback conversation, it could result in forms being completed weeks later with fading memories. Faculty may be less willing to complete a long form leading to forms being completed less frequently, by a fewer number of faculty and for a fewer number of clinical encounters. This will adversely impact analysis of the assessment ratings, provide less written feedback for learners, and track learners' activities less well. Another WBA form may be brief, focus on only one assessment goal, and lend itself to more frequent completion while with the learner. However, without added design structure it may require more faculty training in order to be used properly or could run the risk of being misused. Without specific rating scales or checklists to act as memory aids and with pressure to complete the brief WBA quickly and frequently, faculty may not include meaningful written assessment or feedback comments. This could adversely impact the learning potential of the WBA and risk it being viewed as a checklist exercise. There are no perfect WBA forms so these trade-offs must be chosen wisely to align with the intended goals for the assessment.

A reasonable strategy to accommodate trade-offs in assessment tool design is to select two or more WBA tools. We would encourage reviewing the potential combination for redundancies and bottlenecks. For example, in terms of addressing assessment goals it would be useful to identify which WBA tools are providing tracking, feedback, and/or assessment information. From the learner's perspective, what information are they receiving about their performance? How much of it is documented in open text, on rating scales, and in checkboxes? How often do they receive assessment information? From the faculty perspective, it is useful to determine who is completing the WBA forms and how many different forms a given individual may need to complete. For example, a program may implement a WBA tool focused on feedback such as multisource feedback where patients, peers, other health professionals, and faculty complete forms that provide written feedback. In addition, they may implement a WBA tool that focuses on collecting assessment judgments, such as the Mini-CEX. Questions we encourage Kirsty to ask herself include: Will a given learner need to ask a single supervisor to complete both a MSF form and a Mini-CEX form during the same one-week period? If so, does she anticipate any adverse effects on the quality of comments that are provided, completion rates, or assessment ratings?

WBA tools commonly include a written comment box. However, it is often unclear if the box is meant for feedback comments or for assessment comments or both (Watling and Ginsburg 2019). There is overlap between the two as well as some clear differences. The information included to justify an assessment judgment and to help support progression decisions is different from the information included to help a learner further improve their clinical skills. Depending on the goal it may be helpful to have separate comment boxes with distinct instructions. This issue also raises the challenge of having multiple audiences for workplace assessment: there are the learners and the decision-makers. Decision-makers may consist of one or two key program directors or a panel of faculty (sometimes called a clinical competency committee) who determine whether the learner has achieved expected levels of clinical competency for their stage of training. There may be written feedback that could help the learner change their behavior, but faculty do not include it because they are concerned it could be damaging if viewed by a program director or competency committee. Conversely, faculty may not want to include information on the form that would be helpful to a program director or competency committee if it might be harmful to the learner's confidence or to the supervisor–learner relationship (Ginsburg et al. 2020). A design that includes "blind" assessment comments seen only by decision-makers and not the learner, similar to blind comments to an editor during publication manuscript review, may allow information to be formally shared with decision-makers. However, this approach could be detrimental to ongoing faculty–learner relationships if it resulted in faculty providing one message to the decision-makers and a discrepant message to the learner.

The Implementation of WBAs

Implementing workplace-based assessments can appear deceptively straightforward. Because learners and supervisors are already in the workplace it may seem like the addition of some forms is a relatively simple enhancement. However, the administration of WBA is a massive undertaking and cannot be overlooked in the planning stages. Both electronic and paper collection approaches pose challenges for those receiving, submitting, reviewing, collating, and reporting on who has completed which forms. There are also challenges with interpreting the information contained in the forms. Kirsty will need to think about how data from the numerous WBAs is aggregated and presented to both learners and the decision-makers. The turnaround time from submission of the form to when the learner can access it can impact the educational value of the information. Learners may view their assessments, reflect on their learning gaps, and identify learning goals for performance improvement. However, enlisting the help of a coach, peer, or mentor can aid in the reflective and future goal setting process (Buis et al. 2018). The program director or competency committee's interpretation of the assessment information is aided when the WBA forms are organized, easily searchable, summarized, and/or prescreened and highlighted for gaps and salient details. The time required to compile the forms for an entire cohort will affect the timeline for scheduling review points for portfolios and competency committee meetings. Since data collection systems are continuously changing and improving, we will not discuss any in detail but would advise Kirsty to seek out the experiences of programs similar to hers before committing to an administration strategy. In this respect, portfolios are a possible means of collating assessment data for each learner and are discussed in the chapter "Portfolios in Health Professions Education."

Another important consideration for Kirsty is faculty training and the resources required to help faculty engage with WBAs. Faculty development is critical to the change in culture that is often necessary when introducing WBAs (Holmboe et al. 2011). Shifting assessments to the workplace requires a lot of explanation, orientation in how to complete the forms, training in how to engage in feedback conversations, and education about assessment literacy for clinicians. The duration, format, and technology needed for busy clinicians to access faculty training must be given ample consideration, continually evaluated, and refined to help increase its success. It is important for both faculty and learners to be clear about the purpose, expectations, and standards regarding WBAs. Assessment activities require time and attention from faculty and learners. It is a priority that competes with health care service provision and the two commitments can come into tension.

Quality Improvement Issues for WBAs

In this section we will discuss some of the quality improvement issues particular to WBAs, including limitations of the process, variable judgments, quality of assessment information, and differing end user perspectives.

A strength of WBAs is the authenticity of collecting assessment information in the workplace with real patient cases (Van Der Vleuten and Schuwirth 2005). The authenticity of the assessment information contributes strong validity evidence for workplace-based assessments – evidence that the assessment information that is collected represents the learner's clinical abilities (Wilkinson et al. 2002). However, there are downsides to collecting assessment information in the workplace. A big one is that a given learner can receive varying scores on consecutive assessments. In real life, patient cases are unstandardized and the variation in case difficulty can affect the scores that are assigned. The variation can be problematic for analyzing ratings but is fine for the goals of providing feedback and tracking clinical activities. It is also difficult to control the case mix and it may not be possible for all learners to be assessed on the same clinical encounters. For example, a learner with a paediatric rotation at a small urban hospital in the summer will encounter a different patient mix than a learner with a comparable rotation at large tertiary hospital in the winter.

Variability is also added into WBAs by the faculty who complete them (Gingerich et al. 2014). WBAs require clinicians to engage in assessment activities while also providing patient care in dynamic settings where time pressures, cognitive overload, and other demands compete for available time. The lack of dedicated time available for direct observation, completion of the assessment form, and conversation with the learner has an impact on the quality of the assessment information. There are many factors that can influence how assessors translate their observations into judgments and then into scores and feedback for learners. Such factors include the use of heuristics or shortcuts; the influence of recognized and implicit biases; and the use of our own perceived level of clinical competence as the criteria for judging the competence level in others, personal performance schemas, or personal exemplars (Kogan et al. 2011). In addition, there are contextual factors such as prior interactions with the learner, prior knowledge of learner performance, and anticipated learner responses to feedback (Lee et al. 2019). As such, poor reliability and excessive subjectivity are often cited limitations of WBA.

A strategy commonly used to improve reliability and accommodate subjectivity is the collection of many assessments from many different assessors in many different contexts. WBAs tend to be designed as short assessments, usually taking less than 20 minutes to complete. The briefer duration is intended to enable assessors to complete forms more frequently than when a longer form is used. More frequent assessments allow the learner to be assessed in a greater number of varying contexts to increase the breadth of assessment information. This is analogous to obtaining more pixels (or data points) to form a clearer picture of a learner's overall performance (e.g., a crisp higher-resolution versus pixelated blurry picture), as well as their abilities in differing contexts and time points (e.g., like a travel journal). It is also important to ask the right people (assessors) the right questions (constructs) about the right things (competencies) when making use of multiple expert judgments (Crossley and Jolly 2012). This feature allows for independent pieces of information to increase rigor from both a psychometric and qualitative perspective that aligns with the concept of the wisdom of the crowds (Surowiecki 2005). It also allows for differences in context to be accommodated along with changes over time to be documented. Even though the assessments will have variable information and judgments, when used collectively and longitudinally, they map the progression of learner competence and enable a defensible judgment of overall performance.

Differing Perspectives of WBAs

Although workplace-based assessments have the potential for encouraging more frequent feedback in authentic clinical contexts, perceptions from learners and faculty can vary and current research supports this difference. Often there is real tension between the formative and summative aspects of WBAs and how much focus is given to each aspect. We shall next examine some of the potential issues from both learner and supervisor perspectives.

Even though workplace-based assessments are promoted as learner centered, we have found that there is insufficient evidence in the current literature that learners are using them effectively to self-regulate their own learning and/or seek out feedback to improve their own performance. Learners are encouraged to develop a growth mindset (Dweck and Yeager 2019) and ask for feedback from their supervisors in order make these assessments more purposeful and valuable. However, at times they are overwhelmed by the regulatory and administrative requirements of submitting their assessments by the end of the term or rotation. This in turn can lead to the perception that these tools are merely tickbox exercises used to meet training requirements in order to progress. Therefore, less heed is paid to the content and quality of the formative aspects of the assessment. Negative factors relating to workplace culture and context may also result in these assessments not being valued by the learners or their supervisors. The learner's own motivation, autonomy, and agency also influence how they view workplace-based assessments for their own learning.

From the faculty's perspective, administrative burdens in completing the assessment forms and accreditation requirements can also result in perceptions of ticking boxes with little educational benefit (Bindal et al. 2011). In addition, contextual factors such as time pressures to complete the assessment and give feedback, frequent work interruptions and anticipated learner responses to more stringent performance feedback may result in poor-quality feedback (Yepes-Rios et al. 2016). Another aspect is the burden of real-time assessment and its perceived impact on concurrent service provision and patient care (McQueen et al. 2016). In some cases, supervisors may be less stringent or water down their feedback because of the realities of managing complex or undifferentiated patients in variable and dynamic circumstances. As a result of shifting assessments from exam halls or OSCE stations to the workplace, there may be a clash in purpose because clinicians now have to juggle patient care and safety while providing contemporaneous assessment documentation and specific, timely feedback to learners. These added contextual tensions are unique to this form of assessment compared with OSCEs, for example, where the setting is more standardized, controlled, and there is often no face-to-face feedback.

Final Considerations

WBAs can also be used to inform remediation since they can indicate when learners need more clinical experiences and report on learners' performance while engaging with targeted clinical encounters. Kirsty and her faculty may view clinical learning as a series of cycles where learners engage with clinical experiences, reflect on their performance and feedback, and attempt to implement feedback in subsequent experiences. Some learners progress faster than others, some require more experiences than others, and some seem unable or unwilling to apply feedback to future encounters (Gingerich et al. 2020). If clinical learning is about making progress, then WBAs can serve as markers of that progression. If Kirsty was to imagine each WBA as a progress marking data point, similar to the GPS coordinates used by satellite maps, learner progress can be mapped. Assessment decisions and remediation could then be viewed as directions to help re-route learners back onto a more informative route. WBAs have benefited from focus on their design and could be further improved through focus on how their information is synthesized, reviewed, interpreted, and used to guide learners in their learning.

From the examples given above, there is still more work to be done in terms of faculty and learner utilization and engagement with workplace-based assessments.

Managing these tensions is important to progressing and enhancing workplace-based assessments as authentic tools which are meaningful and purposeful for measuring routine performance and facilitating workplace learning. Kirsty should think about how to improve both assessment and feedback literacy (Carless and Boud 2018) for her learners and faculty in order to reach higher levels of mutual engagement and joint enterprise in the use of workplace-based assessments. Affording learners, the autonomy and agency to be in control of their own assessment portfolio and its constituent elements can help them to achieve relevant competency-based outcomes and maximize their learning goals. Making sure learners and faculty understand both the purpose of and how to tailor workplace-based assessments to align with each individual's learning goals may help Kirsty to overcome the anticipated perception of the burdensome nature of these assessments.

Conclusion

In conclusion, WBAs are uniquely authentic assessments that enable direct observation and feedback while delivering professional health care services. They have taken many forms to serve multiple purposes, of which the most important are tracking, feedback, and assessment judgments. The concept of programmatic assessment has pushed us to strategically design assessment forms and intentionally incorporate them into programs of assessment so that their strengths align with the purpose and best inform the assessment decisions. There continue to be differing perceptions of their utility. Ultimately, developing a greater understanding of assessment and feedback literacy for learners and faculty will help engender mutual engagement and better utilization of these as assessments for learning.

Cross-References

▶ Programmatic Assessment in Health Professions Education

References

Al-Wassia H, Al-Wassia R, Shihata S, Park YS, Tekian A. Using patients' charts to assess medical trainees in the workplace: a systematic review. Med Teach. 2015;37(Suppl 1):S82–S7.

Bindal T, Wall D, Goodyear HM. Trainee doctors' views on workplace-based assessments: are they just a tick box exercise? Med Teach. 2011;33(11):919–27.

Buis CA, Eckenhausen MA, ten Cate O. Processing multisource feedback during residency under the guidance of a non-medical coach. Int J Med Educ. 2018;9:48.

Carless D, Boud D. The development of student feedback literacy: enabling uptake of feedback. Assess Eval High Educ. 2018;43(8):1315–25.

Crossley J, Jolly B. Making sense of work-based assessment: ask the right questions, in the right way, about the right things, of the right people. Med Educ. 2012;46(1):28–37.

Donnon T, Al Ansari A, Al Alawi S, Violato C. The reliability, validity, and feasibility of multisource feedback physician assessment: a systematic review. Acad Med. 2014;89(3):511–6.

Donoff MG. Field notes: assisting achievement and documenting competence. Can Fam Physician. 2009;55(12):1260.

Dweck CS, Yeager DS. Mindsets: a view from two eras. Perspect Psychol Sci. 2019;14(3):481–96.

Gingerich A, Kogan J, Yeates P, Govaerts M, Holmboe E. Seeing the 'black box' differently: assessor cognition from three research perspectives. Med Educ. 2014;48(11):1055–68.

Gingerich A, Sebok-Syer SS, Larstone R, Watling CJ, Lingard L. Seeing but not believing: Insights into the intractability of failure to fail. Med Educ. 2020;00:1–11. https://doi.org/10.1111/medu.14271. Early view online.

Ginsburg S, Kogan JR, Gingerich A, Lynch M, Watling CJ. Taken out of context: hazards in the interpretation of written assessment comments. Acad Med. 2020 95(7):1082–1088.

Holmboe ES, Ward DS, Reznick RK, Katsufrakis PJ, Leslie KM, Patel VL, et al. Faculty development in assessment: the missing link in competency-based medical education. Acad Med. 2011;86(4):460–7.

Khanghahi ME, Azar FEF. Direct observation of procedural skills (DOPS) evaluation method: systematic review of evidence. Med J Islam Repub Iran. 2018;32:45.

Kogan JR, Conforti L, Bernabeo E, Iobst W, Holmboe E. Opening the black box of clinical skills assessment via observation: a conceptual model. Med Educ. 2011;45(10):1048–60.

Lee V, Brain K, Martin J. From opening the 'black box' to looking behind the curtain: cognition and context in assessor-based judgements. Adv Health Sci Educ. 2019;24(1):85–102.

Lörwald AC, Lahner F-M, Nouns ZM, Berendonk C, Norcini J, Greif R, et al. The educational impact of Mini-Clinical Evaluation Exercise (Mini-CEX) and Direct Observation of Procedural Skills (DOPS) and its association with implementation: a systematic review and meta-analysis. PLoS One. 2018;13(6):e0198009.

McQueen SA, Petrisor B, Bhandari M, Fahim C, McKinnon V, Sonnadara RR. Examining the barriers to meaningful assessment and feedback in medical training. Am J Surg. 2016;211(2):464–75.

Miller GE. The assessment of clinical skills/competence/performance. Acad Med. 1990;65(Suppl 9):S63–S7.

Norcini JJ, Blank LL. The mini-CEX (clinical evaluation exercise): a preliminary investigation. Ann Intern Med. 1995;123(10):795–9.

Norcini J, Burch V. Workplace-based assessment as an educational tool: AMEE guide no. 31. Med Teach. 2007;29(9):855–71.

Norcini JJ, Blank LL, Duffy FD, Fortna GS. The Mini-CEX: a method for assessing clinical skills. Ann Intern Med. 2003;138(6):476–81.

Pangaro L, ten Cate O. Frameworks for learner assessment in medicine: AMEE guide no. 78. Med Teach. 2013;35(6):e1197–e210.

Ross S, Poth CN, Donoff M, Humphries P, Steiner I, Schipper S, et al. Competency-based achievement system: using formative feedback to teach and assess family medicine residents' skills. Can Fam Physician. 2011;57(9):e323–30.

Schüttpelz-Brauns K, Narciss E, Schneyinck C, Böhme K, Brüstle P, Mau-Holzmann U, et al. Twelve tips for successfully implementing logbooks in clinical training. Med Teach. 2016;38(6):564–9.

Schuwirth LWT, van der Vleuten CPM. General overview of the theories used in assessment: AMEE Guide No. 57. Med Teach. 2011;33(10):783–97.

Sebok-Syer SS, Goldszmidt MA, Watling CJ, Chahine S, Venance SL, Lingard L. Using electronic health record data to assess residents' clinical performance in the workplace: the good, the bad, and the unthinkable. Acad Med. 2019;94(6):853–60.

Starmer DL, House CL, Langworthy KM. Student exposure to cancer patients: an analysis of clinical logbooks and focus groups in clinical year medical students. J Canc Educ. 2020;35:760–765.

Surowiecki J. The wisdom of crowds. Anchor Books. New York. 2005.

ten Cate O, Hart D, Ankel F, Busari J, Englander R, Glasgow N, et al. Entrustment decision making in clinical training. Acad Med. 2016;91(2):191–8.

Van Der Vleuten CPM, Schuwirth LWT. Assessing professional competence: from methods to programmes. Med Educ. 2005;39(3):309–17.

Watling CJ, Ginsburg S. Assessment, feedback and the alchemy of learning. Med Educ. 2019;53(1):76–85.

Wilkinson TJ, Challis M, Hobma SO, Newble DI, Parboosingh JT, Sibbald RG, et al. The use of portfolios for assessment of the competence and performance of doctors in practice. Med Educ. 2002;36(10):918–24.

Yepes-Rios M, Dudek N, Duboyce R, Curtis J, Allard RJ, Varpio L. The failure to fail underperforming trainees in health professions education: a BEME systematic review: BEME guide no. 42. Med Teach. 2016;38(11):1092–9.

Focus on Selection Methods: Evidence and Practice

65

Louise Marjorie Allen, Catherine Green, and Margaret Hay

Contents

Introduction: An Overview of Selection	1252
Where to Start with Selection: A Mission Statement	1254
Taking Your Mission Statement and Applying It to Your Approach to Selection	1255
Applying the Evidence to Selection Practice: Choosing Your Selection Methods	1258
Academic Attainment	1258
Letters of Reference	1259
Traditional Interview	1260
Multiple Mini-Interview (MMI)	1261
Situational Judgment Test (SJT)	1262
Personality Testing	1263
Personal Statements and Curriculum Vitae (CVs)	1264
Summary of the Evidence Base for Quality Selection Methods	1265
Implementing a Quality Selection Process	1265
Aligning Mission, Tools, and Process	1266
Training, Standardization, and Moderation	1268
Evaluating the Selection Process	1268
Selection Challenges	1269
Conclusion	1270
Cross-References	1270
References	1271

L. M. Allen (✉)
Monash Centre for Professional Development and Monash Online Education, Monash University, Clayton, VIC, Australia
e-mail: louise.allen@monash.edu

C. Green
Royal Victorian Eye and Ear Hospital, East Melbourne, VIC, Australia

M. Hay
Faculty of Education, Monash Centre for Professional Development and Monash Online Education, Monash University, Clayton, VIC, Australia
e-mail: margaret.hay@monash.edu

© Springer Nature Singapore Pte Ltd. 2023
D. Nestel et al. (eds.), *Clinical Education for the Health Professions*,
https://doi.org/10.1007/978-981-15-3344-0_122

Abstract

Selection plays an essential role in shaping the future of the healthcare workforce and therefore healthcare delivery. As the selection process is essentially responsible for determining who makes up the healthcare workforce, it is crucial that selection methods and processes are defensible, and that they help shape the healthcare workforce to be more representative of our populations. In recent decades, there has been a significant increase in scholarship on the processes and outcomes of selection that allow for the use of selection methods and processes that are defensible and enable widening access to health professional courses. Much of the focus of this scholarship relates specifically to selection into medical courses and subsequent speciality training, with increasing representation of selection into health professions more broadly. Although the content of this chapter draws mostly on the literature in medical education, the processes and issues discussed apply to selection across a range of health professions and literature relating to other health professions has been included where available.

This chapter is for anyone new to selection in the health professions. It aims to provide insights on the current state of selection discourses, what you need to know about selection, and how to approach selection, providing practical considerations and summarizing the available evidence base on selection methods. The chapter concludes with a review of the future challenges in selection and potential scholarship opportunities for educators interested in this important area of health professions education.

Keywords

Selection · Admissions · Selection tools · Widening participation

Introduction: An Overview of Selection

Selection into health professions courses, once based solely on academic achievement, has in recent decades undergone significant changes as the skills and attributes needed for practice in healthcare systems have been recognized to expand beyond academic capability. There has been a significant increase in scrutiny of, and scholarship on, the processes and outcomes of selection in the health professions, with an increasingly sophisticated commentary on the role of selection in shaping the future of the healthcare workforce and therefore healthcare delivery. More recently, the challenges of undertaking selection across all levels of education and training in the health professions for applicants and institutions have been magnified by the COVID-19 pandemic, forcing a rethink of selection methods that require applicants to attend in person. For these reasons, now is an exciting time for educators in the health professions with an interest in the selection of future health professionals to have an understanding of contemporary best practice and dominant discourses in selection. In this chapter, we provide an overview of selection processes and methods to equip the reader with sufficient knowledge to effectively engage in the process of selection, and to understand the complex contexts in which it occurs. We recommend the paper by Patterson et al. (2016a) for an in-depth understanding of selection methods and their reliability and validity, and Patterson et al. (2018) for a comprehensive overview of the policies and procedures required for a quality and defensible selection process.

The salient purpose of selection into the health professions is to admit students with the desired attributes to successfully complete their training and to practice as competent and safe health professionals after graduation or completion of training. Selection processes should also exclude those who are likely to be unsuccessful or problematic (Rosenstein and O'Daniel 2008) and enable wider access to health professions education for underrepresented groups (Ballejos et al. 2015; Coyle et al. 2021; Razack 2021). The World Health Organization (WHO) has outlined the obligation of medical schools to produce a healthcare workforce that meets the needs of the communities in which they are placed (Boelen and Heck 1995; Boelen 1999). Training institutions, especially those in countries where training is subsidized by taxpayers, have an obligation to direct their education, research, and service activities towards addressing the priority health concerns of the community, region, and the nation that they have a mandate to serve. This accountability mandate, along with the shift to patient-focused and team-based care in complex healthcare systems, have led to significant changes in selection processes. Historically, selection into the health professions was largely unscrutinized, with academic merit being the sole determinant at all levels of education and training. While academic meritocracy in selection remains, selection processes have necessarily adjusted to enable admission of students with both academic and personal characteristics that ensure they succeed through their education and graduate with the competencies required for effective practice.

In medicine, and many other health professions, selection into both undergraduate and specialty postgraduate training is a high-stakes and often costly process for applicants and their families, training institutions, patients, and society (Foo et al. 2020). There are many more applicants than available places leading to intense competition and significant domestic and international relocation of students to gain entry into medical, nursing, and allied health courses. Education and training is expensive and lengthy, with non-completion of training representing a sunk cost for both institutions and trainees. However, low attrition rates, especially in medical education, mean that admission to a course or speciality training program is effectively admission to the profession (Morrison 2016). Selection is therefore the first step in determining the future healthcare workforce of a nation. Globally, the number of commencing medical students has significantly increased (Medical Schools Council 2014; Medical Training Review Panel 2015; Rigby and Gururaja 2017), with an additional 5000 places recently called for in the UK (Medical Council UK 2021) and an 18% increase in the USA (AAMC 2020). This has resulted in the largest number of applicants applying for speciality training ever encountered and prompted a renewed focus on selection into speciality training in addition to the existing focus on undergraduate selection.

Table 1 Key points from the Ottawa Conference consensus on selection statements

Ottawa 2010 consensus statement – Prideaux et al. (2011)	Ottawa 2018 consensus statement – Patterson et al. (2018)
Focus: the adoption of principles of good assessment and curriculum alignment, use of multi-method programmatic approaches, development of interdisciplinary frameworks, and utilization of sophisticated measurement models • Proceeding from a clear blueprint of the content for selection • Using evidence from psychometric studies and a theory base to inform the selection process • Developing congruity between selection, curriculum, and assessment • Using clear standard-setting and decision-making procedures • Providing a focus on the impact of selection (a variant of the adage that assessment drives learning)	Broader systems perspective of selection focusing on four areas: 1. Philosophy and policies 2. Effectiveness of selection methods 3. Diversity and globalization issues 4. Selection theory and evaluation

Selection is more important than ever due to the increasing volume of applicants and the need to have the health workforce better represent our diverse populations. As a reflection of this, research in selection has significantly increased in the last two decades and now represents a substantial topic of scholarship. The vast majority of the available literature pertains to selection into medical training at both undergraduate, postgraduate, and speciality training, with a significantly smaller but emerging literature on selection into other health professions (Kudlas 2006; Paynter et al. 2022; Kale et al. 2020; Haavisto et al. 2019). While literature on selection in the health professions outside of medical training is still emerging, a consensus statement on selection for the healthcare professions and speciality training was developed at the Ottawa 2010 Conference (Prideaux et al. 2011). A revised consensus statement was developed at the Ottawa 2018 Conference (Patterson et al. 2018) to reflect the changes in selection discourse and approaches since the original statement. The key points of both the 2010 and 2018 consensus statements are summarized in Table 1.

These statements along with the evidence for selection in the health professions are used in this chapter to provide a "how to" approach for novices in the area of selection. Our goal is that the reader understands the complexity of selection and obtains sufficient knowledge to actively contribute to and engage in quality selection processes across all levels of admission to health professions education and training.

Where to Start with Selection: A Mission Statement

The starting point for the development or refinement of a selection process involves understanding the philosophy, usually in the form of a mission statement, of the health professions course or specialty into which the selection process will admit.

The mission statement provides a description of the skills, attributes, perspectives, and behaviors that can be expected of graduates from the course. Mission statements, many of which are widely available on the internet, tend to be highly variable (Lewkonia 2001). In addition to the standard statements of highest-level clinical skills and knowledge, ethical behavior, and evidence-based informed practice, contemporary mission statements for courses in the health professions are increasingly focused on the broader aspects of patient focused care; for example, advocacy for those less advantaged, and awareness of diversity along a range of dimensions including culture and sexuality. Policy, such as the Federal Government of Australia's requirement that universities admit 25% of commencing medical students from rural areas to increase the rural healthcare workforce (Hay et al. 2017a), must also be understood to ensure selection processes meet these stated and often mandated outcomes. This policy, also adopted in other countries (Tesson et al. 2005), assumes that students from rural areas will return to rural areas after graduation. However, evidence from rural (Hay et al. 2017a) and lower socioeconomic status (SES) (Griffin et al. 2016) applicants suggests that this is not universally the case.

Policy can also be driven by specific values of the university; for example, a set quota for Indigenous student selection to increase the Indigenous healthcare workforce, inclusion of students from lower SES contexts, again premised on the assumption that future practice will be in the communities from whence they came (Fielding et al. 2018; Mian et al. 2019). Selection methods and processes are tasked with admitting students who have the potential to develop into the graduate described in the mission or policy statements. Diversity and globalization issues can inform selection philosophy in the broader context of global health movements, and have become increasingly important with increased geopolitical insecurity (Sladek and King 2018), a detailed analysis of which is beyond the scope of this chapter but an area the reader should be aware of nonetheless. This process of defining the competencies and graduate attributes in a mission statement should involve people who are highly familiar with the requirements of the work the health professional will perform and the context in which it is performed (Patterson et al. 2008; Hertel-Waszak et al. 2017; Hudak et al. 2000).

Taking Your Mission Statement and Applying It to Your Approach to Selection

The effectiveness of selection processes, methods, evaluation, and selection theory are aligned, with selection theory and evaluation informing selection processes and methods. This alignment of the selection process is the focus of this chapter. Despite key insights into selection processes and policy since the initial consensus statement, Patterson et al. (2016a) acknowledge that much remains to be done to refine the so-called science of selection in the health professions. Patterson et al. (2018) identify three approaches to selection in the health professions which provide a useful framework for reviewing selection methods and processes. Each approach is operationalized by fit-for-purpose selection methods, tools, and processes that align with the stated graduate outcomes (i.e., as contained in the mission statement), a sample of which are contained in Table 2. The three approaches of Patterson et al. (2018) are:

1. **Individually focused processes** – typically focuses on academic success with little if any consideration of nonacademic traits.
2. **Competency-based framework processes** – focuses on a range of behaviors and attitudes thought to be associated with success as a student or health professional.
3. **Social accountability and workforce planning processes** – focuses on widening participation and aims to "mitigate the impact of institutionally or societally determined barriers to their achieving the same academic success" (Patterson et al. 2018, p. 1092).

Historically, selection has involved a largely individually focused process, with academic attainment previously the only method considered when selecting for health profession programs (Patterson et al. 2016a). However, the past two decades have seen a shift to competency-based selection involving assessment of a range of attributes beyond the academic (Garrud 2018). This has followed on from the implementation of competency-based assessment within health professions

Table 2 Overview of selection tools and processes for the three levels identified by Patterson et al. (2018) at undergraduate, postgraduate, and speciality training selection

Selection philosophy	Tools used at the undergraduate level	Tools used at the postgraduate level	Tools used at the specialty training level
Individually focused processes	Academic achievement • ATAR/A levels/SATs Aptitude tests • UCAT	Academic achievement • GPA Aptitude tests • MCAT • GAMSAT Letters of reference • Personal statements/CV/extracurricular activities	• USMLE • Personal statements and CV • Letters of reference
Competency-based processes	• Interview/MMI • SJT • Personality tests, e.g., big five personality traits or PQA • Extracurricular activities	• Interview/MMI • SJT • Personality tests	• Interview/MMI • SJT
Social accountability processes	Policy and procedures for increased representation of: • Indigenous • Rural • Socially disadvantaged	Policy and procedures for increased representation of: • Indigenous • Rural • Socially disadvantaged	Policy and procedures for increased representation of: • Indigenous • Rural

education (Danilovich et al. 2021). The increased focus on patient-centered care and effective teamwork practice in health professions education has led to the inclusion of competency-based selection methods that can capture personal characteristics such as perspective taking (empathy), ethical reasoning and integrity, communication skills, advocacy for the disadvantaged, and cultural sensitivity (Schreurs et al. 2020). Competency standards or frameworks describe these characteristics, skills, attributes, and attitudes that students and practitioners in their field must possess at an established standard, to be considered as safe and competent healthcare workers. Many competency frameworks exist in the health professions, for example, in Australia, the following health professions have competency or practice standards – Aboriginal and Torres Strait Islander health practitioners, Chinese medicine practitioners, dentists, dietitians, doctors, midwives, nurse practitioners, occupational therapists, optometrists, osteopaths, pharmacists, physiotherapists, podiatrists, psychologists, registered nurses, paramedics, social workers, and speech pathologists. All are freely accessible on the internet through either regulatory or professional bodies. These competency frameworks, in addition to other factors including the mission of a particular institution such as training for research versus practitioners for rural and remote clinical work (Coyle et al. 2021; Hay et al. 2017a), should be considered when developing competency-based selection methods. A range of different selection tools now exist to assess these broader competencies (Patterson et al. 2016a), some of which will be explored in the following section of this chapter.

Despite this broader view of characteristics required to produce a quality and safe health professional, selection processes reliant solely on academic attainment or a combination of academic attainment and competency-based approaches have not achieved the desired diversity within the admitted cohorts to meet the WHO social accountability mandate. Social accountability and workforce planning processes in selection directly challenge the individual meritocracy approach which favors the socially advantaged over the disadvantaged (Boelen et al. 2016). To achieve social accountability, selection must therefore enable admission of students who have the potential to eventually become safe practitioners, but also facilitate the inclusion of people from diverse backgrounds through widening access programs (Razack et al. 2015). Mandated proportional representation or quotas for Indigenous students and/or students from rural areas (Matsumoto et al. 2008; Puddey et al. 2014; Greenhill et al. 2015) are examples of policy driven initiatives to widen access, as are differing admissions requirements for Indigenous (Young et al. 2012; Girgulis et al. 2021) and/or lower SES applicants (Puddey et al. 2017). There are increasing calls for courses in the health professions to admit students with disabilities to further diversify the healthcare workforce (Fitzmaurice et al. 2021). These processes also aim to meet the needs of our populations, by selecting a more diverse cohort of students as future healthcare providers. While social accountability and workforce planning are addressed largely through policy and procedures, a range of selection tools exist to address the individually focused and competency-based framework processes as shown in Table 2. A brief description of the main selection methods are provided below and evidence for their effectiveness is presented. In modern selection processes, a mix of individually focused, competency-based framework focused, and social accountability and workforce planning focused processes are used.

Applying the Evidence to Selection Practice: Choosing Your Selection Methods

Patterson et al. (2016a) offer a comprehensive systematic review of the extensive available literature and their paper is a must read for educators in the health professions with an interest in selection. While there is a lack of prospective longitudinal studies examining predictors of success after qualification (Puddey et al. 2014), there is consensus regarding methods that reliably evaluate nonacademic attributes such as perspective taking, integrity, professionalism, and advocacy for others (via MMIs and SJTs), and an expanding body of evidence on effectiveness of selection methods (Patterson et al. 2016a). Decisions on selection should be based on the extant research evidence. In this section, the evidence base for both individual and competency-based methods included in Table 2 are reviewed. Individual selection methods included are academic attainment, personal statements, CVs, extracurricular activities, and letters of reference. Competency-based methods included for review are interviews (traditional panel and multiple mini-interview [MMI]), situational judgment tests (SJT), and personality tests. We include personality testing as although it is not widely used, there is advocacy for its inclusion in selection into health professions courses (Schripsema et al. 2016; Cantwell 2019; Powis et al. 2020).

Academic Attainment

Selection into many health professions courses is a highly competitive process, with many more applicants than available places. Academic attainment is therefore used as the initial selection tool, to identify a group of eligible applicants for further testing from the larger population of applicants (Mercer et al. 2018). Academic attainment refers to both academic achievement and aptitude tests, both of which have long been and remain a major component of selection into health professions undergraduate and postgraduate degrees. Academic achievement refers to matriculation score or rank (e.g., the Australian Tertiary Admissions Rank - ATAR) for undergraduate entry courses, or grade point averages (GPA) for graduate entry courses. While aptitude tests refer to performance on specifically designed tests to assess knowledge and skill. For school leaver entry selection, these include the University Clinical Aptitude Test (UCAT) for selection into medical schools in Australia, New Zealand, and the United Kingdom (Mercer and Puddey 2011). For graduate entry medical course admissions in the USA, the Medical College Admissions Test (MCAT) is used, and the Graduate Medical Schools Admissions Test (GAMSAT) in Australia, New Zealand, and Ireland (Puddey and Mercer 2014).

When exploring the evidence for selection methods, there is by far the greatest volume of evidence for academic achievement and aptitude tests. When looking at the effectiveness of selection methods, a key indicator is the predictive validity, that is the extent to which performance on a selection tool predicts subsequent academic performance, most often summative assessment tasks, during education. There is considerable evidence in all levels of medical training (i.e., medical school and speciality training), as well as other health professions that there is a correlation between prior academic achievement and academic performance scores during education (Mercer and Puddey 2011; Maan et al. 2012; McManus et al. 2013; Patterson et al. 2016a, Anderton 2017; Roberts et al. 2018; Crawford et al. 2021; Alhurishi et al. 2021; Paynter et al. 2022; Russell et al. 2021). While there is a correlation with academic performance, the evidence for performance on clinical assessments is less clear. However, it is worth noting, particularly in medical school, that academic achievement scores and aptitude scores usually sit in a narrow range at the high end of the scale (known as restriction of range). And that while correlations have been shown between prior academic achievement and academic performance, prior academic achievement is not predictive of failure or attrition. In addition, there is research that shows SES and type of school (i.e., public/government or private/independent) are associated with prior academic achievement, that is, having a higher SES is associated with higher prior academic achievement, as is attending a private school (Razack et al. 2015).

Aptitude tests have good reliability in a medical education context (Patterson et al. 2016a). There is evidence that scores on aptitude tests predict scores on subsequent written assessments within a course, and at the beginning and end of the course across two medical schools in Australia (Mercer et al. 2018). Overall, the evidence of predictive validity is mixed (Patterson et al. 2016a); however, there is evidence that using aptitude tests helps to select students with higher abilities and motivation to study medicine (Patterson et al. 2016a). This mixed evidence is not unexpected given the range of different aptitude tests that exist. If the reader is considering the use of an aptitude test, we encourage deeper investigation into the specific test. The main value that aptitude tests provide to medical education selection is their use in selecting a small number of applicants from a large pool. There is some evidence for the predictive validity of aptitude in nursing (Crawford et al. 2021), where aptitude tests and prior academic achievement were shown to be the most predictive of student success during their course. Academic attainment scores (UCAT/ATAR) at selection also predicted performance on written examinations in physiotherapy students (Paynter et al. 2022).

Letters of Reference

Letters of reference are unstructured written statements, although structured statements do exist, by a healthcare professional who has supervised or worked with an applicant in the healthcare setting, either as a student or during their career. The letters generally contain statements about the qualities, capabilities/competencies, and characteristics of the applicant that qualify them for the health profession they are applying to enter. They are almost exclusively used for post-graduate and specialty training, and rarely used as a selection tool for undergraduate courses in the health professions.

The value of unstructured letters of reference is widely debated (Kreiter and Axelson 2013; Kuncel et al. 2014), but the consensus is that this information is not useful for selection into medical school (Patterson et al. 2016a). As for specialist medical training, unstructured letters of recommendation have low reliability, while structured letters of recommendation have been shown to have mixed reliability and inconclusive validity (Roberts et al. 2018). In nursing, there is limited conclusive evidence (Crawford et al. 2021). There are a number of issues with letters of recommendation which caution against their use. They are perceived to have value because the person writing them is assumed to have had the opportunity to directly observe the trainee's performance in the clinical or another environment and is therefore well placed to make assessments or judgments on their performance. However, the referee may not have directly supervised the applicant; there may be a reluctance by the writer to include negative comments due to concerns about confidentiality or discoverability; and self-selection bias may be introduced through applicants only listing referees who they believe will provide a favorable report. Selectors may be biased through being more likely to be influenced if a reference is from someone they know. There also may be differences in how two or more reviewers' rate or score the information (i.e., poor inter-rater reviewer reliability). The rating or scoring process can be expensive in terms of the time of admissions committee members who must read and interpret each letter (Patterson et al. 2016a). Despite these limitations, letters of reference continue to be used in speciality training selection.

Traditional Interview

Traditional interviews refer to unstandardized interviews usually undertaken by a panel of interviewers. There can be variability in purpose, duration, structure, content, and panel constitution. They may involve some element of standardization, e.g., a list of questions, but as they involve a panel there is potential for interviewers to deviate from the predetermined question structure, which decreases consistency. While some evidence in favor of traditional interviews exists, the majority of evidence shows that traditional interviews lack predictive validity and reliability (Patterson et al. 2016a). There is a range of common concerns about traditional interviews including: that in unstructured interviews content covered for each applicant varies therefore standardized comparisons are difficult; the same information may be interpreted differently by different interviewers; that interviewers tend to make up their minds early in the interview; and, there is an unconscious tendency for interviewers to favor and select people who look and act like themselves (Rivera 2012; Burkhardt 2015). As the name suggests, traditional interviews were traditionally a mainstay of selection. However, structured interviews such as the multiple mini-interview (MMI) have been shown to have superior predictive validity, and to be a more reliable and valid method of selection than traditional interviews (Patterson et al. 2016a).

Multiple Mini-Interview (MMI)

A widely used competency-based selection method is the multiple mini-interview (MMI). The MMI is a structured and standardized interview approach where applicants rotate through a series of stations at specified time intervals answering a set of structured interview questions designed to test applicants' nonacademic attributes that have often traditionally been assessed by panel interviews (Pau et al. 2013). The stations are designed to assess various competency domains which usually link to competency frameworks (as mentioned earlier in this chapter) and which are decided upon prior to development. The majority of MMIs consist of 4–12 independent stations, each of 5–10-min duration, with time allocated to both read the scenario and consider the issues raised in it, and for the interviewer questions and applicant responses (Patterson et al. 2016a; Pau et al. 2013; Rees et al. 2016). Each station contains a different scenario and set of questions and is assessed by a single interviewer (Pau et al. 2013). This enables independent judgments or scores across each different scenario and associated questions, thereby achieving a broad and independent assessment of each applicant. A major strength of the MMI is that the scenarios and questions are flexible and can be molded to assess attributes that best meet the requirements of the particular course or program (Eva et al. 2004) and can be developed fit-for-purpose by experts in a particular field. The inclusion of multiple stations enables a broad range of competencies to be assessed (Roberts et al. 2018). Additionally, specific learnt knowledge is not required, with assessment instead aimed at evaluating an applicant's ability to logically work through a problem, from several possible perspectives, and express their ideas clearly.

Since the MMI was first described by Eva et al. (2004), there has been wide uptake of this selection method with a growing body of evidence supporting its reliability, validity, feasibility, and acceptability in a medical education context (Pau et al. 2013; Patterson et al. 2016a; Rees et al. 2016; Roberts et al. 2018). While there is variation in how MMIs are conducted, for example: the number of stations ranging from 4 to 12, and the length of each station ranging from 5 to 10 min, if well designed, they have been shown to have higher predictive validity and reliability than traditional interviews (Pau et al. 2013; Patterson et al. 2016a; Roberts et al. 2018). MMIs have been shown to predict performance on the objective structured clinical examination (OSCE) for clinical skills assessment in physiotherapy (Paynter et al. 2022) and other examinations in medicine (Patterson et al. 2016a). The evidence for the predictive validity of MMIs in nursing is mixed (Crawford et al. 2021). Using 7–12 stations with one examiner has been shown to optimize reliability in undergraduate health programs (Rees et al. 2016). Similarly, when considering development of MMIs, increasing the number of stations, as opposed to increasing the duration of stations, has a greater effect on reliability in undergraduate health programs (Rees et al. 2016). There is less evidence regarding the number and duration of stations when selecting for specialist medical training; however, there is evidence of reliability and predictive validity in this setting for six station MMIs (Roberts et al. 2018). As multiple interviews are involved in MMIs, a major factor affecting reliability is interviewer subjectivity, highlighting the importance of appropriate interviewer training and standardization (Roberts et al. 2008). There is a small amount of evidence regarding the effect of coaching on MMI performance which shows that applicants who reported being coached did not perform better than those who did not report being coached, and that having the scenarios in advance had no effect on performance (Rees et al. 2016). In addition, evidence shows that MMI results are not biased against applicants regarding age, gender, or socioeconomic status, with more research into First Nations Peoples, those from rural areas and those from different ethnic backgrounds being required (Rees et al. 2016).

Various studies have demonstrated that the MMI is able to measure: professionalism (Hofmeister et al. 2009); legal, ethical, and organizational skills (Eva et al. 2009); motivation, interest, decision-making, and the ability to debate a complex issue (O'Brien et al. 2011); empathy, and moral and ethical reasoning, teamwork, leadership, honesty, and integrity (Till et al. 2013); and advocacy, ambiguity, collegiality and collaboration, cultural sensitivity, responsibility, and reliability (Lemay et al. 2007).

Situational Judgment Test (SJT)

Another competency-based selection method, the situational judgment test (SJT), is designed to assess an applicant's judgment regarding a situation encountered in the workplace, targeting professional nonacademic attributes rather than clinical knowledge (Lievens et al. 2008). Candidates are presented with hypothetical scenarios and asked to identify an appropriate response from a list of alternatives (Pollard and Cooper-Thomas 2015). Responses are generally behaviors or actions that can be taken in response to the situation depicted in the scenario. The SJT enables a range of different formats, two examples being ranking actions in order of appropriateness, e.g., most to least appropriate, or rating the appropriateness of actions independently. They are scored by comparing responses with a predetermined scoring key agreed upon by subject matter experts (SME) (Pollard and Cooper-Thomas 2015). SJTs are derived from behavioral consistency theory, which asserts that past behavior is the best predictor of future behavior (Patterson et al. 2012). They are also believed to be a measure of prosocial implicit trait policies (ITPs), which are shaped by socialization processes that teach the utility of expressing certain traits in different settings (Patterson et al. 2016b). ITP theory proposes that individuals develop beliefs about the effectiveness or costs and benefits of different behaviors in particular situations, which are influenced by the individual's inherent tendencies or traits (Patterson et al. 2016b).

Similarly, to the MMI, the SJT is increasingly being used for selection for both medical school and specialty training. In these settings, the SJT has been shown to be both a valid and reliable selection measure (Patterson et al. 2016b; Roberts et al. 2018). A recent meta-analysis showed "that scores generally demonstrated incremental predictive validity, over and above tests of knowledge and cognitive ability" (Webster et al. 2020, p. 888). The SJT is reported to be highly predictive of performance outcomes relating to the attributes they assess (Lievens and Patterson 2011; Lievens and Sackett 2012; O'Connell et al. 2007; Patterson et al. 2009, 2016a). Beyond validity and reliability, the SJT has been shown to have a number of strengths including:

- Being less impacted by socioeconomic, cultural, and gender bias than other selection tools (Lievens et al. 2016; McDaniel et al. 2007; Patterson et al. 2009, 2016b).
- When used in conjunction with cognitive tests and other traditional selection tools, the SJT can produce sizable reductions in the racial inequality of entrance scores (Ployhart and Holtz 2008).
- Coaching has minimal effect on SJT scores due to strategies required to deliver the correct response being more complex than other tests (Cullen et al. 2006; Patterson et al. 2013; Stemig et al. 2015).
- Building complexity into SJT scenarios can reduce susceptibility to coaching effects (Patterson et al. 2013).
- The SJT is acceptable and feasible (Patterson et al. 2016a; Roberts et al. 2018).

There are, however, some important points that should be considered when delivering an SJT. This includes that applicants who are older and have English as a second language may show reduced scores, and be negatively impacted by test time (Hay et al. 2017b). It is therefore important to consider the total duration allowed for applicants to complete an SJT and ensure that this does not disadvantage any group of individuals. While there is some evidence for the cost-effectiveness of the SJT, they are complex to develop, requiring an investment at the start of implementation (Patterson et al. 2016b). Subject matter experts (SMEs) and experts in SJT construction, scoring, and evaluation should be engaged in design and development, with a thorough analysis of the requirements of the job constructed in consultation with SMEs (Pollard and Cooper-Thomas 2015; Patterson et al. 2016b).

Personality Testing

Personality testing aims to capture how people typically think, behave, and feel, that is, capturing their personality traits (Woods and Barratt 2018). One of the most common measures for testing personality is the "Big Five" personality traits: extraversion, agreeableness, conscientiousness, emotional stability, and openness. There are a range of other personality tests that exist (Goffin and Christiansen 2003). The personal qualities assessment (PQA) developed in Australia by Powis et al. (2005) specifically for medical student selection measures the personality traits of:

involvement, self-control, and emotional resilience. Involvement is characterized as high empathy and confidence in dealing with people, and low narcissism and aloofness.

The role of personality tests in selection for medical education has been debated (Ferguson and Lievens 2017; MacKenzie et al. 2017; Patterson et al. 2017). A number of studies have shown the "Big Five" personality traits may correlate with various aspects of medical school performance (Patterson et al. 2016a). However, gaps in the literature of medical selection with respect to personality do exist, for example: lack of data on personality change and its implications for professionals' health and performance; the lack of assessment of trait expression (i.e., distinguishing qualities) and context sensitivity; and no real recognition of the effect of the degree to which a trait is expressed and its effect on performance (the optimal level of a trait) (Ferguson and Lievens 2017). The PQA is not widely used so there is limited information available on its effectiveness as a selection tool (Powis et al. 2020b).

Other concerns about personality testing include:

- Personality traits are believed to be changeable across the lifespan and contexts, and there is no information on how personality changes during health professions education and training (Patterson et al. 2017).
- The predictive validity of personality traits for the required aspects of future practice is often low and poorly understood (Patterson et al. 2017).
- Personality assessment may narrow the diversity of types of individuals entering training (Patterson et al. 2014).

Personal Statements and Curriculum Vitae (CVs)

A personal statement is a written description that provides an indication of a person's achievements, their interests, and their key strengths in the area they are applying to enter (Patterson and Zibarras 2018). Similar to letters of reference, a personal statement or CV can be structured or unstructured. While a CV is a summary of an individual's education, qualifications, achievements, previous employment, and potentially professional development and personal achievements among other things. The use of personal statements and CVs as selection methods are problematic (Patterson et al. 2016a; Roberts et al. 2018). Minimal evidence exists in favor of the predictive validity of personal statements and CVs for medical student performance, with substantial evidence showing that personal statements lack validity and reliability (Patterson et al. 2016a). In nursing, there is limited evidence that is inconclusive (Crawford et al. 2021). They may inadvertently favor those who have social connections that can provide access to prestigious opportunities and with the financial ability to participate in such activities (Dore et al. 2017; Wright 2015). Applicants may present themselves in ways they believe increase their chance of success, but which may not necessarily be accurate (Patterson et al. 2016a; White et al. 2012) and enlist the help of knowledgeable supporters to help write up their experiences (Dore et al. 2017). This risk of coaching or having personal statements written by someone else is extremely concerning (Patterson et al. 2016a), and hence the appropriateness of these tools for selection needs to be strongly considered.

Summary of the Evidence Base for Quality Selection Methods

Patterson et al. (2016a) provide a comprehensive systematic review of the reliability and validity of a broad range of selection methods currently used in selection into medical education and is a must read for any educator engaging in selection. While there is growing evidence in other health professions, there is considerably less than in medical education, hence this review provides a sound starting point regardless of profession. The research shows that the evidence is better for some selection methods than others, for example, MMI, SJT, academic record and aptitude tests (i.e., Universities Clinical Aptitude Test – UCAT, Medical College Admissions Test – MCAT, Graduate Medical Schools Admissions Test – GAMSAT) have enhanced quality over the traditional panel interviews, letters of reference, and CVs (Patterson et al. 2016a). Crawford et al. (2021) found prior academic achievement and selection aptitude tests to be the strongest predictors of course performance in nursing. Paynter et al. (2022) found that selection interview (MMI) was a positive predictor of OSCE and final year clinical performance in physiotherapy students. There is inconclusive evidence for traditional interviews, personal statements, and previous healthcare experience. There is insufficient evidence for a definitive conclusion about personality tests due to their limited use. It should be cautioned, however, that the evidence is mixed and tends to evaluate effectiveness on the basis of student or trainee achievement on assessments, rather than whether they go on to become a successful health professional in the future.

Implementing a Quality Selection Process

Patterson et al. (2019) note that selection processes are often implemented based on a limited evidence base. Also, processes used in one context (e.g., undergraduate selection) may not translate to others (e.g., speciality selection) or to different health professions. The authors suggest three overarching processes to a fair selection system which are presented in Table 3 alongside important considerations for each process. The following sections of this chapter will address each of these important considerations which overall form a multistep fair selection process which has been illustrated in Fig. 1. Selection should be considered as a cycle of continuous improvement, with each step always considered not only in itself but in the context of the system in which it occurs. For each step of the process, it is helpful to have specified what tasks are required and to identify what skills are required for effective implementation. An overview is presented in Table 4.

Table 3 Overarching processes to a fair selection system as advocated by Patterson et al. (2019) with important considerations

Overarching processes	Important considerations
(i) Having objective and valid criteria (developed through an appropriate job analysis)	Align the mission with the tools and processes. Weight tools accordingly. Be transparent on the requirements to all stakeholders
(ii) Accurate and standardized assessment by trained personnel	Training, standardization, and moderation
(iii) Monitoring outcomes	Quality assurance – evaluation of outcomes and processes. Consequences (intended or otherwise) of changes to selection processes, feedback on tool performance, selection outcomes relative to mission and social accountability, and reporting to key stakeholders

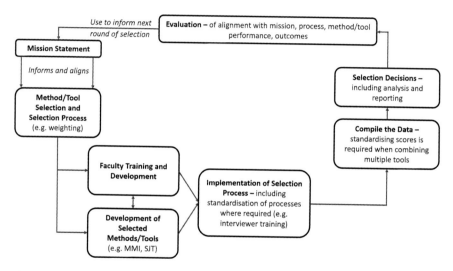

Fig. 1 Main elements of a selection process and relationship between each element

Aligning Mission, Tools, and Process

As shown in Fig. 1, the process begins with alignment of the mission of the course or program (i.e., the desired graduate attributes), which will determine the selection methods used and their relative weighting in the final decision. The mix of selection tools chosen and policies and procedures for aspects, such as widening access, should ultimately reflect the mission statement as should the weighting of each of the selection tools chosen. For example, the scores from the MMI may be weighted higher to ensure applicants who perform well on this selection tool and therefore have the competencies the tool is assessing are ranked higher. This process aligns with the institution's mission of wanting to select those applicants with competencies

Table 4 Broad overview of a selection process and associated tasks and skills for each step

Selection step	Task	Skills
Selection philosophy – aligned with mission	Identify required competencies and their weightings – often informed by competency standard frameworks of the health profession	Knowledge of the competency standard framework requirements for the profession into which the applicant is applying for
Choice of selection methods to align with philosophy	Selection of methods and tools that assess the identified attribute or competency desired in students and graduates	Knowledge of available methods and their validity, reliability, feasibility, etc.
Selection method development	Development of selection tools – e.g., scenario and question development in MMIs, and scenario and item response development in SJTs	Expertise in specific selection method design (i.e., MMI, SJT) Subject matter expertise (i.e., SJT)
Selection implementation	• Process requirements for each method/tool • Standardization and training of interviewers • Applicant briefings	Standardization processes Understanding of factors that impact on decision-making in people making judgment (i.e., MMI – unconscious bias)
Selection decisions	• Determining those who will be offered a place in the course or training program, and those who will not • Usually via ranking of applicants across all methods in the process according to specific and transparent weights of each tool or method • Reporting and evaluation of process for QA	• Statistical analyses expertise, especially in combining data from various sources using different scales, weighting scores, and ranking • Psychometric analysis, including conducting reliability analysis, and other measures of tool performance. • Reporting of selection outcomes, tool performance relative to current and previous years • Evaluation of the process and outcomes, impact of modifications, identification of areas for improvement

that are measured by the MMI (e.g., ethical reasoning, advocacy for the disadvantaged, cultural sensitivity) and not just on academic attainment.

Once selection tools have been chosen to align with the mission statement, a determination can be made as to what, if any, selection tool development is required. Tools that capture academic achievement and aptitude already exist as previously mentioned and therefore development of these is not required. However, if competency-based selection methods such as MMIs and SJTs are used, these will need to be developed specific to the particular selection context. These tools can be developed internally; however, the resources and expertise required to develop valid and reliable MMIs and SJTs have led to the outsourcing of work to independent organizations and SMEs. This can be at considerable financial and opportunity costs, which is an increasing consideration when identifying selection methods at undergraduate, postgraduate, and specialty training selection (Foo et al. 2020).

Training, Standardization, and Moderation

While tools are being developed, it is very important that both training and development of faculty occurs. Faculty may need to upskill in the various processes associated with selection if they are new to the selection process. Currently, this largely occurs informally through mentoring, reading, and gaining understanding of the evidence base, and in some instances, more formal training such as statistics training. Formal faculty development relating to selection is limited, and this is a future challenge for selection, as described later in the chapter. Not only is training of faculty required, but standardization processes are essential to ensure the development and delivery of reliable and valid selection tools. For example, item developers for SJTs and MMIs, and interviewers for MMIs should undergo training. This training should ensure that interviewers, assessors, and all involved in the delivery of the chosen selection methods are familiar with the rationale for the selection methods, their role, and what is required from them. Training should also focus on allowing time for standardization where required, this is particularly the case for MMIs where often there are multiple instances of the one station (due to high applicant numbers), and therefore multiple interviewers rating different groups of applicants on the same station. Therefore, interviewers on the same station must ensure that they are interpreting and scoring applicant responses in a consistent manner. This standardization process is vital to inter-rater reliability. It is extremely important that the interviewers have a shared understanding of the issues involved in the station, and what they would expect of a very good applicant relative to a good, average, or poorer performing applicant. This standardization process usually occurs by having interviewers on the same station meet prior to the delivery of the MMI to discuss the scenario, develop a shared understanding of the key issues and the level of sophistication they expect when assigning scores to each question to determine applicant performance.

Once training, standardization, and moderation processes are complete, the selection process can be implemented. Data collected for each selection tool should be standardized so that the scores from multiple tools can be combined, and the predetermined weightings in addition to any social accountability policies and procedures should be applied. These final weighted scores should then be used for selection decisions, ensuring that any social accountability policies and procedures are adhered to.

Evaluating the Selection Process

Once selection decisions have been made, the final, and possibly most crucial, step is evaluation. Evaluation, also referred to as quality assurance, should aim for continuous improvement and should be a cyclical process – that is, results of the evaluation should feedback into the selection process. It is important that reliability and validity of tools are monitored and that evaluation data of not only individual steps but also the whole process are fed back into the cycle. Evaluation is essential to ensure that methods being used are the right ones, measuring the right qualities, and are valid and reliable. It is also important that institutions delivering healthcare education and training programs can demonstrate that they are meeting the changing needs of society (Dore et al. 2017), and that the goals of their mission statement are being achieved. For example, if targets for the selection of Indigenous applicants are not met, the reason for this should be investigated, and the selection process altered to address this. Or, if an SJT or MMI is determined to have lower than expected reliability, or there is variation across interviewers for the MMI, these issues should be investigated and remedied.

The selection process produces a large amount of data; however, selection remains segregated at each point in the training process and so data is usually only used for ranking applicants. Given the resources allocated to selection, whether it be for undergraduate or graduate entry, or specialist college training, the data collected could be utilized beyond the admission decision. Selection is almost exclusively based on rank order, and this rank is determined through combining scores across the utilized tools. Scrutiny at the tool level is rarely undertaken. For example, both SJTs and MMIs assess multiple domains, and it is possible for applicants to vary in performance across these domains. Differences in patterns of performance could provide valuable information on the needs of those applicants who are selected and also remediation points for those who are not. These could then be used to give feedback to both successful and unsuccessful applicants on how they can improve.

Selection Challenges

Despite decades of widening access initiatives and innovation in selection, the outcome remains a largely homogenous cohort of students and trainees who are not meeting workforce needs, especially in rural areas (Hay et al. 2017a). It is therefore clear that selection approaches to date are not having the desired outcome, that is a diverse cohort of health professions graduates who are representative of the populations they will serve. Future selection processes may focus less on meritocracy (for either academic or nonacademic traits) and may involve different processes, policies, and procedures for selecting a broader and diverse healthcare workforce (Coyle et al. 2021).

As we continue to move towards more competency-based selection tools across all levels of training, additional resources and training are required to ensure appropriate expertise in selection processes. In order to ensure that selection tools are being used appropriately, as part of a quality selection process, there is a need to ensure that there are sufficient resources for both applicants and those involved in selection to create sustainable, high quality processes. Without sufficient resources, there is the risk that the development of competency-based tools, for example, SJTs and MMIs, will be compromised and potentially result in tools with poor validity and reliability.

For applicants, selection is a resource-intensive process that includes a range of costs from preparation costs, travel costs potentially to multiple locations for interviews, and costs for completing aptitude tests, for example, the UCAT, GAMSAT, and United States Medical Licensing Examination – USMLE to name a few (Foo et al. 2020). In response to the COVID-19 pandemic, we have had to change every aspect of health professions education, including selection. During the pandemic, selection had to rely solely on remote or digital methods. Remote selection offers both benefits and challenges. There is a clear financial benefit for applicants with travel costs associated with selection reduced to zero. This has the potential to open selection to a broader range of people. There are, however, some important considerations such as applicants' familiarity with and ability to access the technology being used. As we move towards the COVID new normal and more face-to-face interactions occur, there is a need to consider the pros and cons of the selection tools or methods, and the opportunity that technology, for example, advancements in virtual and augmented reality, offers to improve access to selection and the selection process itself. This is a rich field for scholarship in the field of selection into the health professions.

Finally, selection in the health professions is a complex undertaking; however, very little (if any) professional development exists in this area. This is particularly so regarding tool development and selection ranking. We need to ensure that those involved in selection are provided with opportunities to upskill, but currently this is likely to be done informally. The development of formal professional development in selection would be greatly beneficial for increasing the quality of selection processes. This too is a rich field for scholarship in this area.

Conclusion

This chapter has provided the reader with an overview of the main considerations, method, tools, and processes involved in selection of students and trainees in the health professions. We have provided the main steps involved in a fair selection process, along with a review of the selection methods and tools that are in use today across individual, competency-based, and social accountability aspects. We have provided the steps for a quality and defensible selection process and noted some future challenges and opportunities in the area. We have also noted areas for further research. There is rich and increasing literature on selection into the health professions, and also an extensive community of practice that we encourage readers with an interest in selection to access.

Cross-References

▶ Approaches to Assessment: A Perspective from Education

References

Alhurishi SA, Aljuraiban GS, Alshaikh FA, Almutairi MM, Almutairi KM. Predictors of students' academic achievements in allied health professions at King Saud University: a retrospective cohort study. BMC Med Educ. 2021;21:93. https://doi.org/10.1186/s12909-021-02525-x.

Anderton RS. Identifying factors that contribute to academic success in first year allied health and science degrees at an Australian University. Aust J Educ. 2017;61(2):184–99. https://doi.org/10.1177/0004944117713321.

Association of American Medical Colleges. Enrollment up at US Medical Schools. December 2020. https://www.aamc.org/news-insights/press-releases/enrollment-us-medical-schools. Accessed 27 Mar 2022.

Ballejos MP, Rhyne RL, Parkes J. Increasing the relative weight of noncognitive admission criteria improves underrepresented minority admission rates to medical school. Teach Learn Med. 2015;27(2):155–62. https://doi.org/10.1080/10401334.2015.1011649.

Boelen C. Adapting health care institutions and medical schools to societies' needs. Acad Med. 1999;74:S11–20.

Boelen C, Heck J. Defining and measuring the social accountability of medical schools. Geneva: World Health Organisation; 1995. https://apps.who.int/iris/handle/10665/59441. Accessed 18 Nov 2021

Boelen C, Pearson D, Kaufman A, Rourke J, Woollard R, Marsh DC, et al. Producing a socially accountable medical school: AMEE guide no. 109. Med Teach. 2016;38(11):1078–91.

Burkhardt JC. What can we learn from resident selection interviews? J Grad Med Educ. 2015;7(4):673–5. https://doi.org/10.4300/JGME-D-15-00403.1.

Cantwell P. Personality tests in medical student selection. Australas Med J. 2019;12(7):220–1.

Coyle M, Sandover S, Poobalan A, Bullen J, Cleland J. Meritocratic and fair? The discourse of UK and Australia's widening participation policies. Med Educ. 2021;55(7):825–39. https://doi.org/10.1111/medu.14442.

Crawford C, Black P, Melby V, Fitzpatrick B. An exploration of the predictive validity of selection criteria on progress outcomes for pre-registration nursing programmes – a systematic review. J Clin Nurs. 2021;30(17–18):2489–513. https://doi.org/10.1111/jocn.15730.

Cullen MJ, Sackett PR, Lievens, F. Threats to the operational use of situational judgment tests in the college admission process. Intern J Selec and Assess. 2006;14(2):142–155. https://ink.library.smu.edu.sg/lkcsb_research/5565.

Danilovich N, Kitto S, Price DW, Campbell C, Hodgson A, Hendry P. Implementing competency-based medical education in family medicine: a narrative review of current trends in assessment. Fam Med. 2021;53(1):9–22. https://doi.org/10.22454/FamMed.2021.453158.

Dore KL, Roberts C, Wright S. Widening perspectives: reframing the way we research selection. Adv Health Sci Educ Theory Pract. 2017;22(2):565–72. https://doi.org/10.1007/s10459-016-9730-5.

Eva KW, Rosenfeld J, Reiter HI, Norman GR. An admissions OSCE: the multiple mini-interview. Med Educ. 2004;38(3):314–26.

Eva KW, Reiter HI, Trinh K, Wasi P, Rosenfeld J, Norman GR. Predictive validity of the multiple mini-interview for selecting medical trainees. Med Educ. 2009;43(8):767–75.

Ferguson E, Lievens F. Future directions in personality, occupational and medical selection: myths, misunderstandings, measurement, and suggestions. Adv Health Sci Educ Theory Pract. 2017;22(2):387–99.

Fielding S, Tiffin PA, Greatrix R, Lee AJ, Patterson F, Nicholson S, et al. Do changing medical admissions practices in the UK impact on who is admitted? An interrupted time series analysis. BMJ Open. 2018;8(10):e023274. https://doi.org/10.1136/bmjopen-2018-023274.

Fitzmaurice L, Donald K, de Wet C, Palipana D. Why we should and how we can increase medical school admissions for persons with disabilities. Med J Aust. 2021;215(6):249–251.e1. https://doi.org/10.5694/mja2.51238.

Foo J, Rivers G, Allen L, Ilic D, Maloney S, Hay M. The economic costs of selecting medical students: an Australian case study. Med Educ. 2020;54(7):643–51. https://doi.org/10.1111/medu.14145.

Garrud P. Selecting medical students: we need to assess more than academic excellence. Med J Aust. 2018;208(5):202–3. https://doi.org/10.5694/mja17.01224.

Girgulis K, Rideout A, Rashid M. Performance of Black and Indigenous applicants in a medical school admissions process. Can Med Ed J [Internet]. 2021 Nov 1 [cited 2021 Nov 23]. Available from: https://journalhosting.ucalgary.ca/index.php/cmej/article/view/72121

Goffin RD, Christiansen ND. Correcting personality tests for faking: a review of popular personality tests and an initial survey of researchers. Int J Sel Assess. 2003;11(1/2):340–4.

Greenhill J, Walker J, Playford D. Outcomes of Australian rural clinical schools: a decade of success building the rural medical workforce through the education and training continuum. Rural Remote Health. 2015;15(3):2991. https://doi.org/10.22605/RRH2991.

Griffin B, Porfeli E, Hu W. Who do you think you are? Medical student socioeconomic status and intention to work in underserved areas. Adv Health Sci Educ Theory Pract. 2016;22(2):491–504. https://doi.org/10.1007/s10459-016-9726-1.

Haavisto E, Hupil M, Hahtela N, Heikkila A, Huovila P, Moisio E-L, et al. Structure and content of a new entrance exam to select undergraduate nursing students. Int J Nurs Educ Scholarsh. 2019;16(1):8. https://doi.org/10.1515/ijnes-2018-0008.

Hay M, Mercer AM, Lichtwark I, Hodgson WC, Aretz HT, Armstrong EG, et al. Selecting for a sustainable workforce to meet the future healthcare needs of rural communities in Australia. Adv Health Sci Educ Theory Pract. 2017a;22(2):533–51. https://doi.org/10.1007/s10459-016-9727-0.

Hay M, Lichtwark I, Metcalf J, Henry S. The influence of first language, gender and age on situational judgement test (SJT) scores in nursing interns. In: Research presentation. AMEE conference, innovating in education, 26–30 August, Helsinki. 2017b.

Hertel-Waszak A, Brouwer B, Schönefeld E, Ahrens H, Hertel G, Marschall B. Medical doctors' job specification analysis: a qualitative inquiry. GMS. J Med Educ. 2017;34(4):Doc43.

Hofmeister M, Lockyer J, Crutcher R. The multiple mini-interview for selection of international medical graduates into family medicine residency education. Med Educ. 2009;43(6):573–9.

Hudak RP, Brooke PP Jr, Finstuen K. Identifying management competencies for health care executives: review of a series of Delphi studies. J Health Adm Educ. 2000;18(2):213–43. Discussion 244–9

Kale S, Kamble MW, Spalding N. Predictive validity of multiple mini interview scores for future academic and clinical placement performance in physiotherapy, occupational therapy and speech and language therapy programmes. Int J Ther Rehabil. 2020;27(4):1–13. https://doi.org/10.12968/ijtr.2018.0149.

Kreiter CD, Axelson RD. A perspective on medical school admission research and practice over the last 25 years. Teach Learn Med. 2013;25(Suppl 1):S50–6. https://doi.org/10.1080/10401334.2013.842910.

Kudlas MJ. Effects of radiography program admissions practices on student retention. J Allied Health. 2006;35(3):162–8.

Kuncel NR, Kochevar RJ, Ones DS. A meta-analysis of letters of recommendation in college and graduate admissions: reasons for hope. Int J Sel Assess. 2014;22(1):101–7. https://doi.org/10.1111/ijsa.12060.

Lemay EP, Clark MS, Feeney, BC. Projection of responsiveness to needs and the construction of satisfying communal relationship. J Personality and Soc Psych. 2007;92(5):834–853. https://doi.org/10.1037/0022-3514.92.5.834.

Lewkonia RM. The missions of medical schools: the pursuit of health in the service of society. BMC Med Educ. 2001;1:4. https://doi.org/10.1186/1472-6920-1-4.

Lievens F, Peeters H, Schollaert E. Situational judgment tests: a review of recent research. Pers Rev. 2008;37(4):426–1.

Lievens F, Patterson F. The validity and incremental validity of knowledge tests, low-fidelity simulations, and high-fidelity simulations for predicting job performance in advanced-level high-stakes selection. J Appl Psych. 2011;96(5):927–940. https://doi.org/10.1037/a0023496.

Lievens F, Sackett PR. The validity of interpersonal skills assessment via situational judgment tests for predicting academic success and job performance. J Appl Psych. 2012;97(2):460–468. https://doi.org/10.1037/a0025741.

Lievens F, Patterson F, Corstjens J, Martin S, Nicholson S. Widening access in selection using situational judgement tests: evidence from the UKCAT. Med Educ. 2016;50(6):624–636. https://doi.org/10.1111/medu.13060.

Maan ZN, Maan IN, Darzi AW, Aggarwal R. Systematic review of predictors of surgical performance. Br J Surg. 2012;99(12):1610–21.

MacKenzie RK, Dowell J, Ayansina D, Cleland JA. Do personality traits assessed on medical school admission predict exit performance? A UK-wide longitudinal cohort study. Adv Health Sci Educ Theory Pract. 2017;22(2):365–85.

Matsumoto M, Inoue K, Kajii E. Characteristics of medical students with rural origin: implications for selective admission policies. Health Policy. 2008;87(2):194–202. https://doi.org/10.1016/j.healthpol.2007.12.006.

McDaniel MA, Hartman NS, Whetzel DL, Grubb WL. Situational Judgement tests, response instructions, and validity: a meta-analysis. Person Psych. 2007;60(1):63–91. https://doi.org/10.1111/j.1744-6570.2007.00065.x.

McManus IC, Dewberry C, Nicholson S, Dowell JS. The UKCAT-12 study: educational attainment, aptitude test performance, demographic and socio-economic contextual factors as predictors of first year outcome in a cross-sectional collaborative study of 12 UK medical schools. BMC Med. 2013;11:244.

Medical Schools Council. Selecting for excellence final report. Medical Schools Council. 2014. https://www.medschools.ac.uk/media/1203/selecting-for-excellence-final-report.pdf. Accessed 24 Nov 2021.

Medical Schools Council. The expansion of medical student numbers in the United Kingdom. October 2021. https://www.medschools.ac.uk/our-work/the-expansion-of-medical-student-numbers. Accessed 27 Mar 2022.

Medical Training Review Panel (MTRP) 18th Report. Australian Government Department of Health. Commonwealth of Australia. ISBN (print): 978-1-76007-162-2. 2015. Retrieved 29 June 2015, from http://www.health.gov.au/internet/main/publishing.nsf/Content/work-pubs-mtrp-18

Mercer A, Puddey IB. Admission selection criteria as predictors of outcomes in an undergraduate medical course: a prospective study. Med Teach. 2011;33(12):997–1004.

Mercer A, Hay M, Hodgson WC, Canny BJ, Puddey IB. The relative predictive value of undergraduate versus graduate selection tools in two Australian medical schools. Med Teach. 2018;40(11):1183–90. https://doi.org/10.1080/0142159X.2018.1426839.

Mian O, Hogenbirk JC, Marsh DC, Prowse O, Cain M, Warry W. Tracking Indigenous applicants through the admissions process of a socially accountable medical school. Acad Med. 2019;94(8):1211–9. https://doi.org/10.1097/ACM.0000000000002636.

Morrison J. Selecting for medical education. Med Educ. 2016;50(1):3–5.

O'Brien A, Harvey J, Shannon M, Lewis K, Valencia O. A comparison of multiple mini-interviews and structured interviews in a UK setting. Med Teach. 2011;33(5):397–402.

O'Connell MS, Hartman NS, McDaniel MA, Grubb WL, Lawrence A. Incremental validity of situational judgment tests for task and contextual job performance. Intern J Selec and Assess. 2007;15(1):19–29. https://doi.org/10.1111/j.1468-2389.2007.00364.x.

Patterson BF, Mattern KD. Validity of the SAT for predicting first-year grades: 2009 SAT validity sample. Statistical report no. 2012-2. 2009; College Board. ERIC Number ED563103. https://eric.ed.gov/?id=ED563103. Accessed 24 Nov 2021.

Patterson F, Zibarras L. Selection and recruitment in the healthcare professions research, theory and practice. 1st ed. Cham: Palgrave Macmillan; 2018.

Patterson F, Ferguson E, Thomas S. Using job analysis to identify core and specific competencies: implications for selection and recruitment. Med Educ. 2008;42(12):1195–204.

Patterson F, Ashworth V, Zibarras L, Coan P, Kerrin M, O'Neill P. Evaluations of situational judgement tests to assess non-academic attributes in selection. Med Educ. 2012;46(9):850–68.

Patterson F, Ashworth V, Kerrin M, O'Neill P. Situational judgement tests represent a measurement method and can be designed to minimise coaching effects. Med Educ. 2013;47(2):220–1.

Patterson F, Ferguson E, Knight AL. Selection into medical education and training. In: Swanwick T, editor. Understanding medical education: evidence, theory and practice. Chichester: Wiley; 2014. p. 403–20.

Patterson F, Knight A, Dowell J, Nicholson S, Cousans F, Cleland J. How effective are selection methods in medical education? A systematic review. Med Educ. 2016a;50(1):36–60. https://doi.org/10.1111/medu.12817.

Patterson F, Zibarras L, Ashworth V. Situational judgement tests in medical education and training: research, theory and practice: AMEE guide no. 100. Med Teach. 2016b;38(1):3–17.

Patterson F, Cleland J, Cousans F. Selection methods in healthcare professions: where are we now and where next? Adv Health Sci Educ Theory Pract. 2017;22(2):229–42. https://doi.org/10.1007/s10459-017-9752-7.

Patterson F, Roberts C, Hanson MD, Hampe W, Eva K, Ponnamperuma G, et al. Ottawa consensus statement: selection and recruitment to the healthcare professions. Med Tech. 2018;40(11):1091–101. https://doi.org/10.1080/0142159X.2018.1498589.

Patterson F, Ferguson E, Zibarras L. Selection into medical education and training. In: Swanwick T, Forrest K, O'Brien BC, editors. Understanding medical education: evidence, theory, and practice. 3rd ed. Hoboken: Wiley-Blackwell; 2019. p. 375–88.

Pau A, Jeevaratnam K, Chen YS, Fall AA, Khoo C, Nadarajah VD. The Multiple Mini-Interview (MMI) for student selection in health professions training – a systematic review. Med Teach. 2013;35(12):1027–41.

Paynter S, Illes R, Hay M. An investigation of the predictive validity of selection tools on performance in physiotherapy training in Australia. Physiotherapy. 2022;114:1–8. https://doi.org/10.1010/j.physio.2021.11.001.

Ployhart RE, Holtz BC. The diversity-validity dilemma: strategies for reducing racioethnic and sex subgroup differences and adverse impact in selection. Person Psych. 2008;61(1):153–172. https://doi.org/10.1111/j.1744-6570.2008.00109.x.

Pollard S, Cooper-Thomas H. Best practice recommendations for situational judgment tests. Austral J Org Psych. 2015;8(e70). https://doi.org/10.1017/orp.2015.6.

Powis D, Bore M, Munro D, Lumsden MA. Development of the personal qualities assessment as a tool for selecting medical students. J Adult Contin Educ. 2005;11(1):3–14. https://doi.org/10.7227/JACE.11.1.2.

Powis D, Munro D, Bore M, Burstal A. In-course and career outcomes predicted by medical school selection procedures based on personal qualities. Med Teach. 2020;42(8):944–6. https://doi.org/10.1080/0142159X.2020.1747605.

Powis D, Munro D, Miles Bore M, Eley D. Why is it so hard to consider personal qualities when selecting medical students? Med Teach. 2020b;42(4):366–71. https://doi.org/10.1080/0142159X.2019.1703919.

Prideaux D, Roberts C, Eva K, Centeno A, McCrorie P, McManus C, et al. Assessment for selection for the health care professions and specialty training: consensus statement and recommendations from the Ottawa 2010 conference. Med Teach. 2011;33(3):215–23.

Puddey IB, Mercer A. Predicting academic outcomes in an Australian graduate entry medical programme. BMC Med Educ. 2014;14:31. https://doi.org/10.1186/1472-6920-14-31.

Puddey IB, Mercer A, Playford DE, Pougnault S, Riley GJ. Medical student selection criteria as predictors of intended rural practice following graduation. BMC Med Educ. 2014;14:218. https://doi.org/10.1186/1472-6920-14-218.

Puddey IB, Playford DE, Mercer A. Impact of medical student origins on the likelihood of ultimately practicing in areas of low vs high socio-economic status. BMC Med Educ. 2017;17(1):1. https://doi.org/10.1186/s12909-016-0842-7.

Razack S. "Meritocracy" and "fairness" in medical student selection: comparing UK and Australia. Med Educ. 2021;55(7):772–4. https://doi.org/10.1111/medu.14525.

Razack S, Hodges B, Steinert Y, Maguire M. Seeking inclusion in an exclusive process: discourses of medical school student selection. Med Educ. 2015;49(1):36–47. https://doi.org/10.1111/medu.12547.

Rees EK, Hawarden AW, Dent G, Hays R, Bates J, Hassell AB. Evidence regarding the utility of multiple mini-interview (MMI) for selection to undergraduate health programs: a BEME systematic review: BEME guide no. 37. Med Tech. 2016;38(5):443–55.

Rigby PG, Gururaja RP. World medical schools: the sum also rises. JRSM Open. 2017;8(6):1–6. https://doi.org/10.1177/2054270417698631.

Rivera L. Hiring as cultural matching: the case of elite professional service firms. Am Sociol Rev. 2012;77(6):999–1022.

Roberts C, Walton M, Rothnie I, Crossley J, Lyon P, Kumar K, et al. Factors affecting the utility of the multiple mini-interview in selecting candidates for graduate-entry medical school. Med Educ. 2008;42(4):396–404.

Roberts C, Khanna P, Rigby L, Bartle E, Llewellyn A, Gustavs J, et al. Utility of selection methods for specialist medical training: a BEME (best evidence medical education) systematic review: BEME guide no. 45. Med Teach. 2018;40(1):3–19. https://doi.org/10.1080/0142159X.2017.1367375.

Rosenstein AH, O'Daniel M. A survey of the impact of disruptive behaviors and communication defects on patient safety. Jt Comm J Qual Patient Saf. 2008;34(8):464–71. https://doi.org/10.1016/s1553-7250(08)34058-6.

Russell S, Murley G, Oates M, Li X, Raspovic A. Does the Australian Tertiary Admissions Rank score (ATAR) predict academic performance in a podiatry course? Focus Health Prof Educ. 2021;22(1):68–87.

Schreurs S, Cleutjens KBJM, Cleland J, Oude Egbrink MGA. Outcomes-based selection into medical school: predicting excellence in multiple competencies during the clinical years. Acad Med. 2020;95(9):1411–20. https://doi.org/10.1097/ACM.0000000000003279. PMID: 32134790; PMCID: PMC7447174

Schripsema NR, van Trigt AM, van der Wal MA, Cohen-Schotanus J. How different medical school selection processes call upon different personality characteristics. PLoS One. 2016;11(3):e0150645. https://doi.org/10.1371/journal.pone.0150645.

Sladek RM, King SM. From pipedream to possibility: developing an equity target for refugees to study medicine in Australia. In: Sengupta E, Blessinger P, editors. Strategies, policies and directions for refugee education. Bingley: Emerald Publishing Limited; 2018. p. 249–61.

Stemig MS, Sackett PR, Lievens F. Effects of organizationally endorsed coaching on performance and validity of situational judgment tests. Int J Sel Assess. 2015;23(2):174–81.

Tesson G, Curran V, Pong R, Strasser R. Advances in rural medical education in three countries: Canada, the United States and Australia. Educ Health. 2005;18(3):405–15. https://doi.org/10.1080/13576280500289728.

Till H, Myford C, Dowell J. Improving student selection using multiple mini-interviews with multifaceted Rasch modeling. Acad Med. 2013;88(2):216–23.

Webster ES, Paton LW, Crampton PES, Tiffin PA. Situational judgement test validity for selection: a systematic review and meta-analysis. Med Educ. 2020;54(10):888–902.

White J, Brownell K, Lemay JF, Lockyer JM. "What do they want me to say?" The hidden curriculum at work in the medical school selection process: a qualitative study. BMC Med Educ. 2012;12:17. https://doi.org/10.1186/1472-6920-12-17.

Woods SA, Barratt J. Personality assessment in healthcare and implications for selection. In: Patterson F, Zibarras L, editors. Selection and recruitment in healthcare professions. Cham: Palgrave Macmillan; 2018. p. 51–77.

Wright S. Medical school personal statements: a measure of motivation or proxy for cultural privilege? Adv Health Sci Educ Theory Pract. 2015;20(3):627–43. https://doi.org/10.1007/s10459-014-9550-4.

Young ME, Razack S, Hanson MD, Slade S, Varpio L, Dore KL, et al. Calling for a broader conceptualization of diversity. Acad Med. 2012;87(11):501–1510. https://doi.org/10.1097/ACM.0b013e31826daf74.

Practice Education in Occupational Therapy: Current Trends and Practices

66

Stephen Isbel, Ted Brown, Mong-Lin Yu, Thomas Bevitt, Craig Greber, and Anne-Maree Caine

Contents

Introduction	1278
What Is Practice Education in Occupational Therapy?	1278
The Purpose of Clinical and Practice Education	1279
Clinical and Practice Education: Evidence from the Student Perspective	1279
Clinical and Practice Education: Evidence from the Practice Educator	1280
Clinical and Practice Education: Evidence from the Settings	1281
High-Quality Placements	1282
Promoting Reflective Practice in Practice Education	1283
Reflective Practice in Occupational Therapy	1284
Models of Reflection	1285
Practice Education Models	1286
Competencies in Practice Education	1288
Supervision and Feedback	1289
Best Practice When Evaluating Students on Placement: Theory and Process	1290
Supporting the Development of Professional Reasoning in Practice Education	1292
Trends in Practice Education and Future Directions	1295

S. Isbel (✉) · C. Greber
Faculty of Health, University of Canberra, Canberra, ACT, Australia
e-mail: stephen.isbel@canberra.edu.au; craig.greber@canberra.edu.au

T. Brown · M.-L. Yu
Department of Occupational Therapy, School of Primary and Allied Health Care, Faculty of Medicine, Nursing and Health Sciences, Monash University – Peninsula Campus, Frankston, VIC, Australia
e-mail: ted.brown@monash.edu; mong-lin.yu@monash.edu

T. Bevitt
Faculty of Health, The University of Canberra Hospital, Canberra, Bruce ACT, Australia
e-mail: Thomas.Bevitt@canberra.edu.au

A.-M. Caine
School of Allied Health Sciences – Occupational Therapy, Griffith University, Nathan, QLD, Australia
e-mail: a.caine@griffith.edu.au

© Springer Nature Singapore Pte Ltd. 2023
D. Nestel et al. (eds.), *Clinical Education for the Health Professions*,
https://doi.org/10.1007/978-981-15-3344-0_137

Conclusion 1296
References 1297

Abstract

Practice education is critical in the occupational therapy profession as it is the time when students have the opportunity to apply the theory and skills acquired in a classroom environment to a practice setting. It is seen as an opportunity to allow students to develop critical thinking, to be resilient learners, and become ethical practitioners. This chapter describes key aspects of practice education in occupational therapy including the evidence supporting practice education, the competencies involved in successful practice education, practice reasoning during practice education, the quality of practice education, evaluation of practice education, and future trends and directions.

Keywords

Occupational therapy · Practice education · Practice education · Practice reasoning · World Federation of Occupational Therapy · Competency · Models of practice education · Supervision · Feedback · Quality placements

Introduction

What Is Practice Education in Occupational Therapy?

Practice education is "a process of work based learning which involves a partnership between the practice educator and the student in the practice setting" (National University of Ireland Galway 2020, p. 1). When related specifically to occupational therapy, it is helpful to re-visit the definition of occupational therapy as it helps to frame practice education from an occupational perspective.

> Occupational therapy is a client-centred health profession concerned with promoting health and wellbeing through occupation. The primary goal of occupational therapy is to enable people to participate in the activities of everyday life. (World Federation of Occupational Therapists 2012, p. 4)

Practice education in occupational therapy can take place anywhere that people or communities engage in occupation, which is wide and varied. Hence, practice education can take place in settings such as in hospitals, schools, aged care facilities, subacute rehabilitation centers, private practices, or in fact potentially in any place that people engage in leisure, play, self-care, education, work, sleep/rest, volunteer, or social participation related daily activities. In acknowledging that practice education can occur in these diverse settings, it also acknowledges it can take place in areas that deliver occupational therapy services to individuals, to families, to communities, to organizations, and to populations.

The World Federation of Occupational Therapists (WFOT) (2016) has recommended that all occupational therapy students enrolled in entry-to-practice

WFOT accredited education courses complete a minimum of 1000 hours of practice education. There has been some debate about the need to maintain this practice education requirement since this has remained unchanged since it was established in 1958 (Brown et al. 2016; Thomas and Penman 2019).

The Purpose of Clinical and Practice Education

The World Federation of Occupational Therapists states that "The purpose of practice education is for students to integrate knowledge, professional reasoning and professional behaviour within practice, and to develop knowledge, skills and attitudes to the level of competence required of qualifying occupational therapists" (WFOT 2016, p. 46). In order to gain the experience required to graduate as competent occupational therapists, students are expected to have a breadth and depth of practice education that encompasses people of different age groups, exposure to people with health needs, and using interventions that focus on the person, the occupation, and the environment (WFOT 2016). Professional education should be guided by sound teaching and learning principles, be adequately supervised, documented, evaluated, and at all times informed by evidence-based practice (WFOT 2016).

Practice education experience is significant since it is the context where students can apply the professional foundation knowledge, theories, interventions, and assessments they have learned in the university context. Time management, problem solving, professional reasoning, and communication skills are key abilities that occupational therapy students need to develop and refine in the practice education environment. Students have to be able to accept and act on constructive input from their practice educator (supervisor). They also need to navigate the complex set of skills working with clients and their families and abide by the policies and procedures of the practice education setting. Students need to exhibit professional skills such as privacy, ethical conduct, client safety and respect, cultural awareness and sensitivity, and reflective practice.

Clinical and Practice Education: Evidence from the Student Perspective

Numerous studies have been completed regarding aspects of occupational therapy student practice placements. For example, Kemp and Crabtree (2018) investigated the match between student characteristics and demands of practice education settings. The top six characteristics and abilities practice educators rated that occupational therapy students needed to demonstrate to be successful on placements were time management, communication with supervisor when help was needed, overall professional behavior, ability to make change based upon supervisor's feedback, flexibility with schedule changes, and organizational skills (Kemp and Crabtree 2018).

Hills et al. (2016) delved into Generation Y students' views and preferences about the provision of feedback during practice education. Occupational therapy students stated that feedback while completing placements should be regular and consistent, immediate explicit feedback was welcomed when it identified skills that needed improvement, protected supervision time for feedback was valued, and opportunities for students to self-evaluate prior to receiving feedback were suggested (Hills et al. 2016).

Andonian (2013) explored the relationship between students' emotional intelligence, self-efficacy, and their practice performance and determined that occupational therapy students' emotional intelligence was positively correlated with some aspects of their performance while self-efficacy was not (Andonian 2013). Brown et al. (2020b) studied the relationship between occupational therapy students' resilience and their success on practice education placements. It was found that aspects of resilience (e.g., managing stress, finding one's calling, and living authentically) were strong predictors of a range of students' practice education performance skills including professional behaviors, self-management skills, and communication skills (Brown et al. 2020).

Clinical and Practice Education: Evidence from the Practice Educator

Several studies have been completed that investigated what traits an outstanding and effective practice educator exhibited, the pros and cons related to providing practice education placements from the perspective of practice educators, and why did practice educators decline to supervise students. Rodger et al. (2014) completed a qualitative study that investigated what makes an excellent practice educator. The thematic analysis results indicated that "providing the 'just right' challenge was the overarching theme that symbolised excellence in practice education from students' perspectives" (Rodger et al. 2014, p. 159). Three other themes that underpinned the "just right challenge" were (i) valuing a reciprocal relationship, (ii) facilitating learning opportunities and experiences, and (iii) promoting autonomy and independence (Rodger et al. 2014). In another study, Koski, Simon, and Dooley (2013) investigated the behaviors of practice educators that students and educators considered valuable in American contexts. In general, there was alignment between what students and practice educators viewed as effective behaviors. These were: assess students according to performance standards based on objective information; provide students with prompt, direct, specific, and constructive feedback throughout the practice education experience; demonstrate sensitivity to student learning styles by adapting teaching approaches; and work to establish a collaborative relationship that values the client perspective including diversity, values, beliefs, health, and well-being as defined by the client, and facilitate the learning process (Koski et al. 2013).

Some investigations have examined the positive and negative aspects of supervising occupational therapy students from the viewpoint of practice educators. Thomas et al. (2007) used an online questionnaire to determine the perspectives of occupational therapy practice educators from Queensland, Australia, about the benefits and challenges of providing practice education placements. Challenges identified by practice educators included staffing issues (high staff turnover, only part-time staff), lack of physical resources (e.g., desk space, computer access), and high workload pressures while acknowledged benefits involved the opportunity to vet students for potential future recruitment, students conducting projects, and developing resources for the practice education site, a sense of "giving something" back to the profession, and improving practice educator skills (e.g., supervision, communication, delegation, organization, and time management skills). Based on a survey of 817 practice educators from 41 US states, completed by Evenson et al. (2015) on behalf of the American Occupational Therapy Association (AOTA) Commission on Education, the most frequently reported perceived advantages of providing practice education for students were: the opportunity to update practice/keep current/apply new ideas, research, or theories; gain personal satisfaction/reward; give back to the university/profession; develop practice reasoning; develop supervision skills; and evaluation for future employment potential (Evenson et al. 2015). Conversely, the most often identified challenges linked with practice education were: workload pressures/time, physical space/availability of room/desk/computer, concerns about students' capabilities, and cost of staff time (Evenson et al. 2015).

A number of studies have investigated why occupational therapists decline to supervise students on practice education and these are: decreasing productivity, adversely affecting workload requirements, work environment stress, limited resources, anticipation of challenging student interactions, role strain and the view that requests for student supervision are an additional responsibility and pressure that is not central to their practice role (Barton et al. 2013; Ozelie et al. 2015). Varland et al. (2017) investigated positive and negative factors that influenced practice educator decisions about supervising students completing placements in American environments. The top five positive factors identified by respondents were: being offered continuing education units; if the university practice education coordinator offered educational resources to supervisors that clearly outlined practice education placement requirements and expectations; the supervisor's past experiences as a student; if there was an opportunity to share student supervision with another occupational therapist; and if the university offered access to educational resources for practice educators (Varland et al. 2017). The five most commonly cited factors dissuading practice educators from taking on students were: current job responsibilities, number of clients on caseload, productivity standards, working less than full time, and a fear of having to fail a student (Varland et al. 2017).

Clinical and Practice Education: Evidence from the Settings

One other focus of occupational therapy practice education research is related to the environments where it occurs. Gat and Ratzon (2014) explored the perceptions of two groups of occupational therapy students from the United States who had completed a placement, in either a community setting or a hospital-based environment, about their professional and personal skills. No significant differences were found between students who attended the two settings. Students in the community setting who had a practice educator and those who did not were also compared. It was noted that students who did not have a practice educator in the community setting scored higher on their perceptions of personal responsibility, cultural competence, and overall personal skills. It was recommended that entry-to-practice occupational therapy students be given the opportunity to complete their practice education placements in a variety of agency-based and community contexts. Nielsen, Klug, and Fox (2020) compared the impact of second year graduate-entry masters occupational therapy students completing a nontraditional practice educational experience versus a traditional one on their development of critical thinking using the Health Sciences Reasoning Test (HSRT) (Facione and Facione 2007). The findings indicated that all students demonstrated significant improvements on the HSRT Analysis subscale and that students who completed the nontraditional experience had significantly greater increases on the HSRT total score and on the Analysis subscale. Students who score higher on the HSRT Analysis subscale would typically exhibit a range of aptitudes including the ability to recognize reasons, themes, general ideas, assumptions, and important patterns and details.

High-Quality Placements

A quality placement has been described as one where learning is optimized and individualized to meet the learning needs of students (Kirke et al. 2007). Many researchers in the health professional context have explored the critical elements of a high-quality occupational therapy placement from the perspectives of multiple stakeholders, including students, practice educators, organizations, and universities. Studies have identified various characteristics of a high-quality placement and described a combination of personal attributes of those involved, along with those more related to environmental, educational, and institutional factors (e.g., Grenier 2015; Lalor et al. 2019).

Practice educators can contribute to quality by ensuring thorough planning and preparation for students (Rodger et al. 2011). Educators should ensure students have access to a range of learning experience appropriate to their skill level (e.g., the level of challenge moves from a just right fit to gradually being more demanding and complex so the skill level of the student is challenged and hence increased) and are provided with regular, balanced, and constructive feedback (Grenier 2015; Lalor et al. 2019; Rodger et al. 2011). Communication skills are vital in ensuring feedback to students is both understood and able to be acted on (Brown et al. 2020; Yu et al. 2018).

Students consistently report that educator approachability and ability to provide clear and realistic expectations have a significant impact on the quality of their placement learning and experience (Grenier 2015). Furthermore, collaborative problem solving to develop action plans is seen to enhance student performance and contributes to quality in practice placements (Rodger et al. 2014). From a practice setting perspective, key contributors to placement quality appear to include appropriate resourcing, orientation planning, provision of a welcoming and safe learning environment, and educator training and support (Lalor et al. 2019; Rodger et al. 2011).

Universities can enhance quality in placements by ensuring adequate planning and support for educators and students, including clear communication channels and expectations regarding student performance. The provision of timely support to educators and students is imperative if student performance is to be maximized (Rodger et al. 2011).

Students too have a role to play in ensuring quality in their placement experience. This includes completing necessary preparation set by universities and placement settings, active engagement in observation and learning opportunities, critical reflection on their practice, clarification of understanding and expectations, and seeking feedback on their performance (Lalor et al. 2019).

The Improving Quality in Practice Placements – Allied Health (iQIPP-AH) Guides were developed in 2012 (The University of Queensland 2012), based largely on the work of Rodger et al. (2011) and their exploration of the perspectives of practice educators, students, and university staff with regard to quality in practice education. The iQIPP-AH explores quality at four key stages of the placement process: establishment, preparation, maintenance (during the placement), and review. It not only provides opportunity for critical reflection against key indicators with the use of probe questions, but also encourages action planning and review. Its application can occur at an individual level for students, practice educators, organizations, and university staff, or at a team level as part of quality improvement processes (The University of Queensland 2012).

If we are to reinforce the importance of reflective practice in the education of future occupational therapists, then it makes sense that this reflective practice extends to the provision of quality practice placements for students. All stakeholders have a role to play in maximizing quality in such experiences.

Promoting Reflective Practice in Practice Education

Reflection has been described as a metacognitive process that is active, intentional, cyclical and involves both thoughts and feelings (Boyd and Fales 1983; Schon 1983; Boud et al. 1985). It has been argued that when we return to experiences through reflection, new learning is often revealed (Boud et al. 1985). Epstein (1999) believed that exemplary practitioners have the capacity for critical reflection that "pervades all areas of practice." Health professionals need to be able to critically reflect on theories, evidence, and experiences to inform and improve practice. Student health professionals also need to be able to reflect critically on learning opportunities to optimize outcomes from practice education experiences.

One of the challenges for students, and indeed some practice educators, is understanding the true meaning of critical reflection. There are many models which categorize types and levels of reflection, including that by Kember et al. (2008) who described the first level of reflection, which involves simply describing what happened as in fact, "nonreflection." They argued that critical reflection has only occurred when one can demonstrate how their thinking and perspective have changed as a result. Schon (1983) described two forms of reflection that take place at different stages of an experience: (a) reflection-in-action – as the experience is occurring; and (b) reflection-on action or retrospective reflection – after the experience.

It is vital that practice educators promote and encourage critical reflection on knowledge and experiences by students. This helps link new and existing knowledge; identify learning needs; promote an understanding of professional beliefs, values, and attitudes; contribute to development of professional reasoning; and develop self-aware health professionals (Mann et al. 2009). Key actions to promote reflective practice in occupational therapy students include providing a supportive environment which includes time and space for critical reflection, modeling and describing of practice educators' own reflections, use of structured templates and guides, and the provision of peer reflection opportunities (Mann et al. 2009).

Some students require additional time to reflect and educators can support this in several ways, for example, identifying the topic for reflection prior to en experience, or allowing a short time for a student to think and document thoughts and feelings before debriefing. Expert guidance and support when engaging in reflection is important (Donaghy and Morss 2000), suggesting that critical reflection involves both students and practice educators as vital partners.

Reflective Practice in Occupational Therapy

Reflection is a critical element of occupational therapy practice. For example, The Australian Occupational Therapy Competency Standards (Occupational Therapy Board of Australia 2018) define reflection as:

> ...the process of thinking critically about one's practice. This may involve consideration of assumptions and alternative approaches, comparison to the practice of colleagues, considering the potential relevance and application to practice of new knowledge, acquired through reading, formal learning or other CPD activity. (p. 12)

Historically, many authors have argued that reflection is a key learning tool that informs our professional development (e.g., Clarke 1986; Moon 1999). In essence, reflection is a transformative process that ensures exposure to events leads to personal and professional growth. Without reflection, it has been argued learning does not occur (Schon 1983). For that reason, reflective practice skills are an essential component of occupational therapy education and are a required competency for occupational therapists. For example, the Australian Occupational Therapy Competency Standards (Occupational Therapy Board of Australia 2018) include two specific competencies related directly to reflective practice:

Standard 2.8 – *Reflects on practice to inform current and future reasoning and decision-making and the integration of theory and evidence into practice.*
Standard 3.7 – *Reflects on practice to inform and communicate professional reasoning and decision-making.*

Occupational therapists constantly improve and refine their practice based on thorough reflection on everyday events. Engagement in reflection transforms exposure to events into genuine experience that informs further practice. Therapists continue to engage in reflective practice throughout their entire careers.

Models of Reflection

Developing reflective practice skills can be difficult. Many frameworks and models of reflection exist to support the development of reflective practice skills and each has its own characteristics and applications. Rather than adopt any specific model, occupational therapists are encouraged to draw on those that serve their needs at any point in time. Some common models include:

Kolb's Learning Cycle
Kolb (1984) described a basic learning cycle that incorporated reflective observation as the basis for professional learning and development. In this model, the learning cycle involves four stages: concrete experience, reflective observation, abstract conceptualization, and active experimentation. Importantly, in Kolb's model the learner can enter the cycle at any of those four stages. This means the learner can have an experience, reflect on and understand it, and then try something different. Alternatively, the learner can try something new, observe the outcome, reflect on what happened, and try to understand the reasons for the outcome. The learner can even start from a point of contemplation, decide to try a new way, have the experience, and then reflect upon it. More than anything, Kolb's learning cycle encourages the learner to be an active participant in the learning process, stimulated by curiosity and a desire for self-improvement. It is a useful starting point for those new to reflective practice.

Rolfe's Model of Reflective Practice
Rolfe, Freshwater, and Jasper (2001) developed a more directed reflective process based upon three simple questions: What? So What? Now What? Together these questions provide a clear reflective structure that includes the components of noticing, analyzing, evaluating, and planning. The process starts with a description of the experience and prompts the therapist to consider the implications of the experience, the learnings, and future actions. Rolfe et al.'s model encourages therapists to move beyond mere "noticing" and to use those observations to understand and improve practice. While Rolfe's model provides a simple structure for the reflective process, the questions are broad and sometimes they require further scaffolding to enable the therapist to deeply examine their lived experience.

Driscoll's Model of Reflection

Rolfe et al.'s (2001) model is simplistic and easy to implement, but it doesn't support in-depth analysis and evaluation. Driscoll's (2007) Model of Reflection draws upon the same three questions – What? So what? Now What? – but provides some further signposts to help clinicians embrace each stage more fully. Essentially the model provides a little further direction that can help the therapist contextualize the reflective process.

Gibbs Reflective Model

Detailed reflection requires a more expansive framework. Gibbs' (1988) Reflective Model is a cyclical model that supports in-depth analysis and evaluation in ways that other models of reflection do not. The stages include the identification of both thoughts and feelings (separating these is an important aspect of reflection because we cannot really challenge our emotional responses to an event, but we can legitimately challenge the thoughts on which those emotional responses are based). Gibbs' model challenges therapists to deeply consider what was good and bad about the situation. This helps to make sense of the experience in truly objective ways. By drawing the previous stages together into a conclusion, therapists are able to define specific actions and timeframes that will allow them to respond to the situation by changing their practice for the future.

The other advantage of Gibbs' model is that it prevents therapists becoming fixated on feelings and thoughts, or jumping immediately to conclusions about what to change. The stepwise cycle promotes slow and deep consideration of each stage before moving on. The result is a well-considered response to a trigger event.

Practice Education Models

With new occupational therapy university programs continuing to open and existing university programs expanding their enrolment numbers, greater demands are placed on health care networks, community agencies, and individual clinicians to take students on practice education placements. To creatively respond to these challenges, several alternatives to the *Traditional Apprenticeship Model* of practice education have been proposed. One example is the *Collaborative Model of Fieldwork Education*, also referred to as the 1:2 or 1:3 model, where one educator supervises two or more students (Kinsella and Piersol 2018). Cited advantages of this model include increased collaboration and teamwork, positive peer pressure, greater communication, increased practice competence, and facilitation of active learning (Martin et al. 2004; O'Connor et al. 2012). Furthermore, the *Shared Clinical Practice Model* is where two practice educators share the supervision of one student within a workplace. Evenson et al.'s (2015) study respondents indicated that practice educators preferred model of supervision of occupational therapy students continued to be the traditional one supervisor to one student model, while the next preferred was a 2:1 (supervisor: student) model (Evenson et al. 2015).

In a *Multiple Mentoring Model*, a team of students is supervised by a team of educators (Copley and Nelson 2012), providing students with an opportunity to observe multiple approaches and in some circumstances, multiple caseloads (Farrow et al. 2000). Copley and Nelson's (2012) reported that the challenges of setting up such a placement were worth it in light of student skill development, for example, teamwork and caseload management, and enhanced services to clients.

Another example of practice supervision is referred to as *Near-Peer Assisted Supervision* where a senior student or recent graduate supervises a more junior student in some aspects of their placement (Larkin and Hitch 2019). Some universities have set up onsite campus-based clinics where students provide services to clients and families under the supervision of academic staff (Erickson 2018). A more recent model is labeled the *University-Supported Placement* where students are placed in a setting (e.g., primary school, aged care facility) where no occupational therapists are currently employed, but instead the university contracts a clinician to supervise students at the site on a part time basis.

Another model, the *Role-Emerging Practice Placement Model*, is where a student is placed at an agency where no occupational therapy role exists and the student endeavors to establish or demonstrate what the occupational therapy role might be. In this model, the students are usually supervised by another professional who works on site (e.g., social worker, physiotherapist, psychologist, teacher) and are supported remotely by a university-based educator. In the role emerging practice placement model, generic skills such as communication and professionalism can be taught and modeled by a person from another profession with occupational therapy specific skills being taught and supported by an occupational therapist who is based elsewhere. This usually involves regular supervision sessions either on site or remotely via video conferencing. Dancza et al. (2013) investigated the learning enablers and barriers of occupational therapy students when completing a role emerging placement using a qualitative approach. Four themes emerged: (i) adapting to less doing, more thinking and planning; (ii) understanding the complexity of collaboration and making it work; (iii) emotional extremes; and (iv) realizing and using the occupational therapy perspective (Dancza et al. 2013).

The context of a role-emerging placement boosts opportunities for students' professional growth, autonomy, self-directed learning, time management, and prioritization of tasks. A similar type of model to the role-emerging model is the *Project-Focussed Practice Placement Model* where students work on developing a resource or service for an agency (University of Queensland and Occupational Therapy Practice Education Collaborative – Queensland 2020). The project can take place in traditional or role emerging settings, with or without an occupational therapy practice educator. An example of a Project-Focused Practice Placement Model was when the Australian Capital Territory (ACT) Arthritis Foundation required a business case to employ an occupational therapist in their organization. Two occupational therapy students from the University of Canberra developed a business case that included projected costs and revenues, a risk strategy and a strategic direction for the service based upon the needs of the service users. The business case was accepted by the CEO of the organization who subsequently employed an occupational therapist in the organization.

Simulated Placements are created when "the environment, people, materials, activities and processes of work are simulated to create a facsimile of occupational therapy practice" (Imms et al. 2017, p. 2). Students can use written case studies, videos, computer simulated scenarios and/or engage with actors playing roles of consumers. For example, a case study of a person who has been injured at work can be used. In this simulation, students are asked to review the referral information, role play an initial interview with an actor, determine appropriate assessments, review the simulated assessment results, and develop a return to work plan with a simulated work place. *Simulated Placements* have been found to be as effective in meeting learning outcomes compared to nonsimulated placements (Imms et al. 2018).

Schmitz and colleagues (2016) explored how to provide supervision and support for occupational therapy students completing placements in remote, role-emerging, and overseas locations using a telesupervision approach. Findings indicated that using telesupervision provided students with the chance to debrief and problem solve, increased a sense of connectedness for students, and provided insights of placement experiences for educators. Murphy and Donnelly (2016) examined the use of online learning communities with occupational therapy students to promote synthesis of practice and theory and the development of professional reasoning. Commenting on this study, Matichuk and White (2016) noted that "students in diverse practice settings had the opportunity to reflect with their peers and an occupational therapy preceptor through guided online discussions and weekly Skype interactions" (p. 19).

Competencies in Practice Education

The WFOT developed the Minimum Standards for the Education of Occupational Therapists (2016) to establish international standards for global occupational therapy education, including practice education. Graduates of WFOT approved programs are required to demonstrate achieving competencies in six areas relevant to professional knowledge, skills, and attitudes, which include: (i) the relationship among person-occupational-environment and how it relates to health, (ii) the therapeutic and professional relationships, (iii) occupational therapy processes, (iv) professional reasoning and behavior, (v) professional practice context, and (vi) evidence-based practice.

Professional bodies in countries, such as Australia, New Zealand, the United Kingdom, Canada, and United States, have developed their own national competency standards which in turn guide how practice education is experienced in different countries (Occupational Therapy Board of Australia [OTBA] 2018; College of Occupational Therapist 2016; Association of Canadian Occupational Therapy Regulatory Organizations [ACOTRO] 2011; American Occupational Therapy Association 2015). The expectations of what constitutes appropriate practice education to make up the recommended 1000 fieldwork hours can be varied across countries, are influenced by the local context, and can impact on graduates receiving overseas registrations. For example, project placements are included as part of occupational therapy practice education in some countries, such as the United Kingdom, Australia, and Canada. These placements involve students engaging in project management and relevant activities (e.g., quality assurance and/or services development) to develop the required competencies (Fortune and McKinstry 2012). However, in places such as Hong Kong, Taiwan, and Japan where occupational therapy services are predominantly within the medical model, project placements are not considered as contributing to practice education.

Supervision and Feedback

Supervision in occupational therapy can be described as a relationship-based process of professional support and learning (OTBA 2018). It enables students to develop knowledge and competence, reflect upon the tasks undertaken, the process, and the connections in between, as well as assume responsibility within their professional practice (Davies 2000; OTBA 2018). Often, supervision comprises the normative, formative, and restorative domains (Occupational Therapy Australia 2019). The normative domain focuses on providing supervision on the administrative requirements (e.g., adherence to policies and procedures) of a role. The formative domain of supervision focuses on the educational components (e.g., skills, knowledge, and attitudes relevant to professional practice) of the role. The restorative domain of supervision addresses the emotional demands.

Effective supervision consists of enabling a balance between providing an appropriate level of support while challenging students (Rodger et al. 2014). Elements of effective supervision include having a reciprocal supervisory relationship with students, provision of learning opportunities and experiences, and encouraging autonomy and independence (Rodger et al. 2014). Feedback provision is also a vital component supporting effective practice supervision, through which learners comprehend information received from multiple sources to facilitate positive changes that enhance their practice or learning (Carless and Boud 2018). Feedback can be provided in written or oral formats to an individual or a group and has been classified based on the process, purpose, and source of the feedback (Tuma and Nassar 2019) as described in Table 1.

Feedback should be sufficient, timely, explicit, regular, and consistent (Brehaut et al. 2016) Actions recommended as part of feedback need to be consistent with the placement expectations, specific, and achievable. Feedback is more effective if provided on several occasions, immediately after a placement activity and targeting individual learning needs. Having a comparator or benchmark, such as expected performance at various stages during a placement, to provide feedback in practice education is helpful in supporting desired performance improvement. Using a variety of feedback that supports comprehension of information and ensuring feedback is sufficient but not overwhelming, credible, and actionable are also imperative.

Table 1 Types of feedback (Tuma and Nassar 2019)

Feedback aspect	Feedback types	Descriptions
Process	Formal feedback	A planned structured feedback, usually provided on a regular basis (e.g., weekly or at midway or end of a placement) focusing on supporting students' practice performance improvement to meet the placement expectations
	Informal feedback	Can be provided at any time and often is short and immediate during or right after a placement activity
Purpose	Formative feedback	An ongoing type of feedback provided frequently during placement, focusing on assisting students to improve practice performance and avoiding making the same mistake again. It is usually provided before summative feedback
	Summative feedback	Provided at the end of a placement to evaluate students' performance against placement expectations
Source	Instructor feedback	Feedback given by the supervisor as the expert of a practice area to provide constructive and specific information on student performance
	Peer feedback	Peer students, provided with basic instruction and support, give and receive feedback from each other to develop knowledge and skills and enrich learning experiences
	Self-feedback	A student is supported to use self-reflection and self-assessment to identify learning goals, develop strategies and plan actions to support professional development
	Consumer/client feedback	Feedback provided directly by recipients of health care about their experiences of the services provided by students

Best Practice When Evaluating Students on Placement: Theory and Process

The WFOT (2016) minimum standards state that student practice placements must be supervised and assessed by an occupational therapist. Evaluation of student performance in practice education is a complex and detailed process which serves a number of purposes for all involved (Allison and Turpin 2004). Evaluation can not only certify competence or the meeting of criteria at the completion of a student practical experience, but can also highlight strengths and areas of challenge, promote further development of skills, behaviors, and attitudes, and highlight areas of opportunity for learning still required during a placement (McBurney 2005).

In occupational therapy, evaluation of student performance encompasses both practice (e.g., assessment, intervention planning, service delivery) and nonclinical skills (e.g., communication, professionalism, and self-management). Nonclinical skills are seen as hallmarks of professional practice and may develop in a more linear fashion than specific clinical skills across subsequent placement experiences. Students acknowledge that becoming novices again each time they commence a new placement creates difficulties in terms of graded learning experiences (Rodger et al. 2011) and this has implications for evaluation of their performance.

It is vital that practice educators are familiar with the evaluation tool set by a student's educational institution in order to evaluate performance effectively. Given that practice education is typically undertaken in a broad range of settings, is supervised by practitioners with different educational backgrounds and student evaluation experiences, and may use different supervision models (e.g., peer learning or multiple mentoring schemes), evaluating student performance in a consistent manner can be problematic. The use of standardized evaluation tools can help to address this issue (Rodger et al. 2016). Examples of the tools completed by practice educators include the Fieldwork Performance Evaluation for the Occupational Therapy Student (FWPE) (AOTA 2002), Student Practice Evaluation Form–Revised (SPEF–R) (Division of Occupational Therapy 2008), and the Competency Based Fieldwork Evaluation for Occupational Therapists (CBFE–OT) (Bossers et al. 2007). Many tools offer opportunities for formative feedback at the half-way mark of the placement and summative feedback at completion. While the use of standardized and evidence-based evaluation tools is ideal, some educational institutions have created their own tool for local use. Ongoing research into the reliability and validity of such tools is imperative.

Prior to placements, practice educators and students should become familiar with the appropriate evaluation tool in order to understand what it measures and to consider what individual evaluation items may look like within a specific practice context. This can provide practice educators with information for early planning of learning opportunities for the student and can inform student preparation. At multiple points throughout practice placements, student performance evaluation tools can be used to guide supervision sessions. Identified areas of need can be discussed, strategies for improved performance planned and further opportunities explored. Evaluation tools can also promote student self-reflection (The University of Queensland 2016). This can take place as students reflect on their progress in preparation for meeting with their educator and can provide valuable information about the student's level of insight into their own performance. Together, educators and students can be guided by the requirements of the evaluation tool to plan for and review future goals.

In order for a student's performance to be evaluated fairly and effectively, it is vital that educators gather sufficient, valid evidence of student performance. This evidence not only assists in selection of ratings but can also be used to provide clear examples of student skills and behaviors to substantiate educator decisions (The University of Queensland 2016). Evidence can be gathered from a wide range of sources, including educator observation, student self-report, student documentation, supervision sessions, and practice discussions (The University of Queensland 2016). Educators should also seek feedback from colleagues within multidisciplinary/interprofessional teams, and where appropriate from consumers, to help in creating a clear and valid picture of student performance. Occasionally, feedback from student peers may also be relevant.

Once information has been gathered regarding student performance, it needs to be synthesized in order to select and substantiate the ratings allocated to the student against evaluation tool criteria. Feedback recorded in the evaluation tool should be reflective of the wording used in the rating scales and/or evaluation criteria and should be clear, concise, and constructive to communicate to the student areas of strength and areas for development. Grenier (2015) found students placed value on constructive feedback that enabled them to better understand their strengths and weaknesses. Formative feedback at the halfway point of a placement should provide guidance for continued skill development and assist with setting expectations for the second half of the experience.

The process of support, supervision, and evidence collection is repeated throughout the final half of the placement. During the final evaluation of student performance, feedback should focus on what was achieved by the student during the practice placement and provide direction, such as learning plans, for further development in future placements or first jobs. The final evaluation period is also a time for the practice educator to reflect on what opportunities were presented, what worked and what did not from an organizational perspective, to assist with future student placement opportunities (Rodger et al. 2011).

Supporting the Development of Professional Reasoning in Practice Education

While the evidence is strong that practice education forms an essential part of preparation for occupational therapy students, and the literature supports various approaches to providing those practice education experiences, there is less certainty over how skills in occupational therapy professional reasoning are best learned. Professional reasoning refers to "the process used by practitioners to plan, direct, perform and reflect on client care" (Schell 2014; p. 134). Solving complicated occupational performance problems requires a unique approach to professional reasoning. Experienced occupational therapists balance information generated through a range of reasoning styles, skillfully drawn together using evidence from empirical and practice sources. This process is a difficult one for occupational therapy students to master and equally difficult for practice educators to teach. Schell and Benfield (2018) described varied styles of reasoning that support occupational therapists to approach their work with clients using holistic, collaborative, multimodal thinking. Henderson and Coppard (2017) were critical of educators for not adequately communicating to students the forms of reasoning they used to make practice decisions, highlighting the importance of modeling professional reasoning as a support for student learning.

Practice educators seek to expedite the development of professional reasoning for students in the early stages of their occupational therapy development. Useful instructional techniques can be drawn from the research methods informing our knowledge of professional reasoning processes in occupational therapy. The challenge in understanding professional reasoning is that it exists as an invisible, complex, cognitive process. While the outcome of reasoning can be easily observed, the process by which decisions are made, the information that is used to inform the decision, and the means by which various forms of reasoning are synthesized all remain hidden. Researchers have sought to investigate these tacit processes in three ways:

1. *Retrospective recall* – Much research into professional reasoning in occupational therapy asks clinicians to recount their decision-making following an interaction with a client (e.g., Mitchell and Unsworth 2005; Unsworth 2001). In doing so, therapists are able to articulate the many factors they balance in their decision making, as well as the way their previous experience influenced their decisions. Retrospective recall can help generate network representations of thinking in the form of decision trees (Arocha and Patel 2019).
2. *Concurrent commentary* – Think aloud protocols encourage clinicians to verbalize and explain their thoughts in real time as they work with a client. This commentary overcomes issues of interference and selective recall that are present in retrospective recall and provides an insight into the way therapists engage in professional reasoning. Thinking aloud has been shown to provide a good description of underlying thought processes (Durning et al. 2013).
3. *Implicit investigation* – In retrospective and concurrent recall, clinicians can only describe those factors they are consciously aware of. In 1991, Kelly first proposed that many of the things that influence decision-making occur in the form of implicit or subconscious thoughts, values, and psychological constructs (Kelly 2020). Kuipers and Grice (2009) applied Kelly's theories and used repertory grid technique to investigate implicit reasoning used by occupational therapists in working with children with cerebral palsy. The methodology provided insight into factors influencing reasoning that the therapists themselves were not aware of.

These research methods provide guidance for practice educators looking to make the hidden process of professional reasoning more evident for students. In doing so, students can begin to understand factors that experienced clinicians take into account and ways they draw together information through various styles of reasoning, consider potential actions, and invoke previous experience. Practice educators can be guided by the research methods used to understand professional reasoning and use similar strategies to model and communicate their own professional reasoning to students:

1. *Share your thinking with the student after the session.* Recount your thinking and describe all the parts of your decision-making. Identify the factors that were relevant and how your previous experience helped you integrate information from multiple styles of reasoning.
2. *Think out loud* – Provide the student with a commentary about what you are thinking, as you are thinking it. Model the synthesis of multiple sources of information as well as the questions you are asking yourself. Describe examples of where you have seen this type of problem before and how it shapes your thinking on this occasion.

3. *Draw it* – Try drawing a mind map, or even a decision tree, that represents all the elements you are balancing or considering. Use lines and arrows to connect things that are related, and use an X to identify lines of thinking that can be closed down or are redundant. In this way, it is possible to exhibit the thinking process to the student and identify particular points where specific knowledge or skills are required.
4. *Reflect* – Share with the student your reflections on the session, trying to recognize the sorts of things that might have influenced your thinking, even though you were not aware of them at the time. These could be personal values, theories, knowledge, skills, experiences, or even biases that are such a part of you that you did not realize they affected your thinking.

Students find it equally difficult to articulate their professional reasoning. Using strategies to describe, understand, and reflect upon their reasoning enables discussion between educator and student, enabling students to describe a rationale for their selection of assessment or intervention approaches. This process can be well supported by using planning sheets that enable them to consider the basis of their decisions. In the same way that practice educators can share their decision making using retrospective or concurrent recall strategies, students can be encouraged to describe their thinking as evidence of their understanding of the occupational therapy process. When students draw decision trees and mind maps, it supports collaboration with practice educators by providing an illustration of the student's thinking (Turpin and Hanson 2018). It can become obvious to the practice educator where there are important factors not considered, or where errant assumptions have been made. When the practice educator adds branches or thought bubbles, they model thinking that is more complete and sophisticated. Turpin and Hanson (2018) described the importance of co-constructing professional reasoning through collaborative problem solving between the therapist and student. By combining modeling, teaching, and shared decision-making, practice educators are able to shape the way students synthesize information using varied styles of reasoning (Henderson and Coppard 2017).

Understanding implicit factors that influence student decision-making is more challenging, yet Henderson and Coppard (Henderson and Coppard 2017) cite metacognition as a critical element of professional reasoning. Using models of reflective practice such as Rolfe's Reflective Model (Rolfe et al. 2001) or Gibbs' Reflective Cycle (Gibbs 1988) leads students to develop insight into their own thinking, become aware of their cognitions, and learn from their own experiences. Deep reflections unearth not just the thoughts themselves, but also the hidden values and experiences that lead to those thoughts. Facilitating development of professional reasoning requires practice educators to implement specific teaching and learning strategies rather than assuming students will acquire effective reasoning skills based on observation alone. By modeling reflective practice, providing student guides and templates, and offering students time and support to engage in critical reflection, practice educators can provide students with models of mature professional reasoning while simultaneously giving them a means of explaining their own reasoning to the practice educator.

Trends in Practice Education and Future Directions

As the essential bridge between academic education and professional practice, practice education programs continue to evolve and respond to the everchanging professional and community needs. Roberts et al. (2015) completed an international systematic mapping of occupational therapy practice education literature to assist with identifying areas of strength and further development for research in practice education. The authors challenge the profession to continue to question and develop evidence for the pedagogy of practice education. Roberts et al. (2015) found less than 10% of occupational therapy published research examined learning and assessment during practice education. The call for action to develop research to support pedagogy in practice placements has recently been supported by Beveridge and Pentland's (2020) mapping of models of placements. These authors challenge us to develop evidence to clarify assumptions of new practice education models. Current literature suggests that new models of placements are effective at developing professional skills, particularly advanced professional skills; however, research is lacking empirical evidence to support these claims (Beveridge and Pentland 2020). Students also continue to report a preference for the one-to-one apprenticeship model placement primarily due to perceived concerns of reduced quality and quantity of supervision, reduced ability to observe the supervisor, and ease of demonstrating skills in a one-to-one relationship (Beveridge and Pentland 2020).

As occupational therapy practice contexts expand and the complexity of the health service increases, questions are being raised about transferability of skills developed across innovative practice education models (Syed and Duncan 2019). Medical education and other allied health programs have been developing and exploring programmatic approaches to determining professional competence (Van Der Vleuten et al. 2015). "Programmatic assessment is an integral approach to the design of an assessment program with the intent to optimise its learning function, its decision-making function and its curriculum quality-assurance function" (Van Der Vleuten et al. 2015, p. 641). A programmatic approach often uses a portfolio of evidence to assist groups of people to determine a student's level of competence in various skills and practice contexts. Programmatic assessment has been shown to assist education programs with determining when a student is demonstrating competence and transferability of skills across settings, developing comprehensive educational remediation programs, and creating a trigger to assist students with determining their own level of competence (Heeneman et al. 2015).

A programmatic approach also assists with detangling the potential conflicted roles of practice educator as an assessor as well as an educator. Watling and Ginsburg (2019) pose that for a student to express and demonstrate vulnerability in regard to their gaps in knowledge, skills, and behaviors, we cannot ask one person to educate/mentor and assess simultaneously. Programmatic assessment allows for the education element to sit within the practice placement space and for the formal assessment of competence to be transferred to the university setting.

Internationally, there is a trend towards consumer/service user involvement in student education. The National Health Service reform in the United Kingdom led to a redesign of a service user led health system in the 2000s (McCutcheon and Gormley 2014). The change in policy prompted local universities to increase their engagement of service users within curriculum. The drive to involve consumers in the development and implementation of health professional education programs is developing internationally for most health professions. Within occupational therapy education programs, consumers are providing input into curriculum development, content delivery, and assessment (Arblaster et al. 2015). However, there is a paucity of consumer involvement in practice education. Finch et al. (2018) completed a systematic literature review from the perspective of allied health students seeking consumer feedback while completing practice education, and planned to develop a system that could be used within a site-specific placement perspective. Nursing courses within the United Kingdom have developed service user feedback systems that assist service users to contribute feedback as part of nursing student placement assessment (Gray and Donaldson 2010). Research has indicated that consumer involvement during practice placements assists student health professionals with practice skills, self-perception of changes in knowledge, result in better health outcomes for the consumer, and improve practical examination results for students (Finch et al. 2018).

Conclusion

Practice education in occupational therapy is critical to allow students to apply the skills and knowledge they have learned in a classroom setting to a practice setting. It is a time for students to apply their developing professional reasoning skills and for practice educators to facilitate developing occupational therapy competencies. As the profession of occupational therapy is diverse, so are the settings in which practice education takes place, the people seen within these settings and the models of practice education used. This can sometimes be challenging for students and practice educators. Practice education performance should be evaluated by evidence-based measures and these are applied in many countries that deliver occupational therapy practice education. Finally, emerging models of practice education in occupational therapy will challenge the profession to keep striving to offer high quality practice education to students and support practice educators in delivering meaningful, engaging, and relevant practice education experiences.

References

Allison H, Turpin MJ. Development of the student placement evaluation form: a tool for assessing student fieldwork performance. Aust Occup Ther J. 2004;51(3):125–32. https://doi.org/10.1111/j.1440-1630.2004.00414.x.

American Occupational Therapy Association. Fieldwork performance evaluation for the occupational therapy student. Bethesda; 2002.

American Occupational Therapy Association. Standards for continuing competence. Am J Occup Ther. 2015;69:1–3.

Andonian L. Emotional intelligence, self-efficacy, and occupational therapy students' fieldwork performance. Occup Ther Health Care. 2013;27(3):201–15. https://doi.org/10.3109/07380577.2012.763199.

Arblaster K, Mackenzie L, Willis K. Mental health consumer participation in education: a structured literature review. Aust Occup Ther J. 2015;62(5):341–62. https://doi.org/10.1111/1440-1630.12205.

Arocha JF, Patel VL. Methods in the study of clinical reasoning. In: Higgs J, Jense GM, Loftus S, Christensen N, editors. Clinical reasoning in the health professions. Edinburgh: Elsevier; 2019. p. 147–58.

Association of Canadian Occupational therapy Regulatory organizations [ACOTRO]. Essential competencies of practice of occupational therapists in Canada. 3rd ed. Toronto: Association of Canadian Occupational therapy Regulatory organizations; 2011.

Barton R, Corban A, Herrli-Warner L, McClain E, Riehle D, Tinner E. Role strain in occupational therapy fieldwork educators. Work. 2013;44:317–28. https://doi.org/10.3233/WOR121508.

Beveridge J, Pentland D. A mapping review of models of practice education in allied health and social care professions. Br J Occup Ther. 2020;72(11):515–7. https://doi.org/10.1177/0308022620904325.

Bossers A, Miller LT, Polatajk H, Hartley M. Competency based fieldwork evaluation for occupational therapists. Toronto: Nelson; 2007.

Boud D, Keogh R, Walker D. Reflection: turning experience into learning. London/New York: Kogan Page/Nicholas Publishing; 1985.

Boyd EM, Fales A. Reflective learning: key to learning from experience. J Humanist Psychol. 1983;23(2):99–117. https://doi.org/10.1177/0022167883232011.

Brehaut JC, Colquhoun HL, Eva KW, Carroll K, Sales A, Michie S, Ivers N, Grimshaw JM. Practice feedback interventions: 15 suggestions for optimizing effectiveness. Ann Intern Med. 2016;164(6):435–41.

Brown T, McKinstry CE, Gustafsson L. The need for evidence and new models of practice education to meet the 1000 hour requirement. Aust Occup Ther J. 2016;63(5):352–6. https://doi.org/10.1111/1440-1630.12239.

Brown T, Yu ML, Etherington J. Are listening and interpersonal communication skills predictive of professionlism in undergraduate occupational therapy students? Health Prof Educ. 2020a;6(2):187–200. https://doi.org/10.1016/j.hpe.2020.01.001.

Brown T, Yu ML, Hewitt AE, Isbel ST, Bevitt T, Etherington J. Exploring the relationship between resilience and practice education placement success in occupational therapy students. Aust Occup Ther J. 2020b;67(1):49–61. https://doi.org/10.1080/07380577.2020.1737896.

Carless D, Boud D. The development of student feedback literacy: enabling uptake of feedback. Assess Eval High Educ. 2018;43(8):1315–25. https://doi.org/10.1080/02602938.2018.1463354.

Clarke M. Action and reflection: practice and theory in nursing. J Adv Nurs. 1986;11(1):3–11.

College of Occupational Therapists. Entry level occupational therapy core knowledge and practice skills. London: College of Occupational Therapists; 2016.

Copley J, Nelson A. Practice educator perspectives of multiple mentoring in diverse clinical settings. Br J Occup Ther. 2012;75(10):456–62. https://doi.org/10.4276/030802212X13496921049662.

Dancza K, Warren A, Copley J, Rodger S, Moran M, McKay E, Taylor A. Learning experience on role-emerging placements: an exploration from the students' perspective. Aust Occup Ther J. 2013;60(6):427–35. https://doi.org/10.1111/1440-1630.12079.

Davies M. The Blackwell encyclopaedia of social work. Oxford: Blackwell; 2000.

Division of Occupational Therapy. Student Practice Evaluation Form (SPEF)-revised edition package. Brisbane: The University of Queensland; 2008.

Donaghy ME, Morss K. Guided reflection: a framework to facilitate and assess reflective practice within the discipline of physiotherapy. Physiother Theory Pract. 2000;16:3–14.

Driscoll J. Practising clinical supervision: a reflective approach for healthcare professionals. 2nd ed. Edinburgh: Bailliere Tindall Elsevier; 2007.

Durning SJ, Artino AR Jr, Beckman TJ, Graner J, Van Der Vleuten C, Holmboe E, Schuwirth L. Does the think-aloud protocol reflect thinking? Exploring functional neuroimaging differences with thinking (answering multiple choice questions) versus thinking aloud. Med Teach. 2013;5(9):720–6. https://doi.org/10.3109/0142159X.2013.801938.

Epstein RM. Mindful practice. JAMA. 1999;282(9):833–9. https://doi.org/10.1001/jama.282.9.833.

Erickson K. On-campus occupational therapy clinic enhances student professional development and understanding. J Occup Ther Educ. 2018;2(2) https://doi.org/10.26681/jote.2018.020202.

Evenson ME, Roberts M, Kaldenberg J, Barnes MA, Ozelie R. National survey of fieldwork educators: implications for occupational therapy education. Am J Occup Ther. 2015;69(Suppl.2):1–5. https://doi.org/10.5014/ajot.2015.019265.

Facione N, Facione P. The health science reasoning test test manual. Millbrae: Insight Assessment; 2007. https://www.insightassessment.com/article/health-sciences-reasoning-test-hsrt-2

Farrow S, Gaiptman B, Rudman D. Exploration of a group model in fieldwork education. Can J Occup Ther. 2000;67(4):239–50. https://doi.org/10.1177/000841740006700406.

Finch E, Lethlean J, Rose T, Fleming J, Theodoros D, Cameron A, Coleman A, Copland D, McPhail SM. How does feedback from patients impact upon healthcare student clinical skill development and learning? A systematic review. Med Teach. 2018;40(3):244–52. https://doi.org/10.1080/0142159X.2017.1401218.

Fortune T, McKinstry C. Project-based fieldwork: perspectives of graduate entry students and project sponsors. Aust Occup Ther J. 2012;59(4):265–75.

Gat S, Ratzon NZ. Comparison of occupational therapy students' perceived skills after traditional and nontraditional fieldwork. Am J Occup Ther. 2014;68(2):e47–54. https://doi.org/10.5014/ajot.2014.007732.

Gibbs G. Learning by doing: a guide to teaching and learning methods. Oxford: Oxford Centre for Staff and Learning Development, Oxford Brookes University; 1988.

Gray MA, Donaldson J. National approach to practice assessment for nurses and midwives: a literature reivew exploring issues of service user and carer involvement in the assessment of studnets' practice. Edinburgh Napier University; 2010. Available from https://www.nes.scot.nhs.uk/media/572852/final_-_volume_1_exploring_service_user___carer_involvement.pdf

Grenier ML. Facilitators and barriers to learning in occupational therapy fieldwork education: student perspectives. Am J Occup Ther. 2015;69(Suppl.2):1–9. https://doi.org/10.5014/ajot.2015.015180.

Heeneman, Oudkerk Pool A, Schuwirth LWT, van der Vleuten CPM, Driessen EW. The impact of programmatic assessment on student learning: theory versus practice. Med Educ. 2015;49(5):487–98. https://doi.org/10.1111/medu.12645.

Henderson W, Coppard B. Identifying instructional methods for development of clinical reasoning in entry-level occupational therapy education. Am J Occup Ther. 2017;2:1–3. https://doi.org/10.26681/jote.2017.010201.

Hills C, Levett-Jones T, Warren-Forward H, Lapkin S. Teaching and learning preferences of 'Generation Y' occupational therapy students in practice education. Int J Ther Rehabil. 2016;23(8):371–9.

Imms C, Chu E, Guinea S, Sheppard L, Froude E, Carter R, . . . Symmons M. Effectiveness and cost effectiveness of embedded simulation in occupational therapy clinical practice education: study protocol for a randomised controlled trial. Trials. 2017;18(345):1–16. https://doi.org/10.1186/s13063-017-2087-0.

Imms C, Froude E, Chu E, Sheppard L, Darzins S, Guinea S, et al. Simulated versus traditional occupational therapy placements: a randomised controlled trial. Aust Occup Ther J. 2018;65(6):556–64. https://doi.org/10.1111/1440-1630.12513.

Kelly GA. The psychology of personal constructs. London: Routledge; 2020.

Kember D, Mckay J, Sinclair K, Wong F. A four-category scheme for coding and assessing the level of reflection in written work. Assess Eval High Educ. 2008;33(4):369–79.

Kemp EL, Crabtree JL. Differentiating fieldwork settings: matching student characteristics to demands. Occup Ther Health Care. 2018;32(3):216–29. https://doi.org/10.1080/07380577.2018.1491084.

Kinsella AT, Piersol CV. Development and evaluation of a collaborative model level II fieldwork program. Open J Occup Ther. 2018;6(3):14. https://doi.org/10.15453/2168-6408.1448.

Kirke P, Layton N, Sim J. Informing fieldwork design: key elements to quality in fieldwork education for undergraduate occupational therapy students. Aust Occup Ther J. 2007;54:S13–22. https://doi.org/10.1111/j.1440-1630.2007.00696.x.

Kolb DA. Experiential learning: experience as the source of learning and development, vol. 1. Englewood Cliffs: Prentice-Hall; 1984.

Koski KJ, Simon RL, Dooley NR. Valuable occupational therapy fieldwork educator behaviors. Work. 2013;44(3):307–15. https://doi.org/10.3233/WOR-121507.

Kuipers K, Grice JW. The structure of novice and expert occupational therapists' clinical reasoning before and after exposure to a domain-specific protocol. Aust Occup Ther J. 2009;56(6):418–27. https://doi.org/10.1111/j.1440-1630.2009.00793.x.

Lalor A, Yu ML, Brown T, Thyer L. Occupational therapy international undergraduate students' perspectives on the purpose of practice education and what contributes to successful practice learning experiences. Br J Occup Ther. 2019;82(6):367–75. https://doi.org/10.1177/0308022618823659.

Larkin H, Hitch D. Peer Assisted Study Sessions (PASS) preparing occupational therapy undergraduates for practice education: a novel application of a proven educational intervention. Aust Occup Ther J. 2019;66(1):100–9. https://doi.org/10.1111/1440-1630.12537.

Mann K, Gordon J, MccLeod A. Reflection and reflective practice in health professions education: a systematic review. Adv Health Sci Educ. 2009;14:595–621.

Martin M, Morris J, Moore A, Sadlo G, Crouch V. Evaluating practice education models in occupational therapy: comparing 1:1, 2:1 and 3:1 placements. Br J Occup Ther. 2004;67(5):192–200. https://doi.org/10.1177/030802260406700502.

Matichuk M, White C. 2016 CAOT conference shines a light on fieldwork. Occup Ther Now. 2016;18(4):19–20.

McBurney H. Exploring the roles of the clinical educator. In: Rose M, Best D, editors. Transforming practice in clinical education, professional supervision and mentoring. Edinburgh: Elsevier; 2005. p. 77–85. https://doi.org/10.1016/B978-0-443-07454-7.X5001-1.

McCutcheon K, Gormley K. Service-user involvement in nurse education: partnership or tokenism? Br J Nurs. 2014;23(22):1196–9. https://doi.org/10.12968/bjon.2014.23.22.1196.

Mitchell R, Unsworth CA. Clinical reasoning during community health home visits: expert and novice differences. Br J Occup Ther. 2005;68(5):215–23. https://doi.org/10.1177/030802260506800505.

Moon J. Reflection in learning and professional development. London: Kogan Page; 1999.

Murphy S, Donnelly C. Fostering integration of fieldwork learning through online learning communities. Poster presented at the 2016 Canadian Association of Occupational Therapists Conference, Banff; 2016.

National Univeristy of Ireland Galway. Practice education. 2020. Available from: https://www.nuigalway.ie/medicine-nursing-and-health-sciences/health-sciences/disciplines/occupational-therapy/practiceeducation/

Nielsen S, Klug M, Fox L. Impact of nontraditional level I fieldwork on critical thinking. Am J Occup Ther. 2020;74(3):1–7. https://doi.org/10.5014/ajot.2020.036350.

Occupational Therapy Australia. Professional supervision framework. 2019. Retrieved from https://otaus.com.au/publicassets/2e35a9f6-b890-e911-a2c3-9b7af2531dd2/ProfessionalSupervisionFramework2019.pdf

Occupational Therapy Board of Australia. Australian occupational therapy competency standards. 2018. Available from: https://www.occupationaltherapyboard.gov.au/codes-guidelines/competencies.aspx.

O'Connor A, Cahill M, McKay EA. Revisiting 1:1 and 2:1 clinical placement models: student and clinical educator perspectives. Aust Occup Ther J. 2012;59(4):276–83. https://doi.org/10.1111/j.1440-1630.2012.01025.x.

Ozelie R, Janow J, Kreutz C, Mulry MK, Penkala A. Supervision of occupational therapy level II fieldwork students: impact on and predictors of clinician productivity. Am J Occup Ther. 2015;69(1):1–7. https://doi.org/10.5014/ajot.2015.013532.

Roberts ME, Hooper BR, Wood WH, King RM. An international systematic mapping review of fieldwork education in occupational therapy. Can J Occup Ther. 2015;82(2):106–18. https://doi.org/10.1177/0008417414552187.

Rodger S, Fitzgerald C, Davila W, Millar F, Allison H. What makes a quality occupational therapy practice placement? Students' and practice educators' perspectives. Aust Occup Ther J. 2011;58(3):195–202. https://doi.org/10.1111/j.1440-1630.2010.00903.x.

Rodger S, Thomas Y, Greber C, Broadbridge J, Edwards A, Newton J, Lyons M. Attributes of excellence in practice educators: the perspectives of Australian occupational therapy students. Aust Occup Ther J. 2014;61(3):159–67. https://doi.org/10.1111/1440-1630.12096.

Rodger S, Chien CW, Turpin M, Copley J, Coleman A, Brown T, Caine AM. Establishing the validity and reliability of the student practice evaluation form–revised (SPEF-R) in occupational therapy practice education: a Rasch analysis. Eval Health Prof. 2016;39(1):33–48. https://doi.org/10.1177/0163278713511456.

Rolfe G, Freshwater D, Jasper M. Critical reflection in nursing and the helping professions: a user's guide. Basingstoke: Palgrave Macmillan; 2001.

Schell BAB. Professional reasoning in practice. In: Schell BAB, Gillen G, Scaffa ME, editors. Willard and Spackman's occupational therapy. Philadelphia: Wolters Kluwer Health/Lippincott Williams & Wilkins; 2014. p. 384–97.

Schell BAB, Benfield A. Aspects of professional reasoning. In: Schell BAB, Schell J, editors. Clinical and professional reasoning in occupational therapy. Philadelphia: Wolters Kluwer; 2018. p. 127–44.

Schmitz C, Drynan D, Nagarajan S, Hall M, McAlister L, McFarlane L, . . . Lam, M. Telesupervision for remote & role-emerging fieldwork: student & supervisor experiences. Poster presented at the 2016 Canadian Association of Occupational Therapists Conference, Banff; 2016.

Schon D. The reflective practitioner: how professionals think in action. London: Basic Books; 1983.

Syed S, Duncan A. Role emerging placements: skills development, postgraduate employment, and career pathways. Open J Occup Ther. 2019;7(1). https://doi.org/10.15453/2168-6408.1489.

The University of Queensland. iQIPP-AH – Improving Quality in Practice Placements Guides – Allied Health. Brisbane: The University of Queensland; 2012.

The University of Queensland. Making the most of the SPEF-R. Student practice evaluation form – revised for occupational therapy, 2016. Retrieved 7 July 2020 from: https://spef-r.shrs.uq.edu.au/learn/module-one-student-arrives/part-one-becoming-familiar-spef-r%C2%A9/making-most-spef-r%C2%A9

Thomas Y, Penman M. World Federation of Occupational Therapists (WFOT) standard for 1000 hours of practice placement: informed by tradition or evidence? Br J Occup Ther. 2019;82:3–4.

Thomas Y, Dickson D, Broadbridge J, Hopper L, Hawkins R, Edwards A, McBryde C. Benefits and challenges of supervising occupational therapy fieldwork students: supervisors' perspectives. Aust Occup Ther J. 2007;54:S2–12.

Tuma F, Nassar AK. Feedback in medical education. In: StatPearls [Internet]. Treasure Island: StatPearls Publishing; 2019. Available from: https://www.ncbi.nlm.nih.gov/books/NBK544311/

Turpin MJ, Hanson DJ. Learning professional reasoning in practice through fieldwork. In: Schell BAB, Schell J, editors. Clinical and professional reasoning in occupational therapy. Philadelphia: Wolters Kluwer; 2018. p. 439–60.

University of Queensland & Occupational Therapy Practice Education Collaborative Queensland [UQOTPEC-Q]. 2020. Placement options and models. Available from https://otpecq.group.uq.edu.au/education-placements/placement-options-and-models

Unsworth CA. The clinical reasoning of novice and expert occupational therapists. Scand J Occup Ther. 2001;8(4):163–73.

Van Der Vleuten CPM, Schuwirth LW, Driessen EW, Govaerts MJB, Heeneman S. Twelve tips for programmatic assessment. Med Teach. 2015;37(7):641–6. https://doi.org/10.3109/0142159X.2014.973388.

Varland J, Cardell E, Koski J, McFadden M. Factors influencing occupational therapists' decision to supervise fieldwork students. Occup Ther Health Care. 2017;31(3):238–54.

Watling CJ, Ginsburg S. Assessment, feedback and the alchemy of learning. Med Educ. 2019;53(1):76–85.

World Federation of Occupational Therapists. Definition of occupational therapy. 2012. Available from https://www.wfot.org/about

World Federation of Occupational Therapists [WFOT]. Minimum standards for the education of occupational therapists. 2016. Available from https://www.wfot.org/assets/resources/COPYRIGHTED-World-Federation-of Occupational-Therapists-Minimum-Standards-for-the-Education-of-Occupational-Therapists-2016a.pdf

Yu M-L, Brown T, White C, Marston C, Thyer L. The impact of undergraduate occupational therapy students' interpersonal skills on their practice education performance: a pilot study. Aust Occup Ther J. 2018;65:115–25. https://doi.org/10.1111/1440-1630.12444.

Practice Education in Lockdown: Lessons Learned During the COVID-19 Global Pandemic

67

Luke Robinson, Ted Brown, Ellie Fossey, Mong-Lin Yu, Linda Barclay, Eli Chu, Annette Peart, and Libby Callaway

Contents

Introduction	1304
University Education Provider Response to the COVID-19 Pandemic	1305
Clinical and Practice Education Provider Responses to the COVID-19 Pandemic	1306
Innovative Clinical and Practice Education Models	1307
Tele-placements	1309
An Overview of Tele-placements	1309
Opportunities and Challenges of Health Professional Student Tele-placements	1310
Considerations for Getting Started with Tele-placements	1310
Considerations for Tele-supervision	1311
Tele-placements in Lockdown: A Practice Example from Australia	1312
Simulating Clinical Placements	1313
Adapting Simulated Clinical Placements for Occupational Therapy Students in Lockdown: A Practice Example in Australia	1314
Reflections and Takeaway Messages	1317
Things to Consider When Designing for Implementing an Online SCP	1317
Online Facilitated Reflective Learning	1318
Facilitated Online Learning in Lockdown: A Practice Example from Australia	1318
Conclusions	1319
References	1320

L. Robinson (✉) · E. Fossey · L. Barclay · E. Chu · A. Peart · L. Callaway
Department of Occupational Therapy, Monash University – Peninsula Campus, Frankston, VIC, Australia
e-mail: luke.robinson@monash.edu; ellie.fossey@monash.edu; linda.barclay2@monash.edu; eli.chu@monash.edu; Annette.peart@monash.edu; libby.callaway@monash.edu

T. Brown · M.-L. Yu
Department of Occupational Therapy, School of Primary and Allied Health Care, Faculty of Medicine, Nursing and Health Sciences, Monash University – Peninsula Campus, Frankston, VIC, Australia
e-mail: ted.brown@monash.edu; mong-lin.yu@monash.edu

© Crown 2023
D. Nestel et al. (eds.), *Clinical Education for the Health Professions*,
https://doi.org/10.1007/978-981-15-3344-0_138

Abstract

The COVID-19 global pandemic has had large impacts on practice education opportunities for students enrolled in health professional courses. In response, educators and clinical supervisors have been required to change the ways in which pre-clinical and clinical education opportunities are delivered. This chapter presents several methods (tele-placement, tele-supervision, online simulated placements, and online facilitated reflective learning) which were adopted for occupational therapy students in response to the impacts of COVID-19 and provides practice examples implemented in Australia alongside lessons learned.

Keywords

COVID-19 · Clinical skills · Pre-clinical skills · Telehealth · Tele-supervision · Tele-placements · Simulated clinical placements · Reflective learning

Introduction

COVID-19 is a new and very contagious coronavirus affecting human beings globally. The primary symptoms of COVID-19 include fatigue, dry cough, breathing difficulties, and fever. About 20% of people who contract the virus require hospitalization due to respiratory difficulties (World Health Organization [WHO] 2020). Older adults over the age of 75 years, individuals with compromised immune systems, and people with underlying medical conditions (such as heart or lung problems, high blood pressure, and diabetes) are particularly vulnerable. The virus is spread from person to person via small liquid droplets when a person infected with COVID-19 speaks, sneezes, or coughs (World Health Organization [WHO] 2020). It can also be contracted from touching surfaces (i.e., tables, door handles, keyboards, handrails) followed by contact with a person's eyes, nose, or mouth. There is currently no vaccine to prevent a person contracting the virus. So, the only way to minimize COVID-19 infection at present is to reduce direct contact between people. Current recommended practices include avoiding touching one's eyes, nose, or mouth, frequent handwashing with soap and water, and use of an alcohol-based hand sanitizer to disinfect one's hands. In addition, maintaining at least one-meter distance between people (referred to as social distancing), using masks in public places, and staying home and self-isolating if feeling unwell are recommended to prevent its spread (Department of Health – Australian Government 2020).

COVID-19 is having significant social and economic impacts internationally, with countries closing borders, travel restrictions being put in place, non-essential businesses closed temporarily, workers encouraged to work from home if feasible, schools closed, and restrictions on the numbers of people who can meet or congregate together. Following a decrease in infection rates, some governments have chosen to gradually ease the restrictions while still encouraging social distancing, use of masks, and hand hygiene practices (such as washing your hands for at least

20 s using soap and water or a hand sanitizer that contains at least 60% alcohol when returning home, arrive at other people's homes, at venues, at shopping centers, or at work) (Health and Human Services – Victorian State Government 2020).

The emergence of the COVID-19 pandemic has also put marked financial, resource, and staffing pressures on the health care systems in many countries, particularly hospitals, intensive care units, and residential care settings. For health care professionals, it has required the routine use of personal protective equipment (PPE) such as face shields, masks, eye protection (such as safety glasses or goggles), gloves, and gowns (Department of Health – Australian Government 2020). Despite best efforts, with marked shortages of health care supplies (such as respirators) and PPE for staff in some countries and regions, infections have spread among health care workers and patients for whom they are caring. Many workplaces, stores, and offices have installed Perspex screens to minimize the contact and physical proximity between staff and members of the public (such as in doctors' offices, post offices, and supermarket checkouts).

University Education Provider Response to the COVID-19 Pandemic

The response to COVID-19 in the higher education sector has been varied. Many universities made the decision early in 2020 to distance students from campuses and have them continue their studies by online distance education. University campuses closed (except for essential services) and quickly transitioned to online teaching platforms (Klasen et al. 2020; Leigh et al. 2020). Academic staff were also strongly encouraged to work from home while delivering courses online for students. The need for social distancing as a means to control the spread of COVID-19 meant that gatherings of students on campus in lecture halls, tutorial rooms, and laboratories were stopped. Hence, many courses in which there were previously practical skills sessions, workshops, or tutorials had to be revised for online delivery (Pather et al. 2020). For many health professional courses, such as nursing, medicine, physiotherapy, radiography, dentistry, and occupational therapy, teaching staff have rapidly adapted their academic content using remote learning approaches (e.g., recorded demonstration of hands-on intervention techniques accompanied by descriptive, detailed narratives). To enable this, a number of digital technologies have been adapted for use in teaching, including webinars/virtual classrooms (e.g., Zoom, Microsoft Teams), video, audio podcasts (e.g., SoundCloud), online group work (e.g., Microsoft Teams, Facebook Private Groups, Padlet), and online student engagement (e.g., Kahoot!, online whiteboards, Blackboard Collaborate) (Ferrel and Ryan 2020; Wong 2020).

In relation to assessment tasks, the majority of campus-based assessments have been replaced by combinations of online tests, take-home examinations, and alternative assessments (Leigh et al. 2020). Further, some existing tasks have needed to be re-weighted to reduce the number of required assessments. This rapid move to online delivery of curricula has created some challenges, but creative and innovative approaches to the delivery of teaching and learning activities for health professional students have also emerged (Weiner and American Association of Medical Colleges 2020, April 15).

The move to online delivery of university curricula has had mixed responses from students themselves. Some have reportedly welcomed the opportunity to study from home, manage their own time, attend online tutorials, and listen to recorded lectures at their own pace. However, some students have found it challenging to engage with fully online delivery of their education, with others experiencing anxiety, depression, loneliness and international students being particularly at risk for these issues (Anderson et al. 2020). In health professional education, these issues may be exacerbated by the extra risks and safety concerns posed by undertaking practice education in settings where COVID-19 patients are being cared for (Henry et al. 2020). Indeed, COVID-19 has posed a number of particular challenges for practice education in health care contexts, which will be explored in the remainder of this chapter.

Clinical and Practice Education Provider Responses to the COVID-19 Pandemic

The COVID-19 pandemic has had significant impacts on health care systems and the professional practice contexts where medical, nursing, and allied health students typically complete clinical practicums and practice education. For example, with health care networks and hospitals having to reallocate funding, resources and staff to deal with the real or expected influx of COIVD-19 patients, many service providers made decisions to cancel or greatly reduce the number of practice education placements or clinical internships on offer to universities. In response, "some student placements have been paused or cancelled as health service providers prepare for the pandemic. Students may also be needed as part of the surge workforce depending on the severity of the pandemic" (Department of Education Skills and Employment – Australian Government 2020, para. 2). Likewise, primary and secondary schools closed, and residential aged-care facilities agencies put restrictions on outside visitors in an effort to minimize the transmission of COVID-19, reducing the scope for nursing and allied health placements in these settings too. Many not-for-profit and non-governmental organizations also temporarily discontinued student placements, particularly those providing services to vulnerable populations. Another reason cited for the cancellation of practice education opportunities by agencies is the need to preserve PPE supplies for qualified and supporting health care staff, rather than have it used by students (Ferrel and Ryan 2020). In sum, the impact of response to the COVID-19 pandemic for medical, nursing, and allied health students' practice education opportunities has been that many of the usual clinical education providers have canceled placements and internships. In turn, this has led to additional pressure to provide practice education in other clinical environments and potentially increase competition for a limited pool of student placements between universities (Rose 2020).

Some health, education, and social care agencies have shifted their services from providing direct face-to-face care to clients and families to using approaches variously described as a telehealth, tele-practice, and tele-rehabilitation to continue providing services safely. In hospitals, with student attendance at ward rounds and clinics being reduced as numbers of patients with COVID-19 have grown, a fundamental shift in clinical education from face-to-face to online formats has also occurred (Arandjelovic et al. 2020). This, in turn, presents a challenge of providing authentic patient engagement experiences for health professional students as a key element of their clinical and practice education (Klasen et al. 2020). Yet, according to Arandjelovic et al. (2020) telehealth "offers an avenue for the continuation of parallel consulting by physicians and medical students [and] may preserve the development of interpersonal skills, which may otherwise be difficult to attain solely through online or simulated learning" (p. 2). This is relevant for nursing and allied health students engaged in telehealth and tele-rehabilitation with patients and their families (Peretti et al. 2017). Indeed, a tele-placement approach, where students do not have face-to-face contact with clients and families, but instead collaborate with them using online video conferencing systems or via mobile phone functions, can enable students to complete relevant practice education placement in some settings. While some students may have reacted to this situation by reporting this not being an authentic clinical education learning opportunity, other students view it as a unique skill building and learning opportunity where they can be creative, agile, adaptive, flexible, and collaborative (Kapila et al. 2020). So, while many clinical practicums and practice education placements have been canceled, new educational opportunities have also emerged in this pandemic, including to gain knowledge about infection control measures, public health and community response, and telehealth as a means to provide care (Anderson et al. 2020).

To promote practice education and clinical rotation opportunities for students, the Australian Government Department of Education, Skills and Employment (2020) has proposed a set of eight "Clinical Education Principles for the COVID-19 Pandemic" which are useful to consider. They include (i) safety of patients, students, and staff; (ii) continuation of clinical education; (iii) outcome focused so that accreditation standards are met; (iv) collaborate and innovate involving all stakeholders; (v) prioritize students closest to graduation; (vi) capacity of students to extend service provision; (vii) identify, monitor, and manage risks to students, education providers, and health services; and (viii) maximize recognition of appropriate clinical education. In addition, Anderson et al. (2020) have proposed a framework for pandemic health professions education with four principles: (i) prioritize health system welfare, (ii) promote learner welfare, (iii) maximize educational value, and (iv) communicate transparently. Together, these provide useful guiding principles for planning changes to clinical practicums and practice education in the context of a pandemic.

Innovative Clinical and Practice Education Models

Recent technological advances have had a significant role in the evolution of the higher education environment by providing multiple modes of learning delivery and communication (Al-Samarraie and Saeed 2018). Videoconferencing (VC) technology is a communication medium that allows users to share visual information (e.g., slides, static images) and spoken and written discussions in real time (Al-Samarraie 2019). With the increase of Internet bandwidth capabilities and speed of computers in developed countries and many developing countries, the use of VC has become more feasible, realistic, and reliable for providing health professionals with clinical education and fieldwork placement opportunities. However, to enable success, educators must ensure that the technology facilitates engagement in a learning space that is secure and compatible with the students' abilities, accessibility, and learning requirements. During the COVID-19 pandemic, VC platforms such as Zoom, Microsoft Teams, and Webex have increasingly been used to provide a platform to complete various theoretical, skill-based, pre-clinical, and clinical learning opportunities.

Several creative clinical and practice education models have emerged or been refined in response to the COVID-19 pandemic, in which medical, nursing, and allied health students have been engaged. For example, at Monash University, allied health students are participating in a telehealth program addressing health and wellbeing for community members using a motivational interviewing and coaching approach to promote functional independence and healthy lifestyles. Other groups of students have been running social skills programs with children with Autism Spectrum Disorder via an online delivery, and activity groups for children with sensorimotor delays via online streaming. In addition, some medical and occupational therapy students have been promoting social connectedness for older adults in aged-care facilities through the use of telephone calls or video conferencing using smart devices. All of these approaches, none of which occurred prior to the COVID-19 pandemic, are examples of meaningful and productive practice education learning opportunities for health professional students designed to occur while abiding by the COVID-19 related health protocols, which also offer a community service. While these innovations are novel and student learning outcomes not yet established, previous research has indicated that the use of telehealth technology during the education of undergraduate medical students improved patient care, overall learning, professional competencies, and medical knowledge (Mian and Khan 2020).

Other approaches to clinical and practice education in the COVID-19 pandemic context include the use of simulation, near-peer learning opportunities, and students working together remotely in teams on clinical cases. For instance, a tablet may be used as the communication portal between the patient and respective health professional students and clinical educators in another room. It has been suggested that virtual and augmented reality are the leading edge in health professional education, and that clinical educators should be partnering with video game developers, the military, and IT specialists who are on the frontier of this online technology (Hollander and Carr 2020). Nevertheless, as Woolliscroft (2020) remarked, "while the new technology is promising, simulations can supplement but will never fully replace actual patient encounters in the medical [nursing and allied health professional] education curriculum" (p. 3).

The following sections in this chapter explore tele-placements and tele-supervision, simulated clinical placements, and online facilitated reflective learning in further detail as three methods that have been developed or refined for delivering pre-clinical and clinical education opportunities during the COVID-19 pandemic.

Following a description of each method, a practice example of how it was implemented in Australia during the COVID-19 pandemic is presented.

Tele-placements

The COVID-19 pandemic, escalating government restrictions for preventive health care, and hospital preparations for patient surge, has challenged health systems internationally (World Health Organization 2020). The resulting impact on essential health services has also led to significant reduction in practice education opportunities for health professional students. With COVID-19 restrictions and the need to maintain hygiene and physical distancing measures, the capacity to offer physical space to students has been challenged across the various acute, rehabilitation and community settings in which practice education may occur. This range of factors has led to a need for rapid redesign of practice education, with one option being a growing focus on tele-placements.

Telehealth has been used in health service provision for some time. However, opportunities for health professional students to gain education and new graduate competencies in this area are not yet mainstream and there is limited published evidence to guide telehealth education and training (Edirippulige and Armfield 2017; Smith et al. 2020). Ensuring the health workforce is telehealth-ready will require this mode of practice to be included in student training and education (Smith et al. 2020). One way to do this is by offering tele-placements.

An Overview of Tele-placements

Tele-placement, in this chapter, refers to clinical training provided to health professional students to develop knowledge, skills, and attitudes for the delivery of health services via digital technology platforms to community, clients, families, and other caregivers. Students attending tele-placements are involved in learning about the use of telehealth equipment, legal and ethical issues, funding sources and resource allocation, environment setup, as well as telehealth etiquette (e.g., professional behavior using telehealth, verbal and non-verbal communications) (Gustin et al. 2020). Students are also required to develop their abilities to modify existing models of care delivery from in-person encounter contexts to suit telehealth practice. This is a unique and essential focus of tele-placements.

Tele-placements can be facilitated in acute, sub/post-acute, emergency, and health promotion services within hospital, community, and educational settings as well as with private practice health providers. These placements bring opportunities for health professional students to work with populations of different ages across the lifespan. Various issues or concerns relevant to health, wellbeing, and life participation may be in focus, such as experience of disability, chronic health conditions, mental health and wellbeing, social participation, and child school readiness. Tele-placements can also enhance the potential for interprofessional collaborations and learning through partnerships among health care providers, government sectors, health insurance agencies, and community organizations and facilities concerned with human health, wellbeing, and life participation.

Opportunities and Challenges of Health Professional Student Tele-placements

Tele-placements can offer opportunities for both health professional students and clients to be taught the use of specific technologies, devices, and eHealth services and also assist students to learn to move away from health care provider-centric approaches (Scott and Mars 2020). Students can learn to customize technology-enabled interventions to suit individual goals and also consider closely the settings in which tele-placement support will be provided. Secure telehealth platforms, technical support, and both client and student digital literacy and readiness for tele-placements will, however, be necessary (Gustin et al. 2020; Smith et al. 2020). Tele-placements also require the ability to identify interventions suitable for remote delivery versus those essential services that require in-person engagement and how that may be achieved (World Health Organization 2020). Guidance from supervisors who have both the required clinical and telehealth experience may, therefore, be required. Specific to COVID-19, close attention to changing government guidance is also needed (e.g., Australian Government Department of Health 2020).

Health professional students may need to be assisted to see the value of remote clinical education, in contrast to face-to-face client interactions. Strategies to scaffold remote supervision with peer support, simulated peer practice, and self-directed learning will be necessary. A structured program of telehealth training can also be of benefit to improve knowledge in key areas of telehealth etiquette (Gustin et al. 2020). However, published evidence of telehealth education and training is currently lacking (Edirippulige and Armfield 2017). Further research, evaluation, and practice guidance are required to inform evidence-based tele-placements; document both advantages and limitations identified; and guide associated curriculum redesign (Gustin et al. 2020; Scott and Mars 2020).

Considerations for Getting Started with Tele-placements

Setting up a tele-placement requires many specific considerations. Significant placement resource development may be required, especially when strict physical distancing restrictions apply as in the current COVID-19 pandemic. Considerations include the following:

Space and equipment: Review of space and equipment available for tele-placements within an organization is imperative. This is also relevant to the placement agreement and insurance coverage of each university, which may have different conditions for tele-placements (e.g., whether students need to be onsite within the organization or can work from home; whether students can use their own computer or mobile phone or only organizational devices to protect privacy and security of information).

Students' knowledge, skills, and attitudes toward telehealth: Telehealth training is not as yet core curriculum within all health professional disciplines. Therefore, pre-placement telehealth training may need to be developed and required as part of the tele-placement orientation to adequately prepare students with essential knowledge, skills, and attitudes prior to commencing a tele-placement, especially before client contact.

Supervision model: Supervision can be provided by one or multiple supervisors, on site with student/s or remotely (via various communication methods, including video link, secure online forums established for student groups, email communications, or phone). Remote supervision is one possible way to manage space and physical distance requirements to facilitate tele-placements. To ensure quality and effective remote supervision and optimal student engagement, support for supervisors to provide remote supervision is required. It is also essential to establish effective supervisor-student communication and documentation system for students to record and communicate their placement activities (e.g., secure shared storage of placement timesheets, progress notes, and time use diaries).

Learning opportunities arrangement: Different from in-person placement contexts, incidental learning opportunities do not necessarily happen naturally in tele-placements, especially if students are receiving remote supervision. Client contact in a tele-placement also varies on a daily basis. Therefore, more effort is needed to arrange learning activities for each placement day. Structuring placement activities that facilitate peer-assisted learning and self-directed learning, plus opportunities for conducting small projects with partnered organizations, is an important consideration.

Considerations for Tele-supervision

Tele-supervision (TS), in this chapter, is defined as the use of telephone or VC technology to allow for communication between university-based staff, clinical supervisors, and/or students undertaking clinical placement. While TS has observed a slow emergence as an alternate or supplementary method of providing remote supervision and support to students during off-campus placements, the onset of COVID-19 has resulted in the need to focus on effective TS (Tarlow et al. 2020).

While still a relatively new method of providing supervision, some studies suggest that, if set up well, TS has similar outcomes on a student's capacity to develop and demonstrate their professional competence in comparison with face-to-face supervision (Martin et al. 2018). Tele-supervision has typically involved direct observation of students and their clients using VC; interactions between students and their clinical educators (if only students or clinical educators present on site); or discussions following the review of audio, video, or written materials (Nagarajan et al. 2016). The impact of COVID-19 has meant that new opportunities to provide effective TS-enabled supervision during clinical fieldwork are beginning to be realized (Tarlow et al. 2020).

Tele-placements in Lockdown: A Practice Example from Australia

In 2020, Australia completed implementation of an AUD 22 billion National Disability Insurance Scheme (NDIS) for people who experience significant and permanent disability and are under 65 years of age at the time of Scheme entry. NDIS participants may receive Scheme funding for allied health services, assistive technology, home or vehicle modifications, and disability support aligned with their participation goals. The NDIS necessitates a growing focus on clinical education for various allied health students in preparation for new graduate NDIS practice. Traditionally, this training has been offered face-to-face in group or supported living programs, or via community allied health practices.

Like other countries, the COVID-19 environment in Australia led to a reduction in face-to-face therapy support provision, closure of group services, and restricted public access to supported living environments of residents who may be vulnerable to virus transmission due to disability. For many universities, this led to an immediate reduction in traditional fieldwork education options. With this loss, staff from the Monash University School of Primary and Allied Healthcare pursued the opportunity for rapid conversion of allied health fieldwork with NDIS participants and their supporters to full-time tele-placement education. The redesigned fieldwork included a structured online training program and resource development drawn from the NDIS policies and practice guidance offered by the Scheme's independent regulatory body, the NDIS Quality and Safeguards Commission; existing online NDIS health professional student training resources in the field of neurological disability and the NDIS, developed by our interdisciplinary team (Callaway et al. 2018); and resources established to guide remote service delivery during COVID-19 (Australian Government Department of Health 2020).

The first step in this converted clinical education was to assess the communication skills and digital literacy, as well as technology requirements (e.g., phone, video link) of NDIS participants and their supporters (e.g., family, paid support workers), and to set up secure tele-placement options. Close consideration was given to the privacy and occupational health and safety of both the recipients of the tele-placement services and students. A structured weekly student timetable was established, with a mix of online learning and video link/phone engagement with people living with a disability and their key supporters. Student project work was also established with a peak body that engages with NDIS participants with neurological disability and paid or family supporters.

Due to the technology and learning demands for both NDIS participants and their supporters during an escalating pandemic, a priority focus was taken on student input for allied health assessment and report writing for those NDIS participants about to attend an annual plan review (which is used for reallocation of funding linked to their personal goals and support needs). In collaboration with the disability support provider, participants were invited to consider voluntary participation in the tele-placements based on their goals, needs, and proximity of timing of their NDIS planning meeting. Students worked in pairs to offer peer support and mentoring, and this was coupled with the remote supervision model from an occupational therapist, experienced in NDIS policy and practice and neurological disability. An NDIS participant who was a previously qualified allied health professional and had experienced a stroke was employed by the University for weekly person-centered mentoring to ensure this focus was central to the tele-placement client engagement. Interdisciplinary online supervision from a neuropsychologist and speech pathologist was also offered for the student group on alternating weeks. As the placement progressed, students were required to schedule and implement therapy sessions, documenting each intervention in progress notes on a secure platform. A range of other activity and participation-focused interventions were assessed for feasibility and adapted for tele-placement. These were then implemented using graded supervision and guided by individual client preferences and goals.

The key tele-placement deliverables were finalized allied health assessment reports to be used by clients in upcoming NDIS planning meetings, and practice guides for the peak body to supply to people with disability and their families. Client, support provider, and student experiences of this initial NDIS tele-placement are currently being evaluated. Findings will be reported back to government stakeholders and the NDIS. It is anticipated these findings will inform iterative allied health tele-placement and associated curriculum redesign.

Simulating Clinical Placements

In recent years, accumulated evidence supports that equivalent student performance can be achieved using simulation-based education to substitute clinical placement hours in some health professions (Bogossian et al. 2019; Imms et al. 2018). Simulation is an educational technique that allows for an interactive, and at times immersive, activity by recreating or amplifying all or part of a real-life experience guided by simulation facilitators (Maran and Glavin 2003). Activities can be conducted using mannequins or actors; through simulating authentic environments, such as home and ward environments; and through the use of equipment. Video footage or interactive computer packages can also be used to recreate scenarios that require the use of clinical and professional reasoning skills to solve problems. An additional advantage of simulation is that tasks can be graded to best reflect the student's stage of learning and therefore can focus on specific skill development.

Simulated clinical placements (SCP) assist students to prepare for work-integrated learning and interprofessional practice. When engaged in SCP, students play the role as student practitioners on placement and are guided by clinical supervisors/simulation facilitators to develop professional skills and competencies. In an SCP, a range of simulated activities utilizing multiple simulation methods are designed to replicate issues and activities that students will usually encounter in a real-life placement (e.g., co-morbidities, environmental considerations through the use of equipment and space, and safety concerns) (Chu et al. 2019).

To guide educators and simulation facilitators in the design of such simulations, Chu, Sheppard, Guinea, and Imms (2019) developed the Conceptual Framework for Simulated Clinical Placement (CF-SCP) (refer Fig. 1) as part of their work in

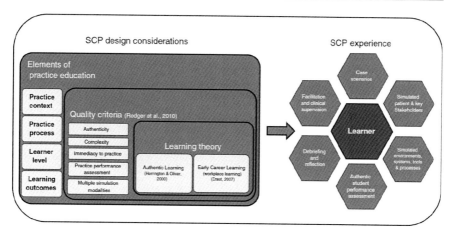

Fig. 1 Conceptual framework for simulated clinical placements (CF-SCP). (With permission from Chu et al. 2019)

pioneering an occupational therapy focused SCP. The framework was developed in an attempt to address the complex learning needs of students while also trying to address shortfalls in the availability of professional practice placements. The CF-SCP incorporates simulation-based learning design principles and concepts (Jeffries et al. 2015; Aebersold and Titler 2014), as well as workplace and authentic learning theories (Herrington and Oliver 2000; Eraut 2007) to inform activities to be included in an authentic simulated clinical placement (Chu et al. 2019). While initially developed with occupational therapy students in mind, the concepts and considerations presented in the framework can be adapted to suit other health care professional disciplines.

Adapting Simulated Clinical Placements for Occupational Therapy Students in Lockdown: A Practice Example in Australia

In response to the reduction in the availability of professional practice placements due to COVID-19, Monash University Department of Occupational Therapy pursued the rapid development of an SCP that could be delivered online and meet student learning and competency outcomes. Students enrolled in a Master of Occupational Therapy Practice (MOTPrac), who were midway through their accelerated full-time graduate entry course that runs across 2 years, were unable to complete their part-time clinical fieldwork placements as a result of COVID-19. To address this shortfall, 4 days of SCP were developed to run in conjunction with academic coursework.

The design of the simulated placement was grounded in the Occupational Therapy Council Accreditation Standards on use of simulation in practice education/fieldwork (Occupational Therapy Council (Australia and New Zealand) Ltd. 2013) and the Conceptual Framework for Simulated Clinical Placements (CF-SCP) (Chu et al. 2019) (Fig. 1). The practice context selected was a fictional health care network with simulated patients receiving services from general medical and neurological wards. Both learner level and learning outcomes were carefully considered when designing the SCP and are outlined in Fig. 2. To meet quality criteria of authenticity, complexity, and immediacy to practice, students completed a range of simulated activities and work processes that replicate practice, progressing from simple to complex tasks, interacting with simulated clients and significant others associated with the case (Fig. 3).

Each student was assigned a clinical supervisor, who was an academic or a clinician employed by the university. This supervisor was briefed prior to commencement of the placement to facilitate students' learning. To provide an environment similar to a professional practice placement, structured and non-structured debriefing and feedback opportunities were provided. Case scenarios were based on the available open access materials (medical history, simulated documentation, and recording forms) developed by clinical experts and experienced simulation designers funded by the Australian Department of Health (Imms et al. 2018). Authentic learning was supported by the actors having filmed video footage of their home environment, which were used to simulate a home assessment, and included a functional task for the students to observe. As part of their experience, students were required to complete initial assessments and interviews via Zoom with the actors portraying the patients, significant others, and other key stakeholders. An authentic student performance assessment was completed using the Student Practice Evaluation Form—Revised (SPEF-R) (Rodger et al. 2016), a standardized tool used for evaluating students' performance on clinical placement in Australia. The SCP, alongside an authentic student performance assessment, enabled the completed experience to be included as part of cumulative fieldwork hours needed to achieve competency for successful completion of the degree.

By the end of the Simulated Clinical Placement, students will demonstrate:

- Professional self-conduct and demonstration of professional behavior
- Time management and organizational skills
- Skills in effective client information gathering through initial assessment and initial interview
- Ability to identify a client's occupational performance issues and assess the impact of environmental and social factors on the client's ongoing participation and engagement
- Ability to identify appropriate client-centered goals
- Documentation skills

Fig. 2 Learning outcomes for the simulated clinical placement

> Activities to simulate work process:
>
> - Students were oriented to a simulated health organization, work processes, their clinical supervisor/simulation facilitator, and activities to be completed over the four days.
> - Each student completed work activity statistics and time sheets each day.
>
> Activities to simulate clinical practice:
>
> - Students received a referral to work with a primary patient in small groups.
> - An initial interview/assessment with a simulated primary patient (a paid actor) in small groups was conducted via Zoom. Each student was required to conduct part of the interview.
> - A simulated home assessment was completed by watching video footage filmed in the simulated patient's home to simulate a home visit.
> - Students observed a patient completing a functional activity (e.g., making a cup of tea, completing a bed transfer) by watching video footage.
> - Students interviewed the patients' primary stakeholders (e.g., ward doctor, neighbor, husband, physiotherapist) in small groups via Zoom.
> - A follow-up interview was conducted with the patient to clarify any issues and to confirm goals and plans moving forward.
> - Students individually completed documentation relating to initial interview, home assessment, progress notes, establishing occupational performance issues, intervention goals, and intervention plan. On the final day of the SCP they were required to present this information verbally to their supervisor/facilitator.
> - Each student was assigned a secondary patient for whom they were required to conduct some investigations around a particular clinical problem.
> - Each student completed specific documentation in relation to the secondary patient which they submitted online to their supervisor/facilitator.
> - A tertiary task was assigned to each small group that involved a brief evidence-based review of a particular area of practice. Students were required to do a short oral presentation to a staff member and fellow students regarding their findings on the final day.
>
> Supervision, debriefing, reflection, and assessments:
>
> - Clinical supervisors/simulation facilitators observed and guided student engagement during the simulated activities.
> - Students participated in structured and unstructured supervision and debriefing sessions to develop clinical reasoning, reflective practice, and practical skills.
> - Clinical supervisors completed placement evaluation with each student and provided feedback on performance at the end of the simulated placement.

Fig. 3 Tasks assigned during simulated clinical placement

Following completion of the 4 days of SCP, the teaching team reflected on the content and running of the program, and feedback was obtained from the students on strengths and weaknesses from their perspective. These reflections are included below:

Reflections and Takeaway Messages

- Health care students in the early stages of their learning can gain important skills from an SCP delivered online, which incorporates quality, authentic learning, and assessment, and is underpinned by a clear conceptual framework.
- Using simulated patients is effective for communication skills training, however, when students practice conducting an interview via Zoom, the camera often does not capture the entire person on the screen, and, therefore, the interviewer heavily relies on verbal communication. This means they may miss out on meanings conveyed through body language and other non-verbal presentations.
  - For example, in the SCP a simulated patient, who had multiple sclerosis, was crying quietly during the interview. Several students engaged in the SCP missed non-verbal cues and therefore did not respond appropriately to her distress.
- When using Zoom or similar platforms, users may find that it is not natural to look at the camera and use eye contact or be impacted by the position and/or angle of the camera. This may lead to misinterpretation of emotions or communications.
- It is still possible for facilitators to guide students' learning by providing immediate feedback, using time out (e.g., pause the activity), providing opportunities for practice, reflection, and debriefing.
- It is possible to develop interprofessional practice skills online in an authentic way by interviewing other health professionals and significant others through phone or Zoom.
- There is reduced opportunity for practicing the use of equipment and other hands-on techniques through online platform.
- Using online technologies to deliver and participate in simulated placement is not intuitive. Additional time is required to adapt an already well-structured program, to provide pre-briefing to orientate staff and students to the program, and to train staff and students to use unfamiliar technologies.

Things to Consider When Designing for Implementing an Online SCP

- Identify the best fit between intended learning objectives and learning activities delivered online.
- Be aware of staff and learners' knowledge and skills in using online platforms and other technologies.
- Consider the benefits and limitations of using online simulated placement when selecting learning objectives.

- Provide clear instructions and procedures for students and staff to follow including procedures for using online platforms.
- Communicate expectation of online etiquette and professional behavior clearly.

Online Facilitated Reflective Learning

The importance of reflection and reflective practice is recognized in the literature of most health care disciplines, with many suggesting reflective capacity is an essential characteristic for professional competence (Mann et al. 2009). A student, or novice health professional, must spend a significant amount of time in novel clinical activities and consequently engage in reflective practice to develop a robust clinical knowledge base that guides the development of their professional/clinical reasoning (Ladyshewsky and Gardner 2008). This development can be supported by peers who learn from one another by sharing ideas and observations, and articulating their professional/clinical reasoning. Peers are a source of compelling, yet safe, discussions that involve clinical practice because of the shared language and biomedical information which can be easily shared and understood by one another (Ladyshewsky and Gardner 2008). Further, communication between peers is often perceived as less threatening than with supervisors, and, therefore, encourages disclosure and discussions and presents deeper learning opportunities. While blogging and discussion forums have historically enabled this process, the advances in VC technology have allowed students to come together while completing their clinical fieldwork and present ideas to one another with or without a university-based educator acting as a facilitator. Such advances have allowed for real-time discussions which also promote social connectedness and peer support.

Facilitated Online Learning in Lockdown: A Practice Example from Australia

While Monash University occupational therapy students complete their final professional practice placements, they are enrolled in an online unit that facilitates reflection on contemporary practice issues, such as evidence-based practice in action and clinical governance. This approach encourages students to reflect and critique professional issues while completing their practice education by presenting their observations to a group of their peers using Zoom. Group members are encouraged to respond to these presentations and provide alternative viewpoints based on literature and their observations. These discussions are facilitated by a university-based educator who provides knowledge, resources, or insights about the practice issue. The quality of these presentations, as well as peer-reviews and contributions, are marked as part of students' academic coursework. Prior to the COVID-19 pandemic, this approach allowed for a positive and effective learning environment where students who were completing fieldwork could learn about different clinical practice areas. In addition, it allowed students to raise with their facilitator any issues encountered during fieldwork as they occur in real time and feel connected to their peers.

During the COVID-19 pandemic, online facilitated reflective learning proved to have additional benefits. First, it allowed students to debrief about the dynamic nature of their fieldwork placements during the pandemic, such as the quick transition to telehealth and its impact on service delivery. Second, it allowed students to articulate shared issues they encountered, such as the stressors associated with completing placements during the pandemic, which encouraged group discussion of strategies on how to address them. Third, it allowed students to learn about the pandemic response from a range of different clinical areas and facilitate discussions about their observations. Finally, it allowed the university-based educator to better understand the pandemic's impact in placement settings and be available for one-on-one consultations with students, who required support while completing their practice education.

While not instigated because of COVID-19, this online approach has highlighted the benefits of facilitating group reflective practice with students while on fieldwork during a pandemic by enabling the sharing of experiences, observations, and responses as well as monitoring student health and wellbeing, providing opportunities for tele-supervision/debriefing outside of the practice placement, and promoting connection. Further, it provided a platform for students to discuss evolving practice issues as they were occurring in real time during the pandemic.

Conclusions

Practice education is an integral part of health professional education in medicine, nursing, and allied health professions. This chapter has identified some of the emerging challenges to providing practice education in health professional education programs during the COVID-19 pandemic. COVID-19 is challenging educators to think differently about how to provide quality learning experiences for students in health professional education programs, and to identify new and meaningful learning opportunities created by the shifting landscape of health care delivery. Here, we have presented tele-placements and tele-supervision, simulated clinical placements, and online facilitated reflective learning as three approaches that have been developed or refined for delivering pre-clinical and clinical education opportunities during the COVID-19 pandemic, with illustrative examples of how each has been implemented.

The COVID-19 pandemic continues to have significant health, social, and economic impacts globally, as well as impacting health care systems and in turn medical, nursing, and allied health students' practice education opportunities. Nevertheless, new educational opportunities have also emerged in this pandemic that can be harnessed to equip graduates with knowledge, skills, and attitudes for more diverse ways of delivering health care.

References

Aebersold M, Titler MG. A simulation model for improving learner and health outcomes. Nurs Clin N Am. 2014;49:431–9. https://doi.org/10.1016/j.cnur.2014.05.011.

Al-Samarraie H. A scoping review of videoconferencing systems in higher education: learning paradigms, opportunities, and challenges. Int Rev Res Open Distrib Learn. 2019;20:121–140.

Al-Samarraie H, Saeed N. A systematic review of cloud computing tools for collaborative learning: opportunities and challenges to the blended-learning environment. Comput Educ. 2018;124:77–91. https://doi.org/10.1016/j.compedu.2018.05.016.

Anderson ML, Turbow S, Willgerodt MA, et al. Education in a crisis: the opportunity of our lives. J Hosp Med. 2020;15:287. https://doi.org/10.12788/jhm.3431.

Arandjelovic A, Arandjelovic K, Dwyer K, et al. COVID-19: considerations for medical education during a pandemic. MedEdPublish. 2020;9. https://doi.org/10.15694/mep.2020.000087.1.

Australian Government Department of Health. Providing healthcare remotely during COVID-19, www.health.gov.au/news/health-alerts/novel-coronavirus-2019-ncov-health-alert/coronavirus-covid-19-advice-for-the-health-and-aged-care-sector/providing-health-care-remotely-during-covid-19. 2020.

Bogossian FE, Cant RP, Ballard EL, et al. Locating "gold standard" evidence for simulation as a substitute for clinical practice in prelicensure health professional education: a systematic review. J Clin Nurs. 2019;28:3759–75. https://doi.org/10.1111/jocn.14965.

Callaway L, Sloan S, Mackey J, Tregloan K, Morgan P, Gee E. My support space: digital and written information resources to build skills and knowledge for supporting people with acquired brain injury, www.mysupportspace.org. 2018.

Chu EMY, Sheppard L, Guinea S, et al. Placement replacement: a conceptual framework for designing simulated clinical placement in occupational therapy. Nurs Health Sci. 2019;21:4–13. https://doi.org/10.1111/nhs.12551.

Department of Education Skills and Employment – Australian Government. National principles for clinical education during the COVID-19 pandemic. 2020, para. 2.

Department of Health – Australian Government. Coronavirus (COVID-19) resources for health professionals, including aged care providers, pathology providers and health care managers, https://www.health.gov.au/resources/collections/coronavirus-covid-19-resources-for-health-professionals-including-aged-care-providers-pathology-providers-and-health-care-managers. 2020.

Edirippulige S, Armfield N. Education and training to support the use of clinical telehealth: a review of the literature. J Telemed Telecare. 2017;23:273–82. https://doi.org/10.1177/1357633X16632968.

Eraut M. Learning from other people in the workplace. Oxf Rev Educa: Learn Across Profess. 2007;33:403–22. https://doi.org/10.1080/03054980701425706.

Ferrel M, Ryan J. The impact of COVID-19 on medical education. Cureus. 2020;12:e7492. https://doi.org/10.7759/cureus.7492.

Gustin ST, Kott SK, Rutledge SC. Telehealth etiquette training: a guideline for preparing interprofessional teams for successful encounters. Nurse Educ. 2020;45:88–92. https://doi.org/10.1097/NNE.0000000000000680.

Health and Human Services – Victorian State Government. Hygiene and physical distancing, https://www.dhhs.vic.gov.au/staying-safe-covid-19. 2020.

Henry JA, Black S, Gowell M, et al. Covid-19: how to use your time when clinical placements are postponed. BMJ. 2020;369:m1489. https://doi.org/10.1136/bmj.m1489.

Herrington J, Oliver R. An instructional design framework for authentic learning environments. Educ Technol Res Dev. 2000;48:23–48. https://doi.org/10.1007/BF02319856.

Hollander J, Carr B. Virtually perfect? Telemedicine for Covid-19. N Engl J Med. 2020;382:1679–81. https://doi.org/10.1056/NEJMp2003539.

Imms C, Froude E, Chu EMY, et al. Simulated versus traditional occupational therapy placements: a randomised controlled trial. Aust Occup Ther J. 2018;65:556–64. https://doi.org/10.1111/1440-1630.12513.

Jeffries RP, Rodgers RB, Adamson RK. NLN Jeffries simulation theory: brief narrative description. Nurs Educ Perspect. 2015;36:292–3. https://doi.org/10.5480/1536-5026-36.5.292.

Kapila V, Corthals S, Langhendries L, Kapila AK, Everaert K. The importance of medical student perspectives on the impact of COVID-19. Lancet Infect Dis. 2020;20:777–8. https://doi.org/10.1002/bjs.11808.

Klasen J, Akschaya V, Burm S. "The storm has arrived": the impact of SARS-CoV-2 on medical students. Perspect Med Educ. 2020;9:181–5. https://doi.org/10.1007/s40037-020-00592-2.

Ladyshewsky RK, Gardner P. Peer assisted learning and blogging: a strategy to promote reflective practice during clinical fieldwork. Australas J Educ Technol. 2008;24:241.

Leigh J, Vasilica C, Dron R, et al. Redefining undergraduate nurse teaching during the coronavirus pandemic: use of digital technologies. Br J Nurs. 2020;29:566–9. https://doi.org/10.12968/bjon.2020.29.10.566.

Mann K, Gordon J, Macleod A. Reflection and reflective practice in health professions education: a systematic review. Adv Health Sci Educ Theory Pract. 2009;14:595. https://doi.org/10.1007/s10459-007-9090-2.

Maran NJ, Glavin RJ. Low- to high-fidelity simulation – a continuum of medical education? Med Educ. 2003;37:22–8. https://doi.org/10.1046/j.1365-2923.37.s1.9.x.

Martin P, Lizarondo L, Kumar S. A systematic review of the factors that influence the quality and effectiveness of telesupervision for health professionals. J Telemed Telecare. 2018;24:271–81. https://doi.org/10.1177/1357633X17698868.

Mian A, Khan S. Medical education during pandemics: a UK perspective. BMC Med. 2020;18:1–2. https://doi.org/10.1186/s12916-020-01577-y.

Nagarajan S, McAllister L, McFarlane L, et al. Telesupervision benefits for placements: allied health students' and supervisors' perceptions. Int J Pract-Based Learn Health Soc Care. 2016:16–27. https://doi.org/10.18552/ijpblhsc.v4i1.326.

Occupational Therapy Council (Australia & New Zealand) Ltd. Occupational Therapy Council Accreditation Standards Explanatory guide: the use of simulation in practice education/fieldwork, https://www.otcouncil.com.au/wp-content/uploads/Explanatory-notes-for-simulation-in-practice-education-updated-March2020.pdf. 2013.

Pather N, Blyth P, Chapman JA, et al. Forced disruption of anatomy education in Australia and New Zealand: an acute response to the Covid-19 pandemic. Anat Sci Educ. 2020;13:284–300. https://doi.org/10.1002/ase.1968.

Peretti A, Amenta F, Tayebati SK, et al. Telerehabilitation: review of the state-of-the-art and areas of application. JMIR Rehab Assist Technol. 2017;4:e7. https://doi.org/10.2196/rehab.7511.

Rodger S, Chien C-W, Turpin M, et al. Establishing the validity and reliability of the student practice evaluation form–revised (SPEF-R) in occupational therapy practice education: a Rasch analysis. Eval Health Prof. 2016;39:33–48. https://doi.org/10.1177/0163278713511456.

Rose S. Medical student education in the time of COVID-19. JAMA. 2020;323:2131–3132.

Scott RE, Mars M. Response to Smith et al.: telehealth for global emergencies: implications for coronavirus disease 2019 (COVID-19). J Telemed Telecare. 2020;26:378–80. https://doi.org/10.1177/1357633X20932416.

Smith AC, Thomas E, Snoswell CL, et al. Telehealth for global emergencies: implications for coronavirus disease 2019 (COVID-19). J Telemed Telecare. 2020;26:309–13. https://doi.org/10.1177/1357633X20916567.

Tarlow KR, McCord CE, Nelon JL, et al. Comparing in-person supervision and telesupervision: a multiple baseline single-case study. J Psychother Integr. 2020;30:383–93. https://doi.org/10.1037/int0000210.

Weiner S, American Association of Medical Colleges. No classrooms, no clinics: medical education during a pandemic, https://www.aamc.org/news-insights/no-classrooms-no-clinics-medical-education-during-pandemic. 2020, April 15.

Wong RY. Medical education during COVID-19: lessons from a pandemic. BC Med J. 2020;62: 170–1.

Woolliscroft OJ. Innovation in response to the COVID-19 pandemic crisis. Acad Med. 2020;95: 1140–2. https://doi.org/10.1097/ACM.0000000000003402.

World Health Organization. Maintaining essential health services: operational guidance for the COVID-19 context: interim guidance, 1 June 2020. 2020. World Health Organization.

World Health Organization [WHO]. Coronavirus, https://www.who.int/health-topics/coronavirus#tab=tab_1. 2020.

Part VI

Evidence-Based Health Professions Education: Focus on Educational Methods and Content

Team-Based Learning (TBL): Theory, Planning, Practice, and Implementation

68

Annette Burgess and Elie Matar

Contents

Introduction	1327
What Is Team-Based Learning?	1328
TBL: Theory and Rationale	1330
Team Formation	1330
Readiness Assurance	1331
Immediate Feedback	1331
In-Class Problem-Solving Activities	1331
The Four S's (Significant Problem, Same Problem, Specific Choice, and Simultaneous Reporting)	1332
Incentive Structure	1332
Peer Review	1333
Current Trends and Evidence for TBL in Healthcare Education	1333
Student Academic Performance	1333
Learner Reaction TBL	1334
Faculty Reaction to TBL	1334
Comparison with Other Learning Approaches	1334
Key Elements of TBL	1334
Key Elements of PBL	1335
Key Elements of CBL	1336

A. Burgess (✉)
Faculty of Medicine and Health, Sydney Medical School, Education Office, The University of Sydney, Sydney, NSW, Australia

Faculty of Medicine and Health, Sydney Health Professional Education Research Network, The University of Sydney, Sydney, NSW, Australia
e-mail: annette.burgess@sydney.edu.au

E. Matar
Faculty of Medicine and Health, Sydney Medical School, Education Office, The University of Sydney, Sydney, NSW, Australia

Faculty of Medicine and Health, Sydney Medical School, Central Clinical School, The University of Sydney, Sydney, NSW, Australia
e-mail: elie.matar@sydney.edu.au

© Springer Nature Singapore Pte Ltd. 2023
D. Nestel et al. (eds.), *Clinical Education for the Health Professions*,
https://doi.org/10.1007/978-981-15-3344-0_128

Planning for TBL in Your Healthcare Faculty 1336
    Curriculum Design 1336
    Backward Design of TBL 1336
    Writing Learning Outcomes 1337
    Writing TBL Cases 1337
    Writing MCQs 1338
Implementation of TBL 1339
    Facilitator Engagement 1339
    Team Teaching 1340
    Facilitation Skills in TBL 1340
    Questioning 1341
    Student Engagement 1344
    Benefits and Challenges of TBL 1344
    Resource Implications for Institutions 1345
    Space/Room Requirements 1345
Emerging Trends in TBL 1348
Concluding Remarks and Future Work 1349
Cross-References 1350
References 1350

Abstract

Team-based learning (TBL) is an effective and resource-wise pedagogical tool with the potential to integrate into a broad range of health educational environments and align student learning outcomes with the knowledge and skills needed by graduates in the workforce. Designed to enhance the quality of student learning, TBL offers a unique approach to small group teaching, providing a resource-efficient strategy to transform small groups into teams. The TBL design provides an effective approach to teach a large number of students in an engaging manner that fosters active small and large group discussion, real-time decision-making, and provision of immediate feedback. Going beyond the simple transfer of knowledge content, TBL focuses on the application of knowledge through conceptual and authentic problem-solving activities. The TBL format offers a feedback-rich learning environment, with opportunities for students to develop critical competencies relevant to healthcare education: teamwork abilities and critical thinking skills.

The purpose of this chapter is to provide readers with an overview of TBL, including the theory and rationale for the use of TBL; the current trends and evidence for TBL in healthcare education; a comparison of TBL with other learning approaches; practical tips for design, implementation, and facilitation of TBL as an instructional strategy within medicine and health education; and emerging trends in the design and application of TBL.

Keywords

Team-based learning · Small group learning · Teamwork · Team teaching · Co-teaching · Collaboration

Abbreviations

IRAT	Individual readiness assurance test
SMP	Sydney Medical Program
TBL	Team-based learning
TRAT	Team readiness assurance test

Introduction

Team-based learning (TBL) is "an active learning and small group instructional strategy that provides students with opportunities to apply conceptual knowledge through a sequence of activities that includes individual work, teamwork, and immediate feedback" (Parmelee et al. 2012). Designed to enhance the quality of student learning, TBL offers a unique approach to small group teaching, providing a resource-efficient strategy to transform small groups into teams (Parmelee et al. 2012; Burgess et al. 2014). Originating from the University of Oklahoma, USA, TBL was developed by Professor Larry Michaelsen in the 1970s for use in graduate business curricula. Faced with increasing class sizes, Michaelson was concerned about the effectiveness of lectures as a teaching method and the alignment of student learning outcomes with the knowledge and skills needed by graduates in the workforce (Parmelee et al. 2012; Burgess et al. 2014). The TBL design provided a strategy to teach a large number of students in an engaging manner that fostered active small and large group discussion, real-time decision-making, and provision of immediate feedback (Burgess et al. 2014). Going beyond the simple transfer of knowledge content, TBL focuses on the application of knowledge through conceptual and authentic problem-solving activities (Michaelsen and Sweet 2008a).

The first reported use of TBL within health professional education was in medicine in 2001, at Baylor College of Medicine, USA, its use expanding to ten US medical schools within just 1 year (Searle et al. 2003). TBL has since gained popularity across the health professions as a teaching pedagogy that is resource-efficient, and student-centered. Currently, TBL is being implemented across the world within the disciplines of medicine, pharmacy, nursing, dentistry, allied health, public health, health sciences, and within interprofessional contexts (Burgess et al. 2014; Fatmi et al. 2013; Reimschisel et al. 2017). Increasingly, TBL is being introduced as an alternative to problem-based learning (PBL). In comparison to PBL, TBL maintains the advantages of small group teaching and learning, without requiring large numbers of teachers. The authors of this chapter were involved in the design and delivery of a new hybrid TBL curriculum that replaced PBL in 2017, across Year 1 and Year 2 of the medical program at The University of Sydney School of Medicine, Australia, following extensive piloting (Burgess et al. 2016, 2017, 2018).

The purpose of this chapter is to provide readers with an overview of team-based learning (TBL), including theory, and the practical implementation of TBL as an instructional strategy within medicine and health education.

What Is Team-Based Learning?

TBL is an interactive, expert-led teaching session that allows a large number of students to work within small teams to apply course content to specific problems (Huggett and Jeffries 2014). TBL provides an innovative approach to student-centered learning, supporting the flipped classroom method of education (Burgess and Mellis 2015). Although traditionally, the aim of face-to-face classes has been to familiarize students with key course concepts, the primary focus of TBL is on the application and practice of these concepts. The student's role shifts from that of a passive recipient of information to taking responsibility for adequate preparation, and engagement in teamwork within their small groups. In turn, this requires that the facilitator's key role shifts from dispensing information to managing a process, and providing timely and accurate feedback. Students are encouraged to self-learn, analyze, communicate, collaborate, speculate, reason, and problem-solve in small teams (Huggett and Jeffries 2014). As an instructional strategy, the effectiveness of TBL is derived from the cohesiveness that is developed within student teams. Michaelsen and Sweet emphasize three distinct phases within the TBL process (Michaelsen and Sweet 2008a):

1. *The preparatory phase,* during which students are provided with learning resources, such as readings, videos, or pre-recorded lectures to complete prior to class.
2. *The readiness assurance phase*, during which students are assessed on their understanding of preparation material and their preparedness for the TBL activities. Traditionally, this requires students to complete a knowledge test on two separate instances – initially on their own to give an indication of "individual readiness" (an "individual readiness assurance test," IRAT) and again as part of their team in class (a "team readiness assurance test," TRAT). Feedback and clarification of concepts is then provided to the students immediately after the TRAT before proceeding to the final phase.
3. *The application phase*, during which students apply their knowledge to clinical problem-solving activities.

These three phases are illustrated in Box 1 along with individual steps within each phase and the respective timeframes. The structured format of TBL provides opportunities for students to apply and build on conceptual knowledge through a sequence of specific steps: preparation, readiness assurance testing, feedback, and clinical problem-solving activities (Burgess et al. 2014; Haidet et al. 2012; Sweet and Michaelsen 2012).

Box 1 The Three Key Phases of TBL: (1) Preparation, (2) Readiness Assurance, (3) Application. Suggested Timings Are Provided for Each Phase Alongside Detail on the Individual Steps within Each Phase

Preparatory phase (1–2 h)

1. Pre-class preparation
This includes pre-reading or viewing pre-recorded lectures online. The material provides students with the relevant background knowledge needed to successfully participate in the TBL session. Student preparation is often reflected through the results of their readiness assurance test scores.

Readiness assurance phase (30–40 min)

2. Individual readiness assurance test (IRAT)
The IRAT is essential in engaging students to take part in the preparation required and is usually undertaken by the student prior to class or at the commencement of class. Questions are typically in the form of a multiple choice/single best answer format. Students are not provided with the answers until step 4.

3. Team readiness assurance test (TRAT)
The TRAT involves the same questions as the IRAT except this time is completed by students in class with their team members. Students will discuss the questions and their responses to come to a consensus on each answer as a team.

4. Immediate feedback and clarification
Using pre-prepared presentation slides, the facilitator provides immediate feedback on team responses. The facilitator can offer clarification, especially on question items and topic areas where teams had difficulty or disagreements on their responses.

Application phase (1.5–2 h)

5. Clinical problem-solving activities
The problem-solving activities allow students to practice making decisions and judgments they would make in the workplace (Sweet and Michaelsen 2012). An authentic clinical case based on the topic of the TBL session is provided to the class for in-depth discussion in student teams. All teams work on the same questions at the same time allowing the entire class to participate in discussion. Student groups are encouraged to work together to solve provided problems and support their responses with clinical reasoning. Each team is expected to contribute to the class discussion.

6. Close (instructor summary)
Facilitators are given the opportunity to reflect on student learning during the TBL session, review key answers, clarify any misunderstandings, and answer student questions (Huggett and Jeffries 2014). Summarizing three key messages or asking each team for one take-home message provides a good way to close the session.

TBL: Theory and Rationale

TBL allows medical and healthcare educators to provide students with resource-effective, authentic experiences of working in teams to solve clinical problems and develop professional competencies (Haidet et al. 2012). Within increasingly complex healthcare systems, excellence in teamwork and communication is essential to improving healthcare and patient safety outcomes (O'Daniel and Rosenstein 2008). The structure of TBL includes elements favorable to preparing students to work in teams, synthesize information, and communicate with each other. Below we explore the theoretical underpinnings of TBL with respect to the "seven core design elements" of the TBL method described by Haidet and colleagues (2012): (1) team formation, (2) readiness assurance, (3) immediate feedback, (4) sequencing of in-class problem-solving, (5) the four S's (significant problem, same problem, specific choice, and simultaneous reporting), (6) incentive structure, and (7) peer review (Haidet et al. 2012).

Team Formation

Three key aspects need to be considered theoretically with respect to team formation for TBL.

Team allocation: Teams need adequate resources to draw from in completing their problem-solving activities, and approximately the same level of resources across teams. Students are assigned to teams using a transparent process that ideally ensures a diverse mix of students and minimizes formation of teams based mainly on pre-existing friendships (Michaelsen and Richards 2005). Random and alphabetical methods of student allocation to teams are likely to prevent teams of friends from self-forming but may not adequately achieve the optimum diversity of learner characteristics. Thus, others have advocated using a combination of random allocation and methods that equalize the expertise and gender mix on each team (Burgess et al. 2014; Thomas and Bowen 2011; Nieder et al. 2005).

Duration of teams: In line with long-standing group dynamics literature (Tuckman 1965; McGrath 1991), TBL guidelines recommend that student teams "stay together as long as possible," to enhance team dynamics, trust, and diversity of knowledge and skills within the team (Parmelee et al. 2012). This would translate to keeping TBL teams constant throughout the duration of at least a subject block or semester.

Team size: Michaelsen and colleagues (2007) suggest that team size should be between five and seven students – small enough to develop teamwork processes and maximize team dynamics, yet large enough to include sufficient intellectual resources (Michaelsen et al. 2007). Burgess and colleagues recommend five to six students per TBL team (Burgess et al. 2017), and there is evidence to suggest that teams of five to seven students perform better academically compared to smaller teams of two students (Wiener et al. 2009).

Readiness Assurance

By testing the knowledge of individuals, and then teams, it is anticipated that students will come to class prepared, motivated by not wanting to let their team down. In turn, class time is freed up for in-class problem-solving activities, and less time is spent covering factual material. The readiness assurance process makes students individually accountable for their preparation, since when they fail to prepare, it affects both their individual and team's learning and performance (Koles et al. 2005). The sequence of formal testing procedures in TBL as a part of the readiness assurance process ensures that students have several opportunities to engage with the content and gauge their own understanding (Michaelsen et al. 2007). Students are able to build on their own learning by comparing their answers to other team members and engaging in discussion to subsequently reach a consensus. Further to this, there is evidence that repeated testing improves better long-term retention of information, increases the regularity of study, and allows the learner to realize gaps in their knowledge (Larsen et al. 2009; Roediger et al. 2011).

Immediate Feedback

Michaelsen and Sweet (2008a) describe immediate feedback following the TRAT as inherent to the TBL process, providing students with an understanding of their content knowledge and application ability (Michaelsen and Sweet 2008a). In TBL, students are never left in doubt. Feedback is received through the readiness assurance process, during and at the end of the clinical problem-solving activities. Where feedback may be sought, it should be given to individuals and groups. Provision of immediate feedback is crucial to knowledge acquisition, application, and retention and enhances students' understanding (Sweet and Michaelsen 2012; Hattie and Timperley 2007; Burgess and Mellis 2015a). Without timely feedback, errors can go uncorrected, and students may feel overwhelmed by new content (Burgess and Mellis 2015a). Additionally, immediate feedback encourages competition between individuals and teams, and team development (Michaelsen and Sweet 2008a; Hattie and Timperley 2007).

In-Class Problem-Solving Activities

During problem-solving activities, students apply their knowledge of course content by working in teams to solve complex, real-life problems. Students must interpret, analyze, and synthesize information to make specific choices during the activity and may be required to defend their choices to the class (Parmelee et al. 2012). Teams are required to use their collective knowledge, ethical views, skills, and values to solve complex clinical problems that apply to real-life situations (Haidet et al. 2012). Evidence suggests that the activation of prior knowledge through small group discussion may have a positive impact on learning (Van Blankenstein et al. 2011), and that increased diversity in learners within groups improves the quality of discussion and learner outcomes (Michaelsen and Sweet 2008a).

The Four S's (Significant Problem, Same Problem, Specific Choice, and Simultaneous Reporting)

The design of the problem-solving activities should promote both student learning and team development. Participation in the clinical problem-solving activities encourages learning and team development through the use of challenging cases (see below). Haidet and colleagues (2012) recommend adherence to "The Four S principle," designed to guide the content, structure, and process of the problem-solving activity phases:

Significant: The problem needs to be significant.
Same: All teams need to have the same problem.
Specific: There needs to be a specific choice in the answer.
Simultaneous: All teams need to report their answers simultaneously.

However, consistent with recent literature, and as noted by Michaelsen himself (Michaelsen and Richards 2005), application of TBL within the healthcare education is constrained by a number of predetermined contextual factors, reducing the benefits of adhering to all traditional TBL design elements. For example, allowing only one "specific choice" within the clinical problem-solving activity phase of TBL may restrict student discussion to predetermined outcomes, and instead, open-ended questions should be incorporated (Burgess et al. 2017; Badget et al. 2014; Burgess and Mellis 2014). One advantage of modifying the "specific choice" element in this way within clinical problem-solving activities is that it averts the difficulty and time-cost of writing specific choice questions (i.e., MCQs).

Incentive Structure

The use of assessment has a large impact on students' achievement of course outcomes. In TBL, assessment is designed to maximize both individuals' pre-class preparation and team collaboration (Haidet et al. 2012). Michaelsen and Sweet (2008a) suggest that an effective grading system is needed to provide rewards for both individual contributions and effective teamwork, and to relieve students' concerns about grading of group work. Grades can be assigned for the IRAT, TRAT, problem-solving, and peer review (Parmelee et al. 2012). A method to assess team performance is to use the clinical problem-solving activities to create a product (such as a mechanistic flow chart) (Burgess et al. 2017) that can be compared across teams and evaluated in real-time by content experts present.

Peer Review

The inclusion of peer review in the TBL process provides an incentive for students to positively contribute to the team's learning and problem-solving (Haidet et al. 2012). Contributions include activities such as pre-class preparation, timely attendance, participating constructively to team discussions, and valuing and encouraging contributions from other team members (Michaelsen and Sweet 2008a). It is recommended that students contribute to the grades of other students by providing both quantitative and qualitative feedback to their team members. Michaelsen et al. (2014) considers peer review to be one of the key components of TBL, because it helps to ensure student accountability (Michaelsen et al. 2014). In addition, the practice of giving and receiving feedback allows students to develop professional competencies in preparation for their professional lives as clinicians with peer review responsibilities (Cushing et al. 2011; Arnold et al. 2007; Burgess et al. 2013).

Current Trends and Evidence for TBL in Healthcare Education

Although TBL gained early popularity in medical education almost 20 years ago (Burgess et al. 2014; Fatmi et al. 2013; Reimschisel et al. 2017), its use has since expanded across the health professions, particularly within the last 10 years. In a recent systematic review of TBL within the health professions, Reimschisel and colleagues reported that from 2001 to 2005, there were only 7 published articles on TBL in the health professions; from 2006 to 2010, there were 24 published articles; and from 2011 to 2016, this number tripled to 87 published articles (Reimschisel et al. 2017). Nearly half (47%) of these 87 studies were from medical curricula, and 19% were from pharmacy. Other disciplines included dentistry (5%), nursing (3%), allied health, public health, and health laboratory science. Reported use of TBL within the health professions derives predominantly from the USA, with the remaining being distributed across 22 countries (Reimschisel et al. 2017). The class size reported varied from 11 to 400 students, with the most common class size reported as being between 101 and 150 students (Reimschisel et al. 2017). The three key reported outcome measures included were: student academic performance; learner reaction; and facilitator reaction to TBL. Each of these areas is discussed below.

Student Academic Performance

Current evidence suggests that participation in TBL is at least as, if not more effective than other methods of teaching at improving academic performance. Regarding the effectiveness of TBL on learning outcomes, Reimschisel and colleagues (2017) found that students' mid- or end-term examination scores either improved or stayed the same for students who had participated in TBL. This systematic review confirmed a finding that has been reported in a number of studies, namely, that TBL seems to help those students who are academically poor performers more than those who are academically stronger.

Learner Reaction TBL

Learner reaction to TBL is mixed. However, Reimschisel and colleagues (2017) reported that generally, learners preferred TBL to more traditional forms of instruction, in particular, lectures. Positive feedback on TBL was around the active learning style, opportunity for peer learning, and application of knowledge to problem-solving, leading to a perceived deeper understanding of the content (Reimschisel et al. 2017).

Faculty Reaction to TBL

Overall, the present studies indicate that faculty generally favored TBL because of the student engagement created through the specific steps of TBL (Reimschisel et al. 2017). Although the additional faculty workload was acknowledged, particularly in early curriculum development of TBL, it was felt that the learner gains made the additional time commitment worthwhile (Reimschisel et al. 2017).

Comparison with Other Learning Approaches

Although a relatively recent addition, TBL is now considered a viable alternative to stand alongside more established learning paradigms in healthcare education such as problem-based learning (PBL) and case-based learning (CBL). TBL, PBL, and CBL all provide learner-centered instructional approaches that are based on the principles of constructivist learning theory. Important characteristics that are similar among the three pedagogies include (1) learning that is based around relevant and authentic clinical problems that students will face in their professional careers, (2) active learning that occurs in small groups, (3) activation of existing knowledge, and (4) application of new knowledge. Within each pedagogy, students are encouraged to apply their new knowledge to authentic clinical problems and to transfer this knowledge through peer learning and discussion in small groups. There are also many differences between TBL, PBL, and CBL. Although there are many variations to the practice of each pedagogy (Burgess et al. 2014; Taylor and Miflin 2008; Thistlethwaite et al. 2012), we have used traditional definitions to provide a summary of each below (see Table 1 for an overview of the comparisons).

Key Elements of TBL

As discussed above, TBL offers a student-centered, instructional approach for large classes of students who are divided into small teams of five to seven students to solve

Table 1 Overview of comparisons between TBL, PBL, and CBL

Key elements	TBL	PBL	CBL
Number of facilitators	1–3	1	1
Class size (students)	100–150	6–10	6–10
Group (team) size	Five to seven students per team	Six to ten students per team	Six to ten students per team
Intergroup interaction	Present	None	None
Resource requirements	One large room	Many small rooms	Many small rooms
Student preparation	Same individual preparation, as directed and generated by the teacher	Different individual preparation, as defined by the students	Different individual preparation, as defined by the students
Thought process	Suitable for problem-solving in basic and clinical sciences. Guided introduction to clinical reasoning	Suitable for problem-solving in basic and clinical sciences	Primarily suited to clinical reasoning. Guided and self-directed
Testing	Individual and team readiness assurance testing	No assessment	No assessment
Peer feedback	Provision of structured peer feedback	No structured peer feedback	No structured peer feedback

professionally relevant problems (Parmelee et al. 2012; Burgess et al. 2014). The TBL format permits one content expert to effectively facilitate a large number of teams (e.g., 12 groups of 6 students in one classroom). TBL distinguishes itself from PBL and CBL through its requirement for pre-class preparation, the sequencing of in-class individual and team activities, its high student-teacher ratio, and the combining of peer learning with immediate feedback and clarification by experts (Burgess et al. 2014).

Key Elements of PBL

PBL offers a student-centered approach wherein professionally relevant problems provide the stimulus for learning. PBL is characterized by small group learning (six to ten students per group) facilitated by one teacher, learning through problem-solving and self-study (Barrows 1996; Barrows and Tamblyn 1980; Hmelo-Silver 2004). During the first meeting and initial discussion, students construct issues requiring further self-study, and all students study the same learning issues. Following self-study, the student group reconvenes (sometimes up to 1 week later) to discuss and synthesize their learnings. Students activate their prior knowledge by discussing a pre-set problem, identifying gaps in their knowledge, and using these gaps to generate issues for additional self-study. During self-study, students are exposed to new content. During the final discussion, students' peers explain content to each other and apply their knowledge to solve the problem. The facilitator encourages students to ask critical questions, engage in reasoning, and discuss disagreements in a constructive fashion, explain new knowledge, and apply new knowledge and insights to solve problems (Dolmans et al. 2015).

Key Elements of CBL

CBL offers a form of inquiry-based learning to link theory to practice, fitting somewhere between structured and guided learning (Thistlethwaite et al. 2012). Real-life, complex clinical scenarios are used to facilitate student discussion in small groups (six to ten students per group) and allow students to develop their skills in analytical thinking and reflective judgment in preparation for clinical practice (Thistlethwaite et al. 2012). Compared to PBL, CBL is less time-consuming and draws the focus of the learners on key points of the clinical case. CBL encourages a structured and critical approach to clinical problem-solving, and in contrast to PBL, makes room for the facilitator (usually a content expert) to correct and redirect students.

Planning for TBL in Your Healthcare Faculty

Curriculum Design

TBL offers a valuable means to integrate the learning and teaching of basic sciences with clinical concepts. However, in order to be successful, TBL needs to form an integral part of the course design that is clearly linked to other course components (Lohman and Finkelstein 2000). Careful consideration should be given to how the TBL classes will sit within the curriculum. For example, if a medical school provides a "system"-based block of teaching, it may be best to include one TBL class at the end of the week, once all of the lectures and lab sessions have been delivered. It is necessary to consider the structure and timeframe of the unit of study, and students' prior knowledge, the size of the student cohort, as well as the learning objectives and the nature of the content being delivered (Parmelee et al. 2012). For instance, units of study aiming to improve students' factual knowledge alone (e.g. basic anatomy) in a short space of time, may be less suited to TBL than more integrated areas of study in which problem-solving can be applied. Additionally, considerable time and expertise of faculty is needed to develop each TBL module (consisting of pre-reading, IRAT/TRAT, answers and feedback, problem-solving activities, and a peer review design). Along these lines, thought also needs to be given to availability of resources including teaching capacity, rooms, and technology.

Backward Design of TBL

The term "backward design" was coined by Wiggins and McTighe (1998), to describe a process of designing a course (Wiggins and McTighe 1998), and can be

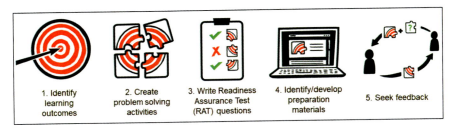

Fig. 1 The process of backward design in TBL (Image Credit: Dr R. Zhou, Ms D. Ayoub)

applied to the design of TBL modules. Traditional forms of education design require faculty to (1) first consider what students need to know, (2) create and deliver relevant lectures, and (3) assess students to test their knowledge. However, "backward design" requires faculty to do the reverse, instead focusing on the outcomes and goals of the unit before designing the learning activities, and assessment tasks. Rather than focusing on what students need to know, "backward" TBL design requires faculty to first consider what they want students to be able to *do* by the end of the TBL session. Initial consideration of the outcomes of a TBL module (depicted in Fig. 1) should therefore motivate the design of the TBL so that all assessments, problem-solving activities, source materials (videos, lectures), and discussions help students to reach these outcomes.

Writing Learning Outcomes

When writing learning outcomes, consider what you want the students to *do* by the end of the unit of study. Rather than just acquiring knowledge, consider instead how students could learn to apply this knowledge to solve authentic clinical problems. Accordingly, verbs should be used whenever possible when writing learning outcomes. Additionally, outcomes should be explicit and assessable (Levine and Hudes 2014). Examples where the verb within each outcome is actionable, are provided in Table 2.

Writing TBL Cases

The clinical problem-solving activities lie at the heart of TBL and consume the majority of in-class time, but are time-consuming to write. The scenario, or patient case, should have added restrictions and complications, as well as consequences if an incorrect decision is made. Although we have acknowledged that a specific choice may not always be relevant when designing TBLs within healthcare education, the four S's (significant problem, same problem, specific choice, simultaneous reporting) should be considered to ensure the clinical scenario is relevant and complex and requires the combined efforts of all team members to solve. An example of a case for Year 2 medical students is provided below.

Table 2 Examples of poorly and improved written learning outcomes

By the end of this unit, you will be able to:

Poorly written outcomes	Improved written outcomes
Review the definition of hyperglycemia	List the differential diagnosis for hyperglycemia
Appreciate how type 2 diabetes is diagnosed	Outline the steps involved in diagnosing type 2 diabetes
Describe the complications of untreated type 2 diabetes	Identify the complications of type 2 diabetes from history and examination
Understand the principles and management of type 2 diabetes	Select and justify the appropriate management option for a patient with type 2 diabetes

> **Box 2 Example of a "Diabetes" TBL Case Appropriate for Year 1/2 Medical Students**
> John Smith, aged 24, has been brought into the Emergency Department by friends from a day out watching a test cricket match. He is drowsy with slurred speech, feels breathless, and has vomited three times today. John says he has consumed two beers (2.6 standard drinks) at the match and denies any recreational drug use. John has had a runny nose and cough for the last few days and said he has been feeling very tired and over the last few weeks which he has put down to a "virus." John also reports he has been losing weight unintentionally (about 5 kg over the past 3 months) and at least a 1-month history of increased urine output and thirst. He takes no regular medications and is currently working as a history teacher at the local high school.

Writing MCQs

Although it seems intuitive to base the multiple choice questions (for the IRAT/TRAT) on the pre-class preparation (readings/lectures/videos/journal readings), it is more important that the questions relate to the clinical problem-solving activities relevant to the TBL, which can be achieved by first asking "what concepts do students need to understand to solve these problems?" Additionally, there should be alignment with the learning outcomes. Normally questions have five possible choices (A–E), with one single best answer. An example of one IRAT is provided in Box 3.

> **Box 3 Readiness Assurance Test Question Relating to a Diabetes TBL Case**
> **Which of the following correctly describes a physiological effect of insulin in humans?**
>
> A. Reduced uptake of glucose into muscle
> B. Enhanced lipolysis by adipocytes

(continued)

Box 3 (continued)
C. Increased synthesis of fatty acids in the liver (Correct answer)
D. Enhanced gluconeogenesis by hepatocytes
E. Inhibition of glycogen synthesis

Identifying and Developing Preparation Materials

The pre-class preparation materials should be identified or prepared after the readiness assurance questions and problem-solving activities have been written. This will allow source material to be updated over time, without requiring significant change to the assessment questions or problem-solving activities. Preparation material might include one or a combination of readings, recorded lectures, lecturers' slides, videos, or journal articles. It is important to ensure that assigned readings are relevant and not too long or difficult. If it is not possible to identify relevant existing material, the material may need to be written or a video lecture prepared.

Seeking Feedback

Before a TBL module is delivered to students, feedback should be sought from a colleague who has expertise in the content to assess accuracy, and from senior students or junior clinicians to assess the level of difficulty and timing. Learning designers are experts in the delivery of content, and their advice should also be sought. Feedback should be continuously gathered throughout the delivery of the TBL to allow constant improvements and updates. The use of validated surveys and focus groups to collect data for analysis can provide a useful means to inform improvements.

Implementation of TBL

Successful implementation of TBL depends on a significant level of engagement from both faculty and students who need to possess a sufficient degree of knowledge of the process itself and be committed to embracing a new learning and teaching method.

Facilitator Engagement

To ensure adequate training of facilitators, faculty development programs will be required. Such a program should encompass theoretical and practical aspects of the TBL process, development of TBL modules (such as writing of outcomes, RATs, and problem-solving activities – previously outlined), and facilitation skills. Importantly, "team teaching" is a popular method within TBL (Burgess et al. 2014) and will require dedicated training, as it can be a new concept to some facilitators, who may be accustomed to teaching alone. This, in addition to other key aspects of any TBL faculty training program, is outlined below.

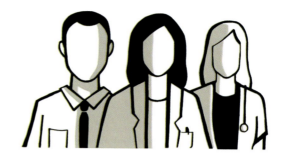

Fig. 2 Team teaching in TBL offers opportunity to educate through role-modeling and allows students to benefit from diverse expertise. The figure depicts a typical example of team-teaching within medicine involving a senior clinician, scientist and junior clinician (Image Credit: Dr R. Zhou, Ms D. Ayoub)

Team Teaching

Team teaching is described as involving two or more educators working together to cooperatively plan, interact, observe, question, and teach while taking advantage of the special competencies of each team member (Singer 1964; Irby and Wilkerson 2003). Healthcare is an interdisciplinary field that is reliant on the sharing of knowledge from various professionals to provide better patient care. Team teaching provides educators with the opportunity to demonstrate through role modeling, with basic scientists, health professionals, and clinicians working together to educate students (Abu-Rish et al. 2012). As an example within health professional education, a TBL facilitation team may include a senior clinician, junior clinician, and basic scientist (Fig. 2), who collaboratively teach and facilitate meaningful learning sessions of theoretical knowledge and clinical application. The benefits for students and facilitators include (Liebel et al. 2017; Crow and Smith 2013):

- Students being provided with more than one explanation of complex cases
- The promotion of teacher development through observation and reflection of teaching and learning
- Exposure to different teaching methods and knowledge for both educators and students
- Increasing diverse interactions within the classroom
- Debate and more active discussions
- Role modeling of interprofessional collaboration
- Less pressure on finding single facilitators with deep levels of expertise in all aspects of a case

Facilitation Skills in TBL

The hallmark of effective facilitation in TBL is being able to actively foster an engaging and meaningful inter-team discussion. Indeed, TBL facilitation differs from other forms of small group teaching largely because of the need for inter-team engagement which ensures accountability for all learners. This is achieved via deliberate and strategic questioning that aims to elicit the students' understanding relating to a topic and, where relevant, generate a safe environment where assumptions can be discussed and challenged. Facilitation in a TBL begins after the TRAT when facilitators are required to probe teams' responses, reveal correct answers, and resolve any misunderstandings (Parmelee et al. 2012; Burgess et al. 2014). To maximize student learning, skilled facilitation is needed to encourage students to ask questions and discuss their uncertainties. During the application phase, facilitators are required to act as a "guide from the side" to ensure students stay on track and stay on time. The aim should be the creation of a dynamic learning environment, with discussion to help students articulate their understanding of difficult concepts or to critique the thought process of clinical problem-solving in others. Through these inter-team discussions, deeper understanding and learning is achieved. In both the feedback session following the TRAT, and the clinical problem-solving phase, the most challenging aspects for facilitators include promoting inter-team discussion, managing questions, and eliciting, rather than freely giving, answers.

Managing the feedback session following TRAT, and the inter-team discussions during the application phase in a large classroom setting, requires a unique set of class management skills. The IRAT and TRAT, and the problem-solving activities, encourage assimilative learning to incorporate new information into existing knowledge (Seel 2012), and transformative learning, where existing knowledge structures are altered through critical thinking (Mezirow 1991). Critical thinking is enhanced through peer learning and teaching in small groups (Meers-Scott et al. 2010). The "elaborative interrogation technique" (Dunlosky et al. 2013) refers to the facilitated learning process that occurs following peer learning and teaching.

Tips to help facilitators provide a TBL platform that promotes a fair and safe learning environment, but still holds students accountable for their own learning and maximizes the student learning experience are provided in Fig. 3.

Questioning

Questioning students can provide an effective method of assessing student knowledge and understanding. There are three types of questions (Lake et al. 2005):

- *Yes/No questions*: basic form of questioning, very simple, and do not stretch the learner.
- *Closed questions*: there is a specific answer, enabling the questioner to check the knowledge of the learner, but not their level of understanding.
- *Open questions*: there is generally no "right" answer and allows for the questioner to probe further asking "why" and "how" type questions. This requires a good understanding of the topic, thinking skills, and problem-solving.

After questioning a learner, it is important to pause to allow the learner to register what you are asking, and to think about their response (see Fig. 4). It is important to allow for this silence and not jump to rephrase the question immediately, or answer the question yourself (Lake et al. 2005). Students need to be encouraged to critically

Timing	It can be difficult to comply with the allocated time. The facilitator needs to make adjustments as time diminishes. This may mean interrupting student teams that are taking an extended period of time to work through each clinical problem-solving activity.
Plan a strategy with co-facilitators ahead of time	It is important to decide before the feedback session who will provide a response to which questions, and which questions need the most attention as not all questions will need an in-depth explanation. Facilitators can decide upon a strategy to respond to each TRAT question while students are working on the questions. Scores for the IRAT will guide the depth of explanations required.
Promote critical thinking during the feedback and problem-solving sessions	Questions need to be asked in order to ascertain the students' understanding of concepts and encourage students to articulate new concepts, and teach each other. At the same time, it is important to remember that students may not trust information from their peers' but may value the expertise of the facilitator.
Allow time to close the TBL session	Providing closure for discussion of difficult concepts assists in ensuring students feel the TBL was valuable, and they are equipped with "take home" messages.
Allow students enough time to think before responding to a question	Students may be nervous when responding to questions, and need time to gather their thoughts. It may be necessary to allow up to 30 seconds for a response.
Ask open-ended questions	The phrasing of questions should force students to critique, analyse, justify and explain their answer Lake et al. (2005). any further elicit a 'yes' or 'no' response, will normally cease any further discussion. Additionally, questions that lead the students to a particular response will limit discussion. However, open ended questions allow students to demonstrate their thought process, and may promote follow-up questions.

Fig. 3 Tips for TBL facilitators

Rephrase student responses to ensure clarity	To help create a safe and engaging learning environment, it may be necessary to repeat and rephrase a students' response. In summarizing and restating what has been said, the facilitator ensures that the class has heard what has been said, unclear information is clarified, complex explanations are simplified, and important principles are repeated to help retention of knowledge.
Hold each individual student accountable	Create an environment where each student knows they may be required to respond to a question. Students will realise that they must be prepared as individuals. They will also realise that they must be prepared to represent their team. Use students' names when possible so that students do not feel they are anonymous. Avoid always choosing the most vocal students to speak.

Fig. 3 (continued)

Fig. 4 The three P's of questioning. (Adapted from Lake et al. 2005)

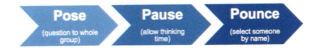

think, and answers should not be discussed too quickly. A helpful mnemonic (three P's of questioning) is shown in Fig. 4 that reiterates this concept.

The Provision of Feedback

Feedback acts as a continuing part of the instructional process that supports and enhances learning (Shepard 2000). It is part of an ongoing unit of instruction and assessment, rather than a separate educational entity (Hattie and Timperley 2007). Feedback promotes learning in three ways (Shepard 2000; Branch and Paranjape 2002):

- Informs the student of their progress
- Informs the student regarding observed learning needs for improvement
- Motivates the student to engage in appropriate learning activities

Barriers to the feedback process:
- Feedback has the greatest impact on students' knowledge and understanding when it is immediate (Burgess and Mellis 2015a).

- The desire to avoid upsetting students with negative feedback can result in inadequate feedback (Burgess and Mellis 2015a).
- Without external feedback, some students may generate their own feedback. However, self-assessment can be wrong, as it has been shown that high performers tend to underestimate their own performance, and lower performers tend to overestimate (Davis et al. 2016).

The role of a TBL facilitator includes:
- Familiarizing themselves with the learning objectives and content for the session
- Facilitating and team-teaching large classes of 60 or more healthcare students
- Providing adequate and timely feedback to students
- Questioning students to encourage critical thinking
- Answering student questions, using knowledge and experience

A good facilitator is someone who:
- Is enthusiastic and encouraging
- Is approachable and makes students feel welcome
- Gives clear explanations and expectations
- Questions skillfully
- Utilizes the knowledge and experiences of students in the group
- Manages group dynamics well
- Encourages and supports all students to be involved
- Gives timely feedback using the positive critique method
- Reflects on their own performance
- Avoids being overly didactic

Student Engagement

It is important that students understand what TBL is and why it is being implemented. Students may resist the implementation of TBL for a number of reasons: additional preparation requirements, previous negative experiences of participating in group work and receiving group grades, and regular testing. A good student orientation can help to alleviate these concerns by educating students on the format of TBL, student requirements, faculty expectations, and the advantages of TBL over other teaching methods. Communication of the benefits of TBL, such as improved preparation for the workplace and higher marks on average received by individuals as part of a team (Burgess et al. 2014, 2016, 2017, 2018; Reimschisel et al. 2017; Ofstad et al. 2013), is likely to make students more receptive to the process, and more enthusiastic about actively participating within their teams and class.

Benefits and Challenges of TBL

Research supports the use of TBL, with evidence indicating positive outcomes for students (Burgess et al. 2014, 2016, 2017, 2018; Reimschisel et al. 2017; Ofstad et al. 2013). For teachers, TBL has the potential to transform their enjoyment and enthusiasm for teaching. Although there are many benefits to TBL for both students and facilitators, it is important to remember that there are also challenges, some of which can be anticipated and overcome. We have provided a summary of both in Table 3.

Resource Implications for Institutions

The design of TBL addresses resource challenges faced by many higher education institutions. The provision of high-quality small group learning is often associated with a high logistical burden, requiring the complex coordination of many individual facilitators across several teaching sessions. A major benefit to TBL is that it provides students with the experience of small group learning in a large group setting, thus reducing the number of teaching sessions and facilitators required (Burgess et al. 2014; Burgess and Mellis 2015; Parmelee et al. 2012). Furthermore, the shift in emphasis from knowledge acquisition to application and assessment of knowledge in a collaborative and competitive environment means students are motivated to complete the pre-reading assigned independently (Burgess et al. 2014; Burgess and Mellis 2015; Parmelee et al. 2012). This allows more time resources in class to be dedicated to developing higher-level skills such as problem-solving and critical thinking (Burgess and Mellis 2015; Ofstad et al. 2013).

Space/Room Requirements

One of the key advantages of TBL is its scalability, that is, it can be scaled up for implementation in large classes, with student numbers of approximately 40–100 per class frequently reported (Burgess et al. 2014). When institutions introduce TBL, existing, conventional learning spaces need to be adapted and new spaces considered. The structure of TBL promotes an active and interactive form of learning. The human factors and architectural principles underpinning the design of active learning spaces are well documented (Oblinger and Lippincott 2006). The benefit of a collaborative approach to the design of learning spaces and alignment with curricula is well recognized (Nordquist et al. 2016). The use of lecture theatres in TBL is likely to detract from the student learning experience, while team-centric learning spaces, designed to optimize communication both within teams and between teams, are ideal (Rajalingam et al. 2018). There is some evidence to suggest that students' attitudes toward TBL improve when they are provided with a comfortable environment that eases communication (Espey 2008).

Tables and seating: The TBL room design should enable small groups seated at round tables to engage in active, intra-team discussion.

Screens: A large screen for each team assists in engaging all team members. Additionally, a computer projector with a very large screen at the front of the class is

Table 3 Summary of the benefits of TBL for students and facilitators

Benefits for students	Challenges for students
Small group experience with facilitators who are experts in their area A clear strength of TBL is having multiple groups in the one room, and having small individual teams of five to six students. Having multiple small groups in one room permits provision of facilitators who have specific expertise within clinical specialties and the basic sciences. This ensures provision of up-to-date, evidence-based guidance and answers (Burgess et al. 2017). **Structured learning** The specific steps of the TBL process help to engage students. Students move beyond active learning as individuals by participating in structured, collaborative learning activities that are interactive and relevant (Handley et al. 2006). Active learning opportunities that engage participants assist in the development of a deeper understanding of knowledge and increased knowledge retention (Graffan 2007). **Students experience the value of working and collaborating in teams** Students compare and reflect on their IRAT and TRAT results, and their peers' contributions to teamwork. Evidence suggests that the worst performing team will usually score higher than the best performing student individually (Michaelsen and Sweet 2008b). **Students are motivated to reflect on their own strengths and weaknesses as members of a team** The peer evaluation prompts students to consider how they can improve as a team member. When implemented correctly, friendly competition promotes student accountability to their "teammates," and to their teachers (Burgess et al. 2016, 2017), encouraging students to prepare for class activities. **Students develop professional attributes, such as giving and receiving feedback through peer review** Peer review is a common requirement among health professionals, yet it is rarely formally taught and practiced at university (Burgess et al. 2013; Silbert and Lake 2012). The ability to give feedback is reported to improve communication skills, problem-solving, decision-making, and responsibility (Ballantyne et al. 2002;	**Orientation to TBL** Students need to be provided with adequate orientation to TBL in order to effectively participate. **Learning style** Students who have experienced and have a preference for passive learning styles, such as lectures, may have difficulty adapting to the active participation requirements of TBL. **Completing pre-class requirements** Students need to complete the assigned readings or pre-class preparation prior to class, and some students report that this is not always achieved (Burgess et al. 2017). Additionally, the assigned preparation may not align well with the problem-solving activities. **Time management during the TBL class** It can be difficult for students to work through each problem within the given time limits and complete all tasks on time (Burgess et al. 2017). Different team members may have different opinions on time management. **Peer review** As reported widely in medical education, students often feel uncomfortable providing feedback to their peers and have difficulty providing honest feedback (Burgess et al. 2013; Thompson et al. 2007).

Cassidy 2006). Similarly, receipt of feedback from peers can provide an effective learning experience for students and create reflective learners, who analyze and reflect on their contributions and performance (Burgess and Mellis 2015a, b).

Benefits for facilitators	Challenges for facilitators
Teaching students who are prepared is more rewarding Staff and students alike value the "flipped classroom" format of TBL. Students are encouraged to prepare for class, and be up-to-date with course content. Rather than "spoon-feeding" content to students, there is time to facilitate meaningful discussion and help students to problem-solve (Michaelsen and Sweet 2008a).	**Facilitator training** Attendance at facilitator training is required, with ongoing exposure to TBL teaching to help become comfortable with the method and understand and apply the TBL method effectively.
Staff work as a team With co-teaching implemented as a strategy in TBL, hospital consultants and university academics come together to develop the students' knowledge and skills in their areas of expertise. Teaching is carried out in a unified manner, bringing together different topics to encourage interaction of the basic sciences with clinical disciplines, enabling students to integrate, conceptualize, and apply this newly acquired knowledge.	**Preparation for class requirements** Facilitators are required to prepare for class and read pre-reading material, the IRAT, the answers, and explanation for answers, the problem-solving activities, and the answers/explanations. **Preparation of TBL material** Preparing the multiple choice questions and answers, the problem-solving activities and the tutor guides for each TBL module is time-consuming and requires input from content experts. **Planning in team-teaching** When team teaching it is necessary to plan together to consider who will take on which role.
Staff learn from each other Evidence suggests that co-teaching is effective in generating student interest, engagement, knowledge acquisition, and retention (Irby and Wilkerson 2003). At the same time, the teachers may build on their own scientific and medical knowledge and further hone their teaching skills by learning from each other during TBL classes, ultimately enriching their teaching experience.	**Classroom management skills** Managing the inter-team discussions during the application phase requires a unique set of class management skills.

needed for facilitators to present material (such as PowerPoint to aid provision of feedback).

Microphones: The use of microphones for inter-team discussion, and facilitator discussion, helps to ensure that each person in the room can hear and engage in the class.

Internet: Wi-Fi connectivity is needed so that students and facilitators can connect with their Learning Management Systems (LMS) where their TBL exercises (including IRAT, TRAT, clinical problem-solving activities) are housed. Students may also use Wi-Fi to research and find evidence to help in their problem-solving activities.

Technology requirements: New technologies, including software specifically designed for the implementation of TBL, streamline the steps involved in TBL, and have the capability to display student results both in real-time and tracked over a period of time. With this information at hand, facilitators are able to better understand student learning needs and focus attention on the more difficult topics that need further explanation to the class (Rajalingam et al. 2018; Gagnon et al. 2017).

Emerging Trends in TBL

Considering its original inception as a tool for teaching graduate business students in the USA, the pervasive implementation of TBL in health professional education speaks to the universality and versatility of this educational format. Accordingly, TBL has capacity to evolve to meet the changing demands and roles of the health professions and has been the basis of new innovations in teaching. An example of this is the emerging use of TBL to promote interprofessional education (Buhse and Della 2017). Modern healthcare is an inherently multidisciplinary endeavor, and an innate understanding of different roles of the health professionals is required to optimize patient outcomes (World Health Organization 2010). The small-group and task-focused nature of TBL lends itself naturally as a means of developing such an understanding and fostering a culture of collegiality among health-professional students. This is done by ensuring a mix of students from different health backgrounds (e.g., pharmacy, nursing, medicine, allied health) within a single team and creating real-world problems that require their diverse input. The application of TBL in this manner has begun to be studied in various health programs (see, e.g., Chan et al. 2017; Lochner et al. 2018; Luetmer et al. 2018). Despite the innate challenges of conducting interprofessional learning activities (Maeno et al. 2019), results so far indicate TBL as an efficacious and promising pedagogical tool for preparing students for collaborative practice.

Another frontier of innovation is the incorporation of health technologies to facilitate team-based learning. Beyond the use of standard Learning Management Systems, many have begun to experiment with the use of blended learning approaches in TBL, such as the use of online survey tools and audience response systems for real-time analytics and feedback during the readiness assurance phase (Willett et al. 2011; Muzyk et al. 2015), the use of social media platforms for engaging students (Wright et al. 2014), and use of interactive online platforms for content delivery (Davidson 2011; Persky 2015). Additionally, technology has enabled the use of TBL in distance learning through live video conferencing across different sites (Corbridge et al. 2013) and even through the use of virtual reality environments to facilitate TBL (Coyne et al. 2018). However, while use of technology in TBL is likely to increase, a systematic review of studies blending technology with TBL in the health disciplines has found evidence for educational benefit and student preference to be lacking (River et al. 2016). Thus, further research regarding the impact of technology-assisted learning in TBL is required to identify best-practice approaches.

Concluding Remarks and Future Work

There are many demands placed on healthcare educators in preparing graduates for future professional practice, where the sheer volume of knowledge in every discipline is expanding and changing rapidly. Constant monitoring and improvements to medicine and health curricula and pedagogy are needed to prepare students for the demands of the increasingly complex healthcare systems in which they will work. The practice of healthcare is increasingly team orientated and interprofessional, requiring coordinated efforts from a number of disciplines to enhance outcomes for patients (Parmelee et al. 2012). Graduate competencies have shifted from knowledge alone, to encompass the ability to solve complex problems, communicate, and collaborate effectively. In this chapter we have provided an overview of TBL as a powerful and resource-effective instructional method that addresses many of these professional, technological, and cultural drivers of change.

As a relatively new instructional format in health professional education, a number of theoretical and empirical questions remain outstanding with respect to TBL. For those considering research in TBL, such questions include:

- How is critical thinking and reasoning promoted through TBL?
- Why are there mixed learner reactions to the TBL process?
- How do generational, cultural, or gender differences affect student response, and the effectiveness of TBL?
- Are all elements of the TBL necessary and are some parts preferred over others?
- What is the optimal timing of a TBL activity and does that change in different contexts?
- What are the characteristics of a good TBL facilitator?
- Does the process of peer review in TBL impact students' behavior, group contributions, and professional development?

The TBL format offers a feedback-rich learning environment, providing opportunities for students to develop critical competencies relevant to healthcare education: teamwork abilities and critical thinking skills (Hrynchak and Batty 2012). While much work remains to be done, the available literature and our own practical experience finds TBL to be an effective, well-received, and resource-wise pedagogical tool with the potential to integrate into a broad range of health educational environments.

Cross-References

▶ Learning with and from Peers in Clinical Education
▶ Supporting the Development of Professionalism in the Education of Health Professionals

References

Abu-Rish E, Kim S, Choe L, Varpio L, Malik E, White AA, et al. Current trends in interprofessional education of health sciences students: a literature review. J Interprof Care. 2012;26(6):444–51.

Arnold L, Shue CK, Kalishman S, et al. Can there be a single system for peer assessment of professionalism among medical students? A multi-institutional study. Acad Med. 2007;82:578–86.

Badget RG, Stone J, Collins TC. The importance of free-text responses in team-based learning design. Acad Med. 2014;89:1578.

Ballantyne R, Hughes K, Mylonas A. Developing procedures for implementing peer assessment in large classes using an action research process. Assess Eval High Educ. 2002;27:427–41.

Barrows HS. Problem-based learning in medicine and beyond: a brief overview. In: Wilkerson L, Gijselaers WH, editors. New directions for teaching and learning. San Francisco: Jossey-Bass; 1996. p. 3–12.

Barrows HS, Tamblyn RM. Problem-based learning. An approach to medical education. New York: Springer; 1980. Borges.

Branch WT, Paranjape A. Feedback and reflection: teaching methods for clinical settings. Acad Med. 2002;77:1185–8.

Buhse M, Della RC. Enhancing interprofessional education with team-based learning. Nurse Educ. 2017;42(5):240–4.

Burgess A, Mellis C. Team-based learning in health care education: maintaining key design elements. J Nurs Care. 2015;S1:007.

Burgess AW, Mellis CM. In reply to Badgett et al. Acad Med. 2014;89:1578–9.

Burgess A, Mellis C. Feedback and assessment during clinical placements: achieving the right balance. Adv Med Educ Pract. 2015a;6:373–81.

Burgess A, Mellis C. Receiving feedback from peers: medical students' perceptions. Clin Teach. 2015b;12:203–7.

Burgess A, Roberts C, Black K, Mellis C. Senior medical student perceived ability and experience in giving feedback in formative long case examinations. BMC Med Educ. 2013;13:79.

Burgess A, McGregor D, Mellis C. Applying established guidelines to team-based learning programs in medical schools: a systematic review. Acad Med. 2014;89:678–88.

Burgess A, Ayton T, Mellis C. Implementation of team-based learning in year 1 of a PBL based medical program: a pilot study. BMC Med Educ. 2016;16(1):1–7.

Burgess A, Bleasel J, Haq I, Roberts C, Garsia R, Robertson T, Mellis C. Team-based learning (TBL) in the medical curriculum: better than PBL? BMC Med Educ. 2017;17:243.

Burgess A, Ayton T, Mellis C. Implementation of team-based learning within a problem based learning medical curriculum: a focus group study. BMC Med Educ. 2018;18:74.

Cassidy S. Developing employability skills: peer assessment in higher education. Educ Train. 2006;48(7):508–17.

Chan LK, et al. Implementation of an interprofessional team-based learning program involving seven undergraduate health and social care programs from two universities, and students' evaluation of their readiness for interprofessional learning. BMC Med Educ. 2017;17(1):221.

Corbridge SJ, et al. Implementing team-based learning in a nurse practitioner curriculum. Nurse Educ. 2013;38(5):202–5.

Coyne L, et al. Exploring virtual reality as a platform for distance team-based learning. Curr Pharm Teach Learn. 2018;10(10):1384–90.

Crow J, Smith L. Using co-teaching as a means of facilitating interprofessional collaboration in health and social care. J Interprof Care. 2013;17(1):45–55.

Cushing A, Abbott S, Lothian D, Hall A, Westwood OM. Peer feedback as an aid to learning – what do we want? Feedback. When do we want it? Now! Med Teach. 2011;33:e105–12.

Davidson LK. A 3-year experience implementing blended TBL: active instructional methods can shift student attitudes to learning. Med Teach. 2011;33(9):750–3.

Davis DA, Mazmanian PE, Fordis M, Van Harrison R, Thorpe KE, Perrier L. Accuracy of physician self-assessment compared with observed measures of competence: a systematic review. JAMA. 2016;296:1094–102.

Dolmans D, Michaelsen L, Van Merrienboer J, Van der Vleuten C. Should we choose between problem-based learning and team-based learning? No, combine the best of both worlds! Med Teach. 2015;37:354–9.

Dunlosky J, Rawson KA, Marsh EJ, Nathan MJ, Willingham DT. Improving students' learning with effective learning techniques: promising directions from cognitive and educational psychology. Psychol Sci Public Interest. 2013;14(1):4–58.

Espey M. Does space matter? Classroom design and team-based learning. Rev Agri Econ. 2008;30:764–75.

Fatmi M, Hartling L, Hillier T, Campbell S, Oswald AE. The effectiveness of team-based learning on learning outcomes in health professions education: BEME Guide No. 30. Med Teach. 2013;35(12):e1608–24. https://doi.org/10.3109/0142159X.2013.849802.

Gagnon P, Mendoza R, Carlstedt-Duke J. A technology-enabled flipped classroom model. In: The flipped classroom. Singapore: Springer; 2017. p. 211–28.

Graffan B. Active learning in medical education: strategies for beginning implementation. Med Teach. 2007;29:86–103.

Haidet P, Levine RE, Parmelee DX, Crow S, Kennedy F, Kelly PA, Perkowski L, Michaelsen L, Richards BF. Perspective: guidelines for reporting team based learning activities in the medical and health sciences education literature. Acad Med. 2012;87:292–9.

Handley K, Sturdy A, Fincham R, Clark T. Within and beyond communities of practice: making sense of learning through participation, identify and practice. J Manag Stud. 2006;43(3):641–53.

Hattie J, Timperley H. The power of feedback. Rev Educ Res. 2007;77:81–112.

Hmelo-Silver CE. Problem-based learning: what and how do students learn? Educ Psychol Rev. 2004;16(3):235–66.

Hrynchak P, Batty H. The educational theory basis of team-based learning. Med Teach. 2012;34(10):796–801.

Huggett KN, Jeffries WB. An introduction to medical teaching. 2nd ed. Dordrecht: Springer; 2014. p. 69–71.

Irby D, Wilkerson L. Educational innovation in academic medicine and environmental trends. J Gen Intern Med. 2003;18:370–6.

Koles P, Nelson S, Stolfi A, Parmelee D, Destephen D. Active learning in a year 2 pathology curriculum. Med Educ. 2005;39:1045–55.

Lake FR, Vickery AW, Ryan G. Teaching on the run tip 7: effective use of questions. MJA. 2005;182(3):126–7.

Larsen DP, Butler AC, Roedigr HL. Repeated testing improves long-term retention relative to repeated study: a randomised controlled trial. Med Educ. 2009;43(12):1174–81. https://doi.org/10.1111/j.1365-2923.2009.03518.x.

Levine R, Hudes P. How-to guide for team-based learning. International Association of Medical Science Educators; 2014.

Liebel G, Burden H, Heldal R, Viktoria, RISE – Research Institutes of Sweden, & IKT. For free: continuity and change by team teaching. Teach High Educ. 2017;22(1):62–77.

Lochner L, et al. Applying interprofessional team-based learning in patient safety: a pilot evaluation study. BMC Med Educ. 2018;18(1):48.

Lohman MC, Finkelstein M. Designing groups in problem-based learning to promote problem-solving skill and self-directedness. Instr Sci. 2000;28(4):291–307.

Luetmer MT, et al. Simulating the multi-disciplinary care team approach: enhancing student understanding of anatomy through an ultrasound-anchored interprofessional session. Anat Sci Educ. 2018;11(1):94–9.

Maeno T, et al. Interprofessional education in medical schools in Japan. PLoS One. 2019;14(1): e0210912.

McGrath JE. Small group. Research. 1991;22(2):147–74.

Meers-Scott D, Taylor L, Pelley J. Teaching critical thinking and team based concept mapping. [Educational]. In: Torres PL, Marriot RV, editors. Handbook of research on collaborative learning using concept mapping. Hershey: IGI Global; 2010. p. 171–86.

Mezirow J. Transformative dimensions of adult learning. 1st ed. San Francisco: Jossey-Bass; 1991.

Michaelsen L, Richards B. Drawing conclusions from the team-learning literature in health-sciences education: a commentary. Teach Learn Med. 2005;17:85–8.

Michaelsen LK, Sweet M. The essential elements of team-based learning. New Dir Teach Learn. 2008a;116:7–27.

Michaelsen LK, Sweet M. Excerpt from Chapter 2 of Michaelsen LK, Parmelee D, Levine R, McMahon K. Team-based learning for health professions education: a guide to using small groups for improving learning. Stylus Publishing, LLC: Sterling; 2008b.

Michaelsen L, Parmelee D, McMahon KK, Levine RE, editors. Team-based learning for health professions education. Sterling: Stylus; 2007.

Michaelsen LK, Davidson N, Major CH. Team-based learning practices and principles in comparison with cooperative learning and problem-based learning. J Excell Coll Teach. 2014;25(3–4):57–84.

Muzyk AJ, et al. Implementation of a flipped classroom model to teach psychopharmacotherapy to third-year Doctor of Pharmacy (PharmD) students. Pharm Educ. 2015;15:44.

Nieder GL, Parmelee DX, Stolfi A, Hudes PD. Team-based learning in a medical gross anatomy and embryology course. Clin Anat. 2005;18:56–63.

Nordquist J, Sundberg K, Laing A. Aligning physical learning spaces with the curriculum: AMEE guide no. 107. Med Teach. 2016;38:755–68.

O'Daniel M, Rosenstein A. Capter 33: professional communication and team collaboration. In: Highes RG, editor. Patient safety and quality: an evidence based handbook for nurses. Rockville: Agency for Healthcare Research and Quality; 2008.

Oblinger D, Lippincott J. Learning spaces (c2006. 1 v). Boulder: Educause; 2006.

Ofstad W, Pharm D, Brunner LJ. Team-based learning in pharmacy education. Am J Pharm Educ. 2013;77(4):70.

Parmelee D, Michaelsen LK, Cook S, Hudes PD. Team-based learning: a practical guide: AMEE guide no. 65. Med Teach. 2012;34:e275–87.

Persky AM. Qualitative analysis of animation versus reading for pre-class preparation in a "flipped" classroom. J Excel College Teach. 2015;26(1):5–28.

Rajalingam P, Rotgans JI, Zary N, Ferenczi FA, Gagnon P, Low-Beer N. Implementation of team-based learning on a large scale: three factors to keep in mind∗. Med Teach. 2018;40(6):582–8. https://doi.org/10.1080/0142159X.2018.1451630.

Reimschisel T, Herring AL, Huang J, Minor TJ. A systematic review of the published literature on team-based learning in health professions education. Med Teach. 2017;39(12):1227–37. https://doi.org/10.1080/0142159X.2017.1340636.

River J, et al. A systematic review examining the effectiveness of blending technology with team-based learning. Nurse Educ Today. 2016;45:185–92.

Roediger H, Putman AL, Sumeracki MA. Ten benefits of testing and their applications to educational practice. In: Psychology of learning and motivation, vol. 55. Oxford; 2011. p. 1–36.

Searle NS, Haidet P, Kelly PA, Schneider VF, Seidel CL, Richards BF. Team learning in medical education: initial experiences at ten institutions. Acad Med. 2003;78(10 Suppl):S55–8.

Seel NM. Assimilation theory of learning. In: Encyclopedia of the sciences of learning. New York: Springer; 2012. p. 324–6.

Shepard LA. The role of assessment in a learning culture. Educ Res. 2000;29:4–14.

Silbert B, Lake FR. Peer-assisted learning in teaching clinical examination to junior medical students. Med Teach. 2012;34:392–7.

Singer IJ. What team teaching really is. Indianapolis: Indiana University Press; 1964. p. 13–22.

Sweet M, Michaelsen LK. Team-based learning in the social sciences and humanities: group work that works to generate critical thinking and engagement. Sterling: Stylus; 2012.

Taylor D, Miflin B. Problem-based learning: where are we now? Med Teach. 2008;30(8):742–63.

Thistlethwaite JE, Davies D, Ekeocha S, Kidd JM, MacDougall C, Matthews P, Purkis J, Clay D. The effectiveness of case-based learning in health professional education. A BEME systematic review: BEME guide no. 23. Med Teach. 2012;34(6):e421–44. https://doi.org/10.3109/0142159X.2012.680939.

Thomas PA, Bowen CW. A controlled trial of team-based learning in an ambulatory medicine clerkship for medical students. Teach Learn Med. 2011;23:31–6.

Thompson BM, Schneider VF, Haidet P, Levine RE, McMahon KK, Perkowski LC, Richards BF. Team-based learning at ten medical schools: two years later. Med Educ. 2007;41(3):250–7.

Tuckman BW. Developmental sequence in small groups. Psychol Bull. 1965;63:384–99.

Van Blankenstein FM, Dolmans DHJM, van der CPM V, Schmidt HG. Which cognitive processes support learning during small-group discussion? The role of providing explanations and listening to others. Instr Sci. 2011;39:189–204.

Wiener H, Plass H, Marz R. Team-based learning in intensive course format for first-year medical students. Croat Med J. 2009;50:69–76.

Wiggins G, McTighe JH. Understanding by design. Columbus: Merrill Prentice; 1998.

Willett LR, Rosevear GC, Kim S. A trial of team-based versus small-group learning for second-year medical students: does the size of the small group make a difference? Teach Learn Med. 2011;23(1):28–30.

World Health Organization. Framework for action on interprofessional education and collaborative practice. Geneva: Health Professional Network Nursing and Midwifery Office, Department of Human Resources for Health; 2010.

Wright KJ, Frame TR, Hartzler ML. Student perceptions of a self-care course taught exclusively by team-based learning and utilizing twitter. Curr Pharm Teach Learn. 2014;6(6):842–8.

Learning with and from Peers in Clinical Education

69

Joanna Tai, Merrolee Penman, Calvin Chou, and Arianne Teherani

Contents

Introduction	1356
Peer Learning Configurations	1357
Episodic Peer Contact Versus Peer Continuity	1357
Same Level or Near-Peers	1358
Peer Learning Activities	1358
Peer Didactics	1359
Peer Mentoring	1359
Peer Observation, Feedback, and Assessment	1359
Discussion and Debriefing	1360
Small Group Learning (PBL, TBL)	1360
Learning Theories Underpinning Peer Learning in Clinical Education	1361
The Zone of Proximal Development	1361
Communities of Practice	1361
Social Comparison Theory	1362

J. Tai (✉)
Centre for Research in Assessment and Digital Learning, Deakin University, Geelong, VIC, Australia
e-mail: joanna.tai@deakin.edu.au

M. Penman
Work Integrated Learning, The University of Sydney, Camperdown, NSW, Australia
e-mail: merrolee.penman@sydney.edu.au

C. Chou
Department of Medicine, University of California, San Francisco and Veterans Affairs Health System, San Francisco, CA, USA
e-mail: calvin.chou@ucsf.edu

A. Teherani
Department of Medicine and Center for Faculty Educators, School of Medicine, University of California, San Francisco, CA, USA
e-mail: Arianne.Teherani@ucsf.edu

© Springer Nature Singapore Pte Ltd. 2023
D. Nestel et al. (eds.), *Clinical Education for the Health Professions*,
https://doi.org/10.1007/978-981-15-3344-0_90

Rationales for Peer Learning 1362
    Educational Benefits 1362
    Practical Benefits 1363
Challenges Encountered in Peer Learning and Strategies to Overcome Them 1364
    Credibility of Peers 1364
    Competition Between Peers 1364
    Logistical Issues 1364
    Student and Staff Skills 1365
Common Clinical Education Scenarios and Peer Learning 1366
    Early Clinical Experiences 1366
    Standard Placement Models 1367
    Longitudinal Integrated Clerkships and Service Learning 1367
Decision-Making Around the Type of Peer Learning to Implement 1368
Conclusion 1370
Cross-References 1370
References 1370

Abstract

Peer learning has a long history yet has only recently attracted wider attention as a formal strategy to improve students' learning experiences within clinical education. This chapter will cover theoretical rationales for the use of peer learning, provide an overview of the potential peer learning configurations in the continuum of clinical education, and outline a range of practical strategies to successfully incorporate peer learning into health professional student education.

Keywords

Peer learning · Peer mentoring · Peer tutoring · Peer assessment · Longitudinal integrated clerkships

Introduction

Peer learning is increasingly used as a formal pedagogical strategy within clinical education and exists in a number of configurations and consists of a wide variety of activities. An overarching definition for peer learning developed within clinical education is:

> "a social practice of mutually beneficial personal and professional development among learners interacting as status equals, characterized by safety, comfort, motivation through relevance, and intellectual risk-taking." (Callese et al. 2019, p. 12)

Peer learning has existed as part of an educator's repertoire for hundreds, if not thousands, of years (Secomb 2008). Historically, informal peer learning has been a part of learning in many educational settings and in various contexts (Sevenhuysen et al. 2015). Peer learning occurs in everyday settings when learners engage in activities such as asking their classmates for answers to questions, drawing on senior students for guidance on resources, or simply observing their peers' interactions and patient care in clinical settings. Formal peer learning occurs when institutions, courses, or programs develop systematic measures by which to encourage, support, and instigate peer learning. While some educators and students value peer learning, others are still concerned about its place within a curriculum. This chapter addresses such concerns through reviewing the theory and evidence for peer learning. It begins by outlining peer learning configurations and activities; discusses a selection of learning theories applicable to peer learning, rationales for peer learning, challenges in peer learning; and finally describes some common implementations of peer learning and provides a framework to design peer learning activities for clinical contexts.

Peer Learning Configurations

Both informal and formal peer learning may occur in episodic or continuous situations. However, when institutions, courses, and programs use formalized, systematic ways to encourage peer learning, the learning value of those activities benefits learners with varied learning needs (Boud et al. 2001; Kucharski-Howard et al. 2019). The following sections discuss characteristics applicable to all peer learning activities, and common types or activities of peer learning. We focus largely on formal peer learning, as they have been relatively well-researched compared to informal peer learning. Formal peer learning is also more likely to be able to be set up and steered by educators.

Episodic Peer Contact Versus Peer Continuity

Episodic peer contact opportunities present when small groups are placed together to work on a task for a short period of time. Examples of such opportunities in health professions education have included team-based learning and small group work within a course (Burgess et al. 2014). By contrast, peer continuity places peers in a longitudinal experience to work, learn, and/or provide support to one another. During this continuity experience, peers usually meet at required formalized times with a concrete focus and faculty guidance (Kucharski-Howard et al. 2019; Chou and Teherani 2017; Mai et al. 2013). They may also partake in informal peer learning throughout the experience.

The concept of peer continuity has emerged relatively recently and harnesses educational theories such as learning communities, social cognitive theory, social comparison theory, and communities of practice (see below; Chou and Teherani 2017).The concept of learning communities, i.e., groups of students who share interests and learning experiences over time, can be applied to clinical education contexts. Through these learning communities, health professional education programs have successfully addressed student well-being, perception of the learning environment, clinical skills instruction, professionalism, advising, and mentoring (Ferguson et al. 2009; Kasper and Brownfield 2018; Collins and Mowder-Tinney

2012). Traditionally, students may be allocated individually to a placement site or organizational unit, corresponding with a decrease in well-being, empathy, and patient-centered behaviors (Chou et al. 2011). Contrastingly, in peer continuity settings, stable cohorts of students can meet frequently (e.g., weekly), perhaps to accomplish some scientific and clinical learning, but also to process and debrief events in the workplace. Other examples of peer continuity may include grouping students in a clinical placement, which requires them to work and learn alongside each other for the duration of the placement. These cohorts emphasize a sense of group belonging, which psychological studies demonstrate is important for well-being and development of trust (Secomb 2008; Haslam et al. 2005; Sevenhuysen et al. 2017; Adachi et al. 2016). Peers provide a support network and enhanced learning environment that counteracts negative aspects of the hidden curriculum commonly encountered in clinical education (Ferguson et al. 2009; Teherani et al. 2013). An example is where medical and allied health programs have developed placement models with continuity, known as "longitudinal integrated clerkships" or service learning, and have found that continuity among peers provides workplace learning, social support, and clinical and professional learning (Mai et al. 2013; Chou et al. 2011; Teherani et al. 2013; Chou et al. 2013).

Same Level or Near-Peers

Near-peer learning or mentoring is a term normally used for a specific type of peer learning where the peers are at differing levels, usually at least one academic year apart (Olaussen et al. 2016). Same-level peer learning may be more realistic to implement, given that students at the same point in the course are more likely to be doing similar placements together (Tai et al. 2018). However, in interdisciplinary or interprofessional learning experiences, peers may be at the same academic year level, but due to the design of their specific educational programs, be at differing ability levels. For example, occupational therapy and physiotherapy students may all be in their final year of their degree, with the physiotherapy students having completed more "hands-on" learning in their earlier placements. Advantages of this model include students reporting increased confidence in describing and understanding their role, and completing certain technical skills such as interviewing a patient (Kucharski-Howard et al. 2019; Larkin and Hitch 2019).

Peer Learning Activities

Under the broad umbrella of peer learning, there are various subtypes. Without promising to be exhaustive, we present here the most common types of peer learning in clinical settings. Assuming a model of predominantly one-way information exchange, Olaussen et al. (2016) presented one heuristic by classifying peer teaching first into a simple system of same-level and near-peer, then on the basis of group size: peer mentoring (1:<3), peer tutoring (1:3–10), or peer didactics (1:>10). However, there are many other opportunities and constructs in which students learn with and from each other and which more fully incorporate social learning models. Within clinical education settings, there are also situations where there is no clear "single" mentor, tutor, or teacher. These situations may include problem-based learning scenarios (even if one student is appointed facilitator or leader, they are likely participating in a similar manner to others and also be a learner rather than just taking on a facilitator role), peer discussion groups, and forms of peer assessment where students receive feedback information from several observers. This section provides a brief description of a range of peer learning activities; further detail is provided for common clinical education scenarios in a subsequent section.

Peer Didactics

Peer didactics is typically a large-group activity, where one or a small group of students are responsible for the content and design of the session, with varying levels of educator support. In addition to clinical knowledge and skills (Adachi et al. 2016; Olaussen et al. 2016), peer teaching has been effective in orienting students to clinical education environments (Masters et al. 2013; Smith et al. 2012). They may be compulsory or voluntary; and between same-level peers (e.g., where one student or group of students are nominated to present on a topic which the whole class must learn) or a senior student might teach a group of junior students.

Peer Mentoring

Peer mentoring, unlike peer didactics, is unlikely to have a fixed curriculum. Mentoring configurations might be one mentor to one mentee, or the mentor may have several mentees. This pairing in the clinical education environment allows for an informal relationship to develop, with the mentee feeling more comfortable to express their uncertainties and seek clarification, and the mentor gaining confidence in their emerging levels of knowledge and skill (Dennison 2010). The mentor usually has more specific experience in the area of mentoring, and is provided with training and/or support to fulfill their role (Kucharski-Howard et al. 2019; Larkin and Hitch 2019). Mentors might provide advice and coaching in a general way, or share their expertise through positive role modeling (Olaussen et al. 2016). Peer mentors may teach specific skills or facilitate the critical thinking of their mentees (Dennison 2010).

Peer Observation, Feedback, and Assessment

There are many ways for students to evaluate peers on some aspect of their work or performance and provide feedback, in formal and informal settings. Peers may be involved in formative assessment through the provision of feedback about their peers' performance in carrying out specific tasks, such as introducing their role to the client, carrying out a functional assessment, or expressing their recommendations in a team case conference. The topic or activity should be one where students have sufficient knowledge and skill to undertake a meaningful judgement (Tai et al. 2016a). The format of pre-existing workplace-based assessments might also be drawn upon to shape a peer assessment interaction and assist with feedback (Mai et al. 2013). Formative Objective Structured Clinical Examinations (OSCEs) can also be used as a vehicle for learning (Chou et al. 2013).

Peers may also contribute to longitudinal evaluations, which usually focus on professionalism and teamwork, and information from these assessments have the potential to contribute to evaluations of performance. A few studies have also incorporated peer grades into final marks; however, this is relatively uncommon due to the likelihood of "gaming" the system (Kovach et al. 2009).

Some activities involving peer observation and feedback have also included the opportunity for students to also take on the patient/service user role. This occurs most commonly in communication skills training. In these situations, it is recommended that the communication task have clear guidelines, including adequate preparation, realistic roles, and tasks which are aligned with learners' current level of ability (Bosse et al. 2015).

Discussion and Debriefing

Discussion activities with peers have focused on debriefing and reflection, with a view to further explore ethical issues, clinical or professional reasoning, and personal values. Some of these activities aimed to aid students in their transition to new clinical learning environments (Crill et al. 2009; Vuckovic et al. 2019). For example, to help students make sense of a new learning environment, or ethical issues they observed during their clinical placements, discussions might occur on a regular basis over a term (Chou et al. 2011; Duke et al. 2015) or as a single session in a shorter rotation (Liu et al. 2016). Where less face-to-face time was scheduled, students might be asked to prepare for the session by submitting a written reflection for discussion.

Small Group Learning (PBL, TBL)

Small group learning with peer continuity is deployed in health sciences professions education most often in settings that prepare students for clinical work. Well-established forms of small group learning include clinical skills and professionalism education, problem-based or team-based learning strategies, and basic science learning (Burgess et al. 2014; Thistlethwaite et al. 2012). More recently, many medical schools have adopted learning communities, groups of students who co-create shared interests and learning experiences over time. In addition to knowledge and skills training, these communities are additionally able to address well-being, assessment of the learning environment, professionalism, advising, and mentoring in a more customized way (Smith et al. 2014).

Learning Theories Underpinning Peer Learning in Clinical Education

Constructivist learning theories tend to best describe the types of learning that occur within clinical placement contexts, where individuals develop, build, or construct their own understanding through interaction with the people and environment around them – and where knowledge is seen to be shared and accessed by a group. We focus on three theories which arise from different traditions within a constructivist framing. Each places a different focus on learning and contributes to an understanding of how peer learning might function within clinical education.

The Zone of Proximal Development

Vygotsky's theory of the zone of proximal development (ZPD) (Vygotsky 1978) contains an explicit role for peer learners. While he described the ZPD in relation to young children learning with each other, the same types of ideas apply to learning at all ages. Essentially, each learner has a "zone of proximal development" of understanding or skills, just beyond their current abilities, which may be more easily reached or attained, with the guidance of another who has already attained that particular ability. Within a clinical context, it is unlikely that all students in a given situation will be at the exact same level of learning: this makes peer learning in the zone of proximal development possible. Those in the role of the "guide" do not need to possess vastly different levels of knowledge or ability, they merely need to be the "more capable other" with skills in assisting other learners. It is also hypothesized that having social and/or cognitive congruence – i.e., that there is a greater shared understanding and ways of thinking – aids peer learning (Rogoff 1990).

Communities of Practice

In their research on learning in workplaces, Lave and Wenger (1991) described the "Community of Practice," where practitioners formed a group with a shared understanding and traditions of practice. Apprentices gradually became part of this group through undertaking tasks and demonstrating competence within that particular field. In the health professions, clinical placements can exemplify this concept. For example, when groups of students are assigned to a clinician-educator for a specified period of time, educators overseeing student learning alongside their normal clinical role. Students generally move along a continuum from initial observation of the educator undertaking their daily tasks, to being entrusted to do parts of the task, through to having a degree of responsibility for a number of the tasks normally assigned to the educator. In their research, Lave and Wenger noted that learning relationships were not solely between the "apprentice" and the "master": apprentices also interacted with each other to learn. Often, learning occurred more efficiently in these peer interactions, as compared to master-apprentice interactions. Within clinical education, this spread of roles might be analogous to clinical staff across the disciplines, who can offer beneficial alternative perspectives on practice, aside from the "master" in one's own discipline.

Social Comparison Theory

Social comparison theory (Raat et al. 2010) has also been applied to peer learning in health professions education. Medical students were found to benefit in their learning by comparing their own performance to those of students better and worse than themselves. Students preferred comparing themselves to their peers, rather than supervisors or tutors, as this gave them the most relevant information regarding the level they needed to achieve in relation to the competency-based standards applicable to themselves. Learning interactions with peers may increase opportunities for comparison of performance and enable students to more clearly see what actions they need to take to achieve an appropriate level of performance. In a near-peer model, the comparison becomes even more evident as the junior students can observe and make sense of the standard they are aspiring to reach within a similar time frame, rather than modeling on the expert practitioner who has achieved that level of expertise through a number of years of practice.

Rationales for Peer Learning

Several systematic reviews have collected evidence for same level and near-peer configurations, across a range of health professions disciplines (Secomb 2008; Santee and Garavalia 2006; Yu et al. 2011; Tai et al. 2016b; Burgess et al. 2013). Tai et al. (2016b) classified these benefits into those for individual students, benefits to the peer group, benefits to educators, and benefits to patients. Studies have largely focused on student learning rather than practical outcomes for educators, service users, and organizational systems: thus, this section will describe educational benefits for learners and discuss some practical advantages.

Educational Benefits

Peer learning has been linked to varied outcomes in the health professions education, including building teamwork and leadership (Chojecki et al. 2010; Ramm et al. 2015), enhancing cognitive skills (Secomb 2008; Christiansen and Bell 2010; Won and Choi 2017), acquiring technical/profession specific skills (Ramm et al. 2015; Ravanipour et al. 2015), and developing affective skills (Christiansen and Bell

2010). These benefits are likely to be similar to those seen in "standard" clinical teaching. However, learning with peers may allow for more co-construction of knowledge and opportunities to explain concepts to others, further identifying gaps in knowledge and deepening understanding (Tawfik et al. 2016; Mills et al. 2017). Cognitive congruence, which refers to possessing a similar knowledge base, may also facilitate learning, as usually learners can explain concepts or assist in the learning of skills at a level a peer can more easily grasp (Mills et al. 2017).

One particular aspect where peer learning may provide benefits is the development of evaluative judgement: the capability to discern and make judgements about quality of the work of oneself and others (Tai et al. 2016a; Tai and Sevenhuysen 2018). Again, this "hands-on" process, where learners are more actively involved in determining content of teaching, likely facilitates learning. Learners must also have some knowledge of the standards in order to make accurate assessments of understanding and skill (for further teaching or assessment). Thus, students' insights into their own competency may develop (Duchscher 2001).

Finally, peer learning experiences may help learners to develop their own skills as educators. Within many health professions, new graduates may be expected to contribute to preregistration teaching almost immediately. Peer learning is a good opportunity to equip learners with education-related skills, such as providing feedback (Tai et al. 2017). These education skills may also support patient education; indeed, students have reported that their clinical communication skills have improved through participation in peer learning (Tai et al. 2016b; McIntyre et al. 2019).

Practical Benefits

Beyond the educational benefits, there are also practical reasons for implementing peer learning within clinical placements. As reported by pharmacy (Smith et al. 2012), occupational therapy and physiotherapy (Sevenhuysen et al. 2017), placement capacity may increase through the use of peer learning placements. Early year placements are generally shorter, so adopting a near-peer mentoring model enables a site to meet their clinical placement targets, with junior students joining their senior peers for a short period of time, using a near-peer mentoring model (Iwata and Gill 2013). Advantages of this type of peer learning exist for the educator, near-peer mentor, and mentee. For the educator, studies have identified either a reduced teaching burden (Cohen et al. 2015; Stenberg et al. 2020), or an enhanced ability for the educator to teach higher level competencies (Sevenhuysen et al. 2015; Tawfik et al. 2016). Other advantages include having the mentor complete the orientation for the mentee (Mills et al. 2017). For later placements, placing same-level peers together may be appropriate and have the effect of doubling effective capacity (Sevenhuysen et al. 2013a).

Peer learning may also provide much wanted social and academic support (Chou et al. 2011; Vuckovic et al. 2019; McIntyre et al. 2019; McPake 2019), and may increase student self-confidence (Secomb 2008; Chojecki et al. 2010; Ravanipour et al. 2015). This is especially crucial in the transition to clinical learning environments (Masters et al. 2013). Students have reported feeling more comfortable learning from their peers (McKenna and French 2011), feeling less anxious, and therefore more confident (Secomb 2008).

Challenges Encountered in Peer Learning and Strategies to Overcome Them

Credibility of Peers

Unsuccessful peer learning is frequently attributed to students not having trust in their peers' abilities, and subsequently privileging the authority of the teacher (Tai et al. 2017). However, it has been argued that student credibility is not an absolute requirement (Boud et al. 2001), as part of the learning process has to do with learners being able to distinguish the quality and accuracy of the information received, and therefore *learning* to make judgements about peers is not necessarily detrimental to learning. However, generally, learners are likely to be wary of peer learning, especially if they have not previously had a productive peer learning encounter. Faculty supervision during peer learning meetings should therefore facilitate the development of ground rules and learning goals. Faculty should have adequate time to oversee peer learning. It is recommended that faculty facilitators create an atmosphere in which students feel like they can learn and grow through open discussion. Part of the success of peer learning also depends on there being additional supervision by a "teacher," i.e., an educator is still present in a more distant capacity to supervise the learning (Chou and Teherani 2017). Care should be taken to select a topic or activity for learners on which they do have sufficient expertise to be successful and useful peer learners (Tai et al. 2017). Establishing confidence is important, so low-stakes situations may help to "ease" students into peer learning.

Competition Between Peers

Social competition in clinical learning settings can be rampant and exacerbated by competition for grades. In fact, there is a recent movement in medical school clerkships to abandon grading altogether, as the practice unduly emphasizes factors that do not necessarily correspond with clinical acumen as much as potential evaluator bias (Hauer and Lucey 2018). One study showed that peer continuity meetings helped to reduce the valence of competition by creating collaborative opportunities for study (Chou et al. 2011). Conversely, a competitive environment may also motivate students' achievement when learning about workplace-based practices and tasks, since co-operation is also valued (Chou et al. 2013).

Logistical Issues

There are logistical and practical needs for peer learning that are vital to creating effective formal peer learning experiences. Peer learning activities should ensure a common conceptual model, including clear guidelines, correspondence to the objectives of the educational intervention, alignment with student needs, and adequate student preparation for the experience (Boud et al. 2001). In addition, designing peer learning must also take context into account. Importantly, group size must allow for ample interaction and learning. For example, peer groups that work together in the clinical setting have ranged in size between 6 and 16 students (Chou and Teherani 2017; Teherani et al. 2013; Poncelet et al. 2011). Most of the research on peer learning has occurred in peer face-to-face interaction, although research on peer interaction via online modalities has increased in the recent years (Koops et al. 2011). The logistical requirements for non-face-to-face peer learning are dependent on the technology involved.

There are mixed opinions about the effect of peer learning on educator workload. Some suggest it has reduced the burden for clinical educators and at the same time increased the learning opportunities as students move in and out of the facilitator/learning roles (Ten Cate and Durning 2007). However, there is still a substantial load for the educator in planning for and managing multiple numbers of students. This can be ameliorated through good planning and communication between education and placement providers, including using workshops to develop a shared understanding (Sevenhuysen et al. 2013b).

Whether learning occurs between two or multiple peers, peers must set early ground rules for group process and participation, and hold to those standards (Ross and Cameron 2007). Peers who create an unsafe or challenging learning environment can hinder learning. Although proponents of peer learning have advocated that peer learning allows for less hands-on faculty involvement in learning (Chou et al. 2011), peer learning occurs ideally when facilitated by a teacher (Chou and Teherani 2017; Tai et al. 2017).

Student and Staff Skills

Faculty supervision during peer continuity group meetings is critical. Within this particular setting, where students may reveal particular dilemmas and concerns about their own performance, faculty with no evaluative role should lead the group meetings, in order to guide student learning appropriately and to provide mentoring (Duke et al. 2015). Learners themselves note that supervision enhances learning and avoids development of bad habits, "illusions of competence," and even unhealthy behaviors (Brydges et al. 2010). Three particular educator skills can enhance learning outcomes: challenging learners when false assumptions or novice perspectives take root; structuring learning to optimize long-term learning; and identifying and responding to situations when learners need stronger support. Skilled educators in these groups refrain from unilateral didactics; instead, they facilitate discussion and reflection to guide trainees toward a path of self-discovery and independent practices (Chou and Teherani 2017). This is particularly important in peer learning situations to ensure that peers see the value the exchange with each other, rather than focusing solely on the educator's input.

For students to participate in peer learning, they are likely to require some educational skills if they are taking on a tutoring, teaching, feedback, or assessment role. Students also need to learn reflective techniques to judge the information shared between peers (Tai et al. 2016a). This may include ways to structure teaching; understanding feedback processes and how to formulate feedback information; and understanding how their particular assessment requirements function. Some of these skills may have been developed prior to clinical placements, while others may have been experienced through encounters with previous educators. Determining students' baseline skills may be necessary to design appropriately targeted supporting materials.

Common Clinical Education Scenarios and Peer Learning

Early Clinical Experiences

The use of near-peer mentoring as a teaching/learning strategy is an innovative solution to the provision of early clinical experiences. For example, Iwata and Gill (2013) found that first-year medical students valued the opportunity to shadow foundation year junior doctors for short periods, although those being shadowed found supervising in this context challenging. Similarly, Harmer et al. (2011) paired senior nursing students with junior students to provide care for a patient. They found that students developed self-confidence and perceived improvements in their ability to time-manage, prioritize care, and make clinical judgements. Maximizing the learning opportunities requires careful planning. For example, in an outpatient midwifery clinic (Cohen et al. 2015), one educator and one senior student were responsible for the clinic appointments, with two novice students responsible for reviewing the patient's notes, providing a short history to the educator prior to the appointment, observing the educator in the appointment, and then completing the patient documentation. The educator retained overall responsibility for service delivery while the senior student guided the novice students outside the clinic with their preparation and documentation tasks. The educator had a critical role in assisting both senior and junior students to maximize the learning opportunities that arose.

Other clinical education scenarios that enable or support peer learning include student-led clinics. Student-led clinics may be stand-alone clinics offering free or reduced fee services, or they may be a specific clinic implemented within a traditional clinical scenario. Regardless of the scenario, the potential for peer learning is extensive. For example, Collins and Mowder-Tinney (2012) outline a pro-bono physiotherapy clinic where senior students assumed an apprentice clinical instructor role with novice students. Here, the senior students were responsible for mentoring the novice students, both facilitating their clinical reasoning as well as providing verbal and written feedback on their performance. In this and similar studies, researchers have identified the importance of preparing the students for their mentee role. Issues to consider are the mentor's perception of their own level of competence and therefore what they can legitimately coach another student to acquire; their judgement around patient and novice student safety – knowing when to intervene or not; and knowing how to engage in useful feedback conversations (Seifert et al. 2016).

In an inpatient environment, student-led care is also possible, for instance, where a pair of nursing students were allocated responsibility for a group of patients, supervised by a rostered preceptor. This developed students' perceptions of independence during their placement and also enabled them to gain a more comprehensive understanding of clinical care (Ekstedt et al. 2019).

Standard Placement Models

There is a large variation in "standard" placement models. In many allied health disciplines, these have been traditionally provided in a 1:1 model where there is one learner and one educator in a single service area. In contrast, some nursing programs allocate a small group of students to a specific ward or department. Students are "buddied" with a registered nurse, and a floating educator assists the nursing student's learning. Medicine has commonly placed multiple learners in a single service area, with multiple staff of various seniorities who are expected to provide some clinical experiences, along with additional specific tutorials from staff. In all of these configurations, peer learning is possible (Olaussen et al. 2016).

Where multiple students are already placed together, it is relatively easy to arrange sessions where a peer learning activity can take place. Space can be booked to ensure a safe learning environment free from interruptions. Students are likely to require direction in terms of the types of activities, which could include peer teaching/tutoring, observation, and feedback. This might occur throughout the placement on relevant topics.

Where students are not yet placed with others, there are several possibilities. First, students across placements might be brought together to participate in joint activities such as tutorial discussions. The success of these groups depends on intentional group formation activities to provide a safe learning environment and establish peers' credibility. Second, placements might be modified to accommodate additional students undertaking similar learning – i.e., same-level peers. This may involve some pre-work for educators in planning the activities that students can undertake in pairs, and time for individual supervision and assessment (Stenberg et al. 2020; McPake 2019). Lastly, near-peer mentoring may be used to expand cross-year level capacity within placements, where senior students contribute to the supervision of junior students through appropriate task selection (i.e., where the senior students are deemed competent to supervise) (McIntyre et al. 2019).

Longitudinal Integrated Clerkships and Service Learning

Longitudinal integrated clerkships (LICs) and service learning place patients at the center of learning and emphasize continuity of care. In these structures, students care for patients longitudinally and across loci of care, rather than placing the healthcare system in the center of learning (e.g., rotations through particular units, wards, or consultation services). These LICs also feature continuity of supervision, where faculty get to know and help develop students' skills over a longer period of time (Poncelet et al. 2011).

Whereas LICs typically refer to medical student education, similar models also exist in allied health, being referred to as service-learning or role-emerging placements. Advantages of this model of learning are numerous. For example, in medical education, when comparing with their counterparts in traditional block clerkships, medical students in LICs demonstrate equal or higher academic achievement, more patient-centered skills, better clinical skills, and rate the quality of faculty feedback more highly (Teherani et al. 2013). A similar integrated model has been used within physical therapy, where students participated in a service-learning clinic over three semesters, moving through the program in a cohort. While students were able to learn and work with their same-level peers, they also benefited from peer mentoring from students in the year above who were also participating in the clinic (Mai et al. 2013).

One of the noted shortcomings of the LIC structure is that students typically rotate through these clinics without sufficient benefit from peer learning; in allied health, students are usually allocated in pairs or small groups. Regardless of discipline, establishing peer continuity groups helps students with advice about workplace norms and expectations, content learning, and logistics (Masters et al. 2013). Therefore, when considering constructing LICs or developing service-learning/role emerging placements, schools must also capitalize on the significant benefits of peer learning in this continuous setting.

Decision-Making Around the Type of Peer Learning to Implement

This chapter has demonstrated there are many different facets to peer learning. The key factor in implementing peer learning is clarifying the purpose and intended learning outcomes of the activity. Following Biggs and Tang's concept of Constructive Alignment (Biggs and Tang 2007), and consistent with the learning theories discussed above, learning occurs when individuals actively construct their knowledge through participation in learning activities. Therefore, learning objectives, learner activities, and assessments must align, so that students clearly know the purpose of the learning activities and can achieve the outcomes through participation in the learning activities.

Since achieving intended learning outcomes can occur in several ways, one must incorporate context and practical considerations. What limits to your resources – both in personnel and equipment – exist? Where and how often might your learners be able to meet? What are your students' peer learning capabilities? Will you need to provide them with training on group discussion, assessment rubrics or standards, feedback, how to use a tool or software, or familiarize them with equipment?

In terms of design, a framework or typology is required. Both peer assessment (Adachi et al. 2018) and peer tutoring (Olaussen et al. 2016) have established frameworks. These frameworks provide a useful guide to designing peer assessment, taking into account the intention/purpose, links to other activities within the curriculum, the type of interaction between peers, the composition of assessment groups, the management of assessment procedure, and contextual elements. On the basis of the framework published by Topping and Ehly (1998), and in alignment with a peer assessment framework which considers context (Adachi et al. 2018), we present a decision-making tool (Table 1), which may help educators decide on the design of

Table 1 Decision-making framework for designing peer learning

Prompting questions	Potential responses
1. What is the purpose or intended outcome of the activity? (what is the curriculum content, are there particular learning objectives?)	Improve content knowledge/skills – > teaching (including reciprocal) or assessment and feedback Improve understanding of standards/required quality – > peer assessment and feedback Improve social cohesion – > discussion/sharing/presentations
2. What are the types of learners you have access to? (will they be within or between institutions, within or across year groups, same or across-ability matching?)	Same-level peers Near peers Interdisciplinary peers
3. What activity, and therefore group size and configuration will you have? (how will they interact with each other, and what are the roles of learners?)	1:1, 1:a few, 1:many Will learners take on different roles throughout the session (e.g., tutor/observer/learner)
4. What skills do your learners already possess/what will you need to upskill them in? (what are the characteristics of the helpers and helped?)	Feedback Assessment rubrics/forms/guides Facilitation/teaching techniques Ethical behavior/honor code

5. What are the temporal arrangements?	Duration
	  Once-off
	  Short term (weeks – month)
	  Medium term (several months)
	  Longitudinal (6 months – year)
	Frequency
	  Daily (if short-term placement)
	  Weekly
	  Fortnightly
	  Monthly
	Location
	  Wards, meeting rooms, breakout spaces

6. Do all learners attend, and are there incentives (will it be voluntary or compulsory? Will you provide rewards or incentives?)	Is it a required activity or an optional extra? If optional, might there be significant barriers to attend for certain groups/populations (e.g., out of hours, long commute from standard placement site) Are there any incentives for learners to attend – e.g., certificate for curriculum vitae, food/drink provided, social gathering afterwards with opportunity for networking
7. What resources do you have or need?	Rooms/breakout spaces Learning materials – Quizzes, problem-based learning cases Equipment – Clinical skills equipment, simulated task trainers, computer/projector, whiteboards, other technology Personnel – Facilitators, simulated patients, clinical academics

peer learning. While we present many options, they may not represent all possibilities. Therefore, while we suggest that educators might find the listed potential responses useful to inform their thinking, there are likely to be additional design outcomes which arise out of a particular context and situation.

Conclusion

Peer learning is not a single educational activity. Rather, it is an umbrella term for a wide range of pedagogical strategies and student configurations which have the potential to significantly enrich student learning. This is particularly true in clinical placements, where the types of tasks and ways of learning are myriad. Research on peer learning in clinical settings demonstrates that it is no different in terms of outcomes, compared to "traditional" methods of supervision, and may provide additional academic and social support. Though both educators and students may be initially skeptical, informal peer learning already has a key place within clinical practice. Therefore, peer learning should be considered as a way of improving clinical placement learning experiences and preparing learners for their future lives as practitioners and educators.

Cross-References

- ▶ Communities of Practice and Medical Education
- ▶ Focus on Theory: Emotions and Learning

References

Adachi C, Tai J, Dawson P. Enabler or inhibitor? Educational technology in self and peer assessment. In: Proceedings of ASCILITE 2016, show me the learning, Adelaide, November 27–30. Adelaide; 2016. p. 11–6.

Adachi C, Tai J, Dawson P. A framework for designing, implementing, communicating and researching peer assessment. High Educ Res Dev. 2018;37(3):453–67.

Biggs J, Tang C. Teaching for quality learning at university. 3rd ed. Maidenhead: Open University Press; 2007.

Bosse HM, Nickel M, Huwendiek S, Schultz JH, Nikendei C. Cost-effectiveness of peer role play and standardized patients in undergraduate communication training. BMC Med Educ. 2015;15 (1):183.

Boud D, Cohen R, Sampson J. Peer learning in higher education. Boud D, Cohen R, Sampson J, editors. London: Kogan Page Ltd; 2001.

Brydges R, Dubrowski A, Regehr G. A new concept of unsupervised learning: directed Self-guided learning in the health professions. Acad Med. 2010;85:S49–55.

Burgess A, Roberts C, Black KI, Mellis C. Senior medical student perceived ability and experience in giving peer feedback in formative long case examinations. BMC Med Educ. 2013;13(1):79.

Burgess AW, McGregor DM, Mellis CM. Applying established guidelines to team-based learning programs in medical schools: a systematic review. Acad Med. 2014;89(4):678–88.

Callese T, Strowd R, Navarro B, Rosenberg I, Waasdorp Hurtado C, Tai J, et al. Conversation starter: advancing the theory of peer-assisted learning. Teach Learn Med. 2019;31(1):7–16.

Chojecki P, Lamarre J, Buck M, St-Sauveur I, Eldaoud N, Purden M. Perceptions of a peer learning approach to pediatric clinical education. Int J Nurs Educ Scholarsh. 2010;7(1)

Chou CL, Teherani A. A Foundation for Vital Academic and Social Support in clerkships. Acad Med. 2017;92(7):951–5.

Chou CL, Johnston CB, Singh B, Garber JD, Kaplan E, Lee K, et al. A "safe space" for learning and reflection: one school's design for continuity with a peer group across clinical clerkships. Acad Med. 2011;86(12):1560–5.

Chou CL, Masters DE, Chang A, Kruidering M, Hauer KE. Effects of longitudinal small-group learning on delivery and receipt of communication skills feedback. Med Educ. 2013;47(11):1073–9.

Christiansen A, Bell A. Peer learning partnerships: exploring the experience of pre-registration nursing students. J Clin Nurs. 2010;19(5–6):803–10.

Cohen SR, Thomas CR, Gerard C. The clinical learning dyad model: an innovation in midwifery education. J Midwifery Womens Health. 2015;60(6):691–8.

Collins J, Mowder-Tinney J. The apprentice clinical instructor (ACI): a Mentor/Protégé model for capstone integrated clinical education (C-ICE). J Phys Ther Educ. 2012;26(3):33–9.

Crill CM, Matlock MA, Pinner NA, Self TH. Integration of first- and second-year introductory pharmacy practice experiences. Am J Pharm Educ. 2009;73(3):50.

Dennison S. Peer mentoring: untapped potential. J Nurs Educ. 2010;49(6):340–2.

Duchscher JEB. Peer learning: a clinical teaching strategy to promote active learning | Ovid. Nurse Educ. 2001;26(2):59–60.

Duke P, Grosseman S, Novack DH, Rosenzweig S. Preserving third year medical students' empathy and enhancing self-reflection using small group "virtual hangout" technology. Med Teach. 2015;37(6):566–71.

Ekstedt M, Lindblad M, Löfmark A. Nursing students' perception of the clinical learning environment and supervision in relation to two different supervision models – a comparative cross-sectional study. BMC Nurs. 2019;18(1):1–13.

Ferguson KJ, Wolter EM, Yarbrough DB, Carline JD, Krupat E. Defining and describing medical learning communities: results of a National Survey. Acad Med. 2009;84(11):1549–56.

Harmer BM, Huffman J, Johnson B. Clinical peer mentoring. Nurse Educ. 2011;36(5):197–202.

Haslam N, Bain P, Douge L, Lee M, Bastian B. More human than you: attributing humanness to self and others. J Pers Soc Psychol. 2005;89(6):937–50.

Hauer KE, Lucey CR. Core clerkship grading: the illusion of objectivity. Acad Med. 2018;1

Iwata K, Gill D. Learning through work: clinical shadowing of junior doctors by first year medical students. Med Teach. 2013;35(8):633–8.

Kasper B, Brownfield A. Evaluation of a newly established layered learning model in an ambulatory care practice setting. Curr Pharm Teach Learn. 2018;10(7):925–32.

Koops W, Van der Vleuten C, De Leng B, Oei SG, Snoeckx L. Computer-supported collaborative learning in the medical workplace: students' experiences on formative peer feedback of a critical appraisal of a topic paper. Med Teach. 2011;33(6):e318–23.

Kovach RA, Resch DS, Verhulst SJ. Peer assessment of professionalism: a five-year experience in medical clerkship. J Gen Intern Med. 2009;24(6):742–6.

Kucharski-Howard J, Babin CJ, Inacio CA, Tsoumas LJ. DPT student perceptions about developing mentoring skills: a progressive model. J Allied Health. 2019;48(2):108–13.

Larkin H, Hitch D. Peer assisted study sessions (PASS) preparing occupational therapy undergraduates for practice education: a novel application of a proven educational intervention. Aust Occup Ther J. 2019;66(1):100–9.

Lave J, Wenger E. Situated practice: legitimate peripheral participation. Cambridge, UK/New York: Cambridge University Press; 1991.

Liu GZ, Jawitz OK, Zheng D, Gusberg RJ, Kim AW. Reflective writing for medical students on the surgical clerkship: oxymoron or antidote? J Surg Educ. 2016;73(2):296–304.

Mai JA, Thiele A, O'Dell B, Kruse B, Vaassen M, Priest A. Utilization of an integrated clinical experience in a physical therapist education program. J Phys Ther Educ. 2013;27(2):25–32.

Masters DE, O'Brien BC, Chou CL. The third-year medical student "grapevine": managing transitions between third-year clerkships using peer-to-peer handoffs. Acad Med. 2013;88(10):1534–8.

McIntyre C, Natsheh C, Leblanc K, Fernandes O, Mejia AB, Raman-Wilms L, et al. An analysis of Canadian doctor of pharmacy student experiences in non-traditional student-preceptor models. Am J Pharm Educ. 2019;83(10)

McKenna L, French J. A step ahead: teaching undergraduate students to be peer teachers. Nurse Educ Pract. 2011;11(2):141–5.

McPake M. Radiographers' and students' experiences of undergraduate radiotherapy practice placement in the United Kingdom. Radiography. 2019;25(3):220–6.

Mills DA, Hammer CL, Murad A. Power of peers: students' perceptions of pairing in clinical dental education. J Dent Educ. 2017;81(1):36–43.

Olaussen A, Reddy P, Irvine S, Williams B. Peer-assisted learning: time for nomenclature clarification. Med Educ Online. 2016;21(1):30974.

Poncelet A, Bokser S, Calton B, Hauer KE, Kirsch H, Jones T, et al. Development of a longitudinal integrated clerkship at an academic medical center. Med Educ Online. 2011;16

Raat J, Kuks J, Cohen-Schotanus J. Learning in clinical practice: stimulating and discouraging response to social comparison. Med Teach. 2010;32(11):899–904.

Ramm D, Thomson A, Jackson A. Learning clinical skills in the simulation suite: the lived experiences of student nurses involved in peer teaching and peer assessment. Nurse Educ Today. 2015;35(6):823–7.

Ravanipour M, Bahreini M, Ravanipour M. Exploring nursing students' experience of peer learning in clinical practice. J Educ Health Promot. 2015;4(1):46.

Rogoff B. Apprenticeship in thinking: cognitive development in social context. New York: Oxford University Press; 1990.

Ross MT, Cameron HS. Peer assisted learning: a planning and implementation framework: AMEE guide no. 30. Med Teach. 2007;29(6):527–45.

Santee J, Garavalia L. Peer tutoring programs in health professions schools. Am J Pharm Educ. 2006;70(3):Article 70.

Secomb J. A systematic review of peer teaching and learning in clinical education. J Clin Nurs. 2008;17(6):703–16.

Seifert LB, Schaack D, Jennewein L, Steffen B, Schulze J, Gerlach F, et al. Peer-assisted learning in a student-run free clinic project increases clinical competence. Med Teach. 2016;38(5):515–22.

Sevenhuysen SL, Raitman L, Maloney S, Skinner E, Haines T, Molloy E, et al. A randomised trial of peer assisted learning in physiotherapy clinical education. J Peer Learn. 2013a;6(1):30–45.

Sevenhuysen S, Nickson W, Farlie MK, Raitman L, Keating JL, Molloy E, et al. The development of a peer assisted learning model for the clinical education of physiotherapy students. J Peer Learn. 2013b;6(1):30–45.

Sevenhuysen S, Farlie MK, Keating JL, Haines TP, Molloy E. Physiotherapy students and clinical educators perceive several ways in which incorporating peer-assisted learning could improve clinical placements: a qualitative study. J Physiother. 2015;61(2):87–92.

Sevenhuysen S, Thorpe J, Molloy E, Keating J, Haines T. Peer-assisted learning in education of allied health professional students in the clinical setting: a systematic review. J Allied Health. 2017;46(1):26–35.

Smith WJ, Bird ML, Vesta KS, Harrison DL, Dennis VC. Integration of an introductory pharmacy practice experience with an advanced pharmacy practice experience in adult internal medicine. Am J Pharm Educ. 2012;76(3):52.

Smith S, Shochet R, Keeley M, Fleming A, Moynahan K. The growth of learning communities in undergraduate medical education. Acad Med. 2014;89(6):928–33.

Stenberg M, Bengtsson M, Mangrio E, Carlson E. Preceptors' experiences of using structured learning activities as part of the peer learning model: a qualitative study. Nurse Educ Pract. 2020;42(November 2019):102668.

Tai J, Sevenhuysen S. The role of peers in developing evaluative judgement. In: Boud D, Ajjawi R, Dawson P, Tai J, editors. Developing evaluative judgement in higher education: assessment for knowing and producing quality work. Milton Park: Routledge; 2018. p. 156–65.

Tai J, Canny BJ, Haines TP, Molloy EK. The role of peer-assisted learning in building evaluative judgement: opportunities in clinical medical education. Adv Heal Sci Educ. 2016a;21(3):659–76.

Tai J, Molloy E, Haines T, Canny B. Same-level peer-assisted learning in medical clinical placements: a narrative systematic review. Med Educ. 2016b;50(4):469–84.

Tai J, Canny BJ, Haines TP, Molloy EK. Implementing peer learning in clinical education: a framework to address challenges in the "real world". Teach Learn Med. 2017;29(2):162–72.

Tai J, Sevenhuysen S, Dawson P. Peer learning in clinical placements. In: Delany C, Molloy E, editors. Learning and teaching in clinical contexts: a practical guide. Sydney: Elsevier; 2018. p. 162–74.

Tawfik SH, Landoll RR, Blackwell LS, Taylor CJ, Hall DL. Supervision of clinical assessment: the multilevel assessment supervision and training (MAST) approach. Clin Superv. 2016;35(1):63–79.

Teherani A, Irby DM, Loeser H. Outcomes of different clerkship models. Acad Med. 2013;88(1):35–43.

Ten Cate O, Durning S. Peer teaching in medical education: twelve reasons to move from theory to practice. Med Teach. 2007;29(6):591–9.

Thistlethwaite JE, Davies D, Ekeocha S, Kidd JM, MacDougall C, Matthews P, et al. The effectiveness of case-based learning in health professional education. A BEME systematic review: BEME guide no. 23. Med Teach. 2012;34(6):e421–44.

Topping KJ, Ehly S. Introduction to peer-assisted learning. In: Topping KJ, Ehly S, editors. Peer-assisted learning. Mahwah: Lawrence Erlbaum Associates Publishers; 1998. p. 1–23.

Vuckovic V, Karlsson K, Sunnqvist C. Preceptors' and nursing students' experiences of peer learning in a psychiatric context: a qualitative study. Nurse Educ Pract. 2019;41(June):102627.

Vygotsky LS. Interaction between learning and development. In: Mind and society. Cambridge, MA: Harvard University Press; 1978. p. 79–91.

Won M-R, Choi Y-J. Undergraduate nursing student mentors' experiences of peer mentoring in Korea: a qualitative analysis. Nurse Educ Today. 2017;51:8–14.

Yu T, Wilson N, Singh P. Medical students-as-teachers: a systematic review of peer-assisted teaching during medical school. Adv Med Educ Pract. 2011;2:157–72.

Simulation for Procedural Skills Teaching and Learning

70

Taylor Sawyer, Lisa Bergman, and Marjorie L. White

Contents

Introduction	1376
Procedural Skills Learning Theory	1377
Characteristics Important in Procedural Skill Learning	1378
Development of Procedural Competency	1379
A Framework for Procedural Skills Teaching	1381
Stage 1: "Learn"	1383
Stage 2: "See"	1384
Stage 3: "Practice"	1384
Stage 4: "Prove"	1386
Stage 5: "Do"	1387
Stage 6: "Maintain"	1387
Barriers to Using Simulation for Procedural Skills Teaching and Learning	1389

T. Sawyer (✉)
Division of Neonatology, Department of Pediatrics, Seattle Children's Hospital, University of Washington School of Medicine, Seattle, WA, USA
e-mail: tlsawyer@uw.edu

L. Bergman
The Office of Interprofessional Simulation for Innovative Clinical Practice, University of Alabama at Birmingham, Birmingham, AL, USA
e-mail: lbergman@uab.edu

M. L. White
The Office of Interprofessional Simulation for Innovative Clinical Practice, University of Alabama at Birmingham, Birmingham, AL, USA

Departments of Pediatric Emergency Medicine and Medical Education School of Medicine, University of Alabama at Birmingham, Birmingham, AL, USA

Department of Health Services Administration School of Health Professions, University of Alabama at Birmingham, Birmingham, AL, USA
e-mail: mlwhite@uab.edu

© Springer Nature Singapore Pte Ltd. 2023
D. Nestel et al. (eds.), *Clinical Education for the Health Professions*,
https://doi.org/10.1007/978-981-15-3344-0_92

Conclusions 1391
Cross-References 1391
References 1392

Abstract

Procedures are a critical part of clinical practice for health professionals. In this chapter, we examine the use of simulation for procedural skills teaching and learning. We start with a review of how technical skills are learned. Next, we examine learner characteristics important in procedural skill acquisition. After that, we review models of procedural competency development. Then, we review a contemporary teaching model for procedural skills teaching consisting of six stages: *learn, see, practice, prove, do,* and *maintain*. We conclude with a review of some barriers to using simulation for procedural skills teaching and learning.

Keywords

Simulation · Technical skills · Procedural skill teaching · Procedural skills learning · Psychomotor skills · Procedural training · Deliberate practice · Mastery learning

Introduction

Procedural skills are a critical part of clinical practice in the health professions. Teaching procedures have been a part of health professions education since its inception (Fulton 1953). Achieving competency with procedures requires knowledge acquisition through teaching and learning and practice. Refining methods to teach health professionals procedural skills is an ongoing challenge (Turner et al. 2007). Instructional approaches must keep pace with contemporary literature on learning and must embrace experiential learning (Kolb 2008). Early methods of procedural skills teaching followed an apprenticeship model, with trainees learning procedures in the clinical environment on patients with coaching from mentors with more clinical experience (Kotsis and Chung 2013; Vozenilek et al. 2004; Lenchus 2010; Rohrich 2006). These methods have come under scrutiny in recent decades due to concerns about patient safety and the ethical implications of using patients as commodities for teaching (Ziv et al. 2006).

Modern methods of procedural skills teaching rely on simulation-based education (Lammers et al. 2008; Wang et al. 2008; Nehring et al. 2001). Simulation-based education is unique because it allows trainees to practice procedural skills in a psychologically safe environment and gain competency without harm to patients. There is a well-documented association between simulation-based procedural teaching with safer patient care and improved patient outcomes (Cook et al. 2011; McGaghie et al. 2011a, b; Schaefer et al. 2011; Zendejas et al. 2013). However, there is still a need for further research into the intricacies of using simulation for psychomotor skill acquisition (Gunberg 2012), and work remains to be done to fully integrate simulation into the organizational context of health professional education and teaching (McGaghie et al. 2010). Additional work is also needed in the area of maintenance of procedural skill competency for expert practitioners, particularly with rarely performed procedures.

In this chapter, we examine the use of simulation for procedural skills teaching and learning. We start with a review of how technical skills are learned. Next, we examine learner characteristics important in procedural skill acquisition. After that, we review models of procedural competency development. Then, we review a contemporary framework for procedural skills teaching that consists of six stages: *learn, see, practice, prove, do,* and *maintain* (Sawyer et al. 2015). We conclude with a review of the barriers to using simulation and some potential ways to overcome these barriers. We hope this chapter will serve as a reference for educators and researchers interested in the use of simulation for procedural skills teaching and learning.

Procedural Skills Learning Theory

Before examining the use of simulation for procedural skills teaching and learning, it is important to understand how procedural skills are learned. One of the most accepted theories of procedural skills learning is Adams' closed-loop theory (Adams 1971, 1987). The closed-loop theory describes a psychomotor feedback loop in which sensory information and perception, obtained while the performance of a motor task, are compared on an ongoing basis to an intended goal or knowledge of results (Adams 1971; Kovacs 1997). In this system, there is automatic correction that takes place in order to align the individual's motor response with the intended goal. Adams conceptually compared his closed-loop theory to a home furnace in which the thermostat setting acts as the intended goal (e.g., knowledge of results) against which the heat output is compared and automatically corrected (Adams 1987). Similarly, as shown Fig. 1, an individual performing a procedure has an intended goal in mind (e.g., knowledge of results) which their motor acts are compared against and corrected in order to successfully complete the procedure.

A key concept of Adams' closed-loop theory is that motor learning is primarily a result of developing the ability to perceive and correct errors. This concept is captured in Adam's axiom *"motor learning is at heart a perceptual process"* (Adams 1987). During the process of learning a new motor skill, the learner must develop the ability to perceive that errors are made in order for learning to take place. This explains how feedback – in the form of error correction – has a critical impact on procedural skills learning. When feedback is provided to a learner, the learner's practice becomes more deliberate through error detection and correction of technique. The concept of directed feedback with the goal of improving performance lies at the foundation of Ericsson's construct of "deliberate practice" (Ericsson 2004). Deliberate practice – when combined with mastery learning – is superior to traditional clinical medical education in achieving specific clinical skill acquisition goals (McGaghie et al. 2011a).

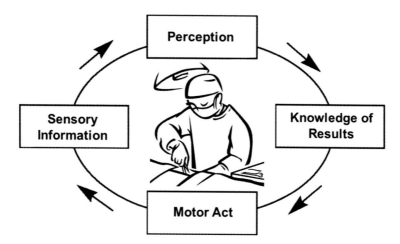

Fig. 1 Adam's closed-loop theory of procedural skills learning. (Figure created by the authors. Open source clip art obtained from http://clipartmag.com/)

Characteristics Important in Procedural Skill Learning

Educators and researchers interested in the use of simulation for procedural skills teaching and learning must be aware of individual characteristics that are important in procedural skill learning. Three characteristics, intrinsic to the learner, have been identified as important in procedural skill acquisition and performance; these include ability, skill, and set (Singer 1972; Harrow 1972; Simpson 1972; Fleishman 1964). Each of these characteristics plays a critical role in an individual's ability to learn and obtain competency with a procedural skill. Given their importance, educators performing procedural skill teaching should have a clear understanding of these learner characteristics. A summary of the three characteristics is provided in Table 1.

Fleishman described an ability as an inherited and intrinsic characteristic that affects movement and the performance of motor tasks (Fleishman 1964). Ability is unique to the individual and difficult to change. Fleishman described 11 different abilities involved in psychomotor tasks, which included: control precision, multi-limb coordination, response orientation, reaction time, rate control, speed of arm movement, manual dexterity, finger dexterity, arm-hand steadiness, wrist-finger speed, and aiming (Fleishman 1964).

In contrast to ability, a skill is a learned capacity to perform a task. Skills, therefore, can be gained through study and teaching (Singer 1972; Harrow 1972). The term *skill* is specific to a given procedure and describes a level of proficiency with that procedure (Singer 1972; Harrow 1972). Skill can be observed and measured. Ability and skills are related, in that ability denotes the inherent propensity to perform procedures and skill describes the level of proficiency to perform a specific procedure, gained after a period of focused teaching and practice.

Table 1 Characteristics important in procedural skill acquisition and performance

Characteristic	Description
Ability	An inherited and intrinsic characteristic that affects movement and the performance of motor tasks
Skill	A learned capacity to perform a task gained through study and teaching
Set	An individual's readiness to act, which includes *mental set, physical set,* and *emotional set*

Set describes an individual's readiness to act (Simpson 1972). Three types of sets have been defined, and include mental set, physical set, and emotional set. A mental set describes an individual's mental state and their unconscious tendency to approach a problem in a particular way in relation to a situation. A physical set describes an individual's physical state, such as heart rate, blood pressure, hand tremors, etc., when confronting a situation. An emotional set describes an individual's emotional state, such as enthusiastic, anxious, scared, etc., when confronting a situation. These sets can be thought of as dispositions that impact a person's performance in a specific situation. When teaching procedural skills, the educator must be cognizant of the mental, physical, and emotional sets of their learners. Educators cannot change these sets directly; however, by changing the environment and context of the learning exercise the educator can optimize their student's sets in order to facilitate learning. For example, educators should appreciate that junior trainees will be nervous about learning a new procedure, especially if their skill is being evaluated. This emotional set will impact their performance.

Using our knowledge of ability, skill, and sets, procedural skill teaching in healthcare should focus on supporting an individual's nascent abilities and work to provide an optimal environment in which to build and develop the individual's skill with the procedures that are needed for clinical care. To optimize student's physical and emotional sets, procedural skill teaching should be done when students are well rested and not distracted by other responsibilities. Additionally, it is important to establish psychologically safe learning environments where the facilitator provides an orientation to the student and provides clear objectives and expectations that students can make mistakes without negative consequences (Rudolph et al. 2014; Turner and Harder 2018; Kang and Min 2019).

Development of Procedural Competency

Before exploring how to use simulation for procedural skills teaching and learning it is important to recognize how competency with procedural skill develops. Several models exist that describe the development of procedural competency. In this section, we will examine two of those models: E. J. Simpson and A. J. Harrow's taxonomy of psychomotor competency and the Dreyfus and Dreyfus five-stage model of skill acquisition. These models provide insight into how individuals develop competency and allow for the classification of learners into different levels along the competency continuum.

E. J. Simpson's taxonomy of the psychomotor domain describes the development of competency with a procedural skill through a continuum of five stages. The stages include guided response, mechanism, complex overt response, adaptation, and origination (Simpson 1972). Guided response indicates the earliest stage in learning a skill and primarily includes imitation and trial and error. *Mechanism* is an intermediate stage wherein learned responses have become habitual and the movements can be performed with some proficiency and confidence. Complex overt response is the stage at which a procedural skill can be performed quickly, accurately, and in a highly coordinated manner requiring a minimum of energy. It is at this stage that performance of a skill has become automatic and can be done without hesitation. In the adaptation stage, skills are so well developed that the individual can modify movement patterns to fit special requirements. Origination is the final step in skill development and describes a phase in which the skill has been mastered to such an extent that new movement patterns can be created to fit a particular situation or unique problem.

The well-known five-stage model of skill acquisition first developed by Dreyfus and Dreyfus and popularized in nursing education by Benner details the development of a learner's scope of vision and range of capabilities along a continuum of stages from novice to advanced beginner, to competent, to proficient, and finally to expert (Dreyfus and Dreyfus 1980; Dreyfus 2004; Benner 1982, 2004). As described by Dreyfus and Dreyfus, the novice must use analytical thinking to solve problems, as they have no practical experience to provide context to the problem. The advanced beginner has some practical experience applying analytical thinking to real situations which enables them to put their experience in context. Competent healthcare professionals rely mostly on past experiences and personal judgment to solve problems, but they can still refer back to analytical processes if needed. Since competent healthcare professionals use personal judgment, they begin to take responsibility for success and failure and develop an emotional investment. This is in contrast to novices and advanced beginners who feel little responsibility and thus lack emotional investment. Dreyfus and Dreyfus theorized that taking responsibility for success and failure and emotional investment fostered a higher level of learning. For proficient healthcare professionals, experiences play an increasingly important role. They start to draw on their emotional experiences from successes and failures to help them focus on and prioritize elements of a situation that are important. Experts reply almost exclusively on experience to arrive at solutions intuitively, rarely using analytical processes, and displaying a high level of responsibility and emotional engagement. According to Dreyfus and Dreyfus, healthcare professionals must draw on their experiences of solving problems in context to reach higher levels of competency. Each time a healthcare professional acquires a new skill in an unrelated domain, they start as a novice where they need to learn the facts and the rules for determining action. As described by Sawyer et al. (2015), the five stages of Simpson and Harrow's taxonomy of the psychomotor domain can be mapped to the five-stage model of skill acquisition described by Dreyfus and Dreyfus (1980). Table 2 provides an outline of this mapping. For more information on competency refer to chapter "The Emergence of Competency-Based Health Professions Education."

Table 2 The development of procedural competency

Level of competency (Dreyfus and Dreyfus 1980)	Descriptions of skills at this level (Simpson 1972)
Novice	Guided response: Skills are learned through imitation and/or trial and error
Advanced beginner	Mechanism: Skills are habitual and movements are performed with some confidence
Competent	Complex overt response: Skills are performed quickly, accurately, and with a high degree of coordination
Proficient	Adaptation: Movement patterns can be modified to address difficult situations
Expert	Originating: New movement patterns can be created to address a unique situation or specific problem

A Framework for Procedural Skills Teaching

To use simulation for procedural skills teaching and learning, it is important to use a standardized **curriculum** framework. Such a framework must comply with the accepted theories of motor learning and competency development discussed above. It must also embrace *experiential learning* as a foundational component (Kolb 2008). As defined by Keeton and Tate (1978), experiential learning is "learning in which the learner is directly in touch with the realities being studied. It is contrasted with the learner who only reads about, hears about, talks about, or writes about these realities but never comes into contact with them as part of the learning process" (p. 2). Many **curriculum** frameworks for teaching procedural skills have been published (Brodsky and Smith 2012; Chiniara et al. 2013; George and Doto 2001; Grantcharov and Reznick 2008; Kneebone 2005, 2009; Kovacs 1997; Lenchus 2010; Motola et al. 2013; Sawyer et al. 2015; Walker and Peyton 1998). Each is unique, but they all share common themes and components. In this section, we will review two of these frameworks: Halsted's "see one, do one, and teach one" framework, and the learn, see, practice, prove, do, and maintain framework proposed by Sawyer et al.

The best-known framework for teaching procedural skills was first proposed by William Stewart Halsted over 100 years ago (Lenchus 2010). Halsted's "see one, do one, teach one" has been widely applied in both surgery and medicine, and is very common approach to teaching procedural skills to physicians in training (Lenchus 2010; Vozenilek et al. 2004). In Halsted's apprenticeship framework, procedural competence is acquired through on-the-job teaching, during the provision of actual clinical care. In the first stage, the trainee watches a senior provider perform a procedure and learns the actions required to perform the procedure through direct observation (see one). After watching the procedure, the trainee is allowed to perform the procedure on a patient with feedback provided by a senior provider (do one). After performing the procedure independently, the trainee then transitions to the teaching role and is tasked with teaching the procedure to others (teach one). While the traditional Halsted mantra is see *one*, do *one*, and teach *one*, some modern interpretations of the framework endorse seeing *many*, doing *many*, teaching *many*, with supervision and learning from the outcomes as important additions. (Rohrich 2006).

The Halsted framework has several positive aspects. First, the framework is highly experiential in nature, and thus embraces experiential learning as a foundational component. The framework also complies with Adams' motor learning theory by providing trainees with mentorship and coaching during procedures in order to ensure they have the correct intended goal in mind (e.g., Adams' "knowledge of results"). In addition, the framework embraces the idea of graduated responsibility, which is the practice of allowing trainees increasing levels of autonomy that culminates in independent practice (Grace et al. 1975). Despite these positive aspects, Halsted's framework has come under scrutiny in recent years due to concerns about patient safety. Critics of the "see one, do one, teach one" framework argue that practice is needed *before* trainees are allowed to perform *the* procedure on patients (Ziv et al. 2006; Cook et al. 2011). Patients express similar concerns, as they fear being "practiced" on (Kotsis and Chung 2013). Therefore, a modern procedural skills teaching curriculum framework needs to embrace the positive aspects of the time-tested Halsted model, but must somehow guarantee a minimum level of competency be developed by the trainee *before* he or she is allowed to perform a procedure on a patient for the first time.

In 2015, Sawyer et al. (2015) outlined a pedagogical framework for procedural skill teaching consisting of six stages. The six stages are: learn, see, practice, prove, do, and maintain (LSPPDM). The LSPPDM framework is based on a critical synthesis review of the literature and was developed as a modern method for procedural skills teaching which overcame the limitations of the Halsted approach. The LSPPDM framework relies on simulation both as an educational technique and as a method of competency assessment. The reliance on simulation stems from the mounting evidence that simulation-based teaching is associated with improved patient care outcomes (Cook et al. 2011; McGaghie et al. 2011a, b; Schaefer et al. 2011; Zendejas et al. 2013). The use of simulation allows for experiential learning and offers the ability to safely develop competency with procedural skills without harming patients (Ziv et al. 2006). The LSPPDM framework requires skills teaching and competency assessment prior to patient care, an experience called "pre-patient" curriculum by Grantcharov and Reznick (2008). The LSPPDM framework also acknowledges the critical importance of continuing to develop competency during patient care and the need for continued practice throughout a career (e.g., lifelong learning). An overview of the LSPPDM framework is presented in Fig. 2. Details on each of the six stages are provided below. Incorporated into the descriptions of each stage of the LSPPD framework are key steps required to teach psychomotor skills described by Nicholls et al. (2016) in their report entitled "Teaching psychomotor skills in the twenty-first century: Revisiting and reviewing instructional approaches through the lens of contemporary literature." The 11 steps outlined by Nicholls et al. are based on contemporary motor learning theory and literature on cognition. They are incorporated here to assist readers in teaching psychomotor skills using the LSPPDM framework.

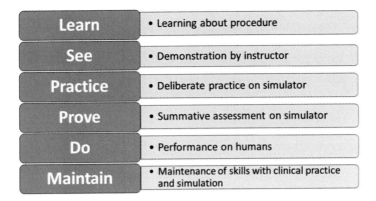

Fig. 2 Learn, see, practice, prove, do, and maintain (LSPPDM) framework for procedural skill teaching. (Figure created by the authors. Adapted from Sawyer et al. (2015))

Stage 1: "Learn"

Learning about the procedure is the first stage of the LSPPDM framework. This step can also be called cognitive conceptualization (Garcia-Rodriguez 2016). In this stage, the trainee learns the technical steps of performing the procedure, as well as the procedure's indications, contraindications, possible complications, patient preparation methods, sterile techniques, and the needs for pain/sedation management during the procedure. While this stage is rudimentary, it is a critical part of teaching procedural skills. Without this stage, the trainee may not fully understand all the steps of the procedure when they move to hands-on practice later in their training. Additionally, without this fundamental knowledge, the learner will not be able to explain accurately the benefits and risks of the procedure to patients.

The *learn* stage can be done using a variety of methods. These include traditional classroom didactic sessions, individual reading, videos, and online modules. At the conclusion of the learning session(s), verification of content knowledge can be performed using multiple choice or fill-in-the-blank exams. Such knowledge testing ensures acquisition of baseline knowledge about the procedure prior to moving to hands-on teaching.

Three of the steps described by Nicholls et al. (2016) can be included in the *learn* stage of the LSPPDM model. These include *identifying learner needs, pre-skill conceptualization*, and *task analysis*. When identifying learning needs, the instructor evaluates the learner's skill and knowledge base in order to focus the skill teaching session (Nicholls et al. 2016). This evaluation could be done in a formal manner using a pretest method or using less formal methods. Using pre-skill conceptualization, the instructor describes all the key information relevant to competent skill execution, taking care to describe what the task should look like, sound like, and feel like in order to establish a sensory norm for the student (Nicholls et al. 2016). Task analysis involves breaking down the task into small "chunks." The specific steps to teach each skill chunk are then itemized and sequenced. Ideally, no more than nine

Table 3 Skill chunks associated with tracheal intubation

1. Position the patient
2. Open the mouth
3. Insert the laryngoscope blade
4. Obtain a view of the vocal cords
5. Advance the endotracheal tube through the vocal cords
6. Check the endotracheal tube depth
7. Secure the endotracheal tube

sequenced steps are covered in any one teaching session (Nicholls et al. 2016). See Table 3 for an example of a skill chunks breakdown for the procedure of tracheal intubation.

Stage 2: "See"

Seeing the procedure performed is the second stage of the LSPPDM framework. As described by Nicholls et al. (2016), this demonstration should include two steps: visualization and verbalization. During visual demonstration, the instructor silently demonstrates the skill with the correct sequence and timing. This provides a visual standard of performance for the learner and allows the learner to get an accurate mental model for performing the entire procedure from start to finish. During verbal demonstration, the instructor repeats the skill demonstration, but this time pauses to describe each skill chunk demonstrated to the learner. During each pause the instructor should explain both correct and incorrect techniques to allow for clearer understanding by the student. After the visual demonstration and before the verbal demonstration, the student should describe all the skill steps to the instructor in the correct sequence. This cognitive strategy is called verbalization execution by Nicholls et al. (2016) and may help to encrypt an error-free motor map for each skill chunk prior to the student engaging in hands-on practice.

The see stage can be done by direct, in-person, demonstration as part of a classroom session, or by using prerecorded educational videos. Virtual or augmented reality are other methods to help learners visualize the relevant anatomy and procedural steps (Sawyer and Gray 2018). Procedural teaching videos used during the see stage are available from a variety of sources including professional organizations, regulatory and governmental bodies, and commercially prepared sources. For institution-specific procedural teaching, producing teaching videos in house may be is an option if resources are available.

Stage 3: "Practice"

Practicing the procedure using simulation is the third stage of the LSPPDM model. In this stage, deliberate practice is used to maximize the educational impact. As defined by Ericsson, *deliberate practice* is a regimen of effortful activity designed to optimize improvements in the acquisition of expert performance (Ericsson 2004). Key factors to move simulation teaching from simple practice to deliberate practice include the identification of well-defined learning objectives, focused and repetitive practice using precise measurements of performance, and the provision of formative feedback (Ericsson 2004). Several reports highlight the benefits of using deliberate practice on both skill acquisition and retention (Kessler et al. 2011; Clapper and Kardong-Edgren 2012; Sawyer et al. 2011). Coaching and mentorship are used heavily at this stage with a focus on sequentially improving procedural skills in specific areas.

Nicholls et al. (2016) identified several steps relevant to the practice stage of the LSPPDM framework. These tips are summarized in Fig. 3. First, Nicholls et al. (2016) recommended that organizing skill practice into multiple, short, practice sessions of 60 min or less is a more effective approach than longer teaching sessions. Second, they suggested that the student verbally describes the skill steps prior to execution – a step they call verbalization performance. This step helps to focus the student's attention on the task, and also improves the creation of mental schema for the skill in the student's motor cortex (Nicholls et al. 2016). Third, they advocated for immediate error correction of all narrated errors during verbalization performance, and all executed errors during simulation-based practice. However, during simulation-based practice, the instructor should limit verbal guidance and coaching.

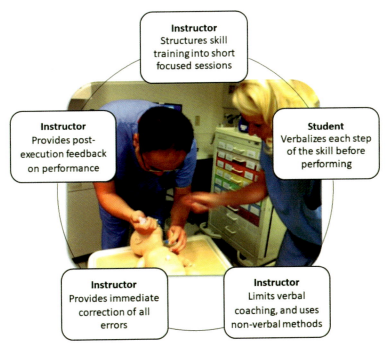

Fig. 3 Important steps in simulation-based practice. (Figure created by the authors)

Verbal feedback should be withheld until the student has completed the task they are practicing. During simulation-based practice, instead of verbal guidance, the instructor should use nonverbal coaching, for example, the instructor uses their hands to correct the student's grip on a piece of equipment, or the instructor manually redirects the student's approach with a needle into the skin. As noted by Nicholls et al. (2016), verbal guidance and coaching during simulation-based teaching are detrimental to skill acquisition for three reasons. First, it takes the learner's focus away from the execution of the task. Second, using verbal guidance may cognitively overload the student's working memory by making the student process multiple domains of information concurrently. Third, the student may become reliant upon verbal coaching and guidance from the instructor to successfully complete the task. Only after the skill has been fully completed should the instructor provide post-skill-execution feedback.

Stage 4: "Prove"

Proving procedural competency on a simulator is the fourth stage of the LSPPDM framework. In this stage, the learner has his/her competency objectively assessed using simulation-based mastery learning (SBML). As defined by McGaghie et al. (2010), SBML includes seven essential characteristics: (1) learning objectives that are clear, (2) an assessment of baseline skill, (3) using a valid assessment tool with a predetermined minimal passing standard, (e.g., "mastery level"), (4) using deliberate practice focused on reaching the mastery level, (5) a test of skill after adequate practice to determine if mastery-level performance has been achieved, (6) additional practice, as needed, until mastery-level performance is achieved, and (7) limiting progression to the next level of teaching until after achievement of the mastery standard with the current task. Research supports the fact that SBML yields better results than traditional clinical education and can lead to improved health for individuals and populations (McGaghie et al. 2011a, b). For more information on SBML refer to ▶ Chap. 28, "Focus on Theory: Emotions and Learning."

Using SBML as an assessment method in the LSPPDM framework ensures that a predefined level of competency (aka "mastery") has been achieved before a student is allowed to attempt a procedure on a patient. The inclusion of a *prove* stage LSPPDM framework sets the curriculum apart from other teaching paradigms (Brodsky and Smith 2012; Chiniara et al. 2013; George and Doto 2001; Grantcharov and Reznick 2008; Kneebone 2005, 2009; Kovacs 1997; Lenchus 2010; Motola et al. 2013; Walker and Peyton 1998). However, the assessment of competency using simulation also increases the challenges in fully implementing the LSPPDM framework (Sawyer and Gray 2018). A specific challenge is the identification, or creation, of valid assessment tools that can be used in this stage of teaching. A full exploration of assessment tool validity and reliability is beyond the scope of this chapter; however, the barrier of using assessment tools is discussed briefly in the next section. Additionally, for more information on performance assessment see ▶ Chap. 60, "Measuring Attitudes: Current Practices in Health Professional Education."

Stage 5: "Do"

Doing a procedure on a patient is the fifth stage of the LSPPDM model. In this stage of procedural skill teaching, the teaching moves from the "pre-patient" curriculum, as defined by Grantcharov and Reznick (2008), to actual patient care. By delaying the performance of procedures on patients until after competency has been proven on a simulator in the *prove* stage, the LSPPDM framework serves as a patient-safety mechanism. In this stage, when the trainee performs the procedure, they are initially under direct supervision by a more experienced practitioner. During these supervised procedures, feedback and coaching are provided using the same basic techniques used in the practice stage (Fig. 3). This type of direct observation during clinical care is commonly known as "workplace-based assessments" or "supervised learning events" (Beard 2011; Ali 2013). It is important to remember that these workplace-based assessments are assessments *for learning*, rather than as assessments *of learning*, and thus are formative, rather than summative. For more information on workplace-based assessments refer to ▶ Chap. 64, "Workplace-Based Assessment in Clinical Practice"

Creating a clinical care environment, where supervised practice and formative assessment of procedural skills can occur in a way that ensures patient safety, is an important aspect of this stage of procedural skills teaching. An example of such an environment is a medical procedure service, where medical trainees can get individualized one-on-one teaching in procedures (Huang et al. 2009; Lenhard et al. 2008; Smith et al. 2004). Evidence suggests that the use of dedicated medical procedure services improves the knowledge, confidence, and experience of trainees, and is also associated with higher levels of patient satisfaction with bedside procedures (Mourad et al. 2011; Mourad et al. 2012). Adequate supervision of trainees on a medical procedure service is critical and should be provided by an attending physician, or other experienced healthcare provider, as opposed another trainee (Mourad 2010; Huang et al. 2006). Most healthcare institutions implement organized preceptorships or residencies to facilitate supervision of procedural skills for onboarding healthcare professionals of all kinds. Over time, as the trainee's skill and competency improve, less supervision is needed to ensure safe patient care, and so the supervisor can gradually decrease the amount of supervision provided. This natural evolution toward less supervision during patient care in the setting of medical education is called "graduated patient responsibility" (Grace et al. 1975). Graduated responsibility allows the trainee increasing levels of autonomy while performing procedures that culminate in independent practice and the conclusion of teaching.

Stage 6: "Maintain"

The final stage of the LSPPDM framework is maintaining procedural competency. This stage starts at the end of teaching and continues for the rest of a healthcare professional's career. The inclusion of this *maintain* stage into the LSPPDM framework acknowledges the fact that all skills are perishable and will degrade with time if not regularly practiced. This gradual loss of skills resulting from infrequent practice has been called "de-skilling" (Levitt 2001). The rate of de-skilling varies based on individual factors (e.g., abilities and skill) and the frequency with which procedures are performed. In general, de-skilling occurs rapidly in healthcare professionals who are novices or advanced beginners and less rapidly in healthcare professionals who are competent, proficient, or experts. However, skill degradation curves, based on learner competency, procedure type, and duration of time without practice, have yet to be developed (Jackson et al. 1993). Thus, a proactive and individualized approach to skills maintenance is needed (Grantcharov and Reznick 2008).

In the *maintain* stage, healthcare professionals supplement their clinical practice experiences with simulation to ensure that competency with the procedures critical for their profession is maintained. Simulation is the only feasible method to practice procedures for those practitioners who do not perform procedures on a regular basis in clinical care, or who have long gaps in clinical time (Kneebone 2004). In the past, various terms have used to describe the intentions and ways that simulation-based teaching could be done to maintain skills. Recently, however, Sullivan et al. (2019) proposed a standardized nomenclature and framework for simulation strategies used to obtain, maintain, or regain skills. The three types of simulation-based teaching used to preserve procedural competency as proposed by Sullivan et al. are "maintenance," "booster," and "refresher" (Fig. 4).

In maintenance teaching, skill deterioration is prevented through low-dose high-frequency (LDHF) simulation teaching (Sawyer and Strandjord 2014). When skills

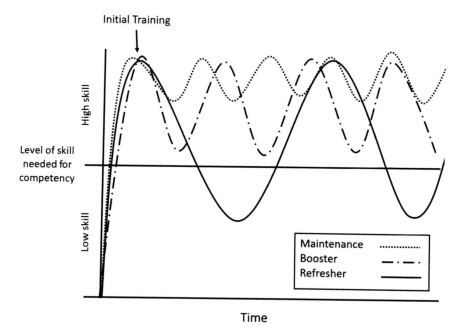

Fig. 4 Maintenance, booster, and refresher teaching. (Adapted from Sullivan et al. (2019))

have begun to wane, booster teaching is used. Booster teaching occurs less frequently than maintenance teaching and involves a higher level of intensity to overcome the decay in skill that has occurred (Matterson et al. 2018). Refresher teaching is aimed at reestablishing skill levels after procedural competency has dropped to unsatisfactory levels (Niles et al. 2009). Refresher teaching is higher in intensity than both maintenance and booster teaching (Sullivan et al. 2019).

The LSPPDM framework can be used for maintenance teaching, booster teaching, and refresher teaching. For maintenance teaching, the learner is evaluated by a trained simulation facilitator on their performance of the procedural skill in the simulated environment as in the prove stage. If the learner is able to meet the previously established benchmark of competency, they can proceed to the do stage, where they perform the procedure in the clinical environment under supervision. If they are unable to attain this benchmark, they are prescribed deliberate practice as the novice learner did in the practice stage, with the expectation of a repeat assessment (prove) before proceeding to the clinical environment (do). For booster teaching, because the skill has degraded further, the learner should refresh their cognitive understanding of the procedure by repeating the learn/see stages first, then proceeding through the framework as described for maintenance training. For refresher training, because it is established that the skill has degraded below the level of competency, the learner should complete the entire LSPPDM procedural skills teaching curriculum as if they were a novice to ensure that they refresh both their cognitive understanding and psychomotor skill (Sawyer et al. 2015).

The use of simulation to maintain procedural competency has been embraced by national regulatory bodies and medical boards. The American Board of Anesthesiology's current maintenance of certification process uses simulation-based practice to satisfy the Maintenance of Certification in Anesthesia (MOCA) 2.0® Part 4: Quality Improvement Requirements (Steadman and Huang 2012). Other health profession specialties are also investigating the use of simulation-based teaching for maintenance of certification (Steadman and Huang 2012). For more information on maintenance of certification refer to chapter "Certification and Revalidation for Health Professions Practice."

Barriers to Using Simulation for Procedural Skills Teaching and Learning

There are a number of barriers to using simulation for procedural skills teaching and learning, especially when using a rigorous curriculum framework like LSPPDM. Some of these barriers include the availability of trained faculty able to teach procedural skills, access to space and equipment needed to perform the teaching, and the availability of assessment tools with evidence of both validity and reliability. In this section, we review these barriers and offer some potential solutions.

One of the key barriers to procedural skills teaching is the lack of faculty or clinical educators who are competent in specific procedural skills and available to provide teaching to trainees, students, and onboarding healthcare professionals

(Norris et al. 1997). This barrier is particularly challenging in small institutions; however, it is sometimes an issue in larger institutions as well. One potential method to overcome this barrier is to implement a train-the-trainer model by conducting simulation-based procedural skills teaching for faculty and clinical educators to train them how to teach others using simulation-based procedural training. Such teaching would ideally use the same methods as the first four stages of the LSPPDM framework: *learn, see, practice,* and *prove*. Requiring facilitators of simulation-based procedural teaching to proceed through these four steps has a few potential advantages. First, it ensures that facilitators have a shared experience of going through the same curriculum their learners will experience. Second, it ensures that all facilitators have proven their procedural competency prior to teaching others. Providing faculty and clinical educators with adequate time to teach procedural skills to others can be a challenge. As previously discussed, establishing dedicated medical procedure services for trainees where faculty have protected clinical time to focus on teaching procedures is one potential solution (Mourad et al. 2011, 2012). Additional solutions include providing simulation training to clinical educators and building procedural simulation activities into institutional onboarding activities for health professionals.

Access to space and equipment needed to perform simulation-based teaching can be a significant barrier. If large group teaching is done with a number of procedures, then a large space is needed to accommodate the teaching. Finding enough task trainers and manikins to use during these teaching sessions can be challenging, depending on local resources. Access to necessary medical equipment, such as needles, syringes, chest tubes, laryngoscopes, endoscopes, etc. can pose an additional challenge. Today, many hospitals have onsite simulation programs (Rutherford-Hemming and Alfas 2017) that can be leveraged for use during simulation-based procedural skills teaching. If the simulation space is limited, other spaces can be used since procedural skills teaching can often be done in a conference room. Additional costs are embedded in the specialized kits needed for procedures and for assuring a level of fidelity in the training. Partnerships with supply chain (for expired kits) and/or suppliers may allow for efficient use of materials in training sessions. For those hospitals without a simulation program the "up-front" costs of space allocation and equipment acquisition for procedural teaching can be high (Norris et al. 1997). If faced with this challenge, educators may be able to negotiate for space and equipment based on evidence showing cost savings to organizations that use simulation to teach procedural skills. As reported by Cohen et al. (2010), an SBML central venous catheter insertion program that costs $112,000 in faculty time and equipment resulted in the prevention of ten central-venous-catheter-related bloodstream infections (CRBSIs). Each CRBSI occurrence prevented saved the institution approximately US$82,000 (Cohen et al. 2010). Thus, the teaching resulted in a net savings of approximately US$700,000, or a 7 to 1 return on investment. Such cost savings evidence can be a powerful tool when negotiating for institutional resources.

As discussed in the prior section, a barrier to using the LSPPDM framework for procedural skills teaching is the identification, or creation, or assessment tool that can be used in the *prove* stage of teaching. To be useful as part of the LSPPDM framework, these assessment tools must have strong evidence of both validity and reliability. References are available that clearly describe the methods used to determine the validity and reliability of assessment tools (Downing 2003; Downing 2004; Cook and Beckman 2006). Assessment tools used to determine procedural competency most commonly take the form of checklists and global rating scales (Lammers et al. 2008). Both of these formats have their own pros and cons. Several assessment tools are available for educators to use, and some have had their psychometric properties reviewed (Jelovsek et al. 2013; Ahmed et al. 2011). Good examples of how to develop and perform validation testing on novel assessment tools are also available (Johnston et al. 2019). Although the process of finding, or developing, and assessment tools can be rigorous, it is not insurmountable.

Conclusions

In this chapter, we examined the use of simulation for procedural skills teaching and learning. We began with a review of how technical skills are learned. Then, we examined learner characteristics important in procedural skill acquisition. Next, we reviewed models of procedural competency development. After that we took the time to review a contemporary framework for procedural skills teaching consisting of six stages – *learn, see, practice, prove, do*, and *maintain* – and we examined each stage in detail. Finally, we concluded with a review of potential barriers to using simulation for procedural skills teaching and learning and explored some potential ways to overcome these barriers. For educators interested in the use of simulation for procedural skills teaching, this chapter should serve as an important reference on teaching methods. For researchers on psychomotor skill acquisition in healthcare, this chapter should provide insight into areas for future research.

Cross-References

- ▶ Coaching in Health Professions Education: The Case of Surgery
- ▶ Developing Patient Safety Through Education
- ▶ Focus on Theory: Emotions and Learning
- ▶ Learning and Teaching in Clinical Settings: Expert Commentary from an Interprofessional Perspective
- ▶ Learning and Teaching in the Operating Theatre: Expert Commentary from the Nursing Perspective
- ▶ Supporting the Development of Professionalism in the Education of Health Professionals
- ▶ Teaching Simple and Complex Psychomotor Skills

References

Adams JA. A closed-loop theory of motor learning. J Mot Behav. 1971;3:111–49.

Adams JA. A historical review and appraisal of research on the learning, retention and transfer of human motor skills. Psychol Bull. 1987;101:41–7.

Ahmed K, Miskovic D, Darzi A, Athanasiou T, Hanna GB. Observational tools for assessment of procedural skills: a systematic review. Am J Surg. 2011;202(4):469–80.

Ali JM. Getting lost in translation? Workplace based assessments in surgical training. Surgeon. 2013;11(5):286–9.

Beard J. Workplace-based assessment: the need for continued evaluation and refinement. Surgeon. 2011;9(Suppl 1):S12–3.

Benner P. From novice to expert. Am J Nurs. 1982;82(3):402–7.

Benner P. Using the Dreyfus model of skill acquisition to describe and interpret skill acquisition and clinical judgment in nursing practice and education. Bull Sci Technol Soc. 2004;24(3):188–99.

Brodsky D, Smith C. A structured approach to teaching medical procedures. NeoReviews. 2012;13(11):e635–41.

Chiniara G, Cole G, Brisbin K, Huffman D, Cragg B, Lamacchia M, Norman D, Canadian Network for Simulation in Healthcare, Guidelines Working Group. Simulation in healthcare: a taxonomy and a conceptual framework for instructional design and media selection. Med Teach. 2013;35:e1380–95.

Clapper T, Kardong-Edgren S. Using deliberate practice and simulation to improve nursing skills. Clin Simul Nurs. 2012;8(3):e109–13.

Cohen ER, Feinglass J, Barsuk JH, Barnard C, O'Donnell A, McGaghie WC, Wayne DB. Cost savings from reduced catheter-related bloodstream infection after simulation-based education for residents in a medical intensive care unit. Simul Healthc. 2010;5(2):98–102.

Cook D, Beckman T. Current concepts in validity and reliability for psychomotor instruments: theory and application. Am J Med. 2006;119(116):e7–e16.

Cook DA, Hatala R, Brydges R, Zendejas B, Szostek JH, Wang AT, et al. Technology-enhanced simulation for health professions education: a systematic review and meta-analysis. JAMA. 2011;306(9):978–88.

Downing S. Validity: on the meaningful interpretation of assessment data. Med Educ. 2003;37:830–7.

Downing S. Reliability: on the reproducibility of assessment data. Med Educ. 2004;38:1006–12.

Dreyfus S. The five-stage model of adult skills acquisition. Bull Sci Technol Soc. 2004;24(3):177–9.

Dreyfus SE, Dreyfus HL. A five-stage model of the mental activities involved in directed skill acquisition. Berkeley: Operations Research Center, University of California. 1980. https://doi.org/10.21236/ada084551.

Ericsson KA. Deliberate practice and the acquisition and maintenance of expert performance in medicine and related domains. Acad Med. 2004;79(10 Suppl):S70–81.

Fleishman EA. The structure and measurement of physical fitness. Englewood Cliffs: Prentice-Hall; 1964.

Fulton J. History of medical education. Br Med J. 1953;2:457.

Garcia-Rodriguez JA. Teaching medical procedures at your workplace. Can Fam Physician. 2016;62(4):351–4.

George J, Doto F. A simple five-step method for teaching clinical skills. Fam Med. 2001;33(8):577–8.

Grace WJ, Sarg M, Jahre J, Greenbaum D. Graduated patient responsibility. JAMA. 1975;231(4):351.

Grantcharov T, Reznick R. Teaching procedural skills. Br Med J. 2008;336(7653):1129–31.

Gunberg RJ. Simulation and psychomotor skill acquisition: a review of the literature. Clin Simul Nurs. 2012;8:e429–35.

Harrow AJ. A taxonomy of the psychomotor domain. New York: David McKay; 1972. p. 14–31.

Huang GC, Smith CC, Gordon CE, et al. Beyond the comfort zone: residents assess their comfort performing inpatient medical procedures. Am J Med. 2006;119(1):71.e17–24.

Huang GC, Smith CC, York M, Weingart SN. Asking for help: internal medicine residents' use of a medical procedure service. J Hosp Med. 2009;4(7):404–9.

Jackson WD, Diamond MR, Jackson DJ. Procedural medicine. Is your number up? Aust Fam Physician. 1993;22(9):1633–6.

Jelovsek J, Kow N, Diawadkear G. Tools for the direct observation and assessment of psychomotor skills in medical trainees: a systematic review. Med Educ. 2013;47(7):650–73.

Johnston L, Sawyer T, Nishisaki A, Whtifill T, Ades A, French H, Glass K, Dadiz R, Bruno C, Levit O, Gangadharan S, Zhong J, Scherzer D, Arnold J, Stavroudis T, Auerbach M. Neonatal intubation competency assessment tool: development and validation. Acad Pediatr. 2019;19(2):157–64.

Kang SJ, Min HY. Psychological safety in nursing simulation. Nurse Educ. 2019;44(2):e6–9.

Keeton M, Tate P, editors. Learning by experience – what, why, how. San Francisco: Jossey-Bass; 1978.

Kessler DO, Auerbach M, Pusic M, Tunik MG, Foltin JC. A randomized trial of simulation-based deliberate practice for infant lumbar puncture skills. Simul Healthc. 2011;6(4):197–203.

Kneebone R. Evaluating clinical simulations for learning procedural skills: a theory-based approach. Acad Med. 2005;80:549–53.

Kneebone R. Practice, rehearsal, and performance: an approach for simulation-based surgical and procedural teaching. JAMA. 2009;23(30):1336–8.

Kolb DA. Experiential learning: experience as the source of learning and development. Englewood Cliffs: Prentice-Hall; 2008.

Kotsis SV, Chung KC. Application of the "see one, do one, teach one" concept in surgical teaching. Plast Reconstr Surg. 2013;131(5):1194–201.

Kovacs G. Procedural skills in medicine: linking theory to practice. J Emerg Med. 1997;15(3):387–91.

Lammers R, Davenport M, Korley F, et al. Teaching and assessing procedural skills using simulation: metrics and methodology. Acad Emerg Med. 2008;15:1079–87.

Lenchus JD. End of the "see one, do one, teach one" era: the next generation of invasive bedside procedural instruction. J Am Osteopath Assoc. 2010;110(6):340–6.

Lenhard A, Moallem M, Marrie RA, Becker J, Garland A. An intervention to improve procedure education for internal medicine residents. J Gen Intern Med. 2008;23(3):288–93.

Levitt LK. Use it or lose it: is de-skilling evidence-based? Rural Remote Health. 2001;1(1):81.

Matterson HH, Szyld D, Green BR, Howell HB, Pusic MV, Mally PV, Bailey SM. Neonatal resuscitation experience curves: simulation based mastery learning booster sessions and skill decay patterns among pediatric residents. J Perinat Med. 2018;46(8):934–41.

McGaghie WC, Issenberg SB, Petrusa ER, Scalese RJ. A critical review of simulation-based medical education research: 2003–2009. Med Educ. 2010;44(1):50–63.

McGaghie W, Issenberg B, Cohen E, Barsuk J, Wayne D. Does simulation-based medical education with deliberate practice yield better results than traditional clinical education? A meta-analytic comparative review of the evidence. Acad Med. 2011a;86(6):706–11.

McGaghie WC, Issenberg SB, Cohen ER, Barsuk JH, Wayne DB. Medical education featuring mastery learning with deliberate practice can lead to better health for individuals and populations. Acad Med. 2011b;86(11):e8–9.

Motola I, Devine LA, Chung HS, Sullivan JE, Issenberg SB. Simulation in healthcare education: a best evidence practical guide. AMEE guide no. 82. Med Teach. 2013;35:e1511–30.

Mourad M, Kohlwes J, Maselli J, MERN Group, Auerbach AD. Supervising the supervisors – procedural training and supervision in internal medicine residency. J Gen Intern Med. 2010;25(4):351–6.

Mourad M, Auerbach AD, Maselli J, Sliwka D. Patient satisfaction with a hospitalist procedure service: is bedside procedure teaching reassuring to patients? J Hosp Med. 2011;6(4):219–24.

Mourad M, Ranji S, Sliwka D. A randomized controlled trial of the impact of a teaching procedure service on the training of internal medicine residents. J Grad Med Educ. 2012;4(2):170–5.

Nehring WM, Ellias WE, Lashley FR. Human patient simulators in nursing education: an overview. Simul Gaming. 2001;32(2):194–204.

Nicholls D, Sweet L, Muller A, Hyett J. Teaching psychomotor skills in the twenty-first century: revisiting and reviewing instructional approaches through the lens of contemporary literature. Med Teach. 2016;38(10):1056–63.

Niles D, Sutton RM, Donoghue A, Kalsi MS, Roberts K, Boyle L, Nishisaki A, Arbogast KB, Helfaer M, Nadkarni V. "Rolling Refreshers": a novel approach to maintain CPR psychomotor skill competence. Resuscitation. 2009;80(8):909–12.

Norris T, Cullison S, Fihn S. Teaching procedural skills. J Gen Intern Med. 1997;12(Suppl 2):S64–70.

Rohrich RJ. "See one, do one, teach one": an old adage with a new twist. Plast Reconstr Surg. 2006;118:257–8.

Rudolph JW, Raemer DB, Simon R. Establishing a safe container for learning in simulation: the role of the presimulation briefing. Simul Healthc. 2014;9(6):339–49.

Rutherford-Hemming T, Alfas CM. The use of hospital-based simulation in nursing education: a systematic review. Clin Simul Nurs. 2017;13(2):78–89.

Sawyer T, Gray M. Simulation-based procedural skill teaching. Intern Med Rev. 2018; https://doi.org/10.18103/imr.v4i9.760.

Sawyer T, Strandjord T. Simulation-based procedural skills maintenance training for neonatal–perinatal medicine faculty. Cureus. 2014;6(4):e173.

Sawyer T, Sierocka-Castaneda A, Chan D, Berg B, Lustik M, Thompson M. Deliberate practice using simulation improves neonatal resuscitation performance. Simul Healthc. 2011;6(6):327–36.

Sawyer T, White M, Zaveri P, Chang T, Ades A, French H, et al. Learn, see, practice, prove, do, maintain: an evidence-based pedagogical framework for procedural skill teaching in medicine. Acad Med. 2015;90(8):1025–33.

Schaefer J, Venderbilt A, Cason C, Bauman E, Glavin R, Lee F, Navedo D. Literature review: instructional design and pedagogy science in healthcare simulation. Simul Healthc. 2011;6(7):S30–41.

Simpson E. The classification of educational objectives in the psychomotor domain: the psychomotor domain, vol. 3. Washington, DC: Gryphon House; 1972.

Singer RN. The psychomotor domain: movement behaviors. Philadelphia: Lea & Febigor; 1972. p. 385–414.

Smith CC, Gordon CE, Feller-Kopman D, et al. Creation of an innovative inpatient medical procedure service and a method to evaluate house staff competency. J Gen Intern Med. 2004;19(5 Pt 2):510–3.

Steadman RH, Huang YM. Simulation for quality assurance in training, credentialing and maintenance of certification. Best Pract Res Clin Anaesthesiol. 2012;26(1):3–15.

Sullivan A, Elshenawy S, Ades A, Sawyer T. Acquiring and maintaining technical skills using simulation: initial, maintenance, booster, and refresher training. Cureus. 2019;11(9):e5729.

Turner S, Harder N. Psychological safe environment: a concept analysis. Clin Simul Nurs. 2018;18: 47–55.

Turner SR, Hanson J, de Gara CJ. Procedural skills: what's taught in medical school, what ought to be? Educ Health. 2007;20(1):9.

Vozenilek J, Huff JS, Reznek M, Gordon JA. See one, do one, teach one: advanced technology in medical education. Acad Emerg Med. 2004;11:1149–54.

Walker M, Peyton JWR. Teaching in theatre. In: Teaching and learning in medical practice. Rickmansworth: Manticore Europe; 1998. p. 171–80.

Wang E, Quinones J, Fithc M, et al. Developing technical expertise in emergency medicine – the role of simulation in procedural skill acquisition. Acad Emerg Med. 2008;15:1046–57.

Zendejas B, Brydges R, Wang AT, Cook DA. Patient outcomes in simulation-based medical education: a systematic review. J Gen Intern Med. 2013;28(8):1078–89.

Ziv A, Wolpe PR, Small SD, Glick S. Simulation-based medical education: an ethical imperative. Simul Healthc. 2006;1(4):252–6.

Simulation for Clinical Skills in Healthcare Education

71

Guillaume Alinier, Ahmed Labib Shehatta, and Ratna Makker

Contents

Introduction	1396
Background	1397
Education in the Healthcare Context	1399
Teaching and Learning Strategies	1400
The Importance of Developing Clinical Skills	1403
Foundation of Clinical Skills	1404
Acquisition of Knowledge	1406
Using Simulation to Prepare for Real-World Situations	1406
Other Benefits of Simulation	1408
Conclusion	1410
Cross-References	1411
References	1411

G. Alinier (✉)
Hamad Medical Corporation Ambulance Service, Doha, Qatar

School of Health and Social Work, University of Hertfordshire, Hatfield, UK

Weill Cornell Medicine Qatar, Doha, Qatar

Faculty of Health and Life Sciences, Northumbria University, Newcastle upon Tyne, UK
e-mail: g.alinier@herts.ac.uk; galinier@hamad.qa

A. L. Shehatta
Medical Intensive Care Unit, Hamad General Hospital, Hamad Medical Corporation, Doha, Qatar

Clinical Anaesthesiology, Weill Cornell Medicine, Qatar, Doha, Qatar
e-mail: ashehatta@hamad.qa

R. Makker
Consultant Anaesthetist, Clinical Tutor, Clinical Director of the WISER (West Herts Initiative in Simulation Education and Research), West Herts Hospitals NHS Trust, Watford, Hertfordshire, UK
e-mail: Ratna.Makker@whht.nhs.uk

© Springer Nature Singapore Pte Ltd. 2023
D. Nestel et al. (eds.), *Clinical Education for the Health Professions*,
https://doi.org/10.1007/978-981-15-3344-0_93

Abstract

Patients are heavily reliant on healthcare providers being knowledgeable and highly competent in a broad range of skills underpinned by sound knowledge. Some of these skills can be very specific, while others are rather general and may apply in combination or in parallel to others. The founding step to providing safe and effective patient care and working collaboratively with the wider clinical team lies in the acquisition of such skills. For learning to be imprinted in memory and then translated into performance, multiple factors come into play, such as the learners, the educators, the teaching methods, and the environment. The process is not the same for everyone, but some key educational principles prevail and some contribute to a better and faster assimilation of those skills. Simulation in particular, of which a broad range of modalities exist, and which are sometimes supported by more or less complex technology, is a particularly interesting approach as it promotes learner engagement, demonstration of competence, collaboration, and reflection. Simulation, in its various forms, has become a key element of the competency-based frameworks increasingly adopted in the educational process of healthcare learners and professionals. Its key aspects are that it is transformative for learners as it contributes to changing their mental frames and behaviors, helps them to assimilate new knowledge and skills, and promotes collaboration and reflection. The latter point is particularly important for non-procedural clinical skills and can be promoted through structured feedback or debriefing phase following each simulation-based activity.

Keywords

Clinical skills · Competency · Practical · Assessment · Communication · Nontechnical skills

Introduction

Healthcare education, in the broadest sense of the term, exists to ensure clinicians continue to acquire, maintain, and improve their skills throughout their careers. With scientific and technological developments, higher patient expectations, and medico-legal legislation, healthcare practitioners are required more than ever to acquire and maintain skills and knowledge. Patients are heavily reliant on them being knowledgeable and highly competent in a broad range of skills underpinned by sound knowledge and professionalism. This repertoire of skills will vary to some degrees between professions and specialties, but the generally accepted commonalities relate to providing effective, high quality, compassionate, safe, and person care. As such, human factors play a critical role in the foundation of a healthcare provider's knowledge and skills and how they will interact with their peers, their patients, and their environment. Healthcare providers are professionals who have qualified by undertaking a staged developmental process that aimed to equip them in an effective manner with the minimum expected knowledge and skills required for their function. Then comes their individual responsibility, often mandated by a professional body to retain their license to practice, to undergo continuing professional development (CPD) on a regular and ongoing basis to ensure that their knowledge and skills are at the required level and updated with the latest evidence-based clinical practices. Clinical skills acquired by healthcare professionals are the heart of proper methodical patient care. They are discrete observable acts within the context of aggregate patient care that may determine the outcome for the patient. Poor clinical skills can influence outcomes significantly. Healthcare is after all a high stake, high risk, often time pressured, and cost constrained industry where patients are very vulnerable. Then there is the challenge of unprecedented media scrutiny. Ironically, the most critically ill patients are often seen first of all by the most junior doctors within the system. Newly qualified practitioners have to learn, but nobody wants a novice practitioner learning on their loved ones, especially when they are unwell. Simulation can be a forgiving answer to these challenges.

Modern health care systems have shifted from mainly individual-based knowledge and skills to a team-based effort and service delivery. A challenge for educators is to deliver effective interdisciplinary team development that meets everyone's needs. Indeed, clinicians must now be prepared to teach and learn across several disciplines, not just within their own profession (Peyton 1998). As such, the increasing scale of information and competencies required from them with limited time availability and financial support for CPD becomes an issue. Rethans and colleagues (2002) argued that progression from theoretical knowledge acquisition to practical skills application, specifically transition from cognitive awareness to behavioral change in real life, is neither straight forward nor linear. The behavior and attitude of healthcare practitioners is influenced by a number of factors which may be individual (e.g., meeting patient expectations) or systemic factors (e.g., government initiatives, medico-legal laws). This chapter concentrates on the acquisition of nonprocedural clinical skills using simulation as an educational approach.

Background

Until recently, the teaching and learning of clinical skills invariably occurred by observation at the patient's bedside or other clinical areas, reinforced by didactic lectures or tutorials. This "apprenticeship model" allowed direct observation and performance of skills overseen by senior clinicians. Historically, a Halstedian adage paved the way for medical education and had become acceptable for many if not all skills. In 1904, Dr. Halsted, a pioneering surgeon proposed the "see one, do one, teach one" approach to medical education (Rodriguez-Paz et al. 2009). Obviously this has several limitations as learners assimilate knowledge and skills at different paces, and not all will attain the required knowledge, skill, and attitude by adopting this approach (McGaghie et al. 2011). However, the patient perspective was neglected to some extent. Skills were taught to novices, beginners, and not so advanced students while the patients accepted being used as experimental models.

The communication and consent issues were disregarded at worst and referred to fleetingly at best, but it is now clearly and rightfully seen as a moral obligation that directly concerns the patients and is ethically mandated (LaRosa and Grant-Kels 2016).

Another aspect to consider is that of "talent," which is a natural endowment or ability of a superior performance in a specific domain (Ericsson 2004). Skills can also be transmitted from one person to another, whereas a talent cannot be taught or transferred as it is part of someone's nature. Thus, it is constant and enduring. Skills in contrast are acquired and nurtured through an educational process and exposure through repetition which provides experience and helps an individual to evolve from novice to master (Buja 2019). The process of mastering a skill takes time and is usually supported by guidance or coaching and the acquisition of good knowledge foundations. As such, a person can learn how to hold a golf club, build a house, write a sentence, or do arithmetic. On the other hand, a talent is based on high natural abilities, innate giftedness, that needs little or no knowledge or effort to maintain, but can still be improved by engaging in deliberate practice to achieve deeper learning (Ericsson 2004). Irrespective of the approach used, such learning process is not linear (Aldrich 2003).

The past 20 years has seen a changing clinical environment and working practices. In 1998, the introduction of a restriction for doctors to a 48-hour working week as a health and safety legislation initiative, known as the European Working Time Directive (EWTD), impacted how nursing services are coordinated (Barton and Mashlan 2011). In fact, the EWTD resulted in developments in nursing roles such as prescribing, nurse led night teams, patient assessments, and nurse educator roles. The shorter working week with reduced opportunities for training, especially in craft specialties such as surgery and acute medicine, and shift systems, has led to the demise of the apprenticeship model in favor of a more structured model focusing on the acquisition of key competencies (Mahesh et al. 2014; Breen et al. 2013). These competencies are then formally tested through high stake examinations such as Objective Structured Clinical Examination (OSCE) (Yune et al. 2018). Such tests need environments that recreate authentic clinical contexts within a *"circle of focus"* (Kneebone 2010) for learners to realistically demonstrate their level of competence (Brightwell and Grant 2013; Houghton et al. 2012). The environmental elements outside the circle of focus are less important to achieving the learning objectives of interest. If competencies are tested too much in isolation of one another, there is an inherent risk of learners never being properly equipped to work competently in the real clinical environment as they may not demonstrate synthesis of competencies. Similarly, if assessments are primarily based on multiple choice questionnaires (MCQ), then it is likely that learners will only focus on the knowledge aspect of skills. However, if an assessment system uses terms such as "demonstrate" or "perform" (linked to OSCEs), then they will be directed towards developing procedural competencies (Boursicot 2010).

For learners to acquire the required experience, while the apprenticeship model is disappearing, has led to the development of alternative training solutions. For experiential learning to still occur, clinical skills laboratories and simulation centers have been created throughout the world (Alinier 2007a; Bradley and Postlethwaite 2003; Riley et al. 2003; Shafiq et al. 2017; Boker 2013). Such facilities are very useful in preparing learners for the real-life clinical environment as long as there is consistency in the way things are done between both settings (Houghton et al. 2013). There is overarching evidence for the success of simulation as an educational modality as it can be supported by a diverse range of tools ranging from part-task trainers, computer-controlled mannequins, virtual-reality and screen-based simulators, augmented and mixed reality solutions, and simulated patients (Alinier 2007b; Chiniara et al. 2013). Simulation technology is advancing rapidly and the sophistication and level of fidelity is increasing; however, the emphasis is sometimes to the detriment of focusing on the educational quality and content of training interventions. Several authors, more or less explicitly, ask for a paradigm shift from technology to learning (Salas et al. 1998; Alinier et al. 2015; Kyaw Tun et al. 2015). They want a learner-centric approach that is holistic and not detracted by the obsession with realism where it may not bring real educationally enriching benefits. This is because the simulation heuristic is mostly derived after the simulated event when the actions are examined, decisions leading to them are explored, and the frame that led to the decision is dissected. Thus, excellence in simulation-based education (SBE) stems often from the postsimulation analysis phase, commonly called debriefing, involving an experienced facilitator guiding learners' reflections (Oriot and Alinier 2018) and not necessarily from the act of participating in the simulation activity itself (Lai et al. 2016).

Education in the Healthcare Context

In the education sector, over the past three to four decades, novel concepts of adult learning and different theories of education have been introduced (e.g., Knowles' Andragogy, self-directed, and transformational learning) (Knowles 1980, 1984; Merriam 2001, 2004). There has been a growing epistemological shift from a teacher-centered model to a learner-centered approach. This is coupled with a transition from the "teacher is the expert," typically seen in didactic, lecture-based, teaching activities to a concept of "educators are the facilitators." Hereby, educators guide learners towards resources for them to acquire knowledge while still being available to facilitate/enhance learning (McKimm and Jollie 2007). Educators are also expected to provide engaging experiential learning opportunities and this is where simulation, in its various modalities, plays a major role for a variety of valid reasons.

A number of elements underpin effective teaching, whether it is in higher education or for CPD of healthcare professionals, and these include the educators, the learners, the teaching methods, and the environment (Alinier and Hssain 2019). Some of the key complementary requirements are about setting clear learning objectives, providing a learning experience that is intellectually challenging to the learners and safe for everyone involved, assessing their learning and level of competence in an appropriate manner, as well as providing feedback and encouraging reflection (Oriot and Alinier 2018; Ramsden 2003). In healthcare, when we refer to learning of clinical skills, we can describe this as an activity when the healthcare providers or learners deconstruct and reconstruct meaning for themselves. This often places considerable demand on educators as many activities are only applicable to small groups of learners at a time.

Healthcare education, at both undergraduate and postgraduate levels, is considered the art and science that drives teaching and learning. It strives to invest in frontline healthcare professionals to enable them to provide safe and patient-centered care within multidisciplinary teams while implementing evidence-based practices, supported by technology (e.g., electronic medical records, diagnostic tools, medical imaging), and applying quality improvement initiatives. The ultimate goal of healthcare education is to support clinicians in their roles and promote safe patient-centered care. At the individual level, this means a more confident and competent practitioner, while at an institutional level this translates into safer, more cost-effective and efficient service provision, and better patient outcomes. At a nationwide scale, this boosts public confidence in the healthcare system and promotes a healthier population and hence can positively impact a country's economy and status (Bedir 2016). There is a significant interplay between education and health to develop human capital at all levels of a society, and hence, governments and healthcare institutions should always strive to put the appropriate resources and regulations in place to deliver the best possible medical care to the population they serve.

Given its critical role, one must wonder what are the "best" means for the provision and evaluation of health care professional education? Are there evidence-based educational approaches for health care professionals which are better than others?

Teaching and Learning Strategies

Teaching and learning are interlinked. Learning can be referred to as a change in knowledge, skills, behavior, values, preferences, insights, or a combination of those (Gross 2015). Learning can also be seen as a "comprehensive activity in which we come to know ourselves and the world around us" (p. 65) (Fish and Coles 2005). It is about adjusting our mental models based on new knowledge and experiences guided by reflection. The outcome may range from mere awareness to understanding and being able to explain, to expanding our memory, influencing our knowledge and behaviors. From a slightly different perspective, learning can also be seen as a cognitive and behavioral process (Aldrich 2003). Learning is an individual responsibility and activity as no one can learn on behalf of someone else; hence, it relies on motivation and different learners have different styles and pace of learning (Alinier and Verjee 2019). Although processes can be put in place and techniques can be shared to promote better learning and assimilation of new knowledge and concepts, people still need to learn for themselves. Perfect learning probably occurs as a consequence of integration of understanding and action. When competency (skill-based) training and competence (holistic education) merge, then learning becomes outstanding. It is possible to envisage that with simulation-based education, both of these objectives can be achieved. Teaching is one of the vehicles to achieve learning and it involves the modification of student's environment according to specific educational needs and to allow for their development and progress (Alinier and Hssain 2019). As such, recreating an authentic clinical context can impact on the skill being learnt as it may or not stimulate the expected behavior or performance of the learner so they can appropriately demonstrate their level of competence (Brightwell and Grant 2013). Furthermore, when we refer to competence, it usually indicates a single individual. There is now a move towards the notion of capability as opposed to competence because then the key themes can be team performance in terms of "working well with others" as opposed to a single individual (O'Connell et al. 2014). Here again, we return to the realm of simulation-based education supplementing other approaches that are used to lay the foundation for prerequisite knowledge and skills.

Traditional educational approaches in healthcare include lectures, interactive presentations, individual or group tutorials, demonstrations, ward rounds, meetings, panel discussions, symposia, and conferences. For example, an instructor may deliver an interactive presentation on a specific topic, engaging learners through questioning so they can share their views and experience. This can be supplemented with different tools such as images, videos, or other illustrated material or even physical artifacts or samples. This method, akin to a masterclass, is primarily used to boost knowledge rather than to assimilate skills or modify attitudes and behaviors. Such an approach, often referred to as a "lecture," allows mass-education at low cost but it has significant limitations. On the other hand, more learner-centric methods include: group learning role play, facilitated case study discussions, workshops, brainstorming, facilitated practice, games, and skill or scenario-based clinical simulation (Ramsden 2003). Such variety of approaches may seem exhaustive, but it is actually beneficial for learners as they all have varying preferences and learning styles that need to be accommodated for (Alinier and Verjee 2019). Similarly, some of the activities are more or less appropriate for different types of learning objectives, whether they are skills or knowledge related.

The main drawback of didactic approaches is poor retention and recall of the educational material presented as highlighted in 1969 by Dale whose key work can be summarized by Fig. 1 which shows the cone of learning (Lord 2007; Dale 1969). Various commonly used educational approaches are ranked in order of information retention by learners. It is suggested that learners typically recall less than 20% of educational material after reading about a subject or attending a verbal lecture and that these figures decline as time goes by (Masters 2013). A combination of verbal and written material as in an illustrated lecture improves the percentage of material recalled. This is in obvious contrast to more than 70% retention of knowledge or skills by actual practice and teaching others, but again a decay would be observable over time once this stops (Lord 2007; Masters 2013). Aspects of this have been demonstrated in a systematic review which identified 14 studies and looked at the impact of various methods of education on patient-centered outcome (Davis et al.

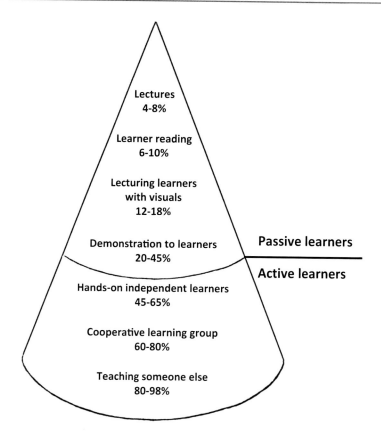

Fig. 1 Approximated learning recall for various types of educational activities 6 weeks post-educational intervention. (Adapted from Dale (1969))

1999). The authors concluded that didactic teaching did not improve physician's performance. On the other hand, interactive education can bring about improvement in physician's clinical practice (Davis et al. 1999).

Other experiments have been conducted to verify Dale's work and validate his established hierarchy of educational approaches in terms of learning retention. Although cited percentages are understandably sometimes variable, especially as what was tested varied or percentages may have been simply estimated, most studies support his claims (Lord 2007; Masters 2013). Other work is sometimes more critical as to the claims made and stated percentages, because they can vary significantly and may not be based on a clearly defined methods as to how they have been determined (Masters 2019). It is also interesting to draw a parallel with the Halstedian adage which promotes observation, doing, then teaching others. It makes this process somehow appear logical if we do not consider the "One" literally as being done during a real patient care episode but as a set of repetitions of a particular skill in a safe and controllable learning environment such as through simulated practice (Der Sahakian et al. 2019).

The Importance of Developing Clinical Skills

The concept of clinical skills is a complex one and is key to the management of patients. A generic definition of "clinical skills" describes the term as being *"a set of knowledge and practices which aim to develop the competencies necessary for the proper professional practice"* (de Oliveira Barbosa et al. 2016) and hence is applicable across all healthcare disciplines. Looking at the etymology of the word "Clinical," one can learn that it is derived from the Greek *"klinikos,"* which means *"of or pertaining to a bed,"* and in a medical context referred to a physician attending to a bedridden patient, although called a *"clinician,"* who is a person who can provide advice and treat patients. The word *"skill"* is rooted from the Greek *"techne"* and hence refers to the skillful way a clinician practices their profession (Athreya 2010). In fact, to execute a particular clinical skill, several types of *"skills"* come into play.

Clinical skills are not only bedside examination skills, but comprise many domains, including one or more of practical procedural skills, physical examination, communication or interpersonal skills, and psychomotor skills (Jünger et al. 2005; Kurtz et al. 2017). To this list, we can also include critical thinking and decision-making skills which are crucial to making an accurate diagnosis and to the care delivered to patients (Benbassat et al. 2005). In more general terms, clinical skills are often said to comprise three key elements which are the clinician's underlying knowledge, the procedural steps, and their clinical reasoning as represented in Fig. 2 (Michels et al. 2012).

The broad domains of clinical skills can be divided into technical and behavioral skills (often referred to as nontechnical skills) (Murphy et al. 2019), both underpinned by a critical cognitive aspect as knowledge and experience will guide their clinical practice. Major technical and/or practical skills are those related to history taking, examination, diagnostic, and procedural skills which range from simple tasks such as suturing, knot tying, and venipuncture, to more complex and invasive ones such as central venous or arterial cannulation, neuraxial blocks, laparoscopic procedures, etc. On the other hand, nontechnical skills are often said to encompass communication, teamwork, leadership, assertiveness, situation awareness, decision-making, and workload management (Kurtz et al. 2017; St Pierre et al. 2008; Duvivier and van Dalen 2012).

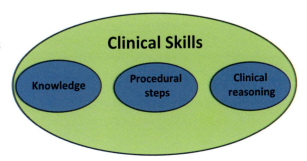

Fig. 2 Representation of the three main clinical skills domains according to Michels et al.(2012) enhanced by interprofessional collaboration

We will explore these aspects and determine that both technical and nontechnical skills are not only meant to be performed in the real patient care settings, but lend themselves effortlessly to first being learnt and practiced using various simulation-based educational modalities in different environments to improve patient care in general and promote patient safety. As evidence, a meta-analysis of 14 studies concluded that deliberate practice using simulation-based techniques was found overall to be a superior method of training compared to the apprenticeship model in the medical field (McGaghie et al. 2011).

Clinical skills have so far been the lifeblood of medical and allied healthcare professionals' work. But, in this era of technological advances and artificial intelligence (Shortliffe and Sepúlveda 2018), do we still need clinical skills? Why do we need to listen to heart sounds or breathing anomalies when we can get a CT scan or an echocardiogram? The literature supports one view or the other depending on what we wish to prove. On balance, a case can be made for learning and retaining skills. In a cash strapped healthcare system, we cannot ignore that over-investigating is not recommended. Effective skills, executed with competence may allow focused and only necessary investigations to be requested and conducted. Further, clinical skills are easy to monitor and impact the effectiveness of treatment instituted. Flegel (1999) suggests that physical examination skills "thoughtfully integrated with new technology" are the bridge between the patient's history and the investigations required to make a diagnosis and will *"continue to be central to clinical practice"* (p. 1118).

Foundation of Clinical Skills

Acquisition of clinical skills requires the learner to have the procedural knowledge, which is how to do things, to understand the basic science knowledge, and to link both through clinical reasoning (Buja 2019; Michels et al. 2012). Clinical reasoning is a key aspect of clinical skills as it can be considered as the cornerstone of patient care. This aspect is usually taught after students have learned history-taking and physical examination skills (Benbassat et al. 2005). Encouraging reflective practice and problem-based learning (PBL) activities can promote clinical reasoning. Thus, acquiring proficiency in clinical skills requires knowledge and understanding of the task at hand, preparation, confidence, actual successful execution, teamwork, communication with the patient, troubleshooting, and record keeping. The term "clinical skills" may seem simple at a superficial glance, but at a deeper level, there is a complex interdependence of many variables as illustrated in Fig. 3. Clinical skills, in many situations, are dependent on the clinician's ability to demonstrate interprofessional collaboration aptitudes. Mastering all of this synchronously requires experience which junior clinicians often cannot acquire at the bedside for evident safety and ethical reasons. Moreover, patients are not sympathetic to delays in management and medical errors and may be unforgiving to learners trying to gain competence by practicing their skills on them. As such, novice clinicians need to be

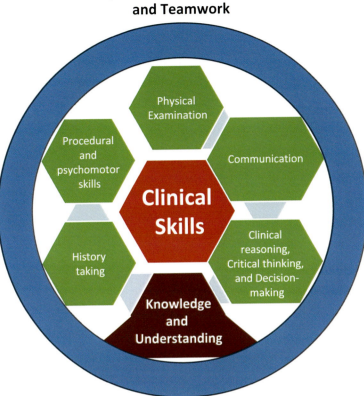

Fig. 3 Extended representation of the clinical skills required of healthcare professionals underpinned by knowledge and understanding and framed by interprofessional collaboration and teamwork.

offered or seek other methods of acquiring clinical skills, and increasingly benefit from substituted rather than augmented clinical experience.

Clinical skills, such as gross motor skills, are not essentially knowledge-based. For example, simple skills such as cannulation can be easily learned without substantial background knowledge. The speed of successful execution of that skill can be improved by repetition so it becomes an automatic action. However, knowledge and understanding become imperative for the mastery of the skill. In the case of cannulation, knowing how to manage a patient when there has been extravasation calls for knowledge-based competency. Sometimes, a practitioner may retain competency in performing a skill but does not retain the knowledge base that accompanies it. For example, an anesthetist may be competent at inserting a central venous cannula into the internal jugular vein using an ultrasound machine to guide them, but they may not remember the anatomical details of all the surrounding structures or identify aberrant structures as a consequence of fade in their knowledge. Skills and knowledge decline at different rates, with their relative decline varying in different studies (Ali et al. 2001; Smith et al. 2008; Yang et al. 2012; Riggs et al. 2019).

Acquisition of Knowledge

Learners are seldom taught a clinical skill without first being given some background information so they can understand why it is required and how it should be performed. "Factual knowledge of medical science is essential for the development of clinical skills" (p. 3) (Buja 2019). Knowledge can be gained or easily recalled in the modern era by accessing the search engines available at one's fingertips, but it is not the same as acquired or memorized knowledge which is immediately accessible and almost instinctively guides clinical decision-making. To translate knowledge into clinical practice that is delivered safely and to a high standard, healthcare providers need a wide repertoire of skills, all of which are underpinned by human factors aspects (Leonard et al. 2004), and this often cannot be improvised using technology and search engines. Medical knowledge, technical expertise, or clinical skill proficiency on their own are not enough to successfully manage patients. It is well described that the combination of knowledge, skills, and attitude are essential for integrated healthcare, whereby all the parts of a wider system work together (Hean 2015). This particularly relies on interprofessional working, which is dependent on the provision of education and training to clinicians that gives them a clear understanding of how their work fits in with the contributions of the other members of the healthcare team (Masterson 2002). It is argued that for interprofessional education to work, it relies on all learners having a solid knowledge foundation and understanding of biomedical sciences (Dow and Thibault 2017). Scenario-based simulation is one of the key modalities that can help learners reflect on and understand the roles of other healthcare professionals (Alinier et al. 2014). It provides an opportunity to engage specific professions to work together by tailoring clinical scenarios around preidentified learning needs and then involving all learners jointly in a facilitated debriefing session that promotes mutual understanding among the various professions involved. It also allows for the observation of more complex and often hidden aspects of professional practice, such as the attitude and behavior of the learners. Scenarios can also be created to get learners to demonstrate their ability to use checklists, implement guidelines and standard operating procedures, and report incidents.

Using Simulation to Prepare for Real-World Situations

Simulation lends itself to skills acquisition not only in healthcare but also in the defense, aviation, and nuclear power industries, as well as other high reliability organizations, so employees can become competent and safe at doing their jobs and are always ready to deal with a variety of potential situations (Birnbach et al. 2013). It is utilized in such organizations to minimize risks due to human factors with an understanding that risks can never be totally eliminated: accidents can still occur because of procedural or organizational factors. It is also commonly used at regular intervals to maintain or evaluate proficiency levels and enable rating of an individual or an organization. Some relevant examples include the international regulations imposing airports to conduct on a regular basis exercises to test their emergency response plan through table-tops and full-scale emergency scenarios (Romig 2015), and the fact that pilots also need to return to a flight simulator and have their general competence assessed every 6 months (Taylor et al. 2014).

Healthcare is fundamentally patient-centric and the scale of complexity within the healthcare system means that delivery of care is fraught with potential errors. Although simulation cannot replace the real-world experience in most instances, it can make the latter safer by allowing the learner to make errors in a relatively safe environment and rehearse skills until competency is achieved. After all, who would like a less-experienced clinician to practice on their loved ones especially for the first time? Rare and critical life-threatening events can be rehearsed and by using various methods of debriefing, the learners can engage in facilitated reflection *in* action and *on* action (Jones and Alinier 2015). Simulation also allows the observation of behaviors that may predict how professionals behave in the real world (Ker and Bradley 2013). It also provides a unique opportunity to help address the issues around consenting patients to be cared for by junior clinicians as they may practice that aspect from a communication point of view. If it is something which is part of their learning objectives and is not discussed during the encounter with a simulated patient or patient simulator, the "patient's" response can bring up the issue or ignore it so it is discussed at the time of the debriefing. However, there is a significant cost involved in SBE, in terms of physical and human resources required to make it happen. It is often dependent on range of up-to-date technology and equipment, a facility, and expert educators and operations specialists (Alinier and Granry 2015).

In terms of readiness for potential real-world situation, simulation is commonly used in most sectors for people to learn to deal with crisis situations. Healthcare demands thoughtful actions and smart decision-making especially during crisis management, and this is an aspect junior clinicians need to be taught and experience in various situations (Buja 2019). When junior clinicians lack experience, face extreme time pressure, the stakes are high, and there is uncertainty, then having a repertoire of knowledge and competence in skills is vital to achieve better patient outcomes. The situation can be exacerbated in the context of organizational deficiencies, changing teams, and variable team dynamics, as is the case in all clinical practice settings.

Clinicians can be exposed to scenarios that require them to perform to their maximum potential followed by expert debriefing that can help identify further knowledge or performance gaps that may not have been directly observable, and address these in a safe environment (Oriot and Alinier 2018). An action is the result of a decision made which can be analyzed by probing into the mental framework of the decision maker. This mental framework is subject to perceptions, thoughts, and emotions which are generally not explicit. A behavior is usually visible and influenced by perceptions, feelings, thoughts, intention, and motivation. Consequently, there are numerous drivers that influence a mental framework and potentiate a decision which then results in an action.

Put into context, skills that encompass high intensity tasks, such as the management plan for a complex trauma or critical care patient, can be rehearsed through simulation at a pace that suits the learner. A variety of scenarios can be created and enacted for learners to develop or exhibit their skills and be provided an opportunity for guided reflection and deepening of their learning. Crucially, simulation can be employed to focus on aspects such as patient monitoring, priority setting, team working, and even mundane aspects such as practicing the implementation of sepsis or blood transfusion guidelines (Breymier and Rutherford-Hemming 2017; Kessler et al. 2016). Further learning opportunities can then be arranged to fine tune identified skills' gaps using complementary strategies and tools which may involve self-study, mental rehearsal, online learning, and practice on part-task trainers or virtual reality simulators (Alinier 2007b; Anton et al. 2017). Different learning strategies may be used to learn different types of skills. It is also said three modes of learning are applicable to medicine, and these are observation, deliberate practice, and learning by dechunking (Sinha 2016). Simulation lends itself to all modes including the third technique of dechunking, which is about breaking down a task into its component steps so the learner can repeat the elements until competence is achieved. Learning through dechunking is unlike intuitive learning when lesser attention span is required. For deeper learning, the context may be as important as the content within the learning as well as the learners' motivation which may be intrinsic or extrinsic (Swanwick 2013).

Although there is no single educational theory that can be attributed explicitly to simulation as an educational tool, behaviorism underpins this concept wherein behavior, environment, and personal factors interact to determine outcomes (Bandura 2001). Different objectives can be achieved by calling into play different theories applicable to simulation (Der Sahakian et al. 2019). Simulation helps overlearning as a means of improving retention and making behaviors automatic (Swanwick 2013) and as such it is a powerful adjunct to learning in the real world, but it also brings other benefits.

Other Benefits of Simulation

What learners are offered to experience through SBE can be very much controlled and tailored to their individual needs and level of experience, and this is one of the key advantages of SBE. For this reason, it has become an integral part of most healthcare curricula. Simulation, as an experiential learning activity, offers the opportunity for experimentation, reflection, and repeated practice so learners' performance can be improved, usually over a protected time window. Learners may gain speed and automaticity, therefore enhance the retention of what they will have practiced and learnt. It helps with their understanding of important concepts and implementation of procedures performed individually or as part of a team.

Another advantage of SBE is that it allows a form of "legitimate peripheral participation" (LPP) (Lave and Wenger 1991) by learners who can benefit in an observer capacity from their peers' participation in a scenario-based activity. This is usually done in an intermittent manner, whereby learners are often split into small teams and take turn in either taking part in the hands-on simulation activity or observing the live-stream of the activity from an adjacent room via an audio-visual system (Alinier et al. 2014). Then all learners, participants and observers, can be involved in the debriefing process facilitated by the educator(s) (Oriot and Alinier 2018). This enables the gradual mastery of skills by learners. This is not dissimilar to Collins et al.'s "cognitive apprenticeship" method for the teaching and learning of cognitive skills, encouraging learners to think and problem solve as a form of reflection, and in which observation plays a key role (Collins et al. 1988). Learners are encouraged to reflect on their own performance or what they observe in comparison to that of an expert. That method also incorporates coaching, modeling, articulation, and scaffolding. Collins et al.'s method is particularly useful to gain confidence in executing skills, whereas LPP is useful for social integration into a team, referred to in that context as a "community of practice" (Lave and Wenger 1991).

There are, however, some caveats to using simulation to achieve proficiency in skills or other aspects of performance. Simulation suites should be safe havens for trainees to practice without fear or embarrassment, irrespective of their level of experience. Kolb's reflection is used widely in SBE as it offers learners a structured basis to reflect, conceptualize, and experiment to improve performance (Jones and Alinier 2015; Kolb et al. 2001). This is where facilitated debriefing can help learners engage in reflection-in-action as well as reflection-on-action. There needs to be expert debriefing which is formative and constructive in nature whereby learners should be helped to identify performance gaps and receive guidance on how to close them and intended to help the learners (Oriot and Alinier 2018; Der Sahakian et al. 2015). This implies that other important aspects of the debriefing are that it occurs in a safe environment and provides an opportunity for emotional recovery from the experience. Another aspect to emphasize is to genuinely reinforce positive behaviors and interventions (Dieckmann et al. 2017). This is easier to achieve if it is done in a structured manner, whereby the debriefing is constituted of phases as proposed by various models, and that the learners have been informed of the debriefing process adopted (Oriot and Alinier 2018). For example, the "RUST" debriefing model includes "Reaction – Understanding – Summarizing – Take away learning points" that will help learners going through a comprehensive analysis of their performance and help improve their skills (Karlsen 2013). Debriefing is hence a dynamic process that requires the educators to be not only good observers, but also adaptable and measured in their facilitation approach to be able to respond to any potential situation and so learners' feelings are well managed while learning can still effectively occur. This implies that educators should also master the art of questioning. Advocacy-enquiry has been proposed as an effective method of understanding mental frames and promoting reflection on the part of learners (Sawyer and Brett-Fleegler 2016). It involves stating an observation and following up with query encouraging the

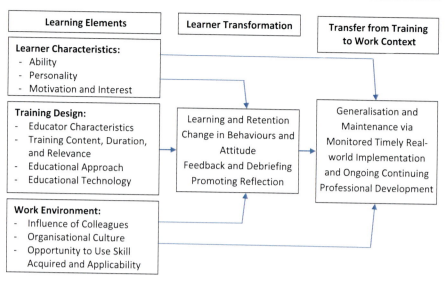

Fig. 4 Adaptation of the model of the Transfer of Training initially proposed by Baldwin and Ford (1988)

learners to justify their action based on the information they had at the time and assumptions they may have made (Oriot and Alinier 2018). Educators also need to be able to deal with learners who are not engaged, too quiet, too vocal, argumentative, and even those who get upset (Oriot and Alinier 2018; Der Sahakian et al. 2015).

Transfer of skills learned through simulation to the real world may not be easy to accomplish. Simulation cannot always replicate the uncertainty, complexity, and dynamism of real situations and settings. Transferability refers to the condition of transfer and is a complex issue confounded by the learners, the training design, and work environment (Liu et al. 2009). As illustrated in a revised version of Baldwin and Ford's Transfer of Training Model (Baldwin and Ford 1988) (Fig. 4), the inputs are multiple but they are also affected by several factors including the duration of the activity and the timeliness of the training versus when the skill will actually be required on the real job and how it will be maintained through actual use during real or simulated patient care.

Conclusion

So that healthcare professionals and students can effectively contribute to patient care delivery, it is very important for them to develop technical and nontechnical skills underpinned by sound knowledge and understanding. This includes skills that they need to master as individuals, as well as many more that relate to teamwork and interprofessional collaboration. The use of simulation in its various forms in healthcare education is dependent on various key factors which are the learners, the educators, the teaching methods, and the environment. Eventually, they all have an impact on the delivery of safe patient care. Various simulation-based teaching and learning strategies can be used to impart new skills, knowledge, and experiences guided by reflection. These contribute to adjusting learners' mental models and behaviors. It is important to recognize that there is no single best evidence-based educational approach to impart nonprocedural clinical skills as there are multiple factors to take into consideration and complex interdependences. Some of the activities are more or less appropriate for different types of learning objectives and levels of learners, whether they are nontechnical skills or knowledge related, and they should aim to prepare learners for real world clinical situations. Some of the key benefits of SBE are that it provides opportunities for controlled and individualized learning experience with protected time for reflection. It may benefit participants as well as observers, especially attributable to the debriefing phase that allows for deepening of the learning and closure of performance gaps.

Cross-References

- ▶ Approaches to Assessment: A Perspective From Education
- ▶ Cognitive Neuroscience Foundations of Surgical and Procedural Expertise: Focus on Theory
- ▶ Critical Theory
- ▶ Debriefing Practices in Simulation-Based Education
- ▶ Focus on Theory: Emotions and Learning
- ▶ Measuring Performance: Current Practices in Surgical Education
- ▶ Simulation for Procedural Skills Teaching and Learning
- ▶ Supporting the Development of Patient-Centred Communication Skills
- ▶ Supporting the Development of Professionalism in the Education of Health Professionals
- ▶ Teaching Simple and Complex Psychomotor Skills
- ▶ Transformative Learning in Clinical Education: Using Theory to Inform Practice

References

Aldrich C. Simulations and the future of learning: an innovative (and perhaps revolutionary) approach to e-learning. San Francisco, CA, USA: Wiley; 2003.

Ali J, Adam R, Pierre I, Bedaysie H, Josa D, Winn J. Comparison of performance 2 years after the old and new (interactive) ATLS courses. J Surg Res. 2001;97(1):71–5.

Alinier G. Enhancing trainees' learning experience through the opening of an advanced multi-professional simulation training facility at the University of Hertfordshire. Br J Anaesth Recover Nurs. 2007a;8(2):22–7.

Alinier G. A typology of educationally focused medical simulation tools. Med Teach. 2007b;29(8): e243–50.

Alinier G, Granry J-C. Fundraising: a potential additional source of income for the research and educational activities of a healthcare simulation program. In: Palaganas J, Mancini B, Maxworthy J, Epps C, editors. Defining excellence in simulation programs. Philadelphia, USA: Wolters Kluwer; 2015. p. 321–8.

Alinier G, Hssain I. Creating effective learning environments: the educator's perspective. In: Chiniara G, editor. Clinical simulation: education, operations, and engineering. 2nd ed. London: Elsevier; 2019. p. 217–27.

Alinier G, Verjee M. Learning through play. In: Chiniara G, editor. Clinical simulation: education, operations, and engineering. 2nd ed: London, Elsevier; 2019. p. 157-169.

Alinier G, Harwood C, Harwood P, Montague S, Huish E, Ruparelia K, et al. Immersive clinical simulation in undergraduate health care interprofessional education: knowledge and perceptions. Clin Simul Nurs. 2014;10(4):e205–e16.

Alinier G, Bello F, Kalbag A, Kneebone R. Space: Potential locations to conduct full-scale simulation-based education. In: Palaganas J, Mancini B, Maxworthy J, Epps C, editors. Defining excellence in simulation programs. Wolters Kluwer; 2015. p. 455–64.

Anton NE, Bean EA, Hammonds SC, Stefanidis D. Application of mental skills training in surgery: a review of its effectiveness and proposed next steps. J Laparoendosc Adv Surg Techn. 2017;27(5):459–69.

Athreya BH. Handbook of clinical skills: a practical manual. Hackensack: World Scientific; 2010.

Baldwin TT, Ford JK. Transfer of training: a review and directions for future research. Pers Psychol. 1988;41(1):63–105.

Bandura A. Social cognitive theory: an agentic perspective. Annu Rev Psychol. 2001;52(1):1–26.

Barton D, Mashlan W. An advanced nurse practitioner-led service–consequences of service redesign for managers and organizational infrastructure. J Nurs Manag. 2011;19(7):943–9.

Bedir S. Healthcare expenditure and economic growth in developing countries. Adv Econ Bus. 2016;4(2):76–86.

Benbassat J, Baumal R, Heyman SN, Brezis M. Suggestions for a shift in teaching clinical skills to medical students: the reflective clinical examination. Acad Med. 2005;80(12):1121–6.

Birnbach DJ, Rosen LF, Williams L, Fitzpatrick M, Lubarsky DA, Menna JD. A framework for patient safety: a defense nuclear industry–based high-reliability model. Jt Comm J Qual Patient Saf. 2013;39(5):233–40.

Boker A. Setup and utilization of Clinical Simulation Center, Faculty of Medicine, KING Abdulaziz University, Saudi Arabia. Life Sci J. 2013;10(1):1079–85.

Boursicot KA. Structured assessments of clinical competence. Br J Hosp Med. 2010;71(6):342–4.

Bradley P, Postlethwaite K. Setting up a clinical skills learning facility. Med Educ. 2003;37(1):6–13.

Breen KJ, Hogan AM, Mealy K. The detrimental impact of the implementation of the European working time directive (EWTD) on surgical senior house officer (SHO) operative experience. Ir J Med Sci. 2013;182(3):383–7.

Breymier T, Rutherford-Hemming T. Use of high-fidelity simulation to increase knowledge and skills in caring for patients receiving blood products. Crit Care Nurs Clin. 2017;29(3):369–75.

Brightwell A, Grant J. Competency-based training: who benefits? Postgrad Med J. 2013;89(1048):107.

Buja LM. Medical education today: all that glitters is not gold. BMC Med Educ. 2019;19(1):110.

Chiniara G, Cole G, Brisbin K, Huffman D, Cragg B, Lamacchia M, et al. Simulation in healthcare: a taxonomy and a conceptual framework for instructional design and media selection. Med Teach. 2013;35(8):e1380–95.

Collins A, Brown JS, Newman SE. Cognitive apprenticeship: teaching the craft of reading, writing and mathematics. Thinking J Philos Children. 1988;8(1):2–10.

Dale E. Audiovisual methods in teaching. New York: Dryden Press; 1969.

Davis D, O'Brien MAT, Freemantle N, Wolf FM, Mazmanian P, Taylor-Vaisey A. Impact of formal continuing medical education: do conferences, workshops, rounds, and other traditional continuing education activities change physician behavior or health care outcomes? JAMA. 1999;282(9):867–74.

de Oliveira Barbosa AP, Sebastiani RL, Bez MR, Flores CD, de Castro MS. Use of a simulator to develop clinical skills for pharmacists. In: Cruz-Cunha MM, Miranda IM, Martinho R, Rijo R, editors. Encyclopedia of E-Health and telemedicine. Hershey: IGI Global; 2016. p. 412–21.

Der Sahakian G, Alinier G, Savoldelli G, Oriot D, Jaffrelot M, Lecomte F. Setting conditions for productive debriefing. Simul Gaming. 2015;46(2):197–208.

Der Sahakian G, Buléon C, Alinier G. Educational foundations of instructional design applied to simulation-based education. In: Chiniara G, editor. Clinical simulation: education, operations, and engineering. 2nd ed. London: Elsevier; 2019. p. 185–206.

Dieckmann P, Patterson M, Lahlou S, Mesman J, Nyström P, Krage R. Variation and adaptation: learning from success in patient safety-oriented simulation training. Adv Simul. 2017;2(1):21.

Dow A, Thibault G. Interprofessional education-a foundation for a new approach to health care. N Engl J Med. 2017;377(9):803.

Duvivier RJ, van Dalen J. Learning in the Skillslab. In: Al Alwan I, Magzoub ME, Elzubeir M, editors. International handbook of medical education: a guide for students. SAGE; 2012. p. 169–75.

Ericsson KA. Deliberate practice and the acquisition and maintenance of expert performance in medicine and related domains. Acad Med. 2004;79(10):S70–81.

Fish D, Coles C. Medical education: developing a curriculum for practice: developing a curriculum for practice. Berkshire: McGraw-Hill Education; 2005.

Flegel KM. Does the physical examination have a future? Can Med Assoc J. 1999:1117–8.

Gross R. Psychology: the science of mind and behaviour 7th edition: Hodder Education; 2015.

Hean S. Strengthening the links between practice and education in the development of collaborative competence frameworks. In: Vyt A, Pahor M, Tervaskanto-Meantausta T, editors. Interprofessional education in Europe: policy and practice. Antwerp: Garant Publishers; 2015. p. 9–36.

Houghton CE, Casey D, Shaw D, Murphy K. Staff and students' perceptions and experiences of teaching and assessment in clinical skills laboratories: interview findings from a multiple case study. Nurse Educ Today. 2012;32(6):e29–34.

Houghton CE, Casey D, Shaw D, Murphy K. Students' experiences of implementing clinical skills in the real world of practice. J Clin Nurs. 2013;22(13-14):1961–9.

Jones I, Alinier G. Supporting students' learning experiences through a pocket size Cue Card designed around a reflective simulation framework. Clin Simul Nurs. 2015;11(7):325–34.

Jünger J, Schäfer S, Roth C, Schellberg D, Friedman Ben-David M, Nikendei C. Effects of basic clinical skills training on objective structured clinical examination performance. Med Educ. 2005;39(10):1015–20.

Karlsen R. Stable Program. Adaptation of the RUS model. Original work from the Center for Medical Simulation (D.R.), Cambridge, MA. 2013.

Ker J, Bradley P. Simulation in medical education. In: Swanwick T, editor. Understanding medical education: evidence, theory, and practice. Chichester: Wiley; 2013. p. 175–92.

Kessler DO, Walsh B, Whitfill T, Gangadharan S, Gawel M, Brown L, et al. Disparities in adherence to pediatric sepsis guidelines across a spectrum of emergency departments: a multi-center, cross-sectional observational in situ simulation study. J Emergency Med. 2016;50(3): 403–15.e3.

Kneebone R. Simulation, safety and surgery. Qual Saf Health Care. 2010;19(Suppl 3):i47–52.

Knowles MS. The modern practice of adult education: from pedagogy to andragogy. 2nd ed. - New York: Cambridge Books; 1980.

Knowles MS. Andragogy in action: applying principles of adult learning. San Farancisco: Jossey-Bass; 1984.

Kolb DA, Boyatzis RE, Mainemelis C. Experiential learning theory: previous research and new directions. Perspectives Thinking Learn Cognitive Styles. 2001;1:227–47.

Kurtz S, Silverman J, Draper J. Teaching and learning communication skills in medicine. 2nd ed. Abingdon, UK: CRC Press; 2017.

Kyaw Tun J, Alinier G, Tang J, Kneebone RL. Redefining simulation Fidelity for healthcare education. Simul Gaming. 2015;46(2):159–74.

Lai A, Haligua A, Bould MD, Everett T, Gale M, Pigford A-A, et al. Learning crisis resource management: practicing versus an observational role in simulation training–a randomized controlled trial. Anaesthesia Crit Care Pain Med. 2016;35(4):275–81.

LaRosa C, Grant-Kels JM. See one, do one, teach one: the ethical dilemma of residents performing their first procedure on patients. J Am Acad Dermatol. 2016;75(4):845–8.

Lave J, Wenger E. Situated learning: legitimate peripheral participation. Cambridge: Cambridge University Press; 1991.

Leonard M, Graham S, Bonacum D. The human factor: the critical importance of effective teamwork and communication in providing safe care. BMJ Qual Saf. 2004;13(suppl 1):i85–90.

Liu D, Blickensderfer EL, Macchiarella ND, Vincenzi DA. Transfer of training. In: Hancock PA, Vincenzi DA, Wise JA, Mouloua M, editors. Human factors in simulation and training. Boca Raton: CRC Press; 2009. p. 49–60.

Lord T. Revisiting the cone of learning: is it a reliable way to link instruction method with knowledge recall? J Coll Sci Teach. 2007;37(2):14–7.

Mahesh B, Sharples L, Codispoti M. Effect of the full implementation of the European working time directive on operative training in adult cardiac surgery. J Surg Educ. 2014;71(4):492–9.

Masters K. Edgar Dale's pyramid of learning in medical education: a literature review. Med Teach. 2013;35(11):e1584–e93.

Masters K. Edgar Dale's pyramid of learning in medical education: further expansion of the myth. Med Educ. 2019.

Masterson A. Cross-boundary working: a macro-political analysis of the impact on professional roles. J Clin Nurs. 2002;11(3):331–9.

McGaghie WC, Issenberg SB, Cohen MER, Barsuk JH, Wayne DB. Does simulation-based medical education with deliberate practice yield better results than traditional clinical education? A meta-analytic comparative review of the evidence. Acad Med J Assoc Am Med Coll. 2011;86(6):706–11.

McKimm J, Jollie C. Facilitating learning: teaching and learning methods. 2007. https://www.academiaedu/download/56698746/Facilitating_learning_teaching_-_learning_methods.pdf. Accessed 09 Apr 21.

Merriam SB. Andragogy and self-directed learning: pillars of adult learning theory. New Directions Adult Continuing Educ. 2001;2001(89):3–14.

Merriam SB. The role of cognitive development in Mezirow's transformational learning theory. Adult Educ Q. 2004;55(1):60–8.

Michels MEJ, Evans DE, Blok GA. What is a clinical skill? Searching for order in chaos through a modified Delphi process. Med Teach. 2012;34(8):e573–e81.

Murphy P, Nestel D, Gormley GJ. Words matter: towards a new lexicon for 'nontechnical skills' training. Adv Simul. 2019;4(1):8.

O'Connell J, Gardner G, Coyer F. Beyond competencies: using a capability framework in developing practice standards for advanced practice nursing. J Adv Nurs. 2014;70(12):2728–35.

Oriot D, Alinier G. Pocket book for simulation debriefing in healthcare. Cham: Springer; 2018.

Peyton JR. Teaching & learning in medical practice. Rickmansworth, UK: Manticore Europe Limited; 1998.

Ramsden P. Learning to teach in higher education. London: Routledge; 2003.

Rethans JJ, Norcini J, Baron-Maldonado M, Blackmore D, Jolly B, LaDuca T, et al. The relationship between competence and performance: implications for assessing practice performance. Med Educ. 2002;36(10):901–9.

Riggs M, Franklin R, Saylany L. Associations between cardiopulmonary resuscitation (CPR) knowledge, self-efficacy, training history and willingness to perform CPR and CPR psychomotor skills: a systematic review. Resuscitation. 2019;138:259–72.

Riley RH, Grauze AM, Chinnery C, Horley RA, Trewhella NH. Three years of "CASMS": the world's busiest medical simulation Centre. Med J Aust. 2003;179(11/12):626–30.

Rodriguez-Paz J, Kennedy M, Salas E, Wu AW, Sexton J, Hunt E, et al. Beyond "see one, do one, teach one": toward a different training paradigm. BMJ Qual Saf. 2009;18(1):63–8.

Romig T. The hijacking of Flight ET 702: the challenges of managing a major security threat, media attention and continuing daily airport operations. J Airport Manag. 2015;9(4):310–6.

Salas E, Bowers CA, Rhodenizer L. It is not how much you have but how you use it: toward a rational use of simulation to support aviation training. Int J Aviat Psychol. 1998;8(3):197–208.

Sawyer T, Brett-Fleegler M, Eppich WJ. Essentials of debriefing and feedback. In: Grant V, Cheng A, editors. Comprehensive healthcare simulation: pediatrics: Springer; 2016. p. 31-42.

Shafiq Z, Mufti TS, Qayum I. Role of clinical skill centre in undergraduate medical education: Initial experience at Rehman Medical College Peshawar encounter. J Pak Med Assoc. 2017;2:4.

Shortliffe EH, Sepúlveda MJ. Clinical decision support in the era of artificial intelligence. JAMA. 2018;320(21):2199–200.

Sinha R. The anatomy of success: management lessons from a surgeon. Noida, India: HarperCollins India; 2016.

Smith KK, Gilcreast D, Pierce K. Evaluation of staff's retention of ACLS and BLS skills. Resuscitation. 2008;78(1):59–65.

St Pierre M, Hofinger G, Buerschaper C. Crisis management in acute care settings: human factors, team psychology, and patient safety in a high stakes environment. Berlin: Springer; 2008.

Swanwick T. Understanding medical education: evidence, theory, and practice. Chichester: Wiley; 2013.

Taylor A, Dixon-Hardy DW, Wright SJ. Simulation training in UK general aviation: an undervalued aid to reducing loss of control accidents. Int J Aviat Psychol. 2014;24(2):141–52.

Yang C-W, Yen Z-S, McGowan JE, Chen HC, Chiang W-C, Mancini ME, et al. A systematic review of retention of adult advanced life support knowledge and skills in healthcare providers. Resuscitation. 2012;83(9):1055–60.

Yune SJ, Lee SY, Im SJ, Kam BS, Baek SY. Holistic rubric vs. analytic rubric for measuring clinical performance levels in medical students. BMC medical education. 2018;18(1):124.

Screen-Based Learning

72

Damir Ljuhar

Contents

Introduction	1418
Context	1419
E-Learning and the Historical Context	1419
Advantages and Challenges of E-Learning and SBL	1419
Content for Screen-Based Learning	1420
Content Development	1421
Content Management	1421
Content Delivery	1422
Developments and Projections	1423
Mobile Learning	1423
Social Learning	1425
Simulation	1426
The Virtual Environment	1427
Serious Games and Gamification	1427
Blended Learning	1429
Conclusion	1430
Cross-References	1430
References	1430

Abstract

As screens become an increasingly more ubiquitous part of our lives, so too does their role in learning. From accessing information on the go, to interacting with experts and other learners from all over the world, learning is increasingly becoming a screen-based activity. It is necessary to understand the forms in which this interaction can take place, and how learners are using their screens

D. Ljuhar (✉)
Department of Surgical Simulation, Monash Children's Hospital, Clayton, VIC, Australia

Department of Paediatrics, School of Clinical Sciences, Faculty of Medicine, Nursing and Health Sciences, Monash University, Melbourne, VIC, Australia
e-mail: damir.ljuhar@monash.edu

© Springer Nature Singapore Pte Ltd. 2023
D. Nestel et al. (eds.), *Clinical Education for the Health Professions*,
https://doi.org/10.1007/978-981-15-3344-0_94

to sift out an often-overwhelming amount of information available. This chapter will aim to introduce screen-based learning (SBL) not only as a modality of e-learning, but any learning that takes place through a screen. It will discuss how the content of SBL can be developed, and the importance of design in an ever-growing design-dependent environment. Some current projections and developments will be discussed, namely, that of mobile and social learning, and the use of screens for simulation, serious games designed for learning, and the role gamification plays in clinical education. Blending learning will ultimately rely on the combination of a number of screen-based and in-person activities to optimized, and often individualize, the continually technology-engaged approach to learning.

Keywords

Screen-based learning · E-learning · Mobile learning · Health technology · Learning management systems · Blended learning · Simulation · Gamification

Introduction

We are exposed to more screens on a daily basis than ever before. However, despite the issues and controversies this often produces, screens remain an important gateway to learning. Students of all ages and disciplines are utilizing their screens for a range of learning activities and understanding how this learning happens, as well as how this differs to 'traditional' methods is necessary to optimize the interaction.

Portable electronic devices, such as smartphones and tablet computers, are almost universally owned by medical students and doctors (Nerminathan et al. 2017). Similar reports have been described in nursing and midwifery students (Achampong et al. 2018). These screens can provide learners with a range of resources to support their learning in a range of environments, both inside the clinical setting and out. At their disposal is a wealth of digital knowledge that at times can be almost overwhelming, and at other times, has even been reported to lead to increased disruptions during teaching (Wu et al. 2013).

For screen-based learning (SBL) to be integrated into clinical education strategies and practices, it is important to understand the context in which it finds itself in modern day education, namely, that of e-learning. Furthermore, practices, institutions, clinicians, and students must understand how the content for SBL is designed, managed, and delivered in order to optimize its effect.

However, it is important to realize that SBL is often likely to happen outside the purposeful intent of e-learning. In this manner, SBL can be considered *any* learning that happens through a screen, and as such is most often learner-centered, flexible, collaborative, and interactive. Similarly, the rate of change in technological innovation is accelerating as never before. The time between invention and mass adoption of technologies has dropped dramatically. Now more than ever, technology-based media and the virtual world need to become an essential part of health-care education. Not only are the technological advances proceeding at an ever-growing pace, but so are the learning needs and expectations of technologically native learners.

Context

E-Learning and the Historical Context

E-learning is a comprehensive concept that involves the use of all kinds of electronic media and screens in education (Merzouk et al. 2014) and it creates the foundation for SBL. To be able to understand the uses and advantages of SBL, it is important to understand the rise of technology in the context of e-learning.

The foundations of e-learning were laid more than 50 years ago by B.F. Skinner, a behavioral psychologist who constructed one of the first teaching machines. This form of SBL involved a computer screen which would present problems in random order to a learner and give feedback after each response (Skinner 1958). In later years, he developed early computer-based training programs that followed the idea of programmed instruction. Here, information was sequenced into smaller parts and delivered to build a bigger picture of description, questions, and answers. Learners were then rewarded and progressed for correct answers, and later, Norman Crowder refined the feedback process such that incorrect answers resulted in review or presentation of reinforcement materials (Crowder and Martin 1962).

The growth of the Internet during the 1990s transformed e-learning with web-based learning becoming the dominant branch. This allowed for centralized content distribution, allowing reduction of cost and easier updating of material (Merzouk et al. 2014). Similarly, within the last decade, one of the most significant changes has been the embrace of smartphones, with over four billion smartphones being owned globally (Ericsson Mobility Report 2019). This ubiquity has resulted in their use in nearly all aspects of life, and health-care education is no exception. From social media, to podcasts, and dedicated applications, the familiarization of technology by both students and instructors has become an expectation for the utilization of these technologies for learning.

Advantages and Challenges of E-Learning and SBL

The major advantages of e-learning can be seen to either target learning delivery or learning enhancement (Ruiz et al. 2006). Learning delivery, which arguably offers the greatest advantage of e-learning, involves increased accessibility to information, ability to update content, and quickness and ease of distribution. In more recent years, the widespread availability of portable electronic devices with intrinsic Internet capabilities, such as in the forms of smartphones, and tablets, has resulted in improved access to educational materials. This is often crucial as learning can often be unplanned. Similarly, it is easier to update electronic material compared to printed, and educators can change and revise their content more quickly. Since the start of the 'digital revolution' educators have shown that giving learners the control of the pace, time, and often the media, of learning content allows them to tailor their experience to meet personal learning objectives (Chodorow 1996). Internet technologies have facilitated the ability for learning delivery to happen to many people simultaneously at anytime, anywhere in the world.

The other major advantage, although more difficult to quantify, is through improved learning enhancement. Undoubtably, e-learning technologies offer a new paradigm in content delivery in which learning is able to be linked to specific needs, and to be applied practically, allowing a more effective and efficient learning process (Ruiz et al. 2006). This learning enhancement allows increased interactivity and promotes a student's efficiency, motivation, and cognitive effectiveness. By allowing learners to be more active in the experience through the learning enhancement offered by e-learning, a well-designed experience can motivate learners to become more engaged with the content (Clark 2002).

From the early days of e-learning, there was evidence to suggest that e-learning results in faster acquisition of knowledge and skills, with this efficiency likely to translate into improved motivation and performance. Furthermore, e-learners demonstrated better achievements of knowledge, skills and attitudes (Clark 2002). In more recent times, the e-learning environment has seen the massive expansion of hundreds of both free and for-profit online open learning initiatives by a number of universities across the world. While there is much variability in what is offered and how it is delivered, there is evidence to show that these open learning initiatives result in faster learning, reduced time to completion and cost savings, and faster completion and improved learning outcomes (Kaufman et al. 2013).

The history of e-learning has been one of rapid technological change and has been written about from a range of perspectives in the last two decades (Fernández-Manjón et al. 2008; Rosenberg 2000; Selwyn 2012; Yang 2013; Cook and Sonnenberg 2014). E-learning, and how it has been offered, has changed with each step. With the ubiquity of technologies such as portable electronic devices and the Internet, screens are an evolving platform on which e-learning happens. Whether screen-based technologies offer static information, or interactive and virtual environments, SBL is most often the end-product of e-learning delivery.

Content for Screen-Based Learning

Content for SBL includes all instructional material a learner is exposed to on any given screen. It can range significantly in complexity, from discrete items of information (for example, a Wikipedia article), to larger modules (for example, an anatomy mobile application, or podcast), to entire virtual environments (for example, a critically unwell patient in a virtual reality simulation). A digital learning object, therefore, is any grouping of digital materials structured in such a way to address an educational objective.

Content Development

Ideally, there are content creators who use pedagogical principles to produce content and instructional material that meets pre-defined and specific learning objectives. While these instructional designers may be available for formal curricula, e-learning modules and courses, this may not be the case for all educational material. Yet even so, every interaction a learner has with a screen possesses the ability to meet a learning need as long as there is the intention of learning. The likelihood of achieving this is partially dependent on ease and ability of the learner finding the required information.

The benefits of improved content delivery and learning enhancement through e-learning and SBL however, can often be lost through poor design. As such, a learner's experience of any screen-based content is highly dependent on the quality of design. This was identified over 20 years ago (Chu and Chan 1998) and much has been written about it since (Riley et al. 2004; Sweller and van Merriënboer 2013; TEDxMaastricht 2011). The migration from the physical to virtual classroom, arguably, has signaled a migration to a design-dependent environment. The particular mix of colors, layout, audio, animation, words per page, and other design elements can make the difference between good and bad experiences for learners whose main interaction with educational content is through their screens (Hampson 2013).

Health education has under-appreciated the role of design in e-learning. The goal should be for greater collaboration and integration between clinicians, educationalists and instructional designers to develop content for a design-dependent environment that is able to meet digital learning objectives.

Content Management

Content management includes all administrative functions needed to facilitate SBL to learners. At times, this is often managed by the learners themselves, who will apply a search term into a search engine, or use their own device to filter, store, index, and catalogue their own learning through any range of electronic or cloud-based programs. In the setting of more formal e-learning modalities, this happens through portals, repositories, digital libraries, e-Portfolios, and learning management systems (LMS).

An LMS is usually an Internet-based software program that facilitates the delivery and tracking of e-learning across an institution. On top of delivery of content to the learner, it can also provide facilitation of communication from student-to-student, student-to-faculty, and faculty-to-faculty. Many studies have reported on the positive use of LMS in both undergraduate (Zakaria et al. 2013) and postgraduate (Mahoney et al. 2016) medical teaching. Similarly, LMS adoption has been shown to improve educational outcomes in resource-poor settings (Tibyampansha et al. 2017). An LMS can also serve a number of additional functions, including automating administrative and supervisory tasks, tracking learners' achievements, and operating as a repository for instructional resources to learners.

At present, there are over two hundred available LMS programs. Broadly speaking these can be open source, such as Moodle™, or they can be considered commercial/proprietary systems, such as Blackboard™. Moodle (originally an acronym for modular object-oriented dynamic learning environment) already supports over 60 million users and six million courses (Mahoney et al. 2016) with extensive plug-in availability. Its core components allow for the creation of courses, uploading documents, creating basic webpages and discussion forums, and the upload of videos, although size limited. While accessible and useful for laptops and computers, the format often however, does not consistently project well on smaller screens such as smartphones and tablets. Blackboard has the largest representation among large universities and has been active for a long time. It has similar abilities to Moodle, with expanded feature set for assignment submission, grading, and scheduling. Similar to Moodle however, it can often be cumbersome on the smaller screen and is often an issue in its use to SBL. Similarly, annual fee licensing varies but is often in the tens-of-thousands of dollars.

Google Classroom is also a system that integrates some of the successful Google design principles into an LMS. While often described as a "virtual classroom," Google Classroom is still more of an individual experience rather than a collective one, where learners join separately and work separately within it, moving at their own pace and uploading documents as they are ready (What is a Virtual Classroom? 2019). While students can collaborate through Google Docs and Slides, Google Classroom supplements a classroom rather than recreating it. Nonetheless, it offers a virtual experience of an LMS that is often easier to navigate.

Finally, personalized achievements may be culminated in the learner's e-Portfolio. An e-Portfolio is a purposeful aggregation of digital items (feedback, reflection, assessments etc.) which represents evidence of a person's learning and/or ability (Merzouk et al. 2014). As medical practice is evolving towards competency-based training (Harris et al. 2017), e-Portfolios can be a robust tool to record evidence of competency by storing them in a private electronic place. In a well-designed e-Portfolio, a student may have a quicker and better understanding of their overall progression in training compared to a traditional paper-based portfolio.

Content Delivery

Similar to e-learning, SBL can be considered either synchronous or asynchronous (Hrastinski 2008). Synchronous content delivery refers to real-time, instructor-led learning that is beamed to a learner's screen and all learners receive information simultaneously and communicate directly with other learners (Merzouk et al. 2014). This includes media such as teleconferencing, where audio and video are shown to all learners either via a central screen or streamed individually and viewed in real-time. Similarly, this occurs when learners engage with each other and their instructors via instant messaging services through their smartphone devices. Additionally, instant messaging, collaboration, and editing through sharable cloud-based platforms such as Google Docs can also be a synchronous form of content delivery.

Asynchronous delivery, on the other hand, refers to the transmission and receipt of information that does not occur simultaneously. The learners are responsible for pacing their own instruction and learning. If there is a formal e-learning component to it, then the learner and instructor communicate via email or feedback technologies, but not in real-time. This may include the uploading of a learner's assignment and receiving feedback via the Blackboard LMS system or the completion of an online module where learner specific feedback is provided at a later date.

It should be noted that in reference to SBL, most modalities can be both synchronous and asynchronous. With technological advancements, real-time communication is becoming quicker, easier, and more accessible. Nonetheless, one of the major advantages of SBL is the learners' abilities to control the pace, volume, and relevance of content they expose themselves to via their screens. In this way, while technology and platforms allow for more synchronicity among a range of learners and instructors, the major approach to SBL is still likely to be asynchronous (Lau and Bates 2004).

Developments and Projections

SBL is often a result of purposeful intention where tailored and designed content is delivered to a learner through their screens. Realistically however, SBL is often likely to happen outside of this purposeful intent. As such, SBL should also include any interaction a learner has with a screen as long as the intention is to learn. This content can come from a range of sources and their development and design will be addressed with brief examples.

Mobile Learning

At the core of SBL is mobile learning and this has become a new approach to traditional learning. While there are a number of definitions of mobile learning, it is considered an independent part of e-learning where educational resources, tools and materials can be accessed anytime and anywhere using a mobile device. In particular, the characteristics than differ mobile learning from e-learning is the spontaneity, privacy, portability, informality, interactivity, and connectivity (View of Defining, Discussing and Evaluating Mobile Learning 2007). It is these features which enable learners to carry them easily and thus access the learning content 'on to go', such as when waiting for courses, tutorials, or lectures, or at 'point of care', such as at the time of interaction with a patient or an instructor. Furthermore, content for mobile learning is usually designed to be shorter, more personalized, and interactive than traditional e-learning materials, which is often made of longer compact units. Mobile learning is designed for one idea per screen, large buttons, simple navigation all allowing learners to take in a small amount of information over a short period of time (Understanding The Difference Between eLearning and mLearning 2018).

Mobile learning has been shown to have a positive effect on the educational process when compared to no intervention (Wu et al. 2012), as well as compared to traditional learning methods (Cook et al. 2008). There is likely a positive motivational role in the whole process of learning because ownership of the device increases commitment to using and learning from it. Likewise, mobile learning is likely to positively affect learning attitudes by improving educational interest and concentration (Ciampa 2014).

A strong argument for the use of mobile learning is the ubiquitousness of mobile devices in health education. A 2017 study showed that 91% of postgraduate doctors owned a smart-phone and 88% used their mobile device frequently in a clinical setting (Nerminathan et al. 2017). Undergraduate medical students were more likely to use their mobile devices, with 100% of students owning a smartphone or tablet. The most common uses for these devices included accessing medical apps during admission/clerkship, followed by improving knowledge, and test taking (Lau and Kolli 2017). Other uses of mobile devices by healthcare students includes assessment, examination, collection of supervisory reports and student feedback, or downloadable course-specific material (Lumsden et al. 2015).

A 2018 review study on the use of mobile learning in medical education showed that overall the use of a mobile device as an educational tool had a positive effect on the acquisition of knowledge and skill among medical students (Klímová 2018). Some of the reasons listed for this positive effect is that medical students, who are usually between the ages of 18–26 years, use mobile devices on a daily basis and are willing to exploit them for their studies. Furthermore, the inherent attractiveness and interactivity that draws people to their mobile devices is what drives their use for educational purposes as well. The review also showed that there is efficient acquisition and retention of new knowledge, learning new medical procedures, acquiring new skills, and improved practice behavior in the management of a new disease. The use of mobile devices has also been linked with improved performance in examinations by both undergraduate internal medicine (Baumgart et al. 2017) and surgery (Smeds et al. 2016) students.

In spite of all the benefits of mobile learning, there are still certain limitations that must be addressed. These include the cost of the device, and who pays for it, the small size of the screen of smartphones, limited memory and battery, technical problems, and security issues (Briz-Ponce et al. 2016). Additionally, while instant messaging (either through SMS or other apps, such as WhatsApp) is a popular method for communication and information dissemination, it is not that effective for teaching (Hoonpongsimanont et al. 2016). This relates back to the more asynchronous nature of SBL. Furthermore, the presence of mobile devices has also been reported to lead to increased disruption during teaching sessions, and higher dependence on seniors for decision making (Wu et al. 2013).

Other studies have identified significant practical and social limitations to the use of mobile devices, such as poor Internet access in clinical areas and a lack of perceived acceptance by patients and clinicians (Chase et al. 2018). However, if the devices are explained and identified for professional use, then patients are amenable to their use (Alexander et al. 2015). Additionally, simple innovative ideas such as university or hospital branded cases can assist in reducing negative reactions.

Overall, given societal changes in the use of mobile devices, mobile learning will be, and already is, a ubiquitous part of medical education. This modality of SBL is likely to be an ongoing and important source of acquisition of new knowledge and skills.

Social Learning

Social learning theory started well before social media, with Albert Bandura stating that behavior is learned primarily by observing and imitating others (Bandura 1977). This is particularly relevant in the modern-day with the complex nature of information exchange via social media. Social media consists of web-based technologies that facilitate idea sharing through collaboration, interaction, and discussion. The term encompasses multiple platforms ranging from blogs/micro blogs (Twitter®), through to wikis, YouTube®, and social network sites such as Facebook®. Invariably, all these platforms are accessed through screens.

Social media is becoming an ever-growing component of screen-time for students, especially the younger digitally native generation. A 2015 review on social media in medical education found that 91% of students aged 18–25 years and 78% of students aged 26–35 years used some form of social media (Pander et al. 2014). As such, it is becoming an increasingly important aspect of health education.

There are two learning theories that underpin the use of social media in medical education: connectivism and constructivism (Whyte and Hennessy 2017). Connectivism explains how Internet technologies have created new opportunities for people to learn and share information across online peer networks. It is easier for learners to connect to one another via social media, allowing for an active learning environment. Learners are able to share information, ideas and feedback outside the classroom, transcending geographical barriers. This increases the speed of access to information and enhances learning efficiency as well as student satisfaction (Pander et al. 2014). It has been shown that increased learner engagement stimulates interactivity between students and leads to better examination results, likely through improved communication (Junco et al. 2011).

Constructivism is an umbrella term for a number of learning theories that centers on the fact that students subjectively construct knowledge themselves (Flynn et al. 2015). The versatility and customizable nature of social media can be tailored to learners' needs, and as such can build on the positive foundations of e-learning. This has helped create Personal Learning Environments (PLEs) which are learner-designed approaches that incorporate various tools selected by learners to match their needs, style, and pace (Johnson et al. 2011). This can include combining procedural videos from YouTube, flashcard apps to learn anatomy, and tweets from leaders in their field of interest. All this aims to give learners an increasing amount of control over how and when they learn. Various studies have shown that Twitter, podcasts, and blogs most frequently engage learners and enhance education, while YouTube and wikis are used for technical skills and improvement of self-efficacy (Sterling et al. 2017).

Conferences and conventions have hashtags and Twitter accounts and at times have more online distant participants that those at the convention Centre (Hillman and Sherbino 2015). While studies have been able to quantify the presence of online participants, it is very difficult to quantify the learning that happens through this screen presence. Nonetheless, it has sparked a number of different projects that include online journal clubs where authors can discuss their work. 'Tweet chats' are able to help flatten hierarchy and allow a multidisciplinary team to participate in online discussion of any topic that can help both disseminated as well as advance a topic relevant to a learners needs (Forgie et al. 2013).

With the integration of social media into medical education, learning has become a more social process where learners are able to build their own knowledge from multiple external sources. Considering the rise of use of social media for communication among experts, it is also a way for learners to identify positive behaviors from which they can base their own approach to online professionalism.

Simulation

Simulation-based education (SBE) is developing an ever-growing body of evidence supporting its benefits and validity in medical education (Weller et al. 2012). Depending on the type of simulator, SBL can play a big role in the simulation-based educational activities.

Firstly, screens are inherently an important interface on which a majority of simulation activities can occurs. Body mannikins can be coupled with sophisticated software, that along with expert-directed feedback, can provide information on a learner's performance. Laparoscopic bench trainers, whether coupled with a smartphone, tablet, or expensive laparoscopic hardware allow for mastery learning and deliberate practice of laparoscopic skills through SBL. Their effectiveness in the acquisition of basic laparoscopic skills has been well documented (Dhariwal et al. 2007), and while traditionally very expensive and inaccessible, they have become cheaper and more available (Hennessey and Hewett 2013).

Secondly, screens can be an important source of feedback for learning to occur. Feedback can be thought of as the information provided to a learner to modify behavior and enhance learning, and has been shown to be the most important factor in learning a skill (Hattie and Timperley 2007). It is central to supporting cognitive, technical, and professional development. Screens themselves can be the source of feedback through simulator-generated feedback (SGF). SGF has the potential to emulate feedback provided by expert clinicians, potentially overcoming the need for constant expert supervision, by offering end-of-task or real-time feedback. End-of-task feedback refers to a summary of a learner's performance, for example at the end of a virtual-reality simulator simulating a laparoscopic cholecystectomy, complete with metrics that identifies a learner's strengths and weaknesses. Real-time feedback involves the simulator providing feedback as the simulated procedure is occurring so that a learner may refine their skills in real-time (Zhou et al. 2013).

Lastly, screens may be a tool through which supervisors and trainers provide experienced feedback. Video-based feedback has been utilized alongside simulated participants (SPs) in order to provide feedback to learners on a range of technical and cognitive skills (Lehmann et al. 2018).

The Virtual Environment

In a similar fashion to smartphones, the landscape of emerging technology has seen an evolution in available wearable technologies. These refer to electronic devices with sensing and computational capabilities that are worn or attached to the body (Slade Shantz and Veillette 2014), and have the potential to be another disruptive force in healthcare (Kolodzey et al. 2017). Microsoft's HoloLens (Microsoft Corporation, Redmond, WA, USA) is a mixed reality (MR) head-mounted display (HMD), which allows the user to interact with their environment using holograms while engaging their senses through an immersive experience. The user wears a headpiece with a screen that is able to compute their 3D environment, and a hologram is projected onto their screen. Virtual, augmented, and mixed reality are related concepts but with significant differences. Virtual reality (VR) is the representation of the real environment on a device such as a computer, television, or mobile screen. Augmented reality (AR) is a combination of the real and virtual environments on a device with a video camera integrated into its interface. Examples include Google's now out-of-service Google Glass (Google Inc., Mountain View, CA, USA), which overlays an image onto the user's glass and blends digital data with the real world. In MR however, users can quickly and more easily interact with those digital objects to enhance their experience of reality or improve efficiency with certain tasks. (Pantelidis et al. 2017). A recent systematic review on the use of wearable devices in medical education, both in clinical and simulation settings, discussed a range of clinical applications including communication, education, safety and efficiency, and information management. (Kolodzey et al. 2017)

Serious Games and Gamification

Serious games and gamification are screen-based strategies that have been used to provide a 'stealth mode' of learning where the educational goal is mixed with an enjoyment factor (Gentry et al. 2019). As with many SBL strategies, these offer "learner centered" approaches to education in which a learner controls the learning process. A serious game is an "interactive computer application that has a challenging goal, is fun to play and engaging, incorporates some scoring mechanism, and supplies the user with skills, knowledge, or attitudes useful in reality" (Bergeron 2006). Learning is mixed with the gaming design of the program, and in doing so, the program incites and encourages the user while at the same time ensuring acquisition of knowledge or skill. This process inherently supports three fundamental educational concepts that are relevant for medical education: mastery learning (Bloom 1968), deliberate practice (Ericsson 2008), and experiential learning (Kolb 1984).

Gamification is the process by which applying the characteristic and benefits of games to real world problems, users are encouraged and rewarded to perform tasks. It differs from serious games in terms of the design intention. Gamification involves the application of game elements to something with a utilitarian purpose while serious games are full-fledged games for a purpose other than just entertainment (Deterding et al. 2011). Both may be experienced by the user as a complete game, and gamification is considered an important element of a serious games. Additionally, however, gamification has the potential to allow for greater involvement of the user in setting their own objectives or outcomes and personalization of the intervention.

Dr. Game: Surgeon Trouble is a serious game where players match colored shapes to gain points, with players having to troubleshoot their surgical hardware to resume playing. A 2017 study found that during minimally invasive surgical practice, students who played the game as part of their curriculum solved almost twice the number of hardware problems as compared with students in a control group who received a games-free curriculum (Graafland et al. 2017). *Night Shift* is an adventure game designed to improve physicians' triage skills by placing the player in the role of a triage doctor working in an emergency department. When participants who played the game were later assessed in a virtual simulator, those who played the game were significantly less likely to underestimate the severity of injuries (Mohan et al. 2017). LevelEx is a company developing video games for physicians simulating endoscopy (Gastro Ex), bronchoscopy (Pulm Ex), endotracheal intubation (Airway Ex), and cardiac interventional therapy (Cardio Ex) (Level Ex 2019). Through a range of timed levels, players perform a number of interventional therapies, getting tips along the way and warnings about the consequences of making mistakes. The games focus on a patient with a specific problem and begin by having the player choose the type and size of device, then proceed with the intervention. Warnings are given when the patient is in danger or if the player has saved a life (Philips 2019). With over 400,000 users (Level Ex 2019), it aims to utilize technology readily available in the game-world industry and apply it to health education.

While serious gaming is an example of screen-based technologies available to engage learners, the foundation needs to remain centered on valid educational theory. At the core, there must be well-defined learning objectives with tasks being based on validated means of testing. While these new technologies have the means to continue revolutionizing health education, they should continue to be considered as adjuncts to, and catalysts for in-person coaching, relationships building and mentorship.

Blended Learning

SBL can not only transcend space and time boundaries but can also provide up-to-date information through use of current and interactive multimedia. However, one of the disadvantages of e-learning in general is the feeling of isolation that virtual environments can create. Traditional teaching in the physical classroom model is considered vital in building a sense of community. Blended learning, often interchangeably used with hybrid, web-enhanced, or mixed-mode learning, is defined as the combination of traditional face-to-face learning and asynchronous or synchronous e-learning (Garrison and Kanuka 2004). It has the potential to combine the advantages of both traditional learning and e-learning.

With the rapid growth and use of blended learning in medical education, there has been increasing research in relation to its effectiveness, showing both improvement in clinical competencies (Rowe et al. 2012) and lack of evaluation (McCutcheon et al. 2015). However, a 2016 meta-analysis showed that blended learning had a large and consistently positive effect when compared to no intervention, as well as in comparison to non-blended group learning (Liu et al. 2016). This means that blended learning may be more effective than non-blended learning including both traditional face-to-face learning and pure e-learning. It has been postulated that the likely source of this benefit comes from allowing students to review electronic materials as often as necessary, at their own pace, and yet are still less likely to experience feelings of isolation or reduced interest in subject matter.

In a continually technology-engaged approach to learning, the challenge becomes one of integrating blended learning with nontraditional ways of teaching, both online and in person. This requires the use of all aspects of SBL – Internet and mobile learning, videos and other multimedia, interactive exercises, and virtual classrooms and communities such as those accessible via social media. Additionally, it also requires the combination of various pedagogical approaches to learning, including constructivism and connectivism, behaviorism, and cognitivism.

There is no one way to blend learning and technologies. Screen and face-to-face instruction can be combined into several blended learning models and not all models are well-suited to all learning objectives and students. Some models, such as laboratory models in which students complete aspects of the coursework online but complete in-person skills training, may be more suitable for certain aspects of medical education. For example, completion of online modules in relation to suture material properties, followed by laboratory time with physical and virtual trainers may be more appropriate for aspects of surgical training. A flipped classroom style of blended learning, where students may listen to or watch a series of modules or a lecture on a relative topic followed by patient bed-side tutorials may be useful for understanding complex medical disease processes. Blended learning, as a pedagogic model, has wide applicability and has the potential to transform health education (Singh 2015). While the technologies available for blending may change, advance, and expand, the need to blend with purposeful intention will remain a priority.

Conclusion

Over the last 70 to 80 years, our screens have changed drastically. Given these and societal changes, SBL is already becoming a ubiquitous part of clinical education and learning. There needs to be a purpose filled plan in incorporating SBL into medical education, while being mindful of how these screens are being used by learners. At the core of SBL is e-learning, and thus there is a fundamental need for universal access to the internet to ensure useful learning can take place. Furthermore, with the current pace of technological advances, screens and how we interact with them, will change. It will be important that we change with them. We must develop and understand the underlying principles of SBL now, such that when technological advances surpass our current expectations, we have the tools to apply them for health education purposes.

Cross-References

▶ Artificial Intelligence in Surgical Education and Training
▶ Developing Patient Safety Through Education
▶ E-Learning: Development of a Fully Online 4th Year Psychology Program
▶ Embedding a Simulation-Based Education Program in a Teaching Hospital
▶ Focus on Theory: Emotions and Learning
▶ Role of Social Media in Health Professions Education
▶ Simulation as Clinical Replacement: Contemporary Approaches in Healthcare Professional Education
▶ Simulation for Clinical Skills in Healthcare Education
▶ Simulation for Procedural Skills Teaching and Learning
▶ Technology Considerations in Health Professions and Clinical Education

References

Achampong EK, Keney G, Attah NO Sr. The effects of mobile phone use in clinical practice in Cape Coast Teaching Hospital. Online J Public Health Inform. 2018;10(2):e210. https://doi.org/10.5210/ojphi.v10i2.9333.

Alexander SM, Nerminathan A, Harrison A, Phelps M, Scott KM. Prejudices and perceptions: patient acceptance of mobile technology use in health care. Intern Med J. 2015;45(11):1179–81.

Bandura A. Self-efficacy: toward a unifying theory of behavioral change. Psychol Rev. 1977;84(2):191–215.

Baumgart DC, Wende I, Grittner U. Tablet computer enhanced training improves internal medicine exam performance. PLoS One. 2017;12(4):e0172827.

Bergeron BP. Developing serious games: Charles River Media. Hingham, Massachusetts, USA: Charles River Media; 2006. 452 p

Bloom BS. Learning for Mastery. Instruction and Curriculum. Regional Education Laboratory for the Carolinas and Virginia, Topical Papers and Reprints. 1968.

Briz-Ponce L, Juanes-Méndez JA, García-Peñalvo FJ, Pereira A. Effects of mobile learning in medical education: a counterfactual evaluation. J Med Syst. 2016;40(6):136.

Chase TJG, Julius A, Chandan JS, Powell E, Hall CS, Phillips BL, et al. Mobile learning in medicine: an evaluation of attitudes and behaviours of medical students. BMC Med Educ. 2018;18(1):152.

Chodorow S. Educators must take the electronic revolution seriously. Acad Med. 1996;71(3):221–6.

Chu LF, Chan BK. Evolution of web site design: implications for medical education on the internet. Comput Biol Med. 1998;28(5):459–72.

Ciampa K. Learning in a mobile age: an investigation of student motivation. J Comput Assist Learn. 2014;30(1):82–96.

Clark D. Psychological myths in e-learning. Med Teach. 2002;24(6):598–604.

Cook CW, Sonnenberg C. Technology and online education: models for change. Contemp Issues Educ Res. 2014;7(3):171–88.

Cook DA, Levinson AJ, Garside S, Dupras DM, Erwin PJ, Montori VM. Internet-based learning in the health professions: a meta-analysis. JAMA. 2008;300(10):1181–96.

Crowder NA, Martin GC. Adventures in algebra. 1st ed. The English Universities Press. London, UK: Hodder & Stoughton General Division; 1962. 360 p.

Deterding S, Dixon D, Khaled R, Nacke LE. Gamification: toward a definition. Presented at: The ACM CHI conference on human factors in computing; 2011 May 7–12; Vancouver.

Dhariwal AK, Prabhu RY, Dalvi AN, Supe AN. Effectiveness of box trainers in laparoscopic training. J Minim Access Surg. 2007;3(2):57–63.

Ericsson KA. Deliberate practice and acquisition of expert performance: a general overview. Acad Emerg Med. 2008;15(11):988–94.

Ericsson Mobility Report June 2019. 2019;36.

Fernández-Manjón B, Sánchez-Pérez JM, Gomez-Pulido JA, Vega-Rodríguez MA, Bravo J. Computers and education: e-learning, from theory to practice; 2008. https://doi.org/10.1007/978-1-4020-4914-9.

Flynn L, Jalali A, Moreau KA. Learning theory and its application to the use of social media in medical education. Postgrad Med J. 2015;91(1080):556–60.

Forgie SE, Duff JP, Ross S. Twelve tips for using Twitter as a learning tool in medical education. Med Teach. 2013;35(1):8–14.

Garrison DR, Kanuka H. Blended learning: uncovering its transformative potential in higher education. Internet High Educ. 2004;7(2):95–105.

Gentry SV, Gauthier A, Ehrstrom BL, Wortley D, Lilienthal A, Car LT, et al. Serious gaming and gamification education in health professions: systematic review. J Med Internet Res. 2019;21(3):e12994.

Graafland M, Bemelman WA, Schijven MP. Game-based training improves the surgeon's situational awareness in the operation room: a randomized controlled trial. Surg Endosc. 2017;31(10):4093–101.

Hampson K. Design and screen-based learning in higher education | Acrobatiq [Internet]. 2013 [cited 2018 Nov 27]. Available from: http://acrobatiq.com/design-and-screen-based-learning-in-higher-education/

Harris P, Bhanji F, Topps M, Ross S, Lieberman S, Frank JR, et al. Evolving concepts of assessment in a competency-based world. Med Teach. 2017;39(6):603–8.

Hattie J, Timperley H. The power of feedback. Rev Educ Res. 2007;77(1):81–112.

Hennessey IAM, Hewett P. Construct, concurrent, and content validity of the eoSim laparoscopic simulator. J Laparoendosc Adv Surg Tech. 2013;23(10):855–60.

Hillman T, Sherbino J. Social media in medical education: a new pedagogical paradigm? Postgrad Med J. 2015;91(1080):544–5.

Hoonpongsimanont W, Kulkarni M, Tomas-Domingo P, Anderson C, McCormack D, Tu K, et al. Text messaging versus email for emergency medicine residents' knowledge retention: a pilot comparison in the United States. J Educ Eval Health Prof [Internet]. 2016 [cited 2019 July 2];13. Available from: http://www.jeehp.org/DOIx.php?id=10.3352/jeehp.2016.13.36

Hrastinski S. Asynchronous & synchronous e-learning. Educ Q. 2008;31(4):51–5.

Johnson L, Adams S, Haywood K. NMC Horizon report: 2011 K-12 Edition [Internet]. The New Media Consortium; 2011 [cited 2019 July 2]. Available from: https://www.learntechlib.org/p/182017/

Junco R, Heiberger G, Loken E. The effect of Twitter on college student engagement and grades. J Comput Assist Learn. 2011;27(2):119–32.

Kaufman J, Ryan S, Thille C, Bier N. Open learning initiative courses in community colleges: evidence on use and effectiveness. Carnegie Mellon University; October 2013 [Internet]. Available from: https://hewlett.org/wp-content/uploads/2013/12/CCOLI_Report_Final_1.pdf

Klímová B. Mobile learning in medical education. J Med Syst. 2018;42(10):194.

Kolb D. Experiential learning: experience as the source of learning and development, vol. 1. Englewood Cliffs, NJ, USA: Prentice Hall; 1984.

Kolodzey L, Grantcharov PD, Rivas H, Schijven MP, Grantcharov TP. Wearable technology in the operating room: a systematic review. BMJ Innov. 2017;3(1):55–63.

Lau F, Bates J. A review of e-learning practices for undergraduate medical education. J Med Syst. 2004;28(1):71–87.

Lau C, Kolli V. App use in psychiatric education: a medical student survey. Acad Psychiatry J Am Assoc Dir Psychiatr Resid Train Assoc Acad Psychiatry. 2017;41(1):68–70.

Lehmann M, Sterz J, Stefanescu M-C, Zabel J, Sakmen KD, Ruesseler M. Influence of expert video feedback, peer video feedback, standard video feedback and oral feedback on undergraduate medical students' performance of basic surgical skills. Creat Educ. 2018;09:1221.

Level Ex: Home [Internet]. Level Ex. 2019 [cited 2019 July 6]. Available from: https://www.level-ex.com/

Liu Q, Peng W, Zhang F, Hu R, Li Y, Yan W. The effectiveness of blended learning in health professions: systematic review and meta-analysis. J Med Internet Res. 2016;18(1):e2. https://doi.org/10.2196/jmir.4807.

Lumsden CJ, Byrne-Davis LMT, Mooney JS, Sandars J. Using mobile devices for teaching and learning in clinical medicine. Arch Dis Child Educ Pract. 2015;100(5):244–51.

Mahoney NR, Boland MV, Ramulu PY, Srikumaran D. Implementing an electronic learning management system for an Ophthalmology residency program. BMC Med Educ. 2016;16(1):307.

McCutcheon K, Lohan M, Traynor M, Martin D. A systematic review evaluating the impact of online or blended learning vs. face-to-face learning of clinical skills in undergraduate nurse education. J Adv Nurs. 2015;71(2):255–70.

Merzouk A, Kurosinski P, Kostikas K. E-learning for the medical team: the present and future of ERS Learning Resources. Breathe. 2014;10(4):296–304.

Mohan D, Farris C, Fischhoff B, Rosengart MR, Angus DC, Yealy DM, et al. Efficacy of educational video game versus traditional educational apps at improving physician decision making in trauma triage: randomized controlled trial. BMJ. 2017;359:j5416.

Nerminathan A, Harrison A, Phelps M, Alexander S, Scott KM. Doctors' use of mobile devices in the clinical setting: a mixed methods study. Intern Med J. 2017;47(3):291–8.

Pander T, Pinilla S, Dimitriadis K, Fischer MR. The use of Facebook in medical education – a literature review. GMS Z Für Med Ausbild. 2014;31(3):Doc33.

Pantelidis P, Chorti A, Papagiouvanni I, Paparoidamis G, Drosos C, Panagiotakopoulos T, et al. Virtual and augmented reality in medical education. Med Surg Educ Past Present Future [Internet]; 2017 [cited 2019 Nov 12]. Available from: https://www.intechopen.com/books/medical-and-surgical-education-past-present-and-future/virtual-and-augmented-reality-in-medical-education

Philips gets into the interventional cardiology video game [Internet]. Medical Design and Outsourcing. 2019 [cited 2019 Dec 2]. Available from: https://www.medicaldesignandoutsourcing.com/philips-gets-into-the-interventional-cardiology-video-game/

Riley JB, Austin JW, Holt DW, Searles BE, Darling EM. Internet-based virtual classroom and educational management software enhance students' didactic and clinical experiences in perfusion education programs. J Extra Corpor Technol. 2004;36(3):235–9.

Rosenberg MJ. E-learning: strategies for delivering knowledge in the digital age. 1st ed. New York: McGraw-Hill Education; 2000. p. 344.

Rowe M, Frantz J, Bozalek V. The role of blended learning in the clinical education of healthcare students: a systematic review. Med Teach. 2012;34(4):e216–21.

Ruiz JG, Mintzer MJ, Leipzig RM. The impact of e-learning in medical education. Acad Med. 2006;81(3):207.

Selwyn N. Education and technology: key issues and debates [Internet]. Continuum International Publishing Group; 2012 [cited 2019 Dec 10]. Available from: https://research.monash.edu/en/publications/education-and-technology-key-issues-and-debates

Singh AK. Blended learning for medical professionals. Harvard office for External Education. [Internet]. 2015. Available from: https://hms.harvard.edu/sites/default/files/assets/Sites/OGE/files/Blended_Learning_for_Medical_Professionals.pdf.

Skinner BF. Teaching machines: from the experimental study of learning come devices which arrange optimal conditions for self-instruction. Science. 1958;128(3330):969–77.

Slade Shantz JA, Veillette CJH. The application of wearable technology in surgery: ensuring the positive impact of the wearable revolution on surgical patients. Front Surg. 2014;1:39. https://doi.org/10.3389/fsug.2014.00039.

Smeds MR, Thrush CR, Mizell JS, Berry KS, Bentley FR. Mobile spaced education for surgery rotation improves National Board of Medical Examiners scores. J Surg Res. 2016;201(1):99–104.

Sterling M, Leung P, Wright D, Bishop TF. The use of social media in graduate medical education: a systematic review. Acad Med. 2017;92(7):1043–56.

Sweller J, Merriënboer JJG van. Instructional design for medical education [Internet]. Oxford University Press; 2013 [cited 2019 Dec 10]. Available from: https://oxfordmedicine.com/view/10.1093/med/9780199652679.001.0001/med-9780199652679-chapter-7

TEDxMaastricht – Lawrence Sherman – "Turning medical education inside out and upside down" [Internet]. 2011 [cited 2019 Dec 10]. Available from: https://www.youtube.com/watch?v=YpSd5u_di9w&t=13m31s

Tibyampansha D, Ibrahim G, Kapanda G, Tarimo C, Minja A, Kulanga A, et al. Implementation of a learning management system for medical students: a case study of Kilimanjaro Christian Medical University College. MedEdPublish [Internet]. 2017 Mar 15 [cited 2019 Jun 20];6. Available from: https://www.mededpublish.org/manuscripts/899

Understanding The Difference Between eLearning and mLearning [Internet]. 2018 [cited 2019 July 2]. Available from: https://www.shiftelearning.com/blog/difference-between-elearning-and-mlearning

View of Defining, Discussing and Evaluating Mobile Learning | The International Review of Research in Open and Distributed Learning [Internet]. 2007 [cited 2019 July 2]. Available from: http://www.irrodl.org/index.php/irrodl/article/view/346/875

Weller JM, Nestel D, Marshall SD, Brooks PM, Conn JJ. Simulation in clinical teaching and learning. Med J Aust. 2012;196(9):594.

What is a Virtual Classroom? Definition from Techopedia [Internet]. Techopedia.com. 2019 [cited 2019 July 1]. Available from: https://www.techopedia.com/definition/13914/virtual-classroom

Whyte W, Hennessy C. Social media use within medical education: a systematic review to develop a pilot questionnaire on how social media can be best used at BSMS. MedEdPublish [Internet]. 2017 May 11 [cited 2019 July 2];6. Available from: https://www.mededpublish.org/manuscripts/984

Wu W-H, Jim Wu Y-C, Chen C-Y, Kao H-Y, Lin C-H, Huang S-H. Review of trends from mobile learning studies: a meta-analysis. Comput Educ. 2012;59(2):817–27.

Wu RC, Tzanetos K, Morra D, Quan S, Lo V, Wong BM. Educational impact of using smartphones for clinical communication on general medicine: more global, less local. J Hosp Med. 2013;8(7):365–72.

Yang HH. New world, new learning: trends and issues of E-learning. Procedia Soc Behav Sci. 2013;77:429–42.

Zakaria N, Jamal A, Bisht S, Koppel C. Embedding a learning management system into an undergraduate medical informatics course in Saudi Arabia: Lessons Learned. Med 20. 2013;2(2):e13.

Zhou Y, Bailey J, Ioannou I, Wijewickrema S, O'Leary S, Kennedy G. Pattern-based real-time feedback for a temporal bone simulator. In: Proceedings of the 19th ACM symposium on virtual reality software and technology [Internet]. New York: ACM; 2013 [cited 2018 Nov 10]. p. 7–16. (VRST '13). Available from: http://doi.acm.org/10.1145/2503713.2503728

Artificial Intelligence in Surgical Education and Training

73

Melanie Crispin

Contents

Introduction	1436
Artificial Intelligence in Surgical Education and Training	1436
Artificial Intelligence Technology Today	1436
Artificial Intelligence Applications Within Surgical Training	1438
Ethics and Accountability	1441
Curriculum	1443
Conclusion	1444
Cross-References	1444
References	1445

Abstract

The landscape of surgical education and training is rapidly changing. Technology is becoming more integrated into learning, practice, and assessment, and with new technologies comes new opportunities as well as responsibilities and ethical considerations. One such technology is artificial intelligence (AI), which has already provided breakthroughs in the automotive industry (Tesla and self-driving cars), tech industry (Google Photos and Google Translate), and is showing promise in big data (IBM Watson) (Hashimoto et al., Ann Surg. 268:70–6, 2018). The four key components of AI are machine learning, natural language processing, artificial neural networks, and visual processing, each of which is relevant to its potential applications in surgical education. It has relevance for clinical diagnosis (particularly in image recognition), audit and risk management, research, and the individualization of both patient care and surgical training. We must approach artificial intelligence responsibly, considering its ethical implications such as culpability, management of error, awareness of algorithms and its weaknesses. Teaching regarding the judicious use and application of artificial intelligence technology needs to begin at the undergraduate level, so that future

M. Crispin (✉)
Monash Health & The University of Melbourne, Melbourne, Australia

© Springer Nature Singapore Pte Ltd. 2023
D. Nestel et al. (eds.), *Clinical Education for the Health Professions*,
https://doi.org/10.1007/978-981-15-3344-0_133

clinicians can be prepared to integrate this promising and inevitable technology into future practice. This chapter aims to address the current state of AI technology; its potential applications for surgical education and training; important considerations such as accountability, ethics, and governance relating to AI; and potential future curriculum changes required to successfully incorporate AI into surgical education and training.

Keywords

Artificial intelligence · Technology · Surgical education · Machine learning · Natural language processing · Artificial neural networks · Visual processing · Big data · Governance

Introduction

Artificial intelligence (AI) is the simulation of intelligent behavior in computers by way of algorithms (Hashimoto et al. 2018). It warrants careful consideration in the field of surgical education and training. The four key components of AI are machine learning, natural language processing, artificial neural networks, and visual processing, all of which are relevant to the potential applications in surgical education (Hashimoto et al. 2018). AI already has applications within other industries including automotive (Tesla), tech (Google), and big data and information technology (IBM Watson). It has important implications regarding surgical education and training, from diagnostic assistance when it comes to interpretation of electrocardiograms and chest radiographs, to trawling electronic medical records (EMR) to conduct audits, risk management and research, to training in laparoscopic surgery with robotic AI assistance. It is important to recognize AI as a tool to be used by a critically thinking clinician who must always remain aware of the pitfalls of AI, for example, gaps within algorithms. Clinicians and trainees must take responsibility for the ethics and governance regarding the application of AI technology into the health care, and lead the way in designing curricula for undergraduate learners to be equipped for the use of AI in their future practice.

Artificial Intelligence in Surgical Education and Training

Artificial Intelligence Technology Today

The information age is transitioning towards the age of artificial intelligence (Wartman and Combs 2018). It is our challenge to harness this new technology to simplify our lives and improve our efficiency, including within the field of surgical education, training, and practice (Hashimoto et al. 2018). This is particularly relevant within the changing landscape of surgical training towards safe working hours, shorter working weeks, combined with increasing demands of public accountability, outcomes-based surgery, and competency-based training (Wong and Matsumoto 2008). Technological changes which have facilitated the growth and development of AI includes the roll out of EMR, increased capacity for greater data storage, image acquisition and processing technology, improved computer processing speeds, and cloud-based rather than fixed-location storage (Kapoor et al. 2019).

Machine Learning

Machines are capable of storing and processing far more information that humans are able to, and therefore, AI will inevitably be integrated into daily clinical decision making to assist clinicians with their work (Hashimoto et al. 2018). AI machines are capable of learning from their own successes and failure in order to improve its future predictions (Hashimoto et al. 2018). Machine learning can be either "supervised" or "unsupervised"; supervised machine learning occurs when the computer is fed labelled data and learns to recognize this data as per its label, thus training an algorithm to predict a known result or outcome, such as the presence of an abnormality on a chest radiograph (Hashimoto et al. 2018). Unsupervised learning occurs when the computer recognizes structures and patterns within big data, large datasets which cannot be analyzed in traditional methods. These data are unlabeled, and AI computers have the ability to detect patterns and connections within medical data, for example, risk factors for development of surgical site infections (Hashimoto et al. 2018).

Natural Language Processing

Natural language processing is the ability of AI machines to understand semantics and syntax within text or speech, and to infer meaning and sentiment from prose (Hashimoto et al. 2018). It involves the machine understanding not only individual words, but also context, and even shorthand or colloquial language. In health care, AI has the potential to "read" and analyze EMR data, and search it to detect adverse events and postoperative complications from documentation (Hashimoto et al. 2018). It can already predict anastomotic leak based on words and phrases used in operation report and progress notes (Hashimoto et al. 2018). It may, therefore, prove to be a useful adjunct to conducting audits for surgical units and individual clinicians, and for quality improvement purposes. It may also allow for AI-assisted documentation of patient–clinician interactions, for example, ward rounds and outpatient clinic notes, potentially saving time and even improving documentation accuracy.

Artificial Neural Networks

Multilayered artificial neural networks are very complex and comprised of multiple layers and interactions. Using artificial neural networks and algorithms AI machines can integrate an entire patient's history to predict ICU mortality more accurately than APACHE II, and accurately predict in-hospital mortality after open abdominal aortic aneurysm repair (Hashimoto et al. 2018).

Visual Processing

Visual processing or computer vision describes the development of AI machine's ability to recognize images and videos. This can be applied to the interpretation of two-dimensional images, such as ECG interpretation, pathology slide interpretation, or chest radiograph interpretation as well as video data, for example, laparoscopic or colonoscopy video image data. Within some image-based specialties such as radiology, pathology, and dermatology, AI may eventually replace some basic diagnostic responsibilities of clinicians (Hashimoto et al. 2018).

Artificial Intelligence Applications Within Surgical Training

AI has the potential to provide meaningful diagnostic assistance when partnered with a well-informed clinician (Kapoor et al. 2019). The components of machine learning and visual processing allows AI to analyze data and recognize patterns in images (Hashimoto et al. 2018; Kapoor et al. 2019). AI has already been shown to be more superior than specialist clinicians when it comes to ECG interpretation, identifying skin cancers on smart phone photos, identifying pathology in ophthalmology retina photos, diagnosing breast cancer lymph node metastases on pathology slides, and interpreting chest x-rays (Hashimoto et al. 2018; Kapoor et al. 2019; Mirnezami and Ahmed 2018). AI can accurately predict the onset of sepsis in ICU patients, as well as select the statistically most beneficial intervention for patients, and detect chronic obstructive pulmonary disease exacerbations early (Kapoor et al. 2019). However, while AI is able to provide a strong statistical and data-driven basis of practice, it is unable to understand and tailor this to the nuanced clinical, psychological, or social context of the individual patient, within which the diagnosis must be interpreted. Therefore, the AI-savvy physician must interpret and communicate the AI's diagnosis appropriately and accurately, and thus aid the patient with the decision making (Kapoor et al. 2019). By assisting in and automating certain tasks such as "straight-forward" diagnosis, AI has the potential to free up specialists' and trainees' time in their busy days, allowing them to focus on both the more complex problem-solving tasks of their job, as well as the human, compassionate side of patient care which has been notably impacted by the advent of electronic medical record (EMR) (Mirnezami and Ahmed 2018; Hodges 2018).

Clinicians must maintain a critical view when it comes to utilizing AI as a diagnostic assistant and be conscious of the risk of automation bias (Kapoor et al. 2019; Hodges 2018). Rather than accepting all of the information provided by AI as completely trustworthy, clinicians must maintain a high index of suspicion for machine learning error, and also understand to some extent the algorithm used by the machine to reach that conclusion (Kapoor et al. 2019). For example, in recognizing a pneumothorax on a chest radiograph, one must ensure that the computer is not simply recognizing a "chest tube" and labelling that as a "pneumothorax" (Hashimoto et al. 2018). The diagnoses and suggestions of AI should always be tested against a clinician's own judgment and assessment. While not every clinician requires in-depth knowledge about AI, there must be at least some within each institution or specialty who are well educated in the area, who can partner with data scientists to provide technical support to clinicians when using and troubleshooting AI in clinical practice (Hashimoto et al. 2018).

The use of AI technology may also prove to be cost-effective, if machines are able to replace some of the time-consuming tasks usually conducted by doctors and other health professionals. Machines are able to process larger volumes of information more rapidly than humans can: for example, DeepMind AI AlphaZero taught itself how to play chess from scratch in 4 hours, and was thereafter able to beat a chess master (Mirnezami and Ahmed 2018; Hodges 2018). By replacing some of the automated duties of clinicians, AI machines can work relatively cheaply around the clock, and they do not become fatigued or hungry, or have "off" days. However, they do still require maintenance (Hashimoto et al. 2018). Due to the sheer volume of data that AI can process and retain, error and bias may be reduced, and there may be fewer missed diagnoses overall (Hashimoto et al. 2018; Hodges 2018). Statistical probabilities of adverse events, for example, postoperative complications can be accurately predicted, allowing surgeons and trainees to make informed decisions in conjunction with patients (Marchalik 2017).

More sophisticated use of AI in clinical decision support includes IBM Watson for Oncology (WFO), which is already in use within the oncology setting, integrating large volumes of knowledge and multiple parameters such as clinical, genetic, and radiological variables, to assist physicians in choosing the best therapy for individual patients with cancer (Mirnezami and Ahmed 2018; Hamilton et al. 2019). By incorporating this big data, AI can provide statistically sound advice regarding multimodal therapy use, surgery timing and type, personal risk data based on their demographics, pathology, and physiology (Mirnezami and Ahmed 2018). These are complex assessments which are beyond the capacity of most human minds. While humans can be prone to biases when making assessments or selecting therapies, WFO is able to provide a bias-free statistically accurate recommendation; however, it should be noted that its "black box" algorithm must always remain transparent and available for analysis. Patient surveys have found that WFO is accepted by patients as part of their care, as long as it is used in conjunction with a physician (Hamilton et al. 2019). AI could, therefore, become a key member of multidisciplinary cancer team meetings and cancer outpatient consultations in the future.

Another key application of AI is in relation to natural language processing. With many doctors citing the EMR as a key source of job dissatisfaction, AI's natural language processing has the potential to act as an intelligent digital assistant, writing notes, providing instant verbal response to queries about patient histories, and more, thus potentially replacing much of the paperwork that surgeons and trainees are tasked with daily, and improving workplace satisfaction (Hashimoto et al. 2018; Mirnezami and Ahmed 2018; Johnston 2018). The intelligent AI assistant could transcribe consultation and ward round notes based on accurately interpreted summaries of the conversations and interactions, write letters to general practitioners saving time on dictation, locate key information in patient histories regarding previous medical conditions, allergies and alerts, surgical procedures, or medications (Hashimoto et al. 2018; Mirnezami and Ahmed 2018; Arora 2018). This may even allow surgeons and trainees to return from the computer screen to the face-to-face interaction and provide more compassionate and mutually satisfying patient care (Mirnezami and Ahmed 2018; Marchalik 2017; Johnston 2018).

AI-driven robots have been shown to perform certain surgical tasks better than surgeons. For example, the surgical tissue approximation robot (STAR) at Johns Hopkins University, Baltimore, USA can perform a small bowel anastomosis with laparoscopic suturing better than surgeons (Hashimoto et al. 2018). Much of surgical practice has already been streamlined using technology, such as stapler devices for bowel anastomosis; could the assistance of a robot for certain steps be a feasible undertaking in the future? AI video image recognition can also accurately identify the individual steps in operations such as a sleeve gastrectomy (Hashimoto et al. 2018). This could open avenues for trainees to have a virtual surgical coach, or an operative "GPS." As trainees learn to perform laparoscopic surgeries, either in simulations or with actual patients, they can be mentored not only by a surgeon, but also by an AI computer which can provide a real-time checklist of steps to perform, and provide warnings if steps are missed, or if important structures are endangered, and even feedback as to individual performance when compared to individual past performance, or expected level of performance for training stage (Mirnezami and Ahmed 2018).

Autonomous surgical robots are still far off on the horizon in terms of development (and may never actually eventuate), but glimpses of this ability have already been seen. For example, the Trauma Pod prototype has the potential to provide lifesaving critical care within military settings. The armored Trauma Pod can be deployed onto a battle field, where an injured soldier can receive immediate resuscitation by a robot remotely controlled by a surgeon, before being evacuated for definitive care (O'Sullivan et al. 2019). A similar beneficial application can be seen in other situations, for example, other difficult-to-access areas where deploying a surgeon may be too risky, such as on the international space station, in Antarctica, or when faced with contagious threats such as SARS. Within every operating theatre, AI technology could provide assistance similar in a way to a robotic theatre technician, automatically adjusting the table height and tilt for surgeon height and the part of the operation, light brightness and focus, insufflation pressures, and theatre temperature (Mirnezami and Ahmed 2018).

Scientific research can also be performed by AI machines by trawling big data and unlocking clinically relevant information within the data (Arora 2018). AI machine learning and artificial neural networks can search these databases and find relevant information based on a clinical question (Hodges 2018). AI has been shown to be able to accurately predict an anastomotic leak based on the types of words used in the operation note and in progress notes, and can, therefore, flag the potential risks to treating clinicians (Hashimoto et al. 2018). It can assist in performing retrospective audits and provide complications data based on coding, freeing up surgical trainees' time when it comes to monthly surgical audits, and improving clinical governance (Arora 2018).

Big data and AI can help to personalize patient care. Combining EMR with wearable technology such as smart watches, together with mobile phone health apps, and social media, means there is potentially a wealth of information available regarding individual patient and collective population health. This may allow treatments to be personalized based on individual patients' disease phenotype and genotype (Krittanawong et al. 2017). The data input needs to be high quality for machine learning and AI to produce meaningful results (Hashimoto et al. 2018; Wartman and Combs 2018; Kapoor et al. 2019). The data also needs to be representative of the population in question, for example, often women and minorities are underrepresented in most studies (Hashimoto et al. 2018). The integration of this information by AI neutral networks has the potential to assist clinicians in providing individualized patient care on a new detailed level (Hodges 2018; Jiang et al. 2017). The cloud-based, rather than paper-based or institution-based, storage of information also means that care can be brought to the patient, for example, in remote settings, rather than the patient coming to the hospital to receive care (Wartman and Combs 2018).

AI technology has the potential to bring individualized health care to the patient, with the clinician taking leadership of the multidisciplinary health care team, as well as managing the interface between humans and machines (Wartman and Combs 2018). Similarly, it can also individualize surgical training by providing individualized feedback on both trainees' technical and nontechnical skills. Big data-driven decision support and decision making will eventually become commonplace, and so physicians and trainees, therefore, must equip themselves with knowledge about AI, and be educated in interpreting the AI-generated probabilities and statistics, determine their validity in each clinical context, and communicate these to patients in a compassionate way (Wartman and Combs 2018; Krittanawong et al. 2017). The growing use of AI in mobile health applications, and accessibility afforded by the Internet means that there is a narrowed knowledge differential between the doctor and the patient than in the past, and so the human qualities of empathy, communication, and building trust become even more paramount, as we guide patients as active collaborators through their treatment decisions (Wartman and Combs 2018).

Ethics and Accountability

It is critically important to consider accountability and governance in relation to AI technology, its decision making, and its performance. There must be strict legal, regulatory, and ethical frameworks for its use. AI computers must be accountable, which means that its actions must be explainable, providing record of all inputs, algorithm calculations, as well as outputs; in other words, the "black box" of AI must be available for analysis in case of error (O'Sullivan et al. 2019). However, providing absolute transparency of AI algorithms and processes may conflict with intellectual property rights. In case of AI error, liability must lie with a person, or persons, as a machine cannot be liable for its actions, and cannot understand blame or culpability. Additionally, machines have no civil liberties and, therefore, cannot be punished (O'Sullivan et al. 2019). There is still uncertainty about who would take responsibility for AI machine error, but key stakeholders and, therefore, possible persons responsible include the manufacturer, the operator, or the person responsible for maintenance (O'Sullivan et al. 2019). Insurance companies will also need to include AI clauses into their policies, including provisions for if the manufacturer went out of business, or if the AI robot behavior becomes unpredictable and outside of its programming (O'Sullivan et al. 2019). It is because of this need for human responsibility that surgical robots may never be fully autonomous, similar to the autonomous car industry, because a human "in the loop" is essential for assigning responsibility in case of adverse event or complication (O'Sullivan et al. 2019).

Within the driver-assist car industry, levels of automation range from level zero to level five; at level zero, the driver is in full control, and the machine provides warnings only. Level one is where the machine is autonomous, but the driver can retake control at any time. Level two is "hands off," with the driver monitoring the vehicle and intervening if there are any errors. Level three is "eyes off," where the drivers' attention can be elsewhere, but can also take over at any time. Level four is "mind off," where the driver can sleep. Level five is fully automatic, where no human intervention is required (O'Sullivan et al. 2019). In robot-assisted surgery, where the surgeon remains in control (level zero), for example, the Trauma Pod in military settings, we must consider the implications if the transmission is lost midway through the operation (O'Sullivan et al. 2019). In that case, should the robot have an autonomous function to continue the operation or resuscitation independently (level five)? In military settings where the risk to life is significant, potentially the ethics surrounding autonomous robot surgeries are less stringent; however, in civilian settings, that risk may be unacceptable (O'Sullivan et al. 2019). It has not been addressed whether the Trauma Pod would be able to triage multiple wounded soldiers on a battlefield like an experienced army surgeon would be able to (O'Sullivan et al. 2019).

While remote-controlled surgical robots may allow for patients in rural settings to receive care closer to home, the risk of technological failure is currently still too great to be ethically justified (Alemzadeh et al. 2016). Even for robot-assisted surgery where the surgeon is present and in control, informed consent must be obtained from the patient with clear details about the level of autonomy the robot has, as well as the added material risks which relate to the technology and robot/AI being used (Alemzadeh et al. 2016). Another important consideration is, if AI can assist trainees in performing operations by providing prompts for the operative steps and anatomical overlay, should AI be able to stop a surgery from continuing if it deems the risk to the patient is too great? And, if so, can this function be overridden if the identified risk is a necessary step to complete the operation, for example, a radical cancer resection that would involve damage to certain important structures? (Mirnezami and Ahmed 2018).

Cybersecurity is another important consideration, as AI computers have the potential to be hacked and algorithms corrupted, and machines instructed to make harmful or even lethal decisions when involved with patient care. This must also be considered and addressed before AI and robot-assisted surgery can become widespread (O'Sullivan et al. 2019). Precautions should be taken, such as video recording of every operation for analysis in case of error, and taking care to not alter software or download new programs or make any changes to the set-up during an operation (O'Sullivan et al. 2019). As always, the focus should be on improving patient care and on patient safety. Clinicians trained in AI need to lead the way in policy writing and implementation.

Big data also has ethical implications of data ownership and privacy (Arora 2018). Written, voice recorded, and video data can all be stored in unlimited quantities in the cloud, and these need to be securely stored and labelled, even encrypted, with protection against privacy breaches and hacking in place (Arora 2018). It is still unclear as to who owns the data, whether it is the patient who owns their own data, or institutions, or governments. With so much personal information available, care must also be taken to not discriminate against people based on their health information, for example, for health insurance, life insurance, or employment opportunities. Clinicians and trainees must also take care to not deskill in the diagnostic tasks with which AI technology can assist; the diagnosis made by AI computers should always be tested against a clinician's own judgment and hypothesis for accuracy and rigor (Kapoor et al. 2019).

Curriculum

Surgical education and training curricula must begin to incorporate teaching regarding the understanding and use of AI technology, as its role in our future (and current) practice is inevitable (Hodges 2018; Johnston 2018). AI has the potential to individualize surgical training, by collecting trainee-specific big data and using that to improve training, feedback, and assessment (Arora 2018). Surgical training is currently often haphazard, variable and difficult to standardize, as patient complexity and case mix varies considerably day to day, and between surgical units and institutions and countries. AI technology has the ability to collect data about trainees' consultations, clinical encounters, patterns of touch during examinations (via haptic data), eye tracking and video recordings during operations particularly laparoscopic surgery, individualized complication data, geolocation, and time spent doing different tasks (Kapoor et al. 2019). These data can then be analyzed in conjunction with clinical supervisors and fed back to the trainees about how they can improve. It can be an additional source of determining competence with certain aspects of surgical training, and a tool used for trainee assessment. By collecting big data about individual trainees to track their progress, AI algorithms could also assess an individual surgeon or trainees' suitability to perform a specific operation based, for example, on video analysis of performance or complications data, which itself has ethical implications (Mirnezami and Ahmed 2018). All of this also raises privacy concerns as to who would have access to this data, and whether it could influence future job prospects for trainees and surgeons (Arora 2018). Within the wider education sphere, AI is already in use for tailoring learning to individual needs, and it seems only apt to apply it to surgical education too (TeachThought Staff 2018).

Changes must also be made to the undergraduate medical curriculum. Medical students must be taught about AI technology, applications, and ethics, and be educated in how to use it effectively and responsibly (Hodges 2018; Johnston 2018). In addition, the rapidly expanding body of medical knowledge combined with AI technology's ability to process and store far more information than a human brain can may mean that rote learning may become increasingly less relevant in medical training. Instead, students should be taught how to interpret and integrate and test information from a variety of sources, including those from AI systems (Marchalik 2017; Johnston 2018). With less need to memorize vast amounts of knowledge, which can be made readily available to them via AI computer systems, students can instead focus more on honing their skills in the more human aspects of medicine, such as communication, empathy, leadership, teamwork, and conflict resolution (Johnston 2018). Perhaps, literature could even be reintroduced into the medical school curriculum, promoting self-reflection and intellectual flexibility, qualities both so valuable in our diverse world (Marchalik 2017).

Clinicians will need to learn the skills to effectively communicate the recommendations of AI machines to patients in a meaningful and relevant way. Educators need to adapt to the AI age, and at the same time cultivate within their students the human qualities which form the cornerstone of medicine (Mukherjee 2017). Barriers to medical education reform may include tradition, accreditation concerns, and faculty resistance to change (Wartman and Combs 2018). However, within big data and AI technology lies the potential to revolutionize and individualize health care and medical and surgical training and practice (Arora 2018).

Conclusion

Artificial intelligence is relevant to surgical education and training in many ways. It can provide diagnostic assistance, decision support, tailor treatment to patients, tailor training to trainees, assist with note writing and audit and research, perform aspects of surgery, and act as a virtual coach during operations. It has the potential to revolutionize the way surgery is taught and practiced, improve our efficiency, and optimize patient care. It is a rapidly developing field which requires careful governance and regulation. It will function best and most safely in the hands of well-educated clinicians who know how to utilize AI and who understand its limitations. It must be implemented within careful legal and ethical frameworks to protect patient and clinician privacy, and to ensure patient safety.

Cross-References

- Artificial Intelligence in Surgical Education and Training
- Focus on Theory: Emotions and Learning
- Future of Health Professions Education Curricula
- Learning and Teaching in the Operating Theatre: Expert Commentary from the Nursing Perspective

► Simulation as Clinical Replacement: Contemporary Approaches in Healthcare Professional Education
► Simulation for Clinical Skills in Healthcare Education
► Simulation for Procedural Skills Teaching and Learning
► Surgical Education: Context and Trends
► Teaching Simple and Complex Psychomotor Skills
► Technology Considerations in Health Professions and Clinical Education

References

Alemzadeh H, Raman J, Leveson N, Kalbarczyk Z, Iyer RK. Adverse events in robotic surgery: a retrospective study of 14 years of FDA data. PLoS One. 2016;11(4):e0151470.

Arora VM. Harnessing the power of big data to improve graduate medical education: big idea or bust? Acad Med. 2018;93(6):833–4.

Hamilton JG, Genoff Garzon M, Westerman JS, Shuk E, Hay JL, Walters C, et al. "A tool, not a crutch": patient perspectives about IBM Watson for oncology trained by Memorial Sloan Kettering. J Oncol Pract. 2019;15(4):e277–e88.

Hashimoto DA, Rosman G, Rus D, Meireles OR. Artificial intelligence in surgery: promises and perils. Ann Surg. 2018;268(1):70–6.

Hodges BD. Learning from Dorothy Vaughan: artificial intelligence and the health professions. Med Educ. 2018;52(1):11–3.

Jiang F, Jiang Y, Zhi H, Dong Y, Li H, Ma S, et al. Artificial intelligence in healthcare: past, present and future. Stroke Vasc Neurol. 2017;2(4):230–43.

Johnston SC. Anticipating and training the physician of the future: the importance of caring in an age of artificial intelligence. Acad Med. 2018;93(8):1105–6.

Kapoor R, Walters SP, Al-Aswad LA. The current state of artificial intelligence in ophthalmology. Surv Ophthalmol. 2019;64(2):233–40.

Krittanawong C, Zhang H, Wang Z, Aydar M, Kitai T. Artificial intelligence in precision cardiovascular medicine. J Am Coll Cardiol. 2017;69(21):2657–64.

Marchalik D. The return to literature-making doctors matter in the new era of medicine. Acad Med. 2017;92(12):1665–7.

Mirnezami R, Ahmed A. Surgery 3.0, artificial intelligence and the next-generation surgeon. Br J Surg. 2018;105(5):463–5.

Mukherjee S. AI versus M.D. The New Yorker. 2017. Available from: https://www.newyorker.com/magazine/2017/04/03/ai-versus-md

O'Sullivan S, Nevejans N, Allen C, Blyth A, Leonard S, Pagallo U, et al. Legal, regulatory, and ethical frameworks for development of standards in artificial intelligence (AI) and autonomous robotic surgery. Int J Med Robot. 2019;15(1):e1968.

TeachThought Staff. 10 roles for artificial intelligence in education: TeachThought: we grow teachers 2018. Available from: https://www.teachthought.com/the-future-of-learning/10-roles-for-artificial-intelligence-in-education/

Wartman SA, Combs CD. Medical education must move from the information age to the age of artificial intelligence. Acad Med. 2018;93(8):1107–9.

Wong JA, Matsumoto ED. Primer: cognitive motor learning for teaching surgical skill – how are surgical skills taught and assessed? Nat Clin Pract Urol. 2008;5(1):47–54.

Coaching in Health Professions Education: The Case of Surgery

74

Martin Richardson and Louise Richardson

Contents

Introduction	1448
What Is Coaching?	1448
What Coaching Is Not	1449
Coaching and Learning Theories	1449
Ontological Perspectives	1450
Coaching Skills	1452
Models of Coaching	1453
Coaching and Culture	1454
Limitations of Current Surgical Continuing Professional Development	1455
Wearable Devices	1456
Surgical Outlier Remediation	1457
Research in Coaching	1457
Concluding Comments	1458
Cross-References	1458
References	1459

Abstract

Coaching has become a very important facet of personal and team development, especially in the business world, over the last few years. An article by Atul Gawande in the *New Yorker* in 2011 highlighted the potential of coaching for surgeons (Gawande 2011). Despite this article, "coaching" still has not been widely adopted by surgeons, compared to other leaders in our community. Like Gawande, we find it difficult to understand why surgeons continue to lag behind the executive world in the uptake of coaching as a self-improvement tool.

M. Richardson (✉)
Epworth Clinical School, University of Melbourne, Melbourne, Australia
e-mail: mrich1@unimelb.edu.au

L. Richardson
Epworth Hospital, Melbourne, Australia
e-mail: drjaz@bigpond.com

© Springer Nature Singapore Pte Ltd. 2023
D. Nestel et al. (eds.), *Clinical Education for the Health Professions*,
https://doi.org/10.1007/978-981-15-3344-0_95

Although Caprice Greenberg and her colleagues have developed a coaching program for surgeons in Wisconsin, in the USA (Greenberg et al. 2018), few others have published in this field. Perhaps it is because surgeons feel they have perfected their craft and have no need for a coach. Alternatively, many surgeons may not be aware of the principles of coaching and accompanying benefits, as a potential method of continuing professional development (CPD). In this chapter, we would like to illustrate many of the positive impacts that a coaching culture can provide to health professionals including surgeons and their patients.

Keywords

Coaching · Psychology · Mentoring · Counselling · Experiential learning theory · GROW model

Introduction

In his 2011 article, Gawande emphasized the importance of coaching, even at the pinnacle of one's career, by referencing two compelling examples. Firstly, he noted that Rafael Nadal, the top world tennis player, had a coach. In fact, he surmised he may have had more than one (forehand, backhand, psychological), to improve various aspects of his game. A similar illustration involved the first violinist of the New York symphony having a coach, which coincidently was his wife, to make him the best violinist in the world. Gawande was so inspired by this account, that he sought out his own coach to help further develop his surgical practice, which turned out to be his former fellowship director. Gawande outlined how, in just a few sessions, his coach was able to enlighten his practice, both in his personal surgical expertise as well as focusing on the teaching of his residents (Gawande 2011).

Like Gawande, we advocate that health professionals should be seeking out a coach to challenge and guide their quest to maximize their potential and excel in their professional journeys.

What Is Coaching?

Coaching is traditionally viewed as the domain of sporting teams. However, more recently many highly successful companies have adopted coaching as an integral development tool for top executives, with a filtering down effect through the organization. Tim Gallwey summarizes coaching as maximizing one's performance by minimizing the interferences that limit an individual's potential, represented by the simple equation, $P=P-I$ (Gallwey 1986).

Different types of coaching are appropriate depending on an individual's ultimate goals, and may include skills coaching, peer coaching, executive coaching, expertise coaching, or team facilitation. Nevertheless, each are based on similar underlying principles, which involve creating a partnership between coach and coachee. This provides the space and time to facilitate introspective and reflective conversations for the development of self and others (Elaine et al. 2014).

What Coaching Is Not

Coaching shares many similarities with activities in traditional medical education, such as teaching and mentoring, but is distinctive from these in its focus on the iterative improvement and refinement of *existing* knowledge, skills, and attitudes. An episode of coaching should be self-limiting, with the goal of empowering the person being coached (sometimes called a *"coachee"*) to become their own agents of change and developing an ability to self-coach throughout their career.

However, it is important to clarify the differences between coaching and other educational approaches, such as mentoring, counseling, teaching, or managing.

Mentoring is usually a longer-term relationship between a more senior partner *"mentor"* guiding a more junior *"mentee"* through career development, opening doors with introductions, and helping to direct a careers trajectory. In contrast, coaching does not necessarily assume expertise in the specialist field and is often a peer-to-peer relationship of shorter duration toward a specific goal (Lin and Reddy 2019).

On the other hand, **counselling** involves guiding a client or colleague through a problem, conflict, or ethical dilemma, using reflective listening. Skillful coaching enquires into people's narratives but invokes even more critical listening and involves challenging perspectives. Coaching aims to inspire the *coachee* to take new and innovative actions but the *coach* should be vigilant and refer on to appropriate clinicians if psychological or emotional issues are uncovered (Griffiths and Campbell 2008).

Teaching, in the traditional sense, or training, involves a *master-apprentice* model with a directing, "telling style," in contrast to coaching with an "asking mindset," promoting curiosity and the natural learning capacity, unlocking the inner potential, and maximizing one's own performance (Hu et al. 2017).

Performance management as organizational command and control, aims to ensure that a job is undertaken in an effective and efficient manner but does not necessarily empower them to go above and beyond the limits of their capacity. This approach can often demotivate them from owning the problem and thinking out of the box. Management rules tend to set limits and erect boundaries in contrast to coaching principles that emphasize potential and promote ideals, fostering a culture of awareness and responsibility (Keller 2020).

Coaching and Learning Theories

Coaching draws on adult learning principles. The concept of self-determination is a central tenet of a coaching relationship and an axiom of andragogy (Spence and Oades 2011). This belief that the *coachee* possesses an inner desire to improve themselves helps to drive further advancement. Adult learners should be encouraged to formulate their own personal learning and development goals. Whitmore proposed a framework depicted by the acronym "GROW" as the model for a coach to facilitate this process, helping the coachee to achieve the self-generated *goals*, based on an understanding of current *realities*, developing *options* to achieve these goals and instituting a plan that *will* be enacted (Whitmore 2017).

The AOTrauma organization has based their seven principles of learning on Knowles' concepts of adult learning (Fox 2012). The learners' needs stimulate an inner motivation to learn relevant material, using interaction, promoting reflection based on appropriate feedback with resultant verifiable outcomes. Their well-considered faculty development coaching program is also based on these principles (Uhlmann 2020).

Many coaching encounters utilize Kolb's Experiential Learning Theory (Kolb 1984), founded on work by Dewey (1910). Kolb's learning cycle focuses on an initial concrete experience which is followed by reflective observation developing an abstract conceptualization, promoting active experimentation to base next actions on initiating a further journey around the learning cycle. Coaches often do this, as a mental exercise, to brainstorm possible options that may achieve the desired goals.

Many forms of coaching tap into Mezirow's Transformative Learning Theory (Mezirow and associates Ma 1990), which through a perspective transformation process with three dimensions, behavioral (lifestyle changes), convictional (revision of belief systems), and psychological (changes in understanding of the self), encourage cognitive dissonance. The accuracy of pre-conceived assumptions and beliefs are challenged through a process coined a "disorienting dilemma," promoting reorientation through critical reflection and revised actions.

Coaching is a method of enhancing the coachee's ascent up Maslow's hierarchy of needs, beyond the lower dependent and impulsive levels, toward seeking esteem of others, self-esteem and ultimately aspiring to self-actualization (Abraham 1943).

Ontological Perspectives

Coaching has evolved as an offshoot from psychology and uses much of its theoretical support based on the literature and learnings of psychotherapy. The coach's ontological perspective will influence their approach to coaching. A coach with a **post-positivist** world view will adopt scientific methodological approaches, to help uncover the general laws objectively described (Mulvie 2015). Surgeons and many other health professionals, due to their training and enculturation, tend to come from a positivist mindset and base their decision making on quantitative studies such as randomized controlled trials (RCTs). However, this approach may constrain the development of a coaching culture.

On the other hand, a coach who believes that reality is not objectively knowable adopts a relativist paradigm. Postmodern **constructivism** considers historical, cultural, and social contexts and beliefs of individuals and groups as they construct their world view (Murphy et al. 2005). Many use **pragmatism** to focus on experiential learning, rather than simple ideas, to develop personal models and experiment with various methods to manage blended learning (Bachkirova and Borrington 2019).

Strategies adopted by coaches are founded on a wide variety of schools of thought. Some theoretical approaches include **cognitive behavioral** models that evaluate the quality of thinking around identified realistic goals. Self-awareness is facilitated, addressing cognitive and behavioral barriers to goal attainment (Palmar and Szymanska 2007). **Gestalt** approaches use the paradoxical theory of change, emphasizing moment to moment awareness from interactions with the external world to engage introspection and achieve creative adjustment in a changing environment (Bluckert 2014). Simon (2009) emphasizes the notions of contact and awareness. The former accentuates growth and development occurring at the boundary of "self and other." Awareness building is key to behavior change emerging from that growth and development.

Psychodynamic models have emerged from the works of Freud and address issues of transference and counter transference, and defense mechanisms affecting unconscious conflicts (Graham 2014). **Solutions-focused** approaches use collaborative thinking to concentrate on present and future solutions rather than past problems (Grant 2006). Coaches with an **existential** approach use descriptive exploration to understand the context of present concerns in their world view. They see the human condition based on three principles of relatedness, uncertainty and existential anxiety (Fusco et al. 2015).

The **person-centered** approach is guided by the actualizing tendency, which is a biological tendency for people to strive toward a constructive and positive pathway (Joseph 2006; Rogers 1962). The coach adopts an attitude of non-directivity and fosters a "growth-promoting climate":

- Congruence – the coach is genuine and authentic.
- Empathy – the coach feels and demonstrates empathy.
- Positive regard – the coach has a warm, positive acceptance attitude.
- Unconditionality of regard – the coach maintains a positive feeling without reservations, evaluations, or judgments.

Coaches using a **narrative** approach leverage the coachee's stories and create new connections between these stories, identities, and behaviors, working experimentally, trans personally, and contextually (Drake 2007).

Whereas developmental trajectories have traditionally been used to inform **psychological developmental** approaches (Bachkirova 2011), **positive psychology (Boniwell** 2008) approaches aim to refocus attention away from problems and weaknesses toward strengths and opportunities, harnessing **transpersonal** awareness, connectedness, and creativity (Rowan 2014).

Transactional analysis was developed by Eric Berne to help understand why we think, feel, and act the way we do. It is gaining traction in the field of coaching, to help coachees recognize outdated and irrelevant ego patterns, life scripts, and interactions; and help them to recalibrate the foundations of their actions (Napper and Newton 2000). The Neurolinguistic program approach (**NLP**) to coaching helps to identify patterns, enablers, hindrances to success, and seeks to change habits and behavior using individually targeted and appropriate techniques (Grimley 2013).

Theories, techniques, and strategies of coaching have a strong foundation in psychology, management theory, organizational development, communication studies, and adult learning/development. These techniques and strategies present a solid foundation on which to develop the field of surgical coaching.

Coaching Skills

Effective coaching is founded on the complementary skills of powerful questions and active listening. In this model, the role of the coach involves fostering an appropriate environment, directed by the four key tenets of coaching: (a) an emphasis on client strengths, (b) a view of clients and therapists as partners, (c) the adoption of a constructionist approach, and (d) an emphasis on the narrative form of meaning, in contrast to the traditional sagacious approach (Polkinghorne 2004).

The coaching mindset assumes the intrinsic learning capacity and resourcefulness of a coachee. In so doing, a coaching ethos is built around a paradigm of respect and trust within a collaborative partnership. Extrapolating from marriage counselling, assertiveness, and curiosity have been suggested as effective in countering Gottman's four horsemen of the apocalypse: Blaming, Defensiveness, Contempt, and Stonewalling (Gottman and Silver 1999).

Coaching is based on a conversation or dialogue guided by exploration, rather than instruction. It is assumed that the coachee holds the answers to their dilemmas, and that the art of appropriate questioning by the coach to aid the coachee to introspect, or to uncover (discover) their own answers to their problems, will cultivate a self-perpetuating ability for growth. This is true continuing professional development (CPD), in contrast to the current "tick box" style of CPD on offer as continuing medical education (CME) to many in healthcare (Friedman and Phillips 2002).

The use of open-ended questions "what," "where," "when," "how many," and "who" invite descriptive answers facilitating the reflective process. Open questioning demonstrates curiosity and fosters trust. Questions should attempt to avoid "why" and "how," which can provoke a defensive response that may impair the coaching relationship. The art of questioning is a skill that takes time and practice to develop a natural flow. Deeper probing, "and what else," helps to uncover blind spots and areas of avoidance can be explored by, "I notice you haven't mentioned...."

Active listening is very important as only 7% of one's message comes from the words used, with 38% gleaned from the tone and rhythm and 55% from the facial expressions and body language observed (Mehrabian 1972; Mehrabian and Ferris 1967; Mehrabian and Wiener 1967).

The coach requires a mindful mindset, engaging social and emotional intelligence, to stay attuned for these cues. Skillful coaching requires the coach to be aware of patterns in their own reactions, as well as the coachee, and reflecting back to clarify, challenge, and offer new perspectives and alternative possibilities. This creates a feedback loop and promotes awareness building self-belief, self-reliance, self-responsibility, and ultimately self-coaching.

Models of Coaching

Sir John Whitmore, one of the founding scholars of the coaching movement, has expounded a GROW (goal, reality, options, will/action) model, which has provided a useful framework on which to base a coaching discussion. Under the model, **Goal setting** and clarification are key to most coaching encounters. These goals need to be SMART (specific, measurable, achievable, realistic, and time-based). They should also aim to be PURE (positively stated, understood, relevant, and ethical) and CLEAR (challenging, legal, environmentally sound, appropriate, and recorded). After identifying their goal, coachees are encouraged to explore their current **reality**. This provides a starting point to base the coachee's perspective of the future and helps them identify the actions required to successfully meet their goal. The **options** step involves brainstorming ideas and actionable steps that might achieve the goals. The final step of this model involves establishing the **way forward** by formulating an action plan which establishes a mechanism for change and assists the coachee to commit to achieving their desired goals (Whitmore 2017).

In a systematic review of RCTs on the role of coaching to improve learner outcomes in surgery, Gagnon and Abbasi were only able to identify five studies on medical students and residents (Gagnon and Abbasi 2018). Two groups used formal coaching models: GROW and PRACTICE (Table 1) (Palmer 2007, 2011; Grant 2011). In an RCT investigation the benefit of video-based coaching for developing

Table 1 Models of coaching

Model	Steps	Reference
GROW	Goal setting Reality check Options Way forward	Whitmore (2017)
PRACTICE	Problem identification Realistic, relevant goals developed Alternative solutions generated Consideration of consequences Target most feasible solutions Implementation of Chosen solutions Evaluation	Palmer (2008)
OSKAR	Outcome Scaling Know-how and resources Affirm and action Review	Passmore and Sinclair (2020)

laparoscopic skills in medical students, Singh et al. (2015) used a modified GROW model to enhance performance. Their study reported that intervention subjects receiving coaching significantly outperformed controls, who only watched recorded surgical lectures, on all global rating scales of surgical performance.

The impact of individualized comprehensive coaching program on surgical technical skill in the operating room was assessed by Bonrath using the PRACTICE model. (Bonrath et al. 2015). Post-training, superior skill acquisition was recorded by the Comprehensive Surgical Training Group in comparison to Conventional Training.

In a systematic review of coaching to enhance surgeons' operative performance, Min et al. concluded that, despite variable quality across studies, "surgical coaching interventions have a positive impact on learners' perception and attitudes, their technical and nontechnical skills, and performance measures" (Min et al. 2015). While they could not demonstrate performance measures that improved patient outcomes, they concluded that coaching provided a safe and efficient way to improve intra operative learning and performance.

Coaching and Culture

Recently, the Royal Australasian College of Surgeons (RACS) has gone through a challenging period of reflection relating to reports of bullying and harassment. An overrepresentation of women dropping out of surgical training was attributed to a toxic culture (Liang et al. 2019). The "Operating with Respect" (OWR) program was developed by RACS in response, incorporating a one-hour online teaching video and an optional face-to-face workshop to counter this ethos (Liang et al. 2017). Coaching may offer a mechanism to help repair this culture with its open transformative style.

A culture of blame inhibits learning and diminishes performance, whereas a high-performance culture uses coaching as an enabler to raise awareness and responsibility. The coaching skill of curiosity is a good antidote to a blame culture, decreasing fear and self-doubt, lowering stress, facilitating self-responsibility which enables flexibility and adaptability. Coaching seeks to meet the person where they are, connecting hearts and minds and encouraging assessment of needs and values (Ibarra and Scoular 2019).

> Transformative leadership begins with questions of justice and democracy as opposed to either transactional or transformative leadership. It is a powerful strategy that can counter toxic cultures (Shields 2010). It uses coaching principles to, motivate people and enhance trust and commitment within a safe environment inspiring growth, learning, and success of teams (Burns 1978; Bass 1985). Operative surgical teams could benefit from this coaching culture to enhance technical performance and improve integrated patient care.

Limitations of Current Surgical Continuing Professional Development

Surgeons' perceptions and potential concerns about coaching and the possible challenges of adopting a coaching model in a culture where values of competency and autonomy are deeply entrenched was evaluated by Mutabdzic. Their study questioned the validity of current continuing medical education (CME) in medicine that relies on self-directed identification of gaps in our knowledge and surgical practices and the ability of traditional lectures and workshops to address these gaps. As an alternative, they propose coaching as a potential paradigm to replace continuing professional development (CPD) which ideally should be learner-centered and self-directed in the continuum of a surgical career (Mutabdzic et al. 2015).

After graduation from a surgical training program, surgeons generally experience a high degree of autonomy. Hospitals conduct surgical audit meetings to review patient outcomes within surgical units. These tend to be a summative process and focuses on complications and occasionally near misses but do not necessarily foster improvement in routine practice. To address this, the New Zealand Orthopaedic Association (NZOA) has introduced a formative peer-to-peer practice observation process, whereby a peer will attend a consulting and operative session and provide in-depth feedback on a colleague's practice (Ballance 2019). CPD in the form of "deliberate practice," as espoused by Ericsson, requires feedback to aid goal setting and mastery of a technical skill (Ericsson 2004). This has been well received and both reviewer and reviewee have reported a beneficial learning experience. Formal coaching training may further enhance this initiative.

To address the need for formal surgical coach training, Greenberg et al. have established the Wisconsin Surgical Coaching Framework as a system to develop surgical coaching interventions. These are based around three domains of goal setting: motivation and encouragement, and development and guiding. They also aim to work in three skill domains namely, technical, cognitive, and non-technical (Greenberg et al. 2015). As noted by Gawande (2011), face-to-face live intra-operative coaching may be not be feasible in many contexts, and so alternatives such as video review may offer a valid alternative. As noted in the existing literature, certain surgeries such as laparoscopic cholecystectomies lend themselves to video-based capture.

The Wisconsin framework was piloted with peer-nominated surgeons, trained as coaches, paired with participant surgeons. Following an initial introductory session where the pair established rapport, set goals, and developed an action plan for forthcoming coaching sessions, select operations were video recorded. Subsequent one-hour sessions reviewed and refined the participants' goals, analyzed the surgical procedure identifying areas to work on, and formulated an action plan for future sessions. While scheduling and audio-visual technology issues posed some challenges, the overall program was felt to successfully prepare coaches for their roles and positively received by participants (Greenberg et al. 2018).

In response to a need for structured surgical coaching in an Obstetrics and Gynecology department, Leung et al. described a pilot program of a structured surgical coaching template. This need arose out of a problem of incremental deskilling as surgeons were expected to teach trainees but had limited opportunities to improve their own skills and attain confidence in these procedures. The structured program involved development of individualized learning objectives, intra-operative teaching, and debriefing to aid reflective learning through face-to-face feedback. Participants reported self-perceived improvement in surgical skill and confidence and a desire to incorporate a more structured approach to their teaching (Leung et al. 2013).

To improve surgical CPD, Hu et al. (2012) attempted to emulate a sport-based coaching methodology using post-hoc video-based reviews, whereby the athlete viewed their performance with a coach in a longitudinal self-directed improvement process. Technology in the operating room (OR) allowed visual capture of the operative field in detail, with the OR as an overview and all conversations in synchrony. The coach's one-hour debriefing sessions were analyzed. The perceived advantages were that it allowed surgeons to view themselves in the third person, and it allowed reflection on better teaching of residents. Furthermore, it allowed tailored feedback and coaching to each individual surgeon's learning needs. The nature of the peer coaching was felt to cultivate a supportive environment, which enabled positive action. The use of video-based coaching affords a few efficiencies compared to a direct observation of surgery. The ability to fast forward to points of interest and learning enhanced time efficiencies. The possibility of videoconferencing of coaching utilizing this methodology was also raised. Post-game analysis is scalable, with current technology making it a cost-effective coaching tool, as well as facilitating the participation of remote surgeons. They recommended that providing the coach with contextual information, including preoperative imaging and patient history, may further enhance the feedback process. They also acknowledged the limitation of the one-off session analysis for each surgeon in their study and suggested an ongoing continuum of analysis would be more valuable. They proposed that linking patients' outcomes with video-based coaching programs would further legitimize the value of this intervention.

Wearable Devices

Effective video-based coaching programs are dependent on the availability and fidelity of appropriate technology. A systematic review undertaken by Kolodzey identified several devices being trialed in the operating room (OR), including Google Glass, wearable GoPro cameras, and head mounted displays (HMDs). Each device exhibited unique strengths. Google Glass provided a lightweight, user-friendly interface and the potential for hands free control. GoPro cameras were notable because the powerful HD camera provided good anatomical definition. HMDs offered the first practical way to introduce augmented reality to the OR, especially useful in minimally invasive surgery (MIS). Limitations included issues with battery life, and confidentiality, which may be alleviated by medicine-specific software (Kolodzey et al. 2017).

Surgical Outlier Remediation

A well-constructed surgical coaching program may be used to provide support strategies for clinicians experiencing performance difficulties. The Australian Orthopaedic Association National Joint Replacement Registry (AOANJRR) has now become sophisticated enough to be able to identify surgeons whose long-term results for joint replacement surgery are well below the expected range (Harris et al. 2019). Underperforming surgeons could be identified and be offered a remediation program to improve their results, and a coaching model provides an appropriate platform to help these surgeons. This obviously needs to be conducted in a sensitive and supportive collegial manner, with appropriate goal setting and action planning.

A coaching methodology also offers an opportunity to tap into the learning from surgeons preforming at the elite end of the performance spectrum, as identified in the AOANJRR data. An analysis such as this could highlight factors that continue to enhance these surgeons' mastery, and potentially these surgeons could be trained in coaching techniques and serve as coaches for others.

Research in Coaching

Efforts to design RCTs have been limited due to difficulties in defining the control variable in what is a very complex and fluid coaching interaction. In an effort to refine interview techniques, some studies, particularly in the health field, have mirrored motivational interviewing in programs aimed to address blood pressure control, weight loss, asthma, and smoking (Garbutt et al. 2012). Similarly, there have been few studies examining interviewing skill effectiveness ratings, and validated tools and attempts to use multisource feedback tools to measure leadership behaviors and emotional intelligence also have had limited application (Kombarakaran et al. 2008). For surgical coaching, it may also be difficult to link interventions to patient outcomes.

The *process* of coaching has demonstrated the mutual contributions of both coach and coachee. For the coach, important attributes include relationship building, communication, and interpersonal skills. Coachee attributes, such as interest in their own development and readiness to change, have also been examined. Critical incident methodology and pre-test post-test measures of self-efficacy have been useful in some contexts, particularly for examining cross-cultural coaching issues, such as communication, coach-client relationship, coaching setting, and role understanding. Some small-scale studies have attempted to look at purpose, sustainability, and the ideal duration of a coaching relationship. While these studies suggest it can take six months to achieve various goals, and further that this is not improved if the relationship is extended beyond 12 months, the results are not generalizable (Grant and Cavanagh 2007). Coaching relationships documented in the surgical literature have been far shorter in duration.

Analysis of the coaching interaction dyad have proven to be difficult. The nuances of the coach-coachee interface, understanding how and when questioning is used, and how it influences the coachee, are not always easy to dissect. The oscillation between linguistically rich and linguistically poor content makes exploration of aspects such as listening, silences, clarifying, challenging, thinking, and reflection challenging. Traditional research methods are intrusive and more innovative qualitative strategies including phenomenology, discourse analysis, systematic self-observation, experience sampling methods and grounded theory may be required. For practitioners in this field, action research methods may be useful to construct an evidence base for surgical practice (Ollis and Sproule 2007). A pragmatic approach, challenging apparent truths by testing actions and practice, across different levels of participation, may provide some insights.

Concluding Comments

Coaching is a human development process using appropriate tools, strategies, and techniques, in structured, focused interactions, which help to promote sustainable and desirable change to benefit the coachee and related stakeholders (Elaine et al. 2014). By considering the context of coaching, and how the philosophy of coaching can be translated to medicine, Watling and La Donna argue that the three core elements of coaching are mutual engagement, ongoing reflection for both learner and coach, and embracing failure as a catalyst to learning (Watling et al. 2016). This helps to provide a framework for the application of coaching to various contexts in medicine.

While substantial progress has been achieved in healthcare education with regard to debriefing and reflection, there is still a need to heed Gawande's plea to advance education to the next level by developing a coaching culture that seeks out coaching opportunities as have executives in the business world, military leaders, and elite athletes (Gawande 2011). This offers the opportunity to maximize technical performance and health outcomes for our patients through improvements in integrated care and allowing individual surgeons to fulfil their innate potential both as practitioners and leaders in health care.

Cross-References

▶ Cognitive Neuroscience Foundations of Surgical and Procedural Expertise: Focus on Theory
▶ Conversational Learning in Health Professions Education: Learning Through Talk
▶ Effective Feedback Conversations in Clinical Practice
▶ Learning and Teaching in the Operating Room: A Surgical Perspective
▶ Mastery Learning in Health Professions Education

▶ Measuring Performance: Current Practices in Surgical Education
▶ Reflective Practice in Health Professions Education
▶ Surgical Education: Context and Trends
▶ Surgical Training: Impact of Decentralization and Guidelines for Improvement

References

Gawande A. Personal best top athletes and singers have coaches should you? The New Yorker 2011.
Greenberg CC, Ghousseini HN, Pavuluri Quamme SR, Beasley HL, Frasier LL, Brys NA, et al. A statewide surgical coaching program provides opportunity for continuous professional development. Ann Surg. 2018;267(5):868–73.
Gallwey T. The inner game of tennis. London: Pan; 1986.
Elaine C, Tatiana B, Clutterbuck D, editors. The complete handbook of coaching. 2nd ed. London: Sage; 2014.
Lin J, Reddy R. Teaching, mentorship, and coaching in surgical education. Thorac Surg Clin. 2019;29:311–20.
Griffiths K, Campbell MA. Semantics or substance? Preliminary evidence in the debate between life coaching and counselling. Coach Int J Theory Res Pract. 2008;1(2):164–75.
Hu YY, Mazer LM, Yule SJ, Arriaga AF, Greenberg CC, Lipsitz SR, et al. Complementing operating room teaching with video-based coaching. JAMA Surg. 2017;152(4):318–25.
Keller C. Performance reviews vs. coaching: Centre for Management and Organisation Effectiveness; [cited 2020 9th Feb]. Available from: https://cmoe.com/blog/performance-reviews-vs-coaching
Spence G, Oades L. Coaching with self-determination in mind: using theory to advance evidence based coaching practice. Int J Evid Based Coach Mentor. 2011;9(2):37–55.
Whitmore J. Coaching for performance. The principles and practice of coaching and leadership. 5th ed. Nicholas Brealey; 2017.
Fox R. AO Foundation History of coaching within the AO 2012.
Uhlmann M. AO Trauma Faculty Development Program Committed to Excellence in Teaching 2020 5 Jan 2020:[20 p.]. Available from: https://www.aofoundation.org/what-we-do/education/topic-areas/faculty-development
Kolb D. Experiential learning: experience as teh source of learning and development. Engelwood Cliffs: Prentice Hall; 1984.
Dewey J. How we think. Lexington: Heath; 1910.
Mezirow J. How critical reflection triggers transformative learning. In: associates Ma, editor. Learning as transformation. San Fransisco: Jossey-Bass; 1990.
Abraham M. A theory of human motivation. Psychol Rev. 1943;50:370–96.
Mulvie A. The value of executive coaching. London: Routledge; 2015.
Murphy K, Mahoney S, Chen C, Mendoza-Diaz N, Yang X. A constructivist model of mentoring, coaching, and facilitating online discussions. Distance Educ. 2005;26(3):341–66.
Bachkirova T, Borrington S. Old wine in new bottles: exploring pragmatism as a philosophical framework for the discipline of coaching. Acad Manag Learn Edu. 2019;18(3):337.
Palmar S, Szymanska K. Cognitive and behavioural coaching: an integrative approach. In: Palmer S, Whybrow A, editors. Handbook of coaching psychology: a guide for practitioners. Hove: Routledge; 2007.
Bluckert P. The gestalt approach to coaching. In: Elaine C, Tatiana B, David C, editors. The complete handbook of coaching. Sage; 2014.
Simon S. Applying gestalt theory to coaching. Gestalt Review. 2009;13:230–40.
Graham L. The psychodynamic approach to coaching. In: Elaine C, Tatiana B, David C, editors. The complete handbook of coaching. Sage; 2014.

Grant A. Solution-focused coaching. In: Passmore, editor. Excellence in coaching: the industry guide. London: Kogan Page; 2006.

Fusco T, O'Riordan S, Palmer S. An existential approach to authentic leadership development: a review of teh existential coachin literature and its' relationship to authentic leadership. Coach Psychol. 2015;11(1):61–71.

Joseph S. Person-centred coaching psychology: a meta-theoretical perspective. Int Coach Psychol Rev. 2006;1:47–55.

Rogers C. The interpersonal relationship: the core of guuidance. Harv Educ Rev. 1962;32(4):416–29.

Drake D. The art of thinking narratively: implications for coaching psychology and practice. Aust Psychol. 2007;42(4):283–94.

Bachkirova T. Developmental coaching; working with the self. Maidenhead: Open University Press; 2011.

Boniwell I. Positive psychology in a nutshell. London: PWBC; 2008.

Rowan J. The transpersonal approach to coaching. In: Cox E, Bachkirova T, Clutterbuck D, editors. The complete handbook of coaching. 2nd ed. London: Sage; 2014. p. 145–56.

Napper R, Newton T. Tactics: transactional analysis concepts for all trainers, teachers and tutors and insight into collaborative learning strategies. Ipswich: TA Resources; 2000.

Grimley B. Theory and practice NLP coaching: a psychological approach. London: Sage; 2013.

Polkinghorne D. Narrative therapy and postmodernism. In: Angus L, McLeod J, editors. Handbook of narratie v and psychotherapy: practice, theory, and research. Thousands Oaks: Sage; 2004. p. 53–67.

Gottman J, Silver N. The seven principles for making marriage work. Crown; 1999.

Friedman A, Phillips M. The role of mentoring in the CPD programmes of professional associations. Int J Lifelong Educ. 2002;21(3):269–84.

Mehrabian A. Non-verbal communication. Chicago: Aldine-Atherton; 1972.

Mehrabian A, Ferris S. Inference of attitudes from nonverbal communication in two channels. J Consult Psychol. 1967;31(3):248–58.

Mehrabian A, Wiener M. Decoding of inconsistent communications. J Pers Soc Psychol. 1967;6:109–14.

Gagnon LH, Abbasi N. Systematic review of randomized controlled trials on the role of coaching in surgery to improve learner outcomes. Am J Surg. 2018;216(1):140–6.

Palmer S. PRACTICE: a model suitable for coaching, counselling, psychotherapy and stress management. Coach Psychol. 2007;3(2):71–7.

Palmer S. Revisiting the 'P' in the PRACTICE coaching model. Coach Psychol. 2011;7(2):156–8.

Grant A. Is it time to REGROW the GROW model? Issues related to teaching coaching session structures. Coach Psychol. 2011;7(2):118–26.

Singh P, Aggarwal R, Tahir M, Pucher P, Darzi A. A randomized controlled study to evaluate the role of video-based coaching in training laparoscopic skills. Ann Surg. 2015;261(5):862–9.

Palmer S. The PRACTICE model of coaching:towards a solution-focused approach. Coach Psychol Int. 2008;1(1):4–6.

Passmore J, Sinclair T. Solution focused approach and the OSKAR model. In: Becoming a coach [internet]. Springer; 2020. p. 139–43.

Bonrath E, Dedy N, Gordon L, Grantcharov T. Comprehensive surgical coaching enhances surgical skill in the operating room a randomized controlled trial. Ann Surg. 2015;262:205–12.

Min H, Morales D, Orgill D, Smink D, Yule S. Systematic review of coaching to enhance surgeons' operative performance. Surgery. 2015;158(5):1168–91.

Liang R, Dornan T, Nestel D. Why do women leave surgical training? A qualitative and feminist study. Lancet. 2019;393:541–9.

Liang R, et al. Operating with respect course. Royal Australasian College of Surgeons; 2017. Available from: https://www.surgeons.org/education/skills-training-courses/operating-with-respect-owr-course

Ibarra H, Scoular A. The leader as coach. Boston: Harvard Business Review Press; 2019.

Shields CM. Transformative leadership: working for equity in diverse contexts. Educ Adm Q. 2010;46(4):558–89.

Burns J. Leadership. New York: Harper Row; 1978.

Bass B. Leadership and performance beyond expectations. New York: Collier Macmillian; 1985.

Mutabdzic D, Mylopoulos M, Murnaghan M, Patel P, Zilbert N, Seemann N, et al. Coaching surgeons is culture limiting our ability to improve? Ann Surg. 2015;262:213–6.

Ballance J. NZOA annual report 2019 practice visit programme report. Wellington: NZOA; 2019.

Ericsson KA. Deliberate practice and the acquisition and maintenance of expert performance in medicine and related domains. Acad Med. 2004;79(10 Suppl):S70–81.

Greenberg CC, Ghousseini HN, Pavuluri Quamme SR, Beasley HL, Wiegmann DA. Surgical coaching for individual performance improvement. Ann Surg. 2015;261(1):32–4.

Leung Y, Salfinger S, Tan JJS, Frazer A. The introduction and the validation of a surgical encounter template to facilitate surgical coaching of gynaecologists at a metropolitan tertiary obstetrics and gynaecology hospital. Aust N Z J Obstet Gynaecol. 2013;53:477–83.

Hu YY, Peyre SE, Arriaga AF, Osteen RT, Corso KA, Weiser TG, et al. Postgame analysis: using video-based coaching for continuous professional development. J Am Coll Surg. 2012;214(1):115–24.

Kolodzey L, Grantcharov PD, Rivas H, Schijven MP, Grantcharov TP, Society obotWTiH. Wearable technology in the operating room: a systematic review. BMJ Innov. 2017;3:55–63.

Harris I, Cuthbert A, Lorimer M, de Steiger R, Lewis P, Graves S. Outcomes of hip and knee replacement surgery in private and public hospitals in Australia. ANZ J Surg. 2019;89(11):1417–23.

Garbutt J, Highstein G, Yan Y, Strunk R. Partner randomized controlled trial: study protocol and coaching intervention. BMC Pediatr. 2012;12:42.

Kombarakaran F, Yang J, Baker M, Fernandes P. Executive coaching: it works! Consult Psychol J Pract Res. 2008;60(1):78–90.

Grant A, Cavanagh M. Evidence based coaching: flourishing or languishing? Aust Psychol. 2007;42(4):239–54.

Ollis S, Sproule J. Constructivist coaching and expertise development as action research. Int J Sports Sci Coach. 2007;2(1):1–14.

Watling C, La Donna KA, Lingard L, Voyer S, Hatala R. Sometimes the work just needs to be done': socio-cultural influences on direct observation in medical training. Med Educ. 2016;50:1054–64.

Developing Health Professional Teams

75

John T. Paige

Contents

Introduction 1464
Team Science and Its Implementation 1464
Applications for Developing Health Professional Teams 1472
Optimizing Implementation of Strategies to Develop Health Professional Teams 1476
Conclusion 1478
References 1479

Abstract

Given the importance of having effective teamwork in contemporary healthcare, developing health professional teams is a new priority for clinical educators. The science of teamwork and advances in educational practice can assist educators with this undertaking. This chapter discusses how to develop health professional teams by addressing the following objectives: (1) identifying key concepts related to team science and its implementation; (2) comparing applications of team development interventions in healthcare; and (3) developing a framework for optimizing implementation of team development initiatives.

Keywords

Teamwork · Teams · Team development interventions · Team science · Team training · Simulation-based training · Implementation science · Change management

J. T. Paige (✉)
Department of Surgery, Louisiana State University (LSU) Health New Orleans School of Medicine, New Orleans, LA, USA
e-mail: jpaige@lsuhsc.edu

© Springer Nature Singapore Pte Ltd. 2023
D. Nestel et al. (eds.), *Clinical Education for the Health Professions*,
https://doi.org/10.1007/978-981-15-3344-0_96

Introduction

In today's constantly changing, complex healthcare system, in which the sum of medical knowledge is doubling every 73 days (Densen 2011) and patients require coordinated care across a range of clinical providers and settings (Kuziemsky 2016), a solitary health professional can no longer rely on individual wit, intelligence, talent, or skill to provide safe, quality care to a patient. Instead, the effective, efficient provision of healthcare requires seamless coordination and communication across smoothly functioning interprofessional teams of healthcare clinicians, each bringing their own particular expertise and skill to a specific patient's care, in order to ensure a successful outcome. This growing emphasis on interprofessional, team-based collaboration and interaction has gained increasing attention since the turn of the millennium. In the United States, the Institute of Medicine (IOM) first designated the ability of healthcare professionals to work in interprofessional teams as a core competency in its landmark *Health Professions Education: A Bridge to Quality* (Greiner and Knebel 2003). It followed this work with *Redesigning Continuing Education in Health Professionals* (IOM 2010), in which the IOM advocated a transformation of continuing education along interprofessional lines. Such attention on interprofessional education (IPE) led to the creation of the Interprofessional Education Collaborative (IPEC) that has worked to identify key components of the interprofessional collaboration competency, a process performed throughout other healthcare systems worldwide (IPEC 2016; Thisthlethwaite et al. 2014).

Given the importance of having effective teamwork in contemporary healthcare, developing health professional teams is a new priority for clinical educators, in addition to the knowledge, skills, and abilities they must already teach to each profession under their tutelage. Fortunately, the science of teamwork and advances in educational practice can assist educators with this undertaking. This chapter discusses how to develop health professional teams by addressing the following objectives: (1) identifying key concepts related to team science and its implementation; (2) comparing applications of team development interventions in healthcare; and (3) developing a framework for optimizing implementation of team development initiatives.

Team Science and Its Implementation

Team science has its roots in the group productivity studies of the 1920s conducted at the Hawthorne Works electrical equipment company that gave rise to the concept of the Hawthorne effect (Macefield 2007). It was not until after World War II, however, that research in the field began in earnest as investigators studied group dynamics related to battlefield experiences during this conflict (Driskell et al. 2018). Since then, the focus of team science has evolved from a social psychological to an applied psychological orientation, leading to an emphasis away from group dynamics and toward team productivity (Driskell et al. 2018).

At its core, a team is a group of two or more individuals sharing the same goals and objectives who work together toward a common outcome (Juneja 2020). Other important characteristics of teams in healthcare include making decisions, possessing specialized skills and knowledge, functioning under high workload circumstances, and having a task interdependency making sequential or simultaneous adjustments of one member to another mandatory in order to achieve a common goal (Baker et al. 2003). Each team member, therefore, has a specific role to fill within the context of the team, and each individual interacts with the other members in a dynamic, interdependent, and adaptive manner in pursuit of the common interest (Shuffler et al. 2018).

Teamwork allows teams to leverage the individual talents and efforts of their members. Often, it is conceptualized as the processes that translate team inputs into team outputs. In this input-process-output (IPO) model (McGrath 1964), various affective states and cognitive orientations emerge out of team behavioral processes to produce effective teamwork. Thus, team composition and team member attributes can have a marked influence on teamwork itself or on the roles of members (Bell et al. 2018).

Effective teams possess key team-based competencies that enable them to perform consistently at a high level of function (Fig. 1).

These competencies are present among teams in all industries. Salas et al.'s (Salas et al. 2015; Tannenbaum 2020) 7C's model is currently one of the more

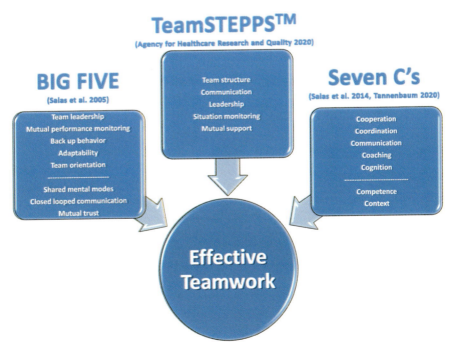

Fig. 1 Models of team-based competencies for effective teamwork

popular models. It incorporates five components, cooperation, coordination, communication, cognition, and coaching, with two influencing factors, competence and conditions. Another model with relevance to healthcare is Salas et al.'s (Salas et al. 2005) Big Five Model of Teamwork. This model has five main traits: team leadership, mutual performance monitoring, backup behavior, adaptability, and team orientation. These five traits pair with three coordinating mechanisms: shared mental modes, closed loop communication, and mutual trust. The Big Five Model served as the foundation upon which the Agency for Healthcare Research and Quality's (AHRQ) TeamSTEPPS™ program developed with its five main domains: team structure, communication, leadership, situation monitoring, and mutual support (AHRQ 2020). TeamSTEPPS™ is one of the more commonly used constructs in healthcare.

In healthcare, as in other industries, teams work in a dynamic environment characterized by unplanned and unpredictable outcomes. Instead of cause and effect, interrelationships between components of the system influence and are in turn influenced by events within the system, creating nonlinear, evolving outcomes. Such characteristics of interdependence, emerging patterns, and iterations are present in complex adaptive systems (CAS). Such systems can put additional strain on teams since small changes can have large impacts (The Health Foundation 2010). Not only is the healthcare environment in which teams operate a CAS, teams themselves have characteristics of a CAS. Team members act autonomously according to their own internalized rules of behavior. An individual member's action can influence the entire team in a nonlinear fashion. Each team can act in parallel, reacting to other members, patient conditions, and the clinical setting. These decisions are dispersed throughout the team, but they end up having an overall impact on the team performance (The Health Foundation 2010). Thus, unpredictable and entirely new team behaviors can arise as the team reacts to past actions as well as the environment in which it is functioning. The team's output, therefore, becomes greater than the sum of its individual components (Pype et al. 2018).

In pursuit of their goals, teams pass through various phases. During the early stages of team formation, teams enter a transition phase in which the mission is analyzed, goals are prioritized, and a strategy is developed. The team then enters the action phase in which it pursues activities to achieve the goal. During this phase, the team monitors progress to the goal, monitors resources and the environment, provides backup behavior to team members as needed, and coordinates activities. During both transition and action phases, the team is also involved in an interpersonal phase in which conflicts are managed, team confidence is built up, and team emotional well-being is promoted (Turner et al. 2018).

Both systems-based and people-focused approaches are available to help educators develop health professional teams (Cafazzo and St-Cyr 2012; Fig. 2).

Systems-based approaches include force functioning, selective automation, process standardization, and reducing complexity (Nolan 2000). Force functioning is one of the most effective systems-based approaches, because it creates a physical constraint that cannot be bypassed by a human. One of the most well-known of these constraints is the anesthesia pin index safety system (PISS) (Weigner and Gaba

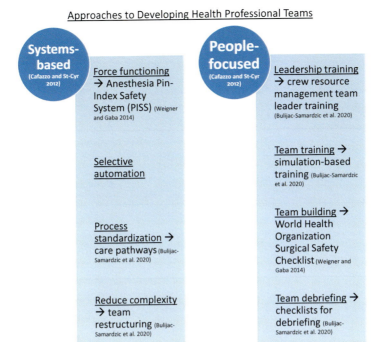

Fig. 2 Approaches to developing health professional teams

2014). Its unique pin orientations ensure that only the right gas cylinder can hook into the corresponding flush valve connector on an anesthesia machine. Other examples of systems-based approaches include organizational redesign. Such redesign can help to standardize care pathways or to restructure teams in order to reduce complexity (Bulijac-Samardzic et al. 2020).

Although systems-based solutions do exist, people-focused approaches are more commonly employed to help develop health professional teams. Such team development interventions can target a particular aspect of the IPO conceptual framework to enhance team effectiveness, or they can have a multifaceted component (Fig. 3).

Team development interventions targeting team inputs include team task analysis, team composition, teamwork design, and team charter. They focus on identifying key behaviors for success, selecting team members based on their attributes, structuring roles and tasks within the broader team, and clarifying team direction, respectively. Team monitoring and assessment of performance is a process-oriented intervention that attempts to determine the degree to which a team is achieving its goals. Finally, team debriefing is an outcome-based team development intervention in which self-reflection leads to process and outcome improvements (Shuffler et al. 2018).

Team training, team building, team coaching, and team leadership are multifaceted development interventions that can target any three aspects of the IPO

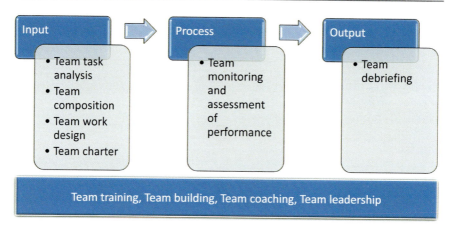

Fig. 3 Team development interventions for enhancing team effectiveness in healthcare

framework. Team training interventions target team-based competencies, whereas team building interventions focus on interpersonal processes. Both focus on the team itself. Team leadership interventions, however, tend to focus on individual team members in an attempt to develop their leadership capabilities. Finally, team coaching is an intervention that can couple with other team development components in order to enhance their effectiveness (Lacerenza et al. 2018; Shuffler et al. 2018).

Clearly, a wide variety of options exists for developing health professional teams. Their success, however, depends on adhering to sound educational principles in their implementation. For example, the development of a team training intervention should follow established curriculum development principles: problem identification and general needs assessment, targeted needs assessment, creation of goals and objectives, development of educational strategies, implementation, and evaluation (Kern 2016). Post-training debriefings should incorporate recognized key elements: approach, establishment of a learning environment, engagement of learners, reaction, reflection, analysis, diagnosis, and application (Arora et al. 2012). Furthermore, facilitators should employ established debriefing techniques to help enhance learning. Advocacy-inquiry is but one of many examples (Rudolph et al. 2006). Finally, faculty development efforts should help prepare facilitators and instructors prior to implementation of an intervention.

Key to any intervention undertaken to improve team effectiveness is the ability to measure accurately the teamwork itself in order to determine if it is working. Without robust, psychometrically sound teamwork assessment tools, adequate evaluation of a particular intervention or a program overall is impossible. Fortunately, a wide variety of teamwork instruments exists in the literature (Table 1), allowing tailoring of a particular assessment tool to the type of intervention.

For example, a simulation-based training intervention focusing solely on surgeons might best employ the nontechnical skills for surgeons (NOTSS) assessment tool for its evaluation. Proper observer training on the use of a tool, however, is

Table 1 Synopsis of recent systematic reviews on assessment tools for teamwork

Target team /assessment tools	Setting	Participants rated	Type of rating
Operating room (Higham et al. 2019, Onwochei et al. 2017, Wood et al. 2017, Wooding et al. 2020)			
Anesthetists' Non-technical Skills (ANTS)	Simulation-based training (SBT) and clinical environment (CE)	Anesthetists	4-point scale
Observational Teamwork Assessment for Surgeons (OTAS)	SBT and CE	Interprofessional operating room (OR) team	7-point scale
Revised Non-technical Skills scale (Revised NOTECHS)	SBT	Interprofessional OR team	6-point scale
Non-technical Skills for Surgeons (NOTSS)	SBT and CE	Surgeons	4-point scale
Oxford Non-technical Skills (Oxford NOTECHS)	SBT and CE	Interprofessional OR team	8-point scale
Non-technical skills for anesthetic trainees	SBT and CE	Anesthetic trainees	4-point scale
Pediatric Cardiac Surgery Teamwork classification tool (PCST)	CE	Interprofessional pediatric cardiac surgery OR team	7-point scale
Scrub Practitioners List of NTS (SPLINTS)	SBT and CE	Scrub practitioners	4-point scale
Nurse Anesthetists' NTS – Denmark (NANTSdk)	SBT and CE	Nurse anesthetists in Denmark	7-point scale
Objective Structured Assessment of Non-technical Skills (OSANTS)	SBT and CE	Surgical trainees	5-point scale
WHO Behaviorally Anchored Rating Scale (WHOBARS)	SBT and CE	Interprofessional OR team for WHO checklist	7-point scale
Anesthetists' NTS Denmark (ANTSdk)	SBT	Anesthetists in Denmark	5- and 7-point scales
Anesthetic NTS – Anesthetic Practitioners (ANTS-AP)	SBT and CE	Anesthetic practitioners	4-point scale
Interpersonal and Cognitive Assessment for Robotic Surgery (ICARS)	SBT	Surgeons for robotic surgery	5-point scale
Communication and Teamwork Skills (CATS)	CE	Interprofessional OR team	Not stated
Adult intensive/emergency care (Boet et al. 2019; Higham et al. 2019; Onwochei et al. 2017; Wooding et al. 2020)			
Team Dimensions Rating Form	CE	Interprofessional emergency department (ED) team	7-point scale

(continued)

Table 1 (continued)

Target team /assessment tools	Setting	Participants rated	Type of rating
Ottawa Crew Resource Management (CRM) Global Rating Scale	SBT	Trainee physicians	7-point scale
Mayo High Performance Teamwork Scale (MHPTS)	SBT	Interprofessional team in CRM training	3-point scale
TeamSTEPPS Teamwork Attitudes Questionnaire (T-TAQ)	SBT and CE	Any hospital resuscitation team	5-point scale
Team Emergency Assessment Measure (TEAM)	SBT and CE	Interprofessional ED team; resuscitation; cardiac arrest; trainees	4- and 10-point scales
Observational Skill-based Clinical Assessment tool for Resuscitation (OSCAR)	SBT and CE	Interprofessional resuscitation team	6-point scale
CARIOTEAM checklist	SBT	Cardiac arrest	Not stated
Simulation Team Assessment Tool (STAT)	SBT	Resuscitation; staff and trainees	3-point scale
Trauma NOTECHS (T-NOTECHS)	SBT and CE	Interprofessional trauma team	5-point scale
Adult Inpatient (Higham et al. 2019)			
Team Functioning Assessment tool (TFAT)	SBT and CE	Interprofessional ward team	7-point scale
Teamwork Mini-clinical Evaluation Exercise (T-MEX)	CE	Medical students; trainee physicians	5-point scale
Pediatric intensive/emergency care (Boet et al. 2019; Higham et al. 2019; Wooding et al. 2020)			
Imperial Pediatric Emergency Training Toolkit (IPETT)	SBT	Trainees	Not stated
University of Texas Behavioral Markers for Neonatal Resuscitation (UTBMNR)	SBT and CE	Interprofessional neonatal team	5-point scale
KidSIM Team Performance Scale	SBT	Trainees	Not stated
Trauma Team Communication Assessment (TTCA)	CE	Pediatric resuscitation teams	4-point scale
Team Average Performance Assessment Scale (TAPAS)	SBT	Neonatal, pediatric (and adult) interprofessional emergency teams	Not stated
Obstetrics (Boet et al. 2019; Higham et al. 2019; Onwochei et al. 2017; Wooding et al. 2020)			
Assessment of Obstetrical Team Performance (AOTP) and Global ATOP (GATOP)	SBT	Interprofessional obstetric (OB) team	5-point scale

(continued)

Table 1 (continued)

Target team /assessment tools	Setting	Participants rated	Type of rating
Perinatal Emergency Team Response Assessment (PETRA)	SBT and CE	Interprofessional OB team	5-point scale
Human Factors Rating Scale (HFRS) and Global Rating Scale (GRS)	SBT	Interprofessional OB team	Not stated
Situational Awareness Global Assessment Technique (SAGAT)	SBT	Interprofessional OB team	Not stated
Prehospital care (Higham et al. 2019)			
Aero-Non-technical Skills (AeroNOTS)	SBT	Doctors on aeromedical teams	5- and 7-point scales
Generic healthcare environment (Boet et al. 2019; Higham et al. 2019; Onwochei et al. 2017)			
Clinical Teamwork Scale (CTS)	SBT and CE	Any interprofessional healthcare team	10-point scale
Undergraduate (Higham et al. 2019; Wooding et al. 2020)			
Standardized Assessment for the Evaluation of Team Skills (SAFE-TeamS)	SBT	Medical and nursing undergraduate students	2-point scale
Individual Teamwork Observation and Feedback Tool (ITOFT)	SBT and CE	Undergraduate interprofessional student teams	3-point scale
Emergency Team Dynamics scale	SBT	Interprofessional student resuscitation teams	Not stated
Operating Room Team Assessment Scale (ORTAS)	SBT	Interprofessional OR student team	Not stated
Team Performance Observation Tool (TPOT)	SBT	Physical therapy and nursing students	Not stated

imperative prior to its implementation as an evaluative piece in order to ensure its accuracy and reliability.

Team science provides valuable information regarding how teams function, what traits make them succeed, which development interventions work, and what assessment tools to use in evaluating an intervention. It can also give insight into the overall effectiveness of team training initiatives across multiple industries. In 2008, Salas et al. (2008) conducted a meta-analysis of the impact of team training interventions involving 2,650 teams across multiple domains, including academia, laboratory experiments, the military, business, aviation, and medicine. They found that moderate, positive relationships existed between team training interventions and cognitive, affective, team process, and team performance outcomes. McEwan et al. (2017) followed with another meta-analysis in 2017 involving 8,439 participants across the domains of academia, laboratory experiments, the military, industry, aviation, and medicine. Like Salas et al. (2008), they found that positive, significant medium-sized effects between training interventions and teamwork and team performance existed. Clearly, training interventions have a positive impact on team effectiveness regardless of domain. The next section examines applications of team development initiatives in healthcare in particular.

Applications for Developing Health Professional Teams

Team science demonstrates that, throughout multiple domains, team development initiatives can improve team processes and outcomes. Although both Salas et al. (2008) and McEwan et al. (2017) included medicine as one of the domains in their meta-analyses looking at the impact of interventions on teamwork and team performance across industries, healthcare only constituted a small percentage of the total number in each. Fortunately, much work has focused exclusively on healthcare and the impact of developing health professional teams. Even more encouraging, Schmutz et al. (2019) have demonstrated a link between teamwork and clinical performance in a meta-analysis looking at 1,390 teams. Their analysis showed a positive medium-sized effect of teamwork on clinical performance across a variety of acute care settings. High team performance was 2.8 times more likely to occur when teams engaged in team processes. Such a finding emphasizes the utility of developing teams in healthcare in order to increase the quality of care patients receive.

Within healthcare, individuals have employed both systems-based and people-focused interventions in order to develop health professional teams. Systems-based solutions have focused on changing organizational structure, mainly through standardizing process pathways, clarifying team roles and responsibilities, and dedicating teams or personnel to a particular area or domain (Bulijac-Samardzic et al. 2020). Such efforts have had positive impacts on teamwork and care. For example, Aeyels et al. (2019) looked at the impact of implementing a care pathway for ST elevation myocardial infarction (STEMI) care across 11 acute care hospitals that covered care from the emergency department through rehabilitation. They found that creating this standardized pathway improved team processes between professions and departments involved in a STEMI patient's care. In addition, the pathway improved such team outputs as patient focused organization, coordination of care, collaboration with primary care, and follow-up care.

Other system-based efforts have attempted to influence teamwork and team performance through the design of the care environment itself. In their systematic review, Gharaveis et al. (2018) found that design layout, visibility, and accessibility were three important influences on teamwork and communication. Thus, spatial arrangements, unit centralization/decentralization, and work station design could all have positive effects on team processes. Additionally, manipulation of the size and configuration of the space layout can help with improving visibility and accessibility between professions, and, consequently, teamwork. For example, Stroebel et al.'s (2019) study of primary clinic designs in the Upper Midwest of the United States demonstrated better teamwork scores among primary care delivery teams who were co-located together in a primary workspace rather than separated from one another. VanHeuvelen (2019) showed that conversion of an open bay configuration to single patient rooms in a neonatal care unit could negatively influence collaboration due to the loss of visibility and accessibility.

Although utilized, systems-based approaches constitute a minority of the interventions employed to develop health professional teams. People-focused approaches are the more popular interventions, particularly team training and team debriefing strategies. For team training, simulation-based practice is common. Additionally, instruction in team-based competencies via a structured curriculum, such as TeamSTEPPS™ or crew resource management (CRM)-based training, is employed. For team debriefing interventions, checklist tools are frequently used (Bulijac-Samardzic et al. 2020).

In general, team training in healthcare successfully improves team processes and behaviors as well as care processes and patient outcomes (Weaver et al. 2014). In their recent meta-analysis, Marlow et al. (2017) found that team training initiatives most often focused on clinicians and less on healthcare students. When students were included, they tended to be medical students. Training frequently addressed communication strategies and incorporated some form of practice-based instruction, such as high-fidelity simulation-based training. Finally, training usually occurred on site and involved feedback opportunities for participants.

Simulation-based training (SBT) of health professional teams has typically concentrated on acute care settings (Bulijac-Samardzic et al. 2020). It is a particularly effective modality for training resuscitation teams in communication, teamwork, and leadership to help improve patient processes and outcomes (Murphy et al. 2016). For example, SBT of interprofessional trauma teams improves their resuscitation knowledge, nontechnical skills, time to task, and task completion (McLaughlin et al. 2019). SBT of obstetrics teams improves intrapartum teamwork and helps reduce morbidity (Wu et al. 2020). Furthermore, SBT can positively influence work place culture, as demonstrated in both the emergency department (Wong et al. 2016) and surgical operating room (Sacks et al. 2015) Finally, SBT is conducive to mass casualty training, helping teams prepare for saturation of resources (Hoang et al. 2020).

Training individuals in CRM principles is another popular strategy to develop health professional teams. Such training typically targets high-risk environments such as the operating room, labor and delivery, intensive care units, emergency rooms, or anesthesia care units (Gross et al. 2019). When combined with SBT, CRM training enhances skill acquisition, improves adverse outcomes, and results in retention of learning on repeat SBT (Fung et al. 2015). Finally, CRM training can enhance acquisition of key resuscitation skills such as advanced life support or airway management (Low et al. 2018).

Another advantage of CRM-based training is that it is well suited for team leadership training. For example, senior medical students undergoing a 10-minute CRM computer-based session were able to perform better as leaders during cardiopulmonary resuscitation (CPR) both in terms of communication and in recognizing poor quality compressions (Haffner et al. 2017). In addition, team leadership training of pediatric rapid response teams using CRM-based principles and SBT resulted in improvements in team performance and processes such as the use of the situation, background, assessment, recommendation (SBAR) format and confirmation of plans (Siems et al. 2017). Finally, team leadership training of individuals in CRM principles as part of CPR training led to more verbalization by the team leader and better overall adherence to advanced life support algorithms by the team itself (Castelao et al. 2015).

Another popular curriculum-based team training program is TeamSTEPPS™. Like CRM-based programs, TeamSTEPPS™ teaches team-based competencies to help develop health professionals. Its curriculum focuses on five main domains: team structure, communication, leadership, situation monitoring, and mutual support. Particularly useful is the many tools it offers to help with team building and interaction. Among the most popular include the SBAR, call back, and call out tools to enhance team communication, the use of "CUS" words (i.e., concerned, uncomfortable, safety issue) to foster mutual support among team members, and the STEP tool (i.e., situation, team members, environment, progress toward goal) to help teams with situation monitoring (Chen et al. 2019). Additionally, it has a variety of measurement instruments to allow instructors to gage training effectiveness. For example, both the TeamSTEPPS™ Teamwork Attitude Questionnaire (T-TAQ) and the Team Performance Observation Tool (TPOT) measure changes in the five domains of the TeamSTEPPS™ curriculum (Chen et al. 2019). Finally, like CRM-based programs, TeamSTEPPS™ is well suited for SBT activities, and the combination has demonstrated improvement in patient process and outcome measures (Welsch et al. 2018). For example, Clapper et al. (2018) reported improvements in team performance and TeamSTEPPS™ course knowledge after an 8-week intervention teaching TeamSTEPPS™ to 547 care providers in a pediatric medicine unit.

Clearly, team training, using SBT and curriculum-based components, is an important and frequently used intervention to develop health professional teams by teaching recognized team-based competencies known to lead to high team performance. Another popular and effective modality for developing teams in healthcare is team debriefing. Unlike team training, it focuses on team processes and outcomes. According to Lacerenza et al. (2018), team debriefings help engage team members in active learning by creating a shared understanding in which the team reviews team priorities, strengths, and weaknesses. Such a review can be self-led by the team or involve guided self-correction using trained facilitators to help the team identify issues with performance. Using a structured debriefing format focusing on performance- or teamwork-related issues enhances the effectiveness of team debriefings. Finally, fostering an open team climate is essential to allow discussion of delicate issues.

When done properly, team debriefings harness the power of team reflexivity. According to Schmutz and Eppich (2017), team reflexivity consists of team level reflection and adaptation of team goals, processes, and strategies. Such collective review and modification of actions can occur during transition or action phases of a team in the form of a briefing before a care event, a huddle/pause during a care event, or a debriefing after a care event. Finally, it is most effective in situations in which teams have complex tasks to perform in a setting with a high degree of uncertainty.

McHugh et al. (2019) have found that team reflexivity in healthcare can take the form of debriefing, video review of in situ events, or peer review. In these forms, it has improved communication and, on one occasion, reduced patient safety events. It also has helped enact process improvements. Finally, equally important, team reflexivity strategies appear well accepted by team members as a means of discussing complexities in practice and exploring solutions (McHugh et al. 2019).

Team debriefings can have a powerful impact on team effectiveness. Tannenbaum and Cerasoli (2013) analyzed a variety of different team debriefing approaches: with and without facilitators, highly or moderately structured, with or without visual aids, within or between group, and real or simulated setting. They found that, overall, these team debriefings improved team performance on average by 25%. In general, team development interventions involving team debriefing strategies in healthcare employ checklists to assist teams with preparation before a care event or after action review following one (Lacerenza et al. 2018). Predominantly, these interventions have focused on the perioperative environment, although they are used elsewhere. Implementation of such briefing and debriefing activities in the operating room (OR) has improved both safety climate and perceived OR efficiency (Leong et al. 2017). It has also helped reduce surgical site infection rates through the identification of issues discovered during debriefings (Hicks et al. 2014).

Checklists and guides for team planning and review also serve as team building tools. In particular, briefings often incorporate several of the four main components found to promote team building: goal setting, interpersonal relationship management, role clarification, and problem-solving. Thus, team building occurs as team members introduce themselves, state their roles, and anticipate problems during a brief before a care event. As a result, trust develops among team members, allowing the team to overcome uncertainty. Finally, team building promotes conflict management and resolution, preventing recriminations among members that impede team performance (Lacerenza et al. 2018).

The World Health Organization's (WHO) Surgical Safety Checklist (SSC) is one of the best-known and widely employed tools to promote team building and debriefing. Patel et al. (2014) have shown that its implementation across a variety of surgical specialties has led to improved communication. In addition, it has resulted in decreases in surgical morbidity and mortality. Furthermore, compliance was high, and staff did not seem to object to its use. Haugen et al. (2019) demonstrated that its use also improved processes of care including antibiotic administration and the use of warming blankets. These improvements led to decreased surgical infection rates. Its use also lowered transfusion costs. Finally, Alidina et al. (2017) found that team members using the SSC found it useful in averting complications related to antibiotic administration, equipment, and surgery side.

Other checklists aid in developing health professional teams. Saxena et al. (2020) found that anesthesia perioperative checklists, including the SSC, improve teamwork, decrease human error, and increase patient safety and the quality of care. In addition, these checklists help with handoffs, routine anesthetic care, and treating emergent situations. Boyd et al.'s (2017) systematic review of randomized controlled trials incorporating checklists in a wide range of settings demonstrated improvements in several patient outcomes. These included improved compliance with evidence-based medication practices, infection precautions, and handover procedures. Finally, they found a decrease in postoperative complications and 30-day mortality (Boyd et al. 2017).

From designing spaces to support teams to checklists for team building and to structure team debriefings, a plethora of applications exist for developing health professional teams. Their success, however, depends on their implementation by overcoming barriers and fostering adoption. The final section will address frameworks and approaches to optimize the development of health professional teams.

Optimizing Implementation of Strategies to Develop Health Professional Teams

Systems-based and people-focused strategies to develop health professional teams are only effective if implemented successfully. Optimizing implementation of a team development initiative, therefore, is essential to ensure widespread adoption of those team-based competencies and processes that lead to superior team performance. This fact is especially true for healthcare, since team function is already less than ideal due to cultural and performance factors. Cultural constraints impeding team performance include a tribalism between professions and specialties that creates an "us" versus "them" dichotomy in which issues and problems shift over to "them" (Mannix and Nagler 2017). This tribalism arises out of the cultural context of the work environment, not innately within the individuals within it (Braithwaite et al. 2016). It combines with a silo mentality born, in part, out of the manner in which patients receive care from discrete entities within the system (Pepler et al. 2018). Such cultural impediments put teams at a disadvantage vis-à-vis functioning cohesively in dynamic situations.

Team processes and performance suffer in this cultural context of tribalism and siloed care. In emergent situations, such as an OR crisis (Davis et al. 2017) or trauma resuscitation (El-Shafy et al. 2018), closed loop communication among team members is limited or completely absent. Instead, individuals infer a task through a question, so-called mixed mode communication, which impairs team performance (Jung et al. 2018). In addition, some, such as nurses and physicians, harbor differing opinions regarding effective collaboration (House and Havens 2017). These differing perceptions can lead to notable variations in how professions within a clinical setting, like the operating room, view the safety climate (Pimentel et al. 2017; Muller et al. 2018). Finally, abusive supervision or overcontrolling leadership can lead to inefficiencies in care (Barling et al. 2018), and incivility and bullying disrupt workflow (Villafranca et al. 2017).

Clearly, successful implementation of team development initiatives is a priority, given the ineffective teamwork in healthcare. Optimizing an intervention's utility requires the use of a change management strategy in order to ensure adoption and cultural change. This approach is especially necessary, given organizational culture and structures can affect team behaviors (Aveling et al. 2018). Fortunately, an emerging field known as implementation science offers theories, models, and frameworks with which to promote change. Defined as the study to promote methods for the systematic uptake of research and evidence-based medicine into practice to improve the quality of healthcare (Nilsen 2015), implementation science, when applied, cannot only substantially increase the effectiveness of an intervention, quintupling it, but it can also slash the time to implementation, decreasing the time to adoption by one sixth (Hull et al. 2017).

Critical elements, as defined by the WHO, for implementation include adequate resources for making change, proper training and education to close gaps in knowledge, necessary oversight and evaluation to measure progress, effective communication strategies for maintaining improvements, and cultural change to promote collaboration (Weiser et al. 2019). Sarkies et al. (2017) confirmed the importance of many of these items in a systematic review of the effectiveness of research implementation strategies. They conceptualized a six-themed unidirectional, hierarchical flow for success: (1) establishing an imperative for change, (2) building trust between stakeholders, (3) developing a shared vision, and (4) actioning change mechanisms while (5) employing effective communication strategies and (6) providing necessary resources to support change.

Sarkies et al.'s six components align with the change management strategy promoted in TeamSTEPPS^{TM}. This approach is the eight-step model formulated by Jon Kotter: (1) establish a sense of urgency, (2) create a guiding coalition, (3) develop a vision and strategy, (4) communicate the change visions, (5) empower employees for broad-based action, (6) generate short-term wins, (7) consolidate gains and produce more change, and (8) anchor new approaches in the culture (Kotter and Rathgeber 2005). Successful implementation of a team development intervention, therefore, requires a systematic approach aiming to embed the changes in the culture.

Measuring progress is an integral component of any implementation project. Hull et al. (2017) have identified eight implementation outcome measures to incorporate into a program in order to determine the effectiveness of an intervention: (1) acceptability, (2) adoption, (3) appropriateness/suitability, (4) feasibility/fit, (5) fidelity, (6) cost, (7) diffusion into practice, and (8) sustainability. By measuring these outcomes in addition to clinical outcomes, the success or failure of an implementation can be more clearly determined.

In addition to having a systematic framework with which to introduce a team development initiative, knowing the barriers to implementation of a particular intervention enables targeted approaches to overcoming them. For example, Bergs et al. (2015) identified several barriers to surgical checklist implementation. These barriers included disruption of routines and workflow within the operating room as well as conflicting priorities and differing perspectives and motivations of stakeholders related to the checklist and patient safety. Questionable usefulness of the checklist itself as well as confusion related to guidelines for its use and surgeon commitment also impeded implementation. Hosny et al. (2017) found different barriers impeding implementation of SBT programs in general surgery. Issues related to cost, practicality, time, motivation, cultural acceptance, access, availability, evidence-base, limited technology, and lack of standards were noted as impediments. The first seven of these issues are rather generic in nature, and, as such, they would likely have applicability to implementations outside the OR environment.

Fiscella et al. (2017) have drawn on team science to recommend several key components of a team training program to ensure its success. First, one must perform a careful needs assessment to determine the need for team training and what tasks should be targeted. Second, one should create a safe, noncritical environment in which to conduct the team training. Third, one should design a training program for maximum availability, usability, and learning. Fourth, one must evaluate the effectiveness of the program in meeting the training needs. Finally, one needs to create a means of sustaining learned teamwork behaviors within the organization and culture.

Jowsey et al. (2019) provide a notable example of applying a systematic approach to implementation of a team development intervention, NetworkZ. NetworkZ is an SBT program for OR teams implemented across New Zealand to enhance patient safety by improving teamwork and communication. Implementation used the Organizing for Quality framework to identify and address six potential challenges to successful adoption. They include the structure of the program and its infrastructure of support, the culture and politics of the target site, and the learning and motivation of the participants. By focusing on and addressing these challenges, the creators of NetworkZ were able to guide implementation of the program. Key lessons learned included the importance of national backing for the program, the need for local ownership and delivery of the program, the utility of multilevel support, the difficulty of promoting cultural change, the impact of quality on acceptance, the necessity of presenting evidence for the need for training, and, finally, the role of ongoing communication to maintain support (Jowsey et al. 2019).

Conclusion

Team science provides key insights into what makes a team, how it can perform well, and the interventions to promote its enhancement. Both systems-based and people-focused approaches are used to improve teamwork and communication in healthcare. Of these, team training using simulation-based techniques and curriculum-based CRM and TeamSTEPPS^{TM} programs are the most popular team development interventions (Bulijac-Samardzic et al. 2020). Team debriefing using checklist tools for structure and guidance is another popular approach to develop health professional teams. Optimizing implementation of a team development initiative requires a systematic approach that addresses key challenges and obstacles to adoption. Drawing on such implementation science can help increase the effectiveness of the intervention and decrease the time to integration of behaviors learned into practice.

References

Aeyels D, Bruyneel L, Seys D, Sinnaeve PR, Sermeus W, Panella M, Vanhaecht K. Better hospital context increases success of care pathway implementation on achieving greater teamwork: a multicenter study on STEMI care. Int J Qual Health Care. 2019;31(6):442–8.

Agency for Healthcare Research and Quality. TeamSTEPPS. 2020. https://www.ahrq.gov/teamstepps/index.html. Accessed 3 Feb. 2020.

Alidina S, Hur HC, Berry WR, Molina G, Guenthner G, Modest AM, Singer SJ. Narrative feedback from OR personnel about the safety of their surgical practice before and after a surgical safety checklist intervention. Int J Qual Health Care. 2017;29(4):461–9.

Arora S, Ahmed M, Paige J, Nestel D, Runnacles J, Hull L, Darzi A, Sevdalis N. Objective structured assessment of debriefing: bringing science to the art of debriefing in surgery. Ann Surg. 2012;256(12):982–8.

Aveling EL, Stone J, Sundt T, Wright C, Gino F, Singer S. Factors influencing team behaviors in surgery: a qualitative study to inform teamwork interventions. Ann Thorac Surg. 2018;106:115–20.

Baker DP, Gustafson S, Beaubien J, Salas E, Barach P. Medical teamwork and patient safety: the evidence-based relation. Agency for Healthcare Research and Quality. Washington, DC. Publication # 05–0053. 2003.

Barling J, Akers A, Beiko D. The impact of positive and negative intraoperative surgeons' leadership behaviors on surgical team performance. Am J Surg. 2018;215:14–8.

Bell ST, Brown SG, Colaneri A, Outland N. Team composition and the ABCs of teamwork. Am Psychol. 2018;73(4):349–62.

Berg J, Lambrechts F, Simons P, Vlayen A, Marneffe W, Hellings J, Cleemput I, Vandijck D. Barriers and facilitators to implementation of surgical safety checklists: a systematic review of qualitative evidence. BMJ Qual Saf. 2015;24:776–86.

Boet S, Etherington N, Larrigan S, Yin L, Khan H, Sullivan K, Jung JJ, Grantcharov TP. Measuring teamwork performance of teams in crisis situations: a systematic review of assessment tools and their measurement properties. BMJ Qual Saf. 2019;28:327–37.

Boyd J, Wu G, Stelfox H. The impact of checklists on inpatient safety outcomes: a systematic review of randomized controlled trials. J Hosp Med. 2017;12(8):675–82.

Braithwaite J, Clay-Williams R, Vecellio E, Marks D, Hooper T, Westbrook M, Westbrook J, Blakely B, Ludlow K. BMJ Open. 2016;6:e012467.

Buljac-Samardzic M, Doekhie KD, van Wijngaarden JDH. Interventions to improve team effectiveness within healthcare: a systematic review of the past decade. Hum Resour Health. 2020;18(1):2.

Cafazzo JA, St-Cyr O. From discovery to design: the evolution of human factors in healthcare. Healthc Q. 2012;15:24–9.

Castelao EF, Boos M, Ringer C, Eich C, Russo SG. Effect of team leadership training on team performance and leadership behavior in simulated cardiac arrest scenarios: a prospective, randomized, controlled study. BMC Med Educ. 2015;15:116.

Chen AS, Yau B, Revere L, Swails J. Implementation, evaluation, and outcome of TeamSTEPPS in interprofessional education: a scoping review. J Interprof Care. 2019;33(6):795–804.

Clapper TC, Ching K, Mauer E, Gerber LM, Lee JG, Sobin B, Ciraolo K, Osorio SN, DiPace JI. A saturated approach to the four-phase, brain-based simulation framework for TeamSTEPPS in a pediatric medicine unit. Pediatr Qual Saf. 2018;3(4):e086.

Davis WA, Jones S, Crowell-Kuhnberg AM, O'Keeffe D, Boyle KM, Klainer SB, Smink DS, Yule S. Operative communication during simulated emergencies: too busy to respond? Surgery. 2017;161:1348–56.

Densen P. Challenges and opportunities facing medical education. Trans Am Clin Climatol Assoc. 2011;122:48–58.

Driskell JE, Salas E, Driskell T. Foundations of teamwork and collaboration. Am Psychol. 2018;73(4):334–48.

El-Shafy IA, Delgado J, Akerman M, Bullaro F, Christopherson NAM, Prince JM. Closed-loop communication improves task completion in pediatric trauma resuscitation. J Surg Ed. 2018;75: 58–64.

Fiscella K, Mauksch L, Bodenheimer T, Salas E. Improving care teams' functioning: recommendations from team science. Jt Comm J Qual Patient Saf. 2017;43(7):361–8.

Fung L, Boet S, Bould MD, Qosa H, Perrier L, Tricco A, Tavares W, Reeves S. Impact of crisis resource management simulation-based training for interprofessional and interdisciplinary teams: a systematic review. J Interprof Care. 2015;29(5):433–44.

Gharaveis A, Hamilton DK, Pati D. The impact of environmental design on teamwork and communication in healthcare facilities: a systematic review of the literature. HERD. 2018;11(1):119–37.

Greiner AC, Knebel E. Health professions education: a bridge to quality. Washington, DC: Institute of Medicine, National Academies Press; 2003.

Gross B, Rusin L, Kiesewetter J, Zottmann JM, Fischer MR, Pruckner S, Zech A. Crew resource management training: a systematic review of intervention design, training conditions and evaluation. BMJ Open. 2019;9:e025247.

Haffner L, Mahling M, Muench A, Castan C, Schubert P, Naumann A, Reddersen S, Herrmann-Werner A, Reutershan J, Riessen R, Celebi N. Improve recognition of ineffective chest compressions after brief crew resource management (CRM) training: a prospective, randomized simulation study. BMC Emerg Med. 2017;17(1):7.

Haugen AS, Woehle HV, Almeland SK, Harthug S, Sevdalis N, Eide GE, Nortvedt MW, Smith I, Softeland E. Causal analysis of world health organization's surgical safety checklist implementation quality and impact on care processes and patient outcomes. Ann Surg. 2019;269:283–90.

Hicks CW, Rosen M, Hobson DB, Ko C, Wick EC. Improving safety and quality of care with enhanced teamwork through operating room briefings. JAMA Surg. 2014;149(8):863–8.

Higham H, Greig PR, Rutherford J, Vincent L, Young D, Vincent C. Observer-based tools for non-technical skills assessment in simulated and real clinical environments in healthcare: a systematic review. BMJ Qual Saf. 2019;28:672–86.

Hoang TN, LaPorta AJ, Malone JD, Champagne R, Lavell K, De La Rosa GM, Gaul L, Dukovich M. Hyper-realistic and immersive surgical simulation training event will improve team performance. Trauma Surg Acute Care Open. 2020;5:e000393.

Hosny SG, Johnston MJ, Pucher PH, Darzi A. Barriers to implementation and uptake of simulation-based training programs in general surgery: a multinational qualitative study. J Surg Res. 2017;220:419–26.

House S, Havens D. Nurses' and physicians' perceptions of nurse-physician collaboration: a systematic review. J Nurs Adm. 2017;47(3):165–71.

Hull L, Athanasiou T, Russ S. Implementation science: a neglected opportunity to accelerate improvements in the safety and quality of surgical care. Ann Surg. 2017;265:1104–12.

Interprofessional Education Collaborative. Core competencies for interprofessional collaborative practice: 2016 update. Washington DC: Interprofessional Education Collaborative; 2016.

IOM (Institute of Medicine). Redesigning continuing education in the health professions. Washington, DC: The National Academies Press; 2010.

Jowsey T, Beaver P, Long J, Civil I, Garden AL, Henderson K, Merry A, Skilton C, Torrie J, Weller J. Towards a safer culture: implementing multidisciplinary simulation-based team training in New Zealand operating theatres – a framework analysis. BMJ Open. 2019;9:e027122.

Juneja P. Understanding team – what is a team? In Team Building. Management Study Guide. https://www.managementstudyguide.com/understanding-team.htm. 2020. Accessed 3 Feb. 2020.

Jung HS, Warner-Hillard C, Thompson R, Haines K, Moungey B, LeGare A, Shaffer DW, Pugh C, Agarwal S, Sullivan S. Why saying what you means matters: an analysis of trauma team communication. Am J Surg. 2018;215:250–4.

Kern DE. Overview: a six-step approach to curriculum development. In: Thomas PA, Kern DE, Hughes MT, Chen BY, editors. Curriculum development for medical education: a six step approach. 3rd ed. Baltimore: Johns Hopkins University Press; 2016.

Kotter JP, Rathgeber H. Our iceberg is melting: changing and succeeding under any conditions. New York: St. Martin's Press; 2005.

Kuziemsky C. Decision-making in healthcare as a complex adaptive system. Healthc Manage Forum. 2016;29(1):4–7.

Lacerenza CN, Marlow SL, Tannenbaum SI, Salas E. Team development interventions: evidence-based approaches for improving teamwork. Am Psychol. 2018;73(4):517–31.

Leong KBMSL, Hanskamp-Sebregts M, van der Wal RA, Wolff AP. Effects of perioperative briefing and debriefing on patient safety: a prospective intervention study. BMJ Open. 2017;7: e018367.

Low XM, Horrigan D, Brewster DJ. The effects of team training in intensive care medicine: a narrative review. J Crit Care. 2018;48:283–9.

Macefield R. Usability studies and the Hawthorne effect. J Usability Stud. 2007;2(3):154.

Mannix R, Nagler J. Tribalism in medicine – Us vs Them. JAMA Pediatr. 2017;171(9):831.

Marlow SL, Hughes AM, Sonesh SC, Gregory ME, Lacerenza CN, Benishek LE, Woods AL, Hernandez C, Salas E. A systematic review of team training in health care: ten questions. Jt Comm J Qual Patient Saf. 2017;43(4):197–204.

McEwan D, Ruissen GR, Eys MA, Zumbo BD, Beauchamp MR. The effectiveness of teamwork training on teamwork behaviors and team performance: a systematic review and meta-analysis of controlled interventions. PLoS One. 2017;12(1):e0169604.

McGrath JE. Social psychology: a brief introduction. New York: Holt, Rinehart and Winston; 1964.

McHugh SK, Lawton R, O'Hara JK, Sheard L. Does team reflexivity impact teamwork and communication in interprofessional hospital-based healthcare systems? A systematic review and narrative analysis. BMJ Qual and Saf. 2019 Jan 7. pii: bmjqs-2019-009921. Epub ahead of print.

McLaughlin C, Barry W, Barin E, Kysh L, Auerbach MA, Upperman JS, Burd RS, Jensen AR. J Surg Ed. 2019;76:1669–80.

Muller P, Tschan F, Keller S, Seelandt J, Beldi G, Elfering A, Dubach B, Candinas D, Pereira D, Semmer NK. Assessing perceptions of teamwork quality among perioperative team members. AORN J. 2018;108(3):251–62.

Murphy M, Curtis K, McCloughen A. What is the impact of multidisciplinary team simulation training on team performance and efficiency in patient care? An integrative review. Australas Emerg Nurs J. 2016;19(1):44–53.

Nilsen P. Making sense of implementation theories, models and frameworks. Implement Sci. 2015;10:53.

Nolan TW. System changes to improve patient safety. BMJ. 2000;320:771–3.

Onwochei DN, Halpern S, Balki M. Teamwork assessment tools in obstetric emergencies: a systematic review. Sim Healthcare. 2017;12:165–76.

Patel J, Ahmed K, Guru KA, Khan F, Marsh H, Khan MS, Dasgupta P. An overview of the use and implementation of checklists in surgical specialties – a systematic review. Int J Surg. 2014;12 (12):1317–23.

Pepler EF, Pridie J, Brown S. Predicting and testing a silo-free delivery system. Healthc Manage Forum. 2018;31(5):200–5.

Pimentel MPT, Choi S, Fiumara K, Kachalia A, Urman RD. Safety culture in the operating room: variability among perioperative healthcare workers. J Patient Saf. 2017; Jun 1. Epub ahead of print

Pype P, Mertens F, Helewaut F, Krystallidou D. Healthcare teams as complex adaptive systems: understanding team behavior through team members' perception of interpersonal interaction. BMC Health Serv Res. 2018;18(1):570.

Rudolph J, Simon R, Dufresne R, Raemer D. There's no such thing as a "nonjudgemental" debriefing: a theory and method for debriefing with good judgement. Simul Healthc. 2006;1 (1):49–55.

Sacks GD, Shannon EM, Dawes AJ, Rollo JC, Nguyen DK, Russell MM, Ko CY, Maggard-Gibbons MA. Teamwork, communication and safety climate: systematic review of interventions to improve surgical culture. BMJ Qual Saf. 2015;24:458–67.

Salas E, Sims DE, Burke CS. Is there a "big five" of teamwork? Sm Group Res. 2005;36(5):555–99.

Salas E, DiazGrandos D, Klein C, Burke CS, Stagl KC, Goodwin GF, Halpin SM. Does team training improve team performance? A meta-analysis. Hum Factors. 2008;50(6):903–33.

Salas E, Shuffler ML, Thayer AL, Bedwell WL, Lazzara EH. Understanding and Improving Teamwork in Organizations: A Scientifically Based Practical Guide. Human Resource Management 2015;54(4):599–622 https://doi.org/10.1002/hrm.21628.

Sarkies MN, Bowles KA, Skinner EH, Haas R, Lane H, Haines TP. The effectiveness of research implementation strategies for promoting evidence-informed policy and management decisions in healthcare: a systematic review. Implement Sci. 2017;12:132.

Saxena S, Krombach JW, Nahrwold DA, Pirracchio R. Anaesthesia-specific checklists: a systematic review of impact. Anaesth Crit Care Pain Med. 2020;39(1):65–73.

Schmutz JB, Eppich WJ. Promoting learning and patient care through shared reflection: a conceptual framework for team reflexivity in health care. Acad Med. 2017;92:1555–63.

Schmutz JB, Meier LL, Manser T. How effective is teamwork really? The relationship between teamwork and performance in healthcare teams: a systematic review and meta-analysis. BMJ Open. 2019;9:e028280.

Shuffler ML, Diazgrandos D, Maynard MT, Salas E. Developing, sustaining, and maximizing team effectiveness: an integrative, dynamic perspective of team development interventions. Acad Manag Ann. 2018;12(2):688–724.

Siems A, Cartron A, Watson A, McCarter R Jr, Levin A. Improving pediatric rapid response team performance through crew resource management training of team leaders. Hosp Pediatr. 2017;7(2):88–95.

Stroebel RJ, Obeidat B, Lim L, Mitchell JD, Jasperson DB, Zimring C. The impact of clinical design on teamwork development in primary care. Health Care Manage Rev. 2019;Aug 1. Epub ahead of print.

Tannenbaum S. The seven C's – cracking the code of teamwork. The group for organizational effectiveness. 2020. https://www.groupoe.com/blog-on-teams/169-the-seven-c-s-cracking-the-code-of-teamwork.html. Accessed 3 Feb. 2020.

Tannenbaum SI, Cerasoli CP. Do team and individual debriefs enhance performance? A meta-analysis. Hum Factors. 2013;55(1):231–45.

The Health Foundation. Evidence scan: complex adaptive systems. London; 2010.

Thisthlethwaite JE, Forman D, Matthews LR, Rogers GD, Steketee C, Yassine T. Competencies and frameworks in interprofessional education: a comparative analysis. Acad Med. 2014;89(6):869–75.

Turner JR, Baker R, Morris M. Complex adaptive systems: adapting and managing teams and team conflict. 2018. https://doi.org/10.5772/intechopen.72344. Accessed 3 Feb. 2020.

VanHeuvelen JS. Isolation or interaction: healthcare provider experience of design change. Sociol Health Illn. 2019;41(4):692–708.

Villafranca A, Hamlin C, Enns S, Jacobsohn E. Disruptive behaviour in the perioperative setting: a contemporary review. Les comportements perturbateurs dans le contexte périopératoire: un compte rendu contemporain. Canadian Journal of Anesthesia/Journal canadien d'anesthésie 2017;64(2):128–140. https://doi.org/10.1007/s12630-016-0784-x.

Weaver SJ, Dy SD, Rosen MA. Team training in healthcare: a narrative synthesis of the literature. BMJ Qual Saf. 2014;23:359–72.

Weinger MB, Gaba DM. Human factors engineering in patient safety. Anesthesiology. 2014;120(4):801–6.

Weiser TG, Forrester JA, Negussie T. Implementation science and innovation in global surgery. BJS. 2019;106:e20–3.

Welsch LA, Hoch J, Poston RD, Parodi VA, Akpinar-Elci M. Interprofessional education involving didactic TeamSTEPPS and interactive healthcare simulation: a systematic review. J Interprof Care. 2018;32(6):657–65.

Wong AHW, Gang M, Szyld D, Mahoney H. Making an "attitude adjustment:" using a simulation-enhanced interprofessional education strategy to improve attitudes toward teamwork and communication. Simul Healthc. 2016;11(2):117–25.

Wood TC, Raison N, Haldar S, Brunckhorst O, McIlhenny G, Dasgupta P, Ahmed K. Training tools for nontechnical skills for surgeons – a systematic review. J Surg Ed. 2017;74:548–78.

Wooding EL, Gale TC, Maynard V. Evaluation of teamwork assessment tools for interprofessional simulation: a systematic review of the literature. J Interprof Care. 2020;34(2):162–72.

Wu M, Tang J, Etherington N, Walker M, Boet S. Interventions for improving teamwork in intrapartem care: a systematic review of randomized controlled trials. BMJ Qual Saf. 2020;29:77–85.

Developing Care and Compassion in Health Professional Students and Clinicians

76

Karen Livesay and Ruby Walter

Contents

Introduction	1486
Philosophical Perspective	1487
Health Ethics	1487
Humanism	1488
Concepts	1488
Care	1489
Compassion	1489
Empathy	1489
Dignity	1489
Inclusion	1489
Perspectives that Inform Practice	1490
Person-Centered Care	1490
Aged Care	1490
Critical Care	1491
End of Life Care	1491
Care of the Carer	1492
Diversity	1492
Identity	1493
Bespoke Care	1494

K. Livesay (✉)
School of Health and Biomedical Sciences, College of Science, Engineering and Health, RMIT University, Melbourne, VIC, Australia
e-mail: Karen.Livesay@rmit.edu.au

R. Walter
School of Nursing and Midwifery, College of Science, Health and Engineering, LaTrobe University, Melbourne, VIC, Australia
e-mail: ruby.walter@rmit.edu.au

© Crown 2023
D. Nestel et al. (eds.), *Clinical Education for the Health Professions*,
https://doi.org/10.1007/978-981-15-3344-0_97

Self-Awareness, Care of Self, Reflection, and Reflexivity 1495
   Self-Awareness 1495
   Reflection and Reflexivity 1495
Care and Compassion Fatigue 1495
Assessing Health Care in the Affective Domain 1496
Conclusion 1497
Cross-References 1497
References 1497

Abstract

The biomedical model of health care is at one end of a continuum while the other end is represented by a psychosocial model. Different health professional disciplines aim to practice at points along this imaginary continuum. Overemphasis on biomedical, technical, and standardized approaches to health care negatively impact care and compassion in health care. Health care perceived to be compassionate from providers who are caring and empathic is associated with improved patient satisfaction and better health outcomes.

Individual perceptions of compassionate care mean that a one-size-fits-all approach is not suitable. Different backgrounds, beliefs, and experiences along with context of care delivery and timing give rise to a layered pattern of preferences for the way compassionate care is enacted. The caring health professional needs to focus on the individual needs of each person from a standpoint of genuine curiosity, desire to be compassionately caring and a foundation of emotional stability. The affective domain is as important as the more objectively measured domains related to skill and competence in quality health care.

Keywords

Care · Compassion · Empathy · Person centered · Perspective · Diversity · Self-care

Introduction

Care and caring are commonly associated with the discipline of nursing and likely emanate from the historical perspectives related to women and healing (Theofanidis and Sapountzi-Krepia 2015). More contemporary literature responding to the professional status of nursing has identified the dual discourses of scientific and technical skills and the caring discourse or feminist critique (Apesoa-Varano 2016). While compassion is linked as a core value to quality health care for all health disciplines, the term is ambiguous. Aspiring to be a caring and compassionate health care provider is a goal enmeshed in many of the standards of health care professions. Opinion is divided among patients and practitioners as to the innate nature of compassion in an individual, but it is suggested that compassion can be awakened and nurtured over time (Sinclair et al. 2016). Positive patient experiences in health care have been linked with health outcomes, patient safety, cost implications, and employee satisfaction. Patient satisfaction is also linked to caring behaviors and person centeredness (Edvardsson et al. 2017). Aspirations for technical skill and efficiency function as measurements of proficiency within the sphere of expert health care practice. Competency and skill often characterize clinician assessment practice overlooking the concepts of person-centered interaction in favor of standardized approaches to delivery (Moore et al. 2017). This exploration of care and compassion will highlight the relevance and importance of the affective domain in person-centered quality health care as well as the influence of context and individual circumstances in providing care and compassion.

For the purposes of clarity in this chapter, we have elected to describe the person receiving care and compassion as "the patient." We are aware of the apparent contradiction, in a chapter that promotes individual person–centered and bespoke care, to consign the person to a reductive role as patient. Similarly, across and within health care disciplines the person receiving care is referred to by a range of different terms. Patient was therefore identified as the most transferable term to encompass all the different contexts and cultures in which a person receives care.

Philosophical Perspective

Health care does not occur in a void but rather each individual requiring care, and indeed the health care system itself, exists within sociopolitical contexts that influence and impact upon care provided and care received. In addition to the clinical knowledge and practical skill required of health care professionals, an awareness and consideration that health and health care exist within a larger context for each presenting individual is important (Stein-Parbury 2018). The practice of health care is strengthened and supported by adopting philosophical perspectives that provide a framework within which to operate, and which protect against discrimination and negligence (Glass 2010). In the following sections, two approaches are introduced, which are not discrete approaches but rather can be used in conjunction.

Health Ethics

Health ethics broadly acknowledge that all health care professionals are focused upon helping and improving the welfare of the patients they work with (Guillemin and Gillam 2006). Ethical standards inform many health professions, particularly those that require registration and are governed by a regulatory authority such as medicine, psychology, and nursing. Most commonly, it is ethical dilemmas that are thought of in relation to ethics in health care, however ethics is broader than this and involves the consideration and application of ethical principles that can guide health care, and more specifically, care and compassion towards the patient (Guillemin and Gillam 2006).

Table 1 Five features of ethical mindfulness. (Adapted from Guillemin and Gillam 2006)

1. The importance of being present to what is going on and paying attention to and being aware of ethically important moments in health care
2. Being prepared to give credibility to moments that do not feel quite right as these may be ethically significant
3. Being able to give voice to why something is an ethical matter
4. Remaining open to others' interpretations and other possibilities in addition to one's own perspective
5. Having the courage to pursue difficult issues that would be more comfortable to leave alone (Sinclair et al. 2016)

Importantly, people seek health care at times when they require information and assistance, and when they simultaneously may be experiencing vulnerability and powerlessness (Johnstone 2014). Health care professionals are in a position to act with care and compassion when they recognize and are party to issues, concerns, questions, possibilities, and sometimes dilemmas within a patient situation.

In their book on Everyday Ethics in Healthcare, Guillemin and Gillam (2006) discuss the concept of ethical mindfulness as being separate to the process of ethical decision-making, and claim its use enables ethical practice. Ethical mindfulness involves the following five features outlined in Table 1.

Humanism

The provision of care and compassion within health care is reliant upon health care professionals being active constructers of a health care environment that considers, supports, and uplifts those receiving care, and their families/caregivers (Kilpatrick 2009). Operating with an ethos that values and respects the experiences of others can provide a framework to guide health care professionals in their caregiving.

Humanism is a philosophy that provides such a framework. Humanistic philosophies within health care place emphasis upon the importance of effective communication and advocate for the expectations and values of the person receiving care being a central consideration of health care provision (Arai et al. 2017). Embedding humanistic philosophies within the practice of care and compassion requires that respect and value of the dignity of each person requiring health care be foundational to health care (Stein-Parbury 2018; Glass 2010; Kilpatrick 2009).

Concepts

Some of the terms used in this chapter have different inflections and meanings according to the way and where they are used in practice environments or written about. The following section provides clarity about the understanding applied to those terms within this chapter.

Care

Care is a noun describing the act of ministration and encompassing the provision of helping or supportive tasks aimed at actions such as treatment, relief of pain, and assistance with activities of living. Care as a verb, centers on the aspect of feeling or concern experienced in a situation. Discourse in health literature may separate the two areas of care to include technical care and nontechnical, or skills and soft skills (Edvardsson et al. 2017).

Compassion

Compassion is described as a deep understanding of the suffering of others coupled with a desire to relieve this suffering (Sinclair et al. 2016). The term is oriented toward action and sometimes compounded with "care" or "practice" as compassionate care, or compassionate practice in order to extend the inference of action. Compassion is regarded as involving both empathy and kindness (McKinnon 2016).

Empathy

An understanding of the emotional state of another is a hallmark of empathy. The distinctive element relates to *pathos* or feeling, often shared with another person, to the extent that meaning and significance of the event is understood, while remaining separate and objective (Harris et al. 2014).

Dignity

The human desire to be recognized as having value is described by Jacobson (2009), as human dignity. It is differentiated in her work from social dignity in which dignity is perceived among people as a mechanism by which worthiness and respect are conveyed. Within interactions, Jacobson (2009) describes the plethora of actions, markers, and behaviors that convey or violate dignity as context-dependant layers. In health care, the context gives rise to professional as well as individual expectations of behavior and attitude that have the potential to promote dignity. These behaviors may be as simple as the manner in which a person introduces themself or the use of a salutation that is appropriate for the culture and setting.

Inclusion

Provision of health care to all is a human right enshrined in law and encompasses suitable care to all whose identities are associated with distinct needs. While focus on cultural diversity and cultural safety training for diverse groups is laudable, performance gaps and societal attitudes such as heteronormative bias still prevail (McCann and Brown 2018). Inclusivity involves adequate education, openness, willingness to examine bias, avoidance of stereotypes, and responding competently with suitable resources to people who identify with a characteristic outside the mainstream.

Perspectives that Inform Practice

If care and compassion embody the elements of context, perspective, and inclusivity to achieve dignity and empathy, then the following viewpoints are presented to develop awareness or at least illustrate the subjectivity of various perspectives.

Person-Centered Care

The term "Person-Centered Care" and its derivations were coined to express the unique needs of the patient in the care equation being foregrounded ahead of treatment or disease. As a recognized part of curriculum in medical education, person centeredness became defined and assessable. Gillespie et al. (2018, p. 1053) suggest that the literature surrounding medicine's response to person centeredness demonstrates greater capacity to define care than to explore the patient's unique experience of it.

In their hermeneutic study of caring, Gillespie et al. (2018) asked outpatients attending a clinic to describe positive and negative experiences of caring. The lived experience of the participants uncovered a range of impressions from facial expression to knowing about the individual and their family as well as willingness to go the extra mile. Reciprocity of relationship, genuine behaviors that avoid predefined conduct instead responding to cues embedded in real life were all described as experiences of caring.

Aged Care

The Australian Government established a Royal Commission into Aged Care Services in 2018 amid questions of care-related failure and service adequacy. In Britain similar issues led to various inquiries and resulted in the Compassion in Practice Vision and Strategy (NHS Commissioning Board Chief Nursing Officer and DH Chief Nursing Adviser 2012). Older adults frequently interact with multiple caregivers associated with increased morbidity and deteriorating health. Independence in care is sometimes compromised through disability and this may be associated with reduced choice in expression of and resultant experiences of caring (Minogue 2015).

Older adults report powerlessness and loss of dignity during hospitalisation. Older adults observed that staff hid impatience and avoided conversation (Minogue 2015). The tension of busy environments and workload pressures contrasted with patients who may have communication deficits associated with loss of hearing or vision or altered cognition suggests the perfect storm of events that may lead to care compromise. Minogue (2015) suggests that in the aged care context, patient discretion and flexibility were more important than knowing the name of the assigned nurse.

Critical Care

In the era of electronic health records and technological advances for assessing and monitoring care, the question of the extent to which the technology obscures the person is a theme to consider. Health professionals are exalted in practice to assess the patient and not the monitoring equipment. Johns' (2005) interesting reflection of the critical care patient questions whether the patient connected to the machine is emotionally isolated in a twilight world of sedation. He further considers the extent to which the health care provider uses the technology as a barrier between themselves and the patient, reducing the person to a list of tasks and measurements. Connected to technology, the patient expresses disquiet, pain, or fear through restlessness and agitation. Is the appropriate response to increase the sedation or consider other nonpharmacologic means to reassure and connect more importantly does sedation subdue distress or only hide its expression (Johns 2005)? Does the caring practitioner ascertain the perspective of the family and patient when sitting with a patient who is sedated with the express purpose of diminishing suffering? Who does this serve, the practitioner, patient, or family?

End of Life Care

In the liminal state at the end of life, as the person transitions from one identity, among the living to another as neither here nor there, the caring compassionate practitioner is separated from the patient (McDermid et al. 2018). The liminal state is not one that is shared and is characterized as alone. Who is the recipient of care and compassion? Is it the family/significant others if present, the patient or is this the opportunity for self-care, compassion for colleagues, how might that be assessed and provided? Minogue (2015) says a better patient experience is related to, and achieved through, mindfulness of the staff experience of the work environment. Mindfulness involves conscious awareness in the moment and therefore an environment that provides support and values staff actively is likely to lead to a better patient experience. In contrast, Sinclair et al. (2016) describe compassion as relational and grounded in emotional resonance and response to suffering. This is a more connected description of compassion than posited by Minogue (2015) and characterizes the importance of connecting with the patient as a person with unique experiences of suffering, beliefs, and desires.

Palliative care patients describe the empathic carer as someone who was understanding, permitted a personal understanding of the patient and their individual needs and relating on an affective level. Compassion was described by these patients as preferred to empathy and differed from empathy through the addition of love, altruism, and kindness (Sinclair et al. 2017).

Care of the Carer

Dr. Kate Grainger, a medical practitioner while living with a terminal illness, documented her experience of caring in the health care system. One of Kate's legacies is the world-wide recognition of the "#hellomynameis" initiative (Hellomynameis n.d.). Kate maintained that introducing oneself to a patient was a fundamental expression of trust and human connection. As an extension to the campaign of introduction, the movement documented a therapeutic ladder of values that demonstrated compassion. These values are summarized as:

- Communication, beginning with an introduction
- Consideration of the so-called "little things" and the impact attention to detail can provide
- Patient influence in decisions expressed as "no decisions about me, without me"
- See me, a concept that encourages the carer to consider the person holistically as a person with a life and important circumstances related to their context (Hellomynameis n.d.)

Diversity

Diverse expectations, manifestations, and interpretations of compassionate care occur as a result of differing norms and beliefs as well as enculturation. Within health care environments the diversity of expectations for compassionate care may be experienced across different discipline groups. The approaches of nursing and medicine to expectations of compassionate care are likely to be different, because practitioners have been enculturated differently. Compassionate care may be directed toward the patient or take the form of support or gestures of concern for colleagues within or between discipline groups. Indeed, staff themselves may identify with characteristics that are diverse compared with the mainstream or dominant culture of the workplace context. Intersectionality describes the dimensions of social and cultural difference that all people present. The various categories of diversity act within our lives simultaneously and to various degrees in different contexts. While traditionally associated with oppression or privlege, intersectionality also assists recognition of the way difference from the dominant or prevailing characteristics changes dynamically in different situations and contexts. This recognition helps to explain the way different life perspectives impact on health care relationships (Livesay 2016). A nurse, doctor, or social worker may be enculturated to expect different methods of peer support. These expectations could surface in alternate ways if the gender or ethnicity of the practitioner was changed. Likewise, the experience may vary with a patient interaction depending on other characteristics of diversity.

Ethnic diversity gives rise to difference in customs, beliefs practices, and language. As we contemplate the range of differences in people's expectations of compassionate care, we are confronted by exponential difference in identity experienced through ethnic diversity. Culturally competent compassionate care is defined as:

> a human quality of understanding the suffering of others and wanting to do something about it using culturally appropriate and acceptable nursing interventions. This takes into consideration both the patients' and the carers' cultural backgrounds as well as the context in which care is given. (Papadopoulos et al. 2016, p. 2)

In order to practice in a culturally competent compassionate manner, health care providers need to demonstrate skills of nonjudgemental assessment of the needs and values of others, while avoiding stereotypes and reflectively uncovering one's own bias.

Identity

While many forms of diversity, such as ethnicity, ability, language, and age are often recognizable by social markers, it is important to note that there are other diverse minority groups that are not. Those identifying as lesbian, gay, bisexual, transgender, intersex, questioning, or asexual (LGBTIQA), for example, may not be recognizable as diverse. This can lead to indirect discrimination where the practices of a health care organization or individual health care professional disadvantage a person or group without intention, but often simply because they are operating from a position of heteronormativity or a binary understanding of gender, rather than consciously adopting inclusive practices (Pedreschi et al. 2013). Examples of indirect discrimination may reflect dominant norms such as an assumption that a woman has a male partner, or that a person identifies as cisgendered (identifies as the sex assigned to them at birth). Discrimination may also be found in the use of institutional forms and routine questioning that do not provide an option for people to self-identify their sex, gender, or sexuality (Zeeman et al. 2018).

Discrimination sends a message of "less than" or "other" to those who do not identify in the offered and expected ways. Discrimination also creates barriers to effective formation of therapeutic relationships if people do not feel seen or understood and therefore trust cannot be established. Actively and intentionally engaging with and valuing diversity can be achieved by consciously enacting inclusive practices (Nivet and Fair 2016) such as using inclusive language and avoiding identity assumptions.

The benefits of diversity and a culture of inclusion can be achieved through the fostering of belonging, respect and the valuing of all persons, and that this in turn improves the quality of care for all (Nivet and Fair 2016). As highlighted in the above section on diversity, health care professionals are also a diverse population. A diverse workforce of health care professionals (including but not limited to race, ethnicity, language, sexual orientation, gender identity, religion, age, and abilities) improves opportunities for learning, understanding, and recognizing difference when caring for patients.

Bespoke Care

The preference for evidence-based care lends credence to standardization of care, while the argument for person-centeredness preferences individual knowledge and negotiated planning and intervention (Bliss et al. 2017). Bespoke care involves developing opportunities for shared decision-making, control, and autonomy to the extent that it is subjectively desired by the individual. Genuinely recognizing that each individual may preference a different degree of autonomy is central to the tenant of person-centredness. The care recipient must be open to care, and the context must be conducive to the care requirements. Finally, the caregiver requires the professional skill and the emotional stability to give of themselves in the care equation and the moral mindfulness associated with interpersonal sensitivity and sophisticated knowledge of self to manage the intimacy, curiosity, and flexibility of the caring relationship (Edvardsson et al. 2017).

Reading examples of compassionate and extraordinary care published across a range of sources, various authors single out behaviors that demonstrate extraordinarily empathic actions in which the carer invests emotionally and develop an intimate care relationship. In Sweeney's (2017) depiction of the care of a preterm infant, the author recognizes the risk of the health care provider in connecting with the baby born at 23 weeks, who could die in the care episode but who ultimately would leave if the care was successful. Either way the health care provider would experience the loss. "On Juniper's 196th day in the neonatal intensive care unit (NICU), Tracy [the carer] came in on her day off and walked us, the three of us, out into the sun" (Sweeney 2017).

Authenticity and genuineness feature as aspects of ideal caring and compassionate care. These notions describe meeting patients on their individual level with a reciprocal sharing of self and engagement in a relationship. Relationship development involves the basics of eye contact where culturally appropriate, deliberate talking and listening and willingness to hear fear or other negative emotion without shying away. Individually mediated behavior is the most significant aspect of bespoke care. Considering research in which patients watched video recordings of health care professionals and rated the behavior as caring or otherwise demonstrated the individual difference in the interpretation of behavior exhibited. The manifestation of the caring behavior is subjective and individually experienced (Quirk et al. 2008).

Self-Awareness, Care of Self, Reflection, and Reflexivity

Self-Awareness

An underpinning concept within caring and compassion is that of self-awareness, and indeed, caring for self. In order for health care professionals to bring care and compassion to their practice, they must firstly be aware of, care for, and understand their own self. This knowing of self (which occurs through examination of the past, present, and through contemplation of the future) is necessary in order to be able to interpret others and their individual contexts in a balanced way (McKinnon 2016). Self-awareness has been linked to emotional intelligence and the notion that the capacity to recognize and deal with one's own emotional responses is intrinsic to being able to recognize and deal with the emotional responses of others (Stein-Parbury 2018).

It is important to recognize that being self-aware, and understanding one's own experiences, beliefs, values, and perspectives, is an ongoing and dynamic process that is never complete. Within a health care context, health care professionals need to commit to a continued practice of examining their own reactions and thoughts in order to remain self-aware and consequently be capable of considering the position and understanding of those in their care. As Glass (2010) posited, heightened levels of self-awareness through continued self-examination on the part of health care professionals leads to increased levels of resilience and greater personal resources to draw upon when delivering compassionate care.

Reflection and Reflexivity

Interwoven within self-awareness/care of self/emotional intelligence is the process of reflection. It is through reflection that examination of thoughts, feelings, and reactions to situations can occur (Jack and Smith 2007). As Daly, Speedy, and Jackson (2017) discuss, engaging in reflection can mediate an increased awareness and sensitivity to the experience of others through the "education of emotions." Reflection, in turn, will influence action and in particular the action of health care practice.

This extension or loop of reflective thought influencing practice or action is known as reflexivity (Redmond 2017). Reflexivity can be thought of as the embodiment of thought/theory into practice where the health care professional consciously draws upon their previous experience, knowledge, their self-awareness, and awareness of others within their practice (Lessard 2012).

Care and Compassion Fatigue

Person-centered health care in which the individual preferences of the patient are foregrounded is beneficial to the patient's perception of quality, and to the financial and clinical outcomes of the organization. Ultimately, caring provides the health professional carer a sense of satisfaction and well-being as well (Edvardsson et al. 2017). Perhaps simplistically, this formula for quality, satisfaction, and well-being appears as a feedback loop that could be established and continue in perpetuity. Yet, that is not the experience of all patients or care providers. Jeffrey (2016) describes the existential neglect that positions patients as objects of intellectual interest. He identified factors including overwork, commercialization of health care, overemphasis of biomedical aspects of health care, lack of continuity of care, and imbalance between scientific-technical aspects of care and psychosocial aspects of care as compassion fatigue causes.

Compassionate care can be cast as a volitional pursuit that is deliberately chosen and of a higher order than mere duty (McCaffrey and McConnell 2015). However, the health care provider does not exercise any choice in when and where suffering occurs. They may need to endure suffering and loss during their work hours without an opportunity for time out of the clinical area. According to Zapac, Moran, and Groh (2017), being denied the opportunity to release emotional distress through ongoing work requirements may lead to the development of compassion fatigue over time. Compassion fatigue, the authors describe, is associated with diminished performance, apathy, callousness, and sleep disturbance. Access to support and debriefing enabled staff at risk of compassion fatigue to acknowledge their own emotional needs.

Empathic distress conceptualized as overactivation of empathic response is a variant of compassion fatigue (Jeffrey 2016). Where the empathic response is self-orientated, the carer understands the patient's position from the perspective of their own experience. Spending time imagining oneself in the position of suffering is exhausting. Additionally, these superimposed feelings lead to assumptions of understanding and personal distress. Ultimately, Jeffrey (2016) predicts that medical staff are likely to distance themselves from the patient in a self-protective manner or eventually become burnt out. Understanding the relationship between providing care, needing care, and care of self demonstrates that health care providers are not merely givers of care and compassion. The emotionally mindful health care provider must care for self and accept care from peers to function well in the care environment. Given the importance of demonstrating individual care and compassion, we finally examine assessment of the affective domain.

Assessing Health Care in the Affective Domain

Use of objective structured clinical examinations (OSCEs) that assess point-in-time care in which health professional students must display attitudes of care, compassion, and empathy while establishing rapport encourage encapsulation of behaviors that may be stereotypical. Gillespie et al., (2018) suggest brief simulated encounters may reassure assessors, rather than measure genuine propensity for caring. Relational skills produced reflexively, and role modeled may be more beneficial to learners that standardized behaviors displayed during assessment episodes.

While assessment related to demonstrations of compassionate care may privilege the behavior that demonstrates caring, at other times, the assessments are embedded in episodes of care that examine technical and disciplinary knowledge alongside rapport and compassion. In these instances, a hierarchy of desirable attributes suggest a tiered approach to the value of compassion compared to technical proficiency. For example, is compassion always required? Certainly, in circumstances where the patient does not appear to be suffering, it is difficult to make an argument for the demonstration of compassionate care. Perhaps for this reason, the assessment of objective, technical, and psychomotor competency is preferenced in many disciplines while hallmarks of quality accreditation favor respect, dignity, empathy, culturally appropriate care, and ethical practice (Franklin and Melville 2015). The tension between assessment of objectively measurable elements and those that are experienced subjectively and prone to individual difference through culture and experience is not going to be resolved simply. This section serves to raise awareness and assist educational developers to think about the qualities of the ideal caring compassionate health care provider.

Conclusion

While care and compassion are documented within the quality standards for health disciplines, many factors impact how those qualities are demonstrated in practice. Busy health care environments and diverse patient needs coupled with economic rationalization and standardization of care have resulted in a call for emphasis on caring being reformed. Conscious effort, emotional maturity, and a willingness to invest time and energy in determining the needs and preferences of individual patients are required. This chapter has presented a range of perspectives on care and recommends curiosity in assessing bespoke needs with persons in our care.

Cross-References

▶ Contemporary Sociological Issues for Health Professions Curricula
▶ Conversational Learning in Health Professions Education: Learning Through Talk
▶ Developing Patient Safety Through Education

References

Apesoa-Varano EC. Not merely TLC: nurses' caring revisited. Qual Sociol. 2016;39(1):27–47.
Arai RJ, Longo ES, Sponton MH, Del Pilar Estevez Diz M. Bringing a humanistic approach to cancer clinical trials. Ecancermedsci. 2017;11:738. https://doi.org/10.3332/ecancer.2017.738.
Bliss S, Baltzly D, Bull R, Dalton L, Jones J. A role for virtue in unifying the 'knowledge' and 'caring' discourses in nursing theory. Nurs Inq. 2017;24(4):e12191. https://doi.org/10.1111/nin.12191.

Daly J, Speedy S, Jackson D. Contexts of nursing: an introduction. Chatswood NSW: Elsevier Health Sciences; 2017.

Edvardsson D, Watt E, Pearce F. Patient experiences of caring and person-centredness are associated with perceived nursing care quality. J Adv Nurs. 2017;73(1):217–27. https://doi.org/10.1111/jan.13105.

Franklin N, Melville P. Competency assessment tools: an exploration of the pedagogical issues facing competency assessment for nurses in the clinical environment. Collegian. 2015;22(1):25–31. https://doi.org/10.1016/j.colegn.2013.10.005.

Gillespie H, Kelly M, Gormley G, King N, Gilliland D, Dornan T. How can tomorrow's doctors be more caring? A phenomenological investigation. Med Educ. 2018;52(10):1052–63. https://doi.org/10.1111/medu.13684.

Glass N. Interpersonal relating: health care perspectives on communication, stress and crisis. South Yarra: Palgrave Macmillan; 2010.

Guillemin M, Gillam L. Telling moments: everyday ethics in health care. Melbourne: IP Communications; 2006.

Harris P, Nagy S, Vardaxis N. Mosby's dictionary of medicine, nursing and health professions-Australian & New Zealand edition-eBook. Chatswood, NSW: Elsevier Health Sciences; 2014.

Hellomynameis [Internet] United Kingdom. n.d. Available from https://www.hellomynameis.org.uk/

Jack K, Smith A. Promoting self-awareness in nurses to improve nursing practice. Nurs Stand. 2007;21(32):47.

Jacobson N. A taxonomy of dignity: a grounded theory study. BMC Int Health Hum Rights. 2009;9(1):3. https://doi.org/10.1186/1472-698X-9-3.

Jeffrey D. Empathy, sympathy and compassion in healthcare: is there a problem? Is there a difference? Does it matter? J R Soc Med. 2016;109(12):446–52. https://doi.org/10.1177/0141076816680120.

Johns C. Reflection on the relationship between technology and caring. Nurs Crit Care. 2005;10(3):150–5. https://doi.org/10.1111/j.1362-1017.2005.00113.x.

Johnstone M. Ethics in nursing. In: Daly J, Speedy S, Jackson D, editors. Contexts of nursing: preparing for professional practice. 4th ed. Sydney: Churchill Livingstone/Elsevier; 2014. p. 157–66.

Kilpatrick A. The health care leader as humanist. J Health Hum Serv Adm. 2009;31(4):451–65. Retrieved from http://www.jstor.org/stable/25790742

Lessard SA. Exploring reflexivity in nursing practice: a concept analysis (Doctoral dissertation) University of New Brunswick, Faculty of Nursing 2012.

Livesay K. Culturally and linguistically diverse simulated patients: otherness and intersectional identity transformations revealed through narrative (Doctoral dissertation) Victoria University; 2016.

McCaffrey G, McConnell S. Compassion: a critical review of peer-reviewed nursing literature. J Clin Nurs. 2015;24(19–20):3006–15. https://doi.org/10.1111/jocn.12924.

McCann E, Brown M. The inclusion of LGBT+ health issues within undergraduate healthcare education and professional training programmes: a systematic review. Nurse Educ Today. 2018;64:204–14. https://doi.org/10.1016/j.nedt.2018.02.028.

McDermid F, Mannix J, Jackson D, Daly J, Peters K. Factors influencing progress through the liminal phase: a model to assist transition into nurse academic life. Nurse Educ Today. 2018;61:269–72.

McKinnon J. Reflection for nursing life: principles, process and practice. London: Routledge; 2016.

Minogue V. "Let me back into the world"–compassionate care in practice: a career and patient's view. Q Ageing Older Adults. 2015;16(2):75–82. https://doi.org/10.1108/QAOA-10-2014-0028.

Moore L, Britten N, Lydahl D, Naldemirci Ö, Elam M, Wolf A. Barriers and facilitators to the implementation of person-centred care in different healthcare contexts. Scand J Caring Sci. 2017;31(4):662–73. https://doi.org/10.1111/scs.12376.

NHS Commissioning Board Chief Nursing Officer and DH Chief Nursing Adviser. Compassion in practice nursing midwifery and care staff our vision and strategy. Leeds: National Health Service Commissioning Board; 2012. 29p.

Nivet MA, Fair M. Defining diversity in quality care. In: Martin ML, Moreno-Walton L, Heron SL, Walker Jones A, editors. Diversity and inclusion in quality patient care. Cham: Springer; 2016.

Papadopoulos I, Shea S, Taylor G, Pezzella A, Foley L. Developing tools to promote culturally competent compassion, courage, and intercultural communication in healthcare. J Compass Health Care. 2016;3(1):2. https://doi.org/10.1186/s40639-016-0019-6.

Pedreschi D, Ruggieri S, Turini F. The discovery of discrimination. In: Discrimination and privacy in the information society. Berlin/Heidelberg: Springer; 2013. p. 91–108.

Quirk M, Mazor K, Haley HL, Philbin M, Fischer M, Sullivan K, Hatem D. How patients perceive a doctor's caring attitude. Patient Educ Couns. 2008;72(3):359–66.

Redmond B. Reflection in action: developing reflective practice in health and social services. New York: Routledge; 2017.

Sinclair S, Norris JM, McConnell SJ, Chochinov HM, Hack TF, Hagen NA, ... Bouchal SR. Compassion: a scoping review of the healthcare literature. BMC Palliat Care. 2016;15(1):6. https://doi.org/10.1186/s12904-016-0080-0.

Sinclair S, Beamer K, Hack TF, McClement S, RaffinBouchal S, Chochinov HM, Hagen NA. Sympathy, empathy, and compassion: a grounded theory study of palliative care patients' understandings, experiences, and preferences. Palliat Med. 2017;31(5):437–47. https://doi.org/10.1177/0269216316663499.

Stein-Parbury J. Patient and person. Interpersonal skills in nursing. 6th ed. Chatswood: Elsevier Australia; 2018.

Sweeney CD. The DAISY Award: a patient-family perspective of compassionate and extraordinary care. J Nurs Adm. 2017;47(9):415–7. https://doi.org/10.1097/NNA.0000000000000506.

Theofanidis D, Sapountzi-Krepia D. Nursing and caring: an historical overview from ancient Greek tradition to modern times. Int J Caring Sci. 2015;8(3):791.

Zajac LM, Moran KJ, Groh CJ. Confronting compassion fatigue: assessment and intervention in inpatient oncology. Clin J Oncol Nurs. 2017;21(4):446–53. https://doi.org/10.1188/17.CJON.446-453.

Zeeman L, Sherriff N, Browne K, McGlynn N, Mirandola M, Gios L, Davis R, Sanchez-Lambert J, Aujean S, Pinto N, Farinella F. A review of lesbian, gay, bisexual, trans and intersex (LGBTI) health and healthcare inequalities. Eur J Pub Health. 2018;29(5):974–80.

Developing Patient Safety Through Education

77

David Pinnock

Contents

Introduction and Background	1502
Developing Patient Safety Through Regulation	1504
Developing Safety Through Professional Curricula	1505
Developing Safety Through Specific Curricula	1506
Patient Safety Development in Practice and Context	1511
Conclusion	1515
References	1515

Abstract

This chapter discusses approaches to the development of patient safety. It begins by recognizing patient safety as a relatively new, still evolving, field of practice that has become an important and central part of professional practice in healthcare. The role that professional regulation plays in shaping safety practices is discussed from an international perspective. The way that curricula are shaped by these same regulators is analyzed to begin to illustrate the way safety is intended to develop.

Accepting the limitations of the advice on curricula to shape patient safety from regulators, a selection of three other frameworks to guide the development of patient safety are identified and analyzed. A synthesis of these three guiding frameworks is proposed to offer a comprehensive and rounded view of what constitutes efforts at safer care.

Finally, this view of the constituents of patient safety development is considered in the complicated context of practice, and a further layer of skills for improvement is offered for developers of safety to work with, along with advice to draw in learning from other disciplines, recognize the value of case studies of patient safety improvement, and engage in social learning processes.

D. Pinnock (✉)
School of Health Sciences, University of Nottingham, Nottingham, UK
e-mail: david.pinnock@nottingham.ac.uk

© Springer Nature Singapore Pte Ltd. 2023
D. Nestel et al. (eds.), *Clinical Education for the Health Professions*,
https://doi.org/10.1007/978-981-15-3344-0_99

Keywords

Patient safety · Quality improvement · Education · Curricula · Safety practices

Introduction and Background

The field of patient safety is relatively new – it is less than a quarter century since the publication of the seismic report: To Err is Human (Institute of Medicine 1999). This pivotal report from the USA has now been cited over 25,000 times and is commonly regarded as the beginning of the patient safety movement (Leape 2014). Building on the foundational work of the Harvard Medical Practice Study that estimated the incidence of adverse events and negligence (Brennan et al. 1991) and their nature (Leape et al. 1991), "To Err Is Human" laid out the scale of avoidable harm occurring in the US healthcare system at that time. The report estimated that errors in healthcare, based on the work of Brennan and Leape et al. and other similar studies, could be regarded as the eight biggest cause of death in the USA. Extrapolating from a range of studies capturing the level of harm caused by healthcare systems, 44,000–98,000 people were dying unnecessarily through error, more than died of AIDS, breast cancer, or in motor vehicle accidents. Brennan et al. (1991) examined over 30,000 case notes from 51 hospitals in New York State and their data suggested the higher death rate of 98,000. Based on their extensive investigation, they suggested that, while most errors caused little or no lasting harm, 13.6% of adverse events resulted in death.

Combining this very significant mortality with (relatively) less serious adverse events, like extended stays in hospital, or prolonged disability, a massive human cost of error emerges. While secondary to this human cost, the financial consequence of error was quantified and acknowledged to be huge. Costs accrued represent a significant proportion of overall healthcare expenditure.

Contemporaneous studies from other advanced healthcare systems, such as Australia (Wilson et al. 1995) and the UK (Vincent et al. 2001), suggested very strongly that this was a global rather than simply a US phenomenon. A year after the publication of "To Err Is Human," there followed a UK government report, "An Organisation with a Memory" (Department of Health 2000), that acknowledged again the scale of harm and associated costs, both human and financial, and echoed many of the findings of the American report. Both reports produced overlapping recommendations for practice.

A central recommendation of "To Err Is Human" is the setting of standards for healthcare professionals related to patient safety and incorporating this into professional development. This report challenged professional regulators to develop patient safety curricula and encourage its adoption. However, the US report "To Err Is Human" and the UK report "An Organisation with a Memory" also comprehensively mapped the direction of development for safety that would populate the codes and competencies of professional regulators. Both reports acknowledge the need to learn from other ultrasafe organizations with a human factors orientation, learn from better reported errors, and rethink healthcare systems for safety – themes that will recur in the following discussion.

This rapidly developed consensus and set of accepted recommendations across well-developed healthcare systems began a broad series of actions. Within these continually evolving actions to develop patient safety are discernible efforts of regulation, training, and education for healthcare professionals. However, as the field evolves, it reckons with what can be viewed as a pattern of uneven success, with recognized problems and some notable failures that suggest this is a journey undertaken rather than a destination reached (Leape 2014; Dixon-Woods and Pronovost 2016; Schiff and Shojania 2022).

Positively, there have been in the United Kingdom (UK) notable successes in infection prevention and control, an early concern in the patient safety field. Methicillin-resistant *Staphylococcus aureus* (MRSA) bacteremia incidence is dramatically reduced in number, and *Clostridioides difficile* (*C. difficile*) prevalence is greatly reduced (UK Health Security Agency 2018; 2022). Both of these threats to patient safety were subject to improvement work, and since their peak in 2007–2008, they have dramatically and consistently improved to a level that could almost be described as transformational. These safety initiatives applied safety critical care bundles in the manner of one of the most outstanding examples of safety improvement, the Michigan Keystone Project (Pronovost et al. 2006), which almost eliminated bloodstream infections from central venous catheters. Furthermore, the growing body of safety and improvement literature contains a great many published examples of localized improvements to safety and quality published in quality and safety journals.

On the other hand, there has been, at the same time, a series of broad organizational failures to maintain safety. Most notably, the tragic events at Stafford Hospital (Francis 2013) and the recognition of similar patterns of patient safety failure (being outliers in terms of higher mortality) in 14 other acute hospitals (Keogh 2013). In terms of more specific clinical failures, National Health Service England reported 235 "never events" between the beginning of April 2022 and the end of January 2023 (NHS England 2023). These are serious events and threats to safety that, as their name suggests, should never happen. All have been the subject of efforts to develop safer practices. Looking further afield, an evidence scan (Health Foundation 2011) looking at levels of harm caused to patients in hospitals in the UK, France, and Spain found levels of harm to be similar to those reported when "To Err Is Human" was published. Even more recently, a retrospective survey of 1000 patient records from Switzerland (Haflon, Staines and Burnand 2017) estimated an adverse event rate of 14.1%.

Accepting as Keogh suggested that those engaged in developing patient safety are trying to "undo more than 50 years of accumulated custom and practice that have failed to put the interests of patients first" (NHS England 2013), there is a perception that given the stakes involved, the development of safety and quality needs to quicken (Dixon-Woods and Pronovost 2016; Schiff and Shojania 2022). A major route to resolving these issues is regulation, training, and education, and a first step in that development is understanding what knowledge constitutes the development of patient safety.

Developing Patient Safety Through Regulation

Even within what is a new and developing field, education and the development of curricula for teaching patient safety is one of the newer elements. With a few honorable exceptions, such as the Institute for Health Improvement, whose educational efforts started in 1988 (IHI 2021), and the Australian Council for Safety and Quality in Healthcare, which endorsed a National Patient Safety Education Framework (APSEF) in 2005, the integration of patient safety as a discrete, defined topic has largely evolved in the past 15 years and can be seen to be still evolving. As it has evolved and gained prominence as a part of professional practice, it has become further integrated into regulatory codes of practice and standards of professional competence.

Using the UK healthcare regulatory standards as a first example, it was in 2013 when the General Medical Council (GMC) identified safety and quality as distinct domains in their regulatory framework for medical practice (GMC 2019). Similarly, the UK regulatory body for registered nurses, the Nursing and Midwifery Council (NMC 2018a), identified preserving safety as a domain of professional practice for these professions in 2015.

Globally, however, the demarcation of safety as a distinct domain of practice is less distinct, perhaps as a result of not yet having experienced scandalous failures in healthcare. For example, the Nursing and Midwifery Board of Australia AHPRA do not identify in either their Code of Conduct (2018) or Registered Nurse Standards for practice (2016) A discrete domain of patient safety. They incorporate various points that could be related to the development of safety, such as a duty of candor, but no specific domain. Standards for Medics (Australian Medical Board AHPRA 2020), however, do with a requirement to work within systems to reduce error and improve patient safety, and support colleagues raising concerns about patient safety.

Following the same pattern, neither the New Zealand (NZ) Code of Conduct for Nurses (Council for Nurses for NZ 2012) has no domain mandating that professional practice includes the development of safety. The NZ competences for professional practice require that registered nurses adhere to professional standards relating to safety and quality healthcare, but without discussing the skills required (Council for Nurses for NZ 2022). However, the Medical Council of New Zealand (2021) specifies that medical practice must include the obligation to maintain and improve standards. They, like other medical regulators, outline the skills and techniques that might be used.

Surveying the degree to which the development of patient safety is a mandated part of practice for nurses across North America is more challenging. In Canada, there are 13 different regulators for nurses in the different provinces and territories. Furthermore, each State in the USA has its own regulatory body for nurses, and the Federation of State Medical Boards (2023) advises state boards that regulate practice in their locality rather than mandating practice. However, it would be hard to imagine anything other than a picture as similarly mixed as the other advanced healthcare systems. A picture within which patient safety is most directly mandated as part of medical practice, with varying degrees of integration and direction included in nurse regulation.

The significance of the inclusion of developing patient safety into regulatory frameworks is twofold. First, it positions this new field of practice as an essential part of professional practice in healthcare. Second, regulatory guidance is associated with the parallel development of patient safety training curricula and an embedding of patient safety as a topic in higher education curricula, at both the undergraduate and postgraduate levels. This leads us to understand what we teach to develop patient safety.

Developing Safety Through Professional Curricula

Professional regulatory standards form a vital strand in developing patient safety. However, the contribution of regulators does not stop there; indeed, it would be obtuse for regulators to mandate specific conduct and skills without contributing to curricula to develop these practices in professionals.

Beginning again with the UK as an example, the NMC standards of proficiency for registered nurses (NMC 2018b) stipulate a set of outcomes for training nurses to improve the safety and quality of care as a platform for practice. Most outcomes in this domain of practice aim to develop a practitioner who is aware of their professional and ethical responsibilities to measure risk, respond appropriately, and report concerns, but one outcome addresses patient safety more directly. However, no specific tools or techniques for learners to use are specified in this guidance. The Australian Nursing and Midwifery Accreditation Council (ANMAC 2019) also specifies in their accreditation framework that nursing curricula must instill an integrated knowledge of safety and quality standards as they relate to healthcare, without identifying what that knowledge consists of, or setting it as a discrete domain for learning.

The Australian Medical Council (2012) standards for assessment and accreditation of medical schools also stipulate, as a single course outcome, that graduating doctors should have an understanding of systems to improve healthcare quality but do not advocate specific skills and knowledge. Postgraduate specialist medics have multiple outcomes related to patient safety development in their course but no discrete domain (Australian Medical Council 2016).

In the UK medical curricula, the guidance for universities is much fuller and divided into two distinct phases. First, the outcomes for graduates (GMC 2020) for qualification as a medical practitioner, and second, the generic Professional Capabilities Framework (GMC 2017) for postgraduate elements of training for doctors developing into specific specializations after initial qualification. Logically, the postgraduate framework builds upon the undergraduate framework, being more specific and slightly more detailed in terms of specifying methods for developing patient safety. A significant difference, however, between the requirements of the NMC and the GMC is that the GMC provides a greater number of specific outcomes addressing the fundamentals of delivering patient safety, though both offer distinct domains of outcomes to be addressed by curricula in relation to developing patient safety and quality improvement.

The fullest set of advice comes from the UK regulators. Making the UK a good exemplar of how professional curricula contribute to the development of patient safety, reflecting a national context that *has* reckoned with scandalous failures in care. The relevant sections of the standards for education are set out for comparison in Table 1.

So, these professional regulators, particularly the GMC, set out what might be described as a set of fundamental topics and, to a lesser extent, a set of tools and techniques that should be used to develop quality and safety as part of regulated professional education, cementing the direction of travel towards better developing patient safety. Good and more specific advice, however, comes from other groups with views on how safety should develop in practice. Advice from bodies such as the World Health Organization (WHO 2011) forms an important part of the picture of how patient safety is developed, offering greater specific detail.

Developing Safety Through Specific Curricula

Discussing regulatory advice on developing safety from an international perspective is challenging; offering the same view as other interested bodies offering advice is even more difficult. For example, the discussion widens to include professional bodies such as the Royal College of Nursing (2019), which offers a broad view on developing patient safety, and governmental bodies such as the US Agency for Healthcare Research and Quality (AHRQ 2022), which offers a range of tools such as the TeamSTEPPS that addresses team functioning for safety. There are also healthcare regulators such as the Care Quality Commission (CQC) in the UK, who assess the components of safety for patients in healthcare organizations (CQC 2022). However, the aim here is to illustrate the dimensions of developing safety to understand what we should be considering in a comprehensive way. So at the risk of being arbitrary, a judicious selection is offered.

To fill out our understanding of the fundamental content of developing patient safety, this work will look at three frameworks that shape an understanding of what constitutes patient safety development. First, the slightly dated World Health Organization's Patient Safety Curriculum Guide: Multi-professional Edition (WHO 2011); second, the Safety Competencies (Canadian Patient Safety Institute (2nd Edition) 2020); and third, the NHS patient safety syllabus (The Academy of Royal Medical Colleges, et al. 2022).

The World Health Organization offers transnational guidance, and their works are intended to be as inclusive as possible in terms of what is considered and who is addressed by the guidance. This curriculum was developed with broad-based input from nurses, midwives, dentists, pharmacists, medics, students of all of these professional groups, and a representative advocating for the patient's voice. The Curriculum Guide is based on and supported by published evidence. Indeed, the Curriculum Guide is based on a previous evidence/literature-based educational program developed in Australia (APSEF 2005) and incorporates the Canadian patient safety competencies (CPSI (1st Edition) 2009). It is intended to offer an

Table 1 The UK professional regulators and other selected advisors shaping of professional education around patient safety

Regulators of professional education shaping professional curricula		
Future nurse: Standards of proficiency for registered nurses (NMC 2018a) Platform 6: Improving safety and quality of care	Outcomes for graduates 2018 (GMC 2020) Domain 5: Patient safety and quality improvement	Generic professional capabilities framework (GMC 2017) Domain 6: Capabilities in patient safety and quality improvement
6.1 Understand and apply the principles of health and safety legislation and regulations and maintain safe work and care environments
6.2 Understand the relationship between safe staffing levels, appropriate skills mix, safety and quality of care, recognizing risks to public protection and quality of care, escalating concerns appropriately
6.3 Comply with local and national frameworks, legislation and regulations for assessing, managing and reporting risks, ensuring the appropriate action is taken
6.4 Demonstrate an understanding of the principles of improvement methodologies, participate in all stages of audit activity, and identify appropriate quality improvement strategies
6.5 Demonstrate the ability to accurately undertake risk assessments in a range of care settings, using a range of contemporary assessment and improvement tools
6.6 Identify the need to make improvements and proactively respond to potential hazards that may affect the safety of people
6.7 Understand how the quality and effectiveness of nursing care can be evaluated in practice, and demonstrate how to use service delivery evaluation and audit findings	(a) Place patients' needs and safety at the center of the care process
(b) Promote and maintain health and safety in all care settings and escalate concerns to colleagues where appropriate, including when providing treatment and advice remotely
(c) Recognize how errors can happen in practice and that errors should be shared openly and be able to learn from their own and others' errors to promote a culture of safety
(d) Apply measures to prevent the spread of infection, and apply the principles of infection prevention and control
(e) Describe the principles of quality assurance, quality improvement, quality planning, and quality control, and in which contexts these approaches should be used to maintain and improve quality and safety
(f) Describe basic human factors principles and practice at individual, team, organizational, and system levels and recognize and respond to opportunities for improvement to manage or mitigate risks
(g) Apply the principles and methods of quality improvement to improve practice (for example, plan, do, study, act or action	Raise safety concerns appropriately through clinical governance systems
Understand the importance of raising and acting on concerns
Understand the importance of sharing good practice
Demonstrate and apply basic human factors principles and practice at individual, team, organizational, and system levels
Demonstrate and apply nontechnical skills and crisis resource management techniques in practice
Demonstrate effective multidisciplinary and interprofessional team working
Demonstrate respect for and recognition of the roles of other health professionals in the effective delivery of patient care promote
Participate in interprofessional learning promote patient involvement in safety and quality improvement reviews
Understand risk, including risk identification (clinical, suicide, and system), management, or mitigation
Understand fixation error, unconscious and cognitive biases
Reflect on their personal behavior and practice effectively pre-brief, debrief, and learn from their own performance and that of others

(continued)

Table 1 (continued)

Regulators of professional education shaping professional curricula		
Future nurse: Standards of proficiency for registered nurses (NMC 2018a) Platform 6: Improving safety and quality of care	Outcomes for graduates 2018 (GMC 2020) Domain 5: Patient safety and quality improvement	Generic professional capabilities framework (GMC 2017) Domain 6: Capabilities in patient safety and quality improvement
to bring about continuous improvement 6.8 Demonstrate an understanding of how to identify, report, and critically reflect on near misses, critical incidents, major incidents, and serious adverse events in order to learn from them and influence their future practice	research), including seeking ways to continually improve the use and prioritization of resources (h) Describe the value of national surveys and audits for measuring the quality of care	Make changes to their practice in response to learning opportunities Be able to keep accurate, structured, and where appropriate standardized records

overview of the content that healthcare professionals should understand to develop safety through their practice.

The Curriculum Guide (WHO 2011) outlines 11 topics that should be addressed. Three of these topics address specific aspects of care that are highlighted and prioritized as areas for action (WHO 2011). A further, foundational section defines patient safety, making a case for developing the remaining seven topics. These form the fundamentals of developing safety in professional practice.

The WHO Curriculum Guide (2011) emphasizes the importance of human factors, and this is related to understanding error and human interactions within a complex system as topics. There are also sections addressing risk perception and management, working as a team and engaging with service users and carers. Finally, and crucially, the curriculum advocates a set of methodologies for developing safety, including the Model for Improvement (including the plan-do-study-act cycle (Langley Moen Nolan et al. 2009) and change management techniques to guide improvement. The Curriculum Guide also advocates approaches to understanding variation as a concept to be considered in care systems. Differentiating variation that occurs as a consequence of suboptimal processes from variation that cannot be planned for and corrected. Plotting safety events (safety incidents or achievements) over time on a line graph with a median value, a run chart (Langley Moen Nolan et al. 2009), can show how interventions for safety are working and be a precursor for more sophisticated and nuanced measuring of improvements to safety.

Established quality management strategies for understanding errors are also advocated, including root cause analysis and cause and effect diagrams (WHO 2011). Root cause analysis develops safety through the examination of incidents for contributory factors, causative factors, and root causes so that threats to safety can be managed (Charles et al. 2016). Cause and effect diagrams are used to collect information on causes of error or unwanted variation by examining categories of influence on the processes that lead to the problematic, less safe area of practice such as the people, equipment, and procedures (NHS England 2021). Another commonly applied tool to understanding sources of error advocated by WHO (2011) is a Pareto chart that categorizes errors and then measures how frequently that type of error occurs in order to prioritize actions for developing safety on the most impactful change (Langley Moen Nolan et al. 2009).

It is hard to overstate the importance of these rational tools in the systematic development of actions for safety. These are the nuts and bolts of developing safety. Combined with the other recommendations of the Curriculum Guide that adjust perspectives on risk and error, healthcare systems, and draw attention to the significance of human factors, it provides a sound base that has been built upon by subsequently developed curricula and refined rather than replaced. This is shown in the content of the Safety Competencies (CPSI (2nd Edition) 2020).

The Canadian competency framework has six domains that overlap with the topics in the WHO document, and like the WHO Curriculum Guide, it is intended for all healthcare professionals and has been developed by a multi-professional panel co-chaired by a nurse and a pharmacist. The six domains considered are patient safety culture, teamwork, communication, safety risk and quality improvement, optimize human and system factors, and recognize, respond to, and disclose patient safety incidents. Whereas the WHO framework defines content and tools to be used, the Canadian framework is more flexible, offering many detailed competencies that might be addressed by quality and safety tools and techniques without prescribing which should be applied.

For example, the Safety, Risk, and Quality Improvement domain competency 3.1 asks that healthcare professionals "Lead and engage in the measurement of quality and performance indicators for the people and populations served" (CPSI (2nd Edition) 2020, p. 20). This competency leads the practitioner to apply run charts and statistical process control charting without advocating that. Instead, the framework is supplemented by case studies of exemplars of application of the framework in practice. The most recently developed guiding framework is the NHS patient safety syllabus.

The NHS patient safety syllabus was developed by the Academy of Royal Medical Colleges et al. (2022). The academy is a collective of 24 professional Royal Colleges and includes all the medical colleges. The syllabus was adopted and advocated by NHS England and Health Education England. It is impressively comprehensive (see Table 2), and this, combined with its contemporary development, means that it stands as a definitive exemplar of the topics that we should address to develop patient safety. These topics are linked to the core techniques of safety improvement. Furthermore, the syllabus addresses the need for different levels of understanding by offering a general level of training for all staff and a higher level of insight and understanding for those with a specific focus or deeper interest in safety, which is a weakness of the WHO (2011) framework and the Canadian competencies.

Table 2 The domains and content of each domain for the UK NHS patient safety syllabus (The Academy of Royal Medical Colleges et al. 2022)

Domain	Elements of that domain addressed in the syllabus

Systems approach to patient safety	The systems approach to safety
	  The safety landscape
	  Safety II and resilience
	  Systems approach to patient safety
	  Organizational culture and learning
	Patient safety and its public context
	  Patient and public involvement in safety
	  Patient safety regulations and improvement
	  Medicolegal and professional responsibilities
	  Learning from and managing complaints

Learning from incidents	Investigating patient safety incidents Designing system-based interventions Managing human performance variability in patient safety Avoiding blame and creating a learning culture through a just culture approach
Human factors, human performance, and safety management	Human factors and clinical practice Task analysis and support Nontechnical skills in clinical practice Process reliability and safety assurance
Creating safe systems	Risk evaluation in clinical practice Mapping techniques to identity risks to patients Designing for systems safety Evaluating safety culture
Being sure about safety	Integrating human factors Risk, escalation, and governance in patient safety Creating a culture of patient safety The safety case

If we compare this to the WHO guidance (2011), we can (as well as noting the recurring themes and similarities) chart the development in patient safety in the time between the two documents being published. For example, the landscape of patient safety has developed over time, and the syllabus includes more novel concepts such as the resilience orientation of Safety II approaches. This newer perspective reframes safety as an ongoing achievement of adaptable professionals in a complex system rather than a failure due to human factors (Hollnagel 2014).

However, while this syllabus is comprehensive, detailed, and contemporary, it has been developed by medical colleges alone. As such, it lacks input from other professions. These other professions have a credible stake in developing patient safety, including pharmacists, physiotherapists, radiographers, and the single largest healthcare profession, nurses.

Collected, these frameworks build upon the mandates of professional regulators to develop patient safety and fill in to a great extent the topics that constitute the development of patient safety in healthcare. Looking across the content they provide, we have a rigorous set of domains, topics, and specific skills that help us understand in large part how safety is developed and how we might develop it further. However, while what we should be learning to develop patient safety is clear, how we do that learning remains to be discussed.

Patient Safety Development in Practice and Context

To work out how best to apply the understandings reached as to what constitutes the development of patient safety, we must remember two key issues. We should remind ourselves that the development of patient safety happens in the complex context of practice and recall that the success of these constituent parts in improving safety is, so far at least, mixed. To quote Lucien Leape, who has a long view on the topic, "Despite the compelling evidence that changing systems actually does reduce harm, it turns out to be very difficult to change systems in practice." (Lucien Leape 2015 Patient Safety in the Era of Healthcare Reform p. 1569).

To understand the interaction between the practice context and efforts to improve safety, it is helpful to begin with a broad view of the skills used to achieve improvement in practice. A good example of this that articulates these skills is the work for the Health Foundation (a UK patient safety charity) by Gabbay et al. (2013). The report, Skilled for Improvement? (Gabbay et al. 2013), was based on primary, qualitative, and research. It examined two NHS organizations with a track record of successful improvement, implementing two projects each and offering four evaluations of improvement work to develop safer care related to the required skills. The work was based largely on semi-structured interviews before and after the projects and document reviews (Gabbay et al. 2013). The outcomes of the research are valuable in understanding the development of safety as it happens in practice. The researchers identified three interdependent skillsets used in the practice of improvement: technical, soft, and learning skills.

Learning skills are the skills that were described, observed, and sometimes recognized as missing from improvement efforts and that can be orientated around the sharing of knowledge and the efficacy of networks within organizations. The so-called "soft skills" range from fundamental skills of self-management and regulation through to finely developed interpersonal skills. These are supported by pragmatic skills such as negotiation and the ability to arrange effective meetings. These categories of skills are detailed in Table 3.

The first and most tangible of these subsets are the technical skills. Here we can see a considerable overlap between the frameworks discussed in the previous section. The tools set out in these frameworks (WHO 2011; Academy of Royal Medical Colleges et al. 2022) and advocated by some regulators are used and applied in practice, reinforcing their primacy in improvement work.

While this validation of the applicability of tools to practice is welcome, it is the other two skillsets that are of greater utility in understanding how to develop patient safety. The researchers put equal emphasis on learning skills and a set of soft skills, suggesting that "the relative absence of skills in one area will lead to a lack of progress overall, irrespective of the strengths in other skill areas" (Gabbay et al.

Table 3 Technical (with explanations in brackets by the author), soft, and learning skills proposed by Gabbay et al. (2013)

Examples of the technical skills identified in the research project necessary for improvement science to be successfully applied	Examples of the personal and organizational ("soft") skills necessary for improvement science to be successfully applied	Examples of the learning skills identified in the research project necessary for improvement science to be successfully applied
Plan, do, study, and act (model for improvement) Run charts (plotting data over time) Care bundles (discrete evidence based care packages) Six Sigma Process mapping (understanding processes) Pareto analysis (locating problematic areas of practice) Flow chart (designing processes) Critical appraisal (developing understandings for safer care) Fishbone diagrams (locating cause and effect) Process measures (understanding if a process if working) Benchmarking (equitable comparisons others or standards) Statistical process control (differentiating between normal and special cause variation) Outcome measures (are we making a difference)	Communication Assertiveness Negotiation Time management and prioritizing Stress management Leadership and team skills Organizing and administrative skills (management) Political skills (understanding the system, managing vested interests, navigating and exploiting powerbases, "people reading," timing interventions shrewdly, listening to and taking into account other people's views) Local knowledge Educational and knowledge	Encouraging participation Organizational learning Externalizing tacit knowledge Collective learning skills Learning communities Communities of practice Individual learning skills Knowledge sharing Willingness to learn Action learning skills Critical reflection Group learning

2013, p. 63). Some of these skills are present in the curriculum advice from the WHO (2011), CPSI (2020), and the NHS patient safety syllabus, but many are not. So developing patient safety requires a synthesis of these frameworks, recognizing and valuing the skills set out here by Gabbay et al. (2013) and others who echo some of the themes raised.

Shah (2021) reports on, rather than researches, practical experience of improving safety and quality; he offers an account of developing learning systems within a healthcare organization. Shah discusses the importance of recruiting the right participants in organizational change with a clarity of purpose, nurturing relationships, and creating horizontal connections between teams or teams to enable sharing and learning across different contexts. In the account offered, Shah (2021) summarizes the contributors to developing learning systems as a shared purpose and language of improvement, with collective leadership and significant autonomy for improvers that supports connection and relationships. He also points out the value of technical skills, emphasizing particularly the value of good measurement and a supportive infrastructure that supports improvement.

Looking at organizational change from a different perspective, Waring et al. (2022) recognized micro-politics at work in an ethnographic study of service reconfiguration. Their analysis showed interested parties sought to advance or protect their particular agendas or interests through engaging in political strategies and behaviors to favorably direct or minimize the impact of change. While not exactly replicating the learning and soft skills for improvement proposed by Gabbay et al. (2013), there is discernible overlap in the positive from Shah and in the negative from Waring et al. (2022), showing how on technical skills might be utilized.

In summary, then, the skills set out by regulators and other sources on what constitutes patient safety development should be filtered through an understanding of the context in which improvement happens and how these contextual issues can be negotiated in practice. Practically, this means unpicking the detail and dynamics of these contextual issues, making greater use of case studies of improvement, and bringing together as many of the interested parties together as possible to foster through dialogue shared interprofessional understandings of the nature of the problem. All three can show how the context might be accommodated, mitigated against, or at least better understood, and deserve further discussion.

In terms of understanding the dynamics of context, we can use the work of authors who combine social theory with improvement and safety work. For example, Dixon-Woods and Pronovost (2016) classify patient safety as a paradigmatic example of the problem of "many hands," an explanatory theory developed to explain failures in public administration (Thompson 2014). They (Dixon-Woods and Pronovost 2016) theorize that in situations like healthcare, there are many parties acting in complex networks of interaction and reaction to each other in ways that have evolved over time in an unplanned fashion. Consequently, it can be difficult to define the direction of development and accountability, the complexity of an organization obscures the mechanics and sense of accountability of individuals working within it. Understanding this issue helps direct some of the work of patient safety to better defining organizational activities and unpicking complexity. This could lead to using a second string of tools to understand complex networks of interest such as, for example, stakeholder analysis that considers the legitimacy, urgency, and power of actors associated with the safety issue (Mitchell Agle and Wood 1997).

Case studies take the principle of patient safety development happening in context further. Rather than setting the context as something to be managed or mitigated, the context is viewed as what creates the development of patient safety. A further dimension to the work of Gabbay et al. (2013) is that, even before discussing their specific findings, the researchers were struck by the diversity in approach to improvement that they saw within the different teams. The environment in which the four improvement projects they researched were undertaken shaped the characteristics of the improvements. They were defined by their context; the detailed and rigorous examination of cases in context can lead to learning points that can be reflected upon to guide the development of patient safety.

An outstanding, if slightly older, example is the ethnographic case study by Dixon-Woods et al. (2011). They revisited a lauded example of safety improvement, the Keystone Michigan project (Pronovost et al. 2006), which achieved remarkable results in dramatically reducing central venous catheter-associated bloodstream infections (CVC BSIs). They proposed, based on interviews and ethnographic observations, a set of social processes running alongside the technical processes that explained the success of this project. Their detailed and lengthy analysis suggested the project succeeded because of a set of concurrent processes they observed:

> (1) isomorphic pressures, (2) networked community effects, (3) reframing CVC-BSIs as a social problem, (4) changing practice and culture at the sharp end by using interventions with different effects, (5) using data as a disciplinary force, and (6) skillfully using "hard edges." (Dixon-Woods et al. (2011, p. 176))

Isomorphic pressures were seen by Dixon-Woods et al. (2011) to exist as a mechanism likened to diffusion in the physical sciences, persuasively spreading involvement in the Keystone Michigan project by asking for a level of commitment though formal enrolment. The greater the number of units committing to the project, the larger the pull of the project on others to commit too. The hard edges to be used skillfully reflect a mildly coercive quality of the project that legitimizes concordance with the aims and practices of the project and challenges those that do not adhere to its requirements. A convincing case is made to recognize the other processes at work within an improvement that developers of safety might understand and learn from.

A further ethnographic case study expanded on their earlier work of explaining the development of safer practices in Michigan. Dixon-Woods et al. (2013) examined the UK health service efforts to match the achievements of the Michigan Keystone project. A shorter but still richly detailed examination, again based on short observations of practice and interviews with intensive care professionals, showed a mixed picture of success. While all 19 units in the study improved (including 2 not participating in this piece of improvement), some improved markedly more than others. Again, organizational context and processes were offered as explanation (though not the same set the researchers had found in their analysis of the original Michigan project). The most successful units managed to identify the project as different from preceding work and negotiated better the challenges of imposed, top-down change while attending to the nontechnical dimensions of the project, such as communication and teamwork, which provided clear learning points for developers of improvement.

In isolation, these case studies offer discrete points for reflection, but together they can form a sort of mosaic image of how safety might be developed through critical reflection as a form of vicarious expertise.

The value of teaching and learning inter-professionally is the final point to be discussed in relation to patient safety in context. Going back to the input of professional regulators in shaping the development of patient safety, it is clear that, relative to nurses, for example, doctors are charged with greater specific responsibilities and higher expectations to proactively develop safer practices (GMC 2017, 2020), reflecting their role as leaders of care. However, without working in partnership with other professionals, any development is likely to fail. Other stakeholders in patient safety represent those constantly present with patients (such as nurses) or gatekeepers of specific skills or processes (such as pharmacists or radiographers). Stakeholders potentially may misunderstand, undervalue, or even subvert the efforts of leaders of safety improvements and any input they might have on routes to improvement might be lost. Managing these issues draws on the soft and learning skills proposed by Gabbay et al. (2013) and the prerequisites of a learning system proposed by Shah (2021). Wherein health professionals need to develop a shared language and sense of purpose related to improvement. Developing understandings that bridge the gap between different professions and power hierarchies (Shah 2021), disrupting normal hierarchies by teaching across professions, models and facilitates this. Interdisciplinary safety development can, though, be taken further still.

This need for collaboration and cooperation, for Gabbay et al. (2013), emphasized how their findings fitted to a model of social learning, specifically communities of practice (COPs). These can be defined as groups of people who share a concern for something they do and learn how to do it better as they interact regularly (Wenger 1998). In the purest sense, COPs are relatively enduring groups with complex dynamics and process of legitimizing members (Borzillo et al. 2011), but even a relatively short well-facilitated collaborative activity can produce a community that is more than the sum of its parts in terms of its contribution to developing safety. The Centers for Disease Control and Prevention (2022), looking at public health specifically, emphasize the plurality of approaches that might be considered a community of practice and highlight the benefits of this social approach to learning and problem-solving.

Conclusion

This chapter has unpacked the development of patient safety. Beginning with surveying and analyzing codes of conduct and competence and moving on to look at the incorporation of patient safety into professional curricula. A wider and more comprehensive view of what constitutes patient safety development is offered by drawing on selected guiding frameworks. These are discussed before the chapter ends with a wider empirically derived set of skills that complement the guiding frameworks and emphasize on interprofessional learning and cross-discipline thinking in relation to safety development.

References

Academy of Royal Medical Colleges, NHS Patient Safety Syllabus. Academy of Medical Royal Colleges; 2022. London, UK.

Australian Council for Safety and Quality in Healthcare. National patient safety education framework. Canberra: The Australian Council for Safety and Quality in Healthcare; 2005. https://www.safetyandquality.gov.au/sites/default/files/migrated/framework0705.pdf

Australian Medical Council Medical School Accreditation Committee. Standards for assessment and accreditation of primary medical programmes. Kingston: Australian Capital Territory, Australia. 2012. https://www.amc.org.au/publications/policy-documents/. Last accessed 01 Apr 2022.

Australian Medical Council Medical School Accreditation Committee. Standards for assessment and accreditation of secondary medical programmes. Kingston: Australian Capital Territory, Australia. 2016. https://www.amc.org.au/publications/policy-documents/. Last accessed 01 Apr 2022.

Borzillo S, Aznar S, Schmitt A. A journey through communities of practice: how and why members move from the periphery to the core. Eur Manag J. 2011;29(1):25–42.

Brennan T, Leape L, Laird N, Hebert L, Localio A, Lawthers A, Newhouse J, Weiler P, Hiatt H. Incidence of adverse events and negligence in hospitalized patient: results of the Harvard Medical Practice Study I. N Engl J Med. 1991;324(6):370–7.

Canadian Patient Safety Institute. The safety competencies: enhancing patient safety across the health professions. 2nd ed. Edmonton: Canadian Patient Safety Institute; 2020.

Charles R, Hood J, Derosier J, Gosbee J, Li Y, Caird M, Biermann J, Hake M. How to perform a root cause analysis for workup and future prevention of medical errors: a review. Patient Saf Surg. 2016;10:20.

Dixon-Woods M, Pronovost P. Patient safety and the problem of many hands. BMJ Q Saf. 2016;25: 485–8.

Dixon-Woods M, Bosk C, Aveling L, Goeschel C, Pronovost P. Explaining Michigan: developing an ex post theory of a quality improvement program. Milbank Q. 2011;89(2):167–205. https://www.ncbi.nlm.nih.gov/pmc/articles/PMC3142336/pdf/milq0089-0167.pdf. Last accessed 09 Mar 2023.

Dixon-Woods M, Leslie M, Tarrant C, Bion J. Explaining matching Michigan: an ethnographic study of a patient safety program. Implement Sci. 2013;8:70.

Donaldson L (Chair). An organisation with a memory: report of an expert group on learning from adverse events in the NHS Chaired by the Chief Medical Officer. London: Department of Health, The Stationery Office. 2000.

Francis R (Chair). The Mid Staffordshire NHS Foundation Trust public inquiry report of the Mid Staffordshire NHS Foundation Trust public inquiry executive summary. London, UK: The Stationery Office. 2013. https://assets.publishing.service.gov.uk/government/uploads/system/uploads/attachment_data/file/279124/0947.pdf. Last accessed 09 Mar 2023.

Gabbay J, LeMay A, Connell C, Klein J. Skilled for improvement? Learning communities and the skills needed to improve care: an evaluative service development. London, UK: The Health Foundation; 2013. https://www.health.org.uk/publications/skilled-for-improvement. Last accessed 09 Mar 2023.

General Medical Council. Generic professional capabilities framework. London, UK: General Medical Council; 2017. https://www.gmc-uk.org/education/standards-guidance-and-curricula/standards-and-outcomes/generic-professional-capabilities-framework. Last accessed 09 Mar 2023.

General Medical Council. Outcomes for graduates 2018 (updated 2020). London, UK: General Medical Council; 2020. https://www.gmc-uk.org/-/media/documents/dc11326-outcomes-for-graduates-2018_pdf-75040796.pdf. Last accessed 09 Mar 2023.

General Medical Council. Good medical practice 2019. London, UK: Medical Council; 2019. https://www.gmc-uk.org/-/media/documents/good-medical-practice-english-20200128_pdf-51527435.pdf. Last accessed 03 May 2023.

Halfon P, Staines A, Burnand. Adverse events related to hospital care: a retrospective medical records review in a Swiss hospital. Int J Qual Health Care. 2017;29(4):527–533.

Hollnagel E. Safety-I and Safety-II: the past and future of safety management, Ashgate Publishing, Farnham, UK; 2014

Institute for Health Improvement. IHI milestones. Boston: Institute for Healthcare Improvement; 2021. https://www.ihi.org/about/Documents/IHITimeline2021.pdf. Last accessed 09 Mar 2023.

Institute of Medicine (Kohn KT, Corrigan JM, Donaldson MS, eds.) Washington, DC: Committee on Quality Health Care in America, Institute of Medicine: National Academy Press; 1999.

Keogh B. Review into the quality of care and treatment provided by 14 hospital trusts in England: overview report. NHS England. 2013. https://www.basw.co.uk/system/files/resources/basw_85333-2_0.pdf. Last accessed 09 Mar 2023.

Langley G, Moen R, Nolan K, Nolan T, Norman C, Provot L. The improvement guide: a practical approach to enhancing organizational performance (2nd Edition) Wiley and sons, Chichester,UK.

Leape L. Patient safety in the era of healthcare reform. Clin Orthop Relat Res. 2014;473:1568–73. https://www.ncbi.nlm.nih.gov/pmc/articles/PMC4385369/pdf/11999_2014_Article_3598.pdf. Last accessed 09 Mar 2023.

Leape L, Brennan T, Leape L, Laird N, Hebert L, Localio A, Barnes B, Hebert L, Newhouse J, Weiler P, Hiatt H. The nature of adverse events in hospitalized patients: results of the Harvard Medical Practice Study II. N Engl J Med. 1991;324(6):377–84.

Medical Council of New Zealand. Good medical practice. Wellington: Medical Council of New Zealand; 2021.

Mitchell R, Agle B, Wood D. Toward a theory of stakeholder identification and salience: defining the principle of who and what really counts, academy of management review. 1997;22(4):853–886

National Health Service England. News/Press Release 15th December 2013. https://www.england.nhs.uk/2013/12/sir-bruce-keogh-7ds/. Last accessed 03/05/2023.

National Health Service England. Provisional publication of Never Events reported as occurring between 1 April 2022 and 31 January 2023 NHS England. 2023. https://www.england.nhs.uk/wp-content/uploads/2023/03/Provisional-publication-NE-1-April-31-January-2023.pdf. Last accessed 09 Mar 2023.

National Health Service England and NHS Improvement. Online library of Quality, Service Improvement and Redesign tools Cause and effect (fishbone) NHS England and NHS Improvement. 2021. https://www.england.nhs.uk/wp content/uploads/2021/12/qsir-cause-and-effect-fishbone.pdf. Last accessed 01 Apr 2023.

Nursing and Midwifery Board of Australia. Registered nurse standards of practice. Melbourne: Nursing and Midwifery Board of Australia; 2016.

Nursing and Midwifery Board of Australia. Code of conduct for nurses. Melbourne: Nursing and Midwifery Board of Australia; 2018.

Nursing and Midwifery Council. Future nurse: standards of proficiency for registered nurses. London, UK: NMC; 2018a. https://www.nmc.org.uk/globalassets/sitedocuments/standards-of-proficiency/nurses/future-nurse-proficiencies.pdf. Last accessed 09 Mar 2023.

Nursing and Midwifery Council. The Code Professional standards of practice and behaviour for nurses, midwives and nursing associates. London, UK: NMC; 2018b. https://www.nmc.org.uk/globalassets/sitedocuments/nmc-publications/nmc-code.pdf. Last accessed 09 Mar 2023.

Nursing Council of New Zealand. Code of conduct for nurses. Wellington: Nursing Council of New Zealand; 2012.

Nursing Council of New Zealand. Competencies for registered nurses. Wellington: Nursing Council of New Zealand; 2022.

Pronovost P, Needham D, Berenholtz S, Sinopoli D, Chu H, Cosgrove S, Sexton B, Hyzy R, Welsh R, Roth G, Bander J, Kepros J, Goeschel C. An intervention to decrease catheter-related bloodstream infections in the ICU. N Engl J Med. 2006;355(26):2725–32.

Royal College of Nursing. The patient-safe future: a blueprint for action. London, UK: RCN. 2019. https://s3-eu-west-1.amazonaws.com/ddme-psl/content/A-Blueprint-for-Action-240619.pdf?mtime=20190701143409. Last accessed 09 Mar 2023.

Schiff G, Shojania K. Looking back on the history of patient safety: an opportunity to reflect and ponder future challenges BMJ. Q Saf. 2022;31:148–52.

Shah A. Quality improvement in practice – part 1: creating learning systems. British Journal of Healthcare Management. 2021. https://doi.org/10.12968/bjhc.2021.0032. Last accessed 01 Apr 2022.

Thompson D. Responsibility for failures of government: the problem of many hands. Am Rev Public Adm. 2014;44(3):259–73.

UK Health Security Agency. National statistics National Statistics MRSA bacteraemia: annual data. UK Health Security Agency. 2018. https://www.gov.uk/government/statistics/clostridium-difficile-infection-annual-data. Last accessed 09 Mar 2023.

UK Health Security Agency. National statistics *Clostridioides difficile* (*C. difficile*) infection: annual data. UK Health Security Agency. 2022. https://webarchive.nationalarchives.gov.uk/

ukgwa/20190509150056/https:/www.gov.uk/government/statistics/mrsa-bacteraemia-annual-data. Last accessed 09 Mar 2023.

Vincent C, Neale G, Woloshynowych M. Adverse events in British hospitals: preliminary retrospective record review. Br Med J. 2001;322:517–9.

Waring J, Bishop S, Black G, Clarke J, Exworthy M, Fulop N, Hartley J, Ramsay A, Bridget RB. Navigating the micro-politics of major system change: the implementation of Sustainability Transformation Partnerships in the English health and care system. J Health Serv Res Policy. 2022. https://doi.org/10.1177/13558196221142237. Last accessed 01 Apr 2023.

Wenger E. Communities of practice learning, meaning and identity. London, UK: Cambridge University Press; 1998.

Wilson R, Runciman W, Gibberd R, Harrison B, Newby L, Hamilton J. The quality in Australian health care study. Med J Aust. 1995;163:458–71.

World Health Organization. Patient safety curriculum guide: multi-professional edition. Geneva: World Health Organization; 2011. http://apps.who.int/iris/bitstream/handle/10665/44641/9789241501958_eng.pdf;jsessionid=ACCE896FDE02172AE38C21D267E4153C?sequence=1. Last accessed 09 Mar 2023.

Supporting the Development of Professionalism in the Education of Health Professionals

78

Anne Stephenson and Julie Bliss

Contents

Introduction	1520
Professionalism Education	1523
The Personal and the Professional Journey: Formation of Professional Identity Through Communities of Practice	1523
Learning About Professionalism Through Formal, Informal, and Hidden Curricula	1523
Professional Practice Guidelines	1525
Professionalism in the Curriculum: Learning Outcomes, Educational Methods, and Assessment	1526
Monitoring and Sanctions: Low-Level Concerns to Fitness to Practice Questions	1528
Conclusion	1529
Cross-References	1530
References	1530

Abstract

How can the professionalism of learners be supported and developed in undergraduate and postgraduate education? In this chapter we will cover the formation of professional identity; learning through the formal, informal, and hidden curriculum; professional practice guidelines; the professionalism curriculum in terms of learning outcomes, educational methods, and assessment; and monitoring and sanctions from low-level concerns to fitness to practice questions. Health professional students bring their personal identities and moral standpoints to their training, and the aim of health professional education is to develop their

---

A. Stephenson (✉)
School of Population Health & Environmental Sciences, Faculty of Life Sciences and Medicine, King's College London, London, UK
e-mail: anne.stephenson@kcl.ac.uk

J. Bliss (✉)
Florence Nightingale Faculty of Nursing, Midwifery & Palliative Care, King's College London, London, UK
e-mail: julie.bliss@kcl.ac.uk

© Springer Nature Singapore Pte Ltd. 2023
D. Nestel et al. (eds.), *Clinical Education for the Health Professions*,
https://doi.org/10.1007/978-981-15-3344-0_100

professional identities through formal instruction and participation in communities of practice. Formal curricula, regulation, and employer guidance are important but only part of the process. Situated learning where learners are immersed in real-life practice is essential, and the hidden curriculum, for example, role modeling and the culture of learning environments, is a powerful teacher. Regular reflective practice and discussions with peers and teachers are keys to addressing professionalism learning, particularly informal (opportunistic) learning and the hidden curriculum. Interprofessional learning augments the understanding and practice of professional values, and assessment through reflective portfolios directs learning. Detection and remediation of low-level concerns is crucial from early on in health profession programs and often prevents more serious fitness to practice concerns later in training. This chapter explores these concepts, some of which are developed further in other chapters of the book.

Keywords

Professionalism · Professional identity · Formal curriculum · Informal curriculum · Hidden curriculum · Guidelines · Assessment · Sanctions

Introduction

Professionalism is a challenging concept to define, and yet it is a term that health professionals use frequently. Concrete conceptualizations of professionalism, based on various professionalism frameworks, have been devised for different health professions, as in the following two examples. The UK Royal College of Physicians in their 2018 document "Advancing medical professionalism" (Advancing medical professionalism 2018) describes the professional attributes of a doctor in terms of roles: healer; patient partner; team worker; manager and leader; advocate; learner and teacher; and innovator. These "aim to help doctors improve their professionalism in practical ways" (Advancing medical professionalism 2018, p. 5).

The UK Nursing and Midwifery Council (NMC 2018), on the other hand, defines professionalism as a set of behaviors whereby nurses and midwives have a common set of values which enables autonomous decision making. To achieve this, professional relationships and an environment that supports professional practice are key. The nursing definition includes the importance of the professional environment in supporting professional practice, a concept that will be developed later in this chapter.

Morrow et al. (2014) undertook research to explore other health profession educator and student perceptions of professionalism. Focus groups were conducted across four organizations with a total of 112 participants, a mixture of paramedics, chiropodists/podiatrists, and occupational therapists. The research identified that participants viewed professionalism as a holistic concept which is underpinned by professional attitudes, professional identify, and professional behavior. Included in the sources that inform professionalism for this group were role models in practice and education, and role modeling is explored later in this chapter.

Thinking more widely about health professionals working together, interprofessional professionalism is defined by the Interprofessional Professionalism Collaborative (Interprofessional Professionalism Collaborative 2018) as "consistent demonstration of core values evidenced by professionals working together, aspiring to and wisely applying principals of (Stern 2006, p. 29) altruism, excellence, caring, ethics, respect, communication, accountability to achieve optimum health and wellness in individuals and communities." As an aside, the use of the term "altruism" is contested as an attribute by "asking for ideals beyond which most ... [healthcare professionals] are capable of delivering" (Harris 2018) and perhaps overlooking the importance of caring for oneself in being able to care for others.

A simple and memorable definition, covering the professionalism of individuals, teams, and systems, is that from Shapiro (Shapiro 2018): "Professionalism is an umbrella term to define behaviours that support trustworthy relationships." Encouraging practitioners-in-training to address the notion of trustworthiness when engaged in conversations about professional behavior is often a helpful way to develop insight and understanding as to what acting professionally means and why it is important.

What determines and guides professional behavior comes from several sources including: the moral development and sensibility of individuals and communities; the guidance of regulators; and expectations of employers. The formal, informal, and hidden curricula in undergraduate and postgraduate education provide regulatory frameworks, present health practitioners with employer expectations, and contribute to the learner's moral development and sensibility in explicit and implicit ways which can support or challenge virtue.

A student comes to professional training with their personal identity and moral standpoint. A wide variety of influences contribute to the moral development and sensibility of individuals and communities, where sensibility is "one's moral being in-the-moment" (Sherblom 2012, p. 127). The development of aspects of the moral self, such as conscience and compassion, begins in childhood with its roots in the collective life, socially negotiated. Two frameworks provide examples of moral development that derive from the theories of such great thinkers as Freud, Durkheim, Dewey, Piaget, and Erikson (Kohlberg 1984; Kegan 1982). Both illuminate where learners might be in their professional journeys. Kohlberg (1984) outlined six stages of moral development: the first motivated by how to avoid punishment; the second by conforming to rules and societal norms; the third by conforming to the rules and societal norms of individuals surrounding us; the fourth on maintaining a functioning society; the fifth on the individual's own ethical principles based on fundamental human rights; and the final stage on a compulsion to seek justice with the ability to step into another's shoes. In Kegan's model (1982), also helpful when guiding students through their training and professional identity formation, the individual moves through six stages from childhood to adulthood: the incorporate stage focusing on sensory information and reflexes where the child lacks a sense of self; the impulsive stage directed by perception and impulse where objects begin to have meaning; the imperial stage which is a period of self-centeredness; the interpersonal stage where the individual can see that others have needs that need to be taken into account in order to best satisfy their own needs; the institutional stage where the individual internalizes the moral, ethical, and legal foundations and rules of their society and develops autonomy, acting on principal rather than impulse; and the final interindividual stage which emphasizes both autonomy and tolerance and a recognition of different value systems. Students and healthcare practitioners may be at any of these levels or points on continuums, dependent on their experiences, cultural, and religious background, and stage of personal growth. As educators, we hope to bring ourselves and our learners to a place of valuing and acting upon justice and empathy, autonomous with a recognition of different value systems. The moral development of individuals and communities however, as seen in history (e.g., the move from the perceived rightness of the paternalistic model of the clinician-patient relationship of the twentieth century to the patient-centered approach of more modern times), is a long and unpredictable journey, as much determined by the context of the moment as by the complexities of moral development over time.

Part of our moral development with respect to professionalism (e.g., in the institutional stage of Kegan) comes from internalizing social norms and mores, exemplified by external regulation as a formal process of the promulgation, monitoring, and enforcement of rules. The UK General Medical Council in "Good Medical Practice" (General Medical Council 2019), the UK Nursing and Midwifery Council in "The Code" (Nursing and Midwifery Council 2018), and the UK Health and Social Care Professions Council in "Standards of conduct, performance and ethics" (HCPC 2016), for example, set out the standards that doctors, nurses, and a range of other health professions must uphold. Compliance with these standards is necessary for the granting of registration and licenses to doctors, nurses, and other health professionals.

Compliance with employers is about being a good employee and adhering to employer guidance. Documents such as Staff Responsibilities, Staff Codes of Conduct, and Expected Standards of Behavior outline what is expected of healthcare staff, for example, in terms of general conduct, appearance, treatment of patients, duty of candor, data protection, health and safety, and dignity at work. In return, employers have duties of care toward their employees.

Regulations and Employer Codes reflect normative expectations. They are explicit, implicit, and habitual and may or may not align with our moral values. As Alan Cribb writes in his article on integrity at work (Cribb 2011), "Professional roles can be seen both as a scaffold to support virtue and as a mask to disguise vice ... [there is] the existence of a potential gap between the normative expectations attached to a role and the personal moral compass of the individual role-holder." This can lead to ethical quandaries and opportunities need to be provided either in tutorials or small group work for these to be addressed in discussions with peers and teachers. Coming back to moral sensibility, Kleinman (2011) stressed the importance of considering hidden values and divided selves ("complex personhood that is portrayed as fractured and at odds with itself" (Kleinman 2011, p. 804)) in the education of clinicians to develop a deep understanding of their ethical and moral responsibilities.

Professionalism Education

The Personal and the Professional Journey: Formation of Professional Identity Through Communities of Practice

Our thinking about professional development has developed from one of purely formal instruction, something to be taught and assessed, to include the development of the professional identity. A professional identity, using the example of a physician, is "a representation of self, achieved in stages over time, during which the characteristics, values and norms of the medical profession are internalised, resulting in an individual thinking, acting and feeling like a physician" (Cruess et al. 2014). This identity, for all health professions, is formed through a process of socialization where, in a process of legitimate peripheral participation to full participation, the health professional becomes part of a community of practice (Wenger 1998), a "socially configured space[s] that necessarily involve[s] learning as an aspect of membership" (Tummons 2018). Learners enter this training with their preexisting personal identity and experiences and through socialization and personal negotiation, acceptance, compromise, and rejection to develop their professional identity and their personal identity further (Cruess et al. 2018). For as long as the person is a health professional this is a continual process. It happens though formal programs of learning and through work-based learning where learning opportunities arise from being involved in normal work (Boud and Solomon 2001). As Cruess, Cruess, and Steinert explain (2018), the process of socialization is influenced by role models and mentors, and clinical and nonclinical experiences as well as by formal teaching and assessment, by symbols (e.g., the stethoscope and scrubs) and rituals (such as graduation ceremonies), and by how the learner is treated by patients, peers, healthcare professionals, and the public. It is the educator's task to support learners in all these aspects as they develop professionally through formal, informal, and hidden curricula. Crucial is providing opportunities for conscious reflection rather than unconscious acquisition. Thus, professional development requires the triad (ideally contemporaneous) of formal teaching, experiential learning (Kolb 1984), and reflective (and, more challenging, reflexive) practice. "Reflection in the context of learning is a generic term for those intellectual and affective activities in which individuals engage to explore their experiences in order to lead to new understandings and appreciations. It may take place in isolation or in association with others" (Boud et al. 1985, p. 19). Reflexive practitioners, in addition, "engage in critical self-reflection: reflecting critically on the impact of their own background, assumptions, positioning, feelings, behaviour while also attending to the impact of the wider organisational, discursive, ideological and political context" (Finlay 2008, p. 6).

Learning About Professionalism Through Formal, Informal, and Hidden Curricula

The importance of the curriculum which addresses six aspects of teaching and learning – who and what, why and how, as well as when, and when is to be taught or learned (Hughes and Quinn 2013) – in the development of professionalism in health professions education must not be underestimated. The curriculum for each health profession is informed by relevant professional standards and the Quality Assurance Agency (QAA) benchmark statements, for example, for Dentistry, the General Dental Council "Preparing for Practice" Dental Team Outcomes for Dentists 2015 (General Dental Council 2015) and the QAA Benchmark Statement "Dentistry," 2002 (Quality Assessment Agency for Higher Education 2002). However, it would be foolhardy to assume that the formal curriculum is the sole source of knowledge, skills, and attitudes that inform professionalism. When exploring the assessment of behaviors and attitudes in the UK medical schools, Stephenson and colleagues found that conflicting messages were received by students (Stephenson et al. 2006). The conflict arose between the formal and the hidden curriculum, that is, the influences of the culture and organisation, including institutional "slang," on learning (Hafferty 1998). More recently, a study of physiotherapy and dietetics students found that students felt that observation and incidental learning, for example, interactions between lecturers and students and the way lecturers were dressed, (informal learning) contributed to the development of professionalism alongside formal curriculum activities (Grace and Trede 2013). These studies clearly set out the importance of considering the informal and hidden curricula alongside the formal curriculum in the education of health professionals.

One example of the importance of the informal and hidden curriculum is the NMC statement that "registered nurses and midwives practicing at graduate levels are prepared with the behaviours, knowledge and skills to provide safe, effective, person-centred care and services. They are professionally socialised to practise in a compassionate, inter-professional and collaborative manner" (NMC 2018, p. 3). This statement assumes that these concepts are integral to the delivery of nursing and midwifery education with little or no consideration of informal and hidden curricula. This is within a context where legitimacy as a professional stemmed from competence, with concern that in the curriculum the caring role was being reduced to further develop technical know-how (Scott 2007). It has been argued that the hidden curriculum is the mechanism whereby adult nursing students form a professional identify and develop professional values (Raso et al. 2019). While Raso and colleagues explore this in nursing, the impact of the hidden curriculum on professionalism applies to all health professions. A scoping study that reviewed 18 papers found that the literature which did explore the hidden curriculum in nursing focused on the negative aspects of the hidden curriculum, for example, rather than the clinical learning environment being orientated to education on occasions it was found to have a work-orientated orientation (Raso et al. 2019). It could be argued that there are many positive aspects in hidden curricula, for example, students identified the importance of personalized care, respect, and dignity. Whether aspects are positive or negative, by raising an awareness of the impact of the informal and hidden curriculum it is possible for them to have a positive impact on the development of professionalism. This is explored later in the chapter when considering professionalism in the curriculum.

Jeanne Dart and colleagues undertook a systematic review to identify how professionalism is conceptualized and defined to inform the education of dietitians

(Dart et al. 2019). They identified four themes: personal attributes, interpersonal communication, approach to practice, and a commitment to lifelong learning. This suggests that while professionalism can be taught, individual values and behaviors also play a role in developing professionalism. The Values Based Recruitment (VBR) Framework (HEE 2016) sets out a set of principles to facilitate the recruitment of individuals who have the right skills and are also able to support teamworking and the delivery of excellent patient care, thereby accessing the personal identify and moral standpoint of applicants. However, VBR alone will not result in health profession students understanding professionalism and integrating it into their practice. Role modeling and sharing their own understanding and experiences with peers, academic, and practice staff will further support students to develop as professionals. The contribution of academic and practice staff sharing their own experiences including dilemmas and failures has been described as "intellectual streaking," a mechanism showcasing reflection in action alongside resilience (Bearman and Molloy 2017).

Professional Practice Guidelines

The contribution of professional bodies to the development of programs leading to registration as health professionals has been explored earlier in the chapter. It is important to remember that professional bodies that have responsibility for protecting the public also issue codes of conduct and other guidance. Links to the professional codes, for example, the Health and Care Professions Council (HCPC) Standards of Conduct Performance and Ethics (HCPC 2016 (Morrow et al. 2014)), must be made explicit within the curriculum. The NMC (2018) explores how the application of the Code facilities nurses and midwives to demonstrate professionalism in practice. The importance of ongoing professional development is included in each of the professional codes with reflection identified as an approach that can empower medical students and doctors (GMC 2018). Academic and clinical practice staff are well placed to articulate how reflection in and on action can have not only a positive impact on care delivery but also on professional development. Taking into consideration the influences of the culture including institutional "slang" on learning discussed earlier, this is of importance and should be formally acknowledged in health professions education.

The use of social media features in professional practice guidelines, for example, the HCPC states "You must use all forms of communication appropriately and responsibly, including social media and networking websites" (HCPC 2016 (Morrow et al. 2014, p. 6)). The NMC has taken this a step further publishing guidance which builds on the Code with regard to social media (NMC 2019), and the General Medical Council (GMC) has produced a similar document (GMC 2013). Promoting professional behavior reflecting the codes of practice on social media is an important component of education for health professionals. Rather than seeing social media as a potential pitfall it has been suggested that it could be reimagined as professional media. A systematic review of the use of social media in nursing and midwifery education found that the interactive nature of social media can support student learning, facilitate professional networks, and increase confidence (O'Connor et al. 2018). By increasing confidence with regard to social media from a professional perspective, opportunity for professional development is increased, for example, the use of Twitter as an interactive tool across professional groups (Bliss 2016).

Professionalism in the Curriculum: Learning Outcomes, Educational Methods, and Assessment

There is a plethora of curriculum models and philosophies of teaching that can be utilized to guide and underpin professional education programs. The work of Beattie (1987), pp. 15–34) provides a model to consider the varied types of knowledge, skills, and attitudes required to be a healthcare professional. This includes the technical knowledge and skills alongside the values that support the development of professionalism. The fourfold curriculum model focuses on a map of key subjects, a schedule of basic skills, a portfolio of meaningful experiences, and an agenda of important cultural issues. Although the model was initially developed for nursing, it has much to offer in the education of all health professionals with its explicit focus on aspects reflecting the various health professions' codes of practice. The use of a portfolio of meaningful experiences based on previous experience provides an opportunity to acknowledge the different points on the continuum that students are in relation to their experiences, cultural, and religious background and stage of personal growth discussed earlier in the chapter.

Having identified a curriculum model, it is also important to consider how this will be operationalized. For health professionals who are required to engage in ongoing professional development after registration, the use of discovery learning has much to offer (Bruner 1960). Discovery learning provides a framework for the acquisition of new knowledge, transformation of information and evaluation, that is, the opportunity for heath professional students to build on their experience and knowledge, analyze information for new situations, and evaluate the learning. As such, discovery learning supports health professional students to develop knowledge, skills, and attitudes for registration while becoming familiar with the concept of reflection for ongoing professional development.

The current focus on partnership working with patients, families, and carers, alongside the commitment to interprofessional working, also influences health professions education. The contribution of interprofessional education (IPE) to person-centered care with effective collaboration, trust, and respect has long been recognized and is acknowledged in the CAIPE Interprofessional Education Guidelines (Barr et al. 2017). IPE can also contribute to the development of professionalism, reflecting the values set out in the various professional codes of practice and professional standards discussed earlier in the chapter. McNair (2005) proposed a framework for learning professional and interprofessional practice (Table 1), which has utility across the education of health professionals from the development of programs of learning to individual learning opportunities such as simulated practice.

Table 1 A framework for learning professionalism and interprofessional practice. (Reprinted with permission from McNair R. The case for educating health care students in professionalism as the core content of interprofessional education. Medical Education. 2005;39:456–464. Copyright 2005 John Wiley and Sons)

Areas of capability[a]	Interprofessionalism and interprofessional practice curriculum	Methods of evaluation of outcomes[b]
1. Values	The elements of professionalism which form the joint value system	Observation of interprofessional behavior during shared tasks as measure of value
	Attitudes towards collaboration	
	Attitudes towards other disciplines	Longitudinal tracking by student reflect diary through course
2. Ethic[a]	Interprofessional ethical principles (e.g., Tavistock: rights, balance, comprehensiveness, improvement, safely, openness, and cooperation)	Sell appraisal Peer appraisal
3. Knowledge	Understanding of health care professional roles	Pre- and post-questionnaires of perceived learning
	Principles of effective teamwork	
4. Skills for the process of care	Interpersonal communication between disciplines	Objective structured clinical examination involving interprofessional practice
	Skills for collaboration, and teamwork including dealing with error and joint decision-making	Observation and group appraisal of shared tasks such as problem solving and group presentation of learning task
	Skills for appropriate and respectful leadership including change management	
	Reflectiveness	Reflective diary
5. Application (mostly post-registration)	Adaptability across a range of health care settings and health care teams	Patient satisfaction measures
	Ability to shift personal role in different teams	Teamwork: quality of meetings, leadership, division of roles, measured by peer appraisal, and external observation
		Clinical audit cycle

[a]The capability framework adapted from Sainsbury Centre for Mental Health (2001)
[b]Includes measures of effective teamwork described by Borrill et al. (2000)

Education for health professionals is not restricted to the classroom, but includes learning in clinical practice. Although not part of the workforce, students are part of the health and social care team and are able to develop knowledge, skills, and behaviors within the context of real-life practice. Situated learning provides students with an opportunity to be participants in practice. Lave and Wenger (1991) developed the concept of legitimate peripheral participation as a mechanism to move from the status of beginner by developing competence to becoming a full participant within the cultural and social practices of the community. The contribution of learning in practice to the transformation of professional identity as part of a formal program of study is clearly articulated in research exploring the professional education of community nursing students from the perspective of their practice educators (Sayer 2013).

Assessing professionalism is not easy and is best done longitudinally with multiple trained assessors and multiple methods in different settings. Observed clinical practice is important and the use of portfolios that promote critical reflection in authentic clinical settings with face-to-face review can both enhance and capture professional development (Wilkinson et al. 2009). One example is the Pan London Practice Assessment Document (PLPAD), 2.0 Nursing (Pan London Practice Learning Group 2019), which has been developed by 11 approved education institutions and their practice partners. The PLPAD 2.0 assesses against the NMC 2018 Future Nurse Standards (Nursing and Midwifery 2018) and includes an assessment of professional values for each practice placement. The professional values assessed mirror the four components of the NMC Code (NMC 2018): prioritize people, practice effectively, preserve safety, and promote professionalism and trust. The assessment of professionalism in health profession education need not be limited to the practice setting. Guraya et al. (2016) explore a range of assessment tools used to assess professionalism; these include case-based discussions which could be further developed as an academic assignment contributing to the program.

Monitoring and Sanctions: Low-Level Concerns to Fitness to Practice Questions

How do we ensure that healthcare practitioners have the necessary knowledge, skills, attitudes, and behaviors (professionalism) to provide healthcare safely? At the highest level, health profession regulation is there to "set and promote those standards which, for reasons of safety, everyone in a profession (or branch of a profession) has to meet in publishing a register of those who meet these standards, and ensuring that everyone on the register continue to meet the standards, both by periodic checks for all and by procedures for resolving concerns which a complaint or incident might create" (Professional Standards Authority 2018). At a developmental level, throughout health professional education a process of monitoring and remediation is essential so that professionalism concerns can be detected and addressed early. Low-level concerns such as failure to attend, communicate properly and in a timely manner, or meet deadlines are markers of poor professionalism. Furthermore, professionalism concerns are often markers of personal and health problems that need pastoral care and support. Assessment and support from physical, mental health, disability, and well-being services; occupational health; finance, accommodation, and careers advice; chaplaincy; educational support services; personal tutors, clinical advisers and educational supervisors; and peer support organizations can be sought. Multiple instances of low-level concerns increase the signal that there is a problem. Many health professional courses are developing online monitoring and raising concerns systems to ensure that there are fair and transparent processes to identify, manage, and support those whose behavior calls their professionalism into question. Low-level concerns can be logged and multiple concerns flagged and acted upon, and more serious concerns (such as bullying or dishonesty) can be dealt with swiftly. Monitoring systems can also be used to report and address poor role modeling and behavior from faculty. Professionalism and support teams, through dealing with these issues over time, build expertise and engender trust in their communities and thus promote a culture of reporting and dealing with concerns safely and effectively. Fitness to Practice mechanisms are only brought into effect when a person's professional behavior is significantly different from expected standards and where their behavior might endanger patient and public safety, or the public's trust in the health profession. Showing insight and responding to remediation are critical features that decide whether there is a fitness to practice issue. Where there are health issues, these alone are not usually sufficient to conclude impairment. An example of guidance in this area comes from the GMC in their document "Professional behaviour and fitness to practise: guidance for medical schools and their students" (General Medical Council 2016). They list questions that are helpful when deciding when Fitness to Practice processes may be necessary for a medical student: "Has a student shown a deliberate or reckless disregard for professional or clinical responsibilities towards patients, teachers or colleagues? Have attempts to improve a student's behaviour or health failed and does the medical school identify a remaining unacceptable risk to patient safety or public confidence in the profession? Has a student abused a patient's trust or violated a patient's autonomy or other fundamental rights? Has a student behaved dishonestly, fraudulently or in a way designed to mislead or harm others?" These questions would be appropriate for querying the Fitness to Practice route for any health professional. Finally, those who are engaged in Fitness to Practice processes need to have adequate knowledge of legal requirements and their responsibilities for promoting equality and diversity.

Conclusion

In undergraduate and postgraduate health professions education, the development of professionalism and professional identities of learners is key to ensuring patient safety and public confidence in the health professions. What do we mean by professionalism? Definitions of professionalism are numerous – a simple definition focuses on behaviors that support trustworthy relationships – and conceptualizations, guidance, and regulations have been devised for all health professions, both individually and interprofessional. In practice, education centers around the formal and informal curricula with awareness of the effects of the hidden curriculum (that can be positive or negative and where role modeling is a powerful component) and through being part of a community (or communities) of practice. The development of professionalism builds on the personal identity, values, and moral development of the learner that is formed within social and cultural contexts with the aim of supporting the learner to reach the stage of being trustworthy, autonomous, and tolerant, recognizing different value systems, and with a compulsion to seek justice. In terms of educational methods, the triad of formal teaching, experiential learning, and reflective and reflexive practice (as individuals and in groups) together enable professional development to take place: discovery learning; working and learning in partnership with patients, families and carers; interprofessional learning; and situated learning all provide rich opportunities for the development of professional identities. Assessing professionalism is challenging and is best done longitudinally with multiple trained assessors and using multiple methods in different environments: observed clinical practice, case-based discussions, and the use of portfolios that promote critical reflection (both capturing and enhancing learning) are all important tools in this regard. Systems for the monitoring of low-level professionalism concerns are crucial so that multiple instances of low-level concerns can be detected and addressed, often markers of personal and health problems for which remediation is necessary. Raising concerns processes where concerns can be safely reported by others is also critical and can be used to address the professionalism of both learners and Faculty. Fitness to Practice mechanisms are only brought into effect where there are serious professionalism concerns and lack of insight and failure to engage with remediation are critical features in the decisions about whether the learner is fit to practice. However, it must be kept in mind that the vast majority of our learners, with support and supervision, become trustworthy, knowledgeable, skillful, and caring professionals, themselves becoming teachers of the next generation of health professionals.

Cross-References

- ▶ Communities of Practice and Medical Education
- ▶ Developing Professional Identity in Health Professional Students
- ▶ Focus on Selection Methods: Evidence and Practice
- ▶ Hidden, Informal, and Formal Curricula in Health Professions Education
- ▶ Measuring Attitudes: Current Practices in Health Professional Education

References

Advancing medical professionalism. Royal College of Physicians. 2018. https://www.rcplondon.ac.uk/projects/outputs/advancing-medical-professionalism Accessed19 July 2020

Barr H, Ford J, Gray R, Helme M, Hutchings M, Low H, Machin A, Reeves S. Interprofessional education guidelines London. Centre for the Advancement of Interprofessional Education. 2017. https://www.caipe.org/resources/publications/caipe-publications/caipe-2017-interprofessional-education-guidelines-barr-h-ford-j-gray-r-helme-m-hutchings-m-low-h-machin-reeves-s. Accessed 29 June 2019.

Bearman M, Molloy E. Intellectual streaking: the value of teachers exposing hearts (and minds). Med Teach. 2017;39(12):1284–5. https://doi.org/10.1080/0142159X.2017.1308475.

Beattie A. Making a curriculum work. In: Allan A, Jolly M, editors. The curriculum in nursing education. London: Croom Helm; 1987.

Bliss J. Using twitter as a tool for CPD. Br J Community Nurs. 2016;21(3):117. https://doi.org/10.12968/bjcn.2016.21.3.117.

Boud D, Solomon N. Work-based learning: a new higher education? London: McGraw-Hill Education; 2001.

Boud D, Keogh R, Walker D. Reflection: turning experience into learning. London: Kogan Page; 1985.

Borrill C, West M, Shapiro D, Rees A. Team working and effectiveness in health care. Br J Health Care Manag. 2000;6(8):364–71.

Bruner JS. The process of education. Cambridge, MA: Harvard University Press; 1960.

Cribb A. Integrity at work: managing routine moral stress in professional roles. Nurs Philos. 2011;12(2):119–27. https://doi.org/10.1111/j.1466-769X.2011.00484.x.

Cruess RL, Cruess SR, Boudreau JD, Snell I, Steinert Y. Reframing medical education to support professional identity formation. Acad Med. 2014;89(11):1446–51. https://doi.org/10.1097/ACM.0000000000000427.

Cruess RL, Cruess SR, Steinert Y. Teaching medical professionalism. 2nd ed. Cambridge: Cambridge University Press; 2018.

Dart J, McCall L, Ash S, Blair M, Twohig C, Palermo C. Toward a global definition of professionalism for nutrition and dietetics education: A systematic review of the literature. J Acad Nutr Diet. 2019;119(6):957–71. https://doi.org/10.1016/j.jand.2019.01.007.

Enabling professionalism in nursing and midwifery practice. Nursing and Midwifery Council. 2018. https://www.nmc.org.uk/standards/guidance/professionalism/read-report/. Accessed 29 June 2019.

Finlay L. Reflecting on 'Reflective practice'. The Open University. 2008. https://www.open.ac.uk/opencetl/sites/www.open.ac.uk.opencetl/files/files/ecms/web-content/Finlay-(2008)-Reflecting-on-reflective-practice-PBPL-paper-52.pdf. Accessed 29 June 2019.

General Dental Council. Preparing for practice: dental team learning outcomes for registration. Revised edition 2015. https://www.gdc-uk.org/docs/default-source/qualityassurance/preparing-for-practice-(revised-2015).pdf accessed 23 July 2020.

General Medical Council. Doctors use of Social Media. 2013. https://www.gmc-uk.org/ethical-guidance/ethical-guidance-for-doctors/doctors-use-of-social-media. Accessed 29 June 2019.

General Medical Council. Professional behaviour and fitness to practise: guidance for medical schools and their students. 2016. https://www.gmc-uk.org/education/standards-guidance-and-curricula/guidance/professional-behaviour-and-fitness-to-practise. Accessed 29 June 2019.

General Medical Council. The reflective practitioner: guidance for doctors and medical students. 2018. https://www.gmc-uk.org/education/standards-guidance-and-curricula/guidance/reflective-practice/the-reflective-practitioner%2D%2D-guidance-for-doctors-and-medical-students. Accessed 29 June 2019.

General Medical Council. Good Medical Practice. 2019. https://www.gmc-uk.org/ethical-guidance/ethical-guidance-for-doctors/good-medical-practice. Accessed 26 June 2019.

Grace S, Trede F. Developing professionalism in physiotherapy and dietetics students in professional entry courses. Stud High Educ. 2013;38(6):793–806. https://doi.org/10.1080/03075079.2011.603410.

Guraya SY, Guraya SS, Mahabbat NA, Fallatah KY, Al-Ahmadi BA, Alalawi HH. The desired concept maps and goal setting for assessing professionalism in medicine. J Clin Diagn Res. 2016;10(5):JE01–5. https://doi.org/10.7860/JCDR/2016/19917.7832.

Hafferty F. Beyond curriculum reform: confronting medicine's hidden curriculum. Acad Med. 1998;73(4):403–7.

Harris J. Altruism: should it be included as an attribute of medical professionalism. Health Prof Educ. 2018;4(1):3–8. https://doi.org/10.1016/j.hpe.2017.02.005.

Health & Care Professions Council. Standards of conduct, performance and ethics. 2016. https://www.hcpc-uk.org/standards/standards-of-conduct-performance-and-ethics/. Accessed 29 June 2019.

Health Education England. Values based recruitment framework. 2016. https://www.hee.nhs.uk/our-work/values-based-recruitment. Accessed 29 June 2019.

Hughes SJ, Quinn FM. Quinn's principles and practice of nurse education. Andover: Cengage Learning; 2013.

Interprofessional Professionalism Collaborative. What is interprofessional professionalism. 2018. http://www.interprofessionalprofessionalism.org/. Accessed 29 June 2019.

Kegan R. The evolving self: problem and process in human development. Cambridge, MA: Harvard University Press; 1982.

Kleinman A. The divided self, hidden values, and moral sensibility in medicine. The Lancet. 2011;377(9768):804–5. https://doi.org/10.1016/s0140-6736(11)60295-x.

Kohlberg L. The psychology of moral development: the nature and validity of moral stages. San Francisco: Harper and Row; 1984.

Kolb DA. Experiential learning: experience as the source of learning and development, vol. 1. Englewood Cliffs: Prentice-Hall; 1984.

Lave J, Wenger E. Situated learning: legitimate peripheral participation. Cambridge: Cambridge University Press; 1991.

McNair R. The case for educating health care students in professionalism as the core content of interprofessional education. Med Educ. 2005;39:456–64. https://doi.org/10.1111/j.1365-2929.2005.02116.x.

Morrow G, Burford B, Rothwell C, Carter M, McLachalan J, Illing J. Professionalism in healthcare professions. Health and Care Professions Council. 2014. https://www.hcpc-uk.org/globalassets/resources/reports/professionalism-in-healthcare-professionals.pdf. Accessed 22 Feb 2020.

Nursing and Midwifery Council. Future nurse: standards of proficiency for registered nurses. 2018. https://cec.hscni.net/future-nurse-future-midwife/. Accessed 29 June 2019.

Nursing and Midwifery Council. The code. 2018. https://www.nmc.org.uk/standards/code/. Accessed 29 June 2019.

Nursing and Midwifery Council. Guidance on using Social Media responsibly. 2019. https://www.nmc.org.uk/standards/guidance/social-media-guidance/. Accessed 29 June 2019.

O'Connor S, Jolliffe S, Stanmore E, Renwick L, Booth R. Social media in nursing and midwifery education: a mixed study systematic review. J Adv Nurs. 2018;74:2273–89. https://doi.org/10.1111/jan13799.

Pan London Practice Learning Group. Pan London Practice Assessment Document. 2019. https://plplg.uk/plpad-2-0/. Accessed 29 June 2019.

Professional Standards Authority. Professional healthcare regulation in the UK explained. 2018. https://www.professionalstandards.org.uk/news-and-blog/blog/detail/blog/2018/04/10/professional-healthcare-regulation-explained. Accessed 29 June 2019.

Quality Assessment Agency for Higher Education. Benchmark statement, dentistry. 2002. https://www.qaa.ac.uk/docs/qaa/subject-benchmark-statements/subject-benchmark-statement-dentistry.pdf?sfvrsn=5fe2f781_10. Accessed 29 June 2019.

Raso A, Marchetti A, D'Angelo D, Albanesi B, Garrino L, Dimonte V, Piredda M, De Marinis MG. The hidden curriculum in nursing education: a scoping study. Med Educ. 2019. https://doi.org/10.1111/medu.13911.

Sainsbury Centre for Mental Health. The capable practitioner: a framework and list of the practitioner capabilities required to implement the national service framework for mental health. London: Training and Practice Development Section of the Sainsbury Centre for Mental Health; 2001.

Sayer L. Communities of practice, a phenomenon to explain student development in community nursing. Prim Health Care Res Dev. 2013;15:430–40. https://doi.org/10.1017/S1463423613000455.

Scott SD. 'New professionalism' – shifting relationships between nursing education and nursing practice. Nurse Educ Today. 2007;28:240–5. https://doi.org/10.1016/j.nedt.2007.04.004.

Shapiro J. Confronting unprofessional behaviour in medicine (Editorial). BMJ. 2018;360:k1025. https://doi.org/10.1136/bmj.k1025.

Sherblom SA. What develops in moral development. A model of moral sensibility. J Moral Educ. 2012;41(1):117–42. https://doi.org/10.1080/03057240.2011.652603.

Stephenson AE, Adshead LE, Higgs RH. The teaching of professional attitudes within UK medical schools: reported difficulties and good practice. Med Educ. 2006;40:1072–80. https://doi.org/10.1111/j.1365-2929.2006.02607.x.

Stern DT. Measuring medical professionalism. New York: Oxford University Press; 2006. p. 29.

Tummons J. Learning architectures in higher education: beyond communities of practice. London: Bloomsbury Publishing; 2018.

Wenger E. Communities of Practice: learning, Meaning, and Identity. Cambridge, UK: Cambridge University Press; 1998.

Wilkinson TJ, Wade WB, Knock LD. A Blueprint to assess professionalism: results of a systematic review. Acad Med. 2009;84(5):551–8. https://doi.org/10.1097/ACM.0b013e31819fbaa2.

Supporting the Development of Patient-Centred Communication Skills

79

Bernadette O'Neill

Contents

Introduction	1536
Part 1: Patient-Centredness: Origins, Definitions, and Relation to Clinical Communication	1537
The Emergence of Patient-Centredness as a Relational Model in Healthcare	1537
Defining Patient-Centredness	1538
Clinical Communication and Patient-Centredness	1540
Evidence and Justification for Patient-Centred Clinical Practice and Communication	1540
Part 2: Supporting the Development of Patient-Centred Communication – Approaches to Teaching and Learning	1542
Clinical Simulation	1542
Critical Considerations of Simulation for Developing Patient-Centred Communication	1543
Workplace and Situated Learning	1546
Conclusion	1549
Cross-References	1550
References	1550

Abstract

This chapter critically appraises the main pedagogic approaches used to support the development of patient-centred clinical communication. It begins by tracing the emergence of patient-centredness as a relational model in healthcare and reviews a range of perspectives of what the term has come to mean. The rationale and evidence base for adopting patient-centred communicative practice as core to its delivery are examined, including its role in enhancing clinical outcomes and relationships to provide high quality, humane care. Methods for supporting learners' development of communication through simulated and workplace learning are considered, with reference to the educational theories of behaviourism,

B. O'Neill (✉)
GKT School of Medical Education, King's College London, London, UK
e-mail: bernadette.oneill@kcl.ac.uk

© Springer Nature Singapore Pte Ltd. 2023
D. Nestel et al. (eds.), *Clinical Education for the Health Professions*,
https://doi.org/10.1007/978-981-15-3344-0_101

experiential learning, and social constructivism. These methods are critically evaluated in respect of their strengths and limitations in promoting the skills and ethos of patient-centred communication. Critiques of the transfer model of learning are highlighted, as is the dissonance students experience between simulated and authentic communicative practice. Barriers to the development and sustainment of a patient-centred approach in the clinical environment are considered and interventions informed by research studies and workplace learning theories are proposed to help mitigate these. The pivotal role of patients in helping learners to appreciate and develop patient-centred attitudes and skills, through formal involvement in healthcare education as well as clinically based encounters, is discussed. Finally, additional online resources which can be used to further support patient-centred learning are signposted.

Keywords

Clinical communication · Communication skills · Patient-centredness · Pedagogy

Introduction

The centrality of patient-centredness, allied with skilled communication, for the delivery of high-quality healthcare is well recognized (Pawlikowska et al. 2012; Mead and Bower 2002). Attempts to capture its meaning have yielded a range of definitions (Mead and Bower 2000; Stewart et al. 2006; Brown et al. 1986). Core to these constructs is placing patients' needs, and what is important from their perspective, at the forefront of clinical endeavors. The argument for this approach has been made from a number of standpoints, including its role in enhanced clinical outcomes, increased patient satisfaction, and as a moral imperative in the provision of healthcare (Duggan et al. 2006; Stewart 1995; Mead et al. 2002). Delivering patient-centred care is, however, not without its challenges. These range from macro-level system and organizational barriers (Hower et al. 2019) through to micro interactional level factors (Maynard and Heritage 2005). The need for organisational and governance structures which support such practice is reflected in policy documents internationally (ACSQHC 2010; DoH 2012), and their implementation can be considered a prerequisite to achieving and sustaining its delivery. While acknowledging the impact of the wider systemic healthcare context, the focus of this chapter lies in the interactional domain of clinical care and how patient-centred communicative practice can be developed and supported.

Part 1 of this chapter provides the context from which patient-centred practice and communication have emerged. It does so by tracing the origins of patient-centredness as a relational model in healthcare, with consideration of its key features and its inter-relationship with clinical communication. It also discusses the rationale for why this approach has been widely adopted in modern healthcare systems. Part 2 of the chapter focuses on the development of patient-centred communication through a range of teaching and learning modalities, with reference to relevant educational theory. It examines the strengths and limitations of the pedagogic methods employed in this field and how the patient's voice can be embedded within training and education programs.

Part 1: Patient-Centredness: Origins, Definitions, and Relation to Clinical Communication

The Emergence of Patient-Centredness as a Relational Model in Healthcare

The dynamics of physician-patient relations have been documented since antiquity and should be viewed within the prevailing socio-political and intellectual-scientific contexts of the time (Kaba and Sooriakumaran 2007). Drawing on historians' accounts of medical practice in eighteenth and nineteenth-century Western Europe, we can trace the shifting power balance between practitioners and patients (Jewson 1976; Porter 1997). During this era, medical practitioners, unlicensed and unregulated, plied their trade among the elite classes who had the means to afford their ministrations. Their relationship was marked by a degree of reciprocal regard. The patients selected practitioners for their personal and "healing" qualities, whilst practitioners, wanting to satisfy their patrons' wishes, displayed a personalized interest and concern. The patients' subjective experience of illness was paramount and, in the absence of scientific clinical data, formed the basis for diagnosis and treatment. However, this approach changed radically with the emergence of scientism and the resultant paradigmatic shift to biomedicine as the dominant medical model. The confinement of patients to the newly established hospitals facilitated their "objective" medical assessment using novel diagnostic tools and laboratory techniques. This regime, termed the "medical gaze" by Foucault (1976), saw the separation of the patient's bodily pathology from that of their subjective personhood and negated the previous reliance on their illness narrative to achieve diagnosis. The concurrent professionalization of medical practice further legitimized the doctor's role as "expert" on the patient's condition and arbiter of treatment regimens, based on scientific data rather than subjective experience. This transfer of control to the doctor, now deemed to be acting in the perceived "best interest" of a compliant patient, heralded a new, paternalistic model of care which remained dominant until the late twentieth century (Szasz and Hollender 1956).

By the mid-1900s, the hegemony of the medical model was subject to increasing critique (Friedson 1970) and in the 1960s the term "patient-centredness" entered the medical lexicon. This terminology reflected a realigning of the power dynamic in the patients' favor. It included the reinstatement and primacy of the patients' perspective in the clinical encounter and the adoption of "whole-person medicine" (Balint 1969). This thinking was further advanced by Stewart et al. (2006) who advocated for a "transformed clinical method" espousing the holism of a biopsychosocial perspective, intended to counter the reductive tendencies of the biomedical model. Continuing support for patient-centred practice has led to its endorsement by influential international organizations (ACSQHC 2010; DoH 2012) as central to high-quality healthcare (Epstein and Street 2011), resulting in its adoption as the prevailing model of health service delivery in the twenty-first century.

Defining Patient-Centredness

Despite the increasing espousal of patient-centredness as a model of healthcare, a universal definition of the term remains elusive, perhaps not surprisingly given its scope from conceptual model through to the domains of policy and practice. Illingworth's (2016) review illustrates the range of characterizations attributed to the term through the following three examples.

The first is the UK Department of Health's (DOH 2004) reference to patient-centredness as a "philosophy of care" that encourages:

(a) *A focus in the consultation on the patient as a whole person who has individual preferences situated within social contexts, and/or*
(b) *Shared control of the consultation, decisions about interventions or management of health problems with the patient*

Of note here, and supported by recent health policy guidance (DoH 2012), is the explicit recognition of shared decision-making as central to an egalitarian clinician-patient contract.

The second example is Mead and Bower's (2000) commonly cited conceptual framework which identifies the following five dimensions of patient-centredness:

- Biopsychosocial perspective (including social, psychological, and biomedical factors)
- Patient as person (understanding the personal meaning of the illness)
- Sharing power and responsibility (responding to patient's preferences for information and shared decision-making)
- Therapeutic alliance (developing common therapeutic goals and enhancing the personal bond between doctor and patient)
- Doctor as person (recognizing the influence of personal qualities and subjectivity on medical practice)

This model emphasizes the intersubjective nature of clinical relationships and how these facets may influence the process and outcomes of clinical care.

The final example is Scholl et al.'s (2014) systematic literature review and concept analysis, from which they identify 15 dimensions of patient-centredness, grouped under three themes: Principles, Enablers, and Activities, as set out in Fig. 1.

Scholl's encompassing overview illustrates how original notions of patient-centredness (focusing on individual circumstances, values, and needs) have evolved into an increasingly multidimensional concept. It has expanded beyond the doctor-patient relationship to include important "others," be that family members, carers, or

	Brief description
PRINCIPLES	
Essential characteristics of the clinician	A set of attitudes towards the patient (e.g. empathy, respect, honesty) and oneself (self-reflectiveness) as well as medical competency
Clinician-patient relationship	A partnership with the patient that is characterized by trust and caring
Patient as unique person	Recognition of each patient's uniqueness (individual needs, preferences, values, feelings, beliefs, concerns and ideas, and expectations)
Biopsychosocial perspective	Recognition of the patient as a whole person in his or her biological, psychological, and social context
ENABLERS	
Clinician-patient communication	A set of verbal and nonverbal communication skills
Integration of medical and non-medical care	Recognition and integration of non-medical aspects of care (e.g. patient support services) into health care services
Teamwork	Recognition of the importance of effective teams characterized by a set of qualities (e.g. respect, trust, shared responsibilities, values, and visions) and facilitation of the development of such teams
Access to care	Facilitation of timely access to healthcare that is tailored to the patient (e.g. decentralized services)
Coordination and continuity of care	Facilitation of healthcare that is well coordinated (e.g. regarding follow-up arrangements) and allows continuity (e.g. a well-working transition of care from inpatient to outpatient)
ACTIVITIES	
Patient information	Provision of tailored information while taking into account the patient's information needs and preferences
Patient involvement in care	Active involvement of and collaboration with the patient regarding decisions related to the patient's health while taking into account the patient's preference for involvement
Involvement of family and friends	Active involvement of and support for the patient's relatives and friends to the degree that the patient prefers
Patient empowerment	Recognition and active support of the patient's ability and responsibility to self-manage his or her disease
Physical support	A set of behaviour that ensures physical support for the patient (e.g. pain management, assistance with daily living needs)
Emotional support	Recognition of the patient's emotional state and a set of behaviour that ensures emotional support for the patient

Fig. 1 "Dimensions of Patient-Centeredness." (Reproduced courtesy of Scholl 2014 ©) Scholl et al. (2014)

the wider health/social care team. It may also incorporate how services are structured and delivered to support patient-centred care and include promoting patients' autonomy and self-management capacities.

Clinical Communication and Patient-Centredness

The relationship between clinical communication and patient-centredness has been characterized in a number of ways. Byrne and Long's (1976) seminal study of doctors' audio-recorded General Practice consultations illuminated the impact of their communication style on the extent to which patients were able to actively participate in the consultation, a core requisite of patient-centred practice. The following decade, Mishler (1984) examined medical consultations using a discourse analytic approach. He described how the dynamic of the "voice of the lifeworld" (patients' personal accounts of their illness) and the "voice of medicine" (the doctor's focus on the disease) manifested in the interactions. In doing so he identified communicative acts on the part of the doctor which either facilitated or blocked discussion of "lifeworld" issues. He concluded that interactions dominated by the "voice of medicine" resulted in less humane and less effective patient care.

The findings from such studies have subsequently been used to inform the development of patient-centred consultation models and frameworks. For example, McWhinney's (1989) Disease-Illness Model illustrates the differing agendas of the doctor (with a focus on signs, symptoms, investigations, differential diagnosis) and of the patient (with a focus on ideas, concerns, expectations, and personal experience). The model outlines the doctor's role in integrating these agendas to arrive at a mutual understanding of the patient's problem and enable shared decision-making regarding its management. The Calgary-Cambridge Guide (Kurtz et al. 2003) provides a framework for conducting a patient-centred consultation so that eliciting the patient's perspective and shared decision-making are incorporated in the process. It also identifies a range of evidence-based verbal and non-verbal communication skills which can be drawn upon to build the clinician-patient relationship and achieve the aims of the consultation.

Evidence and Justification for Patient-Centred Clinical Practice and Communication

Studies attempting to provide a clear evidential basis for patient-centred care are hampered by the varied (or lacking) definitions of the concept, thereby undermining their validity and comparability (Illingworth 2016). Rathert et al.'s (2012) systematic review of the literature pertaining to outcomes illustrates this perfectly, with some studies reporting a direct correlation between aspects of patient-centred care and improved outcomes, while others found no clear relationship. Overall, the evidence for greater patient satisfaction and improved self-management was stronger than for other clinical outcomes. Methods for researching the process and effects of clinical communication continue to develop (Roter and Larson 2002; Krupat et al. 2006). A number of studies have reported on health outcomes relating specifically to patient-centred communication. For example, Stewart (1995) reported positive correlations in sixteen studies, such as improvements in patients' emotional health, symptom resolution, and physiologic measures (including blood pressure, glycaemic and pain control). However, Street (2013), recognizing the challenge of identifying direct correlations advocates a more nuanced approach. This involves modeling the pathways that capture both direct and indirect effects that communication may have on patient welfare (Fig. 2). This involves investigating the influence of communication on intervening variables which may lead to improved outcomes. For example, the development of trust in the doctor-patient relationship may increase patient engagement with health services, which in turn enables positive outcomes.

So, despite some inconclusive investigations, a substantial body of research evidence has been amassed to support patient-centred communication as beneficial for both enhanced clinical outcomes and increased patient satisfaction.

In addition to the evidence base outlined above, the case for patient-centredness as a moral imperative in healthcare delivery has also been made. Duggan et al. (2006) draw on the following theoretic frameworks to support this argument:

(i) Consequentialist moral theories – focusing on the positive outcomes of providing patient-centred care.
(ii) Deontological theories – emphasizing how patient-centred care reflects the ethical norms of medicine, such as respect for persons and shared decision-making.
(iii) Virtue-based theories – highlighting the importance of developing patient-centred attitudes and traits, which influence the ways clinicians behave toward their patients.

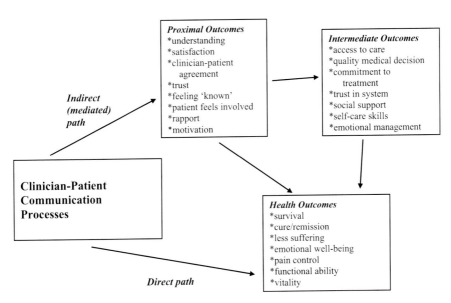

Fig. 2 "Communication pathways to improved health outcomes" (Reproduced from Street 2013). (Reproduced with permission of Elsevier ©)

The authors emphasize the value of these frameworks in legitimizing patient-centredness as a morally valuable concept for clinical practice.

In conclusion, patient-centred communication and practice are evidentially well-supported for their benefits to both clinical outcomes and patient experience. Greater precision, in terms of which definitions of patient-centredness (or its domains) are being used, would enhance future studies. Also, further consideration should be given to the impact of mediating communication variables on health outcomes and how these can be captured. The moral argument for valuing and respecting all those within the healthcare domain as "the right thing to do" has also been posited, along with the empiric justification for patient-centred practice.

Part 2: Supporting the Development of Patient-Centred Communication – Approaches to Teaching and Learning

The history of clinical communication in the practice of medicine, as previously outlined, provides the context from which it has come to be recognized as a discrete discipline in healthcare education. This includes the evolving political and societal backdrop, policy developments, and growing evidence-base relating to improved outcomes resulting from effective, patient-centred communicative practice (Stewart et al. 2006; Brown 2008). In contrast to the previous apprenticeship style of learning in the clinical milieu, involving diverse role modeling and a degree of trial and error, clinical communication is now widely established as a formal and requisite component of healthcare training programs (Bachmann et al. 2013; Noble et al. 2018). Research evidence suggests longitudinal, helical curriculum structures as most effective in supporting learners' development in this area, rather than concentrated or truncated learning episodes (van Dalen et al. 2002). Post-graduate courses of at least one-day duration have also been found to effect positive changes, though this is contingent on training being learner-centred and with a focus on active skills practice (Berkhof et al. 2011).

The following sections review the predominant methods employed in clinical communication teaching and learning, under the broad headings of clinical simulation and work-based learning. These will be discussed with reference to relevant educational theories including behaviourism, experiential learning, and social constructivism, with consideration of how these approaches contribute to the development of patient-centred practice.

Clinical Simulation

Clinical simulation is a commonly used method for the development of communication skills (Hargie et al. 2010), providing learners with the opportunity to conduct consultations with simulated patients (trained actors). It allows students to receive feedback from the patients' perspective, as well as from their peers and tutor. Simulations may be recorded enabling subsequent review and analysis of the interactions. This pedagogic method is primarily informed by behaviourist and experiential learning theories, which will be briefly outlined, before considering their role in developing patient-centred communication.

Simulation and Behaviourism

Behaviourist learning principles have been widely adopted in medical education including clinical communication teaching. Developed by psychologists during the twentieth century (Skinner 1954), the approach aims to bring about behavioural changes in the learner to meet specified standards or competencies. It assumes that "...physical actions such as thinking, acting and feeling can be regarded as behaviours in a teaching and learning setting" (Brown 2016a, p.181) thereby being observable, and for assessment purposes, measurable. When applied to clinical skills teaching this approach centres on breaking down complex tasks into component parts. These can be repeatedly practiced and refined with the aid of feedback. Behaviourist principles continue to inform clinical communication pedagogy. This is illustrated, for example, in the way the Calgary-Cambridge Guide is used for instructional purposes (Hargie et al. 2010; Kurtz et al. 2003). The framework allows for the deconstruction of the consultation into its component phases (opening, gathering information, etc.) and constituent skills (e.g., listening, question styles), which can be honed with the aid of observation and feedback.

Simulation and Experiential Learning

The use of simulation is also informed by experiential learning theory, defined as "... a teaching philosophy that informs many methodologies in which educators purposefully engage with learners in direct experience and focused reflection in order to increase knowledge, develop skills, clarify values, and develop people's capacity to contribute to their communities" (AfEE 2020). Experiential learning sits within a social constructivist paradigm which supports the exploration of how learners understand and construct their views of the world, facilitated through critical reflective practice. As such the role of the teacher becomes that of a facilitator rather than an instructor, whose purpose is to support learners' engagement with, and reflection on, suitable experiences. The case for simulation is supported by recognition that experiential methods are more effective than didactic instruction for clinical communication teaching and learning (Aspegren 1999; Lane and Rollnick 2007).

Critical Considerations of Simulation for Developing Patient-Centred Communication

Behaviourism, Skills Development, and Patient-Centredness

While there is evidence that experiential learning in the form of clinical simulation is effective for developing communication skills, how confident can we be that this method helps to promote *patient-centred* communication? We can begin by considering the effect of the behaviourally informed skills approach. This involves mastering of a range of skills intended to convey interest and respect, facilitate patient involvement and elicit a biopsychosocial understanding of the patient's circumstance. Attainment of these skills through rehearsal, receipt of feedback and reinforcement, may indeed be viewed as a positive leaning outcome, at least in equipping trainees to conduct a patient-centred consultation. However, this approach has been questioned for its role in promoting a restrictive discourse and practice of "communication skills," at the expense of a more encompassing and creative appreciation of "clinical communication" as a subject (Skelton 2008; Salmon and Young 2005). For example, in seeking to demonstrate specified skills such as empathic responses or open questions, there is a risk of developing mechanistic or superficial techniques, to the detriment of genuine responsiveness and engagement with patients. At its extreme, a focus solely on observable and demonstrable communicative acts, without reference to underlying principles and values, may be viewed as a mere training in de-contextualized surface skills (Hanna and Fins 2006). The counter argument is that through deploying patient-centred communication skills learners may come to recognize their effects and benefits, thereby fostering patient-centred attitudes. This is a contention which warrants further focused research (Fernández-Olano et al. 2008). In practice the majority of curricula whilst employing skills-based methods, integrate allied subject areas such as professionalism and medical ethics, and in some instances medical humanities, to promote a rounded consideration of clinical communication. The extent of such integration, however, varies considerably between programs (Hargie et al. 2010; Noble et al. 2018).

A further concern regarding a skills-based approach is that it assumes a transfer model of learning, whereby skills mastered in one context are deemed transferable to another (Brown 2016a). For example, patient-centred communication skills honed in a controlled classroom environment may prove challenging to apply in practice, given the cultural vagaries of the actual clinical setting. The powerful "informal" influence of real-life role modeling and practices, known as the hidden curriculum, is well recognized in undermining the ideals students are encouraged to adopt in formal curricula (Hojat et al. 2009; Hafferty 1998). Bombeke et al. (2012) also identified tiredness and time pressures as detrimental to the transfer of communication skills training to the clinical setting. Despite this, they reported that medical students and junior doctors continued to apply skills learned in training to everyday practice and found them of particular help in challenging situations. The authors concluded that while "best-evidence skills training" remains important, learners need support to incorporate such skills creatively into their personal communication styles. This reflects the notion of "genuineness" as a core attribute of relationship-centred care (Beach and Inui 2006) and its role in countering a mechanistic application of learned communication skills.

Experiential, Simulated Learning, and Patient-Centredness

Though experiential learning theory is relevant to both practice-based and simulated learning, it is considered here in relation to the latter. As previously noted, simulation is commonly used in communication curricula (Hargie et al. 2010) and has a number of advantages. It provides an environment in which learners can prepare to undertake "real-life" consultations without risking harm to patients and with the opportunity to focus in depth on the interactive/relational process rather than medical management. It is also a means to strategically deliver key learning material (Hanna and Fins 2006). Though widely used and recognized as pedagogically effective for skills development, the limitations of simulation for instilling patient-centred attitudes are also recognized.

Yardley et al. (2013) conducted a study of medical students' experiences of simulated and authentic patient interactions. It revealed that students identify a dissonance, or "gap," in their learning between these two spheres. For example, students described feelings of responsibility towards real patients which were lacking in simulated encounters, and of feeling less "judged" in their practice-based interactions than in the performative context of simulation. They also perceived differences between how actual and simulated patients responded, associating the latter with delivering the learning agenda of clinical communication faculty. The authors argue that this dissonance requires recognition and attention if students are to maximize learning from both environments. Rather than viewing the metaphorical gap as a negative source of disconnection, Yardley et al. draw on Vykostsky's (1978) social constructivist approach to reframe it as a valuable opportunity for extending learning, i.e., as a "zone of proximal development." For this to be effective students require support to reflect on and assimilate learning from both contexts, in order to:

(a) Facilitate their active construction of patient-centred communication and practice
(b) Resolve tensions between simulated practice and that witnessed and experienced in the workplace

Hanna and Fins (2006) caution that an over-reliance on simulation, as a proxy for real-life patient engagement, may result in clinicians who are able to "...act out a good relationship with their patients but have no authentic connection with them" (p.265). To counter this potentiality they recommend that simulated learning should be coupled with early clinical exposure, whereby students can experience the communicative challenges of clinical practice first-hand. This, they argue, will promote the relevance of simulated learning in preparing for real-life situations and motivate students to consider their personal and professional responses to these encounters. This view resonates with relational models that highlight the importance of the clinician "as person," cognisant of their values in the context of patient relationships (Mead and Bower 2000).

So far, we have considered simulation as a core pedagogic method for the development of clinical communication through the educational lenses of behaviourism, experiential learning, and social constructivism. We have also considered the strengths and limitations of these approaches in helping to promote patient-centred communicative practice. What emerges is confirmation that skills-based teaching and learning, delivered through credible simulations, is effective for equipping learners with strategies for use in clinical practice.

There is also a sense that these methods work best when complemented by additional pedagogic measures. These may include:

- Supplementing simulation with early clinical exposure and facilitating active reconciliation of learning from both spheres (Bombeke et al. 2012; Yardley et al. 2013).
- Situating clinical communication within a learning paradigm (Rider et al. 2014) which acknowledges the essential presence and impact of values in healthcare which may be personal, professional, cultural, or institutional (Fulford et al. 2012). This encourages the development of learners' self-awareness and "...analytical and communication skills to elicit the values of individual patients and other stakeholders..." (Petrova et al. 2006 p. 5).
- The integration of humanities-based approaches within healthcare curricula as a further means of cultivating learners' awareness of themselves and of others, as a foundation for building caring and authentic patient relationships (Hanna and Fins 2006).

Workplace and Situated Learning

As highlighted previously learners' experience in the clinical workplace plays a crucial role in the development of patient-centred communication. Appreciating the different types of knowledge that students assimilate in formal/university settings and in clinical practice is a useful starting point when considering how best to support workplace learning.

Brown (2016b) refers to clinical communication knowledge as "codified" and "situated." Codified knowledge refers to that which emanates from academic disciplinary sources (e.g., social and behavioural sciences), including published literature and is mainly transmitted via teaching programs. Situated knowledge is generated from real-world working practices in order to meet the needs of service delivery. As students enter the workplace they are challenged to reformulate codified subject knowledge as they assimilate new context-specific knowledge and skills. Evans et al. (2010) are critical of the notion that learning can simply be transferred from one domain to another, i.e., from theory to practice. They describe how different forms of knowledge are contextualized and re-contextualized in diverse sites of learning. This construct of re-contextualization acknowledges the interplay between learner, knowledge formation, and the environment.

Lave and Wenger's (1991) theory of "situated learning" also recognizes that people think and learn differently in different social contexts, reinforcing the notion that knowledge is not a fixed, transferable, entity. They propose that learners engage in a process of "legitimate peripheral participation" within a situated group (e.g., nurses/doctors in a clinical workplace) whereby they become an increasingly involved member of that "community of practice." It is through this process, that their knowledge is thought to be constructed and re-constructed to fit with authentic workplace practices and cultural mores. This emphasis on learning as a social practice highlights the influential role of colleagues, supervisors, and institutional norms in workplace learning.

Challenges to Situated Clinical Communication Development

The challenge of assimilating differing types of knowledge as outlined by Brown (2016b), goes some way to explaining the dissonance experienced by learners between the academic and clinical milieus. As already noted, barriers to patient-centred communication in the clinical area include environmental and human factors such as time pressures and fatigue (Bombeke et al. 2012). Barriers may also be pervasive in terms of institutional cultures and values. Hafferty and Castellani (2009) describe a complex system of influences which may manifest in medical schools, as well as in clinical learning environments, which include:

(a) The informal curriculum (spontaneous and ad hoc teaching and learning) and
(b) The hidden curriculum (organizational and cultural factors)

Messages transmitted to learners through these channels can powerfully influence their perceptions of codified knowledge and how they may re-contextualize it. This is exemplified in the reported erosion of medical students' empathy as their clinical exposure increases (Hojat et al. 2009). Learners/trainees also have difficulty gaining feedback on their communication skills in the workplace, with supervisors tending to focus on the content rather than the process of clinical encounters (Egnew and Wilson 2010). This highlights the importance of an environment in which the value of effective clinical communication is acknowledged and in which trainees are regularly observed and receive feedback from patient-centred role models (van den Eertwegh et al. 2014).

Theories of workplace learning such as re-contextualization and situated learning provide lenses through which to examine the challenges outlined above. They may be used, along with insights from research studies in the field, to inform measures to support the development of patient-centred clinical communication. These include:

- Exploring learners' existing clinical communication knowledge/skills and identifying which areas they seek to develop further
- Providing teaching opportunities in the clinical workplace to meet their learning needs
- Observing trainees'/learners' communication and providing constructive feedback
- Demonstrating and modeling in situ patient-centred practice
- Facilitating reflection, discussion, and the brokering of theoretic and work-based knowledge and practices

These measures capitalize on the opportunities afforded learners within communities of practice and actively assist in the re-contextualization of patient-centred learning as relevant to clinical reality. Evans et al. (2010) also recommend increased partnerships between universities and clinical workplaces to encourage a collaborative approach to teaching and learning, including common goals and values.

The Patient's Voice in Clinical Communication Pedagogy

The pivotal role of patients in helping learners to appreciate and develop patient-centred attitudes and skills, within and beyond clinically based encounters, is well recognized (Spencer et al. 2011; Yardley et al. 2013). The value of early and regular patient contact within healthcare curricula has been discussed earlier and the point that "The patient's voice, as an authentic stimulus, has great authority and is more influential than the teachers" (Van Dalen et al. 1999 p.195) is well made. The introduction of Patient Educators (PEs), i.e., real patients in a formal capacity, have proved a successful means of embedding the patients' voice in healthcare education (Oswald et al. 2014). Their roles vary and may include, for example, supporting students' development of physical examination skills and how to elicit a medical history. PEs bring first-hand insights of their healthcare experiences to the learning encounter, which provides a different perspective to clinician-led teaching. Students also benefit from receiving feedback directly from patients, rather than via the proxy of simulated patients. Learners value the opportunity of hearing the patient's story and their experience of living with their condition. Student evaluations of PE programs suggest they lead to increased empathy and greater awareness of patients' perspectives (Spencer et al. 2011). PEs may also be involved in student assessment and course design/planning, though the latter are dependent on local and institutional initiatives to include patients at a more strategic level (Spencer et al. 2011).

There are additional resources available online, featuring first-hand patient experiences, which can be used to supplement clinical communication teaching. These include:

- "Healthtalkonline" (healthtalk.org 2019) This website hosts the "Database of Individual Patients" Experience of Illness' (DIPEx). People can read about others' experiences of health and illness, watch/listen to patient interviews and find reliable information about conditions, treatment choices, and support.
- "Patient Voices" (patientvoices.org.uk 2020) provides a catalogue of digitized first-person stories including those of patients, medical students, and clinicians. They may be used as reflective prompts in educational programs and as a resource for quality improvement initiatives. The organization also provides support for running locally held workshops for the development and recording of new stories.
- "Picker Institute" (picker.org) is an international charity which draws on patients' experiences to promote compassionate, high-quality care. Their website includes multiple resources aimed at informing and supporting person-centred approaches.

This brief review has outlined some of the ways in which patients actively support learners' development of clinical communication. Without this input, we risk the separation of clinical communication pedagogy from its core purpose and from the key informants of what it means to be patient-centred.

Conclusion

The first part of this chapter briefly traced the emergence of patient-centredness as a relational model in healthcare and considered a range of definitions which attempt to capture its dimensions. This illustrated the breadth of characteristics ascribed to the term both conceptually and operationally. The evidence base supporting the beneficial impact of patient-centred communication on clinical outcomes and patient experience was discussed, along with the case for patient-centredness as a moral imperative. Appreciating the background and rationale for why this model has prevailed provides a substantive foundation for the teaching and learning of clinical communication, and reflects its relation to changing medical practices and societal norms. Recognizing the intersubjective nature of clinical relationships and communication encourages us to pay attention not only to the personhood of patients but also that of clinicians. This allows for consideration of personal and professional values as part of clinical communication pedagogy, providing a rich learning context for the development of necessary skills.

The second part of the chapter reviewed the predominant pedagogic methods employed to support the development of patient-centred communication, with reference to underpinning educational theories including behaviourism, social constructivism, and experiential learning. It confirmed that clinical simulation is widely used and proven to be an effective method for the development of patient-centred communication skills. Supplementing this method with early and concurrent clinical exposure is recommended to provide students the opportunity to assimilate learning from both simulated and authentic patient contact. This can be maximized by facilitating students to reflect on, and make sense of, the dissonances they may encounter between these different learning domains. Theories of situated learning and re-contextualization and have been drawn on to help address the challenges students face in adapting their knowledge to different sites of learning. The influence of supervisors, colleagues and institutional norms as experienced through engagement with communities of practice has also been highlighted.

The crucial role of patients in supporting learners' development of truly patient-centred communication has been highlighted. While simulated patients play an important role in preparing students for (as well as supplementing) clinical practice, the impact of first-hand engagement with authentic patients remains the fulcrum for such learning. In addition to clinically based patient encounters, formalized Patient Educator programs and digitized resources provide further opportunities to learn directly from patients' insights and experiences.

A final consideration in supporting trainees' development in this area, is attending to how they themselves are treated. Creating learning environments which recognize the "Student/trainee as person," mirroring the notion of "Patient as person" can provide a meaningful congruence between clinical education and practice. This can be achieved by valuing and respecting trainees, fostering a sense of purpose and belonging in the clinical environment, actively supporting the attainment of their learning goals, and promoting self-care strategies. These measures may go some way to offsetting the potential erosion of patient-centred attitudes that may result from the challenges and rigours of day-to-day clinical practice.

Cross-References

▶ Arts and Humanities in Health Professional Education
▶ Developing Care and Compassion in Health Professional Students and Clinicians
▶ Hidden, Informal, and Formal Curricula in Health Professions Education
▶ Targeting Organizational Needs Through the Development of a Simulation-Based Communication Education Program

References

ACSQH. Australian safety and quality framework for health care [Online]. Australian Commission on Safety and Quality in Healthcare (ACSQHC) 2010. Available: http://www.safetyandquality.gov.au/wp-content/uploads/2012/04/Australian-SandQ-Framework1.pdf. Accessed 02 Oct 2020.

AfEE. What is experiential education? [Online]. Association for Experiential Education. 2020. Available: https://www.aee.org/what-is-ee. Accessed 04 Oct 2020.

Aspegren K. BEME guide no. 2: teaching and learning communication skills in medicine-a review with quality grading of articles. Med Teach. 1999;21:563–70.

Bachmann C, Abramovitch H, Barbu CG, Cavaco AM, Elorza RD, Haak R, Loureiro E, Ratajska A, Silverman J, Winterburn S, Rosenbaum MA. European consensus on learning objectives for a core communication curriculum in health care professions. Patient Educ Couns. 2013;93:18–26.

Balint E. The possibilities of patient-centred medicine. J R Coll Gen Pract. 1969;17:269–76.

Beach MC, Inui T. Relationship-centred care. A constructive reframing. J Gen Intern Med. 2006;21 (Suppl 1):S3–8.

Berkhof M, Van Rijssen HJ, Schellart AJ, Anema JR, Van Der Beek AJ. Effective training strategies for teaching communication skills to physicians: an overview of systematic reviews. Patient Educ Couns. 2011;84:152–62.

Bombeke K, Symons L, Vermeire E, Debaene L, Schol S, De Winter B, Van Royen P. Patient-centredness from education to practice: the 'lived' impact of communication skills training. Med Teach. 2012;34:e338–48.

Brown J. How clinical communication has become a core part of medical education in the UK. Med Educ. 2008;42:271–8.

Brown J. Behaviourism as a way of learning. In: Brown J, Noble LM, Papageourgiou A, Kidd J, editors. Clinical communication in medicine. Wiley Blackwell; 2016a.

Brown J. Situated and work-based learning. In: Brown J, Noble LM, Papageourgiou A, Kidd J, editors. Clinical communication in medicine. Wiley Blackwell; 2016b.

Brown J, Stewart M, Mccracken E, Mcwhinney IR, Levenstein J. The patient-centred clinical method. 2. Definition and application. Fam Pract. 1986;3:75–9.

Byrne PS. & Long BEL. Doctors talking to patients. London: HMSO; 1976.

DOH Liberating the NHS. No decision about me, without me. London: Department of Health; 2012.

DOH Patient and Public Involvement in Health. The evidence for policy implementation. London: Department of Health; 2004.

Duggan PS, Geller G, Cooper LA, Beach MC. The moral nature of patient-centredness: is it "just the right thing to do"? Patient Educ Couns. 2006;62:271–6.

Egnew TR, Wilson HJ. Faculty and medical students' perceptions of teaching and learning about the doctor-patient relationship. Patient Educ Couns. 2010;79:199–206.

Epstein RM, Street RL. The values and value of patient-centred care. Ann Fam Med. 2011;9:100–3.

Evans K, Guile D, Harris J, Allan H. Putting knowledge to work: a new approach. Nurse Educ Today. 2010;30:245–51.

Fernández-Olano C, Montoya-Fernández J, Salinas-Sánchez AS. Impact of clinical interview training on the empathy level of medical students and medical residents. Med Teach. 2008;30:322–4.

Foucault M. The birth of the clinic. London: Tavistock Publications Ltd.; 1976.

Friedson E. The profession of medicine. New York: Dodd, Mead and Co; 1970.

Fulford KWM, Peile E, Carroll H. Essential values-based practice: clinical stories linking science with people. Cambridge: Cambridge University Press; 2012.

Hafferty FW. Beyond curriculum reform: confronting medicine's hidden curriculum. Acad Med. 1998;73

Hafferty F, Castellani B. The hidden curriculum: a theory of medical education. In: Brosnan C, Turner B, editors. Handbook of the sociology of medical education. Routledge; 2009.

Hanna M, Fins JJ. Viewpoint: power and communication: why simulation training ought to be complemented by experiential and humanist learning. Acad Med. 2006;81:265–70.

Hargie O, Boohan M, Mccoy M, Murphy P. Current trends in communication skills training in UK schools of medicine. Med Teach. 2010;32:385–91.

Healthtalk.Org. Healthtalkonline [Online]. 2019. Available: https://www.healthtalk.org/. Accessed 30 July 2020.

Hojat M, Vergare MJ, Maxwell K, Brainard G, Herrine SK, Isenberg GA, Veloski J, Gonnella JS. The devil is in the third year: a longitudinal study of erosion of empathy in medical school. Acad Med. 2009;84:1182–91.

Hower KI, Vennedey V, Hillen HA, Kuntz L, Stock S, Pfaff H, Ansmann L. Implementation of patient-centred care: which organisational determinants matter from decision maker's perspective? Results from a qualitative interview study across various health and social care organisations. BMJ Open. 2019;9:e027591.

Illingworth R. Patient-centredness. In: Brown J, Noble LM, Papageourgiou A, Kidd J, editors. Clinical communication in medicine. Wiley Blackwell; 2016.

Jewson ND. The disappearance of the sick-man from medical cosmology, 1770-1870. Sociology. 1976;10:225–44.

Kaba R, Sooriakumaran P. The evolution of the doctor-patient relationship. Int J Surg. 2007;5:57–65.

Krupat E, Frankel R, Stein T, Irish J. The four habits coding scheme: validation of an instrument to assess clinicians' communication behaviour. Patient Educ Couns. 2006;62:38–45.

Kurtz S, Silverman J, Benson J, Draper J. Marrying content and process in clinical method teaching: enhancing the Calgary-Cambridge guides. Acad Med. 2003;78:802–9.

Lane C, Rollnick S. The use of simulated patients and role-play in communication skills training: A review of the literature to August 2005. Patient Educ Couns. 2007;67:13–20.

Lave J, Wenger E. Situated learning: legitimate peripheral participation. Cambridge: Cambridge University Press; 1991.

Maynard DW, Heritage J. Conversation analysis, doctor-patient interaction and medical communication. Med Educ. 2005;39:428–35.

Mcwhinney I. The need for a transformed clinical method. In: Stewart M, Roter D, editors. Communicating with medical patients. Newbury Park: Sage Publications; 1989.

Mead N, Bower P. Patient-centredness: a conceptual framework and review of the empirical literature. Soc Sci Med. 2000;51:1087–110.

Mead N, Bower P. Patient-centred consultations and outcomes in primary care: a review of the literature. Patient Educ Couns. 2002;48:51–61.

Mead N, Bower P, Hann M. The impact of general practitioners' patient-centredness on patients' post-consultation satisfaction and enablement. Soc Sci Med. 2002;55:283–99.

Mishler EG. The discourse of medicine: dialectics of medical interviews. Norwood: Ablex Publishing Corporation; 1984.

Noble LM, Scott-Smith W, O'Neill, B. & Salisbury, H. Consensus statement on an updated core communication curriculum for UK undergraduate medical education. Patient Educ Couns. 2018;101:1712–9.

Oswald A, Czupryn J, Wiseman J, Snell L. Patient-centred education: what do students think? Med Educ. 2014;48:170–80.

Patientvoices.Org.Uk. Patients voices [Online]. Pilgrim Projects Limited. 2020. Available: https://www.patientvoices.org.uk/. Accessed 30 July 2020.

Pawlikowska T, Zhang W, Griffiths F, Van Dalen J, Van Der Vleuten C. Verbal and non-verbal behaviour of doctors and patients in primary care consultations – how this relates to patient enablement. Patient Educ Couns. 2012;86:70–6.

Petrova M, Dale J, Fulford BKWM. Values-based practice in primary care: easing the tensions between individual values, ethical principles and best evidence. Br J Gen Pract. 2006;56:703–9.

Picker.Org. Picker Institute [Online]. Picker Institute Europe. https://www.picker.org/. Accessed 30 July 2020.

Porter R. The greatest benefit to mankind: a medical history of humanity from antiquity to the present. London: Harper Collins; 1997.

Rathert C, Wyrwich MD, Boren SA. Patient-centred care and outcomes: a systematic review of the literature. Med Care Res Rev. 2012;70:351–79.

Rider EA, Kurtz S, Slade D, Longmaid Iii HE, Ho M-J, Pun JK-H, Eggins S, Branch WT Jr. The international charter for human values in healthcare: an interprofessional global collaboration to enhance values and communication in healthcare. Patient Educ Couns. 2014;96:273–80.

Roter D, Larson S. The Roter interaction analysis system (RIAS): utility and flexibility for analysis of medical interactions. Patient Educ Couns. 2002;46:243–51.

Salmon P, Young B. Core assumptions and research opportunities in clinical communication. Patient Educ Couns. 2005;58:225–34.

Scholl I, Zill JM, Härter M, Dirmaier J. An integrative model of patient-centredness - a systematic review and concept analysis. PLoS One. 2014;9(9):e107828. Published 2014 Sep 17. https://doi.org/10.1371/journal.pone.0107828

Skelton J. Language and clinical communication - this bright Babylon. Routledge; 2008.

Skinner BF. The science of learning and the art of teaching. In: Skinner BF, editor. The technology of teaching. New York: Meredith Corporation; 1954.

Spencer J, Godolphin W, Karpenko N, Towle A. Can patients be teachers: involving patients and service users in healthcare professionals' education. The Health Foundation; 2011.

Stewart MA. Effective physician-patient communication and health outcomes: a review. CMAJ. 1995;152:1423–33.

Stewart M, Brown JB, Weston WW, McWhinney IR, McWilliam Cl & Freeman TR. Patient-Centred Medicine: Transforming the Clinical Method. Oxford: Radcliffe Medical Press Limited; 2006.

Street RL. How clinician-patient communication contributes to health improvement: modeling pathways from talk to outcome. Patient Educ Couns. 2013;92:286–91.

Szasz TS, Hollender MH. A contribution to the philosophy of medicine: the basic models of the doctor-patient relationship. JAMA Intern Med. 1956;97:585–92.

Van Dalen J, Hout JCHMV, Wolfhagen HAP, Scherpbier AJJA, Vleuten CPMVD. Factors influencing the effectiveness of communication skills training: programme contents outweigh teachers' skills. Med Teach. 1999;21:308–10.

Van Dalen J, Kerkhofs E, Van Knippenberg-Van Den Berg BW, Van Den Hout HA, Scherpbier AJ, Van Der Vleuten CP. Longitudinal and concentrated communication skills programmes: two dutch medical schools compared. Adv Health Sci Educ Theory Pract. 2002;7:29–40.

Van Den Eertwegh V, Van Dalen J, Van Dulmen S, Van Der Vleuten C, Scherpbier A. Residents' perceived barriers to communication skills learning: comparing two medical working contexts in postgraduate training. Patient Educ Couns. 2014;95:91–7.

Vygotsky LS. Mind in society: the development of higher psychological processes. Cambridge, MA: Harvard University Press; 1978.

Yardley S, Irvine AW, Lefroy J. Minding the gap between communication skills simulation and authentic experience. Med Educ. 2013;47:495–510.

Contemporary Sociological Issues for Health Professions Curricula

80

Margaret Simmons

Contents

Introduction	1554
Contemporary Sociological Issues for Health Professions Curricula	1554
Refugee and Asylum Seeker Health	1557
Sustainability	1560
Rurality	1563
Conclusion	1565
Cross-References	1566
References	1566

Abstract

This chapter explores three contemporary sociological issues in health professions curricula in the setting of a graduate-entry medical program in rural Australia using three very topical and political examples. The three issues under sociological investigation are refugee/asylum seeker health, sustainability, and rurality. The chapter seeks to address several key questions in the context of health professions curricula including why sociology is important, what it offers to health professional students, and how it can be appropriately embedded within the health professions curricula.

Keywords

Refugee/asylum seeker · Sustainability · Rurality · Sociology · Health professions curricula

M. Simmons (✉)
Monash Rural Health, Monash University, Churchill, VIC, Australia
e-mail: Margaret.simmons@monash.edu

© Springer Nature Singapore Pte Ltd. 2023
D. Nestel et al. (eds.), *Clinical Education for the Health Professions*,
https://doi.org/10.1007/978-981-15-3344-0_129

Introduction

This chapter explores three contemporary sociological issues in health professions curricula in the context of a graduate-entry medical program in rural Australia: refugee/asylum seeker health, sustainability, and rurality. The chapter will highlight what sociology can offer to the health professions using these three topical and political examples. A social perspective on health is vital for a well-informed health professional and complements the more traditional biomedical model of health. Using key sociological concepts such as C. Wright Mills' "sociological imagination" (Mills 1959) and Foucault's (Germov 2019) notions on power; bringing in authorities on these three learning topics; and utilizing reflective techniques along with media, film, art, and literature, it will be demonstrated how sociology can overlay a health professional's learning in a way which informs, excites, and generates curiosity and discussion. We know historically from the work of Virchow (Mechanic 1990) that social, cultural, economic, and political factors are often the major factors behind disease and ill health. With some of the current complex issues impacting on health, such as climate change and marginalization due to rurality or refugee status, taking a sociological perspective on health is even more important.

Contemporary Sociological Issues for Health Professions Curricula

The context for the work in this chapter is a small (circa 100 student) graduate-entry medical program in rural Australia, and while the chapter's aim is to explore contemporary sociological issues in *health professions* curricula, it will necessarily have a specific focus on *medical* curricula. It is argued, however, that the approaches and ideas used to teach medical students about the contemporary issues of refugee health, sustainability, and rurality are also applicable to other health professions students. In sociological terms moreover, medical students have no claim to a specific or unique body of knowledge in regard to these contemporary issues; these issues are pertinent to anyone working in the field of health care and merit further exploration and engagement.

While a social perspective on health is vital for any well-informed health professional and acts to balance the more traditional biomedical model of health, it *is* frequently argued that the biomedical model of health is limited (Nettleton 2006). Indeed, it is suggested that the biomedical model is reductionist and fails to consider the social determinants of health alongside social injustices and health inequities (Nettleton 2006; Annandale 1998; White 2017; Barry and Yuill 2012). Such inequities and injustices are overlaid by issues of class, gender, ethnicity, ecology, and power in the social worlds of people which thus impact on health outcomes at both the individual and population level and subsequently demand a sociological exploration (White 2017). The Black Report in the United Kingdom in the 1980s demonstrated how socioeconomic status and ethnicity affected health - highlighting the unequal distribution of morbidity and mortality in Britain based on those measures (Gray 1982).

Further back in history, over a century ago, Virchow - in arguing that access to health care is a human right - stated that "medicine is in essence a social science, and politics nothing more than medicine on a larger scale." (p. 67) (quoted in Lahelma 2001). Farmer (2003) concurs with the notion that health is a human right and uses poetry to argue for social justice and equity. Bertolt Brecht's (Farmer 2003) poem "A Worker's Speech to a Doctor" illustrates that disease and illness arise from social conditions:

> When we come to you
> Our rags are torn off us
> And you listen all over our naked body.
> As to the cause of our illness
> One glance at our rags would
> Tell you more. It is the same cause that wears out
> Our bodies and our clothes.
> The pain in our shoulder comes
> You say, from the damp; and this is also the reason
> For the stain on the wall of our flat.
> So tell us:
> Where does the damp come from? (p. 39) (Farmer 2003).

If we accept that disease and illness arise from social conditions, then it is imperative for health professions students to consider the social origins of those diseases, not only in order to try and find solutions to the issues but to better understand and support their future patients. The imperative therefore is to educate health professionals about contemporary sociological issues. However, while the teaching of a social perspective on health, including the social determinants of health, is quite widespread, it is not universal. In a 2014 poll of medical educators through the Association for Medical Education in Europe (AMEE), 77% said that the social determinants of health and social issues *were* taught in their medical programs (Association for Medical Education in Europe (AMEE) n.d.). In the graduate-entry medical program at a rural preclinical teaching site of the Doctor of Medicine (MD) program of Monash University, Australia, teaching a social perspective on health is a compulsory and highly valued part of the curricula, as evidenced by its inclusion in the program's assessment component and its learning objectives. The learning objectives include associations between health, illness, and social influences such as ecology, social position, and place (among others), all of which encompass access to health care and public policy.

Three contemporary sociological issues commensurate with these objectives have been selected for the focus of this chapter as they are considered topical, politically important, and interesting. Anecdotal evidence over many years of teaching these topics demonstrate their usefulness and appeal to students, such as "[t]hanks for sharing your passion with us and teaching us all about the challenges of rural health care"; "[t]hank you for reminding us to think about the whole person and for providing a holistic view to our studies"; "I've loved learning and discussing all the different topics..."; and "[the subject] has been a highlight for me this year. Not only will it make me a better doctor, but a better person as well."

In the medical program, the tool or "template" (Germov 2019) that is used to teach a social perspective on health is the "sociological imagination." It is not necessary for health professionals to become sociologists – although this would make for an interesting health-care sector – but it is useful for them to have some theoretical "tools" in their toolbox to help them make sense of the social world. Taking a sociological perspective; seeing issues through a social lens; or applying the sociological imagination will enable health professional students to better understand the social and health problems and issues that beset their clients and patients.

The sociological imagination is a term first coined by sociologist C. Wright Mills and "enables us to grasp history and biography and the relations between the two within society" (p. 6) (Mills 1959). The sociological imagination moves its user beyond "taken-for-granted" assumptions and requires a critical examination and questioning of the social structures, histories, cultures, values, language, and other practices and ideologies that impact on social dynamics, behavior, and health (Barry and Yuill 2012; Willis and Elmer 2011). With a critical sensibility, as espoused through the sociological imagination, the health professions student is tasked with asking "how can it be otherwise?" and inevitably from there should interrogate where and how power is situated (Willis 1999, 2011).

To grasp the impact of where power lies and the inevitable power imbalances that arise in health care, it is useful for health professions students to appreciate a Foucauldian understanding of power. Michel Foucault's work commands an interrogation of the origins of power, an exploration of the social order, a critique of the medical "gaze" (or the way the body is regulated and viewed in medicine and health care), and a recognition of notions of the "body" and acts of self-surveillance, which are all integral parts of the way society is organized, particularly in relation to the medical experience (Nettleton 2006; Lupton 2012; Cockerham 2001).

Through the interrogation of power and critiquing of the medical experience, the student utilizing the sociological imagination is inspired to learn more and hopefully to make a difference. Indeed, according to Mills, the sociological imagination is both exciting and transformative for its adopters: "[t]heir capacity for astonishment is made lively again. They acquire a new way of thinking....by their reflection and by their sensibility, they realize the cultural meaning of the social sciences" (p. 8) (Mills 1959). The tool of the sociological imagination is a way of thinking, a *quality* of thinking which enables a greater understanding of not only the self but also wider society, a term known as reflexivity (Mills 1959; Willis 2011).

It is argued that sociology differs from other disciplines in health professions education because of this invitation to be reflexive, which demands a step away from clinical and personal practice (Scambler 2012; Turner 2004). Within the subject at the rural education site that is the context of this chapter, students are encouraged to reflect, not only on themselves and their own views of the world but the worlds within which they will practice, thus expanding their knowledge of the social issues they will encounter once they leave the education site.

Reflective techniques and engagement are encouraged in the curricula through forums and questions along with the use of social media, documentaries, film, art, games, and literature. The pedagogy behind the use of these reflective teaching techniques draws on the work of Bolton and Shapiro and Rucker (Bolton 2014; Shapiro and Rucker 2003). As Shapiro and Rucker argue, "[t]he craft and artistry of literature and painting can help learners see clinical situations and patients not only from different perspectives, but also with greater clarity, identifying insights and feelings in ways learners might not be able to fully articulate" (p. 954) (Shapiro and Rucker 2003). The study of the social side of medicine through more humanities-type techniques utilizing reflexivity "creates a welcome zone of safety and relaxation" (p. 954) (Shapiro and Rucker 2003) which is borne out in anecdotal student feedback: "your classes were always a nice breath of fresh air away from the complexities of the [technical and clinical sciences]" and "we could relax in your classes and catch our breath; but you still made us think." In addition to innovative and diverse delivery techniques, the subject of a social perspective on health also includes a raft of expert guest speakers on the various topics explored throughout the year.

Thus, health professions students are taught a social perspective on health; indeed, they need "social theory ...in order to resocialize their understanding of who becomes sick and why, and of who has access to health care and why" (p. 138) (Farmer 2003). As access to health care is a social justice issue, three topics have been selected to focus on in this chapter because they are topical, political, and highly valued by students. Refugee and asylum seeker health, sustainability, and rural health will now be explored in more depth to demonstrate the impact of the issues at the individual and societal level in terms of health and also how the sociological perspective enhances student understanding of these public issues.

Refugee and Asylum Seeker Health

With the topic of refugee and asylum seeker health, it is important for health professions students to appreciate the complex health and social issues faced by refugees and asylum seekers in the community and particularly of those incarcerated in Australian mainland and offshore detention centers. Students should also understand the appropriate clinical resources available in their area, as well as the current political environment regarding the entry of asylum seekers into Australia and their subsequent treatment. An asylum seeker is a person who is seeking refuge or protection but has not yet been granted refugee status (Phillips 2015) and, according to the 1951 United Nations Refugee Convention, may need to breach a country's immigration rules. A refugee, according to the convention, is "someone who is unable or unwilling to return to their country of origin owing to a well-founded fear of being persecuted for reasons of race, religion, nationality, membership of a particular social group, or political opinion" (p. 3) (United Nations High Commissioner for Refugees (UNHCR) UN Refugee Agency 1951). The number of refugees and displaced persons across the world is huge with the World Health Organization estimating there are a billion migrants globally, of whom 68 million are forcibly displaced largely due to war and conflict (World Health Organization: Refugee and migrant health 2019). While Australia has settled around 800,000 refugees and displaced persons since World War II, it is currently granting 13,750 places a year in its humanitarian program (Phillips 2015).

The topic of refugee health is highly amenable to being explored sociologically and in particular through utilizing the tool of the sociological imagination. By understanding the historical, political, and structural ramifications of the issue, the health professions student is better placed to manage the social and health issues of refugees and to think about how the situation might be different at both an individual and societal level. Historically, Australia's treatment of refugees and asylum seekers has been complicated and even criticized by the United Nations Human Rights Commission (UNHRC) which argues that Australian policies do not meet international standards (United Nations Human Rights Commission (UNHRC) 2002). In a 2002 visit to Australian detention centers, the UNHRC was particularly concerned about the indefinite length of detention of asylum seekers along with the conditions in the centers which they likened to prisons. Their report describes closely monitored "inmates," razor wire surrounds, permanent surveillance, handcuffs used whenever asylum seekers are escorted outside, and escapees being prosecuted (United Nations Human Rights Commission (UNHRC) 2002). Under these draconian conditions, the delegation found mental health issues, behaviors including self-harming, and suicide attempts in what they reported as "collective depression syndrome" (United Nations Human Rights Commission (UNHRC) 2002). Meanwhile, the Australian government proclaims that immigration detention is "administrative not punitive" (Australian Border Force 2019).

Moreover, refugees living in the community, as well as those seeking asylum and living either in the community or in detention centers, have specific combinations of health issues which are rarely encountered in other population groups in Australia. Nutrition-related conditions, preventable communicable diseases, and poor mental health arising from histories of torture and trauma are prevalent. Reduced access to health care as a result of linguistic and cultural barriers and limited access to Medicare (Medicare is the Australian government taxpayer-subsidized scheme that provides low- or no-cost access to health care. See https://www.healthdirect.gov.au/what-is-medicare) and the Pharmaceutical Benefits Scheme (The Pharmaceutical Benefits Scheme is a government-sponsored scheme that provides subsidized medicines to Australian citizens. See http://www.pbs.gov.au/info/about-the-pbs) also contribute to poorer health outcomes in comparison with other groups (Australian Medical Association (AMA) 2015; Victorian Refugee Health Network: Asylum Seeker Health 2015).

Australia's history with regard to refugees and asylum seekers has always been murky, intersected as it is with government and structural policies toward immigration and its problematic legacy of the treatment of Indigenous peoples in Australia. Some have argued that Australia has had a continuous history of locking people up in spaces likened to concentration camps such as Aboriginal "reserves," internment camps, quarantine hospitals, psychiatric institutions, and reform schools which have all positioned people in particular deleterious ways (Nethery 2002). It is important to ask the critical question of who is being "protected" from whom in in these spaces and to think about the power relations involved in these situations.

In some cases, history shows that situations improve over time, yet while Australia had supposedly ended the White Australia Policy (The Australian Government in 1901 legislated measures that were racially exclusive with the aim to "... keep before us the noble idea of a white Australia—snow-white Australia if you will. Let it be pure and spotless" – hence the notion of a "White Australia policy." See https://www.aph.gov.au/About_Parliament/Parliamentary_Departments/Parliamentary_Library/pubs/APF/monographs/Within_Chinas_Orbit/Chapterone) in the 1970s, the 1990s saw the introduction of mandatory detention and a more hard-line approach to anyone seeking asylum (Neumann and Tavan 2002). Political, cultural, and social narratives promulgated through the media all combined to deny any welcome to "boat people," "queue jumpers," or "illegals" (Phillips 2015; Burnside 2015) despite the United Nations Convention stipulating that "subject to specific exceptions, refugees should not be penalized for their illegal entry or stay," nor under the principle of non-refoulement, should refugees be returned to a place where they fear for their life (p. 3) (United Nations High Commissioner for Refugees (UNHCR) UN Refugee Agency 1951). Thus, the topic of asylum seekers and refugees has to be understood in its historical, social, structural, and cultural context in order to gain a deeper understanding of the issues. Only by being aware of where power relations lie in relation to these matters can the health impacts of those involved be fully appreciated and then solutions sought.

In terms of solutions, health professions students are often highly motivated to seek and make changes. Encouraging change and challenging the status quo is an important element of the sociological imagination and can be part of an educator's remit. While acknowledging that change can be difficult, it must be reinforced that health professionals are often best placed to make a difference for people at the individual and societal level. Some examples of where this has happened in relation to refugees and asylum seekers include doctors agitating and succeeding in getting the Australian Medevac Bill enshrined in law in 2018 (Refugee Council of Australia 2019). The Medevac Bill states that two independent doctors can recommend that a refugee or asylum seeker in offshore detention (which at the time of writing is Manus Island or Nauru) can be brought to the Australian mainland for treatment. This Bill effectively creates an independent medical process thus removing medical decisions from bureaucrats and politicians (Refugee Council of Australia 2019). However, in December 2019, the Medevac Bill was repealed (see Asylum Seeker Resource Centre: asrc.org.au/medevac/faq).

Another example of where health professionals have made a difference occurred when doctors and other health personnel from the Royal Children's Hospital in Melbourne refused to allow patients to return to offshore detention, arguing that it would be dangerous and unethical to do so (Hatch et al. 2015). While this move to defy laws, which threaten 2 years jail for health workers who "blow the whistle" on detention center conditions (Hatch et al. 2015) is brave, it also aligns strongly with the critique of the sociological imagination in demonstrating how health professionals can make a difference. Further, the Australian Medical Association has expressed the view that detention is deleterious to health and violates people's human rights and seeks as a matter of urgency a solution to indeterminate lengthy stays in detention

(Australian Medical Association (AMA) 2015). Other recommendations to address the issue of refugee and asylum seeker health from the United Nations include reviews of Australian laws and policies, a reduction or elimination of the time spent by asylum seekers in detention, better training for immigration officers, and the provision of legal aid to asylum seekers to ensure that Australia meets its obligations under international law (United Nations Human Rights Commission (UNHRC) 2002).

Further initiatives that highlight the critique of the sociological imagination include the formation of a group, Doctors for Refugees (D4R), who are passionate advocates for the rights and the health of their refugee and asylum seeker patients. Two of their medical student members argue:

> As future healthcare professionals, medical students are stakeholders in all of the same health issues that doctors are. For many of us, the prime impetus behind our desire to practice medicine involves an essential need to leave the world a better place. To achieve this, a broad spectrum of inequalities must be overcome, such that all people truly have access to the fundamental human right of health. One of the most glaring inequalities in Australia is our behaviour towards refugees and asylum seekers. (Betts and Fernandes 2018)

Thus, it is clear that the topic of refugees and asylum seeker should be viewed through a sociological lens in order to better understand and to elicit change on this issue. While the discussion has largely revolved around political refugees seeking refuge from war and conflict, it is also important for health professional students to recognize the increased risk of climate change, forcing many peoples across the world to flee the ravages of rising sea levels and other weather calamities (Doherty 2017). The next section explores the issue of climate change and sustainability in terms of a social perspective on health and what that may mean for health professionals and health professions students.

Sustainability

With the topic of sustainability, there is a need for health professions students to understand how health and sustainability are linked and the implications for the health system from a changing climate and subsequent biodiversity effects. Ecology, place, and access to health care are key areas for greater knowledge, recognizing that it is the most vulnerable, the poor, the elderly, rural, remote, and disadvantaged groups of people who will be more severely impacted by climate change. Just as exploring the issue of refugees through the sociological imagination assists in a deeper appreciation of all the factors involved, the tool can equally help health professions students understand more about the issue of sustainability and climate change. The notion of sustainability is variable and contested and its definition depends on which group is doing the defining. These definitional dilemmas have emerged because different disciplines are all trying to tackle the issue from their different perspectives (Moore et al. 2017). However, we do know that sustainability has impacts on people socially, economically, and environmentally (Moore et al. 2017) and therefore it should be examined from these aspects as well as historically.

Exploring sustainability historically, we learn that the concept arose in Germany in the eighteenth century (translated from the German *Nachhaltigkeit*) and was a term coined in forestry to avoid overharvesting (Kuhlman and Farrington 2010). There are elements of stewardship of the environment involved in sustainability as well as the preservation of resources for future generations (Kuhlman and Farrington 2010). In more recent years, sustainability has increasingly come to be linked with climate change, although the two terms are not necessarily interchangeable. As O'Donnell and MacDougall explain, sustainability is about continuation and meeting the "needs of the present without compromising the ability of future generations to meet their own needs" (p. 185) (O'Donnell and MacDougall 2016).

In terms of climate change specifically, the science is concerning. The United Nations Intergovernmental Panel on Climate Change (IPCC) states that human action across the planet has created a one-degree Celsius rise in temperature. The IPCC predict a rise to 1.5 degrees by the mid-twenty-first century (Masson-Delmotte et al. 2018). The Australian Bureau of Meteorology more direly predicts that over the next 50 years, average temperatures could climb by $5°C$ unless there are significant reductions in greenhouse gas emissions (Australian Government 2018). The outcomes from these temperature rises include rising sea levels from melting sea ice, decreased water quality, more extreme weather events, and fire dangers, and, along with the concomitant increasing air and water pollution from fossil fuel burning, there are risks to biodiversity, water quality, food security, and habitat destruction impacting on agriculture and the entire ecosystem (Masson-Delmotte et al. 2018; Australian Government 2018; Watts et al. 2018). Direct consequences of climate change on human health include an additional "250,000 deaths per year, from malnutrition, malaria, diarrhoea and heat stress" (World Health Organization n.d.). The economic cost to human health is estimated to be up to USD 4 billion dollars by 2030 (World Health Organization n.d.). The cost to the planet is incalculable.

The environmental and health threats of climate change will place health professionals at the frontline of all these events and outcomes. It is imperative therefore that an understanding of the risks and dangers forms part of health professions curricula (Verrinder and Verrinder 2012). And while it is important that health professions students understand the science behind climate change, they also need to consider the social, cultural, political, and economic ramifications of the issue. As previously stated, it will be the poorest and the most vulnerable who will be most immediately and severely affected. Those living in lowest-lying areas (often in developing countries) will fall prey to more frequent and dangerous storms and rising sea levels; the rates of infectious diseases will increase, and floods and famine will have more serious implications including the inevitability of more people being displaced (Masson-Delmotte et al. 2018; Zhang et al. 2018).

In Australia, the Indigenous peoples and people living remotely are also more likely to be affected by climate change, particularly given Aboriginal and Torres Strait Islander peoples' close and sensitive connection with the land. Indeed, Bell (1998) argues that we must recognize that for Indigenous people there is a "complex identification of land as a sentient body and as kin, of damage to land as constituting a desecration... and an injury to the living" (p. 268). This Indigenous ethical and cultural relationship with the land sends two messages, the first that the effects of climate change will be even more impactful for the physical and mental health of Indigenous peoples and second that there is much that could be learned from their successful environmental stewardship of the Australian landscape over many thousands of years (O'Donnell and MacDougall 2016).

For these reasons, understanding the risks of climate change itself is vitally important to health professions students. However, sustainability should also be embraced through a more informed knowledge of the health-care system. It is crucial to recognize that the health system is a heavy consumer of resources including water, carbon, energy, and other materials, so knowledge of how this occurs and how processes can be improved to reduce environmental impacts is important (Cole 2009; Kayak 2011). From small initiatives such as using "keep-cups" for coffee to larger modifications including improved hospital design, recycling equipment and medications, and composting waste, there are many ways in which health professionals can make a difference (45, 46), thus applying the critique of the sociological imagination to their own workplaces. Health professions students are often keen to pursue these measures, and this is evidenced by a guest speaker who returns to talk to the medical students every year about the issue of sustainability and climate change, who was themselves part of the cohort and demonstrates a clear mandate and passion for passing knowledge on.

In response to the risks of climate change and to advance sustainability of the health of the Australian people, the Australian Medical Association has formally declared climate change to be a "health emergency" (Australian Medical Association (AMA) 2019). This move is in-line with the World Health Organization, the British and American Medical Associations, and Doctors for the Environment Australia (Australian Medical Association (AMA) 2019). Of course, if we are to fully explore the issue of climate change, underpinned by understandings of where power lies, it is necessary to examine the ways in which governments respond to climate change and produce policies and demonstrate leadership. According to Doctors for the Environment Australia [DEA], the government has been slow to transition to renewables and low carbon electricity generation, and they are advocating for more government initiatives (Australian Medical Association (AMA) 2019). As an example of how health professionals can make a difference, on 16 September 2019, DEA delivered thousands of pledges to health Minister Greg Hunt calling on immediate and bipartisan action on climate change; these pledges came from over 2000 health professionals as well as the Royal Australian College of General Practitioners (RACGP), The Royal Australasian College of Physicians (RACP), the Australian College of Rural and Remote Medicine (ACRRM), and the Australian Medical Students' Association (AMSA) (Australian Medical Association (AMA) 2019).

A further example of how health professionals can make a difference in terms of responses to climate change includes a working group formed by the medical deans of Australia and New Zealand (MDANZ) (Madden et al. 2018). The working group's aim is to develop resources and curricula to address issues of climate change impacts (Madden et al. 2018). At the nexus between health and climate change, health professionals and health professions students will play a critical role in educating, addressing, and managing the expected effects of climate change. As Zhang et al. (2018) point out, Australia "has an enormous opportunity to take action and protect human health and lives" (p. 474.e1) and has the health professional expertise to achieve this. Yet it appears that few Australian medical schools teach sustainability and/or climate change. To combat this omission, medical students through AMSA have developed their own online short course (Madden et al. 2018), thus applying the critique of the sociological imagination. Another way that health professionals have challenged the status quo is by forming organizations such as Doctors for the Environment Australia (DEA n.d.) and Healthy Futures (n.d.) both of which welcome medical students into their ranks, with the latter accepting other health professionals as well.

Taking a social perspective on the issue of climate change promotes a Foucauldian view of where power lies and a critique of government and even the media on the issue of sustainability and climate change. There is evidence that media items about climate change and health in Australia declined by 50% during the years 2008–2017, in comparison to a large increase globally in the same period (Zhang et al. 2018). These issues are political, and it behooves the health professions student to be informed and engaged with them. Chastonay et al. (2015) argue that health professionals are in the privileged and unique position to be at the forefront in taking action against climate change and its effects and to advocate on behalf of the most disadvantaged in our communities. One of the many groups that will be most severely affected will be those living in rural areas, be that regionally or remotely. The next section will explore rurality in more detail through taking a social perspective on health.

Rurality

Rurality is the final issue that will be explored from a sociological perspective in this chapter. Through this undertaking, health professions students will be better able to understand the range of factors that can impact on health and wellbeing in rural communities; the diversity of rural communities; the need for a community approach to health; and the implications for a rural health workforce. The topic of rural health can be examined through the four elements of the sociological imagination by looking at its history, culture, and structure and then applying a critique to gain a deeper appreciation of rural health issues and potential solutions.

Around one third of Australians live in rural or remote areas of Australia (Humphreys 2012). On the surface, rural and remote areas of Australia might appear to be healthier than metropolitan environments, which have higher rates of pollution, traffic, pedestrian and public transport overcrowding, and housing unaffordability as well as high rates of stress (Hughes 2019). The paradox is that rural people have the worst health outcomes of all Australians despite the apparently "healthier" environment in which they live (Hughes 2019). Some of the reasons for this disparity include lack of access to health care, education, employment; lower levels of health literacy and income; and poorer roads and housing (National Rural Health Alliance 2011). In remote areas of Australia, the differences are even more marked with diabetes rates three times higher, road accidents five times higher, twice the number of suicides, and higher rates of death to lung cancer and cardiovascular disease (National Rural Health Alliance 2016; Bourke et al. 2019).

One of the most serious health-related problems for people living in rural areas is the lack of access to specialist medical services, pharmacists, mental health professionals, rehabilitation services, and allied and dental health care (Bourke et al. 2019). Indeed, there are 80% less specialists in remote areas of Australia compared with metropolitan areas (National Rural Health Alliance 2016). Management of both acute and chronic illnesses is more difficult the further away from major cities people live (National Rural Health Alliance 2016). An example of the disparities between rural and metropolitan access to health care is the very low rates of podiatrists (critical for diabetes management) with only one podiatrist for every 20,000 persons in remote Australia (National Rural Health Alliance 2016). As Smith (2007) argues, rural Australia is "the home of some of the greatest health inequalities in the world" (p. 87).

In terms of understanding more about rural Australia, it is important to explore the multi-dimensions of Australian rurality; often romanticized, particularly in film and by the media, rural Australians have been portrayed as stoic, as "battlers" – but this vision is often aggressively masculinized and stereotyped and thereby leaves out women, Indigenous Australians, and migrants, among others (Bell 2005; Kaino 2000). Indeed, it has even been argued that some places in rural Australia are mythologized as "outposts of racism, poverty, misogyny and environmental vandalism" (p. 176) (Bell 2005). These myths are problematic in that they can flow over to workplaces where rural Australia is viewed as less attractive in terms of health-care practice (Bourke et al. 2010).

It is therefore critical that rural Australia is appreciated for its diversity and its complexities at the same time acknowledging the rural health disadvantages. Health professions students need to understand that avoiding a deficit model is vital; instead the focus should be on the richness, rewards, and opportunities of living and working rurally when they graduate (Bourke et al. 2010). The deficit model is particularly inappropriate when it comes to Indigenous health because it overlooks the strong Indigenous connection to land and its familial and kin relationships (Bourke et al. 2010). As Gary Foley argues, the problem is not in Aboriginal society, nor is it necessary for white people to enter Aboriginal communities to "help" (which has been done in the past with devastating effects) but that non-Indigenous people should be "daily challenging the ignorance and fear that is the greatest obstacle" to Indigenous peoples' wellbeing (p. 87) (Foley 2000). Tackling racism and recognizing the positions of power and privilege and the changes required in non-Indigenous society should be the goal for all, but particularly health professionals and health professions students in addressing Indigenous disadvantage and supporting the healing process (Foley 2000).

Identifying some of the historical, cultural, structural, and political elements that demonstrate the importance for health professions students to learn more about the topic of rurality, it is timely now to explore this topic through the critique of the sociological imagination. Some of the initiatives and solutions to the issues that face rural people, in particular, include the AMA's position on rural health. The AMA stance includes lobbying the government and those in power to make long-term commitments to the renewal and building of rural and regional public hospitals; training and better support for rural health professionals including medical students and doctors; and retaining and sustaining the rural health workforce to ensure that the complex health needs of rural people are not compromised (Australian Medical Association (AMA) 2016).

Other initiatives to support rural people include The National Rural Health Alliance which is Australia's leading nongovernment organization for the promotion and improvement of rural and remote health. This body suggests where there is a shortage of specialists, telehealth and video consultations can be used in diagnosis and treatment (National Rural Health Alliance 2016). Incentives and grants could also be provided to health professionals to overcome the rural health workforce shortages, and the AMA has a package of recommendations for ways to improve the doctor shortage. The AMA stresses that rural Australians deserve to have the same access to high-quality services that their metropolitan counterparts enjoy, and some of the measures they advocate include providing locum support, professional development opportunities, and flexible working hours as well as boosting the number of rural-origin medical students (AMA/Rural Doctors Association Australia (RDAA) 2016). Rural communities themselves can be agents of change where health professionals have the advantage of increased knowledge and understanding of their patients' needs, thus providing more opportunities to make changes; these are considered "ground-up" approaches to caring for rural people (Bourke et al. 2010). By exploring these issues sociologically and with the health professions understanding more about the problems facing rural Australians, it is hoped that change will happen.

Conclusion

Being able to think sociologically, to think independently, to ask questions about where power lies, and to seek solutions to issues are all facets of the tool of the sociological imagination (Willis 1999, 2011). This tool or skill is simple but valuable and can be utilized by health professions students within the curricula and beyond as they try and understand people and populations better. By exploring three contemporary social issues of refugee and asylum seeker health, sustainability, and rurality, it should be clear just how useful a sociological perspective can be in health professions curricula. Mills advises that the sociological imagination can be cultivated through reflexivity and taking another's perspective (Mills 1959). Indeed, rather eloquently, Mills advocates that in order to learn more, the student must allow the mind to "become a moving prism catching light from as many angles as possible" (p. 214) (Mills 1959). By taking another perspective or seeing through a sociological lens, the health professions student will hopefully be able to make a difference for their future clients and patients from an informed position. In a "call to arms" regarding the poor, which also applies to those impacted by refugee status, climate change, and rurality, Gutiérrez reminds us that the disadvantaged "are a by-product of the system in which we live and for which we are responsible. They are marginalized by our social and cultural world ... [h]ence the poverty of the [disadvantaged] is not a call to generous relief action, but a demand that we go and build a different social order" (p. 139) (Farmer 2003). A sociological perspective may just provide the understanding, the knowledge, and the impetus for those changes to occur.

Cross-References

▶ Future of Health Professions Education Curricula
▶ Planetary Health: Educating the Current and Future Health Workforce

References

AMA/Rural Doctors Association Australia (RDAA). Building a sustainable future for rural practice: the rural rescue package. Joint policy statement. 2016; 1-4. https://ama.com.au/system/tdf/documents/AMA-RDAA%20Rural%20Rescue%20Package%20Revision_Final.pdf?file=1&type=node&id=44019. Accessed 15 Sept 2019.

Annandale E. The sociology of health & medicine: a critical introduction. Cambridge: Polity Press; 1998.

Association for Medical Education in Europe (AMEE). Med Ed World. n.d. https://amee.org/getattachment/AMEE-Initiatives/MedEdWorld/38074-Social-Science-in-Med-Education-WEB.PDF. Accessed 12 Sept 2019.

Australian Border Force. Immigration detention in Australia. 2019. https://www.abf.gov.au/about-us/what-we-do/border-protection/immigration-detention. Accessed 14 Sept 2019.

Australian Government. Bureau of Meteorology & CSIRO. State of the Climate 2018. Commonwealth of Australia. 2018. http://www.bom.gov.au/state-of-the-climate/State-of-the-Climate-2018.pdf. Accessed 15 Sept 2019.

Australian Medical Association (AMA). Health care of asylum seekers and refugees – 2011. Revised 2015. https://ama.com.au/position-statement/health-care-asylum-seekers-and-refugees-2011-revised-2015. Accessed 12 Sept 2019.

Australian Medical Association (AMA). Position paper: a plan for better health care for regional, rural, and remote Australia. 26 May 2016. https://ama.com.au/position-statement/plan-better-health-care-regional-rural-and-remote-australia. Accessed 15 Sept 2019.

Australian Medical Association (AMA). Environmental sustainability in health care – 2019. 2019. https://ama.com.au/position-statement/environmental-sustainability-health-care-2019. Accessed 14 Sept 2019.

Barry AM, Yuill C. Understanding the sociology of health. 3rd ed. London: Sage; 2012.

Bell D. Ngarrindjeri Wurruwarrin: a world that is, was, and will be. North Melbourne: Spinifex Press; 1998.

Bell S. The wheatbelt in contemporary rural mythology. Rural Soc. 2005;15(2):176–90. https://doi.org/10.5172/rsj.351.15.2.176.

Betts N, Fernandes B. Medical students' perspective. Doctors for refugees members' publications. Doctors 4 refugees. AMA NSW. 2018. https://www.doctors4refugees.org/members-publications. Accessed 14 Sept 2019.

Bolton G. Reflective practice: writing and professional development. 4th ed. London: Sage Publications; 2014.

Bourke L, Humphreys JS, Wakerman J, Taylor J. From 'problem-describing' to problem-solving': challenging the 'deficit' view of remote and rural health. Aust J Rural Health. 2010;18(5):205–9. https://doi.org/10.1111/j.1440-1584.2010.01155.x.

Bourke L, Humphreys J, Wakerman J, Taylor J. Beyond the workforce crisis: developing contextual understanding of rural and remote health. 2019. https://www.ruralhealth.org.au/2rrhss/files/pre-reading/Bourke_Humphreys_Wakerman_Taylor.pdf. Accessed 13 Sept 2019.

Burnside J. What sort of country are we? The conversation. 2015. https://theconversation.com/julian-burnside-what-sort-of-country-are-we-48162. Accessed 11 Sept 2019.

Chastonay P, Zybach U, Simos J, Mattig T. Climate change: an opportunity for health promotion practitioners? Int J Pub Health. 2015;60(7):763–4. https://doi.org/10.1007/s00038-015-0709-4.

Cockerham WC. Medical sociology and sociological theory. In: Cockerham WC, editor. The Blackwell companion to medical sociology. Massachusetts: Blackwell Publishers; 2001. p. 3–22.

Cole A. Saving the planet as well as lives. BMJ. 2009;38:742–4. https://doi.org/10.1136/bmj.b933.

Doctors for the Environment (DEA). n.d. https://www.dea.org.au/about-dea/. Accessed 15 Sept 2019.

Doherty B. Disaster alley: Australia could be set to receive new wave of climate change refugees. The Guardian. 5/4/2017. https://www.theguardian.com/environment/2017/apr/05/disaster-alley-australia-could-be-set-to-receive-new-wave-of-climate-refugees. Accessed 15 Sept 2019.

Farmer P. Pathologies of power: health, human rights, and the new war on the poor. Berkeley: University of California Press; 2003.

Foley G. Whiteness and Blackness in the Koori struggle for self-determination: strategic considerations in the struggle for social justice for Indigenous people. Just Policy: A J Aust Soc Policy. 2000;9-20:4–88. https://search.informit.com.au/documentSummary;dn=200102959;res=IELAPA. Accessed 15 Sept 2019

Germov J. Imagining health problems as social issues. In: Germov J, editor. Second opinion: an introduction to health sociology. 6th ed. Docklands: Oxford University Press; 2019. p. 2–23.

Gray AM. Inequalities in health. The black report: a summary and comment. Int J Health Serv. 1982;12(3):349–80.

Hatch P, Ireland J, Booker C. Royal Children's Hospital doctors refuse to return children to detention. The Age. 10/10/2015. https://www.theage.com.au/national/victoria/royal-childrens-hospital-doctors-refuse-to-return-children-to-detention-20151010-gk63xm.html. Accessed 12 Sept 2019.

Healthy Futures. n.d. http://www.healthyfutures.net.au/about_us. Accessed 2 Sept 2019.

Hughes C. Rural health. In: Germov J, editor. Second opinion an introduction to health sociology. 6th ed. Docklands: Oxford University Press; 2019. p. 205–27.

Humphreys J. Rural and remote health. In: Willis E, Reynolds L, Keleher H, editors. Understanding the Australian health care system. 2nd ed. Chatswood: Elsevier Australia; 2012. p. 131–47.

Kaino L. Woop Woop(s) and woolly film-making: rural representations of culture in contemporary Australian feature film. Rural Soc. 2000;10(3):319–27. https://doi.org/10.5172/rsj.10.3.319.

Kayak E. Guide to Greening your Hospital. Doctors for the Environment Australia (DEA). 2011. https://www.dea.org.au/images/general/DEA-Guide_to_greening_hosp.pdf. Accessed 11 Sept 2019.

Kuhlman T, Farrington J. What is sustainability? Sustainability. 2010;2(11):3426–48. https://doi.org/10.3390/su2113436. Accessed 14 Sept 2019

Lahelma E. Health and social stratification. In: Cockerham WC, editor. The Blackwell companion to medical sociology. Massachusetts: Blackwell Publishers; 2001. p. 64–93.

Lupton D. Medicine as culture: illness, disease and the body. 3rd ed. London: Sage; 2012.

Madden DL, McLean M, Horton GL. Preparing medical graduates for the health effects of climate change: an Australasian collaboration. MJA. 2018;208(7):291–2. https://doi.org/10.5694/mja17.01172.

Masson-Delmotte V, Zhai P, Pörtner HO, Roberts D, Skea J, Shukla PR et al. IPCC: summary for policymakers. In: Global warming of 1.5°C. An IPCC special report. World Meteorological Organization, Switzerland; 2018. https://report.ipcc.ch/sr15/pdf/sr15_spm_final.pdf. Accessed 14 Sept 2019.

Mechanic D. Commentary: the role of sociology in health affairs. Health Aff. 1990;9(1):85–96. https://www.healthaffairs.org/doi/pdf/10.1377/hlthaff.9.1.85

Mills CW. The sociological imagination. Oxford: Oxford University Press; 1959.

Moore JE, Mascarenhas A, Bain J, Straus SE. Developing a comprehensive definition of sustainability. Implement Sci. 2017;12(110):1–8. https://implementationscience.biomedcentral.com/track/pdf/10.1186/s13012-017-0637-1. Accessed 14 Sept 2019

National Rural Health Alliance. Fact sheet 28: the determinants of health in rural and remote Australia. 2011. https://www.ruralhealth.org.au/sites/default/files/publications/factsheet-determinants-health-rural-australia.pdf. Accessed 9 Sept 2019.

National Rural Health Alliance. The health of people living in remote Australia. 2016. https://www.ruralhealth.org.au/sites/default/files/publications/nrha-remote-health-fs-election2016.pdf. Accessed 20 Aug 2019.

Nethery A. 'A modern-day concentration camp': using history to make sense of Australian immigration detention centres. In: Neumann K, Tavan G, editors. Does history matter? Making and debating citizenship, immigration and refugee policy in Australia and New Zealand. Canberra: ANU E Press; 2002. p. 65–80. Accessed 14 Sept 2019. https://press-files.anu.edu.au/downloads/press/p109651/pdf/book.pdf.

Nettleton S. The sociology of health and illness. 2nd ed. Cambridge: Polity Press; 2006.

Neumann K, Tavan G. Introduction. In: Neumann K, Tavan G, editors. Does history matter? Making and debating citizenship, immigration and refugee policy in Australia and New Zealand. Canberra: ANU E Press; 2002. p. 1–8. https://press-files.anu.edu.au/downloads/press/p109651/pdf/book.pdf. Accessed 14 Sept 2019.

O'Donnell K, MacDougall C. Social determinants and the health of Australia's first peoples. In: Keleher H, MacDougall C, editors. Understanding health. 4th ed. South Melbourne: Oxford University Press; 2016. p. 176–96.

Phillips J. Asylum seekers and refugees: what are the facts? Parliamentary library research paper. 2015. Accessed 14 Sept 2019.

Refugee Council of Australia. Medevac bill: the facts. 2019. https://www.refugeecouncil.org.au/umt-bill-facts/. Accessed 12 Sept 2019.

Scambler G. Teaching sociology to medical students. 2012. http://www.grahamscambler.com/teaching-sociology-to-medical-students/.

Shapiro J, Rucker L. Can poetry make better doctors? Teaching the humanities and arts to medical students and residents at the University of California, Irvine, College of Medicine. Acad Med. 2003;78(10):953–7.

Smith JD. Australia's rural and remote health: a social justice perspective. 2nd ed. Croydon: Tertiary Press; 2007.

Turner B. The new medical sociology: social forms of health and illness. Cambridge: University of Cambridge; 2004.

United Nations High Commissioner for Refugees (UNHCR) UN Refugee Agency. United Nations Convention and Protocol relating to the Status of Refugees. 1951. https://www.unhcr.org/protection/basic/3b66c2aa10/convention-protocol-relating-status-refugees.html. Accessed 14 Sept 2019.

United Nations Human Rights Commission (UNHRC). Economic and social council. Visit to Australia. 2002. https://documents-dds-ny.un.org/doc/UNDOC/GEN/G02/153/91/PDF/G0215391.pdf?OpenElement. Accessed 15 Sept 2019.

Verrinder G, Verrinder A. Climate change: drivers and health impacts, mitigation, and adaptation strategies for the health sector. In: Liamputtong P, Fanany R, Verrinder G, editors. Health, illness and well-being: perspectives and social determinants. South Melbourne: Oxford University Press; 2012. p. 136–53.

Victorian Refugee Health Network: Asylum Seeker Health. 2015. http://refugeehealthnetwork.org.au/wp-content/uploads/Asylum-seeker-health-April-2015.pdf. Accessed 14 Sept 2019.

Watts N, Amann M, Ayeb-Karlsson S, Belesova K, Bouley T, Boykof M, et al. The Lancet countdown on health and climate change: from 25 years of inaction to a global transformation for public health. Lancet. 2018;391:581–630. https://doi.org/10.1016/S0140-6736(17)32464-9.

White K. An introduction to the sociology of health and illness. 3rd ed. London: Sage; 2017.

Willis E. The sociological quest. 3rd ed. Allen & Unwin: St Leonards; 1999.

Willis E. The sociological quest: an introduction to the study of social life. 5th ed. Allen & Unwin: Crowsnest; 2011.

Willis K, Elmer S. Society, culture and health: an introduction to sociology for nurses. 2nd ed. South Melbourne: Oxford University Press; 2011.

World Health Organization. Climate change. n.d. https://www.who.int/health-topics/climate-change#tab=overview. Accessed 14 Sept 2019.

World Health Organization: Refugee and migrant health. 2019. https://www.who.int/migrants/en/. Accessed 12 Sept 2019.

Zhang Y, Beggs PJ, Bambrick H, Berry H, Linnluecke K, Trueck S, et al. The MJA–Lancet Countdown on health and climate change: Australian policy inaction threatens lives. MJA. 2018;209(11):474e1–e21. https://www.mja.com.au/journal/2018/209/11/mja-lancet-countdown-health-and-climate-change-australian-policy-inaction. Accessed 15 Sept 2019

Developing Clinical Reasoning Capabilities

81

Joy Higgs

Contents

Introduction	1572
Further Reading	1572
Clinical Reasoning: Exploring the Phenomenon	1573
Definition	1573
Further Reading	1575
The Changing Context of Professional Health Care Practice and Reasoning	1575
Further Reading	1577
Clinical Reasoning Approaches	1578
A Model of Clinical Reasoning as Encultured Decision-Making Capabilities	1578
Further Reading	1581
Learning, Teaching, and Developing Clinical Reasoning	1581
Facilitating the Development of Clinical Reasoning in Clinical Practice and Education Settings	1583
Further Reading	1584
Conclusion	1585
Cross-References	1585
References	1585

Abstract

This chapter addresses five questions: What is clinical reasoning as a metapractice? What are key elements of context in clinical reasoning and professional decision-making and what impact do they have on these practices? How can we categorize the main clinical reasoning and decision-making approaches? How can the learning and teaching of clinical reasoning and health care decision-making be facilitated and pursued? At the end of the chapter readers are invited to reflect on how the contents of the chapter have stimulated thoughts about their own reasoning practices and capabilities and their clinical reasoning development strategies.

J. Higgs (✉)
Professional Practice and Higher Education, Charles Sturt University, Sydney, NSW, Australia
e-mail: jhiggs@csu.edu.au

© Springer Nature Singapore Pte Ltd. 2023
D. Nestel et al. (eds.), *Clinical Education for the Health Professions*,
https://doi.org/10.1007/978-981-15-3344-0_103

Keywords

Clinical reasoning · Learning approaches · Capabilities · Pedagogies

Introduction

If we were to reduce professional practice in the health sciences to six essential ingredients, these could arguably be: humanity, professionalism (including ethical conduct), clinical reasoning or professional decision-making, reflexivity, effective communication, and profession-relevant technical capabilities. In this list we find what it takes to be:

- A client-centered person governed by a personal commitment to professional ethics in general and to the code of conduct of the given profession.
- A person capable of making sound health care decisions for the client's interest and to meet the performance and outcome expectations of the setting/organization where he or she works.
- An ethical agent of change in terms of health care intervention, education, and enhanced wellbeing outcomes.
- A collaborative partner and good communicator working with clients and colleagues.
- Someone who values others (clients, carers, and colleagues) and works with them to enhance clients' wellbeing.
- A professional in terms of implementing high standard care and pursuing ongoing development to maintain relevance and capability in this age of uncertainty.

In the paragraph above, we began with six core practice ingredients and expanded their significance into the entire scope of health professional practice. The same arguments in different contexts could be made in relation to other professional practice fields ranging from teaching, law, engineering, etc. In most practice spaces, it is usually the visible actions and technologies that can be seen as the practitioner seeks to walk the walk and talk the talk of their profession and workplace. However, we need to move beyond the visible in professional practice in professional practice, and it is the decision-making and resultant ethical conduct that enables practitioners to claim the title of professional and distinguishes them from technicians performing their roles under the supervision of decision-making professionals or within standard frameworks and protocols. This chapter focuses on this core element of professional practice, professional decision-making, and explores what it is and how practitioners (novice and experienced) can develop their clinical reasoning capability.

Further Reading

Recently an international group of highly experienced educators, researchers, and practitioners (Higgs et al. 2019b) released the fourth edition of the multidisciplinary textbook *Clinical Reasoning in the Health Professions*. This book provides an extensive exploration of the practice of clinical reasoning and how it can be learned and developed. It is beyond the scope of this chapter to cover all of these topics in depth so the reader is referred to this book for further reading, particularly around the way clinical reasoning or professional decision-making is interpreted, practiced, and taught across multiple professions.

(Refer to the table of contents here: https://www.elsevier.com/books/clinical-reasoning-in-the-health-professions/higgs/978-0-7020-6224-7.)

Throughout this chapter, the terms "clinical reasoning" and "professional decision-making" are used largely synonymously but at times with specifically nuanced meaning. Similarly, the terms clients and patients are interchanged but with the emphasis on the former to acknowledge the many contexts when the setting is not clinical and/or the client is a health pursuing customer, rather than someone who is necessarily ill or disabled, etc. Readers should apply their own context considerations and choose the words that make most sense to themselves.

Clinical Reasoning: Exploring the Phenomenon

Definition

Clinical reasoning or professional decision-making in the health professions is a context-dependent, complex, encultured, and professional way of thinking and decision-making to guide high-quality, professionally responsible practice actions.

Contextually, clinical reasoning:

- Occurs within health professional practice, meaning it is governed by the purpose of enhancing health and wellbeing, the codes of conduct of professional behavior of the discipline(s) and setting(s) in question, quality standards of health care and the expectations of ongoing professional development in the pursuit of continued high standards of decision-making and practice.
- Is situated directly in decision-making spaces (including the client space, the relevant capacities, knowledge, values, of the clinician(s)/practitioner(s), client(s), carers, work team, and the sociocultural/professional/global/organizational influences of the given setting).
- Occurs with the frame of reference of the practitioner(s) practice model and values.
- Is encultured in various layers of the life cultures of the participants, the context and the professional practice culture(s) of the professions involved; it involves the way each of these players walk, talk, and think as what they value and what motivates them.

Clinical reasoning and decision-making can be considered a metapractice in that it comprises "an interactive of practices and capabilities" (like a pride of lions) that:

- Goes far beyond a process, a skill or set of skills, a protocol or body of rules.
- Addresses the needs of people more than regulations because people require reasoning and decision-making that is person-centered, particular to them, and situation relevant.
- Requires evidence and justification and is informed, but not restricted by research findings or the scientific method in any limited interpretation of evidence-based practice.
- Involves (a) micro, (b) macro, and (c) meta level decision-making, relating to deciding and making judgements (respectively) on such matters as (a) tasks/steps to take in data collection; (b) major decisions or interpretations like diagnoses, prognoses, action plans; and (c) the trustworthiness or relevance of data, the level of client satisfaction, the effectiveness and value of outcomes in relation to goals and interests, etc.
- Comprises multiple complex and encultured capabilities including metacognition (critical self-evaluation), reflexivity, mindfulness, interpretation, emotional intelligence, communication (interpersonal and digital), and practice wisdom as well as a range of "fit-for-purpose and ability" reasoning approaches (e.g., hypothetico-deductive reasoning, pattern recognition, narrative reasoning), patient assessment, and the evaluation of intervention effectiveness and value to stakeholders.
- Involves the construction of narratives and critical conversations to make sense of the multiple factors and interests pertaining to the current reasoning or decision-making task.
- Utilizes core dimensions of practice knowledge, reasoning, and metacognition and typically draws on these capacities in others, being a process that engages others, from clients providing their concerns, interests/motivations, clinical history, and responses to overt engagement of clients, carers, and colleagues in collaborative decision-making. Empowerment and education of clients as well as advocacy in relation to social justice may be required in facilitating collaborative decision-making.
- Involves the ability to communicate the reasoning and decisions to relevant participants and stakeholders in order to facilitate acceptance, participation, justification, and accountability. Such communication needs to be appropriate in terms of language, particularly with regard to jargon use and audience relevance.
- Requires ongoing reflexive appraisal and improvement.
- is enriched by practitioners' expanding expertise and practice wisdom.

As well as being professional, clinical reasoning involves the progressive pursuit of practice wisdom and wise practice (Higgs 2019b). This incorporates making wise decisions and taking actions across all phases of client management (in assessment, intervention, evaluation, and follow-up), that are well judged, critically informed, reflexively appraised, and soundly justified in a specific context to address clients' needs and problems.

Clinical reasoning as a metapractice requires ongoing development, in part because the circumstance, knowledge-base, and interests of the practitioner are evolving but also because the context(s) of professional decision-making places changing demands, and the opportunities and models of reasoning continue to evolve. Practitioners need to continue to seek to understand this complex metapractice, pursue a deeper capacity to perform it more wisely, and manage its wise use in context. Professional practice and its development require understanding, pursuit, and quality management.

Further Reading

For further exploration of these topics see: Costanzo et al. (2019); Higgs (2019c); Higgs and Jensen (2019); Higgs and Jones (2019); Higgs and Trede (2019); Higgs and Turpin (2019); Horsfall et al. (2019); Jensen et al. (2019); Loftus and Higgs (2019); Simpson and Cox (2019); Smith and Higgs (2019); Thomas and Young (2019); Trede and Higgs (2019).

The Changing Context of Professional Health Care Practice and Reasoning

This section examines a number of key contextual changes that have the combined effect of making professional practice and professional decision-making more complex and challenging than ever before. We also face more opportunities for advances in the quality and expansion in modes of providing health care and decision-making due to expanding technical and communication affordances. We are living in the digital age and the age of uncertainty as well as in a global community facing shared challenges and increasing demands for sustainability.

Major changes are happening in the world and these are impacting on health professionals and their practice. These include but go far beyond the commodification of health services and the escalating cost of health care facing people and governments and the expanding possibilities and demands that nations and global societies and organizations are facing in their endeavor to meet the health care expectations and needs of the world's population. Health care as a significant component in many economies is now part of widespread pursuit of commercialization and privatization of health care delivery. Health professionals have to learn how to navigate such economic influences that are often counterproductive and counter-rational to quality clinical reasoning and decision-making.

A cornerstone of globalization is increased accountability and this has many faces. Taking responsibility for the quality of care is not new but in the globalization era it has the added pressures of providing public and often voluminous evidence, which can be narrowly interpreted as largely based in quantitative research with limited space for quality of life and life choices in some interpretations of evidence-based practice. The fiscal demands of cost efficiency can negatively restrict health care decision-making and implementation. The time spent in demonstrating accountability in place of providing health care can be wasteful. On the other hand, setting acceptable standards for health care and seeking equity of health care access and quality delivery is a positive aspect of expanded accountability as are expectations of patient-centered care and putting aside blind faith in the decision-making of professionals, expert, or otherwise.

Significant changes in demography continue to occur. For instance, aging populations in some countries and with increased life expectancy, there can be both positive and negative health effects such as the growth of noncommunicable, chronic diseases and comorbidities. Managing such health conditions creates new forms of complexity in health care and decision-making due to the nature of the conditions but also due to the complications of funding of more complex and long-term care. Advanced technologies in health care does not come cheaply either. Across many countries increasing ethnic and racial diversity comes with the challenge for practitioners to plan interventions and treatments that fit the personal values and cultural customs of clients and communities and address communication issues.

In many areas, there is civil and political unrest, major population displacements, unsettlement and extreme poverty, and environmental disasters. These pose health care challenges. The nature of work today and in the future is dramatically changing with impact on immediate work and with increased numbers of vulnerable and gig economy workers. (The gig economy is characterized by increased temporary work or "gigs," freelancing, job bidding, outsourcing, and lack of job security.) We face wicked problems in society and work, and unpredictable futures (Goodyear and Markauskaite 2019) with concomitant physical, mental, social, and population health issues.

Another pertinent trend is that questions are being raised about whether the responsibilities of the professions in serving society are being met (Susskind and Susskind 2015). Cork (2019) argues that the successors of today's professionals face the challenge of regaining their traditional trusted professional roles and status, as well as the opportunity and responsibility professionalism provides to help society envision and achieve sustainable futures.

> Susskind and Susskind (2015) suggested that the ultimate future for societies will be one in which information is freely available to all people, through the mediation of artificial intelligence (AI). They suggest that AI will make sense of information in ways that all members of society can understand and act upon. Furthermore, they suggest that AI might be in a far better position to apply, impartially, rules based on ethical and moral principles than human decision makers have or could. (Cork and Horsfall 2019, p. 23).

Clinical decision-making is not restricted to the health care of individual clients; it also plays a key role in health promotion programs and projects for local and global communities. The emphasis on sustainable futures by nations, the United Nations, and global players provides an important sphere for health care decision-making and is also a key context in which organizations function, are judged, and create their health care and resourcing directives.

> The Sustainable Development Goals are the blueprint to achieve a better and more sustainable future for all. They address the global challenges we face, including those related to poverty, inequality, climate, environmental degradation, prosperity, and peace and justice. The Goals interconnect and in order to leave no one behind, it is important that we achieve each Goal and target by 2030. (United Nations n.d., n.p.).

The consequences of this changing context for clinical reasoning and professional decision-making are far reaching in terms of demands, challenges, and opportunities:

- There is an increasing need by, and dependence of, professionals and professions on advanced reasoning capabilities as outlined above, as opposed to more simple, uni-layered, operational clinical reasoning processes and protocols.
- Evolving reasoning practices are linked to changes in professional roles, e.g., increasing autonomy of practitioners working without the requirement of medical referrals, the professionalization of health occupations with a shift from procedural to professional decision-making, the more widespread and more deeply integrated use of combined health care practices (e.g., Western and Complementary Medicines) with blended decision-making processes, and the expansion of computer aided health decision-making requiring new behaviors and standards such as new rules and ethics relating to web- and computer-aided interaction and communication.
- Clinical reasoning is becoming an increasingly team-based practice, including shared decision-making with clients. Sound strategies and tools (in terms of decision-making practices and ethics) are needed to facilitate and optimize the ethicality and respectfulness of these expanding collaborations in health care across disciplines and with clients and carers.
- Expanded capacities and strategies are needed to face the challenges of artificial intelligence and the expectations of increasingly well-informed health care consumers whose information may enhance or replace their reliance on the expertise of health professionals or may lead to misinformation, confusion, and unfortunate health care choices. Learning to deal with changing telehealth decision-making practices and opportunities where the collaborative decision maker may be at a distance and may be a computer, is another example.

This section reminds us that clinical reasoning and professional decision-making are not obscured, isolated, or context-free occurrences. They need to be managed with triple bottom line (social, environmental, and economic) mentality and person and stakeholder focused.

> As health care practice occurs in an increasingly complex, diverse and uncertain environment, how clinical reasoning is envisioned, enacted and investigated through models of practice is ... evolving. Importantly, investigative methods for studying clinical reasoning must also evolve. The interdependence of clinical reasoning and clinical practice needs to remain central to both practice and research. Practitioners must engage in a critical practice model that maintains a critical view of current practices along with continual questioning of their clinical reasoning. (Higgs et al. 2019c, p. xii).

Further Reading

Recently an international group of futurists, researchers, and scholars (Higgs et al. 2019a) published a book, *Challenging Future Practice Possibilities*, which provides valuable reading in consideration of the future context of society, health care, and decision-making (Refer to the table of contents here: https://brill.com/view/title/55061).

See also Dyer (2001), Eid and Ward (2009), Wasserman and Loftus (2019), Zubairi et al. (2019).

Clinical Reasoning Approaches

In this section, the main focus is on practitioners working (alone or with colleagues) with individual clients. Some reference will be made to health education and health promotion since these may play a role as part of working with individual clients and groups of clients and a brief mention will be made of decision-making in population health for completeness sake; however, deeper discussion of these topics is beyond the scope of the chapter.

For many decades, health practice abilities, including reasoning and decision-making, were seen to follow a characteristic path from novice to expert practitioners, typically based on the foundational work of Dreyfus and Dreyfus (1980). While the concepts of novice, advanced, and expert practitioners remain, other concepts have taken hold to deal with the complexities of context and practice in health care. Skills and competencies, with their emphasis on isolated and quantitatively measurable elements of practice, are being strongly challenged by the more complex, situated, and interdependent and more complexly assessable constructs of capabilities with their notion and action capacity for enabling agency in situations of unfamiliarity and uncertainty (Higgs 2018, 2019b).

> Whereas being competent is about delivery of specific tasks in relatively predictable circumstances, capability is more about responsiveness, creativity, contingent thinking, and growth in relatively uncertain ones (Scott et al. 2008, p. 12).

A Model of Clinical Reasoning as Encultured Decision-Making Capabilities

A new interpretive model of clinical reasoning (Higgs 2019b) based on hermeneutic investigation of an extensive range of clinical reasoning and professional practice literature, research and experience over 30 years, presents clinical reasoning as encultured clinical decision-making. It builds on the ideas of metapractices, multiple practice capabilities, valuing multiple practice knowledges, epistemic fluency, practice paradigms, and Aristotelian (trans. 1999) intellectual virtues (see Box 1).

> **Box 1 Aristotelian (trans. 1999) intellectual virtues**
> - *Epistêmê* is an intellectual virtue characterized as scientific, universal, invariable, context-independent knowledge. The concept is reflected in the terms *epistemology* and *epistemic*.

(continued)

81 Developing Clinical Reasoning Capabilities

> **Box 1 Aristotelian (trans. 1999) intellectual virtues** (continued)
> - *Téchnê* refers to craft or applied practice. It is an intellectual virtue characterized as context-dependent, pragmatic, variable, craft knowledge, it is governed by a conscious goal and it is oriented toward practical instrumental rationality. The concept is reflected in terms such as *technique, technical*, and *technology*.
> - *Phrónêsis* refers to practical wisdom. It is an intellectual virtue characterized by values and ethics. It involves value-based deliberation and practical judgement. It is reflective, pragmatic, variable, context-dependent, and action-oriented.

The model has four framing influences impacting on the reasoning approach adopted and the major capabilities required. The four influences are the decision-making task (its challenge, complexity), the task context (from highly fluid to more stable), the chosen and habitual decision-making practices (discipline-based, autonomous, interdependence) of the situation and stakeholders, and the decision makers (individual, teams, communities) engaged. The five approach modes (see Fig. 1) incorporated in this model are as follows.

Novice approaches are straightforward and adopted in relatively stable and predictable settings. It is typical of novices who adopt a deliberate, explicit, studied

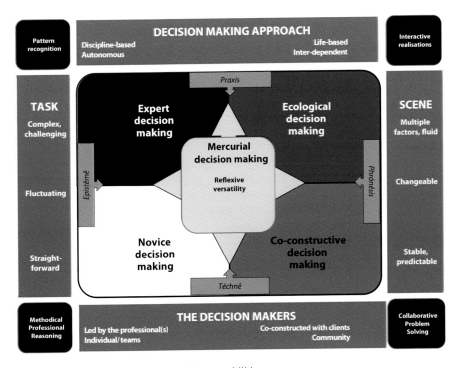

Fig. 1 Encultured clinical decision making capabilities

approach to reasoning and work individually or in professional teams; it relies on emerging disciplinary knowledge. This approach draws on téchnê and epistêmê intelligences. An example is hypothetico-deductive reasoning. This reflects the scientific method, utilizes empirico-analytical cognitive strategies, and involves phases of hypotheses generation (e.g., the establishment of proposed hypotheses and treatment plans) and hypothesis testing (e.g., diagnostic testing and evaluation of treatment effects).

Expert approaches to decision-making in health practice demand more of practitioners who are facing complex and challenging reasoning tasks in relatively fluid settings influenced by multiple factors. Wicked practice problems fit in this category. Expert clinical reasoners adopt complex approaches to reasoning (e.g., pattern recognition), the use of instantiated scripts (see Boshuizen and Schmidt 2019), and deep rich knowledge bases. They may work individually or in professional teams. Such approaches draw on epistêmê and the embedded ethicality, reflexivity, and deeply embodied practice of praxis. They demand high-level reasoning capability that is fluent and rich technical, professional, critical, epistemic, ontological, and interpersonal. Note that expert practice and expert clinical reasoning are not the same thing; they hopefully both occur in the same people.

Co-constructed decision-making approaches emphasize the demands of current times where many clients are better informed and more agentic than ever before. These approaches can work well within the demands of (more) straightforward reasoning tasks in relatively stable and predictable settings and may involve decision-making with individual clients, groups, or communities. The key element that influences such approaches is co-constructed and interdependent decision-making, aiming to pursue life-based decisions rather than focus on purely biomedical, clinically oriented decisions. Co-constructed approaches draw on téchnê and phrónêsis and require a willingness to share expert knowledge and capabilities with clients, and a commitment to valuing the perspectives and input of others.

Ecological decision-making approaches suit the demands of (more) complex and challenging reasoning tasks in relatively fluid settings, influenced by multiple factors including social and environment factors that influence wellbeing, the common good, and social justice, as well as health. Health and wellbeing may well be the secondary effects rather than the primary goals of such programs. These decision-making strategies are typical of highly experienced but nontraditional practitioners who focus on the complexity of practice and community settings where individuals or groups of clients are looking for different narratives and solutions including education and training programs for people and population health projects. The term "ecological" was attached to this approach to highlight the interdependence of the decision-making parties and the need for mutual respect between them for their different perspectives and contributions. The practices of "green" decision-making are inherently dynamic and emergent. Such approaches draw on a strong ability in phrónêsis and the embedded ethicality, reflexivity, and deeply embodied practice of praxis. They demand high-level (individual and collective) epistemic and ontological fluency and rich critical, technical, professional, epistemic, ontologic, and interpersonal capability on the part of practitioners, a willingness to share expert knowledge and capabilities with clients, and a commitment to valuing the perspectives and input of others in order to realize optimal solutions to the challenges posed. Networking of decision-making participants is a key feature of this approach to decision-making.

Mercurial decision-making is placed at the center of the four influence frames (continua) in the model, deliberately emphasizing that some decision-making approaches need to be highly versatile, reflexive, and dynamic. These approaches are included in this model to recognize that clinical decision-making situations and players are not static and the approaches adopted need to be knowingly responsive to these changes – or at times driving context changes. This approach draws on epistêmê, phrónêsis, téchnê, and praxis in varying ways, depending on the task, setting, practice, and players. Such approaches demand a high level of reflexivity; versatility; fluency and rich technical, professional, critical, epistemic, ontologic, and interpersonal capability; a willingness to share expert knowledge and capabilities with clients; and a commitment to valuing the perspectives and input of others.

The categorization of clinical reasoning approaches into these five approaches modes in this model was done to recognize that there are many different disciplinary and collaborative modes and models of clinical reasoning and decision-making, to look at the different users of clinical reasoning and what abilities they bring to reasoning and to recognize that there are many different situations for and in which clinical reasoning occurs. These changing circumstances require clinical reasoning to be adapted and its teaching to be made relevant to those circumstances. See the section below on teaching clinical reasoning. The colors emphasize the differences in the reasoning approach categories and reflect the nature of these different approaches.

Further Reading

For further reading about reasoning in specific professions: medicine, nursing, physiotherapy, dentistry, occupational therapy, emergency medicine, paramedicine, optometry, dietetics, and pharmacy, see Higgs (2019a). See also Benner (1984, 2015), Dreyfus (2004), Gardner (2006), Goodyear and Markauskaite (2019), Stephenson (1998).

Learning, Teaching, and Developing Clinical Reasoning

This section explores ways of developing clinical reasoning capabilities. The foundation of such education is firstly based on understanding what clinical reasoning and decision-making are, secondly on recognizing that it is practitioners who are the focus of these metapractices and require an understanding of clinical reasoning to be able to pursue the development of their reasoning ability and to manage its implementation in varied modes in their practice. Clinical reasoning cannot be rote learned in a one-off fashion. Rather, clinical reasoning is an evolving metapractice and an unending pursuit for desirable practices and enabling capabilities that is dependent on an evolving knowledge base and embedded in the changing context of the practitioner's identity and practice model, the profession's role and practices (e.g., autonomy to practice without medical referral), changing services of organizations (e.g., hospital health education classes and community-based wellbeing health promotion and fitness programs) and the wider health care/possibility environments.

Academic and clinical educators aim to develop novices' clinical reasoning while peers and mentors also support the evolution of more advanced practitioners' clinical reasoning through guidance, support, and feedback. Clinical reasoning development is facilitated by the implementation of pedagogical and assessment strategies, and is grounded in educational theories that are relevant to the teaching and learning of clinical reasoning in educational and practice-based learning contexts. Such teaching strategies can exist within multiple educational contexts (classrooms, online, and in practice settings), knowledge areas, and practice activities. Teaching and learning strategies involve an overt focus on the metapractices and capabilities necessary to implement and communicate clinical reasoning. As well as performing reasoning, novices need to learn to substantiate their decisions with appropriate evidence and also to derive learning about their practice and reasoning from their clinical reasoning experiences.

A critical challenge for educators is how we introduce health professional newcomers to these complex and sophisticated practices. As with many new topics, it is useful for novices to learn about clinical reasoning by relating it to something they already know. For instance, the hypothetico-deductive reasoning model is related to the scientific method that most undergraduates learn in their early research classes and does not require extensive prior practice experience or experience-based knowledge and so it is a suitable strategy for novices to learn about clinical reasoning even if this is not their primary disciplinary reasoning approach. Novices can learn through listening to narratives of health practice reasoning and actions even if narrative reasoning is not to be their primary reasoning strategy. Building on their or their own family's health experiences can utilize practice-based learning strategies such as role plays to explore connections between health problem situations, interventions, outcomes, and critical appreciation of the links between these aspects of clinical decision-making in reality and abstract scenarios and exploring issues such as justification and accountability, differences in the way people value different outcomes, etc.

Clinical reasoning must be recognized as a situated and encultured practice and in its development the novice is learning to walk the walk, talk the talk, and think the think or reason, in the context of their discipline and context. Emergency medicine specialists, paramedics, and surgical teams, for instance, need to swiftly make accurate diagnoses of presenting problems in the sudden-change and critical context of acute settings. Accuracy and speed of diagnosis in these situations can sometimes make the difference between life and death. In contrast, many other health professions, particularly those working in general practices and rehabilitation, are often more concerned with managing long-term relationships with patients. Some practitioners, such as occupational therapists, often work with patients for whom the diagnosis is already established. They work with their clients, such as disabled and elderly patients, to co-create health enhancement and support narratives. The clinical reasoning demands on health professionals who are managing patients with chronic conditions are quite different from those health professionals who are assessing acute conditions. Many health professions (e.g., dentists and optometrists) work in both acute and chronic situations and have to deal with long-term reasoning tasks as well as acute emergency cases.

In addition to learning how to reason in their own profession's practice, practitioners need to learn about the similarities among health professions' reasoning and differences across the professions. The differences reflect the variations in the goals of the health professions and how they conceptualize their work with patients and clients. So reasoning is linked to professional identity and roles. Knowledge of different reasoning practices is necessary for understanding how to work with members of other professions during collaborative reasoning. Speech pathologists, for instance, have found the International Classification of Functioning, Disability and Health (https://www.who.int/classifications/icf/en/), to be a particularly useful framework to organize clinical reasoning and how to teach it to students. This reflects the focus on the diagnosis and remediation of specific disabilities in speech in speech pathology practice. By comparison, nursing education focuses on developing students' clinical reasoning abilities through teaching and learning strategies that foster lifelong critical thinking habits. Medical education typically advocates grounding the teaching of clinical reasoning in medical education in the science of reasoning practice along with biomedical knowledge acquisition and clinical skill building, plus understanding of concepts of clinical uncertainty and diagnostic error.

Facilitating the Development of Clinical Reasoning in Clinical Practice and Education Settings

Consider these situations for instance:

- Two highly experienced paramedics with a trainee are called to a roadside accident involving a seriously injured mother and child.
- A team of medical interns during their fifth week in a presurgical rotation is doing the preliminary admissions of several patients to present their reports to their supervising medical resident.
- An occupational therapy clinical educator is supervising a group of four final year students and is going to watch them one by one, treating their patients in a hand clinic. The students' abilities are quite variable.
- A physiotherapy private practitioner has a senior student doing a clinical education placement at their sports physiotherapy practice and has asked the student to perform a complex technique on the patient. It becomes quickly apparent that the student does not know what they are doing.
- A senior radiographer, the manager of a commercial radiography company has agreed for four radiography students (two second years and two third years) to do

a 4 week clinical education placement at the company's rooms in a busy high street location with many drop-in customers.
- A speech pathologist is working in several schools with speech pathology and occupational therapy students and is helping teachers and teachers' aides to help children who have communication and learning difficulties improve their developmental capacity in the normal environment of the classroom.

What clinical reasoning decision-making challenges to these people face? What challenges are the clinical educators or experienced practitioners/mentors present facing as learning facilitators and in their other roles? How can all parties reflect after the event on the adequacy of their reasoning capability and act to improve it? How would the supervisors or mentors balance their responsibilities as qualified practitioners for the decisions made and actions taken (by practitioners and students/novices) with their role of helping the students/novices learn (which includes learning about their own decisions and learning from less optimal or wrong decisions)? How could the educator or mentor bring issues of ethical and professional conduct and optimal quality of patient care into students' awareness and learning about reasoning?

Perhaps the greatest challenge in helping students learn to do clinical reasoning that is sound is dealing with the fact that much of clinical reasoning is invisible to others (unless it is conducted in a collaborative dialogue mode). In any case, not all of what is being thought about is done in a conscious way, particularly in fast-paced practice situations or during rapid and advanced reasoning situations or strategies such as pattern recognition. And, often inadequate or incorrect knowledge and information can be used without the thinker or observer being aware of the errors occurring. Also, outcomes are often only evaluated from the practitioner's perspective which could mean that the judgement of outcomes from the perspective of clients and their perception of how well the interventions have benefitted them can remain unasked and invisible. These reflections remind us that reasoning cannot be learned by osmosis or copying or demonstration without explanation and justification and that evaluation of the invisibles and different perspective of reasoning can be inadequately assessed. Valuable ways of learning are tutorials, student presentations of their actual patients as cases with teacher and peer review, asking students to discuss their reasoning after their clinical practice treatment/presentation away from the patient, hypothetical role plays and senior practitioners explaining their reasoning and unbundling it to make assumptions and shortcuts visible and defensible to learners. Assessment of reasoning needs to involve explicit not just assumed decisions and their justification and different perspectives, including patients' real opinions.

Further Reading

Ajjawi and Higgs (2019), Ajjawi et al. (2019), Christensen and Jensen (2019), Christensen et al. (2008), Patton and Christensen (2019), Schuwirth et al. (2019).

Conclusion

In summary, the teaching of clinical reasoning involves helping students learn what clinical reasoning is and how to perform it in various practice situations. Learning on campus, online, and in practice settings is required. In addition, learners need assessment of their reasoning capabilities and feedback from their teachers and practice role models, and they need to develop strategies for critiquing and enhancing their own reasoning.

Readers are invited to reflect on how the contents of the chapter have stimulated thoughts about their own reasoning practices and capabilities and their own teaching and learning/development strategies they use.

Cross-References

▶ Supporting the Development of Patient-Centred Communication Skills
▶ Supporting the Development of Professionalism in the Education of Health Professionals

References

Ajjawi R, Brander R, Thistlethwaite J. Interprofessional programs to develop clinical reasoning. In: Higgs J, Jensen G, Loftus S, Christensen N, editors. Clinical reasoning in the health professions. 4th ed. Edinburgh: Elsevier; 2019. p. 397–405.

Ajjawi R, Higgs J. Learning to communicate clinical reasoning. In: Higgs J, Jensen G, Loftus S, Christensen N, editors. Clinical reasoning in the health professions. 4th ed. Edinburgh: Elsevier; 2019. p. 419–25.

Aristotle. Nicomachean ethics. Irwin T, translator. Indianapolis, IN: Hackett Publishing; 1999 (original work published c. 400 BC).

Benner P. From novice to expert: excellence and power in clinical nursing practice. Menlo Park: Addison-Wesley; 1984.

Benner P. Novice to expert: nursing theorist. 2015. http://nursing-theory.org/nursing-theorists/Patricia-Benner.php. Accessed 18 Mar 2017.

Boshuizen HPA, Schmidt HG. The development of clinical reasoning expertise. In: Higgs J, Jensen G, Loftus S, Christensen N, editors. Clinical reasoning in the health professions. 4th ed. Edinburgh: Elsevier; 2019. p. 57–65.

Christensen N, Jensen G. Developing clinical reasoning capability. In: Higgs J, Jensen G, Loftus S, Christensen N, editors. Clinical reasoning in the health professions. 4th ed. Edinburgh: Elsevier; 2019. p. 427–33.

Christensen N, Jones M, Edwards I, Higgs J. Helping physiotherapy students develop clinical reasoning capability. In: Higgs J, Jones M, Loftus S, Christensen N, editors. Clinical reasoning in the health professions. 3rd ed. Edinburgh: Elsevier; 2008. p. 389–96.

Cork S. Our place in society and the environment: opportunities and responsibilities for professional practice futures. In: Higgs J, Cork S, Horsfall D, editors. Challenging future practice possibilities. Rotterdam, The Netherlands: Brill Sense; 2019. p. 79–90.

Cork S, Horsfall D. Thinking the unthinkable: challenges of imagining and engaging with unimaginable practice futures. In: Higgs J, Cork S, Horsfall D, editors. Challenging future practice possibilities. Rotterdam, The Netherlands: Brill Sense; 2019. p. 17–28.

Costanzo C, Doll J, Jensen G. (2019). Shared decision making in practice. In: Higgs J, Jensen G, Loftus S, Christensen N, editors. Clinical reasoning in the health professions. 4th ed. Edinburgh: Elsevier; 2019. p. 181–90.

Dreyfus HL, Dreyfus SL. A five stage model of the mental activities involved in directed skill acquisition. Unpublished report supported by the Air Force of Scientific Research (AFSC), USAF (Contract F49620-79-C—63). Berkeley: University of California; 1980.

Dreyfus S. The five stage model of adult skill acquisition. Bull Sci Technol Soc. 2004;24(3):177–81.

Dyer KA. Ethical challenges of medicine and health on the internet: a review. J Med Internet Res. 2001 Apr–Jun;3(2):e23.

Eid M, Ward SJA. Ethics, new media and social networks. Glob Media J Can Ed. 2009;2(1):1–4.

Gardner H. Multiple intelligences: new horizons. New York: Basic Books; 2006.

Goodyear P, Markauskaite L. The impact on practice of wicked problems and unpredictable futures. In: Higgs J, Cork S, Horsfall D, editors. Challenging future practice possibilities. Rotterdam: Brill Sense; 2019. p. 41–52.

Higgs J. Taking a capability approach to learning for life and work. In: Patton N, Higgs J, Smith M, editors. Developing practice capability: transforming workplace learning. Leiden: Brill Sense; 2018. p. 69–80.

Higgs J. Appreciating practice wisdom. In: Higgs J, editor. Practice wisdom: values and interpretations. Rotterdam: Brill Sense; 2019a. p. 3–14.

Higgs J. Re-interpreting clinical reasoning: a model of encultured decision making practice capabilities. In: Higgs J, Jensen G, Loftus S, Christensen N, editors. Clinical reasoning in the health professions. 4th ed. Edinburgh: Elsevier; 2019b. p. 13–31.

Higgs J, Jensen G. Clinical reasoning: challenges of interpretation and practice in the 21st century. In: Higgs J, Jensen G, Loftus S, Christensen N, editors. Clinical reasoning in the health professions. 4th ed. Edinburgh: Elsevier; 2019. p. 3–11.

Higgs J, Jones M. Multiple spaces of choice, engagement and influence in clinical decision making. In: Higgs J, Jensen G, Loftus S, Christensen N, editors. Clinical reasoning in the health professions. 4th ed. Edinburgh: Elsevier; 2019. p. 33–43.

Higgs J, Trede F. (2019). Clinical reasoning and models of practice. In: Higgs J, Jensen G, Loftus S, Christensen N, editors. Clinical reasoning in the health professions. 4th ed. Edinburgh: Elsevier; 2019. p. 45–55.

Higgs J, Turpin M. Learning to use evidence to support decision making. In: Higgs J, Jensen G, Loftus S, Christensen N, editors. Clinical reasoning in the health professions. 4th ed. Edinburgh: Elsevier; 2019. p. 465–73.

Higgs J, Cork S, Horsfall D, editors. Challenging future practice possibilities. Rotterdam: Brill Sense; 2019a.

Higgs J, Jensen G, Loftus S, Christensen N, editors. Clinical reasoning in the health professions. 4th ed. Edinburgh: Elsevier; 2019b.

Higgs J, Jensen GM, Loftus S, Christensen N. Editors. Preface. In: Higgs J, Jensen G, Loftus S, Christensen N, editors. Clinical reasoning in the health professions. 4th ed. Edinburgh: Elsevier; 2019c. p. ix–xii.

Horsfall D, Tasker D, Higgs J. Clinical decision making, social justice and client empowerment. In: Higgs J, Jensen G, Loftus S, Christensen N, editors. Clinical reasoning in the health professions. 4th ed. Edinburgh: Elsevier; 2019. p. 201–9.

Jensen G, Resnik L, Haddad A. Expertise and clinical reasoning. In: Higgs J, Jensen G, Loftus S, Christensen N, editors. Clinical reasoning in the health professions. 4th ed. Edinburgh: Elsevier; 2019. p. 67–76.

Loftus S, Higgs J. The language of clinical reasoning. In: Higgs J, Jensen G, Loftus S, Christensen N, editors. Clinical reasoning in the health professions. 4th ed. Edinburgh: Elsevier; 2019. p. 129–36.

Patton N, Christensen N. Pedagogies for teaching and learning clinical reasoning. In: Higgs J, Jensen G, Loftus S, Christensen N, editors. Clinical reasoning in the health professions. 4th ed. Edinburgh: Elsevier; 2019. p. 335–44.

Schuwirth LWT, Durning SJ, Norman GR, van der Vleuten CPM. Assessing clinical reasoning. In: Higgs J, Jensen G, Loftus S, Christensen N, editors. Clinical reasoning in the health professions. 4th ed. Edinburgh: Elsevier; 2019. p. 407–15.

Scott G, Coates H, Anderson M. Learning leaders in times of change. Australian Learning and Teaching Council: Sydney; 2008.

Simpson MD, Cox JL. Learning clinical reasoning across cultural contexts. In: Higgs J, Jensen G, Loftus S, Christensen N, editors. Clinical reasoning in the health professions. 4th ed. Edinburgh: Elsevier; 2019. p. 483–90.

Smith M, Higgs J. Learning about factors influencing clinical decision making. In: Higgs J, Jensen G, Loftus S, Christensen N, editors. Clinical reasoning in the health professions. 4th ed. Edinburgh: Elsevier; 2019. p. 445–54.

Stephenson J. The concept of capability and its importance in higher education. In: Stephenson J, Yorke M, editors. Capability and quality in higher education. London: Kogan Page; 1998. p. 1–13.

Susskind R, Susskind D. The future of the professions: how technology will transform the work of human experts. Oxford: Oxford University Press; 2015.

Thomas A, Young M. Evidence-based practice and clinical reasoning: in tension, tandem or two sides of the same coin? In: Higgs J, Jensen G, Loftus S, Christensen N, editors. Clinical reasoning in the health professions. 4th ed. Edinburgh: Elsevier; 2019. p. 137–46.

Trede F, Higgs J. Collaborative decision making in liquid times. In: Higgs J, Jensen G, Loftus S, Christensen N, editors. Clinical reasoning in the health professions. 4th ed. Edinburgh: Elsevier; 2019. p. 159–67.

United Nations. Sustainable Development Goals. n.d.. https://www.un.org/sustainabledevelopment/sustainable-development-goals/ Accessed 2 Sep 2019.

Wasserman JA, Loftus S. Changing demographic and cultural dimensions of populations: implications for health care and decision making. In: Higgs J, Jensen G, Loftus S, Christensen N, editors. Clinical reasoning in the health professions. 4th ed. Edinburgh: Elsevier; 2019. p. 87–96.

Zubairi MS, Mylopoulos M, Martimianakis MA. The context of clinical reasoning across the health professions in the 21st century. In: Higgs J, Jensen G, Loftus S, Christensen N, editors. Clinical reasoning in the health professions. 4th ed. Edinburgh: Elsevier; 2019. p. 79–85.

Part VII

Governance, Quality Improvement, Scholarship and Leadership in Health Professions Education

Professional Bodies in Health Professions Education

82

Julie Browne

Contents

Introduction	1592
What is a Profession?	1593
A Profession Defines Itself Through Its Professional Bodies	1594
Why Do Healthcare Professionals (HCPs) Join Professional Bodies?	1596
What Role(s) Do Professional Bodies Serve?	1597
Is Healthcare Education a Proper Profession?	1600
The Future: Pressures	1601
Conclusion	1607
Cross-References	1608
References	1608

Abstract

Is healthcare education a profession in its own right? What is the position of healthcare educators? And what is the role of professional bodies?

Without professional bodies, there would be no professions. This chapter explores what is meant by "profession" as distinct from a job or an occupation. It argues that a profession's distinguishing features – which include accountability, self-regulation, altruism, and a commitment to continued high standards – are actualized through the work of its professional bodies. Healthcare educators participate in professional bodies for many reasons to do with asserting and maintaining their place as professionals. There are three main reasons why individuals join a professional body: to demonstrate and maintain their membership of a profession; to uphold their profession's ethical standards and enhance its special position within society; and to maintain and develop their professional expertise.

J. Browne (✉)
Centre for Medical Education, Cardiff University School of Medicine, Cardiff, UK
e-mail: brownej1@cardiff.ac.uk

© Springer Nature Singapore Pte Ltd. 2023
D. Nestel et al. (eds.), *Clinical Education for the Health Professions*,
https://doi.org/10.1007/978-981-15-3344-0_109

While each healthcare profession's infrastructure will vary, it is usually possible to observe within each area of professional practice one or more organizations that (1) serve the public by maintaining a register of practitioners and ensuring that standards are met; (2) serve members by offering them opportunities to add to, explore, and communicate their expert knowledge base; and (3) serve the profession by acting as a collective voice, particularly on issues that affect the standing, influence, and organization of its members.

In recent years, health professions education has moved away from its former position as the preserve of interested but untrained enthusiasts. It has developed a growing confidence in asserting its position as a profession requiring specialist expertise and skills, and the professional bodies that serve educators have developed accordingly. They are rising to meet new challenges, developing services to members, speaking on behalf of members with more confidence, and raising their standards to improve public accountability and engagement.

Professional bodies face many challenges. First, they struggle with financial pressures caused by older and outdated models of funding, particularly around subscriptions and publishing. They must also respond to changes in healthcare work structures that are breaking down professional boundaries and hierarchies and contributing to the development of new roles and clinical specialties, resulting in multiple complex (and sometimes bureaucratic and expensive) applications and annual subscriptions for their members. Additionally, there are rapid technological, cultural, and financial shifts in education both within higher education and also in healthcare services, requiring professional bodies to be light on their feet in response to the shifting educational environment.

For professional bodies to survive into the next century, further change will be necessary. Such changes will almost certainly include closer interprofessional working and the development of multi-professional collaborations and mergers.

Healthcare educators, whatever their clinical or academic specialty, need to work together to raise the status of healthcare education as a profession; it is therefore important that individuals support and participate in their professional bodies as a means of developing healthcare education for the benefit of students, patients, and society as a whole.

Keywords

Professionalization · Standards · Membership · Network · Institution · Professional recognition

Introduction

Professional bodies play an important role in the career of every healthcare professional. Regulators, learned societies, and professional organizations ensure that individual healthcare professionals are trained to a particular standard, qualified and licensed to practice, and that they can maintain their knowledge and skills throughout their working life. Professional bodies also serve to reassure the public that members of a profession are properly monitored and accountable for their practice; and they can act as an important collective voice for matters affecting the profession.

Healthcare education has traditionally lacked the status of a profession. It has tended historically to be viewed as an adjunct to clinical practice; but in recent years its status has changed. It is increasingly recognized that healthcare professions education requires the development of specialist expertise and skills, and that dedicated healthcare professions educators need the time, resources, recognition, and career structures that enable them to raise standards across the board.

Professional bodies within healthcare professions education are responding to this new recognition and developing in line with the professionalization of the educator workforce; but they face many challenges. It is essential that individual healthcare professions educators engage with their professional bodies in order to sustain and develop healthcare education as a profession. This will help advance professional healthcare education, but more importantly, will also benefit students, patients, clients, and wider society.

What is a Profession?

The term "profession" is constantly shifting in response to social trends and debates, making it impossible to pin down any single understanding of what it means (Aukett 2017). Sociologists and others have wrangled for decades over its precise nature and functions. Various definitions have been offered, but none has been firmly agreed (see Table 1). It is, however, possible to describe the main characteristics of a profession. Professionals hold a special status in society: they benefit from privileges such as status, public trust, and influence, but, in return for these, they are also expected to fulfil additional responsibilities and duties and commit themselves to high standards of performance.

It is usually accepted that high-status careers such as law, accountancy, university teaching, and veterinary science are professions, whereas work such as advertising, sales work, domestic maintenance, and office administration is more frequently described in terms of occupations or jobs.

Healthcare staff who have specialist training and whose professional practice is overseen by a regulator are also usually described as "professionals." In most cases their names are inscribed on a register from which they may be removed if they fail to carry out their work in accordance with professional standards. In the UK, these individuals usually belong to a body that is overseen by the UK Professional Standards Authority (see Table 2).

In consequence of their professional status, licensed healthcare practitioners hold a special position of respect within society and are among the most trusted occupational groups (IPSOS Mori 2018). Traditionally, they have tended to be more highly paid than colleagues in lower-status occupations within healthcare, such as clerical and domestic staff, where tertiary education is rarely an essential requirement of the post. Collectively, and as individuals, healthcare professionals (HCPs) usually

Table 1 Three definitions of profession

Cruess S, Johnston S, Cruess R. 'Profession': a working definition for medical educators. Teaching and Learning in Medicine. 2004;16(1):74–6.
Profession: An occupation whose core element is work based upon the mastery of a complex body of knowledge and skills. It is a vocation in which knowledge of some department of science or learning or the practice of an art founded upon it is used in the service of others. Its members are governed by codes of ethics and profess a commitment to competence, integrity and morality, altruism, and the promotion of the public good within their domain. These commitments form the basis of a social contract between a profession and society, which in return grants the profession a monopoly over the use of its knowledge base, the right to considerable autonomy in practice and the privilege of self-regulation. Professions and their members are accountable to those served and to society.
Yam BM. From vocation to profession: the quest for professionalization of nursing. *British Journal of Nursing.* 2004;13(16):978–82.

The traits of a profession:
  An extensive theoretical knowledge base
  A legitimate expertise in a specialized field
  An altruistic commitment to service
  An unusual degree of autonomy in work
  A code of ethics and conduct overseen by a body of representatives from within the field itself
  A personal identity that stems from the professional's occupation

Professions Australia. *The Professions, Public Interest and Competition Policy,* 2000. Deakin, Australia: Australian Council of Professions
A disciplined group of individuals who adhere to high ethical standards and uphold themselves to, and are accepted by, the public as possessing special knowledge and skills in a widely recognised, organised body of learning derived from education and training at a high level, and who are prepared to exercise this knowledge and these skills in the interests of others

benefit from considerable autonomy and public confidence in their working lives. Patients, for example, allow healthcare practitioners freedoms (to treat, probe, ask personal questions, and even cause necessary pain and discomfort) that they would never allow to an average person in the street.

However, this special position within society held by healthcare professionals comes with some conditions: anyone who wants to be a healthcare practitioner must first master a complex set of skills and knowledge and must undertake to use these ethically and altruistically in the service of others. Moreover, as a group, healthcare practitioners are allowed some freedom to regulate themselves but only on condition that they hold themselves ultimately accountable to their patients and to society as a whole (Irvine 2006). As William Wickenden argued in the 1930s, ethical commitment to serve the public accountably forms the basis of a social contract with society that turns a job or vocation into a profession (Wickenden 1932).

A Profession Defines Itself Through Its Professional Bodies

For any occupation to be able to call itself a fully fledged profession (and thus for individuals to be able to claim all the privileges and responsibilities that being a member of a profession entails), certain essential functions and structures must be in

Table 2 List of UK professional regulators overseen by the Professional Standards Authority and the professions they regulate

Regulator	Related profession
General Chiropractic Council	Chiropractor
General Dental Council	Dentist, clinical dental technician, dental hygienist, dental nurse, dental technician, dental therapist, orthodontic therapist
General Medical Council	Doctor, psychiatrist, physician associate
General Optical Council	Optician, optometrist, dispensing optician
General Osteopathic Council	Osteopath
General Pharmaceutical Council	Pharmacist, pharmacy technician
Health and Care Professions Council	Arts therapist, biomedical scientist, chiropodist/podiatrist, clinical scientist, dietitian, hearing aid dispenser, occupational therapist, operating department practitioner, orthoptist, paramedic, physiotherapist, practitioner psychologist, prosthetist/orthotist, radiographer, speech and language therapist
Nursing and Midwifery Council	Midwife, nurse, nursing associate
Pharmaceutical Society of Northern Ireland	Pharmacist
Social Work England	Social worker

place. These functions and structures are what allow the profession to fulfil its social contract to serve society and permit its individual members to show that they commit themselves to agreed standards of professional behavior, skills, and knowledge.

Consequently, within any profession one expects to find at least one but usually more professional bodies and associated structures that perform the following functions.

- **High-level specialist training for entry to a profession**, together with university departments and a professoriate to support this. Professions invariably require those who wish to join them to undertake lengthy and demanding study. An academic presence allows learners access to, and the opportunity to demonstrate that they have acquired, the complex body of knowledge and skills they need in order to join a profession; degrees and higher awards offer standardized assessment that is universally recognized.
- **Practice standards against which the profession and its members may be publicly evaluated.** This requires either a regulator or "professional organization" (such as a Royal College, Society, or Academy) to set standards, to make decisions on admission to the profession (including maintenance of a register of licensed practitioners), and to provide professional leadership on matters of policy.
- **Maintenance and development of the expert knowledge base**. A profession needs its own special literature; this is usually in the form of academic journals, textbooks, and evidence that can be used to inform policy and practice and high-level debate about the specialist knowledge that underpins the vocation or

occupation. This is how the profession both constructs and critiques its own knowledge base and ensures that it is applied in the service of others. Many professional bodies own journals, libraries, and even publishing houses producing and archiving the scholarly records that underpin a profession's body of knowledge.

- **Ongoing training for the role**. Professionals usually undertake continuing education and development in order to keep their skills and knowledge up-to-date. As professions usually require an advanced understanding of complex knowledge and practice, it goes without saying that regular education and training must be part of the professional's individual practice.
- **Career paths**. Members of a profession should be able to progress to senior levels based on their demonstrated achievements and competence. Many professional organizations have education departments and recognition schemes through which they offer candidates the opportunity to progress through the stages necessary to achieve mastery of a profession and promotion to more senior roles.
- **Institutional support within the wider professional framework** and context, including recognition by government, other regulators, and other professional bodies. Professional organizations furnish high-level advocacy, networking, and influence in matters concerning their members.
- **Informal networking opportunities**. A support network for those interested in advancing the profession through research, collaboration, funding opportunities, lobbying activity, and social and professional support for individuals. This may be provided by one or several special interest groups, learned societies, research collaboratives, and so on.

Without all these structures and functions in place, a career, occupation, or vocation cannot truly show how it is fulfilling a professional role within society (Pereira 1980). Professional bodies are therefore essential, not just to society's overall confidence in a profession but also at the "coalface": the work of professional bodies fundamentally affects the relationship of trust between patients and clients and the individual professional practitioner.

Why Do Healthcare Professionals (HCPs) Join Professional Bodies?

Nearly all HCPs belong to at least one professional body and many belong to more than one. This is because as individual professionals, they have three key needs:

1. To demonstrate and maintain their membership of a profession
2. To maintain their special position within society as professionals

3. To maintain and enhance their expertise within their chosen profession's complex body of knowledge and practice

These three needs are usually met by membership of at least one, but more usually three, specific type of professional bodies:

1. Regulatory bodies: these primarily maintain the register of qualified practitioners.
2. Professional organizations: these principally undertake to represent the profession, promote professionalism in practice, and lobby on professional issues on behalf of the profession with government and wider society.
3. Learned societies: these chiefly provide a platform for members to discuss issues of interest within the profession, often with the aim of developing awareness of and knowledge about a particular field of professional practice through networking, communication, scholarship, and the maintenance and development of a scholarly archive.

For example, a nurse in the UK may belong to the regulator (the Nursing and Midwifery Council 2019); the professional organization (the Royal College of Nursing or Midwifery 2019); and a learned society such as the Community and District Nursing Association (2019), the British Association of Critical Care Nurses (2019), or similar. An Australian doctor may belong to the regulator (the Medical Board of Australia 2019); a professional organization (such as the Australian Medical Association 2019); and a learned society such as the Australasian Society of Cosmetic Dermatologists (2019) or the Academy of Surgical Educators (2019). The boundaries are not always this clear, however. In some professions, the professional organization is also the regulator; in others, the learned society has developed into the professional organization over time, while many regulators also see it as their responsibility to promote professionalism and scholarship in their field. There is very occasionally a single body which meets all three needs and to which most practitioners belong.

What Role(s) Do Professional Bodies Serve?

Figure 1 shows the overlapping roles of regulators, learned societies, and professional organizations. At the heart of the diagram is the individual healthcare practitioner. Through individual membership of professional bodies, and particularly of professional organizations, HCPs collectively agree on and to make explicit the values that are at the heart of the work they do. Openly expressed adherence to these agreed core values is central to asserting their professional status to their employers, colleagues, and other professionals, those they serve (students, patients, clients, etc.), and to the wider public.

In whatever way an individual HCP's professional bodies are structured, collectively they serve three main constituencies: the public, the profession itself, and the individual practitioner.

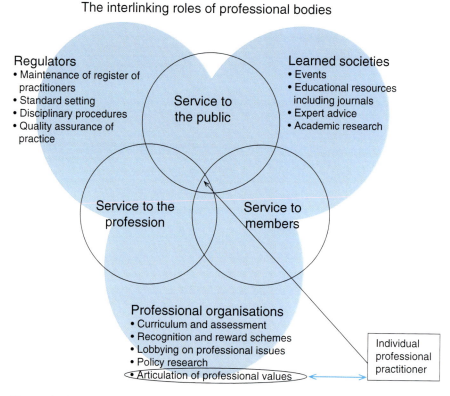

Fig. 1 The interlinking roles of professional bodies

1. *Service to the public*

    This function is principally fulfilled by regulators through their work in maintaining the profession's social contract with those it serves and the wider public, through:
    - Setting transparent and explicit standards for professional conduct against which the profession and its members may be held to account
    - Maintenance of the register of licensed practitioners, to ensure that only those who are properly qualified and can demonstrate that they are maintaining their performance against those standards may practice
    - Complaints and disciplinary procedures both to protect the public but also to allow it to express concerns and grievances in cases where it appears standards are not being upheld
    - Quality assurance of education and training

2. *Service to members*

    Learned societies serve their members, and through them the profession, through their work in offering individual practitioners:
    - Recognition and reward of their professional achievements.

- Opportunities to develop their skills and knowledge through additional voluntary education.
- Opportunities to contribute to and develop the profession's knowledge base through research, peer review, publication, and other academic practices.
- Networking opportunities through meetings, conferences, and increasingly online forums.
- Information about the profession, including raising awareness among potential members, patient or client guidance, careers support, etc.
- Access to professional recognition: in some healthcare professions, candidates sit specialist assessments administered by learned societies in order to demonstrate their advanced capability in a specific area. They may be awarded membership, fellowship, or some other title as a mark of achievement.
- Practitioner insurance, discounts, and other membership perks.

3. *Service to the profession*

  Professional organizations generally undertake the task of serving the profession through their work in promoting and defending the rights and privileges of practitioners and maintaining the profession's influence in matters of policy.
  - The professional organizations often describe themselves as "the voice of the profession," and many have a strong claim to this through their promotion and publication of professional standards (British Medical Association 2019; Association of Optometrists 2019). By joining a professional organization, an individual is not only laying claim to the privileges of professional status but more importantly is showing his or her adherence to its standards – a collectively expressed vision of that profession, its values, duties, and responsibilities.
  - Control of membership: Unlike most learned societies, which usually offer open membership to anyone interested in joining, full membership of professional organizations is contingent upon satisfaction of certain criteria (such as professional licensure, maintenance of practice certificate, a statement adhering to the professional standards, etc.). Many professional organizations award grades of membership (such as associate, membership, fellowship) through examination or assessment processes measured against clear standards. In some healthcare professions, membership of a particular professional organization such as a Royal College is a requirement for certain types of advanced practice; in others membership is desirable and widespread but not mandatory.
  - Curriculum and training: While universities usually award primary healthcare qualifications, it is frequently the profession that sets the curriculum and validates or accredits the course, acting as a guarantor to students and the public of the course's quality. In some cases, matriculation automatically confers licensure to practice. Many healthcare professions, however, also have licensing examinations that may be set by a professional organization such as a college or faculty. For instance, in the UK, Physician Associates may study at any one of a number of universities, but all must pass the Physician Associates' National Certification Exam set by the Faculty of Physician

Associates, before they can be declared fit to practice in the UK (Faculty of Physician Associates 2019).
- Lobbying on behalf of their membership's interests: Some professional organizations perform work similar to that of trade unions, becoming involved in negotiations with employers concerning pay and conditions of their members or supporting them in issues concerning legal indemnity, pension rights, or disputes with employers. In addition, professional organizations may be involved in advising government and employers on wider issues concerning the profession's engagement with public policy by, for example, representing the profession at government inquiries (Mid Staffordshire NHS Foundation Trust Public Inquiry 2013).
- Archive and history: The roots of the oldest surviving healthcare professions organization, the Royal College of Surgeons of England, go back to the fifteenth century. While most other professional organizations are relatively young by comparison, they nevertheless form the collective memory of a profession. Through their archives, including their scholarly publications, the traditions and history of a profession may be preserved, and distinguished practitioners remembered and celebrated (see, e.g., American Optometric Association 2019; British Dietetics Association 2019). While professional bodies are sometimes criticized for having failed to move with the times, it is also accepted that they have a powerful role in establishing a common sense of continuity and professional identity (Mamode 2004; Ackers 2015).

Is Healthcare Education a Proper Profession?

Although healthcare educators (HCEs) are professionals in their own clinical or academic disciplines, and while they fulfil their roles in education in a professional manner, it cannot yet be said that healthcare education is everywhere acknowledged as a profession in its own right. This is because many HCEs still lack opportunities, through dedicated professional bodies in healthcare education, to demonstrate the social contract with society that is essential for every professional practitioner (Wickenden 1932).

For healthcare education to be considered a fully fledged profession, its practitioners all need the same opportunities that they have within their clinical or academic work. They need:

1. Chances to acquire, demonstrate, and maintain their specialist educational knowledge.
2. Through their adherence to an agreed code of conduct or standards, the opportunity to publicly acknowledge and accept their responsibilities to society and those they serve. This includes an undertaking to practice their educational roles competently, ethically, and fairly and a commitment to the promotion of public good.

3. To have a "seat at the table" as part of a professional group – to be able to contribute to and influence educational policy that affects their healthcare profession; to be represented, recognized, and valued at all levels in healthcare; and to have a fair share of the resources and leadership opportunities that other professions take for granted.

Sadly, for many HCEs, these opportunities are lacking. Research among HCEs indicates that many report a lack of clear career paths, training, professional recognition by their peers in education, and explicit lines of accountability for their educational practice; in many cases, institutional support is weak or absent (Sabel and Archer 2014; Beckley 2017; Hartzler et al. 2015). This state of affairs, however, is changing rapidly; and it is largely through its many professional bodies that the professionalization of healthcare education is being brought about.

In terms of the professionalization of the role of HCEs, the picture is becoming clearer and more optimistic over time, and the progress of healthcare education towards full professional status in its own right is accelerating rapidly. This is largely owing to a significant cultural change in our understanding of the importance and value of healthcare educators to improving the overall quality of patient care and in safeguarding the health service of the future. Table 3 assesses the emerging position for HCEs in their progress towards achieving full professional status within their educational roles.

The Future: Pressures

Challenges lie ahead for all professional bodies and particularly for many of the fledgling groupings that have begun to take off in recent years. If healthcare education is to complete its progress towards full professional status, its professional bodies will need to make some difficult choices in the near future.

Financial pressures have always been an issue for professional bodies, but for many, balancing the books is becoming a significant headache (Sontag-Padilla et al. 2012). There are many reasons for this, chiefly to do with the way that such bodies are financed. All professional bodies are "not-for-profit," meaning that if they make a surplus in their operating funds, they must reapply it to their declared benevolent activities. Many receive no government funding at all, relying on membership subscriptions to survive. Some professional bodies are in the fortunate position of being able to charge for the administration of mandatory examinations; some professional bodies oblige individuals to apply for membership in order to practice professionally. Many of the older and more prestigious professional bodies also have alumni support, grant funding, and substantial investment and property portfolios. Even with this additional financial security, however, it is a challenging environment. All professional bodies will have to adapt to survive into the next century.

Nearly all professional bodies rely to some degree on subscriptions from their members; but as we have observed, many HCPs belong to more than one body, and the market is increasingly crowded. Paradoxically, as healthcare education becomes

Table 3 Key indicators of professional status in healthcare education

High-level specialist training for entry to a profession	In many healthcare professions, no training is necessary to become a HCE. Many HCEs still "see one, do one, then teach one" on the job, but it is increasingly common for basic teaching training to be made a requirement in certain occupations. It is rare at present for qualified HCPs to be required to have a formal qualification in education (such as a postgraduate certificate) before they are permitted to teach in clinical settings, but this position is changing rapidly. Some professions include elements of teaching training as part of the primary undergraduate degree. Most HCPs teaching in universities are expected to undertake postgraduate qualifications in education as part of their role, and this is increasingly a condition of appointment, particularly for more senior educational leadership roles.
Practice standards against which the profession may be publicly evaluated	Many healthcare professions have standards for education and training at institutional and organizational level; but fewer have clear statements of standards and guidance against which individual educators may be objectively assessed by their peers, for example, during annual appraisal or membership and fellowship of a college (Bullock and Browne 2013; Academy of Medical Educators 2014).
Maintenance and development of the expert knowledge base	Nearly all healthcare professional groups have academic journals reporting research into best practice within their clinical discipline or specialty. Some of these also report educational research aimed at communicating the latest evidence on the most effective ways of teaching and training. A few of the larger healthcare professions have journals devoted solely to education within that profession (such as nursing, dentistry, and medicine), and there are some interprofessional education journals.
Ongoing training for the role	High-level specialist training in healthcare education, though not yet mandatory, is now widely available, usually as a postgraduate qualification. It is now possible to achieve masters and doctoral qualifications in health education research, and there is a growing professoriate within higher education. Some healthcare specialties and disciplines, if they have not done it already, are considering mandating basic training for some educational roles (General Medical Council 2012). Many are also introducing appraisal and continuing professional development for their HCEs.

(continued)

Table 3 (continued)

Career paths	The route to becoming a HCE is still unclear in many healthcare professions; this is hardly surprising given that nearly all HCEs need to gain substantial expertise in their own professional field before they are considered capable of teaching others. In some professions, it is a requirement that teachers must carry a relevant primary clinical qualification before they can teach; in others, clinical qualifications are not essential, but certificated expertise in some branch of academic study (such as law, ethics, biomedical sciences, or social sciences) is required. For most HCPs, therefore, becoming a teacher requires further levels of commitment, experience, and study; promotion is not inevitable or systematic, and progress usually depends on individuals moving from post to post. Professional bodies have a role to play in promoting their particular profession as a career, and many offer mentoring schemes, prizes, bursaries, and fellowships as a way of supporting individuals to make progress.
Institutional support within the wider professional framework	Many HCEs report that teaching within their profession is considered low status and excellent performance as a teacher is still viewed as less prestigious than success in research or commitment to clinical practice and service delivery [see, e.g., (Flynn and Ironside 2018; Browne et al. 2018). This situation is changing rapidly, however, especially in universities, which are increasingly recognizing the added value that excellent teaching brings to improving the student experience. Furthermore, as many professions seek to bring about changes in response to the rapidly changing environment of healthcare delivery, education and educators are viewed as crucial to introducing and embedding quality improvements. Increasingly, membership of a health professions education professional body is recognized by employers in recruitment and promotion schemes.
Informal networking opportunities	Professional bodies have always offered events such as conferences and meetings where networking can take place, and many are embracing the opportunities offered by modern technology with enthusiasm. HCEs, who are frequently restricted in the amount of time they can devote to face-to-face professional development and training, are benefitting from webinars, LISTSERVs, social media exchanges (both public and members only), and so on.

a focus of growing interest, new learned societies and groups are regularly formed, all seeking the support of the same limited pool of practitioners.

Additionally, commercial interests are increasingly seeking access to areas traditionally occupied by professional bodies. Where once the professional bodies had the lion's share of the market, private companies now offer events, training courses, and publishing opportunities. While most of these commercial "new kids on the block" are entirely respectable and offer good value for money, a small number have been described as "predatory" because they take fees fraudulently, offering little in return (Bowman 2014). The backing of a professional body has currency; its seal of approval on a journal, book, or conference offers purchasers or participants an additional guarantee that the product on offer is legitimate, authoritative, and trustworthy. But although many professional organizations are justifiably proud of the quality of their publications, subscription revenues and conference incomes for many are by no means steady or guaranteed in such a dynamic market (Sontag-Padilla et al. 2012; Waltham 2006; Johnson and Fosci 2015).

Academic conferences and training events, in addition to their educational and networking values, have traditionally offered opportunities to professional bodies for generating much-needed operating funds. Surpluses generated are often then reapplied to the charitable activities of the organization. However, although conference and event organization have traditionally been the prerogative of professional bodies, commercial event organizers, especially in the field of healthcare education, are taking increasing shares of the market.

Publishing is a tried and tested means of raising subscription revenue while at the same time providing a service to members. Many journals are owned by professional bodies or published on their behalf on a profit-sharing basis by commercial publishers. But there is considerable concern about whether traditional models of publishing can remain profitable. With the passing of paper journals to online publications, the explosion in the numbers of (often low quality) online-only journals, and increasing pressure from libraries and universities to move to open access while decreasing their support for subscription-only and author-pays journals, it is clear that professional bodies and their publishing operations will have to adapt if they are to survive in the long term (Waltham 2006; Johnson and Fosci 2015).

Professional bodies traditionally depend on the goodwill of their supporters and volunteer officers. Part of being a professional involves volunteer service to professional bodies (such as reviewing and editorial work for journals; sitting on conference planning and other committees; chairing academic sessions; acting as governing body members, trustees, and directors; assessment, peer review, and exam setting and administration; and so on). This has traditionally been encouraged as bringing reputational value to a professional's employer and as a means of gaining valuable knowledge and leadership experience. In recent years, however, the goodwill has been running thin in healthcare education, for both academics and clinicians. Money to attend conferences and pay for subscriptions is tight; obtaining study leave is a complex and frustrating business. Academics are under workload pressure from multiple sources; a new managerialism within higher education institutions is increasingly reframing academic service "in new ways that serve the administrative interests of the university rather than individual discipline, organisation or network of scholars" (White 2012, p. 61). University demands for service on internal committees are increasingly prioritized over external service on professional bodies. The situation for clinician educators is even more acute. There has never been a time when healthcare practitioners did not have to juggle service delivery with teaching, scholarship, and management tasks, with service to professional bodies usually being squeezed into evenings and weekends (Sholl et al. 2017). But with an unprecedented demand on service that has not been matched by a concomitant increase in staff, it is inevitable that finding time for voluntary work in professional bodies is a decreasing priority for employers and healthcare staff (Sholl et al. 2017).

For many healthcare professions education bodies, there are turbulent financial waters ahead (Sontag-Padilla et al. 2012). The smaller, more specialist, and newer bodies are particularly vulnerable to financial risks; but these are often able to be more responsive and lighter on their feet. While their financial future may be shaky, when it comes to responding to changing societal pressures and expectations surrounding healthcare education, they may be in a better position than their older and more established counterparts.

Over the past few decades, there has been a fundamental shift in the relationship between clinicians and their patients, to which healthcare education has had to respond. Parentalistic approaches to communication have come under increasing criticism, and shared decision-making is both taught and practiced. Patients arrive for consultations better prepared and with higher expectations of the standard of care they want, and most practitioners welcome this new type of partnership working. Likewise, healthcare education has recognized the value of engaging with patients, carers, and the public. Patients are more frequently involved in clinical teaching, not just as learning resources or topics for study but also as consultants and partners in educational decision-making, as teachers and as assessors (O'Malley-Keighran and Lohan 2016). There has also been a perceptible shift in the way in which clinical teachers' relationship with students has developed. The student body is increasingly diverse thanks to energetic widening participation and recruitment activities, coupled with newer types of admission processes aimed at reducing or eliminating old inequities. Old hierarchies are giving way to a more student-centered approach, where students are less subject to passive teaching approaches and punitive assessment regimes and encouraged to develop as self-directed learners (Council of Deans of Health and the Higher Education Academy 2015). This is partly driven by the expectations of the students themselves: healthcare education is an expensive business for them, and they expect – and sometimes demand – increasing levels of support, choice, and engagement as they prepare for their future careers.

In addition to changes in patient and student expectations, educational and workplace barriers between traditional professions have begun to break down. The argument that healthcare practitioners must learn to work collaboratively in teams for the benefit of the patient and that patient care may be compromised where good team communication is lacking is well and truly won (Morley and Cashell 2017). Interprofessional practice and teamwork are seen everywhere in clinical practice. Education, particularly at postgraduate level, is correspondingly addressing the need to educate diverse healthcare practitioners to learn with and from each other for the benefit of patients. Healthcare educators themselves are more than ever working and learning in teams (Hughes et al. 2016). In the UK, for example, with the establishment of Health Education England, NHS Education for Scotland, and Health Education and Improvement Wales as national multi-professional leadership organizations for education, training, and workforce development in the health sector, the pressure to learn to work across traditional professional boundaries has increased (Department of Health 2017).

But while nationally and globally healthcare education and practice have begun to adapt to these changing educational and social expectations, individual health professions education bodies have been racing to catch up (Department of Health 2017). Most now actively seek participation from patients, student, and diverse groups at all levels, and a good deal of excellent work is being undertaken to ensure that professional bodies do not perpetuate systematic bias in their admission processes, standards, governance, assessments, curricula, and other areas of activity. But they still have some way to go. The privilege that has traditionally accrued to white male practitioners (especially in the medical craft specialties) is increasingly being challenged both from outside the professions and within them, and women and minorities are at last beginning to gain leadership positions within professional bodies (Bond and Shapiro 2017).

The issue is one of centuries of healthcare culture. Professional rivalries and traditional "turf wars" between professional bodies may prove hard to eradicate while professions still jostle for influence, esteem, and a fair share of dwindling resource. There are several learned societies that cut across professional divides (examples include the Centre for the Advancement of Interprofessional Education (CAIPE), the Irish Network of Healthcare Educators (INHED), and the Interprofessional Education Collaborative in the USA (IPEC)), but as yet they are additional to, not alternatives to, the big monoprofessional bodies. There is talk in various quarters in the UK of merging some regulators, but progress has been slow (Skinner et al. 2019). Among the professional organizations, there are few that are genuinely interprofessional. The Academy of Medical Educators through its *Professional Standards for Medical, Dental and Veterinary Educators* (Academy of Medical Educators 2014) recognizes the achievements of anyone who teaches in diverse healthcare professions, while Advance HE, although its Professional Standards Framework is not specifically aimed at healthcare educators, recognizes the work of healthcare educators working in universities worldwide (AdvanceHE 2011). Nevertheless, in many cases, generations of unconscious, pro-practitioner protectionism within rigidly defined professional boundaries are so embedded that it may take many years to weed it out (Schuwirth 2004).

Conclusion

Without professional bodies, there would be no professions. Professional bodies serve three main functions, all of which are essential for any occupation which aspires to professional status. Professional bodies usually fall into three categories:

1. Learned societies, which preserve and enrich the evidence base on which their profession is based and which work to engage practitioners in scholarship and quality improvement
2. Regulators, which maintain the register of qualified practitioners and set standards for practice
3. Professional organizations, which unite a profession around its shared values and enable it to have a collective voice on matters of public importance

In performing these functions, professional bodies maintain the profession's contract with society by articulating, promoting, and enforcing professional standards and values; enabling both individual practitioners and professions as a whole to demonstrate both their knowledge and proficiency and their acceptance of accountability to the society they are bound to serve; preserving and enriching the evidence base on which their profession is based; and using their expertise and knowledge to benefit society as a whole. But professional bodies face many challenges, both financial and organizational. The financial challenges threaten the professional bodies' stability and long-term development prospects, while the organizational challenges pose deep-seated threats to public perceptions of the contemporary relevance and values of professions. However, although professional bodies have been criticized for historical protectionism and deeply embedded biases, many are rising to the challenge of adapting to changes in society and healthcare practice with enthusiasm.

There is still a long way to go; in the difficult waters ahead, the culture of monoprofessionalism and even rivalry that has characterized professional bodies for the last few centuries will need to change fundamentally. A more collaborative approach is long overdue. Healthcare education is still waiting to be recognized as a profession in its own right. Such a move would inevitably raise standards across the board; at present nurse educators or doctors running professional development events for dental educators or physiotherapists may be doing a magnificent job – but each professional group is working within a slightly different framework and to slightly different standards and understandings that arise from their individual professions' approach to the support of educators. The potential for misunderstanding and miscommunication is considerable; but it could be mitigated if each profession's professional bodies were to align themselves more closely (Browne et al. 2020). Professional bodies as a group need to look more seriously at how HCEs can be supported as a distinct body with unique expertise and skills rather than as small and undervalued subsets of individual professions. Mergers, collaboratives, and federations, grouped around a shared set of values and understandings, are a long overdue solution to raising the collective profile of all educators in whatever area of healthcare professions education they are working.

Closer alignment is also in the professional bodies' own interests as the field becomes increasingly crowded and what little funding there is becomes more thinly spread. Research funding for educational projects within healthcare is particularly hard to secure, leading to a paucity large-scale and authoritative multi-site, multi-professional studies (Reed et al. 2007). Research collaborations between different professions' learned societies have the potential both to attract more lucrative funding and also to improve our understanding of how healthcare education across professions can be developed for the benefit of the patients, students, and wider public that we all serve.

Healthcare education as a professional practice now has many of the structures in place to allow it to make the move to a fully fledged profession. Many HCEs still lack basic opportunities, but it is through their professional bodies that healthcare educators will be empowered: to express and demonstrate their shared values and standards and have these recognized by their peers; to advocate for their profession and lobby for a fair share of the resources to help them do their work effectively; to develop their knowledge, skills, and expertise; and, crucially, to hold themselves accountable to their students, patients, colleagues, and society as a whole for their performance. It is therefore vital that all HCEs consider joining their professional bodies both for their personal development but also so that they can improve patient care through developing teaching excellence in their chosen profession.

Cross-References

▶ Competencies of Health Professions Educators of the Future
▶ Developing Educational Leadership in Health Professions Education
▶ Health Profession Curriculum and Public Engagement
▶ Surgical Education and Training: Historical Perspectives

References

Academy of Medical Educators. Professional standards 2014. Cardiff: Academy of Medical Educators; 2014.
Ackers P. Trade Unions as professional associations. In: Johnstone S, Ackers P, editors. New perspectives on employment relations. Oxford: Oxford University Press; 2015. p. 95–127.
AdvanceHE UK. Professional standards framework. York: Higher Education Academy; 2011.
American Optometric Association. Optometry history timelines. Available from https://www.aoa.org/about-the-aoa/archives-and-museum/optometry-history-timeline. Accessed 23 Sept 2019.
Association of Optometrists. Voice of the profession. Available from https://www.aop.org.uk/about-aop/aop-news/2017/02/07/voice-of-the-profession. Accessed 21 Mar 2019.
Aukett JW. What is a profession? Br Dent J. 2017;223:323.
Australasian Society of Cosmetic Dermatologists. Homepage. Available from https://www.ascd.org.au. Accessed 23 Sept 2019.

Australian Medical Association. Homepage. Available from https://www.ama.com.au. Accessed 23 Sept 2019.

Beckley ET. Nobody told me there's no supervision manual! Am Speech-Lang-Hear Assoc (ASHA) Leader. 2017;10:44–9.

Bond S, Shapiro G. Diversity and inclusion progression framework. 2017 Benchmarking report: scientific bodies. London: Science Council; 2017.

Bowman JD. Predatory publishing, questionable peer review, and fraudulent conferences. Am J Pharm Educ. 2014;78(10):176. Available from https://www.ajpe.org/doi/full/10.5688/ajpe7810176. Accessed 4 Mar 2019.

British Association of Critical Care Nurses. Homepage. Available from https://www.baccn.org. Accessed 23 Sept 2019.

British Dietetics Association. The history of the BDA and dietetics (web page). Available from https://www.bda.uk.com/about/about_bda/history. Accessed 23 Sept 2019.

British Medical Association. Our collective voice. Available from https://www.bma.org.uk/collective-voice. Accessed 18 Mar 2019.

Browne J, Webb K, Bullock A. Making the leap to medical education: a qualitative study of medical educators' experiences. Med Educ. 2018;52:216–26.

Browne J, Bullock AD, Parker S, Poletti C, Gallen D, Jenkins J. Healthcare educators' values and activities study: final report. Cardiff: Cardiff University Press. Forthcoming 2020.

Bullock AD, Browne J. Advisory group on standards for dental educators. COPDEND standards for dental educators. Oxford: COPDEND; 2013.

Community and District Nursing Association. Homepage. Available from https://cdna-online.org.uk. Accessed 23 Sept 2019.

Council of Deans of Health and the Higher Education Academy. Innovation in teaching and learning in health higher education: final report. London/York: CDH and HEA; 2015.

Department of Health. Promoting professionalism, reforming regulation. Leeds: Department of Health; 2017.

Faculty of Physician Associates. Examinations. Available from https://www.fparcp.co.uk/examinations. Accessed 22 Mar 2019.

Flynn L, Ironside PM. Burnout and its contributing factors among midlevel academic nurse leaders. J Nurs Educ. 2018;57(1):28–34.

General Medical Council. Recognising and approving trainers: the implementation plan. London: General Medical Council; 2012.

Hartzler M, Ballentine J, Kauflin M. Results of a survey to assess residency preceptor development methods and precepting challenges. Am J Health Syst Pharm. 2015;72(15):1305–14.

Hughes AM, Gregory ME, Joseph DL, Sonesh SC, Marlow SL, et al. Saving lives: a meta-analysis of team training in healthcare. J Appl Psychol. 2016;101(9):1266–304.

IPSOS Mori. IPSOS Mori Veracity Index 2018. Available from https://www.ipsos.com/sites/default/files/ct/news/documents/2018-11/veracity_index_2018_v1_161118_public.pdf. Accessed 20 Mar 2019.

Irvine D. A short history of the General Medical Council. Med Educ. 2006;40(3):202–11.

Johnson R, Fosci M. On shifting sands: assessing the financial sustainability of UK learned societies. Learn Publish. 2015;28(4):274–81. Available from https://onlinelibrary.wiley.com/doi/abs/10.1087/20150406. Accessed 19 Mar 2019.

Mamode N. Is the BMA a 21st century organisation? BMJ. 2004;329(7458):161–3.

Medical Board of Australia. Homepage. Available from https://www.medicalboard.gov.au. Accessed 23 Sept 2019.

Mid Staffordshire NHS Foundation Trust Public Inquiry. Final report. London: The Stationery Office; 2013. https://webarchive.nationalarchives.gov.uk/20150407084231/ http://www.midstaffspublicinquiry.com/report. Accessed 16 Dec 2019

Morley L, Cashell A. Collaboration in health care. J Med Imag Radiat Sci. 2017;48:207–16.

Nursing and Midwifery Council. Homepage. Available from https://www.nmc.org.uk/. Accessed 23 Sept 2019.

O'Malley-Keighran MP, Lohan G. Encourages and guides, or diagnoses and monitors: woman centred-ness in the discourse of professional midwifery bodies. Midwifery. 2016;43:48–58.

Pereira GD. Just a GP: the 1979 Gale memorial lecture. J R Coll Gen Pract. 1980;30:231–9.

Reed DA, Cook DA, Beckman TJ, Levine RB, Kern DE, Wright SM. Association between funding and quality of published medical education research. JAMA. 2007;298(9):1002–9.

Royal Australasian College of Surgeons; Academy of Surgical Educators (web page) Homepage. Available from https://www.surgeons.org/fellows/for-educators-trainers/academy-of-surgical-educators. Accessed 23 Sept 2019.

Royal College of Nursing and Midwifery. Homepage. Available from https://www.rcn.org.uk. Accessed 23 Sept 2019.

Sabel E, Archer J. Early careers working group of the academy of medical educators. "Medical education is the ugly duckling of the medical world" and other challenges to medical educators' identity construction: a qualitative study. Acad Med. 2014;89(11):1474–80.

Schuwirth L. Learning by scar formation. Med Educ. 2004;38(8):797–9.

Sholl S, Ajjawi R, Allbutt H, Butler J, Jindal-Snape D, Morrison J, et al. Balancing health care education and patient care in the UK workplace: a realist synthesis. Med Educ. 2017;51(8):787–801.

Skinner H, et al. Gender representation in leadership roles in UK surgical societies. Int J Surg. 2019;67:32–6.

Sontag-Padilla LB, Staplefoote L, Gonzalez MK. Financial sustainability for nonprofit organizations: a review of the literature. Santa Monica: RAND Corporation; 2012. Available from https://www.rand.org/pubs/research_reports/RR121.html. Accessed 17 Mar 2019.

Waltham M. Learned society business models and open access: overview of a recent JISC-funded study. Learn Publish. 2006;19(1):15–30. Available from https://onlinelibrary.wiley.com/doi/abs/10.1087/095315106775122529. Accessed 19 Mar 2019.

White J. Scholarly identity. In: Fitzgerald T, White J, Gunter HM, editors. Hard labour? Academic work and the changing landscape of higher education. International perspectives on higher education, vol. 7. Bingley: Emerald Group Publishing; 2012.

Wickenden WE. The engineer in a changing society. Electr Eng. 1932;51:465–71. Available from https://ieeexplore.ieee.org/stamp/stamp.jsp?tp=&arnumber=6429899. Accessed 5 Mar 2019.

Scholarship in Health Professions Education

83

Lisa McKenna

Contents

Introduction	1612
The Concept of Scholarship	1612
Evolution and Importance of Scholarship in HPE	1613
Challenges in HPE Scholarship	1614
Developing People and Networks to Promote HPE Scholarship	1615
Communities of Practice	1615
Health Professions Education Scholarship Units	1616
Publishing Health Professions Research	1618
Role of Bibliometrics	1618
Social Media and HPE Scholarship	1619
Strategies for Developing as a HPE Scholar	1620
Identify a Mentor	1620
Build Teams and Networks	1621
Read, Develop Research Skills and Academic Writing	1621
Create a Portfolio and Program of Work	1622
Strategies for Supporting and Growing Health Professions Scholarship	1622
Conclusion	1623
Cross-References	1623
References	1623

Abstract

Scholarship has traditionally formed the foundation of all scientific disciplines, building, and supporting their knowledge bases and growth of their scholars. However, this has often been overshadowed in the health professions by primary focus on laboratory and clinical knowledge. As a developing discipline, scholarship is fundamental to health professions education and forms the focus of this chapter. The evolution of the concept of scholarship is outlined and its importance in health professions education discussed. The chapter explores challenges faced

L. McKenna (✉)
School of Nursing and Midwifery, La Trobe University, Melbourne, VIC, Australia
e-mail: l.mckenna@latrobe.edu.au

© Springer Nature Singapore Pte Ltd. 2023
D. Nestel et al. (eds.), *Clinical Education for the Health Professions*,
https://doi.org/10.1007/978-981-15-3344-0_110

within pursuit of scholarship in the discipline, along with the importance of, and strategies for, developing the scholars who will further the discipline into the future. It also examines how health professions scholars can seek academic advancement based on their work in the field and how others can support the development of novice scholars.

> **Keywords**
>
> Academic promotion · Bibliometrics · Boyer · Community of practice · Glassick · Mentor · Publication · Research · Scholarship · Tenure

Introduction

Scholarship has been widely recognized as an important aspect of developing a strong discipline. While slower to develop when compared to other disciplines, recent decades have seen significant growth in health professions education (HPE) as a distinct discipline with many highly regarded scholars globally. Despite this, HPE has been challenged as it has attempted to sit alongside other well established clinical, laboratory, and practice disciplines in health with its own unique body of knowledge.

This chapter focuses specifically on the area of scholarship in health professions education as a distinct discipline. The evolution of scholarship is examined through the foundational work of Boyer and Glassick. This is followed by an exploration of challenges faced by scholars in HPE and strategies for promoting its scholarship. The chapter also examines the importance of research and publication for furthering the discipline and ensuring that its scholars have pathways to career advancement. It concludes with guidance for new scholars entering into health professions education and leaders charged with supporting new scholars as they embark on their professional journeys.

The Concept of Scholarship

In 1990, Ernest Boyer published his foundational work, *Scholarship Reconsidered: Priorities of the Professoriate*. In this work, Boyer argued to that time emphasis had been placed on basic research as the primary form of scholarly activity that was then conveyed to students. He contended that this was not necessarily a one-way path, rather that it could work the other way around whereby, teaching and learning informed research. Boyer went on to define a theoretical model for scholarship comprising "four separate, yet overlapping, functions" that he entitled "the scholarship of *discovery*; the scholarship of *integration*; the scholarship of *application*; and the scholarship of *teaching*" (p. 16). He saw scholarship of discovery as scholarly investigation where new knowledge is discovered. The scholarship of integration entails using and disseminating learnings both within and across disciplines, with scholarship of application enabling it to be applied to new situations and problems. Finally, the scholarship of teaching "both educates and entices future scholars" (Boyer 1990, p. 23).

In 1996, Boyer further developed his work by adding a level of performance to the model. He suggested six goals by which scholarship could be measured, namely "clear goals, appropriate procedures, adequate resources, effective communication, significant results, and careful and thoughtful self-critique" (Boyer 1996, p. 135). In doing so, Boyer introduced the concepts of self-evaluation and peer-evaluation as means for assuring the quality of teaching and learning. Charles Glassick and colleagues (1996) furthered Boyer's work. Their work with granting agencies, scholarly press directors and journal editors identified six key themes around quality and measurement of scholarship, concluding "that for a work of scholarship to be praised, it must be characterised by clear goals, adequate preparation, appropriate methods, outstanding results, effective communication, and a reflective critique" (Glassick 2000, p. 878). Importantly, Glassick (2000) cited the work of Shulman (1999) who argued that for work to be considered scholarship, it must be made available, be peer reviewed and critiqued and able to be reproduced and further developed by other scholars. Hence, the concept of scholarship implores teachers and researchers in the health professions to take on responsibility to evaluate and disseminate their work, as well as apply learnings from other scholars to their practice to continually improve the science into the future.

Evolution and Importance of Scholarship in HPE

Growth in scholarship in the HPE over recent years has been facilitated through expansion not only of unidisciplinary but also multidisciplinary approaches to the education of future health professionals (ten Cate 2021). Recognition of similarity in issues encountered by various health professions, and particularly those with clinical or practice components, has seen traditional fields, such as nursing education and medical education, coming together with other disciplines to forge the field of health professions education and its associated scholarship. This has been furthered through significant publication and research output, all focused towards preparing the best health professionals who together can provide optimal health care (ten Cate 2021).

The evolution of HPE as a science has developed towards enabling understandings of problems encountered, and teaching and learning approaches that are successful (Regehr 2010). Yet, within the clinical environment there has remained some lack of clarity as to whether HPE scholarship activities constitute translational research, implementation science, evidence-based practice, or quality assurance. Importantly, there are subtle differences (Carter et al. 2017).

1. Translational research "seeks to 'translate' research in ways that enable that research to be applied. It also 'closes the circle' by allowing practitioners to provide feedback to researchers based on their experience" (Mitchell 2016, p. 4).

2. Implementation science involves "the scientific study of methods to promote the systematic uptake of research findings and other evidence-based practices into routine practice, and, hence, to improve the quality and effectiveness of health services and care" (Eccles and Mittman 2006, p. 1).
3. Evidence-based practice is defined as that "requires that decisions about health care are based on the best available, current, valid, and relevant evidence. These decisions should be made by those receiving care, informed by the tacit and explicit knowledge of those providing care, within the context of available resources" (Dawes et al. 2005). While the definition is focused on health care provision, it also applies to HPE.
4. Quality assurance in the context of HPE involves "the development, sustenance, improvement, and evaluation of the standard" (Busari 2012) of education.

Challenges in HPE Scholarship

Numerous authors have described challenges associated with developing scholarship in HPE. It can be a particular tension for scholars in disciplines where there is pressure to produce research which directly impacts patient care over research that improves education and producing quality health professionals. This can be further exacerbated where the scholar has clinical responsibilities. Smesny et al. (2007) examined barriers to scholarship for clinical faculty members in the disciplines of dentistry, medicine, nursing, and pharmacy. They found that in all the disciplines pressure to provide clinical services and support clinical teaching for learners limited time for scholarly activities. This, along with not knowing how to document their scholarly activities, often worked against them in seeking academic promotion and/or tenure opportunities. Smesny et al. (2007) also identified a dearth of role models and mentors available for assisting them and building a culture of scholarship in the clinical environment.

Support for HPE scholarship activities has also been recognized as a challenge. Goldszmidt et al. (2008) undertook a study with medical faculty who were interested in medical education to explore their engagement and support needs for pursuing education scholarship. They found that although the majority had been involved in at least one education project in the previous five years, very few had received any funding support or had published their work. Time, accessing support staff and insufficient knowledge of research methodologies were identified barriers to achieving scholarship. The authors concluded that assisting faculty with engagement in education scholarship was complex and recommended provision of institutional supports as needed for faculty, regardless of their level of educational preparation.

More recently, the COVID-19 pandemic has reportedly contributed new challenges for scholarship in health professions education. The initial emergence of the pandemic saw rapid global transfer of face-to-face teaching and learning to online platforms with little supporting evidence about best practice. According to Goh and Sandars (2020), this prompted a need for research approaches that could facilitate "rapid cycles or investigation and implementation" (p.3) such as action research.

Furthermore, these authors suggest that such curriculum changes lead to a vast array of critical new research questions related to teaching and learning than in the past, particularly around equity issues, such as cultural or socio-economic factors, supporting technology employed, instructional and curriculum design. This reinforces a need for institutions to provide necessary support for the required scholarship activities (Nadarajah et al. 2021).

Developing People and Networks to Promote HPE Scholarship

While health professions scholarship is evolving, as the previous section highlighted, it does face a number of challenges. This section proposes strategies for addressing some of these and promoting the science of scholarship in the health professions.

Communities of Practice

Many scholars in the health professions enter the academy with strong clinical expertise and with a focus on the delivery of teaching. Many have limited experience in knowledge development, research methodologies, and knowledge translation. Support is needed to develop these skills and a different focus on the delivery of learning and teaching. Hence, the development of people is fundamental to health professions scholarship. One approach that has been widely implemented is that of communities of practice. Lave and Wenger (1991) introduced the concept of community of practice which they described as constituting a social community where participation enables learning, along with development of ideas, identity, and practices. Wenger (1998) furthered this work identifying components comprising a social theory of learning and suggesting that people are surrounded by communities of practice, often "so informal and so pervasive that they rarely come into explicit focus" (Wenger 1998, p. 7). However, communities of practice have been widely adopted in health professions over recent years in order to bring together like-minded individuals who work together to generate ideas and learn from each other.

Developing communities of practice around HPE scholarship is one fundamental means for developing scholars, ideas, and promoting scholarship. Wenger et al. (2002) advocate seven key principles for cultivating communities of practice that resonate strongly with teams in HPE scholarship, namely:

1. Design for evolution.
2. Open a dialogue between inside and outside perspectives.
3. Invite different levels of participation.
4. Develop both public and private community spaces.
5. Focus on value.
6. Combine familiarity and excitement.
7. Create a rhythm for the community. (Wenger et al. 2002, p. 51)

Health professions workforces are global in nature, and many of the issues they confront are experienced on an international scale. Hence, working collaboratively with international scholars on shared issues can bring broad insights and advantages. With this mind, Ramani et al. (2021a) proposed a set of tips for establishing, growing, and sustaining communities of global scholars to further health professions education:

1. Identify a shared need or vision
2. Develop and disseminate the shared purpose, vision, and work
3. Start to build a community
4. Purposefully cultivate the community
5. Facilitate a variety of leadership, management, and follower roles
6. Establish specific goals, tasks, and projects
7. Welcome and embrace diverse socio-cultural contexts
8. Promote and continuously attend to psychological safety
9. Make space for social interactions – virtual or in-person
10. Celebrate wins – small and large
11. Reflect (in, on and for action) and evaluate what worked, what did not
12. Plan for longer term sustainability. (Ramani et al. 2021a, pp. 967–969)

Meeting like-minded people is fundamental to successfully engaging in meaningful health professions scholarship. Globally, many professional organizations exist that enable scholars in HPE to meet, share learnings and work together; some are uniprofessional while others take a multiprofessional approach. Some examples of these are provided in Table 1. Many offer opportunities for recognizing achievement in scholarship, such as through Fellowship, conferences focused on health professions scholarship, professional publications, and meetings, that can be highly beneficial in enabling connections across organizations, countries, and discipline areas.

Health Professions Education Scholarship Units

Since the early 2000s, health professions education scholarship units (HPESUs) have emerged across many countries including Australia, Canada, New Zealand, the United States (Varpio et al. 2017a), the Netherlands (Humphrey-Murto et al. 2020), and South Africa (Van Schalkwyk et al. 2020). These units provide another mechanism for bringing health professions scholars together. HPESUs are specifically designed functional units, based in higher education facilities or hospitals, that focus on the delivery and scholarship of HPE, bringing together scholars from different health professions to work and develop together. While their individual structures vary, in identifying working definitions around the field, Varpio and colleagues identified key criteria for HPESUs, namely:

Table 1 Professional organizations focused on health professions education scholarship

Organization	Abbreviation	Website
The Academies Collaborative		https://www.academiescollaborative.com/
American Association of College of Nursing	AACN	https://www.aacnnursing.org/
Asian and Pacific Alliance for Nursing Education	APANE	http://www.apanetw.org/e-org.aspx
Association for Hospital Medical Education	AHME	https://ahme.org/
Association for Medical Education in Europe	AMEE	https://amee.org/home
Australian Nurse Teachers Society	ANTS	https://www.ants.org.au/ants/
Australian & New Zealand Association for Health Professional Educators	ANZAHPE	https://www.anzahpe.org/
International Association of Medical Science Educators	IAMSE	https://www.iamse.org/
Nursing Education Association	NEA	https://www.edunurse.co.za/

1. "The unit must stand as a recognizable, coherent, organizational identity within the institution" (Society of Directors of Research in Medical Education 2016).
2. "The unit must be identified as engaging in health-professions education-related scholarship. This scholarship may be conducted at the undergraduate, graduate, and/or continuing education levels. The unit may also house programs that focus on teaching, service provision, professional development program delivery, etc., but these other activities alone are not sufficient for being identified as an HPESU without the scholarship contributions" (Varpio et al. 2017b, p. 208).

In an analysis of eight HPESUs conducted 14 years after their implementation, Humphrey-Murto et al. (2020) found that each had emerged differently but concluded that three key elements were vital to their success, namely people, pipeline, and supporting structures. In regard to people, strong leadership was identified as crucial to enabling the HPESU to develop and be sustainable. Furthermore, a critical mass of scientists/scholars was necessary, along with strategies for unit growth. It was identified that having a centralized physical structure for the unit enabled it to be identified and less vulnerable. There also needed to be a balance between service priorities, and research, and strong messaging about what the unit did. Finally, not relying on a single source, but obtaining funding from a variety of sources was needed for sustainability of the unit.

Publishing Health Professions Research

Disseminating scholarship is an important activity for tenure and promotion, as well as developing the evidence base and science of scholarship. The field of health professions scholarship is growing amidst an increasing number of related journals, both discipline specific and multidisciplinary; yet publishing in the field can still be challenging with a steadily increasing volume of work being produced. Rees et al. (2022) conducted an international survey investigating health professions authors' choices of journals for their work. They identified six key factors influencing journal choice namely, "fit, impact, editorial reputation, speed of dissemination, breadth of dissemination, and guidance from others" (n.p.). They recommended that authors were not disheartened by receiving an editor's decision to revise their work, that journal selection was done early in the research process, and that manuscripts fitted the journal where they were submitted.

In previous decades, securing tenure or promotion could be challenging for academics from health professions whose research was education focused, and continues to remain so in some areas (Wendling 2020). With promotion criteria largely being focused around teaching, research/scholarship, and service, it could be difficult to develop a strong case for promotion around the area of research and scholarship. However, since the emergence of Boyer's work, many universities have begun to view scholarship in broader terms than purely research, encompassing other "scholarly" activities such as development of quality education programs, innovative instructional materials, or researching around teaching and learning (Register and King 2017), and enabling the case for promotion to be made based more on scholarship activities (Hobson et al. 2022).

Role of Bibliometrics

Studies into the science of scholarship, through analysis of bibliometrics, are important in academia (Smith and Hazelton 2011), so have an important role to play in advancing the science of health professions education scholarship. Such analyses will enable gaps in existing knowledge to emerge and guide future scholarship activity. Roberts et al. (2020) conducted a systematic mapping review of entry-level occupational therapy education scholarship in Australia from 2000 to 2019 finding that topics around student characteristics and perceptions had been well researched in the discipline, while there were identified gaps in teaching methods and approaches and learning environment that required further examination. Buffone et al. (2020) conducted a review of authorship in seven health professional journals to explore international representation in the field. They identified from 7793 included articles that 90.4% involved collaborations while 86% were conducted by authors from single region teams, mostly from North America, Northern or Western Europe. Articles led by researchers from Asia, Africa, and South America were low in number. Buffone et al. concluded that diversity in health professions education was low, dissemination was largely unidirectional, and there was a need for greater diversity. This indicates a need for greater international collaborations.

Bibliometric data can also be useful in benchmarking in one's discipline area and may assist with supporting a case for academic promotion or tenure, particularly with a teaching or scholarship focused case. For example, McKenna et al. (2017) conducted an analysis of Australian nursing/midwifery Professors' publication output using the Scopus database. They identified that publications per professor varied from two to 436 and citations from one to 6378. Overall, findings indicated that they compared well with UK colleagues and that performance had escalated since 2010. In a subsequent review, the team examined similar data to determine whether scholarship in nursing or midwifery education could result in a successful research career (Cooper et al. 2018). They found those professors who published in education achieved similar citation levels than those who did not and concluded that focusing on nursing and/or midwifery education did not appear to disadvantage career progression. Such data offers potential for individual benchmarking against peers and strengthening of cases for promotion and/or tenure with a focus on education scholarship.

Social Media and HPE Scholarship

Social media has become a ubiquitous part of everyday life. Increasingly social media platforms, such as Facebook, Twitter, and LinkedIn, are being utilized in academic scholarship as a means of disseminating research and other scholarly activities. Nowadays, most publishers provide authors with links to social media platforms to promote work as soon it is published. While traditionally, success of publication output has been measured by citations counts, the emergence of alternative metrics, or altmetrics, has meant that researchers can have more immediate indications of interest and how their work is being discussed and shared online. By promoting reach, it has the potential to increase subsequent dissemination and citation. A study by Maggio et al. (2017) utilized Altmetric Explorer to search for health professions education work with at least one altmetrics event between 2011 and 2015. They found that over the time, the number of related articles with altmetrics had increased by 145%, reflecting the growing impact of the measure and importance for health professions education.

However, content on social media can vary significantly in its quality and appropriateness. Noting the developments in the area, Sherbino et al. (2015) sought to develop criteria which could support the quality of HPE scholarship disseminated through social media channels. At a professional medical education conference, they undertook to gain consensus from 52 health professions educators from 20 organizations in four countries, identifying four key statements defining and evaluating social media-based scholarship. The criteria suggest that such scholarship must:

1. "Be original
2. Advance the field of health professions education, by building on theory, research, or best practice
3. Be archived and disseminated
4. Provide the health professions education community with the ability to comment on and provide feedback in a transparent fashion that informs wider discussion." (Sherbino et al. 2015, p. 552)

Hence, Sherbino et al. (2015) emphasized that not all social media would meet the standards to be considered scholarship.

Overall, if used well, social media can be a powerful tool for supporting health professions scholarship and supporting academic progression. Identifying a deficit in how to incorporate social media impact into recognized academic accomplishment, such as for promotion or tenure, Acquaviva et al. (2020) employed a crowdsourced approach to the development of guidelines that could assist health professions scholars with documenting contributions. As a result, they developed two sets of guidelines:

1. Guidelines for Listing All Social Media Under Public Scholarship
2. Guidelines for Listing Social Media Scholarship Under Research, Teaching and Service

Hence, their guidelines provide useful frameworks for documentation of scholarly impact via social media that might be considered in supporting academic advancement.

Strategies for Developing as a HPE Scholar

So far, this chapter has explored a number of contributing factors to the success of health professions scholarship, an area that can be daunting for a newcomer. This section provides some guidance on how to get started in developing as a scholar and building a career in health professions education or supporting others in such endeavors.

Identify a Mentor

Mentors have been widely recognized as important for supporting development of scholars in HPE (Crites et al. 2014). Others with prior experience and achievement can be invaluable in helping to navigate pathways towards the development of scholars in a multitude of ways, such as assisting with goal and career development, reviewing proposals, abstracts, or promotion applications. In doing so, they can assist avoid pitfalls and barriers that might present along the way. In an Australian study on nurse scholars' views on contemporary scholarship, the role of mentors was described as focused on "role making," rather than "role modelling" (Stockhausen and Turale 2011). Sullivan (2018) suggests that if a potential mentor is identified that negotiating protected time with them is important for assisting with goal and strategy development towards the mentee's development.

Build Teams and Networks

Building a network of like-minded people is important for developing as a HPE scholar. This can be achieved through joining communities of practice, but if no suitable community exists, it can require time in identifying, building, and growing scholars who can work effectively together. This may require engaging for the first time with HPE scholars in other health disciplines, as professional silos still exist in many places. Directly approaching other scholars may be found to be mutually beneficial if such scholars themselves are seeking opportunities for connecting with other HPE scholars but it may take time to find the mutual middle ground and mutual interest. Scholarly teams may be more likely to produce highly cited research where, according to McGaghie (2009), there are:

1. Shared goals and a common mission
2. Clear leadership that can change and rotate
3. High standards and expectations
4. Sustained commitment and hard work
5. Team members within physical proximity
6. Minimal status differences within the team
7. Promoted and maximized team status
8. Shared activities where trust is fostered (McGaghie 2009, p. 578)

Much scholarship literature is written by teams, rather than individuals. Writing with a team can provide valuable support for less experienced scholars to develop the nuanced skills required in navigating the publication process or grant application development and increase productivity and success. Experienced scholars understand the issues that can arise in publishing, writing styles and the requirements of editors, journals and funding bodies and can provide highly beneficial guidance and support, particularly in newly formed teams.

Ramani et al. (2021b) promote collaborative writing, or writing in teams, as a means of co-creating scholarship in the health professions. This assists with skills and ideas development, provides psychological safety and leadership, and encourages team diversity. These authors recommend regularly reading academic literature, writing workshops and groups, and accessing writing resources to facilitate skills development.

Read, Develop Research Skills and Academic Writing

Many health professionals take on roles requiring scholarship after developing very successful clinical or practice careers. While being excellent practitioners, they may not have broad knowledge of current research and thinking around their area of expertise, and particularly that in learning and teaching. Scholarship requires deep knowledge of existing work in the field, so wide reading is important place to start. It is also vital in facilitating the identification of knowledge gaps for future research. Journals in the relevant field will present the most up-to-date knowledge and research activity in a discipline, so provide an important place to begin. Reading also requires the ability to critique the research being reviewed, that is, the ability to determine levels, quality, and strength of available evidence. It also includes evaluating aspects such as research questions, chosen methodology, ethical and data analysis processes, along with researcher credibility. Working with teams of scholars, as previously described, can assist with refining and developing critiquing skills.

Create a Portfolio and Program of Work

Scholars in HPE should consider developing a learning and teaching scholarship portfolio. Initiating a portfolio early in one's career as a scholar in HPE facilitates the collection of key resources that may be required later for activities such as seeking academic tenure or promotion. While there are many different approaches to developing portfolios, McGaghie (2009) suggests that a professional portfolio "describes and documents professional goals and activities, provides evidence about their quality or impact, and allows for frequent updates of one's academic profile" (p. 586). It should act as a repository for items that demonstrate the scholar's activities and achievements and links between theory and teaching practice. This might include teaching innovations and their evaluations, awards, presentations, reflections on teaching and scholarship, as well as relevant publications or conference presentations.

Reflection plays a key role in developing a HPE scholarship portfolio and can often be used in academic promotion (Crites et al. 2014). In Sweden, Pelger and Larsson (2018) undertook a study with 77 academics who participated in workshops to develop a reflective teaching portfolio. The reflected on three key areas, students' learning processes, their own development as teachers over time and scholarship through activities such as conferences, publications, and collaborations. Participants reported increased their awareness of their teaching, changes in their educational conversations with colleagues, focus on theoretical underpinnings of their teaching practice and enhanced focus on scholarship of learning and teaching.

Strategies for Supporting and Growing Health Professions Scholarship

In addition to individuals implementing strategies to build their careers in health professions education, there is much that education institutions can do to support health professions scholarship. As a focus there is a need to implement institution-wide strategies to support HPE scholarship. Nadarajah et al. (2021) identify the roles of institutions as three-fold, namely supporting individuals to have influence, supporting engagement in HPE scholarship, and identifying scholarship in a range of ways. These can include a range of strategies such as:

- Providing seed funding for learning and teaching project development and innovation or publication support
- Support for internal and external seminars and conference attendance to facilitate skills development and networking opportunities in HPE
- Developing criteria for competence and academic promotion specifically developed around HPE at different academic levels
- Providing recognition of leadership in curriculum development and management
- Annual awards for learning and teaching excellence
- Providing access to expertise for quality assurance and faculty development exercises
- Promoting academics to complete HPE qualifications
- Recognizing achievements in HPE scholarship

Conclusion

Scholarship is a key foundation to the evolution and knowledge underpinning every scientific discipline. As a developing discipline, scholarship is therefore key to health professions education. This chapter has examined the concept of scholarship and what this means for health professions education. It has explored some of the challenges faced in promoting scholarship and has examined strategies for measuring and succeeding in a career in health professions scholarship. The chapter concluded by presenting considerations for new scholars looking to grow their expertise and profiles in the field and strategies for other supporting new scholars in the discipline.

Cross-References

▸ Developing Health Professional Teams
▸ Professional Bodies in Health Professions Education
▸ Reflective Practice in Health Professions Education
▸ Role of Social Media in Health Professions Education

References

Acquaviva KD, Mugele J, Abadilla N, Adamson T, Bernstein SL, Bhayani RK, Büchi AE, Burbage D, Carroll CL, Davis SP, Dhawan N, Eaton A, English K, Grier JT, Gurney MK, Hahn ES, Haq H, Huang B, Jain S, Jun J, Kerr WT, Keyes T, Kirby AR, Leary M, Marr M, Major A, Meisel JV, Petersen EA, Raguan B, Rhodes A, Rupert DD, Sam-Agudu NA, Saul N, Shah JR, Sheldon LK, Sinclair CT, Spencer K, Strand NH, Streed CG, Trudell AM. Documenting social media engagement as scholarship: a new model for assessing academic accomplishment for the health professions. J Med Internet Res. 2020;22(12):e25070.

Boyer EL. Scholarship reconsidered: priorities of the professoriate. The Carnegie Foundation for the Advancement of Teaching; 1990.

Boyer EL. From scholarship reconsidered to scholarship assessed. Quest. 1996;48(2):129–39.

Buffone B, Djuana I, Yang K, Wilby KJ, El Hajj MS, Wilbur K. Diversity in health professional education scholarship: a document analysis of international author representation in leading journals. BMJ Open. 2020;10:e043970.

Busari JO. Comparative analysis of quality assurance in health care delivery and higher medical education. Adv Med Educ Pract. 2012;3:121–7.

Carter EJ, Rivera R, Mastro K, Larson EL, Vose C. Clarifying the conundrum: evidence-based practice, quality improvement, or research? The clinical scholarship continuum. J Nurs Adm. 2017;47(5):266–70.

Cooper S, Seaton P, Absalom I, Cant R, Bogossian F, Kelly M, Levett-Jones T, McKenna L. Can scholarship in nursing/midwifery education result in a successful research career? J Adv Nurs. 2018;74:2703–5.

Crites GE, Gaines JK, Cottrell S, Kalishman S, Gusic M, Mavis B, Durning SJ. Medical education scholarship: an introductory guide: AMEE Guide No. 89. Med Teach. 2014;36:657–74.

Dawes M, Summerskill W, Glasziou P, Cartabellotta A, Martin J, Hopayian K, Porzsolt F, Burls A, Osborne J. Sicily statement on evidence-based practice. BMC Med Educ. 2005;5 https://doi.org/10.1186/1472-6920-5-1.

Eccles MP, Mittman BS. Welcome to Implementation Science. Implement Sci. 2006;1(1) https://doi.org/10.1186/1748-5908-1-1.

Glassick CE. Boyer's expanded definitions of scholarship, the standards for assessing scholarship, and the elusiveness of the scholarship of teaching. Acad Med. 2000;75(9):877–80.

Glassick CE, Huber MT, Macroff GI. Scholarship assessed: evaluation of the professoriate. The Carnegie Foundation for the Advancement of Teaching; 1996.

Goh P-S, Sandars J. Rethinking scholarship in medical education during the era of the COVID-19 pandemic. MedEdPublish. 2020;9(1):97.

Goldszmidt MA, Zibrowski EM, Weston WW. Education scholarship: It's not just a question of 'degree'. Med Teach. 2008;30(1):34–9.

Hobson WL, Gordon RJ, Cabaniss DL, Richards BF. Documenting educational impact in the promotion dossier with an Enhanced Curriculum Vitae. J Contin Educ Health Prof. 2022;42(1):47–52.

Humphrey-Murto S, O'Brien B, Irby DM, van der Vleuten C, ten Cate O, Durning S, Gruppen L, Hamstra SJ, Hu W, Varpio L. 14 years later: a follow-up case-study analysis of 8 health professions education scholarship units. Acad Med. 2020;95(4):629–36.

Lave J, Wenger E. Situated learning: legitimate peripheral participation. Cambridge University Press; 1991.

Maggio LA, Meyer HS, Artino AR Jr. Beyond citation rates: a real-time impact analysis of health professions education research using altmetrics. Acad Med. 2017;92(10):1449–55.

McGaghie WC. Scholarship, publication, and career advancement in health professions education: AMEE Guide No. 43. Med Teach. 2009;31(7):574–90.

McKenna L, Cooper SJ, Cant R, Bogossian F. Research publication performance of Australian Professors of Nursing & Midwifery. J Adv Nurs. 2017;74:495–7.

Mitchell P. From concept to classroom What is translational research? Australian Council for Educational Research; 2016. https://research.acer.edu.au/cgi/viewcontent.cgi?article=1009&context=professional_dev

Nadarajah VD, Lim VKE, Baba AA. Investing in scholarship for health professions education: learning from the past to move into the future. Med Teach. 2021;43(supp.1):S1–4.

Pelger S, Larsson M. Advancement towards the scholarship of teaching and learning through the writing of teaching portfolios. Int J Acad Dev. 2018;23(3):179–91.

Ramani S, McKimm J, Findyartini A, Nadarajah VD, Hays R, Chisolm MS, Filipe HP, Fornari A, Kachur EK, Kusurkar RA, Thampy J, Wilson KW. Twelve tips for developing a global community of scholars in health professions education. Med Teach. 2021a;43(8):966–71.

Ramani S, McKimm J, Forrest K, Hays R, Bishop J, Thampy J, Findyartini A, Nadarajah VD, Kusurkar RA, Wilson KW, Filipe HP, Kachur EK. Co-creating scholarship through collaborative writing in health professions education: AMEE Guide No. 143. Med Teach. 2021b;44:342. https://doi.org/10.1080/0142159X.2021.1993162.

Rees EL, Burton O, Asif A, Eva K. A method for the madness: an international survey of health professions education authors' journal choice. Perspect Med Educ. 2022; https://doi.org/10.0007/s40037-022-00698-9.

Regehr G. It's NOT rocket science: rethinking our metaphors for research in health professions education. Med Educ. 2010;44:31–9.

Register SJ, King KM. Promotion and tenure: application of scholarship of teaching and learning, and scholarship of engagement criteria to health professions education. Health Prof Educ. 2017;4:39–47.

Roberts M, Hooper B, Molineux M. Occupational therapy entry-level education scholarship in Australia from 2000 to 2019: a systematic mapping review. Aust Occup Ther J. 2020;67:373–95.

Sherbino J, Arora VM, van Melle E, Rogers R, Frank JR, Holmboe ES. Criteria for social media-based scholarship in health professions education. Postgrad Med J. 2015;91:551–5.

Shulman L. The scholarship of teaching. Change. 1999;31(5):11.

Smesny AL, Williams JS, Brazeau GA, Weber RJ, Matthews HW, Das SK. Barriers to scholarship in dentistry, medicine, nursing, and pharmacy practice faculty. Am J Pharm Educ. 2007;71(5): article 91.

Smith DR, Hazelton M. Bibliometric awareness in nursing scholarship: can we afford to ignore it any longer? Nurs Health Sci. 2011;13:384–7.

Society of Directors of Research in Medical Education. Membership criteria. Definition of a medical education research unit. 2016. http://sdrme.org/about-criteria.asp. Accessed 22 Sept 2022.

Stockhausen L, Turale S. An exploratory study of Australian nursing scholars and contemporary scholarship. J Nurs Scholarsh. 2011;43(1):89–96.

Sullivan GM. A toolkit for medical education scholarship. J Grad Med Educ. 2018; https://doi.org/10.4300/JGME-D-17-00974.1.

ten Cate O. Health professions education scholarship: the emergence, current status, and future of a discipline in its own right. FASEB BioAdv. 2021;3(7):510–22.

Van Schalkwyk S, O'Brien BC, van der Vleuten C, Wilkinson TJ, Meyer I, Schmutz AMS, Varpio L. Exploring perspectives on health professions education scholarship units from sub-Saharan Africa. Perspect Med Educ. 2020;9:359–66.

Varpio L, O'Brien B, Hu W, ten Cate O, Durning SJ, van der Vleuten C, Gruppen L, Irby D, Humphrey-Murto S, Hamstra SJ. Exploring the logics of health professions education scholarship units. Med Educ. 2017a;51:755–67.

Varpio L, Gruppen L, Hu W, O'Brien B, ten Cate O, Humphrey-Murto S, Irby DM, van der Vleuten C, Hamstra SJ, Durning SJ. Working definitions of the roles and an organizational structure in health professions education scholarship: initiating an international conversation. Acad Med. 2017b;92(2):205–8.

Wendling L. Valuing the engaged work of the professoriate: reflections on Ernest Boyer's *Scholarship Reconsidered*. J Scholar Teach Learn. 2020;20(2):127–42.

Wenger E. Communities of practice: learning, meaning and identity. Cambridge University Press; 1998.

Wenger E, McDermott R, Snyder WM. A guide to managing knowledge: cultivating communities of practice. Harvard Business Press; 2002.

Developing Educational Leadership in Health Professions Education

84

Margaret Hay, Leeroy William, Catherine Green, Eric Gantwerker, and Louise Marjorie Allen

Contents

Introduction	1628
What Is Leadership?	1632
What Is Educational Leadership in HPE?	1634
What Is Educational Leadership Development in HPE Today?	1635
Leader Versus Leadership Development: An Important Distinction	1636
Educational Leadership Development in HPE for Now and the Future	1638
The Primacy of Psychological Safety	1640
What Development of Educational Leadership in HPE Can Become	1645
On Evidence and Scholarship for Educational Leadership Development	1651
Conclusion	1652
Cross-References	1653
References	1653

M. Hay (✉)
Faculty of Education, Monash Centre for Professional Development and Monash Online Education, Monash University, Clayton, VIC, Australia
e-mail: margaret.hay@monash.edu

L. William
Eastern Health Clinical School, Monash University, Box Hill, VIC, Australia
e-mail: leeroy.william@monash.edu

C. Green
Royal Victorian Eye and Ear Hospital, East Melbourne, VIC, Australia

E. Gantwerker
Northwell Health, Lake Success, NY, USA

Zucker School of Medicine at Northwell/Hofstra, Hempstead, NY, USA
e-mail: egantwerker@northwell.edu

L. M. Allen
Monash Centre for Professional Development and Monash Online Education, Monash University, Clayton, VIC, Australia
e-mail: louise.allen@monas.edu

© Springer Nature Singapore Pte Ltd. 2023
D. Nestel et al. (eds.), *Clinical Education for the Health Professions*,
https://doi.org/10.1007/978-981-15-3344-0_111

Abstract

The unprecedented innovations implemented in response to the COVID-19 pandemic confirmed that rapid and successful innovations to health professions education (HPE) and health care are achievable. The pandemic accelerated calls to improve the learning and working environments for all engaged in health care and HPE, where unacceptable levels of stress and burnout were evident even before the pandemic. Contemporary concepts of leadership emphasize distributed collective approaches that focus on developing others to achieve change and innovation, whilst thriving in their workplace. Leadership development is a process that requires considerable time, commitment, and planning across intrapersonal, interpersonal, organizational, and systems dimensions. Currently, educational leadership in HPE is in a position to utilize the insights and experiences of the recent past to create the much heralded, but, as yet unattained, improved future for students, trainees, faculty, clinical teachers, healthcare providers, and patients. Given the inextricable link between education and healthcare provision, investment in educational leadership development in HPE across all levels of training and practice is likely to translate into significant gains in productivity of the healthcare workforce and improved patient care. It is incumbent upon the educational leadership in HPE today to develop the educational leadership of the future. Prioritization, investment, and a renewed focus on a culture of psychological safety and purpose for those at the forefront of health care and education is urgently required from leaders now, to ensure an improved future. The dearth of research on educational leadership development in HPE, and more broadly, confirms that it is a rich area for scholarly enquiry.

Keywords

Leadership · Educational leadership · Leadership development · Health professions education · Leadership and innovation · Psychological safety

Introduction

It is timely to focus on the development of educational leadership in health professions education (HPE). As mentioned in other chapters of this book, the Coronavirus pandemic commencing in 2019 (COVID-19) forcibly motivated many industries globally, including education, to rapidly innovate. HPE, although traditionally slow to change (Frenk et al. 2010; Chunharas and Davies 2016), achieved rapid and substantial new innovations to education alongside the acceleration of other planned ideas. The response enabled an unparalleled agility for educational leadership in HPE, as the focus swiftly turned to new ways of thinking about, planning, and implementing education (Eva and Anderson 2020b; Thomas et al. 2021; Matthew et al. 2021) and healthcare delivery (Jackson and O'Halloran 2021;

Ng et al. 2021; Edmondson 2020). The pandemic response led to an unprecedented global sharing of innovations in HPE, inspired by the reality that everyone was facing the same challenges (Eva and Anderson 2020a). In healthcare delivery the formations of new collaborations and innovations across Australia, including rapid upscaling of intensive care capacity, introduction of virtual care, upscaling of telehealth, and the formation of a National Cabinet to manage the COVID-19 response, were reported (Jackson and O'Halloran 2021). This collaboration and innovation were at least partly inspired by a shared vulnerability that does not usually exist in a hierarchical healthcare system or in educational institutions. No one was immune from COVID-19, nor the uncertainty and anxiety that it caused. The "common enemy" provided a cause for unity, collaboration and broke down existing polarities in society (rich vs poor), health care (medical vs nonmedical), and education (academics vs non-academics). Hierarchies were flattened and what emerged was the essence of education and leadership – of people coming together to solve common problems and using their various skills. This is essentially a merging of professionals and non-professionals, professors, and students to solve the many challenges we all face.

The achievements of educators and practitioners across a broad spectrum of HPE and healthcare delivery have, and continue to be, miraculous. As the world learns to live amidst the pandemic, our global and collective experiences have propelled us along two dimensions of progress and change. First, there is now widespread acceptance that what was initially perceived as short-term pivots to educational practice will in fact endure (Erlich et al. 2021). The immediate focus of leadership in HPE is on the balancing act of determining which of these rapidly implemented innovations will be sustained, revised, expanded, or abandoned while continuing the business of education. In this sense the pandemic response has initiated significant and unprecedented reform of HPE, much of which was called for long before the advent of COVID-19 (Frenk et al. 2010; Chunharas and Davies 2016). This newfound approach to rapid innovation has enabled both educators and healthcare providers to think about and do their work differently. In HPE, it is timely then to focus on how the field will continue to innovate in the face of uncertainty, and to establish a sustainable culture of innovation.

Leadership is all about addressing, creating, and sustaining change (Laksov and Tomson 2017; Sandhu 2019). Achieving successful innovations, especially in times of uncertainty and chaos, is inextricably linked to leadership (Edmondson 2019). Leadership from what we have witnessed during the COVID-19 pandemic can emanate from chaos. Public health HPE are now full of heroes and leaders…but were they considered so before? Leadership, as we explore in this chapter, is about cultivating the environment for curiosity, innovation, and personal and professional development that leads to changes which benefit the many rather than the few. From a healthcare and education perspective, we can each impact the well-being of a sick person but we soon realize that we can do more good for more people by working together. Leaders need to promote that move from internal excellence into an external ability to motivate and sustain similar standards of excellence around a greater good – a worthy cause that gives our personal and professional lives meaning. It is timely then to focus on the development of educational leadership in HPE that will ensure a culture of continued innovation and reform. The complexity of HPE and healthcare provision means that each leadership role has inherently unique challenges, yet relative to the world of commercial business, there has been a long-standing inattention to leadership development in HPE and health care more generally (Gorman and Hay 2017; Sandhu 2019). The enduring interdependencies between healthcare delivery and education also position educational leadership in HPE as significant change agents for healthcare system reform (Sandhu 2019). Past experience, while highly valuable, is no assurance of a preparedness for current or future challenges (Sklar 2018; Souba and Souba 2018). New approaches to HPE and its continued reform require different educational leadership, and therefore new approaches to developing educational leadership in HPE.

Second, the vastness of the pandemic's impact on health, economies, and the social and professional fabrics of populations globally has brought to the fore our human capacity to survive such uncertain times. But it has also unveiled our individual and collective fragility, and accelerated existing calls to humanize many ingrained work practices across all sectors (Ignatius 2020; Dirani et al. 2020). In health care and HPE the fragility of many students, trainees, and practitioners was clearly apparent pre-pandemic with substantial evidence of unacceptable levels of impaired well-being across a range of health disciplines globally (Dendle et al. 2018; Boostel et al. 2018; Zhou et al. 2020), now intensified by the COVID-19 response (Arnetz et al. 2020; Rose et al. 2021; Salari et al. 2020). Informal information via digital platforms from students, trainees, and practitioners sharing their experiences of learning and working through a pandemic further indicates the need for urgent reform. The stress of health professionals, including those in training, has been attributed to the increasingly dysfunctional environments in which they work and learn (Jackson and O'Halloran 2021). Ensuring a safe and positive learning environment for students and trainees in the health professions must be a priority for educational leadership in HPE, despite the complexities of the context in which it occurs. However, the healthcare system of Australia, often heralded as one of the best in the Organisation for Economic Co-operation and Development (OECD) (Dixit and Sambasivan 2018), has recently been described as "... fragmented, inefficient, inflexible, and organisation – rather than person-focussed..." (Jackson and O'Halloran 2021, p. 301). Organizations and rules have a vital place in safety cultures like health care, but have these systems become ossified and, in turn, paralyzed our innovation and ability to change for the better. Healthcare worker job satisfaction and work-related health before the pandemic was known to influence workforce retention and patient care across Europe, the USA, and Australia (Bong 2019; van Diepen et al. 2020). It is pertinent to question whose interests are being prioritized? Patients and students, or the established people in power?

With inauthentic communication and the dehumanization of leadership that has lost sight of healthcare worker vulnerability as "wounded healers," there have been calls for a concerted shift to a person-focused healthcare system (William 2021). We will all become unwell or aged and die. So, what does health, and therefore HPE which prepares the healthcare workforce, mean in this context? Jadad and O'Grady (2008) defined health as: "the ability that we have as individuals or communities to adapt and to manage the inevitable challenges that we face through life - physical, mental, or social." This is an inclusive definition, as opposed to the WHO definition: "Health is a state of complete physical, mental and social well-being and not merely the absence of disease or infirmity" (International Health Conference 2002). If we are to reimagine health care and HPE, then leadership in these areas need to recognize the holistic and collaborative approach that is required. It means looking at the whole person's health, with them and in conjunction with their supporters and the different disciplines that are required for their care. It is health, cared for by professionals and communities together, with a common goal to support each other in our common frailties. Is not this the same in "educational health," i.e., the ability that we have as individuals or communities to adapt and to manage the inevitable challenges that we face through life, the physical, mental, or social. It is all about learning and knowledge and wisdom gained through experience.

Anthropologically, we have learned from stories and the lessons they convey. Health care relies upon obtaining the stories from people and trying to manage what we "diagnose." So, in developing leadership in HPE, do we need to tell stories and develop the art of uncovering and listening and understanding stories? As we tentatively emerge from the pandemic, we have the unique opportunity to listen to the many stories that need to be told, and to reimagine educational leadership and its development to emphasize the human aspects and capitalize on this newfound agility, collaborative spirit, and openness to innovation. Given the long-standing resistance to achieving change in HPE, it is timely to differentiate the leadership of the past, and to consider the qualities and therefore development needs of educational leaders in HPE for the present and future.

In this chapter we appeal to literature on contemporary approaches to leadership to identify the development needs for educational leadership in HPE. Drawing on leadership literature from the business world, social sector, healthcare system, and HPE, we identify key approaches to educational leadership development for sustained educational innovation and positive learning experiences for students, trainees, and educators alike. We acknowledge that the way forward is a long journey requiring significant change and commitment from the leaders of today to prioritize and resource the development of educational leadership that will better serve all engaged in the complex systems of HPE, and by extension, healthcare delivery. We hope that through identifying the significant advantages to students, faculty, and practitioners across all disciplines in the health professions, that educational leadership development can be reconceptualized as a vital aspect of HPE that is critical to achieving continued reforms to both education and health care. We further hope that prioritizing the development of educational leadership may bring a renewed sense of purpose for all engaged in HPE.

What Is Leadership?

Leadership is notoriously difficult to define, largely due to the complexities of the undertaking, and the many and varied contexts in which it occurs. In the business literature and increasingly beyond, the leader has long been reframed from the authoritative and all knowing "boss" who dictates orders to unquestioning subordinates with little regard for their experiences, to a compassionate and visionary conductor of the organization and its resources, with increasing emphasis on the human resource (Collins 2005; Ignatius 2020). In industries and sectors globally, the COVID-19 pandemic has accelerated the sustained recommendations for a shift from authoritative to consultative leadership (Ignatius 2020; McKinsey and Company 2021). It is widely acknowledged that hierarchies and top down decision-making through executive power have limited value in contemporary approaches to leadership (McKinsey and Company 2021; Edmondson et al. 2016). Instead, flattening of hierarchies, breaking down silos in both health care and HPE, and a decentralization of decision-making to achieve the flexibility and agility necessary for survival in contemporary times are encouraged (Dalakoura 2010). Hierarchies inhibit achieving the creativity required for innovation (Edmondson 2019), which may be a contributing factor to the slow reform of HPE (Frenk et al. 2010; Chunharas and Davies 2016). Coltart et al. (2012) call for the medical profession internationally to "... move beyond traditional notions of hierarchy and leadership from an elite minority, and begin investing in the leadership attributes of all its future workforce" (p. 1849). Of course, this applies to health professions more broadly than medicine. Therefore, educational leadership of the future in HPE should strive for nonhierarchical, intergenerational, concentric overlapping circles of function rather than squares on an organizational chart (Sandhu 2019).

Contemporary definitions of leadership encompass cognitive, behavioral, and social aspects. They focus less on the authoritative "command and control" leader as an entity in and of themselves, and more on their ability to positively influence those around them to achieve. While flattening hierarchies is the ultimate aim, nontraditional hierarchies can have an important role in defining leadership capabilities, and this is particularly so in the complex governance and diffuse power structures that feature in social sectors such as education and healthcare. Leadership success, especially at the top levels, is through influence rather than executive power (Collins 2005). Collins (2005) describes a hierarchical pyramid structure of leadership in the social sectors, with level 5 at the pinnacle. The five levels are described in Fig. 1.

Collins (2005) provides the overarching responsibilities of leadership at each of the five levels of his pyramid structure described in Fig. 1. Level 5 leaders epitomize authentic leadership, driven by purpose and mission of the institution rather than their individual gains. There is general consensus on the leadership competencies of priority setting, vision establishment, and capacity to mobilize people and other organizational resources to enact the vision (Green et al. 2019; Reich et al. 2016), which characterize levels 3 and 4 of the Collins structure. McKimm and O'Sullivan

> **Level 5: Executive Leader**, is characterised by personal humility and ambition for the mission of their institution (i.e., the cause) rather than themselves. They are driven to make the right decisions for the long-term high performance of their institution relative to its mission. They consult, however, will make decisions independent of consensus being achieved.
>
> **Level 4: Effective Leader**, stimulates the high-performance standards of others through actions that continuously moves the institution toward a clear and compelling vision.
>
> **Level 3: Competent Manager**, ensures institutional objectives are efficiently achieved through organising the human and other resources.
>
> **Level 2: Contributing Team Member**, is characterised by their individual input into team achievements and their effective ability for teamwork.
>
> **Level 1: Highly Capable Individual**, who contributes productively through their talent, skills, knowledge, and optimal approaches to their work

Fig. 1 Five levels of leadership in the social sector described by Collins (2005)

(2016) conceptualize leadership as a triad, where leaders provide the vision, strategy, energy, and moral compass (Collins levels 4 and 5); managers provide stability, order, and translate the leaders vision to action (Collins levels 3 and 4); and followers both support and challenge the leader (Collins levels 1 and 2). In the McKimm and O'Sullivan model, the productive interdependency of each triad underlies organizational success, reinforcing that leadership is a collective rather than an individual pursuit. This proactive positioning of followers in the McKimm and O'Sullivan model, as distinct from passive subordinates, is a further feature of contemporary leadership, where a culture of active listening and being open to perspectives of others, be they individuals or teams, regardless of their organizational position, defines high-performance leadership (Collins level 5). Hence, our proposed approach to developing educational leadership in HPE requires an understanding of each role and its inherent leadership capabilities, and engenders greater connections in the acknowledgment that everyone is a leader, manager, and follower in their personal or professional roles. However, this first requires the establishment of a culture of psychological safety (which we discuss below), where people feel confident to share ideas without fear of embarrassment or retribution (Edmondson 2019). Inspiring and enabling individuals and teams to perform to their highest ability is a core feature of humanizing work, and is increasingly recognized across industries as critical to the success of organizations and their people, including in health care (Edmondson 2015).

What Is Educational Leadership in HPE?

Educational leadership in the health professions has additional complexity because it involves two inextricably connected yet independently functioning systems: that of healthcare delivery and that of tertiary education. McKimm et al. (2021) note the added and unique sets of challenges for educational leadership in HPE where the education both services and is dependent upon the healthcare sector. Laksov and Tomson (2017) also note the complexity of educational leadership in HPE which involves processes across the three levels of students/trainees, educators/practitioners, and the organizational contexts (hospitals/universities) in which the education occurs. Educational leaders in HPE are required to navigate across environments, sometimes simultaneously as both educator and healthcare provider. Educational leadership in HPE aligns with the organizational structures of teaching institutions (Sklar 2018). Faculty progression is generally from academic and clinical teaching to educational coordinator roles, and to academic or clinical program director and ultimately educational associate dean and dean level positions (Bendermacher et al. 2021). This process engenders a hierarchical task-over-person approach that has proliferated health and educational leadership and has not served either well (Sandhu 2019). In addition, leadership in the context of health care is often used vaguely without reflecting the complexities of the healthcare system and the real world in which this leadership is embedded (Reich et al. 2016). This speaks to the need for the development of educational leadership in HPE that is specific to the conditions in which it takes place (i.e., universities and the healthcare system), and yet is also integrated within the leadership of university/tertiary and healthcare systems in which it occurs (Bendermacher et al. 2021; Coltart et al. 2012; Laksov and Tomson 2017).

The lack of a clear process for leadership development in nursing, in which educational leadership is embedded, beyond the identification of specific competencies with little evidence as to which competencies are critical for success has also been highlighted (Miles and Scott 2019). Tucker (2017) proposes five competencies that educators in the health profession should aspire to obtain, of which leadership is one. These are:

1. Facilitating learning
2. Curriculum design and instruction
3. Assessing learning
4. Scholarship of teaching and learning
5. Educational leadership and administration

Tucker defines the educational leadership and administration competency as the "... knowledge, skills, and abilities that medical educators do to foster collaboration, manage projects, and exhibit integrity" (p. 784). This definition also includes institutional resource management and quality assurance, which better align with the manager role in the McKimm and O'Sullivan (2016) model and level 3 of the Collins (2005) structure. Proficiency in all five competencies is foundational requirements for impactful educational leadership in HPE, and should therefore be developed in all who aspire to educational leadership roles. Expertise in these competencies can be gained formally via additional postgraduate education (Tekian and Taylor 2017; Tekian et al. 2014); informally via the many accredited and unaccredited training programs, and via direct experience opportunities provided through professional development programs for health professionals (Allen et al. 2019); and engagement in communities of practice (Bendermacher et al. 2021).

A qualitative study by Laksov and Tomson (2017) investigated educational leadership through the lens of those in educational leadership positions across a range of health professions. They identified five activities described by educational leaders as inherent to their educational leadership role, and which are somewhat distinct from the models presented thus far. These are:

1. Taking a student-centered approach
2. Leading the development and improvement of students and faculty
3. Embracing the role visionary and inspirer of others
4. Emphasizing organizational learning and creation of a creative learning environment
5. Creating the bridges and networks within the university and externally to learning environments

Bendermacher et al. (2021) studied the role of educational leadership in advancing a positive culture in HPE and concluded that leaders routinely navigate between the intrapersonal, interpersonal, organizational, and managerial aspects of practice. The intrapersonal aspect was defined as creating self-awareness, widely accepted as a requirement at all levels of leadership. The interpersonal aspects included building communities of practice, organizational tasks and goal setting, which align with activities 2, 4, and 5 of Laksov and Tomson (2017), and Collins (2005) level 4. Managerial aspects related to strategy development, which also align with Collins level 4. Bendermacher et al. reported interpersonal aspects as the most influential in enhancing a quality culture in HPE. However, others have reported intrapersonal factors as most influential in nurse technical skill acquisition (Widjaja and Saragih 2018). These contrasting findings confirm an important distinction of focus for educational leadership in HPE when designing a curriculum for technical (so-called "hard") versus human (so-called "soft") skill development, the latter of which has the enablement and support of others at its core.

What Is Educational Leadership Development in HPE Today?

Despite broad acknowledgment of the complexity of educational leadership in HPE, surprisingly little attention has been paid to its development. Leadership development in both health care and HPE is described as a drip-feed (Keijser et al. 2017) haphazard process (Sklar 2018) that is notoriously underdone (Sandhu 2019). Leadership development is often sought post-appointment, as just-in-time training

(Gorman and Hay 2017; Green et al. 2019), usually at senior level (Bendermacher et al. 2021; Sandhu 2019; Keijser et al. 2017). This often results in leaders with no or limited expertise for the leadership aspects of their position, placing them at risk of failure before they commence (Edmondson 2019). The need to move from the current ad hoc leadership training that many leaders in the health professions experience, to an organized and aligned approach has been noted (Sklar 2018). Research has shown that currently the development of educational leadership competencies occurs largely through communities of practice where proactive development of leadership skills and actions (including educational reforms) occur (Bendermacher et al. 2021; Laksov and Tomson 2017). In addition, educational leadership development is self rather than organizationally driven, with limited evidence of a planned systematic educational leadership development program within, across, or external to participants' institutions (Bendermacher et al. 2021; Laksov and Tomson 2017). This may account for leadership in HPE expressing feelings of invisibility as leaders within their organizations (Laksov and Tomson 2017). Addressing the lack of a planned or systematic approach to educational leadership development is essential to achieve a more effective approach (Laksov and Tomson 2017). Advocating for equity in the appreciation of educational leadership roles in health care to those of clinical and research leadership can further advance quality culture in HPE (Bendermacher et al. 2021).

Leader Versus Leadership Development: An Important Distinction

Just over a decade ago Dalakoura (2010) made the prescient and vital distinction between leader and leadership development, arguing that the latter is critical for organizational survival and success in turbulent times. While *leader* development focuses on building the skills of individual leaders, usually senior in their organizational hierarchy, *leadership* development focuses on the broader social context in which leadership is both developed and enacted. The success of leadership development lies in expanding the collective capacity across an organization (Dalakoura 2010). Doing so enables people at all levels of the organization to learn and effectively engage in leadership roles and processes as part of their everyday experience. This focus on upskilling the collective capacity of the organization rather than selected individuals is the crux of the collective social framework, also labeled as integrative (Chunharas and Davies 2016) or distributed (Sandhu 2019) leadership development. Within this framework, to be effective, formal leadership development must be integrated across all levels of the organization, something that is rarely done in educational leadership development in HPE (Bendermacher et al. 2021; Miles and Scott 2019). This collective model enables active engagement in leadership development in the everyday practices of the organization, thereby leading to exceptional leadership practice at "big L" (i.e., leaders with formal titles) and "little l" (i.e., people with no formal leadership role or title) levels (Stoller 2020). It also enables leaders to develop others to be leaders, which is a critical factor to effective leadership and succession planning, again something which is widely reported to be underdone in developing educational leadership in medicine (Gorman and Hay 2017; Sklar 2018; Souba and Souba 2018; Sandhu 2019), nursing (Miles and Scott 2019; Tucker 2020), allied health (O'Donovan and McAuliffes 2020a), and higher education (Cavanaugh 2017).

This collective, integrative, and distributed approach to leadership development uplifts both leader and leadership development capacity across the entire organization with positive outcomes for organizational functioning, and for the people within it. It requires leaders with the skills and expertise to develop future leaders, i.e., leadership educators. Surprisingly, very little is understood about the process of developing leadership educators in any field. The research that does exist explores the professional identity constructions of leadership educators, showing that the leadership development journey contains both cognitive and experiential dimensions (Priest and Seemiller 2018). Procedural aspects such as gaining knowledge, teaching skills, pedagogy, and theories of learning and leadership represent the cognitive dimension. The experiential dimension represents participants' personal growth as both leaders themselves and as leadership educators (Priest and Seemiller 2018). This dimension also contains intrapersonal and interpersonal aspects noted by Bendermacher et al. (2021) and Widjadja and Saragih (2018) Intrapersonal aspects include self-reflection, challenging self-beliefs and biases, learning from successes and failures, with the focus on continual self-growth and improvement of practice as leadership educators (Priest and Seemiller 2018). The interpersonal aspect of the experiential dimension involve enabling the leadership development of others through provision of support and guidance. Modeling leadership as a leader themselves was seen as important to developing leadership ability in others (Priest and Seemiller 2018). Leadership educators held a sub-identity of leader within their identity of leadership educator which impacted on their beliefs about leadership education in the Priest and Seemiller study. They viewed leadership as complex, relational, contextual, and oriented toward change, and therefore leadership education as providing the conditions to develop leaders to lead in these complex, relational, contextual, and change-oriented ways. Consistent with the HPE leadership development literature, much of leadership educator development was reported as on the job experiential learning (i.e., deliver, revise, re-deliver), rather than formal training (Priest and Seemiller 2018). This experiential learning has been described as a continual process of practice, reflection, and refinement that can generate feelings of failure and an imposter syndrome early in leadership educators' careers, as they develop their competency (Priest and Seemiller 2018; Bendermacher et al. 2021).

The identification of educational leadership competencies in HPE is important to ensure their development. The literature reviewed thus far indicates a dearth of research on the required competencies for success and their attainment. The focus is largely on the procedural (training) rather than experiential (developmental) dimensions of leadership development. Given the complexity of educational leadership in HPE, as we emerge from the pandemic there is a clear and urgent need to learn from, plan for, and implement the various approaches to educational leadership development in HPE that support a culture of innovation and lead to a productive learning environment for all engaged in HPE.

Educational Leadership Development in HPE for Now and the Future

We have shown that leadership development requires both training and experience, yet opportunities to gain experience in educational leadership in HPE are rare. There are increasing calls for greater emphasis on collective and distributed developmental approaches to leadership development that have direct applicability to educational leadership development in HPE (De Brún et al. 2019). It has been argued that taking advantage of all of the education years will change perceptions of leadership in nursing from that of a formal role, to that of an influencing process that is used by and taught to all nurses (Miles and Scott 2019). Multiple authors advocate for a shift to collective leadership development that is spread throughout a system (Dalakoura 2010; Laksov and Tomson 2017; Miles and Scott 2019). To achieve this there is a need to develop the knowledge, skills, and competencies to *do* leadership (horizontal development) and development of a sense of *being* a leader (vertical development), both of which require learning leadership through experience (i.e., doing), at all levels of training to truly develop leadership capacity (Dalakoura 2010; Miles and Scott 2019). This should be achieved through a distributed approach to educational leadership development in HPE; however, most existing programs are targeted to those already in leadership positions (Green et al. 2019; Sandhu 2019).

We have noted that the traditional hierarchized organizational structures still highly prevalent in health care and educational leadership today are of limited value and stifle collaboration and innovation. Given that the culture of health care can limit innovation and change (Bendermacher et al. 2021; Keijser et al. 2017; Edmondson 2015), we believe educational leadership in HPE must focus on contemporary approaches to leadership development that encourage a continuation of the newfound culture of collaborative innovation that was a feature of the COVID-19 crisis response. Current leadership in HPE has been called on to pay close attention to the many lessons from the pandemic and to "... seize the moment to facilitate and mobilise real change within their institutions or communities" (McKimm et al. 2021, p. 34). Experience from the past confirms that there is no place for complacency if we are to capitalize on these lessons and not return to the past. For example, Nyenswah et al. (2016) describe a shift to distributed leadership as highly effective in managing Liberia's Ebola virus outbreak of 2014. This shift was necessitated by the inability of the existing hierarchical leadership to appropriately respond to the epidemic, which allowed it to escalate. Distributed leadership was implemented, where responsibilities and authority were shared across all levels of the response. Stakeholders were also engaged, based upon their strategic importance to the response rather than their position on an organizational chart. Despite the success of this distributed approach in managing and ultimately ending the epidemic through unprecedented collaboration and new ways of doing things, the authors describe a rapid return to the previous and ineffectual hierarchical leadership at the declining phase of epidemic, which they conclude leaves Liberia vulnerable to another health crisis. The authors highlight their disheartenment at the "limited appetite for institutional learning" from the experience. This experience confirms the need for immediate diligence to sustain the benefits COVID-19 has provided to HPE as we progress to the declining phase of the pandemic, and the need for active planning to develop educational leadership capacity in HPE for a better future.

We have also noted the increasing requests to humanize the contexts in which HPE occurs given the unacceptable prevalence of impaired well-being, stress, and burnout across many levels of health professions education and practice globally. We believe that creating a safe and productive learning environment for learners and educators in HPE is a significant and salient responsibility of leadership in both health care and HPE of today, and at all levels of the two systems in which it occurs. Increasingly the students and trainees in HPE are anachronistic to hierarchical leadership (Gorman and Hay 2017). Today, people have a heightened expectation of the interpersonal competence of their leaders, and are less tolerant of interpersonal weaknesses in their leadership (Dalakoura 2010). The well-being movement and heightened social and emotional awareness of current students and trainees has underpinned their pleas to humanize their experiences across all levels of their training, and into practice. It is the responsibility of educational leadership in HPE to ensure safe and productive learning environments, and failure to do so is a failure of educational leadership. Given the central place of students, trainees, practitioners, and educators in healthcare systems globally, the known challenges many are facing, and the positive impact educational innovations can have on healthcare practices, it is timely to consider different approaches to developing educational leadership in HPE.

What does the development of educational leadership in HPE need to be, in order to establish at scale educational leadership that addresses the two areas for improvement that we have noted and which are challenging HPE right now? The two areas being:

1. The long and often-noted slowness of HPE to innovate and therefore ensure graduates who have the skills to practice in the environments in which they learn and work
2. The urgent need to humanize the context in which students, trainees, educators, and practitioners learn and perform their work.

The concept of psychological safety first introduced by Edgar Schein in 1965 and popularized by Amy Edmondson helps answer this question by addressing both of these challenges simultaneously.

The Primacy of Psychological Safety

As previously discussed, contemporary frames of leadership development make explicit the link between leadership and innovation. Innovation, by its very nature, requires venturing into novel areas where failure is inevitable. Since our education and reward systems focus on achieving success and avoiding failure, achieving an innovator's mindset goes against much of our learnings and experiences, and requires developing a mindset that misaligns with many existing systems of operation (Dyer et al. 2009). Innovation requires an environment of psychological safety, where curiosity is both encouraged and nurtured, where respectful exchanges of ideas and productive disagreement feature, and where failure is not feared (Edmondson 1999, 2019; Edmondson and Lei 2014). We noted earlier that high-performance leadership creates and enables a culture of active listening – being open to perspectives of others regardless of their status (Collins 2005; McKimm and O'Sullivan 2016). Leadership is first and foremost about helping people and teams succeed to their maximum abilities, which require an environment where psychological safety has primacy (Edmondson 2019). Psychological safety is characterized as the belief that it is safe to ask questions, provide feedback, and voice concerns without interpersonal risk (O'Donovan and McAuliffe 2020b). In the context of HPE, psychological safety requires everyone engaged across all levels to be open to candid and respectful dialogue that is agnostic to status and where all inputs are welcomed. There is a considerable evidence base for psychological safety as a precursor to innovation across individual, team, and organizational levels (McKinsey and Company 2021). Psychological safety is essential for adaptive functioning in the rapidly changing business environment of today, which has clear parallels to health care and HPE (Edmondson 2019; McKinsey and Company 2021). Psychological safety was critical to the creation of safe spaces for experimentation, risk taking, and learning from failure in the COVID-19 response described by Stoller (2020).

Obviously, there is no place for failure in healthcare that risks putting people at harm, but this necessary culture of safety and risk aversiveness in health care may have hindered the establishment of a culture of innovation in HPE, or at least restricted implementation of innovations within the broader system of healthcare delivery. Three levels of failure have been proposed by Edmondson (2019): preventable, complex, and intelligent. Applied to HPE, preventable failures occur due to deviations from defined processes (e.g., the inclusion of concepts/skills not yet learned in a summative assessment task), while complex failures (e.g., stress and burnout in students and trainees) are the result of system breakdown. Intelligent failures result from the exploration of novel ways of doing things through experimentation (e.g., educational innovations in response to COVID-19 that have been less successful than anticipated. For other examples see Norman (2018) and Wilkinson (2018)). Preventable and complex failures produce bad outcomes and are to be avoided, while intelligent failures, because they are thoughtfully planned and have the potential to succeed, do less harm and produce valuable learning. In all cases failures must undergo analysis which leads to tangible changes to ensure they do not reoccur. This process of analyzing failures and implementing change is described as first-order problem solving that is not always evident in responses to failure in health care (Tucker and Edmondson 2003). Intelligent failures can provide insights for further refinement of innovations and learnings applied to continued innovations. As such, there are always learnings to be had from intelligent failures which educational leadership development in HPE can adopt to ensure continual efforts for improvement and reform. This approach is particularly important in the complex and quickly changing volatile, uncertain, complex, and ambiguous (VUCA) environment in which HPE is embedded.

Enabling psychological safety at all levels of an organization, regardless of its importance in achieving a culture of innovation, is a critical role of leaders and leadership, as is actively combatting the many ways it fails (Edmondson 2019). So, which leadership styles are associated with the ability to create psychological safety? Consultative leadership, where leaders actively seek and accept input from team members, and where curiosity, candor, and respectful disagreement are encouraged, not surprisingly directly lead to psychological safety (McKinsey and Company 2021). Consultative leaders model and encourage curiosity by asking thoughtful probing questions, and invite others to speak up, both of which are a feature of psychological safety (Edmondson 2019), collective leadership development (Dalakoura 2010), and the humility of level 5 leaders (Collins 2005). In addition to consultative leadership, supportive leadership, where leaders encourage team members to support each other and model supportive behaviors themselves indirectly contributes to team psychological safety through the establishment of positive team cultures (McKinsey and Company 2021), analogous to level 4 leader capabilities in the Collins (2005) structure. Interestingly a challenging leadership style, where leaders encourage team members to be creative, empower them to initiate change, to self-develop, and to go beyond their self-perceived abilities is strongly related to psychological safety, but requires a positive team climate to be effective (McKinsey and Company 2021). While consultative, supportive, and challenging leadership are all positively linked to psychological safety, authoritative leadership, characterized by command and control behaviors of leaders, is detrimental to psychological safety in teams (McKinsey and Company 2021). Team members tend to be disengaged, unmotivated to provide input into the work of their team, are fearful of interpersonal engagement, and are reluctant to seek help.

Of interest to educational leadership in HPE is the observation that a challenging leadership style, in the absence of consultative or supportive behaviors, causes anxiety and non-help seeking behaviors in team members which stifles collaboration (McKinsey and Company 2021). Team members in this kind of environment "... feel alone and in over their heads but do not feel able to ask for help. They believe their work is important and are challenged by it, but they do not feel supported or enabled to do it well" (McKinsey and Company 2021, p. 6). Given the continued prevalence of authoritative leadership in health care (Sandhu 2019; Keijser et al. 2017), upon which HPE relies, it is possible that challenging students and trainees during their learning in the absence of supportive or consultative behaviors of leaders may account for the unacceptable situation of students and trainees opting out of educational opportunities due to stress (Sandhu 2019). It may also be a contributing factor to high rates of stress and burnout in students and trainees (Zhou et al. 2020). Leaders who challenge and are supportive and consultative create what has been referred to as the learning zone (McKinsey and Company 2021). Here, team members are energized by their work, feel supported and challenged to take risks, freely request and offer input and assistance, and feel capable to achieve. In this environment, innovation is encouraged, and failure is not feared.

In environments like health care and HPE, where the work involves uncertainty, interdependence, and high stakes, psychological safety is critical to success (Edmondson 2019). Given the dependency on teamwork in health care, psychological safety is also necessary for learning and improving how teams resolve functional and constructive conflict (O'Donovan et al. 2021). Furthermore, psychological safety is critical to accomplishing individual and institutional goals in health care and HPE during challenging circumstances, and across all levels, for all professionals (McKimm et al. 2021). Candor, transparency, and learning from reflection on errors (i.e., psychological safety) are essential aspects of both learning and practice in health care (Sandhu 2019). To achieve this, we require leadership that enables learners to question, to freely express divergent views, to seek advice, to find answers to difficult questions, to learn appropriate responses to difficult challenges, and to model these behaviors for others (Sandhu 2019). Given this unequivocal link between leadership styles and psychological safety, educational leadership development in HPE must instill in future leaders the skills and abilities to create positive learning cultures that are not universally evident today, in which all who are engaged can thrive. Large-scale educational leadership development in HPE is needed to achieve this.

Achieving large-scale change is complex because it requires collective action at the intrapersonal, interpersonal, organizational, and system levels (McKimm et al. 2021). Similarly, psychological safety is a complex phenomenon because it is influenced by all levels of the organization across individual, team, organizational, and systems levels (O'Donovan et al. 2021). To alter leadership behaviors, the necessary changes needed to address these complex processes must occur within complex systems (e.g., health care, tertiary education). For this to occur the development of a taxonomy of skills that align to the organizational mission is required (Priest and Seemiller 2018). For example, a mission may be to achieve psychological safety at all levels of the organization, and an aligned skill, a commitment to having an open dialogue. This taxonomy of skills would guide leadership development that is embedded in the day-to-day work of all people across all levels (Priest and Seemiller 2018; Bendermacher et al. 2021; Miles and Scott 2019). Four recommendations for leadership educator development that align with these requirements have been proposed (Priest and Seemiller 2018), which have synergies with recommendations to create psychological safety in the workplace (Edmondson and Hugander 2021), and for developing educational leadership in HPE (McKimm et al. 2021; Miles and Scott 2019; Sandhu 2019). These are:

1. Dedicated time for reflection
2. Engagement in and creation of communities of practice
3. Intentionally designed, developmental approaches to leadership educator development
4. Dedicated practice in being a leadership educator

The first recommendation is for dedicated time for reflection via journaling or other means (Priest and Seemiller 2018). For Sandhu (2019), reflection is at the heart of leadership. Reflection enables leadership educators to constantly consider the evolving concepts of what an effective leadership educator is, and to continually learn from and improve their leadership education practice (i.e., intrapersonal dimension). The importance of both retrospective reflections to identify areas for further development and anticipatory reflection to create visions of and plan for their desired future as a leadership educator have been noted (Priest and Seemiller 2018). Time is also essential for leadership development in psychological safety, where a constant and daily cycle of reflective practice and revision that requires long-term commitment is needed (Edmondson 2019). As part of the reflective process, visualization is an important step to creating and sustaining psychological safety in the workplace (Edmondson and Hugander 2021). This involves leadership visualizing situations in advance of their occurrence (anticipatory visualization). For example, rehearsing individually and with others how they will create an environment that encourages candor and perspective-taking, to enable the internalization of the actions needed to navigate complex discussions or decisions (Edmondson and Hugander 2021).

Consistent with a collective approach to leadership development, the second recommendation of Priest and Seemiller (2018) is engagement in and creation of communities of practice for sharing ideas with others, giving and receiving feedback, and being engaged in dialogue directly relevant to their practice as leadership educators. Communities of practice enable people to learn from others and to safely practice leadership (i.e., interpersonal aspect). Collective workplace learning and communities of practice are important in the creation of a quality culture in HPE (Bendermacher et al. 2021). Deliberate planning for and creation of opportunities for "on the job" networking, communication, and coalition building across departmental and institutional boundaries and subcultures enables the development of educational leaders in HPE who can influence change across a broad range of contexts, via influencing the individuals within them (Bendermacher et al. 2021). Of particular importance is the engagement in communities of practice in the early phase of educator leadership practice (e.g., levels 1 to 3 of Collins (2005), because people can share with and learn from those with more experience (Priest and Seemiller 2018).

The third recommendation is for intentionally designed, developmental approaches to leadership educator development (Priest and Seemiller 2018). These approaches enhance the competence and confidence of leadership educators through provision of skills that match their development, and enable experiences of effective practice. Replacing the trial-and-error approach (Keijser et al. 2017; Sklar 2018) with deliberately planned skill development, especially in the early phase of a leadership educator role, will reduce feelings of inadequacy that many leadership educators report early in their careers (Bendermacher et al. 2021; Priest and Seemiller 2018). In environments characterized by change and uncertainty such as health care, embedding leadership development within the organizational system is essential where "... problems are too many and too complex to be identified and sorted out by one or a few persons" (Dalakoura 2010, p. 436). Such deliberate planning and implementation across all levels of education and training across the system must occur at the organizational level, and is a salient missing element of educational leadership development in HPE today. Health leadership development should consider leadership as evolving within many systems, across many levels, engaging many leaders (Chunharas and Davies 2016). Developing basic educational leadership capacity in HPE at all levels of training will have the greatest possible impact on HPE performance within the complex environment in which it takes place. This approach acknowledges that leadership occurs at all levels regardless of formal leadership titles, and enables expansive contributions that have added value. For example, Sandhu (2019) views students and trainees as the future educational leaders of HPE and health care, and who can provide unique perspectives on HPE. This was confirmed by their active engagement in solutions during the COVID-19 pandemic (Stoller 2020).

The fourth recommendation is for dedicated practice in being a leadership educator (Priest and Seemiller 2018). This involves leaders learning to authentically share with colleagues and students their own shortcomings and successes along their leadership and leadership educator journeys. The existence of intentionally designed curricula across HPE provides unique opportunities for deliberate embedding of educational leadership development learning opportunities and experiences within the curricula during education and training that is currently absent. Given the role of peer (Thomas et al. 2021) and near peer (Tai et al. 2016) teaching in HPE, abundant opportunities for educational leadership development and embedded experience in its practice exist, albeit uncaptured. Embedding these opportunities within the curricula requires a prioritization of educational leadership development in HPE from the leaders of today. It requires dedicated resources for effective planning, implementation (including developing and sustaining communities of practice), mentoring, and evaluation. However, designing and implementing programs that develop leadership at all levels and which focus on creating psychological safety is challenging, requiring extraordinary commitment over time (Dalakoura 2010; Edmondson 2019). These challenges are heightened in healthcare contexts where professional norms of autonomy and organizational structures restrict the free flow of ideas and growth (Edmondson 2019). Integrating leadership development into everyday practices is a solution that has been proposed to address the challenges of leadership development across organizational levels (Dalakoura 2010; Keijser et al. 2017; Miles and Scott 2019; Bendermacher et al. 2021). In practice this includes individuals and teams having regular opportunities to practice skills that promote psychological safety, including perspective-taking, candid inquiry, sharing of ideas, and respectfully exploring disagreements (Edmondson 2019; McKinsey and

Company 2021). For example, having structured and facilitated weekly sessions for both emerging and existing leaders to practice together and to hone these skills (Edmondson 2019). Frequent practice opportunities also serve to normalize these approaches as a standard part of daily work. Given the embedded and integrated nature of educating health professionals in the context of healthcare delivery, leadership development at all levels from the commencement of training should be achievable provided it is appropriately prioritized, planned, and resourced.

What Development of Educational Leadership in HPE Can Become

Despite increasing recognition of its importance as discussed in this chapter, strategic prioritization of educational leadership development in HPE is largely absent. We have outlined in Table 1 tasks, including perspectives and actions, that can lead to immediate change in educational leadership enactment and development, simply by changing mindsets, expectations, and therefore behaviors. We have used the dimensions of intrapersonal, interpersonal, organizational, and system to reflect the collective and developmental approach to educational leadership development we and many others are advocating for. The existing structures and processes of HPE can, with relatively little change, enable a collective and developmental approach to educational leadership development provided it is prioritized as a core competency for students and faculty, with support for effective implementation. This involves a substantial shift in how leadership development in HPE, and health care more generally, is currently undertaken, to focusing on leader*ship* development across all levels rather than leader training for senior leaders, and development of the collective over individual competency attainment. It requires a reframing of educational leadership in HPE as positive change agents across all levels of the system and therefore impacting on health care itself. It involves collective action at the intrapersonal, interpersonal, organizational, and system levels, across the Collins (2005) five levels of leadership in the social sector (see Table 2), and thoughtful consideration of leadership styles that support and encourage learning (see Table 1). It requires establishing a defined purpose for educational leadership that embodies both procedural and experiential leadership competencies and their continued development across all levels of training, and which enables and sustains a primacy of psychological safety.

The complexity of leadership and the urgent need for change in health care and HPE mean that change at all levels, individual (intrapersonal, interpersonal), organizational, and systems, are required to set the stage for a new form of educational leadership development in HPE that is transferable to leadership in health care. Support from senior leadership is important for sustained success, but change can begin immediately through a shared commitment to collective leadership development and psychological safety regardless of position. Three interrelated practices that must be repeatedly applied to enable and sustain psychological safety (Edmondson 2019) are:

Table 1 Educational Leadership Development (ELD) aligned with dimensions of intrapersonal (micro), interpersonal (micro/meso), organizational (meso), and system (macro) levels, leadership style, and required reframe for success

Dimensions	Perspectives and actions	Leadership style	Reframe
Intrapersonal (micro)	Development of educational and educational leadership development (ELD) in pedagogy, procedural skills and competencies (Tucker 2017; Laksov and Tomson 2017) Commitment to regular reflection, visualization, and constant self-development (Priest and Seemiller 2018; Edmondson 2019; Sandhu 2019) ELD takes time over a lifetime and commitment to constant self-improvement (Laksov and Tomson 2017; Sandhu 2019) Understands and contributes to a vision for ELD Commitment to psychological safety for self, self-awareness as a leader (Bendermacher et al. 2021), educational leadership developer (Laksov and Tomson 2017)	Supportive, consultative, challenging	ELD as a long process, over years, never ending, lifelong commitment Personal growth as vital Effective and enabling leadership as vital to positive change Failure as positive
Interpersonal (micro/meso)	Educational leader as leader, coordinator, coach, consultant, and role model (Dalakoura 2010) Frames the work, enabling individuals to develop – communities of practice, mentorship (Priest and Seemiller 2018) Models curiosity, candor, and respect (Edmondson 2019; McKimm et al. 2021; McKinsey and Company 2021) Enables a psychological safe environment and combats ways it fails (Bendermacher et al. 2021; Edmondson 2019)	Supportive, consultative, challenging	Development of others over self as a priority Psychological safety as a right Vulnerability as normal Change as possible Failure as positive

(continued)

Table 1 (continued)

Dimensions	Perspectives and actions	Leadership style	Reframe
	Creates conditions for others' continued learning to achieve excellence, contributes with crucial knowledge and insights (Bendermacher et al. 2021; Edmondson 2019) Acknowledges own and learner's vulnerability and risks through thoughtful questioning (Priest and Seemiller 2018; Edmondson 2019) Provides stability and vision for accomplishing individual and organizational goals (McKimm et al. 2021) Enables both individuals and teams to succeed (Bendermacher et al. 2021; Edmondson 2015) Role models behavioral reinforcement, purpose, motivation (Stoller 2020; Sandhu 2019) Actively enables the collective to achieve organizational vision in ELD (Bendermacher et al. 2021; McKimm and O'Sullivan 2016)		
Organizational (meso)	Organizational reinforcement of ELD as a priority undertaking (Bendermacher et al. 2021) Creates organizational structures that enable an agile developmental collective approach to ELD – space to experiment, take risks, learn from failure (Chunharas and Davies 2016; Edmondson 2019; Stoller 2020) Sets aspirational vision for ELD via consultation with a broad range of stakeholders (Sandhu 2019; Sklar 2018) Ensures a shared mental	Consultative, challenging	ELD as a vital competency for continued reform to both HPE and healthcare practice A culture of innovation and experimentation in HPE as a necessity for continued reform and sustainability Distributed and collective leadership empowers the many Everyone can have valuable contributions if enabled

(continued)

Table 1 (continued)

Dimensions	Perspectives and actions	Leadership style	Reframe
	model of the vision and enables other to enact the vision (Stoller 2020) Provides dedicated and continuing resources for ELD (Bendermacher et al. 2021; McKimm et al. 2021) Monitors alignment with and achievement of purpose and motivation (Bendermacher et al. 2021) Identifies key influences for role modelling. Role modelling from the executive educational and health leadership (Bendermacher et al. 2021; Edmondson 2019) Empowers "big L" & "small l" leadership (Sandhu 2019; Stoller 2020). People who are not bosses are seen as valuable contributors (Edmondson 2019) Identifies high potential future leaders and support for their focused development (Sklar 2018) Shares stories of success (Stoller 2020) and failure (Tucker and Edmondson 2003)		
Systems (macro)	Accountable to all people in the system, organizations, and broader community (Dalakoura 2010) Appreciation of educational leadership on the same level as research and healthcare/clinical leadership (Bendermacher et al. 2021) Empowers educational leadership in HPE Enables synchronized and aligned systems for ELD practice reform, monitoring, policy, governance at all levels (Sandhu 2019; Stoller 2020)	Challenging	ELD as vital to system functioning and reform Enabling intelligent failures Personal growth and development as important as profit Contributions across all levels lead to sustainable reforms

(continued)

Table 1 (continued)

Dimensions	Perspectives and actions	Leadership style	Reframe
	Creation of effective governance structures for innovation and sharing (Stoller 2020) Creation of enabling processes for ELD and implementation – i.e., engaging in innovations, ensuring environment of psychological safety, responding to violations (Bendermacher et al. 2021; Edmondson 2019) Structures that promote innovation and psychological safety, clear protocols for complaints. Actions taken – remediation (Bendermacher et al. 2021; Edmondson 2019) Structures and process that enable collaboration across and within the system (Bendermacher et al. 2021) Acknowledge role in stifling innovation, creativity, and a provision of inhumane workplaces (Sandhu 2019)		

1. Setting the stage through framing (or reframing) the work
2. Inviting participation through humility, inquiry-based questioning and
3. The establishment of structures for input (i.e., discussion forums, communities of practice), and responding productively through appreciation, destigmatization of failure, and sanctioning of violations

Framing the work is the most important skill for leadership to master for achieving psychological safety because it establishes expectations as to why adherence to these expectations matters (Edmondson 2019). A frame is defined as "a set of taken for granted assumptions that powerfully shape how we see a situation" (Edmondson 2019, p. 5). Significant reframing of educational leadership development in HPE is required across all dimensions as listed in column 4 of Table 1. Consistent with the developmental approach we are advocating here, Table 2 identifies the dimensions for individual focus at each of the Collins (2005) levels of leadership in the social sector to progress leadership capabilities of self (intrapersonal), and others (interpersonal, organizational, system). Table 2 enables anyone in health professions

Table 2 Dimension of influence aligned with the five levels of leadership in the social sector described by Collins (2005)

Collins (2005) hierarchical leadership capabilities	Dimension of influence[a]
Level 5: Executive Leader is characterized by personal humility and ambition for the mission of their institution (i.e., the cause) rather than themselves. They are driven to make the right decisions for the long-term high performance of their institution relative to its mission. They consult, however, will make decisions independent of consensus being achieved	Intrapersonal Interpersonal Organizational System
Level 4: Effective Leader stimulates the high-performance standards of others through actions that continuously moves the institution toward a clear and compelling vision	Intrapersonal Interpersonal Organizational
Level 3: Competent Manager ensures institutional objectives are efficiently achieved through organizing the human and other resources	Intrapersonal Interpersonal
Level 2: Contributing Team Member, is characterized by their individual input into team achievements and their effective ability for teamwork	Intrapersonal
Level 1: Highly Capable Individual, who contributes productively through their talent, skills, knowledge, and optimal approaches to their work	Intrapersonal

[a]Refer to Table 1 for specific tasks associated with each dimension

education to locate where they are currently positioned on their educational leadership journey, and the dimensions of their focus (intraprofessional, interprofessional, organizational, or system) to achieve increasing competence as an educational leader and to lead change. Specific perspectives and actions across these dimensions are contained in column 2 of Table 1.

At the intrapersonal level, considerable commitment to development as an educational leader is required, acknowledging the time requirements for learning the educational (pedagogical, etc.) and leadership skills (Collins level 1), reflecting on and modifying approaches through experiential learning (Collins all levels), and continued self-development (all levels). Reframing the role as change agents for system reform (Collins level 5) can instill a sense of empowerment and responsibility that will drive continued innovation and reform (Collins level 3 and 4), where failure is not feared (all levels). At the interpersonal level, reframing psychological safety as a right, and vulnerability as normal (Collins all levels) can empower both emerging and existing educational leadership to ensure and prioritize positive experiences for all involved in HPE. The first step to achieving change is to instill a sense of belief that change is possible (Collins levels 3 to 5). This adds purpose which motivates the change efforts. Reframing educational leadership in HPE is vital to systems functioning (Collins level 5), and to achieve the necessary reform required at the organizational and systems levels (Collins level 4 and 5). Individual actions alone will not achieve the needed changes we are advocating for. Collective action, with organizational and systems support to prioritize educational leadership development (Collins level 5), enabling its enactment through organizational structures and dedicated resources (Collins levels 3, 4, and 5), and ingrained processes to swiftly deal with incursions (Collins levels 3, 4, and 5) are needed, with strong and visible support and role modelling from senior leadership (Collins levels 4 and 5). It requires a renewed focus on the importance of personal growth for both educational leadership and innovation, a prioritization of people over profit, and significantly increased resources for planned educational leadership development for innovation and reform across the lifespan of training.

On Evidence and Scholarship for Educational Leadership Development

In health, professional development education is a multi-billion-dollar industry, with much of the costs borne by individuals, and a focus on clinical (technical) skill development over the human (soft skill) development (Frich et al. 2015; Keijser et al. 2017; Widjaja and Saragih 2018). In the commercial world 8–10% of revenue is re-invested in innovation (Ignatius 2020). Quantifying the added value for the financial and opportunity costs of the collective and developmental leadership approach in HPE we advocate for here is important for engagement across each dimension in Table 1. It is clear from our review that educational leadership development in HPE, and more broadly, is a rich area for scholarship. We have argued for an increased recognition of the importance of educational leadership development in HPE. The concept of leadership often meets with resistance or skepticism within the medical communities, which are traditionally conservative, because its value has not yet been shown (Keijser et al. 2017). The focus of training is on clinical skills (including technical and conceptual knowledge) with leadership development (including personal growth and awareness) underrepresented (Keijser et al. 2017; Frich et al. 2015; Miles and Scott 2019) and "...still in its infancy when it comes to operationalising it in daily clinical practice and education" (Keijser et al. 2017, p. 36). The skepticism toward, and limited focus on, leadership development in medicine and nursing is attributed to the lack of an evidence base needed to convince these healthcare professionals of its added value, and positive return on investment for their time to upskill (Keijser et al. 2017; Sklar 2018; Miles and Scott 2019). Increased scholarship is required to ensure program quality, relevance, and continuous improvement (Sklar 2018). The COVID-19 pandemic provides an opportunity to highlight the need for research into effective educational leadership development. Pertinent research questions to explore include: Who were the leaders that stood out during the pandemic response?; What attributes did they display to become recognized as leaders?; How can we develop those attributes in future educational leadership in HPE?

Developing an evidence base for the value of investment, including opportunity costs, in educational leadership development in HPE of both self and others is a priority to achieve its widespread adoption. Measuring impact and value will also provide evidence for the strategic importance of educational leadership development programs in HPE that is currently lacking (Edmondson et al. 2016). Scholarship opportunities in professional development in HPE are plentiful. A recent scoping review of almost 200 published papers reporting outcomes of continuing professional development (CPD) programs for health professionals confirmed a narrow focus on reporting easily measured outcomes such as knowledge, behavior change, confidence, skills, and attitudes (Allen et al. 2019). Inclusion of the 12 broader categories of impact for evaluating CPD programs reported by Allen et al. (2019) would enable a more accurate capturing of the full range of impacts achieved by those engaging in such programs, beyond the easy to measure. Of particular relevance is the inclusion of interpersonal aspects such as the development of professional relationships, or the personal and organizational changes that have been found to be particularly valuable to educational leadership development. The addition of qualitative methods to capture broader and unanticipated outcomes is also important (Allen et al. 2019). This is particularly pertinent when evaluating the impacts of novel approaches to developing educational leadership in HPE in what remain uncertain times.

Conclusion

Despite two decades of calls for significant reform to HPE globally, change, until recently, has been occurring at a snail's pace. The unprecedented innovations that were implemented in response to the COVID-19 pandemic confirmed that rapid and successful innovations to HPE and health care can be achieved. As we emerge from the experiences and lessons of the pandemic, the capacity to innovate healthcare education and practice has never been more achievable. A challenge for now and the future is to continue this ability for collaborative innovation so that HPE continues to innovate and evolve without the impetus of a destructive global pandemic. New and different approaches to educational leadership development in HPE, as we have presented here, are needed and must begin today. Educational leadership development is a process that requires considerable time, commitment, and planning. Currently, educational leadership in HPE is in a position to utilize the insights and experiences of the recent past to create the much heralded, but as yet unattained improved future for students, trainees, faculty, clinical teachers, healthcare providers, and patients.

Given the inextricable link between education and healthcare provision, investment in educational leadership development in HPE across all levels of training and practice is likely to translate to significant gains in both education and healthcare workforce productivity and improved patient care. As we commence our tentative emergence from a world defined by the COVID-19 pandemic, how we communicate with those around us in our professional work has come to the fore in an unprecedented way across all industries and sectors globally. Previous efforts of industry to build effective leadership only scantily considered achievable in health care and HPE have been escalated. The innovative and agile responses of HPE to the pandemic have opened the door for genuine reform in HPE leadership development. This requires prioritization, investment, and a renewed focus on a culture of psychological safety and purpose for those at the forefront of health care and education. There is much to be done both immediately and in the longer term. It is incumbent upon the educational leadership in HPE of today to develop a fit for purpose educational leadership in HPE of the future. A future that starts now.

Cross-References

▶ Competencies of Health Professions Educators of the Future
▶ Developing Care and Compassion in Health Professional Students and Clinicians
▶ Medical Education: Trends and Context
▶ Optimizing the Role of Clinical Educators in Health Professional Education

References

Allen LM, Palermo C, Armstrong E, Hay M. Categorising the broad impacts of continuing professional development: a scoping review. Med Educ. 2019;53(11):1087–99.

Arnetz JE, Goetz CM, Arnetz BB, Arble E. Nurse reports of stressful situations during the COVID-19 pandemic: qualitative analysis of survey responses. Int J Environ Res Public Health. 2020;17 (21):8126. https://doi.org/10.3390/ijerph17218126.

Bendermacher GWG, Dolmans DHJM, de Grave WS, oude Egbrink MGA. Advancing quality culture in health professions education: experiences and perspectives of educational leaders. Adv Health Sci Educ. 2021;26:467–87. https://doi.org/10.1007/s10459-020-09996-5.

Bong HE. Understanding moral distress: how to decrease turnover rates of new graduate pediatric nurses. Pediatr Nurs. 2019;45(3):109–14.

Boostel R, Felix JVC, Bortolato-Major C, Pedrolo E, Vayego SA, Mantovani MF. Stress of nursing students in clinical simulation: a randomized clinical trial. Rev Bras Enferm. 2018;71(3):967–74. https://doi.org/10.1590/0034-7167-2017-0187.

Cavanaugh JC. Who will lead? The success of succession planning. J Man Pol Pract. 2017;18(2): 22–7.

Chunharas S, Davies SC. Leadership in health systems: a new agenda for interactive leadership. Health Syst Reform. 2016;2(3):176–8. https://doi.org/10.1080/23288604.2016.1222794.

Collins J. Good to great and the social sectors. Boulder: Jim Collins; 2005.

Coltart CE, Cheung R, Ardolino A, Bray B, Rocos B, Bailey A, et al. Leadership development for early career doctors. Lancet. 2012;379:1847–9.

Dalakoura A. Differentiating leader and leadership development. A collective framework for leadership development. J Manag Dev. 2010;29(5):432–41.

De Brún A, O'Donovan R, McAuliffe E. Interventions to develop collectivistic leadership in healthcare settings: a systematic review. BMC Health Serv Res. 2019;19:72. https://doi.org/10.1186/s12913-019-3883-x.

Dendle C, Baulch J, Pellicano R, Hay M, Lichtwark I, Ayoub S, et al. Medical student psychological distress and academic performance. Med Teach. 2018;40(12):1257–63. https://doi.org/10.1080/0142159X.2018.1427222.

Dirani KM, Abadi M, Alizadeh A, Barhate B, Garza RC, Gunasekara N, et al. Leadership competencies and the essential role of human resource development in times of crisis: a response to COVID-19 pandemic. Hum Resour Dev Int. 2020;23(4):380–94. https://doi.org/10.1080/13678868.2020.1780078.

Dixit SK, Sambasivan M. A review of the Australian healthcare system: a policy perspective. SAGE Open Med. 2018. https://doi.org/10.1177/2050312118769211.

Dyer JH, Gregersen HB, Christensen CM. The innovator's DNA. Harv Bus Rev. 2009;87:12.

Edmondson AC. Psychological safety and learning behavior in work teams. Adm Sci Q. 1999;44 (2):350–83. https://doi.org/10.2307/2666999.

Edmondson AC. The kinds of teams health care needs. Boston MA. Harv Bus Rev. 2015 [cited 2021 Jun 1]. Available from: https://hbr.org/2015/12/the-kinds-of-teams-health-care-needs

Edmondson AC. The fearless organization: creating psychological safety in the workplace for learning, innovation, and growth. San Francisco: Wiley; 2019.

Edmondson AC. What hospitals overwhelmed by COVID-19 can learn from startups. Boston MA. Harv Bus Rev. 2020 [cited 2021 Jul 14]. Available from: https://hbr.org/2020/05/what-hospitals-overwhelmed-by-covid-19-can-learn-from-startups

Edmondson AC, Hugander P. 4 steps to boost Psychological Safety at your workplace. Boston MA. Harv Bus Rev. 2021 [cited 2021 Jul 12]. Available from: https://hbr.org/2021/06/4-steps-to-boost-psychological-safety-at-your-workplace. Accessed July 2021.

Edmondson AC, Lei Z. Psychological safety: the history, renaissance, and future of an interpersonal construct. Annu Rev Organ Psychol Organ Behav. 2014;1(1):23–43. https://doi.org/10.1146/annurev-orgpsych-031413-091305.

Edmondson AC, Higgins M, Singer S, Weiner J. Understanding psychological safety in health care and education organisations: a comparative perspective. Res Hum Dev. 2016;13(1):65–83. https://doi.org/10.1080/15427609.2016.1141280.

Erlich D, Armstrong EG, Gooding H. Silver linings: a thematic analysis of case studies describing advances in health professions education during the COVID-19 pandemic. Med Teach. 2021;43(12):1444–9. https://doi.org/10.1080/0142159X.2021.1958174.

Eva KW, Anderson MB. An expression of gratitude to medical education adaptations reviewers. Med Educ. 2020a;54(12):1086–7. https://doi.org/10.1111/medu.14273.

Eva KW, Anderson MB. Medical education adaptations: really good stuff for educational transition during a pandemic. Med Educ. 2020b;54(6):494.

Frenk J, Chen L, Bhutta ZA, Cohen J, Crisp N, Evans T, et al. Health professionals for a new century: transforming education to strengthen health systems in an interdependent world. Lancet. 2010;376(9756):1923–58.

Frich JC, Brewster AL, Cherlin EJ, Bradley EH. Leadership development programs for physicians: a systematic review. J Gen Intern Med. 2015;30(5):656–74. https://doi.org/10.1007/s11606-014-3141-1.

Gorman D, Hay M. Ensuring Australians' healthcare birthright: learning from those we teach. Int Med J. 2017;47(7):725–7. https://doi.org/10.1111/imj.13472.

Green C, Atik A, Hay M. Developing leadership skills in young ophthalmologists. Ann Eye Sci. 2019;44(37):1–8. https://doi.org/10.21037/aes.2019.09.02.

Ignatius A. What is the next normal going to look like? A roundtable with five top executives. Boston MA. Harv Bus Rev. 2020; [cited 2021 Apr 20]. Available from: https://hbr.org/2020/07/what-is-the-next-normal-going-to-look-like

International Health Conference. Constitution of the World Health Organization. 1946. Bull World Health Organ. 2002;80(12):983–4.

Jackson CL, O'Halloran D. Reforming our health care system: time to rip off the band-aid? Med J Aust. 2021;215(7):301–3. https://doi.org/10.5694/mja2.51261.

Jadad AR, O'Grady L. How should health be defined? BMJ. 2008;337(7683):1363–4.

Keijser W, Poorthuis M, Tweedie J, Wilderom C. Review of determinants of national medical leadership development. BMJ Leader. 2017;1(4):36–43.

Laksov KB, Tomson T. Becoming an educational leader – exploring leadership in medical education. Int J Educ Policy Leadersh. 2017;20(4):506–16. https://doi.org/10.1080/13603124.2015.1114152.

McKimm J, O'Sullivan H. When I say … leadership. Med Educ. 2016 Sep;50(9):896–7. https://doi.org/10.1111/medu.13119.

McKimm J, Ramani S, Nadarajah VD. 'Surviving to thriving': leading health professions' education through change, crisis & uncertainty. Asia Pac Scholar. 2021;6(3):32–44. https://doi.org/10.29060/TAPS.2021-6-3/OA2385.

McKinsey & Company. Psychological safety and the critical role of leadership development. McKinsey & Company. 2021 Feb 11 [cited 2021 Jul 14]. Available from: https://www.

mckinsey.com/business-functions/people-and-organizational-performance/our-insights/psychological-safety-and-the-critical-role-of-leadership-development

Miles JM, Scott E. A new leadership development model for nursing education. J Prof Nurs. 2019;35(1):5–11.

Ng NBH, Chiong T, Lau PYW, Aw MM. Delivering medical education amidst COVID-19: responding to change during a time of crises. Asia Pac Scholar. 2021;6(3):111–3. https://doi.org/10.29060/TAPS.2021-6-3/PV2375.

Norman G. Lies, damned lies, and statistics. Perspect Med Educ. 2018;7:24–7. https://doi.org/10.1007/s40037-018-0425-x.

Nyenswah T, Engineer CY, Peters DH. Leadership in times of crisis: the example of Ebola virus disease in Liberia. Health Syst Reform. 2016;2(3):194–207. https://doi.org/10.1080/23288604.2016.1222793.

O'Donovan R, McAuliffe E. A systematic review of factors that enable psychological safety in healthcare teams. Int J Qual Health Care. 2020a;32(4):240–50. https://doi.org/10.1093/intqhc/mzaa025.

O'Donovan R, McAuliffe E. Exploring psychological safety in healthcare teams to inform the development of interventions: combining observational, survey and interview data. BMC Health Serv Res. 2020b;20:810. https://doi.org/10.1186/s12913-020-05646-z.

O'Donovan R, De Brún A, McAuliffe E. Healthcare professionals experience of psychological safety, voice, and salience. Front Psychol. 2021;12:626689. https://doi.org/10.3389/fpsyg.2021.626689.

Priest KL, Seemiller C. Past experiences, present beliefs, future practices: using narratives to re (present) leadership educator identity. J Leader Educ. 2018;17:93–113. https://doi.org/10.12806/v17/i1/r3.

Reich MR, Javadi D, Ghaffar A. Introduction to the special issue on "effective leadership for health systems". Health Syst Reform. 2016;2(3):171–5. https://doi.org/10.1080/23288604.2016.1223978.

Rose S, Hartnett J, Pillai S. Healthcare worker's emotions, perceived stressors and coping mechanisms during the COVID-19 pandemic. PLoS One. 2021;16(7):e0254252. https://doi.org/10.1371/journal.pone.0254252.

Salari N, Hosseinian-Far A, Jalali R, Vaisi-Raygani A, Rasoulpoor S, Mohammadi M, et al. Prevalence of stress, anxiety, depression among the general population during the COVID-19 pandemic: a systematic review and meta-analysis. Glob Health. 2020;16:57. https://doi.org/10.1186/s12992-020-00589-w.

Sandhu D. Healthcare educational leadership in the twenty-first century. Med Teach. 2019;41(6):614–8. https://doi.org/10.1080/0142159X.2019.1595555.

Sklar DP. Leadership in academic medicine: purpose, people, and programs. Acad Med. 2018;93(2):145–8.

Souba W, Souba M. How effective leaders harness the future. Acad Med. 2018;93(2):166–71. https://doi.org/10.1097/ACM.0000000000001955.

Stoller JK. Reflections on leadership in the time of COVID-19. BMJ Leader. 2020;4:77–9. https://doi.org/10.1136/leader-2020-000244.

Tai JHM, Canny BJ, Haines TP, Molloy EK. The role of peer-assisted learning in building evaluative judgement: opportunities in clinical medical education. Adv Health Sci Educ. 2016;21:659–76. https://doi.org/10.1007/s10459-015-9659-0.

Tekian AS, Taylor DCM. Master's degrees: meeting the standards for medical and health professions education. Med Teach. 2017;39(9):906–13. https://doi.org/10.1080/0142159X.2017.1324621.

Tekian A, Roberts T, Batty H, Cook D, Norcini J. Preparing leaders in health professions education. Med Teach. 2014;36(3):269–71. https://doi.org/10.3109/0142159X.2013.849332.

Thomas AT, Gilja S, Sikka N, Ogechukwu O, Kellner R, Schussler L, et al. Peer-to-peer COVID-19 medical curriculum development during the pandemic. Med Educ. 2021;55(11):1302–3. https://doi.org/10.1111/medu.14639.

Tucker CA. If medical education was a discipline, she would have five core competencies. Med Teach. 2017;39(7):783–4. https://doi.org/10.1080/0142159X.2016.1270435.

Tucker CA. Succession planning for academic nursing. J Prof Nurs. 2020;36(5:334–42.

Tucker AL, Edmondson AC. Why hospitals don't learn from failures: organizational and psychological dynamics that inhibit system change. Calif Manag Rev. 2003;45(2):55–72.

van Diepen C, Fors A, Ekman I, et al. Association between person-centred care and healthcare providers' job satisfaction and work-related health: a scoping review. BMJ Open. 2020;10: e042658. https://doi.org/10.1136/bmjopen-2020-042658.

Widjadja A, Saragih EJ. Analysis on the effect of hard skills, intrapersonal and interpersonal skills toward the performance of nurses (a case study on the alumni of husada hospital nursing academy, Jakarta, Indonesia). Res J Bus Manag. 2018;6:31–8.

Wilkinson T. How not to put the O into an OSCE. Perspect Med Educ. 2018;7(Suppl 1):28–9. https://doi.org/10.1007/s40037-018-0424-y.

William L. Humanising future leadership in healthcare. Monash Lens. 2021 Sept 23 [cited 2021 Oct 3]. Available from: https://lens.monash.edu/@medicine-health/2021/09/23/1383814/the-search-for-humanity-in-healthcare-leadership

Zhou AY, Panagioti M, Esmail A, Agius R, Van Tongeren M, Bower P. Factors associated with burnout and stress in trainee physicians: a systematic review and meta-analysis. JAMA Netw Open. 2020;3(8):e2013761. https://doi.org/10.1001/jamanetworkopen.2020.13761.

On "Being" Participants and a Researcher in a Longitudinal Medical Professional Identity Study

85

Michelle McLean, Charlotte Alexander, and Arjun Khaira

Contents

Introduction	1658
"Data" Collection: Questions, Responses, and Comments	1659
Findings: On "Being" Participants in a Six-Year Longitudinal Study	1659
On "Being" a Researcher in the Six-Year Longitudinal Study	1663
Conclusions	1669
References	1669

Abstract

Challenges of longitudinal qualitative research (LQR) include participant motivation and researcher continuity. Following a six-year study of two medical students (Arjun and Charlotte) from Year 1 to their first year as interns, this submission explores our motivations and experiences of "being" participants and a researcher in LQR. To explore our experiences in different roles in the professional identity study, we used what we have called a textual conversational approach. We posed questions to each other and responded individually. I (the researcher) collated and recirculated the responses for further comment. This final working document (a written conversation) became the "data."

Our "conversation" as participants and researcher highlighted a range of LQR considerations. From participants' perspectives, initial participation in a study may depend on intrinsic motivation (i.e., a sense of responsibility) and continued participation may depend on perceived personal benefit (i.e., therapeutic in this

M. McLean (✉)
Faculty of Health Sciences & Medicine, Bond University, Gold Coast, QLD, Australia
e-mail: mimclean@bond.edu.au

C. Alexander
Emergency Department, Gold Coast University Hospital, Gold Coast, QLD, Australia

A. Khaira
Psychiatry Department, Canberra Hospital, Canberra, ACT, Australia

© Springer Nature Singapore Pte Ltd. 2023
D. Nestel et al. (eds.), *Clinical Education for the Health Professions*,
https://doi.org/10.1007/978-981-15-3344-0_139

case). Who the interviewer is matters, with Charlotte and Arjun initially preferring an independent person with no "power." As the interview location needs to be safe and familiar, it should be the participant's choice. From a researcher perspective, our conversation identified the pros and cons of a researcher's status, i.e., being an "insider" (interviewer) or an "outsider" (listening to recordings and reading transcripts). Since being a qualitative researcher can be emotional, emotional intelligence is important. In LQR, cognizance thus needs to be taken of a range of considerations both in terms of participants and the researcher.

Keywords

Longitudinal qualitative research · Narrative · Participant · Professional identity · Researcher · Storytelling · Trajectory

Introduction

In "becoming" and eventually feeling like a doctor, an individual navigates sometimes emotional transitions during medical school and in clinical practice (Helmich et al. 2012; Balmer et al. 2015; Barrett et al. 2017; Busing et al. 2018; Rees and Monrouxe 2018; Atherley et al. 2019). This "becoming" can be viewed as a journey or trajectory which takes place over several years and possibly throughout an individual's professional life (Wenger 1998). While a range of qualitative methodological approaches has been used to study this "becoming" (i.e., professional identity formation), only a handful of researchers have, however, followed individuals longitudinally. There are several reasons for this, not least being the difficulty of recruiting participants and then maintaining their motivation to return. Researcher or research team continuity is also a challenge as personal circumstances change (Miller 2000; Thomson and Holland 2003). Notwithstanding, longitudinal studies that have tracked students' journeys have provided valuable insight into their lived experiences of "becoming" doctors and include, for example, the impact of longitudinal integrated clerkships (Konkin and Suddards 2012), emotional socialization (Bolier et al. 2018), "capital" acquisition for transitions, and the use of audio diaries (Monrouxe 2009; Wong and Trollope-Kumar 2014) and portfolios (Adema et al. 2019) to study professional identity development.

During a phenomenological study across a five-year undergraduate medical program that explored students' perspectives of professional identity development, it became clear that in viewing the "becoming" of a doctor as a trajectory during which individuals undergo personal and professional development, their journeys needed to be studied longitudinally over several years. The original cross-sectional study was amended and the first-year students who were interviewed were approached for follow-up. Two students, Arjun and Charlotte, who are co-authors on this submission, thus became participants (and later co-researchers) in a six-year study that culminated in 2017 when they became first-year interns (junior doctors).

During the first few years of the study, Arjun and Charlotte were interviewed by a research assistant (RA) as the University's Human Research Ethics Committee recommended that academics should not interview research participants who they assess as students. I thus had to listen to interview recordings, read transcripts, and then discuss my perspectives with the RA. Once they became clinical students, I was no longer involved academically and so was able to interview them, becoming more of an "insider" (Granek 2017; Ross 2017), listening and responding first-hand their personal, and sometimes emotional, stories of their very different journeys of "becoming" and eventually "being" doctors.

In attempting to document Charlotte's and Arjun's six-year journeys, I became curious as to why, as new first-year students, they had initially volunteered for the study and why they had persisted for the duration of the study as maintaining participant motivation in LQR is a reported challenge (Miller 2000; Thomson and Holland 2003). In fact, one year, Charlotte contacted the RA to remind her that she was due for an interview. Considering the duration of the study and the fact that they had experienced two interviewers, I was sure that Arjun and Charlotte had questions for me, the principal investigator, whose status changed from "outsider" to "insider" in terms of the interviews. This small follow-up "study" was thus designed to explore our various motivations and commitments to the LQR as participants and researcher.

"Data" Collection: Questions, Responses, and Comments

In 2018, while rereading six years of transcripts, I believed that we could contribute to the qualitative methodological literature by exploring our experiences of "being" participants and "being" a researcher. As Arjun and Charlotte were fully immersed in "being" doctors in different parts of Australia, we used what we have called a textual conversational approach. Individually, we posed questions to each other in terms of "being" participants and "being" a researcher. I then collated the responses, inserting comments to their responses. This document was then circulated for further comment. This became the final working document. We present our results in terms of our experiences (with discussion) of "being" participants and "being" a researcher in a longitudinal study followed by some discussion which we hope adds value not only to the qualitative research discourse but also to the medical education community's understanding of professional identity.

Findings: On "Being" Participants in a Six-Year Longitudinal Study

In this section, Arjun and Charlotte's responses to my questions about their experiences as research participants across the five years of their medical degree, and then as first-year interns, are presented.

Researcher (PI): What made you sign up for the original cross-sectional study?

Arjun: *I liked participating in research and felt it important to participate. A lot of people conduct research but are reluctant to participate. If you expect people to help you, you should help them as well. Adding to this, I also felt that my journey as a medical student might be interesting to progress. I was never the top kid who always knew they were going to be a surgeon from the age of 10 - and I think this is to my advantage. Medicine, like the rest of the world, is changing. What may have made an adequate doctor a generation ago certainly does not now. I hoped by participating in research I could provide some insight into medical education and identity as a health professional for my generation.*

My response: *Throughout the study, you were always very open about who you were, Arjun. I think sometimes, you may have doubted yourself. I found that when I spoke to you as an intern, there had been a big transformation. You had become a doctor.* 😊.

Charlotte: *It was an early stage in my medical journey and everything seemed new and exciting. I wanted to be involved in everything I could. I had signed up to every committee and multiple clubs. I was excited to be interviewed to share why I was so passionate about becoming a doctor.*

My response: *That's how I came to know you, Charlotte, as a student who was fully immersed and engaged in medicine. I am very glad that you joined the research study as your stories, like Arjun's, will contribute to our understanding of professional identity development.*

Viewing research participation as a responsibility reflects Arjun and Charlotte's altruism for wanting to become doctors in the first place as well as their exuberance as "new" students (Sarpel et al. 2013; Walsh 2014). Those authors have, however, alluded to the potential vulnerability of students as participants as they are a captive audience and may feel pressured to participate if the research is being conducted by faculty with whom they interact as students. For Walsh (2014), the gold standard to protect potentially vulnerable students in educational research is obtaining ethics committee approval to conduct the research.

Researcher: *The study tracked you for six years. Why did you continue with the annual interview?*

Arjun: *In the beginning, I thought that was what was required but after the first couple of interviews being nice catch-ups and reflection on a year that had passed, I looked forward to it each year.*

Charlotte: *There are a couple of elements. The first is that each time the interview came around, I felt as though I had grown and I had something to share. I was often excited to share what had happened through the year and how it had impacted me, as well as have the feeling of getting things off my chest. Secondly, the interviews were casual and easy. I never saw them as an inconvenience and in fact I often felt invigorated leaving them.*

My response: *This was a good outcome for you. I enjoyed them as much as you did. Your stories tell of defining moments, validating that you were on track and that you could be a doctor. Charlotte, I found that you did a lot of self-calibration which* led to confidence and self-efficacy. Arjun, you were searching for where you belonged and found 'your people' in psychiatry.

Researcher: *Was participating in the study personally and/or professionally rewarding?*

Charlotte: *Yes. The study provided a platform in which I felt compelled to reflect on how I had changed and grown over the year and to think critically about what had caused those changes. It helped me to cultivate the practice of reflection and be cognisant of the forces around me and their impact.*

My response: *A good outcome, Charlotte. Even though this was a research project, it did become a form of informal support even though it was only once a year.*

Arjun: *I enjoyed participating in the study. It helped me reflect on the year gone by and my own progress and identity as a person. It was nice to speak to someone unbiased, objective and who was genuinely interested in the experiences I had been through. That was a rewarding feeling in itself.*

My response: *You have expressed the same sentiments as Charlotte, Arjun, that participating in this study was a personal development exercise.*

For Arjun and Charlotte, the annual interviews became more than data collection (i.e., the research agenda). In telling their stories and sharing their highs and lows, interviews provided an opportunity for validation, self-calibration as well as some venting. For Ibarra and Barbulescu (2010), *"Stories help people articulate provisional selves, link the past and the future into a harmonious, continuous sense of self, and enlist others to lend social reality to the desired changes"* (p. 138). Storytelling is thus powerful as it reinforces perceptions of "self" through confirmation and validation (Wong and Trollope-Kumar 2014; Bleakley 2005; Wang and Geale 2015; Clandinin et al. 2016). Through their engagement over the six years, but particularly towards the latter part of the study, Arjun's and Charlotte's figured worlds and their future or provisional selves became reality (Ibarra 1999). Their narratives were part of their "becoming" and that their experiences of "being" participants were sufficiently rewarding to return each year is an important message for those involved in longitudinal qualitative research.

Arjun's comment about researchers being genuinely interested in listening to and exploring their stories highlights the importance of the interviewer's disposition in such research. The work of Glesne (2011) and Collins and Cooper (2014) on the emotional intelligence of the qualitative researcher provide insight into the interpersonal skills required of researchers such that participants feel safe rather than vulnerable. The emotionally intelligent qualitative researcher enables participants to learn about themselves, the research, and the researcher such that the interactions become therapeutic (Collins and Cooper 2014). This appeared to be the case for Arjun and Charlotte in this study.

Researcher: *Did you experience any anxiety about participating in this longitudinal study?*

Arjun: *Initially, I was also worried about making the appointment times and being committed but that was about it. I was also worried about letting the* *researchers down and not providing the type of knowledge they were after. I just hoped what I said was useful for the study. Otherwise, I had no other issues.*

My response: *You were very open and honest, Arjun, and I appreciated this. Hopefully, your experiences in this study have made you realise that this study was more about you than it was about me, the researcher.*

Charlotte: *I never felt anxious. The only negative feelings I can remember from the interviews is that sometimes I looked back at what I had said in previous interviews and thought how naïve I must have looked. I felt embarrassed of my earlier 'self'.*

My response: *We all do this, Charlotte, but we are all on a journey and so looking back is part of growing and developing both personally and professionally as we move forward. As a researcher, there was no judgement on my part.*

Arjun raised a good point about "whose agenda," which could lead to participants feeling anxious to deliver. In discussing potential student vulnerability, in addition to students feeling pressured to participate, Walsh identifies the possibility of students answering questions to meet the academic researcher's anticipated agenda [20]. In addition, Charlotte's point about being judged is also an important consideration for qualitative researchers conducting interviews. Anxiety to deliver and meet the researcher's agenda is likely to impact the authenticity of the data. To overcome this, being open and transparent with participants about the research intentions at the outset, including assuring confidentiality, as well as discussing both researcher and participant expectations, would help in develop rapport and trust. Sarpel and colleagues confirmed some of these considerations in their study about students' research participation. Students in that study identified the following in terms of their motivation to participate: A desire to contribute, no coercion (i.e., volunteers' consent) and a perception of minimal risk research (Sarpel et al. 2013).

For Collins and Cooper (2014), an emotionally intelligent researcher (i.e., with personal and social competence) is sensitive to the dynamics and creates a safe space so that participants feel comfortable to share personal information. In addressing Charlotte's concern about "looking naive," Glesne (2011) wrote that *"A good interviewer never does anything to make respondents look or feel ignorant"* (p. 126). Being a good listener is therefore an important skill as a qualitative researcher (Glesne 2011; McClelland 2017).

Researcher: *You were interviewed by two individuals (Heather, an unfamiliar research assistant) and then, with your permission, the Principal Investigator (Michelle, a familiar faculty member). Did this impact on what you said or how you said it?*

Charlotte: *Having a lot of interaction with the interviewer outside of the project runs the risk of having answers filtered, even unconsciously. I think I did feel a little more cautious when Michelle started doing the interviews. Having the [academic] distance of being based at the hospitals was, however, important as I felt free to talk about the teaching, people, etc. without feeling as though she was involved.*

My response: *Hopefully, that concern dissipated after the first interview, Charlotte. Notwithstanding, you raise an important issue about power relations in studies such as these. The Ethics Committee is probably correct in terms of the criterion for* academics not to interview students when they directly involved in assessment. You also raise an important point about 'filtered' information when the researcher is not the interviewer. As an 'outsider', I received second-hand information. This will be a good discussion point in this methods paper.

Arjun: *At the beginning, yes. Whereas with Heather I was quite open and free about my experiences and thoughts, when it switched to Michelle, I was initially a bit hesitant to discuss some things as I knew she was part of the faculty, etc. Michelle was, however, more involved in the junior years and not the senior years that I was in at the time and furthermore she made it very clear that the interview was purely in the role of researcher rather than any member of faculty and quickly put me at ease. I was then able to be honest and open about my thoughts and experiences. To add to this, the question style, etc. was very similar to Heather so there was very little difference.*

My response: *Important points here, Arjun. Glad that I was able to clear this up early when I replaced Heather.*

While Charlotte's and Arjun's preference was for an independent third party, they did indicate, however, that once they were "clinical," when I was no longer involved academically, they were comfortable sharing their stories. Their initial preference for an independent person is line with the University Ethics Committee's recommendation that academics should not interview students who they assess because of the potential power differential which could lead to undue pressure to participate or provide "desirable" answers (Walsh 2014). For Walsh (2014), "best practice" is to ensure that research team faculty members are blinded to the participation of students they might supervise, thus requiring the need for a third party, but he does not consider different types of research or discuss the merits of a researcher being an "insider" or "outsider." This is discussed in the next section (i.e., "being" a researcher). An emotionally intelligent qualitative researcher should, however, be aware of power and hierarchy and what would minimize it (Glesne 2011).

Table 1 provides further conversation about "being" participants, offering insight into Arjun and Charlotte's preference for where their interviews took place. I posed this question as they had chosen to return to campus for the first four years.

On "Being" a Researcher in the Six-Year Longitudinal Study

In this section, I respond to the questions Arjun and Charlotte posed to me as a researcher.

Charlotte: *What made you stick with the study for six years?*

My response: *Once I commit to something, I see it through to the end. That is my personality.*

Arjun's comment: *This is a big factor why a lot of people both researchers and participants do the things they do. I think it is the inherit quality of research.*

My response (cont.): *Having said that, I am genuinely interested in students' experiences. Studying medicine is tough and we feel responsible for you while you are with us. Once you leave the campus, it is more difficult to keep track. I see how*

Table 1 Participants' perspectives of the location of interviews in qualitative research

On "being" a participant: *Familiar setting with familiar faces; returning to where it all began*
When you were contacted for the follow-up, you could choose the location of your choice. Mostly, you chose to return to Bond University to be interviewed. Why was this?   **Charlotte:** *Meeting at the hospital always seemed like the harder option. I felt that I couldn't guarantee when or where we could meet if we made it during the day while on rotations. Bond [University] was not only conveniently located to where I live but also provided some routine and familiarity. We could book a room at a time and stick with it. It also felt like the place where it all started and just felt natural to return there.*   **My response:** *Thanks for this. I had an idea that Bond [University] was a 'safe' place and that is why you came back. Your comment validates this.*
Arjun: *It is a frequent and well-known spot for both the participant and the researcher, and, at times, I would be studying at Bond [University] regardless, so it was convenient. Upon reflection, it was also a comfortable place to meet. There was an element of formality and familiarity rather than a park or a cafe where it may not have felt as private or formal.*   **My response:** *Your comment echoes the same sentiments as Charlotte, Arjun. I would like to believe that we make Bond friendly and comfortable for you to return.*
A recommendation would thus be that participants choose where they wish to be interviewed as it would appear that familiar surroundings (physical space and people) would assist with creating a safe place.

students mature and develop professionally in the 18 months they spend with us on campus. As the Ethics Committee recommends that I not interview students early in the curriculum (a potential power difference), an independent research assistant (Heather) conducted the interviews.

Arjun's comment: *This was very appropriate and gave a lot more merit to the study even though in time it was not an issue. In the beginning, I would have been more apprehensive to share my views if the researcher was directly involved in my teaching.*

My response (cont.): *Heather and I met before and after each interview to discuss issues you may have raised until I was then able to conduct the annual interviews with your permission. This study allowed me to travel with you on your individual and emotional journeys, experiencing the joys as well as your trials and tribulations. I looked forward to catching up with you each to see how much you had progressed. I knew both of you reasonably well as first and/or second year students. Arjun, you were in my first ever PBL group at Bond [University] and Charlotte, you were always so interested in learning more.*

Arjun's comment: *Ha, Ha, Ha! Yes, I remember this still very clearly and the entire PBL group feels like such a journey looking back. In some way, it feels still very fresh.*

Researchers genuinely interested in the lives of participants will ensure longevity of the study. As a researcher exploring the personal journeys of individuals who have invested time and emotions into participating, I have an ethical obligation to complete the research. In participatory research, which this study became, ensuring that the research adds to the research community's understanding is an imperative.

Charlotte: *Did you find the interviews you conducted yourself to be of more value than the transcripts?*

My response: During this study, because of the University's Human Research Ethics Committee requirement, I could not conduct the early interviews. Immediately after the interviews, Heather relayed information to me and we updated your journeys as well as looked for overarching ideas about identity development. Prior to each annual interview, I would prompt Heather her in terms of what might need to be clarified from the previous year and how to facilitate the discussion. In the latter part of the study, once there was no power issue, I was able to explore first-hand your experiences as clinical students and interns. Experiencing some of your stories first-hand was more rewarding than being on the 'outside' listening in. Most of your experiences were positive and I could see how your 'doing' contributed to your 'becoming' of a doctor. Other experiences were, however, emotionally taxing. In hearing first-hand your 'lived' journeys, we could take a deeper dive into what these meant for you in 'becoming' a doctor. An independent interviewer may not have the same interests in your personal and professional development. In reading the transcripts and listening to the recordings, I had to imagine your facial expressions and body language. I would thus consider not being the interviewer a methodological limitation but understand your trepidation about the interviewer being someone you know and the power differential.

Hearing Arjun's and Charlotte's stories first-hand allowed me to explore their experiences in real time. This was more meaningful than listening to audio files and the RA's recollection or reading transcripts. As Charlotte and Arjun indicated, early in the study, their choice was for an independent interviewer, confirming Walsh's (2014) "best practice" of faculty members as researchers being blinded to participants they might supervise, teach, or assess. The choice should, however, always rest with the participant who needs to feel "safe." The potential "power" should always be considered and discussed prior to the research commencing. Notwithstanding, such "objectivity" may compromise data authenticity in qualitative research.

Arjun's next two questions, plus a question from Charlotte (pros and cons of the researcher being emotionally invested), open the door for a discussion about the researcher's emotions in qualitative research, which is not often discussed. Granek's (2017) editorial in a special issue of *Qualitative Psychological* addressing "emotional aspects of qualitative research" highlights how psychology has *"historically taken its epistemological cue from the Western philosophical tradition that has not looked kindly upon the emotional aspects of the research trajectory [and which has been] systematically removed from reporting of our research to academic audiences"* (p. 281). Ross' (2017) article in this special edition is particularly pertinent as she examines the emotional impact of qualitative research through the lens of "insider" research. As a "total insider," she described how her emotional investment in the researcher–participant relationship influenced her role as a research instrument (interviewer) and the challenges she faced in terms of role boundaries and self-disclosure (Ross 2017). McClelland's (2017) reflective article on vulnerable listening, written in the context of interviewing women with Stage V breast cancer, is also a useful read in terms of the vulnerability and emotions of the researcher in studies that may involve, for example, pain, illness, and abuse. These considerations transition into Arjun's next question.

Arjun: *Did you feel like a therapist with my ramblings?*

My response: *No, Arjun. 😊 I felt like someone who was accompanying you (and had the privilege of sharing) on your journey as you negotiated your way through the various hiccups and transitions.*

Arjun's response: *I'm glad to hear!*

My response: *As you were in my first PBL group back in 2012, it was a privilege to read and then hear about your experiences each year as you described your aspirations and goals and how you were finding your way around clinical practice. Over the study period, you were trying to find where you fitted best, i.e. what area of medicine best suited your personality and your values. Your experiences have shaped where you saw yourself eventually practising. By the time of your Year 5 interview, you had found where you fitted, which explains why you have already in a residency program while most of your peers are still thinking about where they might like to specialise. I do think that, however, that these annual catch-up sessions were somewhat therapeutic for you. You often spoke about confidence (lack of) to some extent because of self-doubt but also because of some of your experiences. The very act of telling someone about experiences (positive or negative) is therapeutic and often validation-seeking. Validation is an important part of self-concept. I remember our conversation last year when you were at the end of your first year of internship. I saw a considerable transformation of your confidence from Year 5 to intern. I remember saying "You are a doctor". Although you had the piece of paper to prove you were a doctor, you had 'become' a doctor as you believed in yourself and your ability.*

Arjun's comment: *Yes, I agree. I really do feel like I have found my people doing psychiatry and with this comfort, I feel more like a doctor as well. The knowledge is not even close to a specialist but it comes with time. I think the confidence and identity comes from not feeling helpless, but rather from feeling that I am making a difference in my patient's life for the better and objectively seeing this is part of that validation.*

Returning to the emotionally intelligent qualitative researcher, attributes would also include being non-threatening, therapeutic, and caring among other such that participants feel safe to say what they feel (Glesne 2011; Collins and Cooper 2014). Being therapeutic is, however, not the same as being a therapist. While there may be therapeutic value for participants in telling their stories, as alluded to by Arjun and Charlotte, the researcher's role is not a counsellor or therapist but a listener, learner, and observer (Rossetto 2014). Caring for participants, the research project and oneself as the researcher should thus be an integral part of qualitative research as the researcher is not *"a mere receptacle for a participant's words"* (McClelland 2017; p. 9). Researchers, like participants, are emotional beings. Conducting research with a caring ethic may thus require self-care during the research process.

Arjun: *Were you surprised by what we said?*

My response: *An 'issue' in qualitative research is the 'position' of the researcher. In conducting qualitative research, the researcher needs to declare his/her background, experience and expertise (i.e. be reflexive) so that any potential bias* *is transparent. As a non-clinician, having not worked in clinical practice or not having any family members in the health profession, I would declare that I had no preconceptions about what you or Charlotte said. As a researcher interested in how one becomes a doctor (and not being a doctor myself), and with the view that no two journeys are the same, nothing should really have 'surprised' me. What did surprise me, however, were my own emotions when both of you described some of your experiences, both positive and negative, the ups and downs in 'becoming' doctors. Charlotte described the ride as 'bumpy'. You were open in describing how emotional some experiences were and how this had impacted on you personally and professionally. I am grateful to have shared your journeys.*

Arjun's comment: *I don't think I expected this type of emotional journey when I started medicine either and this is part of what makes medicine quite unique. Although the positives are fantastic, I still think there is huge room for improvement to fix the negatives associated with not only medical school but also junior doctors. There is a pervasive culture that seems to somehow become inherited and this is very unfortunate given the high-risk high-seriousness environment in which a doctor works. There is literally no more serious job than dealing with life. This is part of the increased static mental health risk that health professionals have.*

Charlotte's comment: *Do you think being emotionally invested in the project is a positive or a negative?*

My response: *Good question, Charlotte. I don't know how to answer this. It is not something that is often addressed in the qualitative literature. I do think that being invested in and emotionally responsive to participants' experiences is a form of empathy and this develops trust. I feel that through your narratives, I was able to 'put myself in your shoes'.*

With the Western epistemology viewing emotion with suspicion, it has generally been avoided as a potential source of information for the qualitative researcher (Granek 2017). Ross, reflecting on the benefits and challenges of the emotional impact of being a "total insider," i.e., with multiple identities or profound experiences in common with participants, concluded that more explicit consideration of researchers' emotional selves could enrich the research data, research relationships, and as individuals who are privileged to engage in emotionally important research topics (Ross 2017). While "outsider" status is usually considered the ideal, objective norm, with "insider" status introducing potential bias (Merriam et al. 2001), working within a critical or interpretative paradigm, Chavaz (2008) acknowledges potential value in the knowledge arising from the lived experience. For Ross (2017), her emotional investment allowed her to establish rapport with a participant, be genuinely empathetic as well as grow personally and learn. In terms of my researcher positionality in this study, although not sharing sufficient in common to be considered a "total insider" in that as a non-clinician, I have no shared identity or experiences with Arjun and Charlotte, I have an inherent interest and personal investment in students' well-being as they navigate "becoming" doctors which for many is emotionally challenging (Barrett et al. 2017; Bolier et al. 2018; Busing et al. 2018; Rees and Monrouxe 2018). The above-average incidence of depression and suicide among medical students is a reflection of this long and often difficult journey (Rotenstein et al. 2016).

Table 2 provides further responses to other questions posed by Charlotte (managing data) and Arjun (my interest as a researcher). Arjun's question continues the conversation about the importance of an "invested" researcher.

Table 2 Additional questions and responses from Charlotte and Arjun in terms of the longitudinal management of qualitative data and my interest as a researcher

On "being" a researcher: *Managing "data" (transcripts)*
Charlotte: *Data from the interviews seems immense. What tips would you have for coping with such large quantities of qualitative data?* **My response:** *Indeed. Some transcripts were 30+ pages. I would have read each transcript at least three times, with the earlier ones being read up to six times. I also listened to the audio-recordings when I received the transcriptions as the transcribers could not understand every word. Listening and following the text is good way of getting to grips with the data but it is laborious. There is software, such as NVivo that keeps track of assigned codes. With this longitudinal research, however, I preferred to use the traditional approach of reading, highlighting, inserting notes and codes (what qualitative researchers call 'immersing oneself in the data') and then looking at each of your personal journeys. It requires a lot of time as one needs to be focused. The most recent read of each of your transcripts from Year 1 to first year intern took me all weekend. I kept track by mapping events, stories and with the themes and subthemes that I had identified. In terms of tips, each researcher works out a way of keeping track of data. Longitudinal research data runs the risk of 'getting lost'. For instance, because audio-recordings are large files, I used Dropbox. It allowed the transcriber to access and also accidently delete a file. Electronic back-ups are crucial. As notes were made and diagrams drawn, they were digitised and added to a master file of your journeys.*
On "being" a researcher: *Researcher interest*
Arjun: *Did you find the difference in experiences of the two participants interesting or surprising?* **My response:** *Your very different experiences reinforced for me the uniqueness of each student's journey. It allowed me to appreciate some of the difficulties that individual students may experience along the way. There is a lot of navigating that happens as you negotiate the various transitions and micro-transitions as context, teams and individuals can have a major influence on how one might one day practice medicine. Your journeys were very different and because of who you are and where you want to be, you will end up practicing medicine very differently. I did, however, identify some commonalities. One I have already mentioned (micro-transitions and context). Other commonalities were that notion of a 'persona', i.e. how you wanted others to see you. Sometimes this was to protect yourselves and other times, this was to get things done (e.g. patient trust). Both of you spoke about the hierarchy and tribalism. Over the study period, both of you came to the realisation that doctors can't do and know everything. This is impossible.* **Charlotte's comment:** *Yes, I think the closer I came to 'becoming' a doctor, the less I expected of doctors. When I came closer to finishing, I also saw more of a doctor's imperfections and flaws.* **My comment (cont.):** *I think this was somewhat as a relief for you as it allows for mistakes and makes accepting responsibility easier. Both of you felt that you needed to earn the title 'doctor'. Charlotte, you spoke about introducing yourself as a junior doctor so that the patient (and you) knew that there was room for error, with the opportunity to ask a more experienced colleague. For both of you, being a doctor came with hard work and with meeting the expected level of competence. You were thus reluctant to use titles with 'doctor' (e.g. doctor-in-training in Year 5). You were both 'students' and then 'medical students' for a long time. I think this was for your own protection as you both recalled stories of family and friends calling you 'doctor' even in Year 2 or 3 and asking medical advice, treating you as if you were already doctors.*

Conclusions

In exploring our emic perspectives of "being," we have identified several considerations as participants and as a researcher in LQR. These include the motivational considerations of participants to initially volunteer (i.e., a sense of responsibility) and then to continue participating (i.e., perceived personal benefit and therapeutic). We also identified that it matters who the person is who interviews participants. There is a need for the person to be genuinely interested in participants' stories with no "power" over the students. To ensure participants, particularly if they are new (and so often young) students, do not feel pressured to deliver, the purpose of the research should be clarified at the outset, including assuring participants in terms of anonymity.

From my own perspective as a researcher (and an interviewer), while being an "insider" (i.e., listening to and exploring their narratives firsthand) was more authentic than being an "outsider" (i.e., reading transcripts and listening to audio files), Arjun's and Charlotte's (and Walsh's (2014) reservation about "power" is acknowledged. Our conversation about emotion and the qualitative researcher has highlighted a neglected area in qualitative research (Granek 2017; Ross 2017).

References

Adema M, Dolmans D, Raat J, Scheele F, Jaarsma AD, Helmich E. Social interactions of clerks: the role of engagement, imagination, and alignment as sources of professional identity formation. Acad Med. 2019;94(10):1567–73.

Atherley A, Dolmans D, Hu W, Hegazi I, Alexander S, Teunissen PW. Beyond the struggles: a scoping review of the transition to undergraduate clinical training. Med Educ. 2019; early online https://onlinelibrary.wiley.com/doi/10.1111/medu.13883

Balmer DF, Richards BF, Varpio L. How students experience and navigate transitions in undergraduate medical education: an application of Bourdieu's theoretical model. Adv Health Sci Educ. 2015;20:1073–85.

Barrett J, Trumble SC, McColl G. Novice medical students navigating the clinical environment in an early medical clerkship. Med Educ. 2017;51:1014–24.

Bleakley A. Stories as data, data as stories: making sense pf narrative inquiry in clinical education. Med Educ. 2005;39:534–40.

Bolier M, Doulougeri K, de Vries J, Helmich E. 'You put up a certain attitude': a 6-year qualitative study of emotional socialization. Med Educ. 2018;52(10):1041–51.

Busing N, Rosenfield J, Rungta K, et al. Smoothing the transitions in Canadian medical education. Acad Med. 2018;93(5):715–21.

Chavaz C. Conceptualizing from the inside: advantages, complications, and demands on insider positionality. Qual Report. 2008;13:474–94.

Clandinin DJ, Cave MT, Berendonk C. Narrative inquiry: a relational research methodology for medical education. Med Educ. 2016;51:89–96.

Collins CS, Cooper JE. Emotional intelligence and the qualitative researcher. Int J Qual Meth. 2014;13(1):88–103.

Glesne C. Becoming qualitative researchers. Boston, MA: Pearson; 2011.

Granek L. Emotional aspects of conducting qualitative research on psychological topics. Qual Psych. 2017;4(3):281–6.

Helmich E, Bolhuis S, Laan R, Koopmans R. Entering medical practice for the very first time: emotional talk, meaning and identity development. Med Educ. 2012;46:1074–87.

Ibarra H. Provisional selves: experimenting with image and identity in professional adaptation. Admin Sci Quart. 1999;44:764–91.

Ibarra H, Barbulescu R. Identity as narrative: prevalence, effectiveness, and consequences of narrative identity. Work in macro work role transitions. Acad Man Rev. 2010;35(1):135–54.

Konkin J, Suddards C. Creating stories to live by: caring and professional identity formation in a longitudinal integrated clerkship. Adv Health Prof Educ. 2012;17(4):585–96.

McClelland SI. Vulnerable listening: Possibilites and challenges of doing qualitative research. Qual Psych. 2017;4:338–52.

Merriam SB, Johnson-Bailey J, Lee M-Y, Kee Y, Ntseane G, Muhamad M. Power and positionality: negotiating insider/outsider status within and across cultures. Int J Lifelong Educ. 2001;20:405–16.

Miller R. Researching life stories and family histories. London: Sage; 2000.

Monrouxe LV. Negotiating professional identities: dominant and contesting narratives in medical students' longitudinal audio diaries. Curr Narr. 2009;1:41–59.

Rees CE, Monrouxe LV. Who are you and who do you want to be? Key considerations in developing professional identities in medicine. MJA. 2018;209(5):202–3.

Ross LE. An account from the inside: examining the emotional impact of qualitative research through the lens of "insider" research. Qual Psych. 2017;4(3):326–37.

Rossetto KR. Qualitative research interviews: assessing the therapeutic value and challenges. J Soc Pers Rel. 2014;31:482–9.

Rotenstein LS, Ramos MA, Torre M, et al. Prevalence of depression, depressive symptoms, and suicidal ideation among medical students. A systematic review and meta-analysis. JAMA. 2016;316(21):2214–36.

Sarpel U, Hopkins MA, More F, et al. Medical students as human subjects in educational research. Med Educ Online. 2013;18:19524. https://nyuscholars.nyu.edu/en/publications/medical-students-as-human-subjects-in-educational-research-2

Thomson R, Holland J. Hindsight, foresight and insight: the challenges of longitudinal qualitative research. Int J Soc Res Meth. 2003;6(3):233–44.

Walsh K. Medical education research: is participation fair? Pers Med Educ. 2014;3:379–82.

Wang CC, Geale SK. The power of story: narrative inquiry as a methodology in nursing research. Int J Nurs Sci. 2015;2:195–8.

Wenger E. Communities of practice: learning, meanings and identity. New York: Cambridge University Press; 1998.

Wong A, Trollope-Kumar K. Reflections: an inquiry into medical students' professional identity formation. Med Educ. 2014;48:489–501.

Health Care Practitioners 'Becoming' Doctors: Changing Roles and Identities

86

Michelle McLean and Carla Pecoraro

Contents

Introduction	1672
Study Details	1673
Study Setting	1673
Participants	1674
Transcript Analysis	1674
Findings	1674
Anticipated Role Change, With a Hint of a Nascent Emerging Identity	1677
Deliberate Role Boundaries	1678
A Mindset Shift: 'Becoming' a Clinical Student and Future Doctor	1679
Role and Identity Congruence: Self-tailored Interprofessional Identities	1680
Role and Identity Dissonance: 'Being' a Physiotherapist While 'Being' a Clinical Medical Student	1683
An Unusual Scenario: From 'Being' a Trainee Surgeon (With Two HP Degrees) to 'Being' an Undergraduate Medical Student	1684
Discussion	1684
Limitations	1687
Conclusions	1687
Cross-References	1688
References	1688

Abstract

Despite a rich medical professional identity literature, little has been specifically documented about how individuals from different health professions 'become' doctors. This chapter explores this 'becoming' for health care practitioners (HPs) studying medicine in a five-year undergraduate program. Eleven students (seven females; four males) from seven health professions (pharmacy, physiotherapy, radiography, occupational therapy, nursing, dentistry, orthoptics) across four years of the medical program were interviewed. Two Year 1 students were

M. McLean (✉) · C. Pecoraro
Faculty of Health Sciences & Medicine, Bond University, Gold Coast, QLD, Australia
e-mail: mimclean@bond.edu.au; carlapec1997@gmail.com

© Springer Nature Singapore Pte Ltd. 2023
D. Nestel et al. (eds.), *Clinical Education for the Health Professions*,
https://doi.org/10.1007/978-981-15-3344-0_140

1671

followed up in their final year (Year 5). Using narrative analysis, the intersection between 'being' HPs and 'becoming' doctors was explored.

In terms of their different roles and identities as HPs, medical students, and future doctors, several factors influenced their sense of 'self' and their 'becoming', including their health profession and practice context, how long they had worked as HPs, whether they continued to work as HPs and the alignment between roles and existing and emerging identities. There was also an interplay between their various roles (e.g., HP, medical student, future doctor) and identities (existing and emerging) in this 'becoming', such as a newfound awareness of events or occurrences with potential future relevance, through deliberate role and identity boundaries, cognitive switching to future roles, and the construction of self-tailored hybrid, interprofessional identities. For one student, there was role and identity dissonance.

Individual journeys of 'becoming' doctors are personal and context-dependent. 'Being' HPs generally added value to 'becoming' doctors in terms of, for example, patching perceived deficiencies, leading to interprofessional identities, which challenges the traditional view of a uniprofessional model of identity.

Keywords

Health professional · Professional identity · Interprofessional socialization

Introduction

In 'becoming' a doctor, an individual reputedly develops a professional identity. Jarvis-Selinger and colleagues (2012) definition of identity development – "an adaptive developmental process that happens simultaneously at two levels: (1) at the level of the individual, which involves the psychological development of the person and (2) at the collective level, which involves a socialization of the person into appropriate roles and forms of participation in the community's work" (p. 1186) – highlights that individuals' conceptions of who they are is influenced by the 'doing' and the 'being' within the sociocultural context of the workplace.

While much has been written about professional identity in medicine over the past few years (e.g., Goldie 2012; Trede 2012; Cruess et al. 2014, 2016, 2018, 2019), Volpe et al. (2019) recently highlighted the omission of demographic factors in professional identity research. Considering that the *graduate-entry* (vs. undergraduate) medical education model prevails in North America and increasingly so in Australia, many medical school applicants are likely to be practicing health care practitioners (HPs). It is surprising that little attention has been paid to how such individuals, who are likely to have existing individual and professional group identities and belong to one or more professional communities of practice (McLean 2017; Sharpless et al. 2015; Wong and Trollope-Kumar 2014), 'become' doctors.

The five- or six-year *undergraduate* medical education model which admits largely school-leavers still predominates in Europe, the United Kingdom, Africa, and the Middle East. It is within such a context that the present study set out to explore HPs' constructions of 'self' in 'becoming' doctors. In the Bond University Medical Program, graduates (mostly HPs) comprise about 20% of the cohort, with the remaining 80% being 'school-leavers'. This study was initiated after earlier research identified the challenges facing three highly experienced registered nurses (RNs) as they navigated 'being' medical students in an undergraduate program (McLean 2017). To further explore our primary research question – *How do HPs in an undergraduate medical program 'become' doctors?* – medical students who had already qualified as HPs were recruited.

Based on prior research involving RNs who were 'becoming' 'different' doctors (McLean 2017), this study drew on both developmental and sociocultural theoretical and conceptual considerations. The professional identity literature, particularly in terms of role transitions (Pratt et al. 2006; Ibarra and Barbulescu 2010; Trede 2012), the concept of 'provisional' selves (Ibarra 1999), and the construct of hybrid or interprofessional identities (Sims 2008; Frost and Regehr 2013; Langendyk et al. 2015; Rees and Monrouxe 2018) informed this study. In the current uniprofessional model of health care, in 'becoming' doctors, these HPs would be leaving one community (either of *practice* or of *practitioners*) to legitimately (*albeit* peripherally initially) become participants in another (Wenger 1998; Cruess et al. 2018; Buckley et al. 2019). *Situated learning* as a construct is thus relevant (Artemeva et al. 2017). Since these students were already HPs, this study also drew on Wenger's (1998) development view of identity as "work in progress, shaped by efforts – both individual and collective – to create a coherence through time that threads together successive forms of participation in the definition of a person incorporating the past and the future in the experience of the present" (p. 45).

Study Details

This cross-sectional study involving HPs studying medicine in an undergraduate program took place at Bond University, Gold Coast, Australia. It also involved a longitudinal element as two of the original Year 1 HPs were followed up in their final year (Year 5) of medicine.

Study Setting

The five-year undergraduate program comprised a three-year 'pre-clinical problem-based and case-based phase' and a two-year 'clinical phase'. HPs began Year 1 with mostly 'school-leavers' and received no recognition for any prior learning or professional practice experience. History-taking and procedural skills began in Year 1, with physical examination skills added in Year 2. In Year 3, students relocated to a facility adjacent to a local public hospital where the Bond Virtual Hospital 'app' introduced them to patient management (McLean et al. 2014). They also interacted with patients during supervised ward visits and undertook a General Practice placement. Year 4 comprised clerkship rotations (e.g., Mental Health, Surgery, General Practice, etc.), while Year 5 involved a critical care rotation, a GP placement, selectives, electives, and an MD project. Following graduation, as junior doctors, they would complete an internship.

Participants

Approval to undertake the original study was granted by the Bond University Human Ethics Research Committee (RO1537) in 2012. An application to extend the study to recruit students who had already qualified as health professionals (HPs) was approved in 2015. Following recruitment via email, eleven (11) students representing seven health professions (HPs) – five Registered Nurses (RNs; 4 females, 1 male), a female Pharmacist (PA), a male Sonographer (SO), a male Physiotherapist (PH), a male Periodontist (with a prior Pharmacy (PA) degree), a female Occupational therapist (OT), and a female Orthoptist (OR) across Years 1–4 – were interviewed. The male physiotherapist and the female pharmacist were followed up in their final year (Table 1). In 2015, all but one, a female Year 3 RN (RNY3F), were working.

Transcript Analysis

Narrative analysis of transcribed interviews was used to explore HPs' narratives or 'stories' (Bleakley 2005) of 'being' medical students (as well as practicing HPs) who were 'becoming' doctors (Kelly and Howie 2007; Wang and Geale 2015; Clandinin et al. 2016). Framed by the main research question – how do HPs, who belong to a professional community and presumably with personal and professional identities, 'become' doctors? – both researchers independently read four transcripts (four professions, one from Years 1–4). With 11 students representing seven professions and at different stages of their medical studies, and, acknowledging the uniqueness of individuals' and journeys (Joynes 2018), the *breadth* of their experiences and identity constructions were explored. After discussion of the four transcripts, a coding template was designed to analyze all transcripts. Regular meetings were held.

Findings

HPs' collective narratives of 'becoming' junior doctors while studying medicine in an undergraduate program span a five-year trajectory. Viewing the development of an individual's professional identity as a complex and unique personal journey which starts at a very different place (Joynes 2018), HPs' experiences of 'becoming' doctors were explored (Bandura 1977). Although 'starting from scratch' as undergraduate medical students with no recognition of prior learning or experience, having worked clinically for several years (except RNY3F, A Year 3 female RN

Table 1 Demographic details of the 11 HPs (now medical students) who participated, with two followed up in their final year

Participant (± age)	Sex	Year of study	Occupation and years worked (2015)	Working as HP while studying: Reasons
RNY1M (± 27)	M	1	Registered nurse (mental health): three years	Yes: financial; practice clinical skills
SOY1M (28)	M	1	Sonographer: five years	Yes: financial
PAY1F (± 24)	F	1 Followed up Y5	Pharmacist (hospital-based): three years	Yes, Y1-Y5: financial, enjoys working; maintaining professional contacts
PHY1M (28)	M	1 Followed up Y5	Physiotherapist (hospital-based): about two years	Yes, but stopped early Year 4: financial; in the system with patients
PAY2M (± 42)	M	2	Periodontist (private): several years	Yes: financial
RNY2F1 (mid-30s)	F	2	Registered nurse (hospital-based)	Yes. Part-time/casual Y1–2: financial, enjoys working with patients, accruing long service leave, clinical experience
RNY2F2 (± 29)	F	2	Registered nurse (ICU): about two years	Yes: financial
OTY3F (± 26)	F	3	Occupational therapist (hospital-based): several years	Yes: financial, interaction with patients
ORY3F (late-20s)	F	3	Orthoptist (private): about six years	Yes. Part-time but full-time during holidays: financial, experience in health care system
RNY3F (± 55)	F	3	Registered nurse: 15 months	No
RNY4F (36)	F	4	Registered nurse: 10 years	Yes: financial

with 15 months of nursing practice only), they had acquired considerable 'capital' (e.g., established professional networks; familiarity with the health care system) and 'habitus' (= disposition, e.g., interpersonal and intrapersonal skills) (Bourdieu 1977). With a sense of agency in terms of achieving long-standing goals of 'becoming' doctors, this capital and disposition facilitated their 'becoming' clinical students and future doctors. Using a Year 1 female pharmacist's (PAY1F) description of the intersection of her two identities as a Venn diagram, this was used to depict individual HPs' constructions of 'self' (Table 2). These constructions, however, depended on several considerations: Their particular health profession (which

Table 2 HPs' conceptions of 'self' in terms of how they saw themselves and/or what they tell others and how our depictions of these conceptions

HP	What do you call yourself when someone asks?	Venn diagram
RNY1M	I say "I'm a registered nurse and I'm studying" at the moment. Certainly in my work context, I don't try and blurt out that I'm studying medicine because sometimes that can be taken out of context or I think sometimes nursing staff often is a bit of a tribal thing and there is that historical nursing and medical staff rivalry and division. Sometimes I choose to withhold that information... to friends and family..., I would still introduce myself as my professional role that I'm a nurse, but I would say I'm also a student. RN = registered nurse	
SOY1M	Mainly I'm still saying sonographer and if people keep prying then I might say I'm also studying medicine, but it's not the first thing I say to people. SO = sonographer	
PAY1F (followed up in Y5)	I say, "I'm a hospital pharmacist" and often many people don't know what that is....... I also say that I am a medical student... I'm studying to be a doctor.... I am a pharmacist at a hospital, but I'm also a medical student. PA = pharmacist	
PHY1M (followed up in Y5)	I see myself as a doctor in training more than anything. I know that I am a medical student, I feel like that I've got a lot of knowledge that I bring to the table. Physio is the thing I do for money right now. PH = physiotherapist; DIT = doctor-in-training	
RNY2F1	I'll say "I'm a nurse"... I'll say I am a medical student, but I'm not open about it. I never tell anyone at work.	
RNY2F2	I just tell them I'm a nurse..... If you said you were a student, I'd kind of feel like you might be judged a bit [being a wife and a new mother].... I think the nurse might disappear when I stop that profession.	
PAY2M	I say "I'm a periodontist, but I'm also studying medicine". M-F = maxillary-facial; PER = periodontist	
ORY3F	I still call myself an orthoptist because I think that's what I earn money in. So, on my Facebook... I've got my profession listed as an orthoptist. But I've now changed it, I see myself now more as an orthoptist/medical student now that we're sort of getting a bit more clinical and it feels a bit more real... I'm defining myself now more as a med student, it's changing. OR = orthoptist	
OTY3F	I'm a doctor in training. .....Yes, the money is great [working as an OT], but the main reason is to continue to keep up my communication skills and to have that refinement.... To continue to keep learning instead of removing myself completely from the hospital environment until fourth and fifth year. OT = occupational therapist	

(continued)

Table 2 (continued)

HP	What do you call yourself when someone asks?	Venn diagram
RNY3F	I say "I'm a medical student". But, I don't know if I see myself totally as a medical student... I probably see myself as a mature-aged medical student, not in a bad way..... I just think that I'm expecting that of myself because I've had life experience..... I probably said I was a nurse in the beginning [of medical studies].	RN / Medical student
RNY4F	I'm still a doctor in training. "I'm a medical student in my fourth year and that I want to be a real GP" is what I normally tell people. ..... "I want to be a country doctor". I see myself as a country doctor in training, because I have really made up my mind that that's the pathway I'm going to take.	RN / Country GP in training
PAY1F [Y5]	I'd probably say I'm 70% medical and maybe 30% pharmacist. It's still a big part of me.. it's the sheer amount (sic) of hours that I'm working in that space ..... It can't not be part of me... but I'm definitely moving forward on to the more medical side now.	PA, DIT
PHY1M [Y5]	I'm a doctor in training.... Yeah. I don't consider my [physiotherapy]... I put it there for the capital ... It's just capital.	capital / DIT

included clinical context, scope of practice, professional networks), how long they had been working professionally, whether they were still working professionally while 'being' medical students and the alignment between their HP roles and identity and their roles and emerging identity as future clinical students and doctors. How others saw them was also important. In exploring their various narratives of 'self' across the five years, we highlight how their varied experiences as HPs have informed their current 'being' and 'becoming' as they 'transitioned' from one role, profession, identity, and/or community of practice without having fully left it, while simultaneously entering another without being fully part of it (Levinson 1981). Below, we describe the continuum of various HP 'positions' in terms of how they 'saw' themselves. This begins in Year 1 with, for example, a perceived role change (e.g., a newfound awareness of potentially relevant medical events or occurrences) to 'being' doctors-in-training (i.e., an emerging identity). For most, this involved customizing how they would eventually practice. For one HP, dissonance in terms of 'being' both an HP and a clinical student culminated in abandonment of his physiotherapy practice.

Anticipated Role Change, With a Hint of a Nascent Emerging Identity

Not unexpectedly, as new medical students for three months only, the Year 1 male sonographer (SOY1M) and the Y1 male RN (RNY1M) were very much still HPs, referring to themselves first by their HP title then as 'medical students'. RNY1M 'imaged' that once he was a clinical student (i.e., 'doing'), he would start to feel less like a nurse and more like a 'real medical student'. A defining moment for him would be when he could no longer be registered as an RN once he graduated as a junior doctor:

> "I expect that will happen [feel like a medical student 'becoming' a doctor] when I'm out on clinical rotations.... Probably fourth year... when .... I can truly get my hands dirty and teeth into it .... I'll feel like a real medical student. I do suspect that I'll still be a nurse at that stage, but I think that is certainly when that medical student identity will be flourishing and growing. It's hard to say exactly when that will happen but around that time, I imagine... I'm only hypothesizing but I'm aware that as soon as I have to register with AHPRA [Australian Health Practitioner Regulatory Agency] also as a medical practitioner, I can no longer register as a registered nurse. That might be very cathartic sort of thing to do".

Although there appeared to be little congruence between what he was learning as a first-year medical student and being a mental health nurse, he was nonetheless thinking about his changed status: "[There are] a range of things [from my medical studies] that I'm not necessarily employing when I'm interacting with patients, but I'm certainly thinking about them when I'm out there on the wards".

The Y1 male sonographer (SOY1M), who worked mainly with radiologists, found himself paying attention to medical 'things' because they might potentially be relevant as a future clinical student or doctor. They had previously been of little interest to him as a sonographer:

> "...I'm much more perceptive of what's going on around me at work, because now things at work that normally didn't bother me ... like the transfusion devices.... When they start beeping, you normally just push 'Silent' and forget about it. They're these annoying things. I never really had to learn to use them so I never asked questions, but now I find myself asking the nurse "Why is it beeping? What can we do to fix it?" because I know one day I'll be in a ward and I'll be looked at to probably help fix it. I think my perception of working at the hospital and other jobs people do, I'm opening my eyes up to a lot more. Especially... in resus [resuscitation] situations, just watching what different doctors do. Everyone has their little roles".

In 'being' a medical student, however, he expressed a sense of loss, almost grief, in having to 'let go' of his HP identity: "That's hard .... you're cancelling out your identity of your previous life and when you say you're a medical student, sometimes they just go "Oh, okay, good on you for doing medicine". But I've just wiped out the last six years of hard work".

Deliberate Role Boundaries

In 'being' medical students as well as practicing RNs, the two Year 2 female RNs (RNY2F1 and RNY2F2) used metaphors of 'different hats' and 'different brains' to describe how, while working as RNs, they consciously had to 'be' nurses, deliberately not crossing the nurse/medical student boundary. Although they were considering clinical decisions or events from a new perspective while working as RNs, 'being' RNs, however, invoked their strong 'nurse' identities:

> "I feel like sometimes I fall into different roles...If I go to work, ... even though I've got more insight to some things [as a medical student], I feel like I just put my nursing hat on..... I've got jobs and tasks to do. I do those nursing things... It wouldn't be professional to step ... out of my scope of practice. ... Sometimes I'll just think in my nursing brain, but .... it's difficult because I still sometimes think of a nursing perspective [as a medical student] or I'll really focus on really clinical aspects ..... I sometimes think too far ahead of study as well. I don't know what I identify as.... It changes.... [Working] as a nurse, I am a nurse" [RNY2F1]

> "When I'm working [as an RN], I'm a nurse because ... the patient is the focus and I can so easily get lost in reading a doctor's notes or working out why they're on all of these different medications ... I've got to remember...It's a conscious decision to be a nurse when I'm a nurse at work, when I'm in that role. It's kind of like a scope of practice thing as well. I don't want to do anything outside of that". [RNY2F2]

RNY2F2 went on to describe context-dependent multiple roles (and perhaps identities) which were also related to who asked: "While I'm here [on campus], I am a medical student and when I'm at home, I'm a mother.... I feel like I do [have different identities] and it depends on the person who asks me as to how I reply".

The three preclinical practicing RNs (RNY1M, RNY2F1, RNY2F2), however, disguised their 'medical student' status, mainly to avoid reprisal from some nursing colleagues (Table 2). This may, in part, explain the Year 1 male RN's (RNY1M) comment about being a 'real medical student' (i.e., legitimate) in the clinical years and the two Year 2 female RNs (RNY2F1 and F2) needing to 'stay in role', in addition to AHPRA requirements (Table 2).

A Mindset Shift: 'Becoming' a Clinical Student and Future Doctor

All three Year 3 HPs appeared to have made a psychological or cognitive shift in terms of how they saw their provisional future selves as clinical students and doctors. Least advanced was the female Year 3 RN's (RNY3F) self-concept perhaps because she was a late starter, qualifying as an RN in her late 40s and having worked clinically for about 15 months only before starting her medical studies. She was also the only HP not working. Although she could now 'see' herself as a doctor, she acknowledged that her circumstances may have contributed to this development of her sense of 'self':

> "In the beginning, it took some time for me to be able to see myself as a doctor. I think especially coming from a no-science background and then nursing and then this [studying medicine]...really hard. But, as the years go by and as it gets closer, I can see myself .... I can actually see myself even though I've had to say to myself "You can't know everything, but you know you can aspire to know as much as you can".

The Year 3 OT's (OTY3F) and orthoptist's (ORY3F) professional practice context influenced how they 'saw' their future selves. Like the Year 1 sonographer (SOY1M) who worked mainly with radiologists, the orthoptist (ORY3F) too was somewhat isolated from mainstream clinical practice as her medical colleagues were private practice ophthalmologists (who appreciated her scarce skills). She had thus taken deliberate measures (a psychological shift) to prepare her 'medical student' self for 'being a 'clinical student' in a few months: "I've cut down on my continuing education as an orthoptist. In that part of my life, I used to go to conferences and speak ..... I don't do that anymore ... I'm more motivated to spend time trying to figure things out and go through it [as a medical student] ... a lot more time as a self-directed learner".

'Being' an OT in a public hospital not only allowed the Year 3 female OT (OTY3F) to 'see' her HP practice through a different set of lenses but with her 'medical' knowledge, she was now able to rationalize doctors' decisions. She was, however, '*split*' in terms of her complementary identities (Table 2):

> "I've continued to hold onto it [OT] because it gives me the opportunity to stay in the hospital system to get that clinical experience. . ... You do get a lot of exposure to the medical side... I'm kind of split as a [Year 3] medical student and an OT each time I go back to work. Because I'm still learning things as a med student, I'm flicking through the chart, reading the med notes. "Oh, okay, so that's why they've called for this test...". Previously, ... as an OT, I would just glance over that... I [now] know where the doctors are coming from.... how they're treating the patient .... Having both perspectives is good".

Role and Identity Congruence: Self-tailored Interprofessional Identities

Along the same lines of 'staying in the role' (Year 2 RNs) but in reverse, the Y4 female RN (RNY4F) described how as a clinical student she had to deliberately 'be' the medical student on the wards. With years of nursing practice and still working as an RN while 'being' a clinical student, she instinctively did the 'nurse' thing first, that is, attend to patients' needs:

> "Sometimes I have to re-prioritise in my head how I'm going to do something. So, the nurse in me walks into a room ... sees the patient in the bed .... the pillow not comfortably placed under the head ... the patient ... awkwardly sitting upright or their buzzer out of reach or their little table with their water out of reach. ....As a nurse, I want to fix them all up before I start firing away the doctor questions".

Also using a 'hat' metaphor, she described her customized, hybrid, interprofessional future 'self' in which she patched a perceived deficiency in medicine (i.e., not person-centered) with her caring nursing ethic. She acknowledged, however, that it might not always be her future doctor 'self' who personally provided this 'care':

> "I would classify myself as someone who's going to be a doctor with the nursing care factor. . ... I was told once . .... to take off my nursing hat and put my medicine hat on. I went home and mulled over that... I remember thinking to myself, "No, I'm not taking my

nursing hat off. I'm just going to add my doctor's hat". I don't think I could ever be a health professional that went in, saw a patient, did a history, did a physical exam and walked out without adding in the nursing aspect which is "You look like you're shivering, should I give you a blanket? You've been sitting here in emergency for four hours. Have you been offered a cup of tea?".... There are the nursing things that I would have done to have made that patient extra comfortable. I don't want to take that hat off and stop thinking about the patient from that angle. I want to do both.... Even if I am pushed for time and can't be the one who goes and makes the tea like the nurses would do in A&E... I would hope that I'm still a doctor who would make sure that someone did it for them...... I still see myself as being a nurse and the doctor".

In a similar vein in terms of role congruence, the Year 1 female pharmacist (PAY1F) described the intersection of two identities, that is, her existing pharmacist identity and her emerging medical student and future doctor identity, as a Venn diagram (Table 2):

"They are two separate identities, but they are coming together in a bit of a Venn diagram.... I am sort of pulling back from the pharmacy identity... I'm sort of half... one foot in each camp... I think there is a lot of negatives with this whole Venn diagram situation, but there are also a lot of positives, like I love what I do [as a Pharmacist], so I'm not trying to get away from that".

Her account below highlights the complexity of 'being' a HP as well as a medical student and how others 'see' HPs. She described a situation in which she was undertaking voluntary General Practice experiential learning as a Year 1 medical student. The GP first addressed her as '[Name], the pharmacist', before reminding himself that she was there as a 'medical student': He [the GP] would be like "Oh, [NAME] is a pharmacist. Let's ask her some questions about the drugs, but then "Oh, no. She is a med student as well. That's why she's here". So, it was again this Venn diagram of me". Five years later, as the 'medical student' on a health care team, she recalled how she was sometimes called upon to 'be' the pharmacist:

"All the doctors know my background... There are times when they've actually asked me [as the student] to use my pharmacy knowledge... There has been a couple of complex palliative care patients who have had very poorly controlled pain. They've had a lot of other symptoms ... refused palliative care input. So, the team has actually said "Do you mind going in and sitting having a good chat about everything and going though it and see if... [there is] anything we can do?"... I'm more than happy to do that".

A few years later, as a final year student, PAY1F [Y5]'s narrative below describes an unusual situation in which she was on the same ward for several months in two roles – pharmacist and clinical student. Like the Year 4 female RN (RNY4F), the pharmacist described patching a perceived deficiency (i.e., doctors not providing patients with sufficient information about their medication) by switching between her two complementary roles to improve the patient experience:

"Really handy [being in both roles] because there were times when I'd see the patient on the weekend [as a pharmacist]... They were being admitted and I do their initial medication history and have a chat with them... Part of the role .... reviewing the medications and checking that everything is clinically right and appropriate. You have to know the patient's background and what they've come in with and their medical problems. I guess I probably was a bit more thorough with looking at the medical side of things when I go through their notes and checking their imaging and their blood tests. .... coming from the medical side. So, I was spending a lot more time on the medical things because I had more knowledge on that side. ..... The next day .... that patient was on my team. As the medical student, I was actually giving the hand-over a lot of time to the doctors, because they didn't actually know the patient. I knew the patient best, just because I happened to see [the patient] the day before... The patients would look at me as I was there [again] and then I'd say "Oh, I'm actually a medical student as well. ... Do you mind if I examine you?" And they're like "Oh, yeah, that's fine. We met you yesterday..."

Positive patient responses to her 'being' a pharmacist and 'being' a clinical student validated her 'becoming' a doctor:

"Patients ... because when I speak to them as a pharmacist, I don't know why, but it seems that a lot of them have picked up that maybe I'm not just a pharmacist anymore. ... A lot of people say... "Oh, is there any reason you didn't go and do medicine? Why aren't you a doctor? You've told me more than what the doctors told me" or "You've discussed this in a better way"... Then, I'd be like "Oh, I'm actually studying [medicine]".... I don't know whether it is maybe the way that I communicate in that I'm recognising perhaps some deficiencies in the system...Whether it's time and the doctors don't have the time to explain everything. ... I'm kind of feeling a bit of a responsibility because I'm in that sort of I guess 'club' now or on 'that side of the fence' that I really want this patient to know what's going on. So, I'll sit and I'll spend the time while I have it... as a pharmacist. I'll be going through things and giving them more background about the medical-related things and often that evokes some sort of comment ... I don't know whether it is at a certain confidence or a communication change".

Although PAY1F [Y5]'s 'medical' identity prevailed as a final year student, 'being' a practicing pharmacist, however, reinforced her 'pharmacy' identity (Table 2): "... 70% medical and maybe 30% pharmacist. It [pharmacy] is still a big part of me... I think it's the sheer amount (sic) of hours that I'm working in that space ... It can't not be part of me... But I'm definitely moving forward onto the more medical side... I guess maybe before I was focusing more on medications, whereas now I'm sort of having a bit more of a holistic view on things and not just focusing on medication but talking to them about other things." Notwithstanding, because of the complementarity of pharmacy and medicine, it was not surprising that she (PAY1F [Y5]) was ready to move on and 'be' a doctor: "I haven't really full identified with it [being a medical student] as a journey. I guess I see med school as a bit of a ends to a means which probably sounds terrible but I'm just really looking forward to being qualified... I felt like I've been ready for probably two years now... 100% ready... That's not because I knew everything or because I knew everyone. I think it was that I was very aware of what I knew and what I didn't know and I felt that I could be a safe practitioner, functioning as an intern. ...For me, I just feel like I'm checking boxes until I get that final piece of paper and then that's when the real journey starts for me."

Role and Identity Dissonance: 'Being' a Physiotherapist While 'Being' a Clinical Medical Student

The case of the Year 1 male physiotherapist who was re-interviewed as a Year 5 student (PHY1M [Y5]) is the antithesis of the Year 1 female pharmacist in Year 5 (PAY1F [Y5]) in terms of role and identity alignment. As a first-year student, PHY1M spoke about the usefulness of his particular expertise (Anatomy) to his medical studies and to his peers. He had continued to work clinically to earn an income but also to maintain his skills and engage with patients. Early in Year 4, however, his frustration with his limited scope of practice as a physiotherapist and his inability to apply his extensive medical knowledge led him to abandon 'being' a physiotherapist (Table 2). Below is his description of physiotherapy being of minor importance in the 'big picture' of medicine:

> "I gave it [physiotherapy] up because I was super, super, super annoyed by the lack of scope of practice and the fact that I had all this additional knowledge [from medicine] that I wanted to apply... but I couldn't actually utilise it [as a physio]... It wasn't that it was conflicting. It was more just like this [physiotherapy] was just such a small aspect of this whole entire bigger picture that opened up and I realised that really in the big picture of who I was dealing with that [physio] was a very small minor aspect... If I was to write out a problem list of this particular patient... top 10 problems... I [as the physio] didn't fit in the top 10 problems that I [as the medical student] needed to deal with... That was happening over and over.... I was just like "I can't deal with this"... One patient that I remember so clearly and it burned a hole through my entire career going forward... There was a patient that had a fall and had a really bad swollen knee and I went in there with the physio hat on and I was dealing with it and had a really good idea of what I thought was going on and then the blood test results came back. Previously [as a physiotherapist], I had never read blood results... because I didn't have that skillset to do so and do it accurately.... I did it and I realised that their INR was completely off the planet. They were on Warfarin and I was thinking "Oh, this patient has a bleed in their joint." So, I spoke to one of the orthopaedic surgeons and I said.... "I just had a look. You thought it was a joint thing, but I think that they've actually got bleeding in the joint."... I realised just then that actually none of that I [as a physio] was doing mattered really because this was the problem... That same situation started happening all over the shop... I was like "I can't do this anymore".

Notwithstanding, physiotherapy was 'capital' that opened doors for him as a clinical student: "What I started from there onwards is I used 'physio' as the capital just to gain respect with nurses or random GPs or random clinicians. When you come in [as a medical student], they don't want to let you do something because they don't know who you are. They have to suss you out ... as a med student.... If I said to them, "Oh yeah, I used to work here as a physio. I worked down the street as a physio. I worked with blah, blah, blah as a physio", all of a sudden, they give you a little bit of [leeway]".

Allowing his physiotherapy registration to lapse suggests a conscious psychological and behavioral shift from 'being' a physiotherapist to 'being' a clinical student *en* route to 'becoming' a doctor: "When people ask me to do physio-related things, I use a blanket statement most of the time... *"I'm sorry, I've let my insurance lapse, so I don't do any physio-related work. I only do medical-related work... But I could recommend this...*" Not surprisingly, at the start of his final year, he had fully transitioned to 'becoming' a doctor: "I view my identity now as a doctor-in-training...about to finish medical school. I almost don't view myself as a physio at all. It's completely gone. You can't do both and have the same mentality, because the mentality required to do physiotherapy is totally different to the mentality required to be a doctor."

An Unusual Scenario: From 'Being' a Trainee Surgeon (With Two HP Degrees) to 'Being' an Undergraduate Medical Student

The Year 2 male periodontist's (PEY2M) situation was highly unusual. After graduating with two HP degrees (pharmacy and dentistry), he worked as a trainee maxillary-facial surgeon. Changed regulations, however, forced him to return to medical school. Although working as a periodontist to support his young family and his aging and ailing immigrant parents, he would tell people he was a 'medical student' who was working as a periodontist. When asked why he had 'changed' professions, he responded: "It's not a change, it's a progression. I need two degrees to do head and neck surgery, so that's why I am here [studying medicine]". When asked what he was able to bring from his previous studies and clinical work to 'being' a medical student, his response was: "Coming from a hospital background... everything I have learnt, to be honest... [In studying medicine] there is nothing new in a sense. It just reinforces..." Table 2 thus depicts his pharmacy and dentistry/periodontist identities as well as 'being' a medical student within his overarching identity (due to prior experience) as a future maxillary-facial surgeon.

Discussion

This study explored how 11 HPs representing seven health professions who were studying medicine in an undergraduate program saw themselves 'becoming' doctors. Their 'becoming' clinical students and future doctors was influenced by having 'been' but generally still 'being' HPs, i.e. the context in which they practiced their health profession (e.g., a hospital-based pharmacist on multi-professional teams vs. a sonographer interacting mainly with radiologists), how long they had been HPs, their relationships with members of one or more professional communities, the stage of their medical studies, the alignment between their HP roles and identities and their emerging identities as future clinical students or doctors in terms of how they imagined practicing medicine (e.g., nursing 'care' adding value; physiotherapy mentality different from medical mentality), and whether they still worked as HPs while 'being' medical students, particularly as clinical students.

Both their roles (external, linked to positions in social structures – what they did) as HPs and as medical students, and their existing and emerging identities (internalized meanings and expectations associated with the role – who they were), were influenced by how they 'saw' themselves (Stryker and Burke 2000; Sims 2008; Ibarra and Barbulescu 2010) on their 'becoming' doctors trajectories (Table 2) (Wenger 1998). Role (and presumably identity) congruence and dissonance of roles and identity are exemplified by PAY1F [Y5], who was able to integrate her complementary pharmacy role and identity into 'being' a clinical student, while 'being' a physiotherapist frustrated PHY1M [Y5] as he perceived his work as a physiotherapist as relatively insignificant in terms of the 'big picture' of medicine.

Deliberate role boundary maintenance (or wearing metaphorical hats) was evident for Year 2 RNs who stayed in their nurse role and did not disclose their 'medical student' status to nursing colleagues for fear of criticism. Such a situation probably reflects the documented horizontal violence in nursing (Ditmer 2010) as well as a long-standing animosity between the nursing and medical profession (McKay and Narasimhan 2012; Leong 2014; Romano and Pangaro 2014; Langendyk et al. 2015). In terms of Roccas and Brewer's (2002) social identity complexity framework, while psychologically and cognitively the two Year 2 RNs were merging elements of two roles and identities, challenging situations forced them to compartmentalize how others 'saw' them. PAY1F's narrated experiences in a GP practice as a Year 1 medical student and then as a clinical student, in terms of her interactions with patients (i.e., dual roles) and members of health care teams (asked to be a pharmacist while a medical student) reinforces that how others see us impacts on how we see ourselves (Monrouxe 2009; Sloane and Bowe 2014; Rees and Monrouxe 2018). Her narrative, as did others in this study, also confirms that 'being' (including the 'doing') in the role (either an HP or a clinical student) reinforces an existing identity or strengthens an emerging identity (Cruess et al. 2019). Where there is little or no alignment (i.e., dissonance) between an existing and an emerging identity, the HP identity might be abandoned (Konkin and Suddards 2012; Frost and Regehr 2013; Wong and Trollope-Kumar 2014; Rees and Monrouxe 2018), as was the case for PHY1M.

As practicing professionals who had worked with patients in multi-professional teams and who were now 'being' medical students, it was not surprising that some HPs, especially RNs, had customized or enriched their existing and emerging identities such that they were hybrid and interprofessional (Sims 2008; Frost and Regehr 2013; Langendyk et al. 2015; Rees and Monrouxe 2018). This reflects the dual socialization of individuals in Sims' (2008) study who, in undertaking joint professional training in learning disability nursing and social work, constructed new interprofessional identities which enabled them to cross boundaries in practice. For Rees and Monrouxe (2018), "...a strong shared identity (eg, interprofessional identity) with an understanding of different roles and responsibilities of others can foster trust and facilitate teamwork performance in high intensity situations" (p. 203). RNs were particularly vocal about incorporating person-centeredness into 'being' a doctor, much like the three RNs in a previous study who wanted to be 'different' doctors (McLean 2017). HPs' narratives thus reflect the *patching* of their emerging medical student/future 'doctor' identities with elements from existing identities not as a temporary *splint* as Pratt et al. (2006) described for residents' work-integrity violations to provide confidence moving forward, but rather to address a perceived deficiency (i.e., patient-centeredness) in medicine (MacLeod

2011; Konkin and Suddards 2012; Langendyk et al. 2015; Rees and Monrouxe 2018). Phillips and Dalgarno (2017) recently described medical residents' personal and professional identity dissonance, that is, as caring, empathetic individuals who were working as detached experts. Although PHY1M [Y5] saw no role for his physiotherapy identity as a doctor-in-training, having *been* a physiotherapist was, however, 'capital' (Bourdieu 1977) to secure experiential learning as a clinical student, much like the students in Balmer and colleagues study seeking capital for securing residency positions (Balmer et al. 2015).

For most, their descriptions of their future provisional 'selves' in which they would incorporate professional capital (Bourdieu 1977) as well as identity capital (Goldie 2012), challenges the notion of a uniprofessional identity (Kaiser 2002; Baker et al. 2011; Frost and Regehr 2013; Khalili et al. 2013; Langendyk et al. 2015), which is reinforced by a uniprofessional model of health care, medical education and conceptions of a medical professional identity. Merton (1957) wrote that the purpose of medical education is to "transmit the culture of medicine and... to shape the novice into an effective practitioner of medicine, to give him the best available knowledge and skills, and to provide (him) with a professional identity so that he comes to think, act, and feel like a physician." Cruess et al. (2014) recent definition of a medical professional identity – "A representation of self, achieved in stages over time during which the characteristics, values, and norms of the medical profession are internalized, resulting in an individual thinking, acting, and feeling like a physician" (p. 1447) reinforces a uniprofessional view of identity development, which serves to protect an exclusive area of knowledge, work practices and tightly regulates professional entry which effectively isolates future health care professionals who will need to work together on health care teams (Kaiser 2002; Baker et al. 2011). The impact of this is borne out in Weaver and colleagues (2011) identity study of first- to third-year students at an Australian medical school. Professional inclusivity (i.e., legitimate participation and socialization) and social exclusivity (i.e., peer unity and a strong shared sense of identity) both contributed to students' sense of [uni]professional identity.

RNY4F's description of her self-tailored and personalized interprofessional identity reflects congruence of the past, the present, and the future in her 'becoming':

"The professional identity ... moving from 'being' a nurse to 'being' a medical student to 'being' a doctor. I think they have to respect where you've come from and incorporate that into your journey and not try to tell you to stop wearing the nurse's hat and put on the doctor's hat. . . . . I don't think it's possible to take off a hat that you have worn for 10 or 15 years. I don't understand how someone could do that. It's part of you. . . When you [have] spent so much time in that role to just cut it out, you can't. . . I can't walk into a room and not look at the patient's pillow not being under their head properly. That's ... the professional identity of a nurse... How do you unlearn seeing that? You can't. All you can do is add to your professional identity. Now that you're a doctor, make the patient comfortable and diagnose what the problem is... because there are doctors who don't see it... They'll actually push the table out of the way to get up to the patient, listen to their chest, then walk out the room and leave the patient without their buzzer handy. So that's a doctor-doctor who just doesn't see the nursing side and then there's the nurse who doesn't see the diagnosing side and then, I guess, there's the lucky ones who maybe have a bit of both".

This personalized 'self' supports Trede's (2012) view that "Professional identity is interdependent with the structural context and the situations of others. Critics of explicitly addressing professional identity development [and] formation argue that focusing explicitly on professional identity formation aligns too closely with social engineering (Barnett 2010). Professional identity cannot be forced onto students, as students form their own professional identity" (p. 162). This challenges Cruess et al.'s (2016) proposal to amend Miller's pyramid to include professional identity at the apex (i.e., IS above DOES), suggesting that 'it' can (and should) be assessed. With the construction of identity "a constant process.... combining the elements from the past with the present ones, our expertise in the field of interest, in order to obtain the desired stability, both at a personal and a professional level" (Bulei and Dinu 2013; p. 257), it would not be possible to 'assess' HPs' personal and unique (inter)-professional identities.

Limitations

One limitation of this study is that only 11 (of ±70) HPs representing seven professions were recruited. Notwithstanding, and taking into consideration Volpe et al. (2019) recent comments regarding the absence of demographic considerations in professional identity research, this study has not only added value in terms of starting a research conversation about prior HP identity as one of many factors that influence 'becoming' a doctor but it has reinforced the individual nature of 'becoming' a doctor.

Conclusions

In Khalili et al. (2013) interprofessional socialization framework, preparing health professional education students to work in clinical practice involves a three-stage iterative process, that is, breaking down barriers, interprofessional role learning, and dual identity development. For most HPs in the present study, as professional members of one or more health care teams, the barriers had already been broken down and they generally had clear ideas of the roles of different members of the teams on which they worked, had worked, or will work as clinical students and future doctors. As largely self-efficacious HPs who had worked or were still working in clinical practice, HPs were generally not journeying from 'lay person to physician' which is how 'becoming' a doctor has sometimes been described (Holden et al. 2012). Rather, with appropriate 'habitus' and personal and professional (including identity) (Goldie 2012) 'capital' from life in general and from clinical practice (Bourdieu 1977), most had well-defined concepts of current as well as future 'selves'. Being at different stages of their medical studies, there was a spectrum of constructions of 'self', ranging from a heightened awareness of potentially relevant 'events' to their future roles, through having made a psychological shift to 'become' doctors to acknowledging being ready (confident and safe) to 'be' doctors. Rather than having dual identities (Khalili et al. 2013), there was generally an alignment between their current HP practice and their current and future clinical student and doctor 'selves', with some patching or integrating of emerging future roles and identities with elements from existing roles and identities. This resulted in self-tailored hybrid, interprofessional identities (Pratt et al. 2006; Sims 2008; Frost and Regehr 2013; Rees and Monrouxe 2018). Where there was dissonance, the HP identity was discarded, but nonetheless served as capital as a medical student. As context, culture and personal and professional experiences influence the 'becoming', no single, homogenous experience of professional identity formation thus exists (Joynes 2018). This study has begun to address Volpe and coauthors' concern that professional identity research has not taken into consideration individuals' intersectionality (Volpe et al. 2019). We believe that we have started a conversation about what 'being' HPs in different professions bring to 'becoming' doctors.

Cross-References

▶ Developing Professional Identity in Health Professional Students

References

Artemeva N, Rachul C, O'Brien B, Varpio L. Situated learning in medical education. Acad Med. 2017;92(1):134.
Baker L, Egan-Lee E, Martimianakis MA, Reeves S. Relationships of power: implications for interprofessional education. J Interprof Care. 2011;25:98–104.
Balmer DF, Richards BF, Varpio L. How students experience and navigate transitions in undergraduate medical education: an application of Bourdieu's theoretical model. Adv Health Sci Educ. 2015;20:1073–85.
Bandura A. Self-efficacy: toward a unifying theory of behavioural change. Psychol Rev. 1977;84(2):191–215.
Bleakley A. Stories as data, data as stories: making sense of narrative inquiry in clinical education. Med Educ. 2005;39:534–40.
Bourdieu P. Outline of a theory of practice. Nice R, trans. Cambridge, UK: Cambridge University Press; 1977.
Buckley H, Steinert Y, Regehr G, Nimmon L. When I say ...community of practice. Med Educ. 2019. Early online 11 Feb. https://onlinelibrary.wiley.com/doi/10.1111/medu.13823
Bulei I, Dinu G. From identity to professional identity – a multidisciplinary approach. Paper presented at: 7th international management conference, 7–8 Nov 2013, Bucharest, Romania.
Clandinin DJ, Cave MT, Berendonk C. Narrative enquiry: a relational research methodology for medical education. Med Educ. 2016;51:89–96.
Cruess RL, Cruess SR, Boudreau JD, Snell L, Steinert Y. Reframing medical education to support professional identity formation. Acad Med. 2014;89(11):1446–51.
Cruess RL, Cruess SR, Steinert Y. Amending Miller's pyramid to include professional identity formation. Acad Med. 2016;91:180–5.
Cruess RL, Cruess SR, Steinert Y. Medicine as a community of practice: implications of medical education. Acad Med. 2018;93(2):185–91.

Cruess SR, Cruess RL, Steinert Y. Supporting the development of a professional identity: General principles. Med Teach. 2019;41(6):641-9.Please delete this reference as it is now a duplication. I have amended one of the references so that if reflects the 2019 reference requested.

Cruess SR, Cruess RL, Steinert Y. Supporting the development of a professional identity: general principles. Med Teach. 2019. 42(6):641–9.

Ditmer D. A safe environment for nurses and patients: halting horizontal violence. J Nurs Regul. 2010;1(3):9–14.

Frost HD, Regehr G. "I am a doctor": negotiating the discourses of standardization and diversity in professional identity construction. Acad Med. 2013;88(10):1570–7.

Goldie J. The formation of professional identity in medical students: considerations for educators. Med Teach. 2012;34:e641–8. https://www.tandfonline.com/doi/pdf/10.3109/0142159X.2012.687476

Holden M, Buck E, Clark M, Szauter K, Trumble J. Professional identity formation in medical education: the convergence of multiple identities. HEC Forum. 2012;24:245–55.

Ibarra H. Provisional selves: experimenting with image and identity in professional adaptation. Adm Sci Q. 1999;44:764–91.

Ibarra H, Barbulescu R. Identity as narrative: prevalence, effectiveness, and consequences of narrative identity work in macro work role transitions. Acad Manage Rev. 2010;35(1):135–54.

Jarvis-Selinger S, Pratt D, Regehr G. Competency is not enough: integrating identity formation into the medical education discourse. Acad Med. 2012;87:1185–90.

Joynes VCT. Defining and understanding relationship between professional identity and interprofessional responsibility: implications for educating health and social care students. Adv Health Sci Educ. 2018;23:133–49.

Kaiser R. Fixing identity by denying uniqueness: an analysis of professional identity in medicine. J Med Humanit. 2002;23(2):95–105.

Kelly T, Howie L. Working with stories in nursing research: procedures used in narrative analysis. Int J Ment Health Nurs. 2007;16:136–44.

Khalili H, Orchard C, Spence HK, Farah R. An interprofessional socialization framework for developing an interprofessional identity among health care practitioners. J Interprof Care. 2013;27(6):448–53.

Konkin J, Suddards C. Creating stories to live by: caring and professional identity formation in a longitudinal integrated clerkship. Adv Health Sci Educ. 2012;17:585–96.

Langendyk V, Hegazi I, Cowin L, Johnson M, Wilson I. Imagining alternative professional identities: reconfiguring professional boundaries between nursing students and medical students. Acad Med. 2015;90(6):732–7.

Leong J. From nurse to doctor: the career path less encouraged. The Doctor's Tablet blog web site. 2014. http://blogs.einstein.yu.edu/from-nurse-to-doctor-the-career-path-less-encouraged/. Published 2014. Accessed 30 Mar 2019.

Levinson DJ. Explorations in biography. In: Rabin AL, Aronoff J, Barclay AM, Zucker RA, editors. Further explorations in personality. New York: Wiley; 1981. p. 44–79.

MacLeod A. Caring, competence and professional identities. Adv Health Sci Educ. 2011;16:375–94.

McKay KA, Narasimhan S. Bridging the gap between doctors and nurses. J Nurs Educ Pract. 2012;2(4):52–5.

McLean M. From being a nurse to becoming a 'different' doctor. Adv Health Sci Educ. 2017;22:667–89.

McLean M, Brazil V, Johnson P. How we "breathed life" into problem-based learning cases using a mobile application. Med Teach. 2014;36:849–52.

Merton RK. Some preliminaries to a sociology of medical education. In: Merton RK, Reader LG, Kendall PL, editors. The student physician: introductory studies in the sociology of medical education. Cambridge, MA: Harvard University Press; 1957.

Monrouxe LV. Negotiating professional identities: dominant and contesting narratives in medical students' longitudinal audio diaries. Curr Narrat. 2009;1:41–59.

Phillips SP, Dalgarno N. Professionalism, professionalization, expertise and compassion: a qualitative study of medical residents. BMC Med Educ. 2017;17:21. https://bmcmededuc.biomedcentral.com/articles/10.1186/s12909-017-0864-9

Pratt MG, Rockmann KW, Kaufmann JB. Constructing professional identity: the role of work and identity learning cycles in the customization of identity amongst medical residents. Acad Manage J. 2006;49:235–62.

Rees CE, Monrouxe LV. Who are you and who do you want to be? Key considerations in developing professional identities in medicine. Med J Aust. 2018;209(5):202–3.

Roccas S, Brewer MS. Social identity complexity. Pers Soc Psychol Rev. 2002;6(2):88–106.

Romano CA, Pangaro LN. What is a doctor and what is a nurse? A perspective for future practice and education. Acad Med. 2014;89(7):1–3.

Sharpless J, Baldwin N, Cook R, Kofman A, Morely-Fletcher A, Slotkin R, Wald HS. The becoming: students' reflections on the process of professional identity formation in medical education. Acad Med. 2015;90(6):713–7.

Sims D. Reconstructing professional identity for professional and interprofessional practice: a mixed methods study of joint training programmes in learning disability nursing and social work. J Interprof Care. 2008;25:265–71.

Sloane A, Bowe B. Phenomenology and hermeneutic phenomenology: the philosophy, the methodologies, and using hermeneutic phenomenology to investigate lecturers' experiences of curriculum design. Qual Quant. 2014;48(3):1291–303.

Stryker S, Burke PJ. The past, present, and future of an identity theory. Soc Psychol Q. 2000;63(4):284–97.

Trede F. Role or work-integrated learning in developing professionalism and professional identity. Asia Pac J Coop Educ. 2012;1(3):159–67.

Volpe RL, Hopkins M, Haidat P, Wlopaw DR, Adams NE. Is research on professional identity formation biased? Early insights from a scoping review and metasynthesis. Med Educ. 2019;53:119–23.

Wang CC, Geale SK. The power of story: narrative inquiry as a methodology in nursing research. Int J Nurs Sci. 2015;2:195–8.

Weaver R, Peters K, Koch J, Wilson I. 'Part of the team': professional identity and social exclusivity. Med Educ. 2011;45(12):1220–9.

Wenger E. Communities of practice: learning, meanings and identity. New York: Cambridge University Press; 1998.

Wong A, Trollope-Kumar K. Reflections: an inquiry into medical students' professional identity formation. Med Educ. 2014;48:489–501.

Part VIII

Future Directions for Health Professions Education

Health Professional Education in 2020: A Trainee Perspective

87

Karen Muller and Savannah Morrison

Contents

Introduction	1694
Tick-Tock, Tick-Tock	1694
Beep. Beep. BEEEEEP	1694
References	1703

Abstract

This vignette illustrates the daily struggle faced by junior doctors in order to demonstrate the importance of medical education and mentorship in preparing them for the varied demands of their profession. These include but are not limited to technical skills, time management and triage, administrative tasks, active listening, critical thinking, and providing emotional support to patients and their families. Executing these duties in a high pressure environment with limited time and resources can take a heavy mental and emotional toll on even the brightest in the field which excellent medical education and mentoring can aim to mitigate.

Keywords

Junior doctor · Mentor · Rural health · Telehealth · Compassion fatigue · Decision-making

K. Muller (✉)
Orthopaedic Surgery, John Hunter Hospital, Newcastle, NSW, Australia
e-mail: karen.muller@health.nsw.gov.au

S. Morrison
General Medicine, John Hunter Hospital, Newcastle, NSW, Australia
e-mail: savannah.morrison@health.nsw.gov.au

© Springer Nature Singapore Pte Ltd. 2023
D. Nestel et al. (eds.), *Clinical Education for the Health Professions*,
https://doi.org/10.1007/978-981-15-3344-0_131

Introduction

This book chapter has been constructed to imaginatively display the moral, ethical, and social struggles young doctors may come to face in the early years of their careers. Often functioning on little sleep, a terrible poor intake of macronutrients, and sometimes without adequate guidance or support from seniors, it can be a hostile environment to make a career in. Surgical and medical training can be best compared to learning a trade, in which education, support, and access are pivotal. As two junior doctors who are navigating Australian training programs, we have written a "sliding doors" scenario that demonstrates how education and mentoring can entirely change a trainee's career choice, outlook, ethos, and ultimately the care of their patients. We see the protagonist, Piper, and face situations or people that can lead her life and learning down one path or another. The two are often highly contrastable demonstrating the difference that just one interaction can have on a person in a vulnerable situation.

Tick-Tock, Tick-Tock

Piper's head snaps back up and she glances around hastily making sure no one has witnessed her brief sleep. She rubs a drop of saliva from the corner of her mouth as she spots the sweaty brown head of her supervising resident straining fruitlessly to hear the consultant through leagues of medical bodies. None of the copiously eager to please registrars, advanced trainees, and national or international fellows noticed, phew, but also disappointingly the same, sigh. As a final year medical student, boredom is Piper's most loyal friend. This is not quite the learning experience she thought she would get at clinical school. Self-directed learning was more than just a buzz word here.

"Pippa!" the consultant, Professor Magister, at the front of the pack, waves vaguely at a clinical sign she did not hear, cannot see, and has no hope of feeling from the back of the medical pack.

Piper smiles vaguely, as the consultant says; "Loitering all the way back there is no way of getting a good report on your assessment card."

Her dirty-haired and slightly more senior resident, Wayne, smirks around at her and elbows her to the front, happy to be out of the firing line for once. She stumbles forward, each step an ache in her shoddily made clinical shoes, and looks down at the patient, an emaciated old man who struggles to take a breath. Slowly, he strains his neck up to look at this fresh new face of unexplained torture. He opens his mouth as if to speak before the ticking clock morphs suddenly into an insistent beeping sound.

Beep. Beep. BEEEEEP

"It's a code blue" Wayne chokes out, the sweat seeming to dry in a crust along his receding hairline.

Piper tries to remember if code blue is an external emergency, a bomb threat, or a fall and realizes it is none of the above as the consultant rolls his eyes and waves dismissively at Wayne asking him to "Go sort out that pesky arrest, we're doing real work here."

Sliding Door 1
Wayne glances nervously at the stagnant team, appealing with his sad brown eyes for help. All either look officiously away or feign deep interest in the mysterious clinical sign (which feels strangely like an emperor's new clothes moment), and, feeling too proud to ask for help, Wayne slinks away alone.

Piper is torn. Should she go and provide her help, such as it is, to this unlikable senior? Or should she keep her lips shut, lay low, and hope no extra work, difficulty, and remonstrances find their way to her.

"Yes I do see that sign" she lies to the consultant, turning her attention to the anxious patient, who was busy straining to see his own neck, and gesturing vaguely toward his chest-neck-head area.

Professor Magister's dark eyes gleam knowingly for an instant before he turns abruptly on one shiny brown brogue and swaggers out of the patient's bay and asks jokingly where his next victim is.

Piper bobs along in his wake, trailing away from the nervous patient bleating "Are you coming back? What do I have??"

They pass by the code blue, and through the thinnest crack in the curtains, Piper catches a 2-second view of Wayne's face freshly beaded with perspiration, his jaw set in grim determination as his eyes dart from the insistent red screen to the patient. His shoulders are rounded defensively, and his voice wavers uncertainly as he asks for the noninvasive ventilation machine to be set at 10 and 5, his voice catching on the last syllable. He is not sure. He does not know. He is out of his depth, and he does not ask for help.

Later, she hears that Beryl died shortly after that moment, her alveoli drowning in fluid her heart could not pump away. Some jokingly said Wayne drowned her with his own sweat. It was a joke that died as quickly as Beryl after the aftermath played out.

Wayne endured the repeated questioning on his character and competence during a root/cause/analysis investigation on this incident. Eventually, his license was pulled from general to provisional, an extra year in the hospital not working for the medical consulting company he aspired to work for – another year of cold hatred for all those around him and coarse apathy for those underneath him. With no one willing to listen, no debriefing, no feedback, and no self-reflection or systems change, Wayne continued to flounder in self-doubt and hatred. This was not the life he envisioned for himself, and it was not the life sold to him on medical school brochures. It was not what he saw on Grey's Anatomy or even what his lecturers described in medical

(continued)

school. It seemed that this big grey cloud of a system was good at talking the talk but not walking the walk: Everyone waxing lyrical about a collaborative, open and respectful approach but all the while blaming others for the insufficiencies or mistakes.

Piper knew this was not Wayne's fault. He had been punished for doing the wrong thing by a system that refused to help him to do the right thing. But mainly, she was glad she was not him and made sure to revise acute pulmonary edema management often, hiding behind the feeble approach that this was an isolated incident.

Sliding Door 2

Wayne glances nervously at the stagnant team trying to resuscitate Beryl, avoiding Piper's darting eyes. No, the injustice of the situation suddenly boils up inside her and starts to steam out of her ears she steps forward with her chest puffed out to help him, spreading a trickle of betadine on the newly mopped floor, much to the mirth of the glaring cleaner.

Piper knows her own limits and, unlike Wayne, calls for help from an unwilling but infinitely more knowledgeable consultant. Beryl is revived, moved to the ICU ward for strict cardiac monitoring and vasopressors, and everyone breathes a sigh of relief. Professor Magister recognizes her skill in escalating the situation and commends her on it. They use the SHARP five-step feedback and debriefing tool (Ahmed et al. 2013) to review the situation, and Piper feels empowered and ready for the next crisis she sees at the Lady Alere Hospital. She and her friends mull the situation over at dinner that night. They make fish tacos and talk about how weird it will be when they are all chatting together like this as consultants in their respective fields 20 years from now. Piper also reflects on this moment in her next communication tutorial (Joyce-McCoach and Smith 2016). All the students discuss scenarios they have seen on placement and learn how to tackle difficult situations and conversations with language and expert negotiation skills.

The final year of medical school draws to a close, and Piper graduates feeling exalted and energized to make a difference in her local community. "We both got Bona Loca Hospital!!" screams her best friend Sarah running across the green lawn, academic gown and sash trailing behind her. They embrace and jump around with grins as broad as the Cheshire cat while Piper's parents snap pictures of this momentous occasion. They have waited so long for this moment and do not dare have their dreams dashed by the Medical Dean who warns of challenges ahead in their graduation speech. They giggle their way through the outdated hippocratic oath and derobe into their teary parents' arms, shouldering hiking packs to spend a "last summer" without responsibility in South America.

The first few weeks of being a junior doctor is a whirlwind. Medical school never prepared these two glowing junior doctors for the use of the online medical chart system called "Powerchart" or archaic-written pathology request forms. Who knew you had to call the radiology registrar after finally struggling to figure out the CAT scan electronic-order request and get a green cannula into that dehydrated little old Beryl at 2 am? Despite the challenges, Piper and Sarah take it all in their stride and try to help each other make sure they work hard and play hard. They take time to enjoy their newly earned cash and study-free moments. Piper, unlike some of her colleagues, is aware that if she cannot take care of herself there is no hope in her ability to take care of others. She prioritizes her list of jobs and never compromises patient care nor self-care.

Both Piper and Sarah have luckily landed cardiothoracic rotations together. They are on different teams, and each has full lists of 20 plus patients each day. After a long day of Sunday roistered overtime, as each is working their 85th hour of the week, Piper turns to Sarah with a mischievous grin.

"After this cannula is in, and those packed red blood cells are running I am out of here!"

Sarah looks surprised, "What's on tonight?" she asks.

"Going to find some inner peace with a well-earned yoga class and plenty of downward dog and then..," she looks conspiratorially around the ward, "I've got a hot date with Andy!"

Sarah looked perplexed, "Aren't you interested in surgery? If we don't stay back and prep the handover list, none of the consultants will like us. They will never give us a job next year."

> **Sliding Door 1**
> "Yeah, you're right. Move over a bit so I can get to this computer and help." Piper slides into the worn-out chair and focuses her attention to the bland list on the archaic computer trying to ignore the buzzing of her phone. When she sneaks a look at the screen, her heart cools as she sees a text from Andy which reads, "Can't wait to see you tonight."
>
> Winky face. WINKY FACE!! But she has made her decision, and she knows a few grunt hours now will save her years of disappointing job offers and heartache later. Piper sighs and reaches over Sarah to the jumbo party mix of lollies and takes a fistful.
>
> The following morning, Piper and Sarah stand waiting at the corner of the cardiology ward with just the right amount of anxiety and focus in their blood to lead the cardiothoracic ward round without a hitch. The bosses leave looking somewhat pleased and mildly impressed before they head upstairs for their theatre lists. Piper and Sarah quote repeatedly the snippets of praise they thought they might have heard and wish they were offered an opportunity to scrub in but scurry back to the ward instead. They need to alert the nurses of the bosses' requests and start prepping discharge summaries.

(continued)

The surgeons are well aware that there is a bottleneck of junior doctors vying for training roles. They do not envy their position but think to themselves "we had it tough in our day too. When I was a young junior doctor, I used to sleep here, night after night. Only way to really get any experience I always say." Somehow, this excuses them from the responsibility to nurture their future trainees or advocate for their ongoing career progression. At the end of the day, if they aren't willing to put up with this, then someone else, who looks, speaks, and works similarly, will be.

On the drive home, Piper thinks about the last few weeks and their busy 2 days. Yeah, things ran smoothly today, but she is still not really sure what she could do to be better. She wonders if the teaching and feedback should be her responsibility. She wishes she was not left in the dark so often. She resolves to ask a senior registrar or mentor about it next week, or maybe the week after when things are not so busy. Hmm, there is another task on the bucket list – find a mentor – a difficult task when everybody is rushing around just trying to keep their own head above water, let alone a deadweight junior doctor.

To be fair, there does not really seem to be time for anything, let alone feedback, and certainly not her personal life. She feels herself slipping into an unreactive, bland, and listless state. Is this what it is like to be tired, or is this what it is like to be a surgeon, she wonders? She is losing the drive to learn and ask questions, to care what her patients say back to her, or even to respond to crises on the ward. After all, her seniors do not seem to care that much either. Her friends outside of healthcare call and ask "Is everything alright? I never see you anymore!" and her first response is to hang up, for it is easier not to have the conversation. Life is filled with frozen meals, a notebook with patient stickers, darkness on the drive into work, and darkness on the way out. Her whole life feels a bit like darkness at the moment, and she is not sure when it will lift. She wants to take a day off just to figure it out, but that would be career suicide.

Sliding Door 2

"Naaah as if they'll care about an updated list. They probably won't realise we've been here late! I'm totally exhausted." She sees Sarah's sense of propriety rising around her like a hen settling into a dust nest. "You can stay if you like, but I don't think it will make that patient any safer and some things are more important than impressing the bosses." Piper says decisively.

She knows colleagues who live and die by a word of praise from a lofty surgeon or physician they admire. She remembers Tang that surgical wannabe she dated in medical school, how he dropped hobby after hobby and picked up kilo after kilo until they could hardly have a conversation over brunch that was

(continued)

not related to medicine, the surgical program, or a cool operation he had stayed back late to watch.

Sarah looks dubious for a moment as she thinks it over, until a single shattered wail from one of the long-stay delirious patients near the nursing bay brings her back to the present. She quickly asks if she could come to yoga too, as she pushes the lollies at the nurses station. The young doctors giggle their way through a series of wobbly Downward Dogs and failed Killer Praying Mantis poses, before parting ways outside the yoga studio, with a wave and promises of juicy gossip tomorrow.

Piper swans sweaty and unapologetically late to her date and meets Andy, a previously bored young lawyer from Strasser and Yolkein, a new law firm in the CBD. His eyes light up as soon as they catch sight of the passionate, vibrant, and challenging young doctor who speaks of her work with a spark in her eye.

As to how he will slot into her already hectic schedule and a future that promises a period of distance relationship angst, missed dates, and late-night debriefs, he does not care. This is someone who is passionate, well-rounded, and interesting, someone he could love and support in the long-term.

As a balanced, well-supported young individual, Piper manages to dodge a serious breakdown in her early career, though does develop a splash of anxiety around job interviews. She progresses through her junior registrar years with as open an attitude as possible, though like most, the road behind her is inevitably littered with small mistakes that help her learn big lessons. She pursues intensive care, likely after developing an interest in the acute care she witnessed one boring morning on medical ward rounds. She listens actively to her seniors, reflects insightfully on her successes and failures, values the team around her, and tells them so. She gets involved in simulation-based education, and the more she teaches, the more she seems to learn (Rees et al. 2016). Like pasta thrown at the wall to assess al dente status, every memory made twice has a better chance to stick. Her reference reports for new jobs are always glowing and highlight Piper's leadership, education, and teamwork abilities. She is drawn to further good mentors and does the same to those more junior much like a reverse Catch 22.

In a bid to better understand rural medicine, Piper takes a 6-month secondment away from her then fiancé Andy to Boondabarabranaloo, a rural town in the geographical wasteland of Australia. It boasted a single large-scale Bilby statue in the middle of town as the main recommendation for visiting. Boondabarabranaloo was a washed-out old town that used to have a river coursing through the middle which the people used to amuse themselves with fishing golden carp, or swimming in. But, the droughts had dried it up to a trickle, and, like the river, morale was low on the ground. The people were mainly farmers and miners, and health literacy was thought to be a deity potentially worshipped by people in the Far East.

Her first day in the Intensive Care Unit (ICU) found Piper taking the ward round alone, her supervising consultant busy on his beef farm, known to be highly resistant to coming in for anything short of a planned cardiac massage. The rest of the medical personnel working in here, the largest trauma center west of the coast, are almost entirely hollow-eyed dementors pursuing a quick buck with week-on, week-off locum work.

Piper is also "on" for rapid response calls for the entire hospital; she is understandably quite stressed and can feel panic rising up her throat as she surveys the multidisciplinary team arrayed at the middle desk waiting for her.

Allied health professionals are thin on the ground in rural areas of Australia, and this hospital is no exception. While Bona Loca had an array of physiotherapists, social workers, occupational therapists, dieticians, and psychologists, Boondabarabranaloo has only managed to secure two full-time physiotherapists and a single social worker this year.

The results are not good.

Piper sucks in a deep breath and arrays her face in what she hopes is a disarmingly confident smile as she walks into the first patient bay. Mr. Westworth startles back in his bed despite the pain in his lungs, frightened by the fiery eyed doctor who appears at the end of his sponge cake like bed.

Piper assesses him expertly and then turns to ask the medical student, Julia, to pull up the most recent X-ray. Julia haltingly chokes through the process, as though she has never been addressed by any of the doctors, let alone asked to participate in the clinical diagnosis and decision-making process.

"What do you think about this chest X-ray Julia?" asks Piper as they peered at the films. She enjoys taking the time to teach her more junior colleagues and involve them in the day-to-day tasks this regional ICU offers. "Well. ummmm. ahhhh. It doesn't look normal" are the words that splutter out of Julia's mouth. "Well what would normal look like?" They carry on working through the problem and recognize that this patient has significant issues which cannot be fixed with ventilators and medications alone. They need a speech pathologist's assessment, chest physiotherapy, and further tests which may need to be done in a bigger tertiary center. But, transport is costly and very dangerous for such an unstable patient.

Piper glances around at the medical, nursing, and scant physiotherapy staff who all blink back at her apathetically.

"Well, do we have the facilities to assess this patient fully?" She asks with what she hopes to be authority.

A bolshy nursing unit manager standing in the front row barks out a humorless laugh as she adjusts her rectangular pink-rimmed glasses. "Facilities? Staff? Jeez you must be fresh!"

Sliding Door 1

Piper thinks it over for a second before the advice of one of her surgical registrars whispered past her ear. Do not rock the boat, Piper, the path of least

(continued)

resistance is easier and will help you get out on time. *She lowers her eyelashes and fixes her stare on the peeling lick of linoleum struggling to pull away from the floor.*

"Right. Hah. Very fresh. So what can we offer this man in the way of rehab then?" Her capitulation is met with a smug smirk from the NUM who promptly squares her stocky shoulders, steps forward, and proceeds to claim rights to the ward round and smother all attempts at teaching or innovation.

Piper passed a frightfully boring and unchallenging 6 months in Boondabarabranaloo, often feeling as though she was leading a very well-stocked palliative care ward, where her main hurdles included avoiding confrontations with the senior staff and attempting to work out a route to the hospital that avoided the ridiculously oversized Bilby.

She got out on time most days and complained about the whole situation to Andy on the phone who could not figure out what had so affected his vibrant young spark. They were both relieved when the 6 months was over and she could return safely to the city hospital with high-hoping standards and well-staffed wards.

Sliding Door 2

Piper sends a swift prayer before adjusting her stance.

"Are you telling me that we would sacrifice optimal patient care simply due to a paucity of care? If you tell me we simply do not have the resources, that is an environment we have to work within," she took a deep breath and fixed the NUM with a cold stare.

"But if you're telling me that we will not offer this middle-aged father of four a full multidisciplinary assessment simply because we cannot be bothered to work out the fully functional, if glitchy, telehealth network intended for this exact purpose then, That. Is. Simply. Unacceptable."

With each word, her audience seems to blink faster, shift their positions uncomfortably, and, she feels, she can almost see their brains begin to tick faster.

For the moment, they just want to keep this patient as safe as possible so they call as many of their regional allied health colleagues as possible and organize a telehealth appointment with the St Helen's respiratory and infectious diseases departments the following day.

Piper is pleased with herself and goes home to read up a little more on the topic before tomorrow's telehealth call to the Brockhampton ear nose and throat service. She prepares a few slides for the medical student teaching session and finishes the day with a glass of red wine and a fantasy novel which is reaching its climax.

(continued)

> A few weeks later, just prior to returning to Bona Loca Hospital for her final term, Piper gets the letter she has been waiting for. She successfully completed all the training requirements for her ICU fellowship and will be admitted to the college next month. She calls some of her fellow trainees and bosses to let them know of the news and thanks them for their help and support along the way. Dr. Leggen urges "Well I do hope you take a role with us here at the Bona Loca, Piper, you know you are the wind in the sails of our teaching program and I don't think the Multidisciplinary Team Meetings would be the same without you." "Only if I can make a few extra changes!" she quips as she starts thinking about implementing her perfect code blue team and improving the simulation training lab.

Some months later, Piper rushes up to a four-bed bay on the medical ward with the resuscitation trolley, ICU nurse, cardiology registrar, and medical student in tow. The situation seems eerily familiar, almost deja vu. There is an older man in the bed, straining to see his head-neck-chest area, a sweaty resident with panic in her eyes, and a timid medical student avoiding everyone's glances and the responsibility of having to do anything active in this scenario. There are a few conscientious nurses plugging in cables, pumping IV tubes, drawing up medications into 10 ml syringes, and explaining to their nursing students how to measure the doses. And, at the end of the bed, there is a consultant gastroenterologist in a suit with a look of distaste on his face. How dare this measly old patient try and die on their watch? How frustrating to have to watch this flurry of poorly organized activity!

After a deep breath and 3 s of stillness to compose herself, Piper walks in, introduces herself to all, and stands directly next to the patient to ask what the situation is. She calmly hands the lead to her registrar whom she has trained to handle such a situation and she watches keenly so as to provide detailed and accurate feedback and debriefing at the end. After catching the eye of the medical student who is trying to slink away, she asks them if they will help her gather the equipment for a cannula. Before she even realizes what is going on, the doctor-in-training has put it in herself, with a broad pearly white smile that says it all.

Piper's story comes full circle in the final sliding door which demonstrates how receiving and delivering quality and compassionate teaching can positively impact both parties. These sliding door scenarios have highlighted contemporary drivers in medical and surgical education including: duty hour restriction (Jamal et al. 2011), burn out and compassion fatigue (Coverdill et al. 2011), feedback, multidisciplinary team training, technology, rurality, and a bottleneck in training opportunities (Yang et al. 2018). Addressing these issues now will help to create a more well-rounded cohort of health professionals who strive not only to deliver excellent patient care, but also to teach others to do the same.

References

Ahmed M, Arora S, Russ S, Darzi A, Vincent C, Sevdalis N. Operation debrief: a SHARP improvement in performance feedback in the operating room. Ann Surg. 2013;258:958–63.

Coverdill J, Bittner J, Park MA, Pipkin W, Mellinger J. Fatigue as impairment of educational necessity? Insights into surgical culture. Acad Med. 2011;85:s69–72.

Jamal M, Rousseau M, Hanna W, Doi S, Meterissian S, Snell L. Effect of the ACGME duty hours restrictions on surgical residents and faculty: a systematic review. Acad Med. 2011;86(1):34–42.

Joyce-McCoach J, Smith K. Teaching model for health professionals learning reflective practice. Procedia Soc Behav Sci. 2016;228:265–71.

Rees E, Quinn P, Davies B, Fotheringham V. How does peer teaching compare to faculty teaching? A systematic review and meta-analysis. Med Teach. 2016;38:829–37.

Yang Y, Li J, Wu X, et al. Factors influencing subspecialty choice among medical students: a systematic review and meta-analysis. BMJ Open. 2018;9 https://doi.org/10.1136/bmjopen-2018-022097.

Future of Health Professions Education Curricula

88

Eric Gantwerker, Louise Marjorie Allen, and Margaret Hay

Contents

Introduction	1706
Problem Identification and General Needs Assessment	1707
Artificial Intelligence	1709
Biosensors and Big Data	1711
Robotics	1712
Digital Therapeutics and Telehealth	1712
Quality, Patient Safety, and Value-Based Care	1713
Targeted Needs Assessment	1713
Goals and Objectives	1714
Educational Strategies and Implementation	1714
Active Learning	1715
Adaptive Learning	1717
Technology	1717
MOOCs and Online Learning	1718
Virtual Reality/Augmented Reality	1719
Game-Based Learning	1719
Assessment	1720

E. Gantwerker (✉)
Northwell Health, New Hyde Park, NY, USA

Zucker School of Medicine at Northwell/Hofstra, Hempstead, NY, USA
e-mail: egantwerker@northwell.edu

L. M. Allen
Monash Centre for Professional Development and Monash Online Education, Monash University, Clayton, VIC, Australia
e-mail: louise.allen@monash.edu

M. Hay
Faculty of Education, Monash Centre for Professional Development and Monash Online Education, Monash University, Clayton, VIC, Australia
e-mail: margaret.hay@monash.edu

© Springer Nature Singapore Pte Ltd. 2023
D. Nestel et al. (eds.), *Clinical Education for the Health Professions*,
https://doi.org/10.1007/978-981-15-3344-0_134

Conclusion 1721
Cross-References 1721
References 1722

Abstract

This chapter discusses the future of health professions education (HPE) curricula using David Kern's six steps of curriculum development as an organizing principle. It discusses several problems that future healthcare professionals (HCPs) will face including challenges of greater scope, less time, and less resources to promote health and provide patient care. It also discusses the transition from declarative knowledge and rote memorization to more application of information and problem-solving while leveraging the technology at HCPs' fingertips. There will also be highlights of future technologies that enhance and transform patient care, the massive amounts of data that will be generated, and the future of technology-enabled learning, teaching, and assessment.

Keywords

Technology · Virtual reality · Augmented reality · Digital therapeutics · Artificial intelligence · Robotics

Introduction

Health professions education, and specifically medical education, has been under the magnifying glass ever since Abraham Flexner's scathing report in 1910 entitled *Medical Education in the United States and Canada* (Cooke et al. 2006). The Flexner Report, as it came to be known, and a number of other influential events led to a complete overhaul of the medical education system in North America in the coming decades. These changes, in part, were due to an influx of educational funding (medical school budget in 1910 was US$100,000 which rose to US$20 million by 1965) and a large expansion in the amount of time required to become a physician (four 16-week lectures in the mid-1800s increased to 8 years of formal education by the early 1900s) (Ludmerer 2005). The Flexner Report was revisited for a new generation by Cooke et al. (2006). This fresh look refocused health professions education (HPE) on the task "to transmit knowledge, impart the skills, and inculcate the values of the profession in an appropriately balanced and integrated manner" (Cooke et al. 2006, p. 1341). Since then, the changing paradigm and the expanded role of the 2025 physician that includes diagnostic assessor, content curator (not creator), technology adopter, learner-centered navigator and professional coach, clinical role model, and learning environment designer, engineer, architect, and implementer has been recognized (Simpson et al. 2018).

Nursing deserves special mention as they provide the foundation of the world's healthcare workforce, accounting for 59% of all healthcare professionals or about 28 million nurses worldwide as of 2020 (World Health Organization 2020). But to be practice ready, they must be agile and equipped to deal with increasing complexity, changing care needs, technological advances, changing settings of care, and managing multiple transitions (Bouchaud et al. 2017). Nurses are being asked to multitask between managing higher acuity patients while bearing the brunt of increased documentation and regulatory requirements through electronic health records (EHRs) that deprioritize user experience (Needleman 2013).

Beyond nurses and physicians, healthcare in general is facing a workforce shortage, yet the training paradigm of paraprofessionals continues to be inefficient with increasing training times and paradoxical limited career opportunities and narrow pathways (Nancarrow et al. 2014). To address these educational paradigms, need to shift to more online and community-based models that are based on milestones with multiple career pathway exit points (Nancarrow et al. 2014). In addition, healthcare of the future will be a partnership between doctors, allied health professionals, machines (software and hardware), and patients (Wartman and Combs 2018, p. 1108). As discussed below, the future of health professions education will therefore be a dynamic flux of changing and expanding roles married with advances in technology to both drive changes and assist professionals in dealing with those changes.

Along with these shifts, we also know more about how people learn and the settings in which they will be practicing healthcare. We live in an era where most of the declarative knowledge lives on a device in our pockets that is accessible at all times. This has shifted the burden to healthcare professionals (HCPs) to appropriately problem solve utilizing this information through clinical reasoning and sound judgment to make informed decisions. These just-in-time reference materials were not readily available even four decades ago. Taking these factors into account sets the context as we think about the future of HPE curricula. As this is a large topic that we could dedicate an entire book to, we look to David Kern's six steps of curriculum development to provide a framework to think about and discuss the HPE curricula of the future. Kern's framework involves several steps: problem identification, needs assessment, goals and objectives, educational strategies, implementation, evaluation, and feedback (Thomas et al. 2015). Importantly, all good curriculum development starts with understanding the learners and the gaps you are trying to address. True to Kern, we will focus on the learners and their needs first and then move to the methodology and delivery mechanisms to achieve the goals and objectives of the curricula. Finally, we will focus on the future of assessment and feedback (Table 1).

As has been noted in this eBook, we are seeing truly unprecedented effects on health systems and health professions education globally due to the COVID-19 pandemic. Due to the pandemic, we have seen forced adoption of various technologies and improved remote health access and the silver lining may be the opportunity to completely transform every aspect of the structure and function of education and curriculum in higher education (Moldoveanu 2020).

Problem Identification and General Needs Assessment

Densen (2011) described many of the challenges facing HPE in the twenty-first century, including the exponential growth of medical knowledge, societal factors impacting health, workforce implications, technological advances, and healthcare

Table 1 Kern's framework with considerations for HPE curricula of the future (Thomas et al. 2015)

Step	Summary of considerations for HPE curricula of the future
Problem identification	Challenges facing HPE education: Exponential growth of health and medical knowledge, societal factors impacting health, workforce implications, technological advances, and healthcare reforms (Densen 2011)
Needs assessment	Students need to be able to meet these challenges, including incorporating technological advances (artificial intelligence, augmented and virtual reality, biosensors and big data, robotics, digital therapeutics, telehealth, etc.) into practice (clinical education and research)
Goals and objectives	The ultimate goal of the future curriculum will be to prepare students for their future careers in healthcare
Educational strategies	Utilizing adult learning theories to inform curricula that are adaptive, contextual, respects and activate prior knowledge, introduce autonomy and choice in what and how they are learning, and are problem-oriented, focusing on the application of knowledge
Implementation	Co-creation of practical and relevant personalized learning that seamlessly integrates technology
Evaluation and feedback	Learner-focused assessment, incorporating co-assessment, as well as leveraging technology for more objective learner assessments

reforms. With the entire corpus of medical knowledge is estimated to be doubling about every 73 days as of 2020, as compared to a doubling time of 50 years in 1950, resulting in the first 3 years of clinical education accounting for only 6% of what is known by the end of that decade (Densen 2011). Thus, the educational focus on rote memorization and knowledge attainment is destined to fail. Albert Einstein was famously asked by a New York Times reporter a question from a Thomas Edison job screening questionnaire about the speed of sound, and he aptly responded, "I don't know...I don't burden my memory with such facts that I can easily find in any textbook" (Frank et al. 1947, p. 185). He was also quoted as saying "that the value of an education...is not the learning of many facts but the training of the mind to think something that cannot be learned from textbooks" (Frank et al. 1947, p. 185). It is clear that focusing HPE on attainment of declarative knowledge, as education traditionally has, will fall severely short of preparing health professionals for their future careers. It also ignores the fact that traditional written medical textbooks are generally out of date the second they are published.

Current and future health professionals have ready access to information at their fingertips that offloads a great portion of what they need to memorize, saving cognitive powers for manipulation and problem-solving with that information. In HPE, this translates as focusing education on equipping students with the essential language, foundational knowledge, deep conceptual understanding, and the skills to source, critically appraise, and assimilate information to best enable them for their careers. As such, all educational materials and assessment tools in a curriculum should focus on the application of knowledge, higher order thinking skills, and problem-solving over declarative knowledge and rote memorization. This will become important as we discuss pedagogy and content delivery later in this chapter. Future health professionals will have a plethora of technology-enabled tools at their disposal at the point of care, only some of which are beginning to surface. Besides the skill sets that we need to inculcate in students, we also need to be cognizant of the tools they will have at their disposal and prepare them to integrate these into their workflows. This does not mean that students should be solely reliant on these tools, but they should be facile in how and when to use them properly.

Finally, the COVID-19 pandemic has likely changed education forever, and this is especially profound in HPE. As the pandemic loosens its grip on the world, we should see much of the synchronous, in-person education return to some semblance of normal. We will also see new adaptations based on collective learnings on how technology can enable remote synchronous and asynchronous education to augment in-person curricula. Technologies such as software-based simulation, video game-based learning, and extended reality such as virtual reality (VR) and augmented reality (AR) that saw tremendous interest during the pandemic will likely be leveraged post-pandemic. Although it is not a given that these will be fully embraced, institutions that adopt and adapt these solutions will likely outpace those that do not. The following sections provide a needs assessment for a range of technologies that are likely to impact HPE curricula of the future.

Artificial Intelligence

One technology that will have immediate and long-lasting implications will be artificial intelligence (AI). Artificial intelligence is defined as "a system's ability to correctly interpret external data, to learn from such data, and to use those learnings to achieve specific goals and tasks through flexible adaptation" (Kaplan and Haenlein 2019, p. 15). Artificial intelligence is a large umbrella term that encompasses many different technologies including, but not limited to, natural language processing, neural networks, machine learning, predictive analytics, and robotics. Artificial intelligence is demonstrated using intelligent agents which can be hardware or software based (think IBM Watson). As the human race, we must grapple with the fact that AI-enabled devices will increasingly outperform us in both cognitive and psychomotor tasks (Wartman and Combs 2018). In healthcare, AI has vast use cases including diagnostic assistants, decision support tools, natural language processing, big data analysis and predictive analytics, and intelligent tutoring systems, for example (Topol 2019). We are seeing AI being used to assist in activities of daily living (ADLs) and improving care for patients with Alzheimer's disease and related dementias (ADRD) (Xie et al. 2020). In addition, a recent systematic review found 31 studies with the use of conversational AI agents in a variety of healthcare settings (Milne-Ives et al. 2020).

Calls for reform in recent years have also focused on producing well-rounded and humanistic HCPs. As we advance into a world where society is using more electronic means of communication, there is a distinct worry that future HCPs will lack the interpersonal skills and empathy to maintain the human touch. Instead of looking at the negative aspects of technology, we can recognize the advantages that innovations will bring to the HCP-patient relationship. Artificial intelligence has the potential to enhance and facilitate clinicians' abilities to go from interpretation of digital data to establishing diagnoses and prognoses (Han et al. 2019). As such, AI will enable HCPs to return their focus on the patients, enabling them to engage the humanistic and communication skills that technology cannot easily replace (Han et al. 2019; Topol 2019). Estimates show that physicians spend only about 27% of their time seeing patients while 49.2% of their time is spent documenting and interacting with the EHR (Sanders 2005). Similarly, nurses spend about 26.2–41% of their time documenting in the EHR or paper charts and only about one-third of their time is spent in direct patient care (Schenk et al. 2017; Butler et al. 2018; Roumeliotis et al. 2018; Yen et al. 2018; Baker et al. 2019). With technological advances in big data and analytics, predictive modeling, and AI, the hope is that much of the menial documentation and tasks will be eliminated and HCPs can focus on the real task, caring for and engaging with patients and families. Instead of detracting from the soft skills of HCPs, some companies are even creating AI virtual avatars to teach students how to improve their communication and empathy skills. Maybe, 1 day virtual AI avatars can replace some of the standardized patients that are currently used to assess students given the impartiality, standardization, and analytical data core to these systems (Brown 2021).

Artificial intelligence has tremendous promise but what use cases are going to be most beneficial and actualized has yet to be determined. Imagine if AI could assist radiologists through clinical image analysis to best fit diagnoses and maybe even analyzing histopathology slides to minimize the error in diagnosing malignant lesions. We have already seen AI doing image analysis of patient submitted dermatological images to assist in diagnosing diseases and studies on how AI can analyze and diagnose based on pill endoscopy images, minimizing the onerous task of human analysis of hours of images. Recently, evidence is mounting on the use of the Rothman Index that analyzes 26 different variables and 11 nursing assessment elements to help identify patients at risk for acuity changes and need for intervention (Finlay et al. 2014; Robert 2019). Instead of fearing AI and worrying it will replace clinicians, akin to sentiments during the industrial revolution, we should embrace it in HPE curricula and teach students how to properly leverage it in patient care.

Yang and Veltri (2015) point out the many data sources that will be generated including EHR and clinical text, biomedical imaging, healthcare sensor data, genomic and pharmaceutical databases, spontaneous reporting systems, biomedical and healthcare literature, and social media data. Artificial intelligence may assist in managing this massive amount of data, mining the massive amount of patient level data, to not only predict potential complications (i.e., ED visits, decompensation, complications) but also recommend mitigation steps and auto-schedule clinic visits. In addition, AI can help to translate this data to promote preventative medicine and leverage it for predictive modeling and precision healthcare (Yang and Veltri 2015; Wartman and Combs 2018). From a curriculum standpoint, future health professionals need to understand how these technologies source and analyze data, how data are stored and accessed, and how to appropriately manage, or ignore, recommendations from the systems.

Healthcare systems across the world have different priorities and organizational structures. The Institute of Medicine's (IOM) 1999 landmark report, *To Err is Human,* forced a widespread refocusing on the role of HCPs in medical error and quality. In this report it was estimated that as many as 98,000 people died a year from in-hospital medical errors, setting in motion a giant magnifying glass on patient safety and quality improvement (Institute of Medicine 2000). In response, healthcare began to revive efforts on a culture of safety and collaboration of HCPs to engage in elements of continuous quality improvement (CQI), borrowing from trades such as the automotive industry (Cohen 1999; Leape and Berwick 2005). With this in context, we have seen a refocusing of the curriculum on the role of the HCP in a much wider health system. As discussed above, we can see how technologies such as AI can help reduce the human error in systems, but we also see a greater focus on the healthcare system as a whole beyond just clinical learning.

Biosensors and Big Data

Luckily, tomorrow's HCPs will have some unique technology tools at their disposal. Besides the traditional EHR and all the big data that AI can assist with, we also have the rapidly advancing world of patient level data being generated by biosensors and personal wearables. Think about the data that gets collected from continuous glucose monitors (CGMs), sleep apnea machines, activity monitors, and smartphone and wearable heart rate monitors, for example. All of these will generate massive amounts of data expanding the purview of the clinician to truly get a snapshot of a patient's health and activity. Enormous consumer level data alone is generated through smartphones, wearables, and in-home smart devices that may lead to health insights for tomorrow's clinicians. With the Internet of Things (IOT) and devices all communicating massive amounts of data, HCPs will have information regarding all aspects of daily life of patients including purchasing and dining habits, variations in emotional states based on sentiment analysis, medication ordering, and even wearable data such as daily activity, heart rate, blood pressure, and ECG tracings. Integration of these data using different AI applications can actually create predictive algorithms about patients who are at risk of anything from heart attacks and strokes to cancer. Physical therapists/physiotherapists will also have access to technology that uses inexpensive biosensors to monitor balance and gait and assist in biofeedback and rehabilitation (Huang et al. 2014; Horak et al. 2014). Again, focusing on patient health, and how the person behaves outside the clinical setting, may allow clinicians to prevent disease instead of just treating it. As Wartman and Combs (2018) discuss, it is important to understand the four Vs of big data: volume (the amount of data generated); variety (multiple data sources); velocity (the acceleration of data generation); and veracity (the need to assess the quality of data generated). Curricula of the future may include how to validate, incorporate, and manage these types of data, and utilizing these various sources of information to drive and monitor patient care.

Robotics

We are starting to see more robotics in the clinical realm going beyond just prosthetics, for example, in the world of rehabilitation. Recent articles have noted the use of robotic arms to do range of motion and rehabilitation without the need for a physical person to be present. This self-guided or auto-guided therapy could revolutionize care across the continuum (Bruni et al. 2018). Starting in 2014, the National Science Foundation (NSF) has invested $3 million in robotics being able to perform various nursing tasks (Robert 2019). Collaborations at Duke University have even developed the Tele-Robotic Intelligent Nursing Assistant (TRINA) that is a remote-controlled robot meant to operate inside hazardous clinical areas that can perform 60% of predefined nursing tasks, albeit at a much slower pace (Li et al. 2017; Robert 2019). From a surgical or procedural standpoint, we already have robotic-assisted surgical devices to help perform difficult procedures that give unparalleled visualization, dexterity, and precision. These systems even have tremor dampening technology that can make up for gross errors or inaccuracies from surgeons. With time, we will start to see more autonomous surgical applications where simple, rote procedures may be performed without human input and only with human supervision. This means that students may have much more advanced procedural tools at their disposal, requiring them to know how to interact and problem solve with these systems.

Digital Therapeutics and Telehealth

Clinicians will also have access to patient care tools that are just now starting to emerge. There are already AI avatars that are assisting in cognitive behavioral therapy for soldiers returning from war settings and even a new robot called Moxie that assists children with emotional processing and autism-related issues (Rizzo et al. 2010; Begum et al. 2016). Virtual reality is also leading the way for digital therapeutics (DTx) for everything from treating post-traumatic stress disorder (PTSD) to managing pain to phobia desensitization (Chad et al. 2018; Gupta et al. 2018; Difede et al. 2007; Rizzo et al. 2010; Wechsler et al. 2019). Almost daily, we have new apps for teaching people how to manage their diabetes, asthma, and chronic kidney disease.

The year 2020 saw the first video game approved as a digital therapeutic tool for treating children with attention-deficit/hyperactivity disorder (ADHD) (Kollins et al. 2020). Digital therapeutics (DTx) is a field that is rapidly expanding using both software and hardware-based solutions to help prevent and treat diseases. We also have smartphone applications that can actually deliver coaching messages, analyze dietary choices, provide alternative recommendations, and send reminders for compliance with medications and other therapeutics to assist in disease management. Business leaders estimate the DTx space will reach $56 billion by 2025 underlying the rapid investment, development, and deployment of solutions (Insider Intelligence 2021).

In addition, one thing we saw during the COVID-19 pandemic was meteoric rise of virtual and telehealth. This is likely one area that will remain and strengthen long after the pandemic frenzy concludes. The Australian Federal government recently extended Medicare-subsided telehealth, following its success as a response to COVID-19 (Curtis 2021). The future of virtual care and telemedicine will increase access to care and help usher in technologies such as Bluetooth-enabled patient monitoring devices to assist in care. We are even starting to see teletherapy solutions in virtual care in the home (Huang et al. 2014; Horak et al. 2014). Today's HCPs are already dealing with how to change their practices on the fly to accommodate caring for patients remotely. Tomorrow's HCPs will have to be trained on using these platforms and deciding what patient evaluations and care needs to be done in-person versus done remotely and how to integrate this into their daily workflows. They will need to learn how to integrate these technologies with traditional prescriptions and therapeutic interventions and ultimately how to drive their development and implementation, as well as how to troubleshoot them.

Quality, Patient Safety, and Value-Based Care

The United States and several other countries have seen a strong move toward value-based care which essentially asks clinicians to be stewards of cost, while also increasing quality of care. Tomorrow's HCPs will need a better understanding of health systems science and the role that population health, social determinants of health (SDOH), informatics, patient safety, quality improvement, diversity, inclusion, and health equity have in patient health (Skochelak and Stack 2017). Health system science "refers to the critical competencies that are necessary for us to deliver the highest quality value-based health care in a manner that is both patient and population centered" (Mann 2019, para. 2). As the focus moves outside the walls of the traditional healthcare environment, future HCPs will need to incorporate these concepts while refocusing not just on patient care, but also promoting patient health on the continuum of care, including patients in their home environments, not just in the clinic or hospital.

Targeted Needs Assessment

Healthcare students of tomorrow will have tremendous barriers to overcome and tremendous tools at their disposal. As time goes on, we see the responsibility of HCPs extending beyond just the clinic or the hospital and following patients across the continuum of their lives. They must practice in a healthcare system that is asking them to do more with less and be cognizant of the business of healthcare. To get students ready for the tall task that awaits them, we need to prepare for the myriad of technologies and data they will utilize, including DTx, robotics, biosensor data, and the plethora of AI applications.

Understanding that future HCPs will spend greater time in larger interprofessional teams, we also see a huge need to introduce interprofessional education (IPE) as early as possible. Interprofessional education "occurs when two or more professions learn with, from and about each other to improve collaboration and the quality of care" (Ford and Gray 2021, p. 3). IPE has historically been difficult due to limited opportunities, institutional logistics, coordination of schedules, varying clinical expertise, and limited time (Lee et al. 2020). However, studies on IPE have shown that there can improved overall collaboration among different disciplines and, ultimately, improved overall patient quality of care and outcomes by reducing medical errors and hospital length of stay (Curran et al. 2008; Renschler et al. 2016; Gary et al. 2018; Lee et al. 2020). Interprofessional education can also change attitudes toward patient care, enthusiasm among HCPs, and better and more efficient patient care (Smith 2014).

Goals and Objectives

The ultimate goal of future healthcare professionals training curricula will be to prepare students for their future careers in healthcare. In addition to their clinical skills, knowledge, procedural skills, and problem-solving abilities, they need to be ambassadors of healthcare quality and value, leaders in diversity, inclusion, and healthcare equity, practice patient-centered care, and be patient advocates. We also need to create a workforce that meets the needs of the systems of healthcare across the world which will require creative and flexible solutions.

Hence, the goals of future curricula are to enable future health professionals to:

- Provide optimal patient care and greater focus on prevention of disease
- Optimize the use of healthcare teams to facilitate the optimal care of patients in a variety of healthcare settings
- Lead efforts to maximize physical, emotional, and psychological health of patients and society
- Leverage data and technology to their fullest extent in the service of ensuring patient health
- Be shepherds of healthcare quality and value-based care while minimizing medical error and inefficiencies of healthcare systems
- Convey leadership and teamwork through effective IPE

Educational Strategies and Implementation

In addition to the content that was discussed from the needs assessments, goals, and objectives, we should have a heavy focus on how we should be teaching. We know so much more about how people learn and strategies to improve skill and knowledge attainment and retention that go way beyond traditional HPE pedagogy. Having faculty develop a greater understanding and appreciation of various theories of motivation and learning can enhance teaching by making it more efficient and effective which is so needed in an era where faculty are being asked to do more with less.

The core principle of self-determination theory (SDT) is that humans innately want to learn, and they have basic needs including competency, autonomy, and relatedness (Ryan and Deci 2000). Knowles et al. (2011), on adult learning theory (ALT), noted that adult learners are different from children in that they want to be responsible for their own decisions on education, bring a wealth of prior knowledge to the educational experience, want to learn things that have immediate relevance to their work, respond better to internal motivations, have a need to know the reasoning behind learning something, and learn better when the application of knowledge is immediate and problem focused. What this means for the HPE curriculum is that we need to be mindful of these needs and wants as we develop educational content.

In this respect, the HPE curriculum should:

- Respect and activate prior knowledge
- Introduce autonomy and choice in what and how they are learning
- Provide the context, reasoning, and relevance for the learning
- Focus on the application of knowledge and be problem oriented

We also see the need for faculty to create environments of co-creation of learning and de-emphasize rote memorization of declarative facts. In this sense, we must embrace that students have literal computers in their pockets at all times that can access more facts than any preceding human had the ability to access. Thus, education should instead focus on teaching a foundation of knowledge so that students can recognize, categorize, and utilize any new information that gets presented to them. They can build upon this prior knowledge as they gain expertise and mastery. They need to be encouraged to be lifelong learners, seeking out new knowledge and integrating with their existing knowledge.

Many HPE schools have started to provide greater context and proximal application of content by providing for earlier clinical exposure. The benefits of including early clinical exposure for medical students have been shown to persist throughout students educational years and include improved student satisfaction, confidence in patient care, and sense of patient-centeredness (Hirsh et al. 2012).

Active Learning

We know that knowledge retention is facilitated by conversion of short-term memory to medium-term and ultimately, to long-term memory (Jonides et al. 2008). The context and learning environment are major factors that affect conversions such that, the more active the learning process, the better the knowledge will be retained. We know that the better one understands, connects, and manipulates information, the better they will retain said knowledge. Thus, learning needs to be practical and problem focused. It is not coincidental that case-based and, specifically, problem-based learning (PBL) has taken HPE by storm. Although, some of the data on the effectiveness of these methods is somewhat lacking, Albanese and Dast (2013) point out that some of these findings may be due to lack of expertise and consistency in the quality of PBL across institutions. Changing from pure lecture-based curricula to more active, problem-solving has seemed to be a growing trend, but multiple schools have tried different techniques to achieve this, and yet reversion to the mean of lectures at many institutions continues. Some factors include fear of innovation, lack of technology expertise or investment, lack of faculty competency, and lack of faculty motivation or time (Stevens 2018). Institutions need to be more deliberate about where didactics fit in the grand scheme of the HPE curriculum of the future.

To enable better utilization of PBL, several guiding theories and principles have been proposed including contextual learning, constructive learning, self-directed learning, and collaborative learning (Dolmans 2019). These guiding theories can help us to understand how PBL applies in certain situations and how it can be a value-add. Again, respecting adult learning theory, contextual learning where "learning preferably starts by engaging students in tasks derived from a professionally relevant context in order to stimulate transfer of learning to new situations" (Dolmans 2019, p. 880). Learning tasks should enable students to integrate these skills into practice and facilitate transfer.

Constructive learning is an active process where learners construct and reconstruct networks of knowledge in order to create meaning and ultimately gain a deep understanding (Dolmans 2019, p. 881). While constructivism is a theory, through the work of Jean Piaget, that states that knowledge develops when learners are able to construct their understanding through experiences and how those experiences interact with their own ideas (Wadsworth 1996). Evidence exists that students learn better through the constructivist model, which is mediated by deeper understanding, better cognitive strategies, and improved motivation for learning and have improved retention rates for information (Hickey et al. 1999; Dogru and Kalender 2007; Minner et al. 2009). Problem-based learning facilitates this type of experiential learning and technology, and game-based learning may have a role to play as well, as will be discussed later in this chapter. There is also evidence for simple solutions such as retrieval practice, distributed practice, and spaced education on learning outcomes (Kerfoot 2010). Retrieval practice allows for learners to deliberately access the knowledge gained, and this can be done through relevant questions or even flashcards. Distributed practice and spaced education is when these retrieval sessions are spaced out over time (Kerfoot 2010). Spaced retrieval practice can easily be used by allowing students to synthesize their newly acquired knowledge over specified periods of time to blunt the forgetfulness curve and improve learning comprehension (Kerfoot 2010; Versteeg et al. 2019).

Self-directed learning is where "students take the initiative to determine their own learning needs, set goals and strategies to achieve these goals and evaluate their learning" (Dolmans 2019, p. 881). Faculty need to face the reality that some students, if given access to all the relevant content and time set aside, would come out learning just as much if not more than those going through set curriculum. However, not all learners are oriented this way. We need to encourage self-regulation and self-direction among students and provide opportunities for self-directed learning. Some schools have integrated time for self-study in the curriculum in which afternoons are dedicated to reflection and integration.

As opposed to self-study, we see much more collaborative learning opportunities in PBL. Collaborative learning proponents state that learning as a group has distinct advantages over individualized learning with certain complex learning tasks (Dolmans 2019). This is built on the theory of connectivism in which knowledge is gained by connecting multiple nodes from multiple individuals to create a greater connected understanding (Downes 2014). Thus, we know that we can share and refine knowledge through learning and teaching with each other. This is heavily relied upon in small group PBL spaces. We also know that these can facilitate learning between multidisciplinary teams (MDT), an area that future curricula should consider. In schools where MDT learning was integrated, participants reported improved working relationships among interprofessional teams and better team (Samuriwo et al. 2020).

Adaptive Learning

One of the great applications for technology will likely be in adaptive learning. Healthcare professions students of the future will have grown up in an era of technology and will have experienced a world that is focused on personalization. We personalize everything from our mobile phone covers to our face masks during the pandemic era. There is a reasonable expectation that learners will have that their education should be personalized and leverage technology, including increased use of their personal devices. With integrated assessments and better predictive analytics, we will see students get personalized learning plans and coursework based on their skills and abilities and less so on the time of the year. We know that not all students progress at the same rates, and as we try achieving mastery for learners corralling all students together, hinders the development of mastery in some and leaves some students behind in the dust. Imagine if all biomedical science and content knowledge was instead customized for each student. As Harden (2018) foresee, "there will be an adaptive curriculum with the pace, duration and strategies for each learner's experiences to be continuously adapted to their individual unique and evolving characteristics and readiness for learning" (Harden 2018, p. 1012). We may see a flexible curriculum based on pretests that would provide more scaffolding and resources for those coming in with lower pre-curriculum testing and personalized plans specifically focusing on areas of weakness (Hays 2018).

Technology

There is much discussion around technology in HPE. Currently, many HPE schools still ban certain technology use in the classroom and during assessments. If we truly want to prepare students for the future, we should embrace technology and integrate it seamlessly into classrooms and assessments, just as it will be in real life. Just as Einstein said about the speed of sound, students will have a tremendous resource at their disposal and to deprive them of that during their training is not practical and can be a detriment to their growth. Classroom sessions and assessments should instead focus on what cannot be Googled. Things that require deeper understanding, and transfer of knowledge and skills that can leverage declarative knowledge found on just-in-time online resources, would be best serving future health professionals. Hughes et al. (2006) give us a great model to think about technology integration in the classroom that is referred to as the replacement, amplification, and transformation (RAT) model, which discusses how technology can replace, amplify, or transform educational experiences. Replacement refers to how a technology can simply replace without altering the core educational experience. Amplification refers to how technology can enhance the efficiency or effectiveness of an educational experience. Transformation is reserved for when technology reinvents an entirely new way of learning or thinking about a subject (Hughes et al. 2006).

Health professions education faculty need to think critically about how they themselves can create personalized learning spaces and use the RAT model to appropriately leverage technology. Faculty preparation is the focus of the chapter by Allen et al., so will not be focused on in this chapter, but creating competent and expert faculty in all the areas above will be vital to preparing students for the world in which they will be practicing. Likely, we should also educate students to enable them to be teachers themselves. We have a tremendous responsibility to professionally develop educators of tomorrow and focus on the ultimate goal, to prepare students for their future healthcare careers. We should strive for ways to engage learners through active problem-solving and leverage technology appropriately.

MOOCs and Online Learning

In an effort to overcome the time and funding issues that currently plague medical education reform, technology has been heralded as the Panacea (Hollands and Tirthali 2014). Education at all levels has undergone a massive evolution over the last decade to incorporate technology into current curriculum as well as developing new innovations to help improve educational experiences and outcomes. Massive open online courses (MOOCs) are one solution for providing educational content to large audiences in a systematic way. This educational forum has been introduced and popularized by large, prominent universities intending to provide learning experiences to the masses (Mullaney 2014). Also, as the COVID-19 pandemic has taken hold across the world, we have seen much of the educational system go near completely online. As we come out of this era, the likely result will be more hybrid curricula that include self-directed online learning that is asynchronous, as well as synchronous online learning through teleconferencing software, thus saving synchronous in-person education for those skills and knowledge that cannot be taught elsewhere. Design for online learning requires curriculum development skills that are different from face-to-face development, and basic competency in educational technology will be increasingly a requirement of educators in the health professions.

Virtual Reality/Augmented Reality

Much has been talked about the advanced technologies such as extended reality (XR) and what the potential can be in HPE. Extended reality encompasses a myriad of technologies including AR, VR, and mixed reality (MR), each with its own varying amount of digital versus real-life data that is viewed and interacted with. Extended reality brings another layer of complexity to the well-established world of simulation and in some ways can replace, amplify, or transform learning, respecting the RAT model. When done well, these technologies can enhance the experience and embed learners in real-life scenarios that may have not seen or experienced firsthand to help contextualize their learning and spark curiosity. Whole books could just be dedicated to XR in HPE, but for the purpose of thinking about future curricula, we can imagine all the ways that XR can contextualize knowledge, enhance skill development, serve as integrated assessment tools, enhance empathy, and spark curiosity if done well.

Game-Based Learning

Games are as old as time and interest in using games for learning has existed for decades. Recent interest has been sparked in the power of games for learning spawning an entire industry termed "serious games" and even a new word, "gamification." We look to games because beyond just being entertaining and tapping into our intrinsic motivation, they slyly teach us everything it is to know and succeed at playing the game (Schell 2014; Mayer 2019). Games also have a tremendous knack at onboarding new players to the domain without rule books or reading chapters of content. One learns how to play by...well by just playing. If we could tap into those motivations, and the secret sauce of games to help HCPs to learn their craft well, then we have achieved something special. Many schools and institutions have been trying to tap into games as a recent systematic review revealed over 27 randomized controlled trials (RCTs) suggesting moderate to large effect on knowledge improvement for serious games as compared to traditional learning methods and that it may improve learner satisfaction, and, most importantly, can result in improved patient outcomes (Gentry et al. 2019). Stanford introduced a game called *Septris* that actually helped teach principles of ICU resuscitation in a game format (Tsui et al. 2014). This is not limited to medical content; Teresa Chan and colleagues created a game called GridlockED to teach about healthcare systems and "the intricacies of managing multiple patients simultaneously and about working in a resource-limited environment" (Tsoy et al. 2019, p. 66). A recent systematic review of gamification in health professions found over 5000 articles and analyzed 44 studies in a wide array of programs and products targeting medical and dental students,

students, nursing, pharmacy students, speech and hearing students, and medical and surgical resident trainees (van Gaalen et al. 2021). We will continue to see games and, specifically video games, make a stronger presence in healthcare education, just as they are making waves in the digital therapeutic and patient engagement space.

Assessment

Learner assessment has undergone a transformation over the last several decades. There has been a greater focus on competency-based education and introduction of milestones and entrusted professional activities (EPAs) to improve the assessment process. Both facilitate translating learner behaviors into more objective criteria but still require faculty or clinicians to rate students, introducing subjectivity and potential bias. To widen the available data for assessments, we have seen a push for 360 evaluations, self-assessments, and portfolios which introduce multiple perspectives on the learner's performance. One principle we have seen more is the learner-focused assessment, when learners are encouraged to reflect and provide insight into their own performance. These can be done in isolation or with the guidance of a faculty member to facilitate conversations and frank discussions of their progress. These have always been difficult conversations to have, but in self-regulated learning and optimal feedback, allowing the learner to genuinely reflect and then incorporate external feedback can create more meaningful conversations. This more co-assessment technique makes learners feel more responsible for their learning and more receptive to feedback (Dochy et al. 1999).

One major shift recently was the determination in the United States to make the United States Medical Licensing Exam (USMLE) Step 1 exam pass or fail as of 2022. This test was considered the highest stakes test for medical students and often was used as the primary screening for residency applicants. As has been discussed, "this exam (Step 1 USMLE), and the weight that residency programs continue to place on test scores, remains the single greatest barrier to substantive pre-clerkship curriculum improvement" (Stevens 2018, p. 1426). Many institutions and medical students are scrambling to figure out how to properly assess students on paper prior to interviewing them. We need more authentic assessments that can both capture objective measurements of performance and ability and possibly predict future performance. This would also require collaboration among different levels of training to communicate and provide data to build out these predictive analytics. One thing we will see in the future is the ability to better leverage technology for more objective learner assessments. Software-based simulation and online learning platforms create massive amounts of data. Although no information on intent or thinking are collected, this data tracks every action and decision made by users and gives objective evidence of performance. As discussed above, these data can then inform adaptive learning platforms to dynamically serve content that is relevant to that learner. More importantly, this data can be used as objective evidence of behavior, and the more integrated the assessment with the learning experience, the better the data will be. As opposed to high or low stakes testing, these assessments are seamless with experiences and may provide more accurate data on knowledge and skills. Now, with more advanced technology-enabled learning such as virtual and augmented reality, actual hand motions and gestures can be analyzed to see fluidity and efficiency of movement that improve as learners gain expertise (Harvey et al. 2021). We also have technology that can provide accurate information regarding attention through eye tracking on simple webcams. Through eye tracking, we can actually analyze what information learners are paying attention to and in which order they do so (Tien et al. 2014; Ashraf et al. 2018; Brunyé et al. 2019). Experts are able to better filter information quickly to determine relevance of information and see patterns much quicker than novices, and we may be able to see this transition based on attention data (Borys and Plechawska-Wójcik 2017). Finally, we may be able to better extract learner-based data from EHRs and analyze learner behavior in the actual patient care setting.

Conclusion

The future of HPE curricula will be the culmination of many different forces and factors including changing healthcare systems, more learner-centeredness, better evidence-based instruction, better application of the cognitive science of learning, and rapidly advancing technology. Learners will demand, and receive, more personalized learning plans adapted to their own needs and career goals. Passive content knowledge transfer will transition to more conceptual understanding and problem-solving in a more active and interesting way leveraging technology and games. We will see advanced technologies in both the practice of healthcare delivery as well as the education of future HCPs. Healthcare will continue to evolve as the purview of the HCP moves outside the hospital and clinic, necessitating new skill sets and data-informed interventions. Finally, assessment will include more objective behavioral data from our myriad of technology-enable learning experiences to give a more holistic perspective on learner performance and behavior.

We may not be able to predict all the changes that future HCPs will encounter, but we know that they will have a daunting task to manage an aging and rapidly growing population, large-scale trauma from natural disasters, and potentially further pandemics. They will have at their disposal a plethora of tools and technology that we are only starting to see and realize. As the world of genomics and gene therapies, nanoparticles, robotics and microbotics, bionics, and precision medicine evolve, future HCPs will make great medical advances, and we will see completely different knowledge and skills to inculcate into future students. Their preparation for this future lies in our actions of today. What a world we will live in.

Cross-References

▶ Team-Based Learning (TBL): Theory, Planning, Practice, and Implementation

References

Albanese MA, Dast LC. Problem-Based Learning. In T. Swanwick (Ed.) 2013;(pp. 61–79). John Wiley \& Sons, Ltd. Retrieved from http://onlinelibrary.wiley.com.ezp-prod1.hul.harvard.edu/doi/10.1002/9781118472361.ch5/summary

Ashraf H, Sodergren MH, Merali N, Mylonas G, Singh H, Darzi A. Eye-tracking technology in medical education: a systematic review. Med Teach. 2018;40(1):62–9. https://doi.org/10.1080/0142159X.2017.1391373.

Baker KM, Magee MF, Smith KM. Understanding nursing workflow for inpatient education delivery: time and motion study. JMIR Nurs. 2019;2(1):e15658. https://doi.org/10.2196/15658.

Begum M, Serna RW, Yanco HA. Are robots ready to deliver autism interventions? A comprehensive review. Int J Soc Robot. 2016;8(2):157–81. https://doi.org/10.1007/s12369-016-0346-y.

Borys M, Plechawska-Wójcik M. Eye-tracking metrics in perception and visual attention research. Eur J Med Res. 2017;3(16):11–23.

Bouchaud M, Brown D, Swan BA. Creating a new education paradigm to prepare nurses for the 21st century. J Nurs Educ Pract. 2017;7(10):27–35. https://doi.org/10.5430/jnep.v7n10p27.

Brown D. Hospitals turn to artificial intelligence to help with an age-old problem: doctors' poor bedside manners [Internet]. Washington, DC: The Washington Post. 2021 [cited 2021 Feb 24]. Available from: https://www.washingtonpost.com/technology/2021/02/16/virtual-ai-hospital-patients/?arc404=true

Bruni MF, Melegari C, De Cola MC, Bramanti A, Bramanti P, Calabrò RC. What does best evidence tell us about robotic gait rehabilitation in stroke patients: a systematic review and meta-analysis. J Clin Neurosci. 2018;48:11–7. https://doi.org/10.1016/j.jocn.2017.10.048.

Brunyé TT, Drew T, Weaver DL, Elmore JG. A review of eye tracking for understanding and improving diagnostic interpretation. Cogn Res Princ Implic. 2019;4:7. https://doi.org/10.1186/s41235-019-0159-2.

Butler R, Monsalve M, Thomas GW, Herman T, Serge AM, Polgreen PM, Suneja M. Estimating time physicians and other health care workers spend with patients in an intensive care unit using a sensor network. Am J Med. 2018;131(8):972.e9–972.e15. https://doi.org/10.1016/j.amjmed.2018.03.015.

Chad R, Emaan S, Jillian O. Effect of virtual reality headset for pediatric fear and pain distraction during immunization. Pain Manag. 2018;8(3):175–9. https://doi.org/10.2217/pmt-2017-0040.

Cohen J. Letter to medical school deans. Washington, DC: Association of American Medical Colleges; 1999.

Cooke M, Irby DM, Sullivan W, Ludmerer KM. American medical education 100 years after the Flexner report. N Engl J Med. 2006;355(13):1339–44. https://doi.org/10.1056/NEJMra055445.

Curran VR, Sharpe D, Forristall J, Flynn K. Attitudes of health sciences students towards interprofessional teamwork and education. Learn Health Soc Care. 2008;7(3):146–56. https://doi.org/10.1111/j.1473-6861.2008.00184.x.

Curtis K. Federal budget: government to extend telehealth funding until end of 2021 [Internet]. Sydney: The Sydney Morning Herald. 2021 [cited 2021 May 2]. Available from: https://www.smh.com.au/politics/federal/government-to-extend-telehealth-funding-until-end-of-2021-20210425-p57m97.html

Densen P. Challenges and opportunities facing medical education. Trans Am Clin Climatol Assoc. 2011;122:48–58.

Difede J et al. Virtual reality exposure therapy for the treatment of posttraumatic stress disorder following. J Clin Psychiatry. 2007.

Dochy F, Segers M, Sluijsmans D. The use of self-, peer and co-assessment in higher education: a review. Stud High Educ. 1999;24(3):331–50. https://doi.org/10.1080/03075079912331379935.

Dogru M, Kalender S. Applying the subject "cell" through constructivist approach during science lessons and the teacher's view. Int J Environ Sci Educ. 2007;2(1):3–13.

Dolmans DHJM. How theory and design-based research can mature PBL practice and research. Adv Health Sci. 2019;24(5):879–91. https://doi.org/10.1007/s10459-019-09940-2.

Downes S. Connectivism as learning theory [Internet]. Casselman: Half an Hour. 2014 [cited 2021 Oct 12]. Available from: https://halfanhour.blogspot.com/2014/04/connectivism-as-learning-theory.html

Finlay GD, Rothman MJ, Smith RA. Measuring the modified early warning score and the Rothman index: advantages of utilizing the electronic medical record in an early warning system. J Hosp Med. 2014;9(2):116–9. https://doi.org/10.1002/jhm.2132.

Ford J, Gray R. Interprofessional education handbook. Centre for the Advancement of Interprofessional Education. 2021. https://www.caipe.org/resources/publications/caipe-publications/caipe-2021-a-new-caipe-interprofessional-education-handbook-2021-ipe-incorporating-values-based-practice-ford-j-gray-r. Accessed 12 Oct 2021.

Frank, P., Rosen, G. and Kusaka, S. Einstein, his life and times. 1st edn. Edited by S. Kusaka. New York, NY, USA: Alfred A. Knopf: 1947.

Gary JC, Gosselin K, Bentley R. Health science center faculty attitudes towards interprofessional education and teamwork. J Interprof Care. 2018;32(2):231–4. https://doi.org/10.1080/13561820.2017.1376626.

Gentry SV, Gauthier A, L'Estrade Ehrstrom B, Wortley D, Lilienthal A, Tudor Car L, et al. Serious gaming and gamification education in health professions: systematic review. J Med Internet Res. 2019;21(3):e12994. https://doi.org/10.2196/12994.

Gupta A, Scott K, Dukewich M. Innovative technology using virtual reality in the treatment of pain: Does it reduce pain via distraction, or is there more to it?. Pain Medicine (United States), 2018;19(1):151–159. https://doi.org/10.1093/pm/pnx109.

Han E, Yeo S, Kim M, Lee Y, Park K, Roh H. Medical education trends for future physicians in the era of advanced technology and artificial intelligence: an integrative review. BMC Med Educ. 2019;19(1):460. https://doi.org/10.1186/s12909-019-1891-5.

Harden RM. Ten key features of the future medical school – not an impossible dream. Med Teach. 2018;40(10):1010–5. https://doi.org/10.1080/0142159X.2018.1498613.

Harvey C, Selmanović E, O'Connor J, Chahin M. A comparison between expert and beginner learning for motor skill development in a virtual reality serious game. Vis Comput. 2021;37:3–17. https://doi.org/10.1007/s00371-019-01702-w.

Hays R. Establishing a new medical school: a contemporary approach to personalizing medical education. Med Teach. 2018;40(10):990–5. https://doi.org/10.1080/0142159X.2018.1487048.

Hickey DT, Kindfteld ACH, Horwits P, Christie MA. Advancing educational theory by enhancing practice in a technology-supported genetics learning environment. J Educ. 1999;181(2):25–55.

Hirsh D, Gaufberg E, Ogur B, Cohen P, Krupat E, Cox M, et al. Educational outcomes of the Harvard Medical School–Cambridge integrated clerkship: a way forward for medical education. Acad Med. 2012;87(5):643–50. https://doi.org/10.1097/ACM.0b013e31824d9821.

Hollands FM, Tirthali D. MOOCs: expectations and reality. Center for Benefit–Cost Studies of Education, Teachers College, Columbia University. 2014. Available from: http://cbcse.org/wordpress/wpcontent/uploads/2014/05/MOOCs_Expectations_and_Reality.ppd. Accessed: 12 Oct 2021.

Horak F, King L, Mancini M. Role of body-worn movement monitor technology for balance and gait rehabilitation. Phys Ther. 2014;95(3):461–70. https://doi.org/10.2522/ptj.20140253.

Huang K, Sparto PJ, Kiesler S, Mailagic A, Mankoff J, Siewiorek D, et al. A technology probe of wearable in-home computer-assisted physical therapy. In: Proceedings of the SIGCHI conference on human factors in computing systems. Toronto: Association for Computing Machinery; 2014. p. 2541–50. https://doi.org/10.1145/2556288.2557416.

Hughes J, Thomas R, Scharber C. Assessing technology integration: the RAT – replacement, amplification, and transformation – framework. In: Crawford CM, Carlsen R, McFerrin K, Price J, Weber R, Willis DA, editors. Society for Information Technology & Teacher Education international conference 2006. Orlando: Association for the Advancement of Computing in Education (AACE); 2006. p. 1616–20.

Insider Intelligence. [Internet]. New York: Insider Intelligence. 2021 [updated 2021 Jul 29; cited 2021 Oct 11]. Available from: https://www.businessinsider.com/digital-therapeutics-report

Institute of Medicine. In: Donaldson MS, Corrigan JM, Kohn LT, editors. To err is human: building a safer health system. Washington, DC: National Academies Press; 2000.

Jonides J et al. The mind and brain of short-term memory. Annual Review of Psychology, 2008;59:193–224. https://doi.org/10.1146/annurev.psych.59.103006.093615.

Kaplan A, Haenlein M. Siri, Siri, in my hand: who's the fairest in the land? On the interpretations, illustrations, and implications of artificial intelligence. Bus Horiz. 2019;62(1):15–25. https://doi.org/10.1016/j.bushor.2018.08.004.

Kerfoot BP. Adaptive spaced education improves learning efficiency: a randomized controlled trial. J Urol. 2010;183(2):678–81. https://doi.org/10.1016/j.juro.2009.10.005.

Knowles MS, Holton EF, Swanson RA. The Adult Learner. The Adult Learner (Vol. 24). 2011.

Kollins SH, DeLoss DJ, Cañadas E, Lutz J, Findling RL, Keefe RSE, et al. A novel digital intervention for actively reducing severity of paediatric ADHD (STARS-ADHD): a randomised controlled trial. Lancet Digit Health. 2020;2(4):e168–78. https://doi.org/10.1016/S2589-7500(20)30017-0.

Leape LL, Berwick DM. Five years after to err is human: what have we learned? JAMA. 2005;293(19):2384–90. https://doi.org/10.1001/jama.293.19.2384.

Lee AL, DeBest M, Koeniher-Donohue R, Strowman SR, Mitchell SE. The feasibility and acceptability of using virtual world technology for interprofessional education in palliative care: a mixed methods study. J Interprof Care. 2020;34(4):461–71. https://doi.org/10.1080/13561820.2019.1643832.

Li Z, Moran P, Dong Q, Shaw RJ, Hauser K. Development of a tele-nursing mobile manipulator for remote care-giving in quarantine areas. In: IEEE International Conference on Robotics and Automation (ICRA); 2017. pp. 3581–6. https://doi.org/10.1109/ICRA.2017.7989411.

Ludmerer KM. Time to heal American medical education from the turn of the century. Oxford, UK: Oxford University Press; 2005.

Mann S. Health systems science: the future of medical education and the solution to improving health care. Boston: Harvard Macy Institute. 2019 [cited 2021 Oct 12] Available from: https://www.harvardmacy.org/index.php/hmi/health-systems-science.

Mayer RE. Computer games in education. Annu Rev Psychol. 2019;70(1):531–49. https://doi.org/10.1146/annurev-psych-010418-102744.

Milne-Ives M, de Cock C, Lim E, Shehadeh MH, de Pennington N, Mole G, et al. The effectiveness of artificial intelligence conversational agents in health care: systematic review. J Med Internet Res. 2020;22(10):e20346. https://doi.org/10.2196/20346.

Minner DD, Levy AJ, Century J. Inquiry-based science instruction-what is it and does it matter? Results from a research synthesis years 1984 to 2002. J Res Sci Teach. 2009;47(4):474–96. https://doi.org/10.1002/tea.20347.

Moldoveanu M. How our response to COVID-19 will remake higher ed. Boston: Harvard Business Publishing Education. 2020 [cited 2021 Mar 17]. Available from: https://hbsp.harvard.edu/inspiring-minds/how-our-response-to-covid-19-will-remake-higher-ed

Mullaney T. Making sense of MOOCs: a reconceptualization of HarvardX courses and their students. 2014. Available at SSRN: https://doi.org/10.2139/ssrn.2463736.

Nancarrow SA, Moran AM, Graham I. Preparing a 21st century workforce: is it time to consider clinically based, competency-based training of health practitioners. Aust Health Rev. 2014;38(1):115–7. https://doi.org/10.1071/AH13158.

Needleman J. Increasing acuity, increasing technology, and the changing demands on nurses. Nurs Econ. 2013;31(4):200–3.

Renschler L, Rhodes D, Cox C. Effect of interprofessional clinical education programme length on students' attitudes towards teamwork. J Interprof Care. 2016;30(3):338–46. https://doi.org/10.3109/13561820.2016.1144582.

Rizzo AS, Difede J, Rothbaum BO, Reger G, Spitalnick J, Cukor J, et al. Development and early evaluation of the Virtual Iraq/Afghanistan exposure therapy system for combat-related PTSD. Ann N Y Acad Sci. 2010;1208(1):114–25. https://doi.org/10.1111/j.1749-6632.2010.05755.x.

Robert N. How artificial intelligence is changing nursing. J Nurs Manag. 2019;50(9):30–9. https://doi.org/10.1097/01.NUMA.0000578988.56622.21.

Roumeliotis N, Parisien G, Charette S, Aprin E, Brunet F, Jouvet P. Reorganizing care with the implementation of electronic medical records: a time-motion study in the PICU. Pediatr Crit Care Med. 2018;19(4):e172–9. https://doi.org/10.1097/PCC.0000000000001450.

Ryan RM, Deci EL. Self-determination theory and the facilitation of intrinsic motivation, social development, and well-being. Am Psychol. 2000;55(1):68–78.

Samuriwo R, Laws E, Webb K, Bullock A. "I didn't realise they had such a key role." Impact of medical education curriculum change on medical student interactions with nurses: a qualitative exploratory study of student perceptions. Adv Health Sci Educ Theory Pract. 2020;25(1):75–93. https://doi.org/10.1007/s10459-019-09906-4.

Sanders JH. How much paperwork is too much? Fam Pract Manag. 2005;12(1):12.

Schell J. The art of game design: a book of lenses. 2nd ed. New York: A. K. Peters/CRC Press; 2014. https://doi.org/10.1201/b17723.

Schenk E, Schleyer R, Jone CR, Fincham S, Daratha KB, Monsen KA. Time motion analysis of nursing work in ICU, telemetry and medical-surgical units. J Nurs Manag. 2017;25(8):640–6. https://doi.org/10.1111/jonm.12502.

Simpson D, Marcdante K, Souza KH, Anderson A, Holmboe E. Job roles of the 2025 medical educator. J Grad Med Educ. 2018;10(3):243–6. https://doi.org/10.4300/JGME-D-18-00253.1.

Skochelak SE, Stack SJ. Creating the medical schools of the future. Acad Med. 2017;92(1):16–9. https://doi.org/10.1097/ACM.0000000000001160.

Smith KA. Health care interprofessional education: encouraging technology, teamwork, and team performance. J Contin Educ Nurs. 2014;45(4):181–7. https://doi.org/10.3928/00220124-20140327-01.

Stevens CD. Repeal and replace? A note of caution for medical school curriculum reformers. Acad Med. 2018;93(10):1425–7. https://doi.org/10.1097/ACM.0000000000002219.

Thomas PA, Kern DE, Hughes MT, Chen BY. Curriculum development for medical education: A six-step approach. Curriculum Development for Medical Education: A Six-Step Approach, Third Edition (3rd ed.). 2015. https://doi.org/10.7326/0003-4819-130-10-199905180-00028.

Tien T, Pucher PH, Sodergren MH, Sriskandarahaj K, Yang G, Darzi. Eye tracking for skills assessment and training: a systematic review. J Surg Res. 2014;191(1):169–78. https://doi.org/10.1016/J.JSS.2014.04.032.

Topol E. Deep medicine: how artificial intelligence can make healthcare human again. New York: Basic Books; 2019. https://doi.org/10.5555/3350442.

Tsoy D, Sneath P, Rempel J, Huang S, Bodnariuc N, Mercurri M, et al. Creating GridlockED: a serious game for teaching about multipatient environments. Acad Med. 2019;94(1):66–70. https://doi.org/10.1097/ACM.0000000000002340.

Tsui J, Lau JY, Sheih L. Septris and SICKO: implementing and using learning analytics and gamification in medical education. Educase. 2014 [cited 2021 Oct 12]. Available from: https://library.educause.edu/resources/2014/3/septris-and-sicko-implementing-and-using-learning-analytics-and-gamification-in-medical-education

van Gaalen AEJ, Brouwer J, Schönrock-Adema J, Bouwkamp-Timmer T, Jaarsma ADC, Georgiadis JR. Gamification of health professions education: a systematic review. Adv Health Sci Educ. 2021;26(2):683–711. https://doi.org/10.1007/s10459-020-10000-3.

Versteeg M, Hendricks RA, Thomas A, Ommering BWC, Steendijk P. Conceptualising spaced learning in health professions education: a scoping review. Med Educ. 2019;54(3):205–16. https://doi.org/10.1111/medu.14025.

Wadsworth BJ. Piaget's theory of cognitive and affective development: foundations of constructivism. 5th ed. White Plains: Longman Publishing; 1996.

Wartman SA, Combs CD. Medical education must move from the information age to the age of artificial intelligence. Acad Med. 2018;93(8):1107–9. https://doi.org/10.1097/ACM.0000000000002044.

Wechsler TF, Mühlberger A, Kümpers F. Inferiority or even superiority of virtual reality exposure therapy in phobias? A systematic review and quantitative meta-analysis on randomized controlled trials specifically comparing the efficacy of virtual reality exposure to gold standard in vivo exposure in agoraphobia, specific phobia, and social phobia. Front Psychol. 2019;10:1758. https://doi.org/10.3389/fpsyg.2019.01758.

World Health Organization. State of the world's nursing 2020: investing in education, jobs and leadership. Geneva: World Health Organization; 2020. License: CC BY-NC-SA 3.0 IGO

Xie B, Yao C, Li J, Hilsabeck RC, Aguirre A. Artificial intelligence for caregivers of persons with Alzheimer's disease and related dementias: systematic literature review. JMIR Med Inform. 2020;8(8):e18189. https://doi.org/10.2196/18189.

Yang CC, Veltri P. Intelligent healthcare informatics in big data era. Artif Intell Med. 2015;65(2):75–7. https://doi.org/10.1016/j.artmed.2015.08.002.

Yen P, Kellye M, Lopetegui M, Saha A, Loversidge J, Chipps EM, et al. Nurses' time allocation and multitasking of nursing activities: a time motion study. AMIA Annu Symp Proc. 2018;2018:1137–46.

Competencies of Health Professions Educators of the Future

89

Louise Marjorie Allen, Eric Gantwerker, and Margaret Hay

Contents

Introduction	1728
Changing Health Professions Education Landscape	1728
Changing Health Professions Educators	1730
Changing Faculty Competencies	1731
Changing Faculty Development	1732
Challenges to Transforming Health Professions Educators of the Future	1733
Conclusion	1734
Cross-References	1735
References	1735

Abstract

The practices of health professionals can and do change rapidly. Whether this be in response to technological developments, to the changing healthcare needs of the population, or to extreme events such as the current COVID-19 pandemic. This chapter discusses the changing health professions education (HPE) landscape and the need to ensure that we are producing health professionals who are adaptable and prepared for a changing healthcare landscape. It details the

L. M. Allen (✉)
Monash Centre for Professional Development and Monash Online Education, Monash University, Clayton, Vic, Australia
e-mail: louise.allen@monash.edu

E. Gantwerker
Northwell Health, Lake Success, NY, USA

Zucker School of Medicine at Northwell/Hofstra, Hempstead, NY, USA
e-mail: egantwerker@northwell.edu

M. Hay
Faculty of Education, Monash Centre for Professional Development and Monash Online Education, Monash University, Clayton, VIC, Australia
e-mail: margaret.hay@monash.edu

© Springer Nature Singapore Pte Ltd. 2023
D. Nestel et al. (eds.), *Clinical Education for the Health Professions*,
https://doi.org/10.1007/978-981-15-3344-0_135

changing health professions educator competencies that are needed to facilitate this, changing faculty development required to develop these competencies, challenges to transforming health professions educators of the future, and provides suggestions for how these challenges may be overcome.

Keywords

Health professions education · Health professions educators · Educator competencies · Faculty development

Introduction

As we enter 2022, we can look back and see just how much health professionals' practice has changed over the last decade. Several technological developments such as the widespread use of electronic medical records, increased use of wearable technologies, remote monitoring of devices, and the rapid expansion of telehealth due to the global COVID-19 pandemic have dramatically changed the way health professionals' practice. As such, health professions educators need to adapt and change to ensure the delivery of health professions education (HPE) is relevant (McKimm et al. 2020). As we look to the next decade, with the advancement of digital health technologies such as artificial intelligence (AI) in health care, the effects of the global COVID-19 pandemic likely to be felt for some time, and the push toward HPE to focus on health promotion rather than treatment of disease, we can expect even more influential changes to occur. These changes will need to be reflected in HPE, and will therefore require health professions educators to continue to evolve to ensure that we are training health professionals who are equipped to work in this changing healthcare environment. The focus of this chapter is on the competencies of health professions educators of the future. We have projected a decade forward, to discuss the anticipated context of health professions educators in 2032. This chapter explores the changing educational landscape and how as a result, the role of health professions educators will change. It focuses on the changing competencies that health professions educators will require to enact these changes and the inherent changes to faculty development to equip health professions educators with these competencies.

Changing Health Professions Education Landscape

Before considering health professions educators of the future, we must first consider the changing HPE landscape as this will significantly impact health professions educators of the future. COVID-19 has been the catalyst for perhaps the largest and, without a doubt, the most accelerated change in HPE in recorded history. The mandated social distancing measures resulted in a near overnight shift from face-to-face to remote learning utilizing a range of technologies that were previously underutilized, and reduced in-person clinical learning opportunities (McKimm

Table 1 Examples of advances in technology at point of care and in education

Point of Care	Education
AI enabled decision support tools	Virtual and augmented reality
Patient level data tools and biosensors	High tech virtual patients
Big data informing algorithms that create reminders for patient care	Personalized content using adaptive learning software
Patient controlled electronic medical records	Integrated analytics to report performance and ultimately competency

et al. 2020). Many of these changes are likely to have permanency, and in addition to the technologies embraced at the height of the pandemic, advances in technology, both at the point of care and for educators are likely to lead to further changes in HPE of the future. Table 1 provides some examples of advances in technology in both of these settings.

While advances in technology will continue to influence the HPE curriculum of the future, as described in ▶ Chap. 88, "Future of Health Professions Education Curricula" Chapter, so too will a move toward flexible and personalized competency-based education (CBE). Currently CBE is employed by a broad range of health professions (Ash et al. 2019; Hodges et al. 2019; Wu et al. 2019), but the curriculum is still largely a one size fits all approach. Future CBE curriculum can enable personalized self-directed education, with progress informed by the learner's past experiences and previously obtained competencies, rather than delivering the same curriculum to all students, concurrently (Institute of Medicine National Academies of Sciences, Engineering, Medicine 2016; Bajis et al. 2020; Berghman et al. 2019). Competencies too are likely to change to address a shift to primary prevention rather than tertiary care (Institute of Medicine National Academies of Sciences, Engineering, Medicine 2016).

Not only is CBE curriculum changing, so too are the learners and the volume of required knowledge. School leavers now and of the future only know an internet connected world with rapidly advancing technology. They have innate technological literacy and skills. For example, in the Australian state of New South Wales, computer coding is compulsory for primary school children, and students in years 7 and 8 (equivalent to 7th and 8th grade in the USA, Years 8 and 9 in the UK) are required to learn a coding language (Baker, 2018). In addition to advances in technology and the increased technological skills of learners, the volume of medical knowledge is rapidly and vastly increasing. In 2011 it was estimated that by 2020 the doubling time of medical knowledge would be 0.2 years, or 73 days, down from 7 years in 1980 and 3.5 years in 2010 (Densen 2011). This trend is likely to continue meaning that available medical knowledge will become increasingly voluminous.

As such, CBE curriculum will be altered to accommodate the changes in healthcare (see ▶ Chap. 88, "Future of Health Professions Education Curricula"), so that future health professionals are competent to work in changing and increasingly technology-driven health professions. It will need to reflect both these changes in practice, but also more importantly than ever it will need to consider cognition (how we learn) and pedagogy (the theory, concepts, and principles of education) to deal with the rapidly increasing volumes of knowledge. For example, health professions educators will need to employ, via the use of technology, evidence-based strategies from the learning sciences such as spaced repetition and interleaving to optimize knowledge retention (Weinstein et al. 2018). Health professions educators will be responsible for these curriculum changes, but as technology advances and becomes more involved, they may require interprofessional collaboration from those outside the healthcare field, or from those within the healthcare field with expert knowledge of new and emerging technologies. As learners become increasingly more knowledgeable in technology, educators need to be adaptable to meet their learners' needs. Health professions educators will need to continuously upskill in technology and appropriate pedagogy, so that with the ever-increasing use of cloud-based e-learning, education can be provided in an efficient and effective manner. It is therefore clear that health professions educators will need to upskill in the required competencies in order to meet the needs of their future roles. These changes to health professions educators' competencies require faculty development to ensure attainment of these required competencies. But before we consider health professions educators changing competencies and their required faculty development, it is important to consider who health professions educators of the future will be.

Changing Health Professions Educators

The traditional view of health professions educators is faculty employed by universities, or clinical educators who assume the role of educators in various clinical settings. These educators often act as the sage on the stage, with a focus on knowledge provision. With the changing competencies of HPE in the future as described previously, particularly the focus on personalized, self-directed and peer-learning, health professions educators of the future will assume the role of "guide on the side" to facilitate learner achievement. Health professions educators need to therefore rapidly upskill in advancing technologies, but also shift their focus to aiding learners with knowledge management, rather than knowledge provision.

While shifting their focus to knowledge management, health professions educators need to be cognizant of their learner's professional identity development. The forced shift to increased online learning, and reduced clinical contact for both patients and practitioners, means that traditional interactions that aid professional identity development are reduced. Health professions educators need to be innovative in how they aid learners' professional identity development in this changing landscape (see the Developing Professional Identity in Health Professional Students, On "Being" Participants and a Researcher in a Longitudinal Medical Professional Identity Study, and Supporting the Development of Professionalism in the Education of Health Professionals Chapters for more on professional identity development). A range of examples have been described such as introducing students to public health through assistance with COVID-19 swab collection (Klasen et al. 2020) or telephone COVID-19-risk triage (Casas et al. 2020), promoting interprofessional identity through coordinated volunteer efforts (Edelman et al. 2020; Kratochvil et al. 2020), and guided social media engagement to help distribute accurate COVID-19 information (Coleman et al. 2020; Villela et al. 2020) all of which enable "a more community focused, interprofessional, interconnected and inclusive conceptualisation of professional identity formation" (Stetson and Dhaliwal 2020, p. 133).

Health professions educators of the future are likely to form part of a learning community (Talib et al. 2017), where educators include patients, families, communities, other health professionals, and other professionals such as IT professionals and engineers. Faculty-based health professions educators of the future need to be equipped to perform as part of this diverse team and understand their role within it.

Changing Faculty Competencies

Six core teaching competencies have been proposed that describe the attributes and skills appropriate for medical educators (Srinivasan et al. 2011) that are applicable to health professions educators more broadly. While these competencies are likely to be relevant to some extent in the future, there are changes required to ensure that health professions educators of the future have the required competencies. These changes

Table 2 Required changes to health professions educators of the future competencies

Core competencies (from Srinivasan et al. 2011)	Description (from Srinivasan et al. 2011)	Required future changes
1. Content knowledge	Teach content and assess each learner's abilities within their field of expertise	Shift from knowledge provision to assisting with knowledge management, and shift to preventative health focus
2. Learner-centeredness	Demonstrate a commitment both to learners' success and well-being and to helping learners grow into their professional roles	Shift to development of learners' professional identity in online and nontraditional settings
3. Interpersonal and communication skills	Flexibly tailor teaching and communication styles to facilitate learning	Shift to guide on the side, facilitating self-directed and peer learning that is personalized to the learner
4. Professionalism and role modeling	Demonstrate best educational and content-related practices, and role model those behaviors for learners	Continuing best educational practice with an increased shift to embracing appropriate technologies (in education, and at point of care)
5. Practice-based reflection	Demonstrate continuous self-assessment and lifelong learning to improve their effectiveness and capacity as educators	Unchanged
6. Systems-based practice	Utilize resources within the larger system of medical education to advocate for learners and to provide optimal teaching and learning	Shift to broader and more holistic view of the larger system of HPE – coordination and incorporation of other nontraditional health professions educators

are summarized in Table 2, alongside Srinivasan et al. 2011 original core competencies and descriptions.

Changing Faculty Development

Faculty development is essential to ensure that faculty health professions educators develop these required competencies that will better equip them as educators of the future. Faculty development refers to "all activities health professionals pursue to improve their knowledge, skills, and behaviours as teachers and educators, leaders and managers, and researchers and scholars, in both individual and group settings" (Steinert 2014). In addition, it also enables faculty to develop their identity as educators. There are a range of types of faculty development interventions identified in a 2016 review which reported that longitudinal programs (36%) and workshops (29%) are the most common, followed by short courses (14%), other intervention types (13%) such as web-based modules, peer observation and coaching and CD-ROMs, and seminar series (9%) (Steinert et al. 2016). Historically, it is clear that a substantial amount of faculty development is being delivered face-to-face. However, with the COVID-19 global pandemic, like education in general, faculty development has had to adapt from a significant proportion being delivered face-to-face, to being largely delivered online. With the global pandemic continuing, it is likely that for the foreseeable future faculty development will be delivered electronically, and in the long term this will presumably result in a greater portion of faculty development remaining in an online format. Not only this, but the global pandemic has meant that many university resources, especially financial resources, have been significantly reduced. The effects of this reduced funding for faculty development will likely be felt for years to come, and has occurred at a time when faculty development is most needed. It is therefore imperative that the faculty development of the future is effective, both in terms of cost and outcomes.

The social process of learning has been shown to be crucial to the development of a range of impacts of continuing professional development (Allen et al. 2020), the broader umbrella of professional development that faculty development falls under. With the shift toward online learning, it is imperative that the design, development, and implementation of this type of learning considers how this social process of learning can be fostered without face-to-face contact. Rather than just considering how content can best be delivered, consideration needs to be given to how communication, collaboration, and networking can be fostered in the online learning environment. One such approach may be developing faculty development communities of practice (de Carvalho-Filho et al. 2020).

With these considerations, faculty development of the future will need to focus on the cognition and pedagogical principles that can optimize learning in a technologically advanced, knowledge dense world (Hays et al. 2020). Greater knowledge and application of cognition and learning science will be essential in effective education. It will also need to focus on leadership and management as our concept of who health professions educators are evolves to encompass a broader learning community. To have the greatest benefit, faculty development should be delivered in a way that ensures learnings are practically relevant and immediately applicable, delivered in a way that enhances social learning, and readily accessible for flexible engagement.

Challenges to Transforming Health Professions Educators of the Future

It is clear that for existing health professions educators to develop these new competencies, faculty development is a salient requirement. While ensuring that sound pedagogical development of faculty development programs that help educators develop these competencies is essential, there are many challenges to the implementation of appropriate and effective faculty development. Education is a complex system and health professions educators can exist in one or multiple parts of the system. For example, an academic faculty member is expected to teach students, to develop curriculum, to supervise junior faculty, to apply for grants, to conduct research, and to sit on university and external committees. As such, health professions educators have competing demands. As a result of the many "hats" that health professions educators wear, there are a number of barriers to undertaking faculty development.

First, because health professions educators wear many "hats," they have competing priorities. Research-related tasks are often prioritized above education-related tasks, as research metrics are prioritized for promotion decisions with lesser, or in some cases no consideration given to educational accomplishments (McGrail et al. 2006). Second, the cost of faculty development is often a significant barrier (Samuel et al. 2021). This can be viewed as both the cost to the educator to undertake further training in education, for example a postgraduate degree in HPE, and also the opportunity cost to the institution to develop effective and appropriate faculty development (Samuel et al. 2021). Third, education is not valued as highly as research, as it does not attract revenue for universities to the extent that research does. Finally, perhaps because traditionally health professions educators are often clinicians or scientists with no educational background or training, there is a lack of understanding of the required competencies of educators, and a lack of awareness of the need for training and upskilling in education (Chen et al. 2017). As such, rather than having received formal or informal training in regards to educational best practice, health professions educators rely on role-modeling teaching behaviors that they have been subjected to, whether it is effective or not. We therefore need to consider how we engage all faculty, and how we promote the importance of faculty development in educator competencies.

This range of barriers can result in a lack of formal education and training for health professions educators. In order to incentivize individuals to engage in career development in education, there is a need to establish and reward careers in education, with clear career outcomes developed to encourage engagement in faculty development and best practice in HPE. Ultimately, it would be of greatest benefit if these principles were introduced into health professions degrees (both undergraduate and postgraduate), so that future health professionals have a basic understanding of education theory and principles. Given the significant amount of "on-the-job" learning that occurs in HPE, and the identified challenges to this traditional approach both now and in the near future, equipping current students with educator competencies prepares them well for their future roles as health professions educators and bodes well for a quality health professions educators workforce into the future.

Even if faculty are engaging in faculty development, there are a lack of measures to show that these professional development programs are working. A large amount of research has shown that when looking at professional development more broadly, outcomes such as knowledge, skills, attitudes, confidence, and behavior change are measured far more frequently than student/learner/trainee outcomes, patient outcomes, organizational outcomes, and broader society outcomes (Steinert et al. 2016; Allen et al. 2019; Yardley and Dornan 2012; Leslie et al. 2013). Furthermore, changes to the individual participating in the professional development are often neglected such as the development of personal and professional identities, the development of connections and collaborations and the impacts these can have (Allen et al. 2019). Evaluation measures need to be developed that can capture the full range of impacts of professional development program, not just those that are convenient. Furthermore, if we focus solely on measuring intended outcomes, we may miss important and positive outcomes of training programs that were unintended (see the chapter "Hidden Curriculum"), such as improved educator identity and reduced feelings of isolation that can lead to improved job satisfaction and ultimately improved performance.

Conclusion

As the COVID-19 pandemic has demonstrated, healthcare can rapidly change, and how we deliver healthcare and education can change overnight. Health professions educators of the future therefore need to be equipped to deal with the changing healthcare delivery and education landscape that includes: increased use of a range of technologies both at the point of care, and in the delivery of education; moving from tertiary care to primary prevention; a shift to individualized curriculum and self-directed learning that recognizes prior learning and previously obtained competencies; a broadening in the consideration of who health professions educators are to include a broader learning community such as patients, families, and other professionals; and the exponential growth of accessible knowledge. As a result, health professions educators competencies need to evolve to meet the changing needs of learners, shifting from a focus on knowledge provision to knowledge management, fostering professional identity in nontraditional settings, and leading and managing the learning community. Faculty development is essential to ensure that educators of the future develop these competencies. However, there are a number of barriers to the implementation of effective faculty development. In order to minimize these barriers universities need to invest in and prioritize education, providing stronger career pathways and incentives that will encourage faculty to engage in faculty development so that they can achieve the new educator competencies required to effectively educate future healthcare professionals.

Cross-References

▶ Developing Professional Identity in Health Professional Students
▶ Hidden, Informal, and Formal Curricula in Health Professions Education
▶ Supporting the Development of Professionalism in the Education of Health Professionals

References

Allen LM, Palermo C, Armstrong EG, Hay M. Categorising the broad impacts of continuing professional development: a scoping review. Med Educ. 2019;53(11):1087–99.

Allen LM, Hay M, Armstrong E, Palermo C. Applying a social theory of learning to explain the possible impacts of continuing professional development (CPD) programs. Med Teach. 2020;42(10):1140–7.

Ash S, Palermo C, Gallegos D. The contested space: the impact of competency-based education and accreditation on dietetic practice in Australia. Nutr Diet. 2019;76(1):38–46.

Bajis D, Chaar B, Moles R. Rethinking competence: a nexus of educational models in the context of lifelong learning. Pharmacy. 2020;8(2):81. https://doi.org/10.3390/pharmacy8020081.

Baker J. Coding to be mandatory in primary, early high school: the Sydney Morning Herald; 2018 Aug 21 [cited 2020 June 19]. Available from: https://www.smh.com.au/national/nsw/coding-to-be-mandatory-in-primary-early-high-school-20180817-p4zy5d.html

Berghman J, Debels A, Van Hoyweghen V. Prevention: the cases of social security and healthcare. In: Greve B, editor. Routledge handbook of the welfare state. Oxon: Routledge; 2019. p. 46–57.

Casas RS, Cooper JL, Hempel EV. COVID-19 risk triage: engaging residents in telephonic screening. Med Educ. 2020;54:670.

Chen HC, Wamsley MA, Azzam A, Julian K, Irby DM, O'Sullivan PS. The health professions education pathway: preparing students, residents, and fellows to become future educators. Teach Learn Med. 2017;29(2):216–27. https://doi.org/10.1080/10401334.2016.1230500.

Coleman CG, Law KL, Spicer JO. #EducationInTheTimeOfCOVID: leveraging social media to teach during the COVID-19 pandemic pandemonium. Med Educ. 2020;54:852–3.

de Carvalho-Filho MA, Tio RA, Steinert Y. Twelve tips for implementing a community of practice for faculty development. Med Teach. 2020;42(2):143–9.

Densen P. Challenges and opportunities facing medical education. Trans Am Clin Climatol Assoc. 2011;122:48–58.

Edelman DS, Desai UA, Soo-Hoo S, Catallozzi M. Responding to hospital system and student curricular needs: COVID-19 student service corps. Med Educ. 2020;54:853–4.

Hays R, Jennings B, Gibbs T, Hunt JM. Impact of the COVID-19 pandemic: the perceptions of health professions educators. MedEdPublish. 2020. https://doi.org/10.15694/mep.2020.000142.1.

Hodges AL, Konicki AJ, Talley MH, Bordelon CJ, Holland AC, Galin FS. Competency-based education in transitioning nurse practitioner students from education into practice. J Am Assoc Nurse Pract. 2019;31(11):675–82.

Institute of Medicine National Academies of Sciences, Engineering, Medicine. Envisioning the future of health professional education: workshop summary. Cuff PA, editor. Washington, DC: The National Academies Press; 2016. 174 p.

Klasen JM, Meienberg A, Nickel C, Bingisser R. SWAB team instead of SWAT team: medical students as frontline force during the COVID-19 pandemic. Med Educ. 2020;54:860.

Kratochvil TJ, Khanzanchi R, Sass RM, Caverzagie KJ. Aligning student-led initiatives and incident command system resources in a pandemic. Med Educ. 2020;54:1–2.

Leslie K, Baker L, Egan-Lee E, Esdaile M, Reeves S. Advancing faculty development in medical education: a systematic review. Acad Med. 2013;88(7):1038–45.

McGrail MR, Rickard CM, Jones R. Publish or perish: a systematic review of interventions to increase academic publication rates. High Educ Res Dev. 2006;25(1):19–35.

McKimm J, Gibbs T, Bishop J, Jones P. Health Professions' Educators' adaptation to rapidly changing circumstances: The Ottawa 2020 Conference Experience. MedEdPublish. 2020. https://doi.org/10.15694/mep.2020.000047.1.

Samuel A, Cervero RM, Durning SJ, Maggio LA. Effects of continuing professional development on health professionals' performance and patient outcomes: a scoping review of knowledge syntheses. Acad Med. 2021;96(6):913–23.

Srinivasan M, Li ST, Meyers FJ, Pratt DD, Collins JB, Braddock C, et al. "Teaching as a competency": competencies for medical educators. Acad Med. 2011;86:1211–20.

Steinert Y. Faculty development: core concepts and principles. In: Steinert Y, editor. Faculty development in the health professions: a focus on research and practice. Innovation and change in professional education. Dordrecht: Springer; 2014. p. 3–25.

Steinert Y, Mann K, Anderson B, Barnett BM, Centeno A, Naismith L, et al. A systematic review of faculty development initiatives designed to enhance teaching effectiveness: a 10-year update: BEME guide no. 40. Med Teach. 2016;38(8):769–86.

Stetson GV, Dhaliwal G. Using a time out: reimagining professional identity formation after the pandemic. Med Educ. 2020;55:131–4.

Talib Z, Palsdottir B, Briggs M, Clithero A, Cob NM, Marjadi B, et al. Defining community-engaged health professional education: a step toward building the evidence. NAM Perspectives. 2017;Discussion Paper. https://doi.org/10.31478/201701a.

Villela EFM, de Oliveira FM, Leite ST, Bollela VR. Student engagement in a public health initiative in response to COVID-19. Med Educ. 2020;54:763–4.

Weinstein Y, Madan CR, Sumeracki MA. Teaching the science of learning. Cognitive Res Princ Implications 2018;3:2.

Wu W, Martin BC, Ni C. A systematic review of competency-based education effort in the health professions: seeking order out of chaos. In: Management Association, Information Resources, editor. Healthcare policy and reform: concepts, methodologies, tools, and applications. Hershey: IGI Global; 2019. p. 1410–36. https://doi.org/10.4018/978-1-5225-6915-2.ch064.

Yardley S, Dornan T. Kirkpatrick's levels and education 'evidence'. Med Educ. 2012;46(1):97–106.

Index

A
Abilities, 1378, 1379
 (skills) assessment, 1186
Aboriginal and Torres Strait Islander people, 1257, 1561
Abusive supervision, 1476
Academic(s), 1269
 achievement, 1252
 attainment, 1258–1259
 and clinical educators, 1150
 integrity, 1139, 1140, 1142, 1143
 journals, 1602
 rationalism, 592
 standards, 577
Academy of Medical Educators, 1606
Acceptance, 532
Accountability mandate, 1253
Accreditation, 321, 577, 1444
Accreditation Council for Graduate Medical Education (ACGME), 1188
Accrediting Council for Pharmacy Education (ACPE), 618
Achievement emotions, 527
Action, 1407
Action-based IPL approach, 854
Action observation network (AON), 342
Action plan development, 1064–1065
Active learning, 1715–1717
Active listening, 1633
Activity systems, 422
 community, 424
 contradictions, 425, 426
 dialectics, 425
 division of labor, 424
 instruments, 423, 424
 object, 424
 outcome, 423
 rules, 424
 subject, 423
Activity theory (AT), 228, 405, 419, 581, 704, 1076
 analysis, 430, 431
 CL method, 431, 432
 complex activity, 427, 428
 data collection, 429, 430
 educational development, 434
 emergencies, 420
 first generation, 421
 HPE, 419, 429
 in-situ simulation, 435
 medical emergencies, 435
 origins, 420
 practical change, 433
 second generation, 421
 sense-making tool, 435
 system, 421 (*see also* Activity systems)
 theoretical framework, 420, 429
 third generation, 421
 tools, 419
Actor-network theory, 174
Actual practice performance, 62
Adams' closed-loop theory, 1377, 1378
Adaptation, 1380
Adaptive-adjustment/utilitarian function, 1152
Adaptive functioning, 1640
Adaptive learning, 1717
Adaptive motivation, 483
Admissions, 1254, 1257, 1258, 1260
Adult learning theory (ALT), 174, 1399, 1715
Advance care plan, 683, 684
Advanced beginner, 1380
Advanced Cardiac Life Support (ACLS), 1182, 1187
Advanced Life Support Course (ALS), 75
Advanced nurse practitioners (APNs), 616
Advanced practice, 290, 946
Advanced Practice Nursing (APN), 290

© Springer Nature Singapore Pte Ltd. 2023
D. Nestel et al. (eds.), *Clinical Education for the Health Professions*,
https://doi.org/10.1007/978-981-15-3344-0

Advanced Surgical Skills for Exposure in
    Trauma (ASSET), 1189
Advanced Trauma Life Support (ATLS), 1187
Advanced Trauma Operative Management
    (ATOM), 1189
Adverse events, 1193
Advisory College, 1007
Advocacy, 155, 161, 162
Advocacy-enquiry, 1409
Affective assessment, 1190
Affective behaviors, 487, 493
Affective control strategies, 1191
Affective dimension, 1179, 1187, 1190, 1191
Affective learning, 227
Affective (perceptions) dimensions, 1190–1191
Affective responses, 1152
Affective states, 522, 527
Affect labeling, 533
Affordances, 901
Aged care, 1490–1491
Agents of change, 1033
Alcohol
    and drugs policies, 1003
    use, 1003
Allied health
    definition of, 136
    practice and education, 137–139
    professions, 136
Allied health education
    business, marketing, and entrepreneurial
        skills, 146
    consumer and patient involvement,
        144–145
    cultural competency and safety, 142–143
    future trends, 145–147
    ICF, 140–141
    internationalization, 142
    interprofessional education, 141–142
    microcredentials, 146–147
    professional practice, 139–140
    simulation-based, 143–144
Allied health professionals, 137
    qualification levels, 137
Altmetrics, 770, 1619
Altruism, 1521, 1660
American Association of Dental
    Schools, 264
American Dental Association (ADA), 263
American Dental Educators Association
    (ADEA), 264
American Society of Dental Surgeons, 262
Amphetamines, 1003
Amygdala, 523

Anesthesia education
    academic anesthesia, 81
    clinical training, 70
    earlier pre-clinical training, 70
    emerging technologies, 79, 80
    examination, 75
    in-situ simulation, 77, 78
    in low resource countries, 76, 77
    maintenance of clinical skills, 78
    practical skill acquisition, 80
    professional roles, 70
    provision, 71
    quality improvement, 78, 83
    role of anesthetist, 71
    social media platforms, 82
    traditional approaches, 72
    training program, 71
    on wellbeing, 81
Anesthesia training, 71
    assessment during specialty training, 74
    clinical skills, 72
    rotation-based system, 72
    selection and early vocational training,
        73–74
    service delivery, 72
    traditional methods, 72
    WBAs, 74, 75
Anesthetic care, 76
Anesthetic nurse, 939
Anesthetic team
    anesthesia nurses, 937
    anesthetists, 936
    recovery nurses, 937
Anticipatory visualization, 1643
Anti-racist approach, 515
Anxiety, 487
ANZCA Educators program, 76
ANZCA's CPD Program, 78
AOTrauma organization, 1450
Apothecaries, 269–272, 276, 277
Application of theory, 407
Apprenticeship, 54, 57, 59, 270, 272–278, 288,
    289, 292, 296
    model, 1397
Aptitude tests, 1259
Aristotle, 687
Arracheurs des dents, 257
Artificial intelligence (AI), 424, 1436, 1576,
    1709–1711, 1728
    application within surgical training,
        1438–1441
    artificial neural networks, 1437
    autonomous surgical robots, 1440

curriculum, 1444
  as diagnostic assistant, 1438
  ethics and accountability, 1441–1443
  machine learning, 1437
  in mobile health applications, 1441
  natural language processing, 1437
  robots, 1440
  visual processing, 1438
Artificial neural networks, 1437
Aseptic technique, 940
Assertive communication, 901
Assessment(s), 38–43, 493, 905, 965, 966, 1136–1140, 1144, 1224, 1225, 1386
  of ethics, 599–600
  instrumentation, 1191, 1193
  judgments, 1240
  for learning, 1247
  tools, 1391
Assessment, of thresholds
  EPA, 376
  programmatic, 376
Assistants in nursing, 885
Associate Nurse Unit Managers (ANUM), 938
Association of American Medical Colleges (AAMC), 1225
Association of Southeast Asian Nations (ASEAN), 110
Assumptions, 465–469
Asynchronous delivery, 1423
Asynchronous education, 207
Attitude object, 1151
Attitude rigidity, 1154
Attitude(s), 671, 1150, 1545
  approaches for gathering and measuring data, 1154–1156
  description, 1151–1152
  features of quality, 1162–1163
  flexibility, 1154
  to health professional education, 1166–1171
  importance of, 1152
  measurement scales, 1163–1164
  practice-based education, 1166
  research with health professional students, 1169
  simulation-based education, 1165–1166
  types of measurement scales, 1156–1160
  ways to develop, 1153
Attributes, 671
Attributional training, 493
Attributions, 486
Audience response technology, 759–760
Audio-diaries, 370, 372
Audit trail, 1161

Augmented reality (AR), 80, 744–746, 1384, 1709, 1719
Australian Government Rural Clinical School Program, 14
Australian Medical Council (AMC), 824, 1505
Australian Medical Students' Association (AMSA), 824
Australian National Safety and Quality Health Service Standards, 1043
Australian Orthopaedic Association National Joint Replacement Registry (AOANJRR), 1457
Australian Tertiary Admissions Rank (ATAR), 1258
Authentic assessment, 1205
Authenticity, 326, 372, 1244, 1662
Authentic leadership, 1632
Authentic learning, 902, 1315
Authentic performance assessment, 1194
Authoritative leadership, 1641
Automatic assessment, 208
Automatic correction, 1377
Automation bias, 1438
Autonomous surgical robots, 1440
Autonomy, 917, 1715
Avicenna, 254
Awake fiber-optic intubation, 80

B

Balance, 1025
Balint groups, 1011
Baltimore College of Dentistry, 263
Barber-surgeon, 255
Behavioral tradeoffs, 1190
Behavioral measures, 1155
Behavioral process, 1400
Behavioral responses, 1152
Behavioral shift, 1683
Behavioral skills, 672
Behaviorism, 1408
  and simulation, 1543
  skills development and patient-centeredness, 1543–1544
Behaviorist learning, 1543
Belonging, 876
Benner, P., 1380
Bespoke care, 1494
Bias, 1263
  to middle responding, 1163
Bibliometrics, 1618
Big data, 1708–1711
Big Five Model of Teamwork, 1466

Big Five' personality traits, 1264
Billett's work-place pedagogy, 1076, 1077
Binge drinking, 1004
Biographical narrative interview, 1002
Biomedical engineers, 937
Biomedical equipment, 937
Biomedical knowledge, 687
Biomedical model, 800
Biomedical safety
    pathology, 951
    specimens, 951
Biomedicine, 1537
Biopsychosocial perspective, 1537
Biosensors, 1708, 1711
Blackboard Collaborate web conferencing platform, 306
Black box algorithm, 1439
Blended IPL approach, 854
Blended learning, 747, 1429
Block placements, 900
Blogging, 1318
Blogs, 766
Booster teaching, 1388, 1389
Bootcamp program, 206
Bottlenecks in learning, 368
Boyer, E.L., 1612
BRAIDE, 809–810
Brain drain, 185
Briefing, intraoperative teaching, debriefing (BID) model, 924
Briefing/debriefing, 923
British Dental Association, 263
Broaden and build theory, 529–530
Bronfenbrenner, U., 538
    concepts, 542
    early life, 540
    ecological model, 656

C

Calgary Cambridge framework, 1049
Campus-based support, 1009
Canadian competency framework, 1509
Canadian Federation of Medical Students (CFMS), 824
Canadian Interprofessional Competency Framework, 170
Canadian medical schools, 13
Cancelled placements, 1306
Capacity, 975
    building, 884
Cardiopulmonary resuscitation (CPR), 1473
Care and compassion, 1396, 1489
    aged care, 1490–1491
    care of carer, 1492
    critical care, 1491
    diversity, 1492–1493
    end of life care, 1491
    health ethics, 1487
    humanism, 1488
    identity, 1493–1494
    person-centered care, 1490
    philosophical perspective, 1487
    reflection and reflexivity, 1495
    self-awareness, 1495
Career development, 1733
Care pathway, 1472
Care Quality Commission (CQC), 1506
Caring ethic, 1666
Caring for self, 1495
Carnegie Foundation, 264
Carnegie Foundation for the Advancement of Teaching, 8
Case-based collaborative learning (CBCL) method, 162
Case-based discussion, 74, 568, 1236
Case-based learning (CBL)
    elements of, 1336
    vs. TBL, 1335
Cases-based learning, 100–101
Cavadenti, 257
Central venous canula blood stream infections (CVC BSIs), 1514
Certifications, 1182
Certified registered nurse anesthetist (CRNA), 616
Certifying exam, 1183
Champions, 994
Change, 1629
Change laboratory (CL), 431, 432
Change management, 1033, 1477
Chart-stimulated recall (CSR), 1192
Cheating, 1142, 1143
Checklists, 1238, 1391, 1475
Childhood obesity, 579
Child protection, 977
Chirurgia Magna, 257
Christian Albrecht University, 259
Chronosystem, 544
Chunking, 309
Churchill, E., 278
Circadian rhythms, 319
Circulating nurse, 939
    skill, 940
Circumplex model of affect, 526
Citizen control, 563
Classical conditioning, 1153
Classroom teaching, 596
Climate change, 817, 1560–1563
    impact of, 817
    toll of, 821

Index

Clinical anatomy, 323
Clinical Assessment and Management Exam-Outpatient (CAMEO), 1192
Clinical communication, 1536, 1540, 1542–1546
   development, 1547
   faculty, 1545
   history, 1542
   knowledge, 1546
   and patient-centeredness, 1540
   pedagogy, 1543, 1548
Clinical competency committee, 1243
Clinical conference, 101
Clinical context, 490–493
Clinical education, 399–400, 718
   and SBE (*see* Simulation based education (SBE))
   and technologies (*see* Technology, in health professions and clinical education)
   transformative learning in (*see* Transformative learning)
   underperformance in, 1123
   zones in, 1121
Clinical Education Principles for the COVID-19 Pandemic, 1307
Clinical educator, 986
Clinical educators supporting students, 987
Clinical environment, 491, 493–495
Clinical ethics committee (CEC), 975
Clinical evaluation, 88, 104
Clinical facilitation, 878
Clinical facilitator, 879, 882
Clinical fieldwork, 1318
Clinical judgment, 90
Clinical learning, 88, 89, 94, 96, 99, 102–103, 1238, 1246
Clinical Learning Environment Inventory (CLEI), 876
Clinical learning environments, 296, 948
Clinical learning outcomes, 668
Clinical note review, 1085
Clinical nurse educator, 89, 92, 94, 100, 103
Clinical nursing education
   cases-based learning, 100–101
   clinical learning and performance, assessment of, 102–103
   collaborative cluster model, 97
   competencies, 89
   cultural competence, 91
   discussions and clinical conferences, 101
   knowledge and development of clinical judgment, 90
   partnership/collaborative models, 94–95
   patient care assignment, 100
   preceptorship/mentoring model, 95–97
   principles, 89
   professional identity formation, 91
   quality and safety, in health care, 92
   skill development, 90–91
   technology, 98–100
   traditional model, 93–94
   written assignments, 101–102
Clinical placement, 877
   See also Professional practice
Clinical practice outcomes, 90–92
Clinical reasoning, 686, 902, 905, 1404, 1572
   co-constructed decision-making approaches, 1580
   definition, 1573–1575
   ecological decision making approaches, 1580–1581
   expert approaches, 1580
   learning, teaching and developing, 1581–1584
   mercurial decision making, 1581
   novice approaches, 1579
   occupational therapy clinical educator, 1583
   physiotherapy private practitioner, 1583
   senior radiographer, 1583
   speech pathologist, 1584
Clinical reflective skills (CRS) framework, 455, 456
Clinical simulation, 18–19, 1542–1543
Clinical skills, 70, 72, 77, 83, 1397
   acquisition of knowledge, 1406
   foundation, 1404–1406
   importance, 1403–1404
   real-world situations, 1406–1408
Clinical teaching practices, in nursing, *see* Clinical nursing education
Coach-coachee interface, 1458
Coaching, 879, 924, 1263, 1382, 1385
   AOTrauma organization, 1450
   approach, 1308
   and culture, 1454
   definition, 1448
   Kolb's experiential learning theory, 1450
   limitations of current surgical continuing professional development, 1455, 1456
   Mezirow's transformative learning theory, 1450
   models of, 1453
   ontological perspectives, 1450, 1452
   research, 1457
   skills, 1452
   surgical outlier remediation, 1457
   wearable devices, 1456

Co-assessment, 1720
Cocaine, 1003
Co-creation, 1715
Code of ethics, 1166
Codified knowledge, 1546
Cognition, 483–486, 525, 1729
Cognitive and behavioral theories, 10
Cognitive apprenticeship method, 1409
Cognitive assessment, 1178
Cognitive behavioral models, 1451
Cognitive conceptualization, 1383
Cognitive control, 485
Cognitive dissonance, 1154
Cognitive expertise, 337, 339–340
Cognitive (knowledge) dimension, 1181
Cognitive load, 309, 323, 325
Cognitive overload, 904
Cognitive process, 404, 1400
Cognitive reappraisal, 532, 1191
Cognitive responses, 1152
Cognitive structure, 1153
Cognitive tests, 1263
Cognitive workload, 525
Cohen and Bradford's influence without authority (IWA) model, 1034
Collaboration, 963, 1028, 1332, 1340
Collaborative cluster, 97
Collaborative educational models, 876
Collaborative environment, 989
Collaborative learning, 1717
Collaborative learning in practice (CLIP) models, 879
Collaborative model, 94–95
Collaborative Model of Fieldwork Education, 1286
Collaborative practice, 168, 170, 171, 175, 177
Collaborative problem solving, 1294
Collateral learning, 669
Collective leadership, 1641
Collectivist discourse of competence, 10
Collège du Saint Côme, 257
College of Physicians, 263
College of Surgeons, 263
Columbia University, 264
Communicable diseases, 1558
Communication, 221, 386, 394, 397–398, 672, 873, 874, 935, 1403, 1536
  breakdowns, 1100
  framework, 1046–1048, 1051
  principles, 1045
  skills, 1540, 1542–1544, 1546, 1547, 1549
  skills training, 1041, 1042
  strategy, 1044
Communication simulation-based education program, 1043
  communication and immersive simulation models, 1048
  communication framework, 1046–1048
  communication models, 1048–1049
  evaluation, 1049–1051
  program content, 1043–1044
  program structure, 1044–1045
Communication training, 76, 82
  organizational needs, 1041
  simulation-based education training, 1041–1043
Communicative competence, 1100
Communities of practice (CoP), 176, 404–408, 412, 549, 769, 876, 968, 992, 1077, 1078, 1086, 1092, 1103, 1361, 1515, 1549, 1635, 1672
  application of theory, 407
  challenges and barriers, 410
  critiques of, 411
  effectiveness of, 408
  in healthcare, 407–408
  in health professions education, 409–410
  identity formation, 406
  online, 409
  participation in, 409
  professional identity, 406
  in simulation, 410–411
  structural, economic, and cultural factors, 408
  theory, 174
  virtual, 410
Community, 424
Company of Barbers of London, 256
Compassion, 1489
  fatigue, 1496, 1702
Competence, 38, 39, 42, 44, 171, 883, 950, 1279, 1282, 1286, 1289, 1290, 1295, 1296, 1443
Competencies, 88, 89, 91, 96, 100, 102–104, 167, 169, 170, 173, 616–619, 1180, 1223, 1243, 1253, 1266, 1382, 1386, 1398, 1407, 1634, 1715, 1731
  committee, 1243
  frameworks, 224, 1225, 1257
  objectives, 1194
  quality and safety, in health care, 92
  standards, 1257, 1288
Competency-based curriculum, 56
Competency-based education (CBE), 560, 1223, 1729

Index

Competency Based Fieldwork Evaluation for Occupational Therapists (CBFE–OT), 1291
Competency based learning, 348
Competency based medical education (CBME), 8, 18, 1138
Competency-based selection, 1256
Competing priorities, 1733
Complex adaptive systems (CAS), 1466
Complex dimensional abilities, 1194
Complex failures, 1640
Complexity, 367, 799, 806, 808, 809
    of assessment, 1180
    of healthcare provision, 159
    theory, 174
Complex overt response, 1380
Complex skill, 627–629, 632, 636, 641
Comprehensive assessment, 1194
Computer-assisted instruction, 321
Computer-assisted learning, 321
Computer vision, 1438
Concept maps, 375, 377
Conceptual framework, 483–486
Conceptual framework for simulated clinical placement (CF-SCP), 1313, 1314
Concrete thinking, 879
Concurrent commentary, 1293
Confidence, 883, 916, 988
Confidentiality, 1662
Confirmability, 1161
Conflict, 1642
Conflicting responsibilities, 916
Congruence, 1685
Connectivism, 769, 1425
Connectivity optimization, 323
Consensus statement, 1254
Consent, 976
Consequences of disclosure, 1004
Consequentialist moral theories, 1541
Consistency, 1399
Constant-sum scale, 1158
Constructive alignment, 326, 1139–1141, 1368
Constructive feedback, 1292
Constructive learning, 1716
Constructivism, 10, 1425, 1450, 1716
Constructivist grounded theory methodology, 1104
Constructivist learning theories, 1361
Consultation assessment, 1086
Consultation models, 1540
Consultation observation, 1085, 1086, 1088
Consultation schemas, 1086
Consultative leadership, 1632, 1641

Consumer/client feedback, 1290
Consumer/service user involvement, 1296
Consumers in health education, 144
Contact hypothesis, 174
Contemporary approaches, 1631
Content analysis, 1161
Context, 1027
Contextual control, 489
Contextual fidelity, 1193
Continuing medical education (CME), 1189, 1452, 1455
Continuing professional development (CPD), 295, 766, 946, 1397, 1452, 1455, 1732
    OT practice, 946
    programs, 78, 79
Continuity of care, 895
Continuity of care experience (CCE), 897
Continuity of education, 903
Continuous quality improvement (CQI), 1711
Contract cheating, 1142, 1143
Contractual agreements, 877
Contradictions, 425
Control appraisal, 529
Control-value theory, 527
Conversation, 1102
Conversational learning, 1112
Co-production, 231–233
Core competencies for interprofessional collaborative practice, 93
Co-regulation, 492
Coronavirus pandemic, 1628
Corporate businesses, 53
Corridor
    consultations, 1005
    conversation, 1084
Cost-effectiveness, 1051
Co-teaching, 1347
Counselling, 1449
Coursera, 619
Covert processes, 1178
COVID-19 pandemic, 304, 1304, 1614, 1728, 1734
    anatomy learning, 322
    clinical practicums and practice education, 1306–1307
    digital technologies, 323
    disruption, 304, 327
    economics, 327
    entry-level programs, 305
    higher education, 327, 1305
    innovative clinical and practice education models, 1307–1309
    MMD, 306

COVID-19 pandemic (*cont.*)
   politics, 327
   primary symptoms of, 1304
   social, 327
   trends in technology, 327
   university programs, 305
Credentialing system, 993
Credibility, 1161
Crew resource management (CRM), 1473
Critical care, Resuscitation and Airway Skills in High Fidelity Simulation (CRASH) Course, 79
Critical care nursing, 943
Critical conversations, 468
Critical reflection, 227, 451, 454, 457, 465–469, 472, 477
Critical sensibility, 1556
Critical theory
   anti-racist approach, 515
   in clinical education, 504–505
   colonialism and post-colonial oriented projects, 512–513
   description, 500
   feminist and gender approach, 514–515
   hidden curriculum, 511–512
   intersectional theory, 515–516
   Marxist and Neo-Marxist perspectives, 513
   paradigms, 501
   reflexivity, 502
Critical thinking, 465, 466, 469, 470, 491, 1403
Cross-cultural efficacy model, 803
Cross-dimensional competencies, 1194
7C's model, 1465
Cultural beliefs, 873
Cultural competence, 91, 142, 797, 801
   education, 671
Cultural diversity, 884
Cultural-historical activity theory (CHAT), 174, 419
Cultural humility, 802
Cultural safety, 142
Cultural sensibility model, 803
Cultural sensitivity, 802
Cultural web, 671
Culture, 798, 1020, 1027
Curricular planning grid, 657
Curriculum, 32–36, 39, 589, 1444, 1501, 1502, 1504–1509, 1515, 1542
   Guide, 1508
   public engagement, health profession (*see* Public engagement, in health profession curriculum)
   as technology, 592

Curriculum design, TCF-informed spiral, 377
Curriculum vitae (CV), 1264
Cybersecurity, 1442

D

Data
   authenticity, 1665
   collection, 429, 430, 1659
   ownership, 1443
Database of Individual Patients' Experience of Illness (DIPEx), 1548
Day release, 54, 55
Day surgery nurses, 936
Debriefing, 917, 1107, 1108, 1110, 1112, 1319, 1399, 1468
   analytical categories, 702–703
   application of analytical categories to practices, 709–710
   case study, 701–709
   content, 705–707
   description, 700
   interaction patterns, 707–709
   organizational context, 709
   people involved in, 703–705
   physical context, 709
   practices, 701
de Chauliac, G., 257
Decision making, 1238, 1403, 1538, 1700
   skills, 99, 101
Decisions, 1240
   support tools, 1709
   tree, 1294
Declarative knowledge, 1708
Decoding the disciplines approach, 368, 375
Dedicated education unit (DEU) model, 94, 95, 103, 876
Dedicated practice, 1644
De Humanis Corporis Fabrica, 255
Deliberate attentional focus, 1191
Deliberate practice, 91, 350, 351, 355, 902, 964, 1186, 1384–1386, 1389
Delphi process, 372
Dementia, 1166
Demonstrated competence, 1189
Dental Cosmos, 262
Dental education, 154, 252
   apprenticeship as a form of training, 257–259
   attempts to regulate the practice of dentistry, 256
   dental practitioner-author, 255
   dental societies, 263

first dental journals, 262
first dental school, 259–262
Hesy-Ra, 252
holistic approach for patients and learners, 159–163
learner context, 157–159
patient context, 156–157
reform, 263–264
regulation for dentistry practice, 263
self-taught practitioner, 252
societal and regulatory context, 155–156
written record, 253–255
Deontological theories, 1541
Dependability, 1161
Design-dependent environment, 1421
Design of peer learning, 1370
De-skilling, 1388
Dewey, J., 442, 448
Diagnostic assistance, 1438
Dialectical materialism, 420
Dialectics, 420, 425
Dialogue, 465, 468, 476
Didactic teaching methods, 596
Difference, 798, 807
Diffusion tensor imaging (DTI), 338
Digital health technologies, 1728
Digital learning object, 1420
Digital literacy, 583, 584, 1310
Digital open-door, 319
Digital privacy, 209
Digital scholarship, 770
Digital story telling, 454
Digital technology, 308, 317, 323, 325, 1305
Digital therapeutics (DTx), 1712, 1713
Digital upskilling, 306
Digital workbook, 325
Dignity, 1489
Dimensionality, 1163
Directed feedback, 1377
Direct-entry, 297
Direct-entry midwifery' program, 297
Direct learning theory, 309
Direct observation, 1236, 1237, 1239, 1244, 1247
Direct Observation of Procedural Skills (DOPS), 74, 966, 1192, 1236
Direct supervision, 1387
Disciplinary code, 1004
Disclosure of mental illness, 1004
Discordance, 911
Discourse, 508–510
analysis, 1161
Discursive work, 1102

Discussion forums, 1318
Discussions and clinical conferences, 101
Disguised feedback, 1106
Disjuncture, 466
Disorienting dilemma, 465, 466, 469, 470, 472, 476, 1450
Disparity, 1563
Disruption, 304, 327
Dissonance, 1685
Distance education
advantages, 204
challenges of, 209–210
difficulty with longitudinal progress monitoring, 209
digital privacy, 209
education centered workplace, 210
faculty support and development, 209
reduced communities, 209
skills teaching in, 204
suggestions for improving, 211
surgical training, 204
Distractions, 915
Distributed leadership, 1638
Diverse healthcare workforce, 1269
Diverse settings, 993
Diversity, 1255, 1492
Diversity in healthcare education
BRAIDE, 809–810
conceptual clarity, 797–800
evaluation and curriculum, 805–806
institutional requirements and policies, 804
intersectional transdisciplinarity, 806–809
theoretical clarity, 801–805
Division of labor, 424
Djoser, P., 252
Doctor of Physiotherapy (DPHTY), 309
Double gloving, 952
Dreyfus, H.L., 1380
Dreyfus, S.E., 1380
Driscoll's model of reflection, 1286
Duty of care, 942
Dynamic learning community, 310

E
Early clinical experiences, 1366
Education, 493, 1503–1507
psychomotor skills (see Psychomotor skills)
Educational alliance, 1088
Educational assessment
alignment, 1139–1140
cheating and academic integrity, 1142–1143
feedback as a process, 1140–1141

Educational assessment (*cont.*)
  feedback literacy, 1141–1142
  formative assessment, 1138–1139
  health professions, 1144
  standards-based assessment, 1136–1137
  summative assessment, 1137–1138
  sustainable assessment, 1139
Educational games, 237, 240
Educational leadership, in HPE, 1634
  competencies, 1634
  distributed leadership, 1638
  empowerment, 1650
  evidence and scholarship, 1651–1652
  experiential learning, 1650
  hierarchical leadership, 1639
  horizontal development, 1638
  interpersonal aspects, 1637
  intrapersonal aspects, 1637
  leadership style, 1646
  leader *vs.* leadership development, 1636–1638
  proactive development, 1636
  professional identity, 1637
  psychological safety, 1640–1645
  roles, 1635
  self-development, 1650
  strategic prioritization, 1645
  succession planning, 1637
  vertical development, 1638
Educational skills, 1366
Educational strategies, 1708
Educational supervisor, 1008
Educational theory, 174, 568, 963
Education
  models, clinical nursing (*see* Clinical nursing education)
  programs, in allied health professions, 136
  staff, 938
Educator competencies, 1733, 1734
Educator training programs, 76
Educator workload, 1365
Edutainment, 310, 315
Effective communication, 1040, 1041, 1047, 1050
Effective feedback, 925, 1058, 1065
Effectiveness of team training, 1471
Ego-defensive function, 1152
e-Health
  building digital capabilities, 145–146
  telepractice, 145
e-learning, 758–759, 1418–1423, 1429
Electroencephalography (EEG), 338
Electronic medical record (EMR), 1030, 1031, 1438
Electronic resources, 205

Emancipatory pedagogy, 162
Embed, 1019
Emergencies, 420
Emergency medical services (EMS), 615
Emerging technologies, 79, 80, 83
Emic, 1669
Emotional intelligence (EI), 9, 530, 987
Emotional investment, 1665
Emotionally intelligent researcher, 1662
Emotional modulation, 532
Emotional regulation, 530
Emotional set, 1379
Emotions, 522
  in learning, 367
Empathy, 1167, 1489, 1667
Empowerment, 884, 886, 1033, 1650
Enablement, 1635
Encounter cards, 1239
Endoscopy nurses, 936
Engagement, 884, 995, 1028, 1296
  activities, 317
  of trainee, work community, 1080–1082
Enrolled nurse, 292, 293, 872
Entrenched attitudes, 1168
Entrustable professional activities (EPAs), 17, 731, 1222, 1241, 1720
  clinical education relationship, 1228
  in health care, 1223
  training improvement, 1228
Entrustable tasks, 925
Entrustment, 915, 916, 1090
Environment, 1187, 1191–1193
Environmental and health threats, 1561
Epistemological education, 686, 687
e-Portfolio, 1422
Equality Act, 799
Equitable manner, 310, 311, 316
Erosion, 1550
Essential Pain Management course, 77
Essentials in Clinical Simulation Across the Health Professions, 619
Ethical obligation, 1664
Ethical responsibilities, 1505
Ethical thinking, 565
Ethics, 11, 773, 1487
Ethics in healthcare education
  assessment of, 599–600
  challenges, 600–601
  curriculum, 591–593
  for healthcare professionals, 589–590
  informal and formal curricula, 588
  multi-disciplinary team, 598
  syllabus, 593–595
  teaching format, 595–597
  at undergraduate or pre-clinical level, 597

Index

European Academy of Teachers in General Practice (EURACT), 51, 62, 64
Eustachi, B., 255
Evaluation, 1041, 1043, 1049–1051, 1153, 1266, 1268
    and feedback, 1708
    criteria, 1291
    measures, 1734
Evaluative judgement, 1363
Evidence-based dentistry (EBD), 161
Evidence-based management, 687
Evidence-based practice, 89, 1614
eWorkbooks, 783, 785–787, 790, 792
Excellent practice educator, 1280
Exchange, 1035
Exchange-based IPL approach, 853
Executive support, 1029
Existential approach, 1451
Exosystem, 544
Expansion of the object, 425
Expansive learning, 426, 427
    cycle, 432
Experiential learning, 226, 876, 967, 986, 1376, 1381, 1382, 1543, 1544, 1650, 1686
Expert, 1380
    surgeons, 340
Expertise, 32, 33, 37, 38, 44, 1181, 1188
    and automaticity, 1191
    cognitive, 339–340
    and experts, 336–338
    factors, 343–344
    neural implementation of, 338–339
    perceptual, 340–341
    psychomotor, 341–343
Extended reality, 1719
Extrinsic motivation, 487, 525, 920
Eye tracking, 1443, 1721

F

Face-to-face instruction, 1429
Face-to-face teaching, 321
Facilitated debriefing, 1409
Facilitating group reflective practice, 1319
Facilitation, 904
Facilitator role, 618–619
Faculty, 1238, 1242–1247
    competencies, 1731
    development, 925–926, 1028, 1728, 1730, 1732–1734
    training, 1242, 1244
    workload, for SBE, 615
Fair selection process, 1265
Faith-based organizations (FBO), 188
Family, 51, 53, 58, 64

Family Medicine Program (FMP), 193
Family nurse practitioners (FNP), 616
Fatigue, 16
Fauchard, P., 257, 258
Federation of State Medical Boards, 1504
Feedback, 89, 91, 102, 104, 905, 911, 914, 990, 1087–1089, 1108, 1137–1141, 1183, 1184, 1187, 1189, 1237–1247, 1279, 1280, 1282, 1283, 1289–1292, 1296, 1377, 1399, 1426
    conversations, 1059
    effective, 1058
    emotionality associated with, 1121
    error correction feedback, 636
    extrinsic feedback, 640
    fading feedback, 640
    for future learning, 1129, 1130
    and guided reflection, 1127
    in-task feedback, 637
    interactions, 1056
    intrinsic sensory feedback, 640
    learner-centered, 1058
    problems with, 1057–1058
    processes, 1125
    relative feedback frequency, 640
    role of, 1056–1057
    terminal/end-task feedback, 640
    vanishing, 1120
Feedback literacy, 1141–1142
Feedback Quality Instrument, 1059–1068
Feedforward, 720
Fellowship of Surgeons, 256
Feminist approach, 514–515
Fidelity, 971, 1399
Field notes, 1240
Fieldwork Performance Evaluation for the Occupational Therapy Student, 1291
Fieldwork, see Professional practice
First generation activity theory, 421
First points of contact, 1008–1009
Fitness to practice, 1002, 1529
Flattening, 1632
Flexner Report, 264
Flipped classroom, 205, 325, 1429
Focus group discussions, 1160
Formal curriculum, 595, 880
Formal equality, 799
Formal ethics education, 594
Formal feedback, 1290
Formal learning, 1104
Formal peer learning, 1357
Formative assessment, 1138–1139, 1178, 1182, 1188, 1192
Formative evaluation, 103, 104
Formative feedback, 1290, 1385

Forms, 1236, 1237, 1239, 1241–1243, 1245
Fostering relationships, 992
Foucault, M., 1556
Foundation for Advancement of International Medical Education and Research (FAIMER), 6
Four Habits Communication Framework, 1049
Fragmented healthcare systems, 219
Frank, P., 259
Fritsche, B., 259
Functionalist theory of attitudes, 1152
Functional magnetic resonance imaging (fMRI), 338
Fundamentals of Endoscopic Surgery™ (FES), 1188
Fundamentals of Feedback' training program, 76
Fundamentals of Laparoscopic Surgery™ (FLS), 1187
Fusiform face area (FFA), 341
Fusiform gyrus (FG), 339, 341

G

Galen of Pergamon, 254
Gallwey coaching equation, 1448
Game-based learning, 1719–1720
Game-informed principles, 315
Gamification, 1428, 1719
Gender
    bias, 993
    differences, 918
Generalists, 52, 63
General Medical Council (GMC), 1504, 1525
General practice (GP)
    apprenticeship relationship, 54
    build trusting relationships, 54
    early assessment, 58
    family medicine, 1074
    increasing competition, 56
    in-practice learning, 59
    in-practice teaching, 60
    Irish training programs, 56
    junior doctors, 52
    lengthen training, 63
    major educational environments, 52
    medical students, 52
    organization, 62–63
    post-graduate junior GP trainee, 1079
    pre-fellowship GP trainee, 1079–1080
    primary care, 1074
    programmatic assessment, 61–62
    senior medical student in, 1078–1079
    specialty training, 53–54
    summative assessment, 62
    training schemes, 55, 59
    vision of quality, 58
    work-based assessments, 61
    workshops, 60–61
General practitioners (GPs), 51
    clinical supervision, 59
    competency-based curriculum, 56
    educational resources, 60
    graded introduction to consulting, 59–60
    in-practice teaching, 60
    jurisdictions supervision, 59
    medical educators, 54
    multi-morbidity, 52
    need for, 52
    organization, 62–63
    programmatic assessment, 61–62
    ReCEnT project, 57
    registrar's work/funding, 59
    relationship-based care with, 51
    summative assessment, 62
    supervisors and practices, in teaching, 57
    workshops, 60–61
Gestalt approaches, 1451
Gibbs cycle, 567
Gibbs' model, 448–449, 456
Gibbs reflective model, 1286
Gies, W.J., 264
Glassick, C.E., 1613
Global environmental changes (GECs), 818
Global performance dimensions, 1192
Global rating scales, 1391
Global surgery
    comprehensive analysis, 183
    definition, 182
    Lancet Commission, 192
Goal orientations, 487
Goal-oriented activity, 424
Good practice, 1090–1091
Google Glass, 1456
Governance, 877, 1441
Grade point averages (GPA), 15, 1258
Graduate Diploma of Psychology Advanced (GDPA), 780, 791, 792
    academic and work-integrated assessments, 789
    content structure and organization, 784–787
    online course content, 781–783
    online course structure, 781
    students and student support, 784
    student satisfaction, 790
    synchronous and asynchronous interaction, 787–788

Index

Graduated patient responsibility, 1387
Graduated responsibility, 1382
Graduate-entry, 1672
Graduate Medical Schools Admissions Test (GAMSAT), 1258, 1265
Graduate outcomes, 1256
Graduate Outcome Statements (GOSs), 824
Graphic rating scales, 1158
Grounded theory, 1161
Group dynamics, 319
Group learning activities, 316
GROW model, 1454
Guided response, 1380
Guy's Hospital, 259

H

Habitual action, 444
Halo effect, 1163
Halsted, W., 277, 278
Halstedian apprenticeship model, 35
Happy-face scale, 1159
Haptic data, 1443
Harris, C., 260, 261
Harris, J., 260
Harvard Medical Practice Study, 1502
Hawthorn effect, 1163
Hayden, H., 260, 261
Head mounted displays (HMDs), 1456
Health advocacy, 919
Health and Care Professions Council (HCPC) Standards, 1525
Healthcare
  assistants, 885
  CoP in, 407–409
  delivery, 1634
Healthcare educators (HCEs), 1600–1602, 1605–1608
Healthcare professionals (HCPs), 957, 1593, 1594, 1596, 1597
  See also Health professionals
Healthcare professions
  effects of applicant population, 1001
  mental illness, 1005
  public engagement in (*see* Public engagement, in health profession curriculum)
Healthcare profession(al) education
  advantages of tools of philosophy in, 566
  applied ethics, 565
  changing paradigms in, 561–564
  landscapes in, 559–561
  macro level drivers in, 559
  philosophy for, 558–559
  reflective practice, 558
  SBE in US (*see* Simulation based education (SBE))
  undergraduate and postgraduate curricula, 566
  values and identity, 567–568
  values-based philosophic approach, 568
Health humanities, 682
  advance care plan, 684
  clinical encounter, 682–683, 693–694
  clinical placements, 684
  content and methods, 684
  health professional curricula, 685
  humanities-type teaching, 685
  journals, books and medical humanities associations, 685
  learning and practicing empathy, 691
  learning and teaching strategies, 688–691
  medical and health professional training, 683
  medical curricula, 686
  pedagogical and professional development perspective, 684
  professional aspects and clinical complexities, 684–685
  professional education, 686
  teachers and practitioners, 684
  tolerance of ambiguity, 691–692
  unstructured learning, 692–693
Health literacy, 873, 1564
Health professionals, 1674
  conceptions, 1676–1677
  demographic detail, 1675
  education, 856, 1066, 1224–1228
  mindset shift, 1679–1680
  role and identity congruence, 1680–1682
  role and identity dissonance, 1683–1684
  role boundaries, 1678–1679
  role change, 1677–1678
  transcript analysis, 1674
Health professional teams
  care pathway, 1472
  checklists, 1475
  CRM, 1473
  implementation of strategies, 1476–1478
  people-focused approaches, 1473
  simulation-based training, 1473, 1474
  systems-based solutions, 1472
  team building tools, 1475
  team debriefing, 1474, 1475
  team reflexivity, 1474

Health professional teams (cont.)
  team science and implementation, 1464–1472
  TeamSTEPPS™, 1474
  team training, 1473, 1474
Health professions curricula
  refugee and asylum seeker health, 1557–1560
  rurality, 1563–1565
  sustainability, 1560–1563
Health professions education (HPE), 176, 348, 354–356, 358, 404, 411, 419, 427, 435, 668, 672, 1612, 1728
  changing landscape, 1728–1730
  CoP in, 409–410
  educational leadership in (see Educational leadership, in HPE)
Health professions education (HPE) curricula
  assessment, 1720–1721
  educational strategies and implementation, 1714–1720
  goals and objectives, 1714
  Kern's six steps of curriculum, 1707
  problem identification and general needs assessment, 1707–1713
  targeted needs assessment, 1713–1714
Health professions education scholarship units (HPESUs), 1616
Health professions educators, 1730–1731
  challenges, 1733–1734
  faculty competencies, 1731–1732
  faculty development, 1732–1733
Health professions students, 548
Healthtalkonline, 1548
Hegemony, 506
Help-seeking strategy, 488
Henry VIII, 256
Hesy-Ra, 252
Hidden curriculum, 19–20, 511–512, 590, 658
  and behavioral skills, 672
  in clinical practice, 676
  clinical settings, 673–674
  definition, 668
  peer interactions, 673
  positive aspects of, 675–676
  professionalism and role modelling, 670–672
  risks and challenges, 674–675
  role of patient, 674
Hierarchical leadership, 1639
Hierarchy, 1663
Higher education, 293–295
Higher order thinking skills, 1708

Holism of practice, 874
Holistic approach, 159–163, 1292
Holistic education, 1401
Horizontal attitude configuration, 1153
Horizontal development, 1638
Hospital-based training, 288–289
Hospital politics, 1027
Human factors, 944, 1406
Humanism, 224
Humanistic pedagogy, 160, 162
Human rights, 1559
Hunter, J., 259
Hybrid education, 306
Hypothetico-deductive reasoning model, 1582

I
Ideal teacher, 913
Identification of gap areas, 1190
Identity, 371, 1077–1079, 1083, 1085–1087, 1095
  alignment, 1683
Illness scripts, 57
Imbalance of capabilities, 1194
Implementation
  outcome measures, 1477
  science, 1021, 1477, 1478
  of team development initiative, 1476
  of WBAs, 1243–1244
Implicit investigation, 1293
Implicit trait policies (ITPs), 1262
Imposter syndrome, 1637
Improvements, 1503
Improvement science, 1021
Improving Quality in Practice Placements–Allied Health (iQIPP-AH) Guides, 1283
Incidental learning, 1311
Incivility, 1111
Inclusion, 657, 660, 1028, 1489
Inclusivity, 320, 321
Incremental achievement, 1194
Independent practice, 910
In-depth interviews, 1160
Indicator behaviors, 1179
Indigenous students, 1257
Individualized feedback, 1441
Individually focused process, 1256
Individual readiness assurance test, 1328
Informal curriculum, 669
Informal feedback, 1290
Informal learning, 1104
Informal networking opportunities, 1596

Index

Information literacy, 371
Infrastructure investment, 328
Innovations, 963, 1629
In-practice learning, 59
In-practice teaching, 60
Input-process-output (IPO) model, 1465
Insider, 1663
Institute of medical ethics, 595
Institute of Medicine (IOM), 1464
Institutional support, 1596, 1601
Instructional design(ers), 315, 320, 323, 327, 1421
Instructional support, 492, 493, 495
Instructor feedback, 1290
Instrument (scrub) nurse, 939, 941
    duty of care, 942
    skill, 942
Integrated models of care, 219
Integrated threshold concept knowledge (ITCK), 375
Integration, 363, 375
Integrity of measurement, 1192
Intelligent digital assistant, 1439
Intelligent failures, 1640
Intended learning outcomes (ILOs), 1137–1140
Interactive patient scenarios, 234, 239
Intercultural maturity model, 803
Interdependent, 1191
Interests, 1151
Inter-institutional relationships, 994
International Classification of Functioning, Disability and Health (ICF), 140–141
International Confederation of Midwives (ICM), 286
International Council of Nurses (ICN), 286, 822
International Federation of Medical Students (IFMSA), 823
International Health Humanities Network, 686
Internationalization, 294
    cultural diversity, 108
    of curriculum approach, 142
    at home approach, 143
International mobility, 110–112
International Pharmaceutical Federation (FIP), 823
Internet, 583–584
Internet-based learning, 758
Internet of Things (IOT), 1711
Internet technologies, 1420
Internships, 1306
Interpersonal aspects, 1637
Interpersonal skills, 1511
Interpretative paradigm, 1667

Interprofessional activities, 902
Interprofessional collaborative practice, 93, 168, 170, 171, 176, 1405
    competencies for, 848–849
Interprofessional communication, 944
Interprofessional competencies, 171
Interprofessional Education Collaborative (IPEC), 1464
Inter-professional education (IPE), 19, 141–142, 228–231, 1464, 1526, 1714
    CAIPE, 168
    challenges, 171, 172
    competencies and frameworks, 170
    at curriculum level, 170
    evidence, 171, 172
    exposure-level IPE strategies, 170
    facilitators, 173, 175
    facilitator skill, 174
    health challenges, 176
    immersion-level IPE strategies, 171
    impact of intervention, 172
    implementation, 176
    interprofessional collaboration, 168
    interprofessional competencies, 171
    interventions, 172, 173
    mastery-level IPE strategies, 171
    movement, 850
    mutual trust, 169
    practice settings, 175
    pre-licensure IPE, 169
    presage factors, 173
    principles of effective IPE, 169, 170
    programs, 615
    research, 169
    shapes and forms, 168
    theories, 174
    timing of delivery, 169
    at undergraduate level, 168
Interprofessional health education, 428
Interprofessional identities, 1673, 1680–1682
Interprofessional learning, 170, 173–175, 596
    benefits of, 851–852
    challenges of, 856
    characteristics of, 851–853
    in clinical practice settings, 857–862
    4B and 4P approach to, 861
    modified Kirkpatrick evaluation for, 860
    teaching types and learning approaches, 853–856
Interprofessional practice, 175, 176
Interprofessional socialization framework, 1687
Interprofessional staff, 1019
Interprofessional training wards (ITWs), 855

Interprofessional working, 1406
Interrelatedness, 883
Intersectionality, 652, 799–800, 807–809
    critical reflexivity, 808
    transdisciplinarity, 808
Intersectional theory, 515–516
Intersubjective, 1538
Interviews, 1155
Intraoperative environment, 939
Intra-operative teaching, 911
Intrapersonal aspects, 1635, 1637
Intraprofessional learning, 864
Intrinsic motivation, 920
Intrinsic traits, 989

J
Jefferson College of Medicine, 261
Journal of Dental Research, 264
Judgments, 1240
Junior doctors, 51–53, 55, 56, 63, 1694, 1697, 1698
Just-in-time reference, 1707

K
Kegan's stage model, 568
Kern, D., 1707
Keystone Michigan project, 1514
King Ashurbanipal, 253
Knowledge
    alien, 366
    function, 1152
    inert, 366
    management, 407
    Nettlesome, 366
    proactive, 371
    ritual, 366
    structures, 1181
    tacit, 366, 375
    troublesome, 366
Knowledge-based teaching approach, 593
Kolb's experiential learning theory, 1450
Kolb's learning cycle, 1285

L
Landscapes of practice (LoP), 406, 408, 410, 412
Language, 1103
Language barriers, 194–195
Large classes, in SBE, see Simulation based education (SBE)

Lay midwives, 296
Leadership, 1022, 1629, 1632–1633, 1650
    development, 1630, 1631, 1634–1638, 1640–1645, 1651, 1652
    and innovation, 1640, 1651
    qualities, 1020
    styles, 914
Learn, see Practice, Prove, Do, and Maintain (LSPPDM) framework, 1381–1387, 1389–1391
Learned societies, 1596, 1607
Learner
    agency, 1067–1068
    clinical learning, 1239
    control, 206
    engagement, 880
    future considerations, 884
    model, 406
    participation, 917
    personal characteristics, 882
    preparation, 920
    preparedness, 880–881, 914
Learner-centric approach, 1399
Learning, 1241
    coach, 1208, 1209, 1212, 1213
    conversations, 1108–1110
    cultures, 1642
    cycle, 1285
    by doing, 1102
    environment, 926
    goals, 901, 925
    needs, 1084, 1085, 1090
    points, 919
    science, 1732
    skills, 1511
    strategies, 483, 486
    by talking, 1102
Learning and teaching
    clinical environment and culture of workplace, 875–877
    education and communication experience, 879–881
    organizational structures and policies, 877–879
    privacy and respect, 872–873
    safety and quality, 874–875
    sociocultural characteristics of patients, families and clinicians, 881–883
Learning-as-acquisition, 404
Learning-as-participation, 404
Learning for Mastery (LFM), 354
Learning-in-context models, 404
Learning management systems (LMS), 1421

Le Chirurgien Dentiste, 257
L'École Dentaire, 262
Legitimate peripheral participation (LPP), 410, 1409
LEGO Pictorial scale, 1159
Leininger's theory, 801
Lemaire, J.J-F., 262
Letters of reference, 1259–1260
Leverage, 1024
Libellus de Dentibus, 255
Licensed practical nurse (LPN), 293, 938
Life and death matters, 1004
Lifeworld, 1540
Likert scales, 1156
Liminality, 367, 369, 373
Liminal space, 364, 367, 369, 373, 375
Listening, 1631
Lived experience, 1667
Live simulation, 235–236, 239
Local program directors, 61
Logbooks, 1241
London School of Dental Surgery, 262
Longitudinal integrated clerkships (LICs), 17, 1367
Longitudinal qualitative research (LQR), 1659, 1661, 1669
Longitudinal studies, 1658
Long Lives, Healthy Workplaces (LLHW) initiative, 81
Long-term doctor-patient relationship, 53
Long term memory (LTM), 337–340, 344, 345
Louis XIV of France, 257
Low achievers, 493
Low income countries and lower-middle income countries
 cultural diversity of students and faculty, 116–117
 international collaboration, 112–114
 international mobility, 110–112
 online learning models, 114–115

M

Machine learning, 1437
Macrosystem, 544
Maintenance, 1387–1389
Maintenance of certification (MOC), 1185
Maintenance of surgical expertise, 343
Major educational environments, 52
Management and administration staff
 clerical staff, 938
 education staff, 938
 NUM, 938

Managerialism, 1605
Manual dexterity, 1378
Marxist perspectives, 513–514
Maslow's hierarchy of needs, 1450
Massive open online courses (MOOCs), 1718
Mastery, 1178, 1186, 1194, 1409
Mastery learning, 963, 1194
 advantages, 351, 357
 articulated curriculum, 349
 assessments, 351, 353
 barriers, 357
 challenges, 358
 competency based education, 350
 competency based learning, 348
 concept of variables, 349
 and deliberate practice, 355
 education framework, 348
 empirical research, 355, 356
 essential elements, 350, 351
 history, 348
 learners' ability and rate of progression, 352, 353
 learning objectives, 349–352, 357
 LFM, 350, 354
 for medical education, 350
 PSI, 354
 randomized control trial, 356
 self-regulation, 357
Materialism, 420
Measurements of performance, 1720
Mechanism, 1380
Media, 1035
Mediation, 421
Medical and digital technology, 947
Medical and midwifery education
 characteristics, 122
 clinical interpretation and decision-making skills, 127
 course structure, 123
 gender imbalances and biases, 123
 hands-on learning affordances, 125–126
 interprofessional education, 130–131
 learning by simulation, 129
 learning skills, 124–125
 pre-vocational training, 122
 professional relationships, 128–129
 public/private sector, 131
 simulation, 130
 unpredictable emergencies, 126
 work-based placements, 122
Medical College Admissions Test (MCAT), 1258, 1265

Medical Deans of Australia and New Zealand (MDANZ), 824
Medical discourse, 871
Medical education, 4, 21, 350, 569, 748–750, 754, 755, 757, 758
  Asia, trends in, 9–10
  climate change, 17
  clinical simulation, 18–19
  educational theories and trends, in curriculum design, 10–11
  hidden curriculum, 19–20
  history, 7
  integration, 17–18
  IPE, 19
  North American medical education, trends, 8–9
  number and distribution of medical schools, 5
  regulation and accreditation, 5–6
  role of medical schools, 6–7
  socially accountable medical schools, 12–14
  students and faculty, changing demographics of, 14–16
  student well-being, 16–17
Medical educators (MEs), 54, 63
Medical emergencies, 435
Medical ethics, 588
  education, 590–591
Medical school, 469, 472, 473, 475
Medical school sources of support, 1009
Medical students, 51–53
  alcohol and drugs policies, 1003
  barriers to accessing medical care and support, 1004
  disclosure, 1004
  illness behavior, 1005
  mindfulness, 1006
  pass/fail system, 1006
  prevalence of mental illness, 1001
  sources of support, 1008–1011
  stigma, 1001
  use of recreational drugs and alcohol, 1003
Medicine, 749
Medic Support, 1007
Membership, 1597, 1599–1601
Mental health, 1558
  curriculums, 144
Mental health education, 218
  co-production, 231–233
  interprofessional education, 228–231
  learning outcomes and pedagogical paradigms, 224–226
  models of learning, 226–228
  technology-enhanced learning, 233–239

Mental Health First Aid, 1008, 1009
Mental illness, 1001, 1166
Mental set, 1379
Mentor(ing), 95–97, 877, 879, 949, 1007, 1449, 1694
Mentorship, 878, 1087, 1092–1094, 1382, 1385
Meritocracy, 1253
Mesolimbic dopamine system, 523
Mesosystem, 543
Metacognition, 225, 371, 482, 483, 485, 495, 1294
Metacognitive knowledge, 483
Metacognitive strategies, 1181
Metaphors, 1678
  learning, 1103
Methods of assessment, 1193
Meyer and Land's criteria for, 364
Mezirow, J., 443–446
Mezirow's transformative learning theory, 1450
Microanalysis, 493
Microblogging services, 207
Microcosm, 1027
Microcredentials, 146–147
Microsystem, 543
Midwifery
  early education, 296–297
  education governance, 896–905
  evidence for care, 895–896
  evolution of higher education, 297–298
  maternity care, 895
  philosophy, 893–894
  scope of practice, 894–895
Milestones, 1720
Miller's Pyramid, 612
Mills, C.W., 1556
Mimicry, 373, 377
Mindfulness-based interventions (MBIs), 1006
Mindfulness-based stress reduction (MSBR), 1006
Mind map, 1294
Mini clinical evaluation exercise (Mini-CEX), 12, 74, 966, 1192, 1236
Minimum Standards for the Education of Occupational Therapists, 1288
Mission statement, 1254
Mixed ability-trait model, 531
Mixed-methods approach, 1162
Mixed reality (MR), 744, 746–747, 1719
Mobile learning, 1423–1425, 1429
Mobile technology, 99
Modelling, 1637
  of clinical nursing education (see Clinical nursing education)
  mathematical, 375

Index

role-modelling, 372
of practice education, 1296
spatiotemporal, 375
Moderation, 1266
Modern dentistry, 252
Monash University (Australia), 831
Monitoring, 1087–1089
Monoprofessionalism, 1607
Moods, 522
Moral erosion, 591
Motivation, 483, 486, 487, 490, 492, 494, 495, 525, 529, 1151
Motivational interviewing, 1308
Motor behavior (abilities), 1179, 1186–1190
Motor learning theories, 631–633
Motor programs, 1186
Motor task, 1377
Multidisciplinary simulated ward, 1165
Multidisciplinary teams (MDT), 871, 1717
Multifaceted roles, 990
Multi-modal delivery (MMD), 305–309, 323, 327
  anatomical material, 322
  clinical anatomy, 321, 323
  cognitive load, 325
  connectivity challenges, 319, 320
  connectivity optimization, 323
  constructive alignment, 326
  digital technology, 325
  DPHTY, 309
  edutainment, 315–317
  flipped practical approach, 325
  learner engagement, geographical location, 319
  learning outcomes, 320
  lectures, 310, 311, 316
  live stream, 324
  outdoor practical session, 318
  pandemic/teaching adaptation, 310
  post-sessions, 326
  practical skills sessions, 317, 319
  remote, 323
  student learning, indirect factors, 311
  traditional delivery approaches, 309
  virtual anatomy, 324
Multimodality, 399
Multimodal thinking, 1292
Multiple learners, 613
Multiple level learners, 60
Multiple mentoring model, 1287
Multiple mini-interview (MMI), 9, 1258, 1261–1262, 1268
Multiple modes, 325
Multiprofessional approach, 1616
Multi-skilled allied health professional, 147

Multisource feedback (MSF), 74, 1192, 1236, 1242
Multi-voiced object, 425
Mutual interest, 1621
Mutual trust, 882

N
Narrative(s), 376, 1661, 1669
  analysis, 1161, 1674
  approach, 1451
  stories, 919
Nascent abilities, 1379
National Academies of Sciences, Engineering, and Medicine (NASEM), 6
National Board of Certification and Recertification for Nurse Anesthetists (NBCRNA), 616
National Council of State Boards of Nursing (NCSBN), 98, 610–611
National Dental Hospital, 262
National disability insurance scheme (NDIS), 1312
National Health Service (NHS), 821
National Institute for Clinical Excellence (NICE), 874
National Institute of Academic Anaesthesia (NIAA), 81
National Organization of Nurse Practitioner Faculty (NONPF), 616
Natural language processing, 1437
Near-Peer Assisted Supervision, 1287
Near-peer learning, 1358
Needs analysis, 1019
Needs assessment, 1708
Negative attitudes, 1167
Negative motivation, 490
Netiquette, 308
Networking, 177, 1603
NetworkZ, 1478
Neurocircuitry, 523
Neurolinguistic programming (NLP), 76, 1451
Neuropsychology, 524
New media, 206–207
New Zealand Medical Students' Association (NZMSA), 824
New Zealand Orthopaedic Association (NZOA), 1455
Nightingale, 287
Non-academic, 1256
Non-clinical skills, 1290
Non-communicable diseases, 17
Non-reflective action, 444

Non-technical skills, 943, 1403
　eye contact, 944
　human factors, 943, 944
　nonverbal communication, 944
　OT settings, 944
Non-Technical Skills for Surgeons (NOTSS), 1468
Non-verbal coaching, 1386
Nonverbal communication, 944
Normative and applied ethics, 565
Northern Ontario School of Medicine (NOSM), 15
Novice, 1380, 1398
Novice learner, 491
Numerical rating scale, 1158
Nurse anesthetists, 947
Nurse manager (NUM), 938
Nurse practitioners, 290, 616
Nursing, 470
　aides, 292
　roles, anesthetic nurse, 939
　students, 88, 91, 92, 94, 95, 97, 99
Nursing and Midwifery Council, 1504
Nursing education
　advanced practice, 946
　challenges for, 295–296
　higher education in, 293–295
　hospital-based training, 288–289
　Nightingale model, 287–288
　operative nurses, 946
　postgraduate, 946
　second level nurse, 291–293
　specialty education, 289–291
　undergraduate nursing, 945
Nutrition-related conditions, 1558

O

Oasis Coffee Lounge, 319
Objective-attribute linkages, 1153
Objective clinical opinion, 1005
Objective structured assessment of technical skills (OSAT), 1189
Objective structured clinical examination (OSCEs), 12, 618, 1189, 1238, 1246, 1398, 1496
Object-oriented activity, 424
Observable practice activity (OPA), 1227
Observation, 1161, 1291
Observational learning, 1153
Observational ratings, 1155
Observations of performance, 102
Observer role, SBE, 613

Occupational therapy, practice education, see Practice education
Odontological Society of London, 262
Oeuvres, 255
One-way' mode of feedback, 724
Online
　delivery, 1306
　journal clubs, 768
　learning, 1718
　lecture, 208
　professionalism, 771
　worlds, 237, 240
Open access, 1604
Operant conditioning, 1153
Operating room (OR), 910, 1456
Operating theatre (OT), 926
　antisepsis, 935
　army surgical teams, 935
　communication, 951
　environment, 948
　healthcare systems, 947
　learning and teaching, 952
　medical and digital technology, 947
　nurse educators, 947
　nurses, 934, 935
　objectives for working, 948
　operating and teaching, 935
　operative environments, 948
　patient safety, 950, 951
　perioperative nursing, 947
　positive learning environment, 935
　risks, 951
　safety of new learners, 950
　skills, 948
　surgery and surgical methods, 935
　surgical procedures, 948
　teamwork, 935
　transitional staff, 936
　workforce, 947
Operating time, 915
Operating with respect (OWR), 1454
Operational budget, 1023
Operational complexity, 917
Operationalization, 1163
Operative care, 934
Operative environment, 945
Operators for the teeth, 257
Optimal environmental, 324
Opuscula Anatomica, 255
Organizational failures, 1503
Organizational needs, 1040–1041
Organizational communities of practice (OCoPs), 408

Index

Orientation, 948, 1077, 1080, 1081, 1089, 1093
Origination, 1380
Orthobullets, 1183
Oscillation, 369
Osler, W., 8
Ottawa clinical assessment tool (OCAT), 1192
Outcomes of clinical education, in nursing, *see* Clinical nursing education
Outsider, 1663
Ownership, 1028

P

Pain management, 70
Pan London Practice Assessment Document (PLPAD), 1528
Pan-tilt-zoom (PTZ), 306
Papyrus, E.S., 253
Parahippocampal gyrus (PHG), 339
Paralanguage, 1101
Paralinguistic cues, 1101
Paré, A., 255
Parmly, E., 260
Participants, 1658–1667, 1669
Participation, 1660, 1662, 1663
Participatory practices, 901
Partnership model, 94–95
Part Zero course, 73
Pass/fail system, 1006
Pathology, 951
Patient(s), 1548
　advocacy, 871
　care assignment, 100
　future considerations, 886
　participation, 576
　permission, 873
　personal characteristics, 883
　voices, 1548
Patient and public involvement (PPI), 578
Patient-centered care, 580, 1714
Patient-centered clinical communication, 1540
　behaviorism, skills development and patient-centeredness, 1543–1544
　challenges, 1547
　clinical communication pedagogy, 1548
　clinical simulation, 1542–1543
　emergence, 1537–1538
　evidence and justification, 1540–1542
　experiential, simulated learning and patient-centeredness, 1544–1546
　simulation and behaviorism, 1543
　simulation and experiential learning, 1543
　workplace and situated learning, 1546–1547

Patient-centeredness, 1536, 1538–1539
Patient-driven care model, 157
Patient educators (PEs), 1548
Patient safety, 880, 915, 916, 944, 946, 950, 988, 1387, 1443, 1711, 1713
　and medical error awareness, 612–613
Patient safety development
　in practice and context, 1511–1515
　professional curricula, 1505–1506
　regulation, 1504–1505
　specific curricula, 1506–1511
Patient service attendants (PSAs), 937
Pattern recognition, 337, 339, 343, 1181
PEARLS framework, 1049
Pedagogical and assessment strategies, 1582
Pedagogy, 1026, 1543, 1548, 1729
Pedagogy–Andragogy–Heutagogy continuum, 309
Pediatric Advanced Life Support (PALS), 1182, 1187
Pediatrics education, 957
　assent, 977
　assessment, 965, 966
　best interests, 975
　capacity, 976
　carer responsibilities, 973
　clinical ethics committee, 975
　communities of practice, 968, 969
　consent, 976
　definition, 957–959
　deliberate practice, 964
　disclosure, 977
　experiential learning, 967
　feedback, 964, 965
　flexible training, 974
　general *vs.* subspecialty, 962, 963
　interactions with parents, 978
　key qualities, 961, 962
　long-term illness, 973
　mastery learning, 963, 964
　psychomotor skills, 970
　reflective practice, 967
　research time, 973
　scenario-based simulation, 972
　simulation-based education, 969, 970, 973
　specialist college frameworks, 959, 961
Peer Assessment Tool (Mini-PAT), 1192
Peer(s), 1318
　continuity, 1357
　didactic, 1359
　feedback, 1290
　learning, 494, 1356
　led education, 207

Peer(s) (cont.)
　mentoring, 1359
　networks, 1094
　observation, feedback and assessment, 1359
People-focused approaches, 1467, 1473
Perceptions, 1190–1191
Perceptual expertise, 340–341
Performance, 33, 37–39, 41–44, 1236, 1237, 1240, 1243, 1245–1247
　analysis, 1058, 1060–1064
　assessment, 1189, 1191, 1192
　criteria, 1189
　dimensions, 1180, 1192, 1194
　enhancement, 1066
　improvement, 1057
　management, 1449
　rating, 103
　requirements, 1180, 1193
　standards, 1193
Peri-operative nurses, 936
Perseverance, 1026
Persistence, 1026
Personal agency, 901
Personal epistemologies, 901
Personality testing, 1263–1264
Personalized system of instruction (PSI), 354
Personal journey, 1674
Personal judgment, 1380
Personal learning environments (PLEs), 1425
Personal protective equipment (PPE), 944, 951
　double gloving, 952
　eye protection, 952
　use, 951
Personal relevance, 592
Personal statement, 1264
Personal tutors, 1008, 1010
Person-centered approach, 1451
Person-centered (models of) care, 156, 222, 1490
Person-focused feedback, 718
Person-focused healthcare system, 1631
Personhood, 1549
Pharmacy programs, 617–618
Philanthropy, 1024
Phobia desensitization, 1712
Phronesis, 687
Physical guidance, 637
Physical set, 1379
Physical therapy (PT) programs, 618
Physician assistant (PA) programs, 616–617
Physician Associates, 1599
Physiological tests, 1155
Picker Institute, 1548

Pin index safety system (PISS), 1466
Planetary health
　becoming mainstream, 819–820
　contributions, 819
　inclusion of, 824
　incorporate, 824
　and sustainability, 829
Planning sheets, 1294
3-P model, 859
Podcasts, 207, 766
Point of care, 1423
Point of care ultrasound (POCUS), 80
Portfolios, 903, 1295
Positive learning experiences, 949–950
Positive psychology, 1451
Post-anesthesia care unit (PACU), 942
Postconferences, 101
Postgraduate, 946
　diploma, 297
　education, 203
Postmodern constructivism, 1450
Postoperative care, 934
Post-positivist world view, 1450
Post-registration qualification, 298
Potentially shared object, 425
Power, 1563, 1564, 1663
　differential, 1663
　as hegemony and oppression, 506
　as ideology, 507–508
　as linguistic and discursive power, 508–510
　theoretical alignments, 510
Practical nurses, 292
Practice-based education, 1166
Practice-based learning approaches, 855
Practice curricula, 902
Practice education, 1279, 1295, 1296
　competencies, 1288–1289
　decline to supervise students, 1281
　definition, 1278
　evidence from settings, 1281–1282
　excellent practice educator, 1280
　high-quality placements, 1282–1283
　practice education models, 1286–1288
　(see also Professional practice)
　professional reasoning, 1292–1295
　reflective practice, 1283–1286
　student perspective, 1279–1280
　student placement, 1290–1292
　supervision and feedback, 1289
Practice educator, 1279–1284, 1286, 1287, 1291–1294, 1296
Practice pedagogies, 902
Practice reasoning, 1281

Index

Practitioners' Health Programme (PHP), 1012
Pragmatism, 1450
Preceptors, 949
Preceptorship, 95–97, 878
Preconferences, 101
Predictive modeling, 1710
Predictive validity, 1259
Prehabilitation, 71
Pre-licensure IPE, 169
Preparation for clinical practice, 1010
Preparedness, 988
    of learner, 880–881
Pre-patient curriculum, 1382
Presenteeism, 1002
Pre-skill conceptualization, 1383
Preventable failures, 1640
Primary contradictions, 425
Printing press, 254
Privacy, 1443
Proactive development, 1636
Proactive knowledge, 371
Probationers, 288
Problem-based learning (PBL), 8, 371, 373, 1138, 1716
    elements of, 1335
    vs. TBL, 1327, 1335
Problem identification, 1708
Procedural based assessments (PBA), 1192
Procedural competency, 1387
    development of, 1379
    maintaining, 1387, 1389
    proving, 1386
Procedural expertise, 337, 338, 341–343
Procedural knowledge, 1404
Procedural performance acquisition, 343
Procedural skills, 1403
Procedural skills learning
    ability, 1378, 1379
    Adams' closed-loop theory, 1377, 1378
    barriers, 1389–1391
    characteristics, 1378–1379
    emotional set, 1379
    mental set, 1379
    physical set, 1379
    skill, 1378, 1379
Procedural skills teaching, 1381–1383
    barriers, 1389–1391
    doing, 1387
    learning, 1383–1384
    maintenance, 1387–1389
    practicing, 1384–1385
    proving, 1386
    seeing, 1384

Procedural training, 1390
Procedural variations, 919, 925
Process-Person-Context-Time (PPCT) model, 542, 545
Profession
    definition, 1593, 1594
    functions, 1595, 1596
    HCEs, 1600, 1601
    HCPs, 1594
    high status careers, 1593
    services, 1599, 1600
    standards, 1595
Professional behaviors, 671
Professional bodies, 823, 1004
    categories, 1607
    education and networking, 1604
    financial pressures, 1601
    healthcare educators, 1607, 1608
    healthcare professionals, 1596, 1597
    interlinking, 1598
    internal committees, 1605
    interprofessional practice and teamwork, 1606
    members service, 1598
    non-profit making, 1601
    privilege, 1606 (*see also* Profession)
    public service, 1598
    society, 1607
    volunteer service, 1604
Professional boundaries, 771
Professional competence, 1504
Professional development, 176
Professional development of supervisors, 1094
Professional discourses, 871
Professional doctorates, 298
Professional education, 1506, 1507
Professional identity, 406, 893, 1600, 1637, 1658–1660, 1672, 1674, 1686, 1730
    access to role experiences and role models, 656
    assessment practices, 660–661
    communities of practice and activity theory, 659
    as copying strategy, 649
    culture and identity, 650
    curricular planning and positioning, 654–656
    development, 671
    as an expression of status, 649
Professional identity formation, 91
    formation, 652–654
    idealized views, 648
    mentoring and role modelling, 660

Professional identity formation (*cont.*)
  multi-professional simulation, 657–658
  responding to hidden curriculum, 658
  and role fluidity, 651
  safe reflective spaces and protected time, 658
  as self and other, 648–649
  socio-cultural perspective, 650
  student engagement, 645
  as transcendent attribute, 652
Professional inclusivity, 649, 1686
Professionalism, 11, 471, 668, 773, 987, 1396
  assessment, 1528
  community of practice, 1523
  concerns systems, 1528
  curriculum, 1524, 1526
  definition, 1520
  discovery learning, 1526
  education, 1523–1525
  employer codes, 1522
  employer guidance, 1522
  external regulation, 1522
  hidden curriculum, 1524
  identity, 1523
  informal learning, 1524
  interprofessional collaborative, 1521
  and interprofessional practice, 1527
  Kegan's model, 1521
  moral development, 1521
  partnership, 1526
  portfolios, 1526, 1528
  practice guidelines, 1525–1526
  reflection, 1523
  regulations, 1522
  role modelling, 1525
  situated learning, 1527
  social media, 1525
  stages of moral development, 1521
  standards, 1524
Professionalization, 294, 1601
Professional organizations, 1595, 1596, 1599, 1607
Professional practice, 139–140, 446–448, 1192
  placements, 1314
Professional proficiencies, 1180
Professional reasoning, 1292–1295
Professional recognition, 1599, 1601
Professional regulation, 1501
Professional rivalries, 1606
Professional roles, 671
Professional silos, 1621
Professional socialization, 671
Profile of mood states, 1007

Program development and delivery, 1094
Program-level learning outcomes, 1206
Programmatic approaches, 990
Programmatic assessment., 61–62, 376, 1231, 1241, 1247, 1295
Programmatic assessment for learning (PAL), 1209, 1212
  agentic learners, 1212
  assessment database, 1208
  assessment-for-learning, 1214
  case study, 1213
  community of practice, 1213
  definition, 1204
  empower, 1211
  engagement, 1209
  feedback, 1209
  hidden curriculum, 1218
  informative assessment, 1209
  integrated curriculum, 1206
  longitudinal assessment tools, 1207
  meaningful feedback, 1210
  mentoring, 1212
  narrative reports, 1216
  online curriculum database, 1207
  peer feedback, 1206
  portfolio report, 1209
  portfolios, 1207
  progression, 1214
  progress tests, 1207
  remediation, 1214
  self-evaluating, 1215
  self-regulated learners, 1211
  self-regulated learning, 1210
Program to Enhance Relational and Communication Skills (PERCS) model, 1046
Progression, 1239–1241, 1243, 1245, 1246
  decisions, 1010
Progressive entrustment, 916
Progress Review Board (PRB), 1215
Project-Focussed Practice Placement Model, 1287
Projective or implicit assessments, 1155
Proximal processes, 545
Psychiatry, 236
Psychocritical transformation, 467
Psychodevelopmental transformation, 467
Psychodynamic models, 1451
Psychodynamic theories of learning, 227
Psychological debriefing, 1110
Psychological developmental approaches, 1451
Psychological First Aid, 1046, 1051

Psychologically safe learning environments, 1065–1067, 1379
Psychological safety, 1111–1113, 1640–1645
Psychology education, 779, 780
Psychometric rigor, 1191
Psychomotor expertise, 341–343
Psychomotor skill acquisition, 1376, 1391
Psychomotor skills, 626–628
  attributes, 628, 629
  consolidation, 639
  definition, 627
  development, 924
  encoding, 639
  features, 628
  pre-skill conceptualization, 635
  relative feedback frequency, 640
  retrieval, 639
  skill acquisition motor learning theories, 631–632
  skill demonstration, 635, 637–639
  task analysis, 634, 635
  task deconstruction, 634
  terminal/end-task feedback, 640
Psychotherapeutic skills, 221
Psychotherapy, 238
Public consultation, 579–580
Public engagement, in health profession curriculum
  curriculum development and implementation, 577
  experts by experience, 580
  internet, 583–584
  limitations, 582
  models, 578–579
  public as partners, 580–581
  public consultation, 579–580
  sociocultural theories, 581–582
Publishing, 1604

Q
Qualifying exam, 1182, 1183
Qualitative thematic analysis, 1106
Quality, 1242
  assurance, 1266, 1268
  of clinical learning, 884
  culture, 1635
  improvement, 435, 1244–1245, 1505, 1507–1509, 1713
  placement, 1282–1283
  and safety in health care, 92
  of training, 63
Quality and Safety Education for Nurses (QSEN), 92
Quality Assurance Agency (QAA), 1524
Quaternary contradictions, 426
Questioning, 1409
Questionnaires, 1155

R
Randomized controlled trials (RCTs), 1450
Ranking, 1156
Rapid deployment, 327
Rapport, 1112, 1662
Rating scales, 1242, 1291
Realism, 971, 1399
Real-life clinical environment, 1399
Real World Anesthesia Course (RWAC), 77
Recertification, 1185
Reciprocity, 1035
Re-contextualization, 1547
Record keeping, 1161
Recovery nursing, 937, 942
  knowledge, 943
  skills, 942
Recreational drugs, 1003
Recursiveness, 369, 377
Reflection, 221, 465–472, 477, 879, 902, 1318, 1400, 1643
  frameworks and models, 448–451
  phase, 488
  types of, 444–446
Reflective action, 444
Reflective activities, 1168
Reflective discourse, 465, 469
Reflective discussion, 1048
Reflective learning groups, 452–453
Reflective modes, 722
Reflective practice, 967, 1283–1284, 1318
  Driscoll's model of reflection, 1286
  Gibbs reflective model, 1286
  Kolb's learning cycle, 1285
  Rolfe's model of reflective practice, 1285
Reflective practice theories
  dimensions of reflection, 444–445
  meaning perspective, 443
  professional practice and Schön, D., 446–448
  types of reflection, 444–446
Reflective techniques, 1556
Reflective thought, 442
Reflectivity
  levels of, 444
  pedagogical approaches for developing, 452

REFLECT model, 450
Reflexivity, 162
Reform, 1629
Refresher teaching, 1388, 1389
Refugee and asylum seeker health, 1557–1560
Registered nurse, 871
Registrars Clinical Encounters in Training (ReCEnT) project, 57
Regulation of context, 483–486
Regulation of motivation and affect, 486–487
Regulators, 1595, 1607
Regulatory codes, 1504
Rehearse skills, 1407
Relatedness, 1715
Relational elements of learning, 926
Relational skills, 221
Relationship-based care, 51
Relationships, 1112
Reliability, 1032, 1162, 1164, 1253, 1386
Reliable assessment, 1216
Remedial action, 492
Remediation, 874, 1246
    definition, 1120, 1121
    feedback processes, 1125
    processes, 1129
    and underperformance, 1121, 1126
Remote clinical education, 1310
Remote-controlled surgical robots, 1442
Remote learning, 1728
Remote supervision model, 1312
Renaissance, 254
Replacement, Amplification, and Transformation (RAT) model, 1718
Report cards, 722
Reports of others, 1155
Research, 494–495
Researcher, 1658–1669
Research-related tasks, 1733
Residency, 1181, 1183, 1187, 1192, 1194
Resident in-training examinations, 1182
Resilience, 901
Resistance to change, 1444
Response set, 1163
Responsibilities, 1632, 1660
Retention, 1182, 1186, 1194
Retrieval practice, 1716
Retrospective recall, 1293
Return on investment, 1024
Revenue raising, 1025
Rigor, 1161
Ringelmann, K.J., 259
Risks, 951, 1505
Rituals, 1003

Robotics, 1712
Robots, 1440
Rogerian theory, 1049
Role boundaries, 1665, 1685
Role-emerging practice placement model, 1287
Role modelling, 372, 882, 885, 904, 926, 1087, 1525
Rolfe's model of reflective practice, 1285
Royal Australasian College of Physicians (RACP), 822, 959
Royal Australasian College of Surgeons (RACS), 1454
Royal College of Surgeons, 262, 263
Rural areas, 1012
Rural clinical schools (RCSs), 14
Rural communities, 1563
Rural health, 1699, 1700
Rurality, 1563–1565
Rural settings, 1442
RUST debriefing model, 1409

S
Safety, 1075, 1080–1083, 1090, 1091
    patient, 1510
    practices, 1501
Salient beliefs, 1153
Same-level peer learning, 1358
Satisfaction, 1541
SBE scalability, *see* Simulation based education (SBE)
Scaffolding, 309, 369, 375, 1310
Scaling, 1163
Scenario-based simulation, 972, 1406
Scholarship, HPE, 1254, 1270
    academic promotion/tenure, 1619
    of application, 1612
    benchmarking, 1619
    bibliometrics, 1618
    build network, 1621
    build team, 1621
    challenges, 1614
    community of practice, 1615
    critical mass, 1617
    critique, 1622
    discipline, 1612
    disseminating, 1618
    evidence-based practice, 1614
    health professions workforces, 1616
    HPESUs, 1616
    identify mentors, 1620
    implementation science, 1614
    of integration, 1612

like-minded individuals, 1615
multidisciplinary approaches, 1613
multiprofessional approach, 1617
peer-evaluation, 1613
portfolio, 1622
publication, 1612, 1613, 1616, 1619, 1621–1623
publishing health professions research, 1618
quality assurance, 1614
read, 1622
roles of institutions, 1622, 1623
scholarship of discovery, 1612
self-evaluation, 1613
social media, 1619, 1620
sustainable, 1617
of teaching, 1612
tenure or promotion, 1618
translational research, 1613
Schön, D., 446–448
School vs. university services, 1009
Schwarz rounds, 1011
Scope of practice, 1677
Scoring validity, 1192
Screen-based learning
  advantages and challenges, 1419–1420
  blended learning, 1429
  content development, 1421
  content management, 1421–1422
  e-learning and historical context, 1419
  mobile learning, 1423–1425
  serious games and gamification, 1427–1428
  simulation-based education, 1426–1427
  social learning theory, 1425–1426
  virtual environment, 1427
Secondary contradictions, 426
Second generation activity theory, 421
Second level nurse, 291–293
See one, do one, and teach one framework, 1381
SEGUE communication framework, 1049
Selection, 1252–1254
  academic attainment, 1258–1259
  aligning mission, tools and process, 1266–1268
  challenges, 1269–1270
  evaluation, 1268
  letters of reference, 1259–1260
  mission statement, 1254
  MMI, 1261
  Ottawa Conference consensus on selection statements, 1254
  philosophy, 1255, 1256
  personality testing, 1263–1264
  personal statements and curriculum vitae, 1264–1265
  quality selection process, 1265
  SJT, 1262–1263
  tools, 1256–1260, 1263, 1264, 1266–1270
  traditional interviews, 1260–1261
  training, standardization and moderation, 1268
Self-actualisation, 225, 227
Self-awareness, 1635
Self-calibration, 1661
Self-categorization theory, 227
Self-determination theory (SDT), 1128, 1715
Self-development, 1650
Self-directed learning, 206, 596, 1716
Self-disclosure, 1665
Self-distraction, 533
Self-feedback, 1290
Self-judgements, 488
Self-management, 1511
Self-promotion, 1029
Self-referring, 1005
Self-regulated learning (SRL), 371, 482
  adaptive motivation, 483
  in clinical context, 490–493
  cognitive control, 485
  cognitive forethought, planning and activation, 483
  cognitive monitoring, 485
  cognitive reaction and reflection, 485–486
  conceptual framework, 483–486
  contextual monitoring, 489
  contextual reaction and reflection, 489
  health professional education and research, 493–495
  motivational control, 487
  motivational forethought, planning and activation, 486–487
  motivational monitoring, 487
  motivational reaction and reflection, 487
  phases and areas for, 484
Self-report, 1291
  of attitudes, 1154
Semantic-differential scales, 1157
Semantics, 1437
Semiotic mediation, 421
Semiotics, 918
Sensory semiosis, 918
Serious games, 744, 756, 1719
Service learning, 1367
Set, 1378, 1379
Shared clinical practice model, 1286

Shared decision making, 580, 1605
Shared understanding, 918
Siebold, K.C., 259
Sierra Leone, 186
Sign making, 387–388
SimLab, 436
Simulated clinical placements, 1313
Simulated learning, 1544
Simulated participants, 874
Simulated patients (SPs), 972, 1407
Simulated placement, 1288, 1314
Simulation, near-peer learning, 1308
Simulation, 744, 950, 1542
   and behaviorism, 1543
   CoP in, 410–411
   and experiential learning, 1543
Simulation-based educational IPL approach, 855
Simulation based education (SBE), 143–144, 410, 874, 884, 969, 970, 1018, 1165–1166, 1313, 1376, 1399, 1426–1427
   actual time and activities, academic and hospital-based, 619
   advanced practice providers, 616
   barriers and enablers to implementation of, 1021–1022
   champions and promotion of, 1028–1029
   clinical placement substitute, 609
   2:1 clinical placement to SBE ratio, 612
   CRNA, 616
   early adopters, 610
   executive support, 1029
   facilitator role, 618–619
   faculty workload for, 615
   fiscal challenges, 1020
   funding challenges in, 1023
   hospital programs, 1025
   implementation, 1019–1020
   innovation and research in, 1026–1027
   introductory SBE education training modules, 619
   leadership and change management, 1033
   NCSBN National SBE study, 610–611
   observer role, 613
   paramedics SBE utilization, 617
   for patient safety and medical error awareness, 612–613
   pharmacy programs, 617–618
   physical therapy programs, 618
   physician assistant programs, 617
   programs, 1024
   purpose and shared purpose, 1026
   quality and safety, 1030
   safe practitioners, 618
   substitution with, 610
   telesimulation, 614–615
   traditional clinical experiences, effective substitute for, 611
   traditional clinical placement, 609–611
   translational simulation, 1030–1031
   TTS approach, 613–614
   undergraduate medical education, 617
   virtual reality, 614
   visionary leadership, 1029
   workload for faculty, 620
Simulation-based learning, 700, 701
   See also Debriefing
Simulation-based mastery learning (SBML), 1386
Simulation-based training (SBT), 1468, 1473, 1474, 1478
Single-item direct attitude scales, 1158
Situated knowledge, 1546
Situated learning, 405, 408–410, 412, 581, 876, 917, 1673
Situational awareness, 945
Situational factors, 917
Situational judgement test (SJT), 1258, 1262–1263
Situationally appropriate, 1191
Situation Background Assessment Recommendation (SBAR), 1474
Skill(s), 88–92, 96–98, 100–103, 1378, 1543
   acquisition, 879
   chunk, 1383
   classification, 628, 630
   deterioration, 1388
   development, 90–91
   simple skill, 628, 630, 632, 637, 640, 641
Skilled migration schemes, 295
Small group learning, 1335, 1345, 1360
Social accountability, 1257
Social adaptation and social reconstruction, 592
Social beliefs, 1151
Social cohesion, 227
Social comparison theory, 1362
Social connectedness, 1318
Social constructivist, 562, 1545
Social contract, 1594, 1600
Social desirability effect, 1163
Social distancing, 1304
   restrictions, 322
Social emancipatory, 467
Social exclusivity, 649, 1686
Social identity theory, 227

Index

Socialization, 406, 653, 1104
Social justice, 1555
Social learning, 465, 472, 1515
    theories, 174
Socially accountable medical schools, 12–14
Social media, 82, 723, 748–749, 1425
Social media, in health professional education
    clinical and educational scholarship, 769–770
    clinical learning, 766–767
    clinical teaching, 767–769
    doctor–patient interaction, 773
    ethical and professionalism issues, 773
    faculty development, 769
    health advocacy, 770
    measures of quality, 772
    organizational promotion, 770
    personal social media reputation, 771–772
    research, 772
Social network analysis, 772
Social norms, 1153
Social participation, 404
Social practice, 702, 705
Social process of learning, 405, 1732
Social semiotics, 386
    doing clinical work, 388–395
    projecting clinical work, 397–399
    review of clinical work, 396–397
    sign making, 387–388
Socio-cultural aspects of patient care, 155, 161
Sociocultural learning theory, 55, 405, 411
Sociocultural theories, 419, 421, 426, 581–582
Socioeconomic diversity gap, 14
Socioeconomic status (SES), 14, 1255
Sociological imagination, 1556, 1563, 1565
Sociology, 1556
Socio-material theory, 174
Sociometric techniques, 1155
Solutions focused approaches, 1451
Sorting, 1156
Space and equipment, 1390
Spaced education, 1716
Specialization, in nursing, 294
Specialized anesthetic training, 70
Specialty postgraduate, 289
Specimens, 951
SPIKES, 1049
St. George's Hospital, 259
Stakes, 1240–1241
Standardization, 1266
Standards-based assessment, 1136–1137
Standards for Medics, 1504
Stapel scale, 1159

ST elevation myocardial infarction (STEMI), 1472
Sterilization, 938
Stigma, 222, 1001
Stigmatization, 1001
Storytelling, 1661
Strategic prioritization, 1645
Structural validity, 1162
Student Evaluation of Teaching Units (SETUs), 790
Student leadership, 175
Student-led clinics, 1366
Student practice evaluation form–revised (SPEF-R), 1291, 1315
Student-run clinics, 175
Student Wellness Committee, 1007
Study environments, 488
Subjective norms, 1153
Subjectivity, 1245
Subject matter experts (SME), 1262
Substantive equality, 799
Succession planning, 1637
Suicide prevention, 1009
Sumerian clay tablet, 253
Summative assessments, 62, 897, 1137–1138, 1178, 1186, 1188
Summative evaluation, 103, 104
Summative feedback, 1290
Supernumerary, 877, 902
Supervised learning events, 1387
Supervision, in general practice setting
    ad hoc supervisory call-in, 1082–1084
    assessment, 1089–1090
    consultation assessment, 1086
    consultation observation, 1085
    formal teaching, 1084
    good practice, 1090–1091
    informal learning, 1084
    learning needs, 1085
    mentorship and role modelling, 1086–1087
    monitoring and feedback, 1087–1089
    new supervisors, 1093
    peer networks, 1094
    proactive learning, 1085
    program development and delivery, supervisor engagement, 1094
    reactive teaching, 1084
    shared supervision, 1091–1092
    supervisor professional development, 1094
    supervisor recruitment, 1092–1093
    supporting supervisors, 1093
    trainee engagement, in working community, 1080–1082

Supervision
  of students, 221, 1280, 1281, 1286–1289, 1291, 1292, 1295
  level, 1078, 1082, 1090, 1091
  model, 1311
Supervision and Nurse Teacher Evaluation Scale, 876
Supervisory capability, 991
Suppression, 533
Surgeons, 936
Surgical abilities, 1186, 1187
Surgical care, 939
Surgical Council on Resident Education (SCORE), 1183
Surgical culture, 1180
Surgical education, 203
  challenges at distance, 203–204
  new media, 206–207
Surgical education and training, 276–277, 280–281
  apprenticeship system, 272–273
  Churchill, E., 278
  in Great Britain and Ireland, 278–280
  Halsted, W., 277, 278
  medical education and universities, 274–275
  new opportunities for learning, 273–274
  role of surgeons, 270
  Royal Charters for physicians, surgeons and apothecaries, 270
  surgeon-apothecaries, pure surgeons and practices, 272
  transformations, in teaching and learning, 275–276
Surgical first assistant, 947
Surgical outlier remediation, 1457
Surgical performance acquisition, 343
Surgical Safety Checklist, 939, 1475
Surgical skills, 1187
Surgical trainees, 1182
Surgical training, 202, 910, 924, 1436
  in Australia and New Zealand, 30
  bootcamps and intensive face to face teaching, 206
  challenges in low-and middle-income countries, 185–190
  competency-based training, 31–32, 42–43
  curriculum design, 32–34
  educational faculty, 186
  educational theory, 34–35
  equipment and infrastructure, 187–188
  high-and low-income countries, 188–190
  and hybrid distant and direct, 203
  institutions, 185–186
  local *vs.* overseas, 185
  in low-and middle-income countries, 184–185
  peer led education, 207
  rethinking assessment, 39–42
  role of assessment, 38–39
  self-directed learning, 206
  surgical training program development, 186–187
  technology enhanced learning, 204
  virtual environments and simulation, 35–38
Surgical workforce, 183–184, 191
Sustainability, 1560–1563
Sustainable assessment, 1139
Synchronous content delivery, 1422
Syntax, 1437
Systemic family theory, 703
Systems-based approaches, 1466

T

Tactile modelling, 637
Tag team SBE (TTS) approach, 613–614
Talent, 1398
Talk as work, 1102
Taxonomy of skills, 1642
Teachable moments, 925
Teachable steps, 914
Teacher
  behavior, 926
  confidence, 917
  future considerations, 885
  patient, learner and, 881
  personal characteristics, 882
  preparation, experience and expectations, 879
  role, 871
Teaching, 1449
  behaviors, 914
  formal and informal, 1084
  proactive learning, 1085
  reactive, 1084
Teaching and learning knowledge (TALK), 308
Teaching model, 632, 641
  contemporary models, 633–634
  instructional steps, 635
  master-apprentice skill teaching approach, 632
  skill demonstration, 635, 637–639
  task analysis, 634–635
  task deconstruction, 634

Team, 1465
   building tools, 1475
   debriefing, 1467, 1474, 1475
   development interventions, 1464, 1467, 1475, 1477, 1478
   inclusiveness, 1108
   interactions, 1107
   readiness assurance test, 1328
   reflexivity, 1107, 1474
   science, 1464–1472, 1478
   teaching, 1340
   training, 1467, 1468, 1471, 1473, 1474, 1478
Team-based healthcare, 409
Team-based learning (TBL), 1327
   application phase, 1328
   backward design, 1336–1337
   benefits and challenges, 1344–1345
   vs. case-based learning, 1335
   case studies, 1337–1339
   current trends and evidence in healthcare education, 1333–1334
   curriculum design, 1336
   description, 1328
   design, 1327
   emerging trends in, 1348–1349
   facilitation skills, 1340–1341
   faculty reaction to, 1334
   future work, 1349–1350
   health care faculty, 1336–1339
   immediate feedback, 1331
   implementation, 1339–1348
   incentive structure, 1332
   in-class problem-solving activities, 1331
   learner reaction to, 1334
   peer review in, 1333
   phases, 1328
   preparatory phase, 1328
   vs. problem-based learning, 1327, 1335
   questioning students, 1341–1344
   readiness assurance, 1331
   readiness assurance phase, 1328
   significant problem, same problem, specific choice and simultaneous reporting, 1332
   student academic performance, 1333
   student engagement, 1344
   team formation, 1330
   team teaching, 1340
   writing learning outcomes, 1337
Team Reflection Behavioral Observation System (TuRBO), 1107
TeamSTEPPS™, 1466, 1474, 1477, 1506
Teamwork, 672, 935, 945, 1100, 1328, 1330, 1332, 1405, 1410, 1464–1466, 1468, 1472, 1473, 1475, 1476, 1478
Teamwork assessment tools, 1468
Technical expertise, 919
Technical skills, 1377, 1391
Technological failure, 1442
Technology, in health professions and clinical education, 98–100, 1706, 1708, 1709, 1711, 1714, 1717–1718
   audience response, 759–760
   e-learning, 758–759
   holograms and mixed reality, 746–747
   mobile applications/devices, 749–750
   online-hosted video, 753–754
   serious games, 756
   social media, 748–749
   technology enhanced learning, simulations with, 754–756
   3D printing, 750–751
   virtual and augmented reality, 745
   virtual dissection tables, 747–748
Technology-enabled tools, 1709
Technology enhanced learning, 204–205, 744, 754–756
Tele-education, 236, 239
Telehealth, 1307–1309, 1701, 1708, 1713, 1728
   training, 1311
Telemedicine, 1713
Telemonitoring, 204
Tele-placement
   approach, 1307
   considerations for tele-supervision, 1311
   description, 1309
   incidental learning, 1311
   in lock down, 1312–1313
   opportunities and challenges of health professional student, 1310
   review of space and equipment, 1310
   supervision model, 1311
Telepractice, 145
Telesimulation, 614–615
Tele-supervision, 1288, 1311
Tensions, 885, 1110
Terminology, discipline-specific, 364
Tertiary contradictions, 426
Tertiary education, 1634
Tertiary Education Quality and Standards Agency requirements (TEQSA), 326
Textual conversational approach, 1659
The American Journal of Dental Science, 262
The Australian and New Zealand College of Anesthetists (ANZCA), 73

The Bass model of holistic reflection, 450
The British Journal of Dental Sciences, 262
The Dentists Act of 1878, 263
The Flexner Report, 1706
The Gies Report, 264
Thematic analysis, 1161
The National Rural Health Alliance, 1565
The New York Dental Recorder, 262
Theoretical awareness, 174
Theoretical framework, 495
Therapeutics, 1661, 1666
Thermometer scale, 1159
Think aloud technique, 904, 1293
Third generation activity theory, 421
Thought-action tendencies, 530
Three-dimensional (3D) printing, 750–751
Three-dimensional (3D) virtual reality simulation, 99
Threshold capabilities, 368
Threshold capability integrated theoretical framework (TCITF), 368
Threshold concepts, 653
  active inaction, 370
  affective dimensions, 374
  bias, stigma, 370
  blood pressure regulation, 374
  burden of responsibility, 370
  care, 370
  characteristics, 363, 368
  client-centered approach, 370
  clinical reasoning, 370
  communication management, 370
  complexity of medical care, 370
  contextual care, 370
  vs. core concepts, 363
  cycle of enquiry, 371
  deficit thinking, 370
  definition, 363
  embodied shared care, 370
  embracing uncertainty, 370
  emotional engagement, 370
  empathy, 370
  ethical challenges, 370
  evidence-based practice, 370
  health as politically and socially determined, 370
  holistic approach, 370
  hormonal control, 367
  immune response, 370
  inclusionary othering, 370
  inequalities in health, 370
  and learning theories, 369
  Meyer and Land's criteria for, 364
  nature of evidence, 370
  patient-centeredness, 370
  population perspectives, 370
  probability, 371
  professional culture, 370
  purposeful action, 370
  race, 370
  reflective practice, 370
  spatial relationships in anatomy, 370
  stigma, 370
  troublesome knowledge, 366–367
  variability, 371
Threshold epistemes, 367
Thurstone scales, 1156
Timely access to surgery, 192
Timor-Leste
  background, 190
  career pathways, 195–196
  challenges in surgical education and training in, 194–197
  equipment and infrastructure, 196–197
  health system, 190
  language barriers, 194–195
  postgraduate diploma in surgery, 192–194
  surgeons as educators, 194
  surgical care, 191
  in surgical education and training, 192–194
Tomes, J., 262
Tools, 1236, 1237, 1239, 1241–1243, 1246, 1247
Tracking, 1238–1239
Tradition, 1444
Traditional apprentice/mentor relationships, 72
Traditional apprenticeship model, 1286
Traditional group facilitation model, 878
Traditional interviews, 1260–1261
Traditional medical education, 71
Traditional paper-based texts, 206
Traditional uni-professional knowledge, 169
  programs, 78, 991
  requirements, 1182
Train-the-trainer model, 1390
Traite sur les Dents, 262
Trajectory, 1658, 1665
  in GP, 1077–1080
Transactional analysis, 1451
Transactional curriculum enquiry, 372
Transdisciplinarity, 806–807
  BRAIDE, 809–810
  intersectionality, 807–809
Transfer, 1544, 1716
Transferability, 1161, 1410

Transformation, 464, 466–472, 475–477
   ontological shift, 364, 369
   perspective transformation, 369
Transformational leadership, 1028, 1034
Transformative leadership, 1454
Transformative learning, 227, 472, 476, 653
   academic/clinical learning environment, 468
   accommodative learning, 466
   assimilative learning, 466
   challenges, 469
   critical conversations, 468
   critical discourse, 469
   critical reflection, 465, 469
   critical thinking, 469
   dialogue, 468
   disorienting dilemma, 465
   evaluation, 472
   faculty development and engagement, 472
   implications and recommendations, 476–477
   reflective discourse, 465
   STAR framework, 470
   theory of change, 472
Transitional surgical staff
   biomedical engineers, 937
   CSSD, 938
   medical device company representatives, 938
   pharmacist role, 937
   radiographer, 937
   theatre technicians, 937
Transition(s), 918
   of nurse education, 289
Translational simulation, 1030–1031
Transparency, 1188
Transpersonal awareness, 1451
Tribalism, 1476
Troublesome knowledge, 366–367, 375, 653
Trust, 916, 1087, 1091, 1228, 1231, 1662
Trusting relationships, 54
Trustworthiness, 1161

U
UK Professional Standards Authority, 1593, 1595
Ultrasound training, 80
Uncertainty, 1020
   during liminality, 367
   managing as a threshold concept, 370
Uncovering, 1631

Undergraduate, 1261
   medical education, 617
   nursing, 945
Underperformance
   boosting learner autonomy during, 1121
   clinical educators, 1120
   clinical educators' experiences of, 1122–1123
   in clinical environment, 1121
   educator-learner relationship, 1120
   five program level strategies, 1123
   levels of, 1121
   literature, 1121
   redressing, 1121
   types of, 1120
   working with, 1120
   zones, 1121
Undifferentiated doctor, 73
Unintended curriculum, 669
United Nations Convention, 1559
United Nations Human Rights Commission, 1558
University Clinical Aptitude Test (UCAT), 1258, 1265
University of Maryland, 261
University of Michigan, 264
University of Pennsylvania, 264
University of Toronto, 262
University-Supported Placement, 1287
US Agency for Healthcare Research and Quality, 1506

V
Validation, 1391, 1661, 1666
   Validity, 1164, 1205, 1253, 1263, 1386
   reliability, 1188
Value(s), 1024, 1151, 1546
   in healthcare, 1546
   of investment, 1651
Value-based (health) care, 176, 1713, 1714
Value-expressive function, 1152
Values-based philosophic approach, 568
Values based recruitment (VBR) framework, 1525
Vanderbilt program, 854
Vanishing feedback, 1120
Variation
   as promoting conceptual change, 375
   in understanding, pre-liminal/liminal/post-limina, 376
Verbal communication, 630

Verbal demonstration, 1384
Verbal guidance, 918
Verbalization execution, 1384
Verbalization–performance, 1385
Verbal self-report questionnaires, 1155
Vertical attitude structure, 1153
Vertical development, 1638
Vesalius, A., 255
Vicarious learning, 669
Video-based coaching programs, 1456
Video-based interventions, 234, 239
Videoconferencing (VC) technology, 1307
Video game-based learning, 1709
Virchow, R., 1555
Virtual anatomy, 324
Virtual and augmented reality, 1308
Virtual classroom, 1422
Virtual CoPs, 410
Virtual dissection, 747
Virtual learning environment, 1010
Virtual reality (VR), 80, 99, 238–240, 324, 614, 745, 746, 755, 1384, 1708, 1709, 1712, 1719
Virtual SPs, 237, 239
Virtue-based theories, 1541
Visionary leadership, 1029
Vision of quality general practice, 58
Visual arts-based educational programs, 688
Visual cues, 918
Visual demonstration, 1384
Visualization, 375, 1643
    See also Modelling
Visual literacy, 688, 689, 692
Visual processing, 1438
Visual thinking strategies (VTS), 689
Vocational nurse, 293
Vocational training, 73
Voice-over PowerPoint (VoPP's) lectures, 325
Voxel-based morphometry (VBM), 338
Vulnerability, 1660, 1662

W

Ways of thinking and practicing, 369, 377
Wearable GoPro cameras, 1456
Web-based learning, 758, 1419
Webinars, 1603
Weight tools, 1266
Welfare officer, 1007
Wellbeing, 1000, 1639
Wellness, 286
Widening participation, 1256
William, D.F., 257
Wisconsin framework, 1455
Wisconsin Surgical Coaching Framework, 1455
Witnessing rudeness, 1111
Woman-centered care, 287, 893, 897
Work-based assessments, 40, 61
Work-based learning, 1076–1077, 1092, 1095
Workflow disruptions, 915
Work-integrated learning, 938
    See also Professional practice
Work integrated learning (WIL), 986
Workloads
    for faculty, 620
    clinicians, 993
Workplace
    curriculum, 1104
    learning, 1066, 1102, 1106, 1107, 1547
    and situated learning, 1546–1547
Workplace assessments (WPA), 1192
Workplace-based assessments (WBAs), 74, 75, 1236–1238, 1387
    assessment judgments, 1240
    feedback, 1239–1240
    implementation, 1243–1244
    learner-centered, 1245
    perspectives, 1245–1246
    quality improvement issues for, 1244–1245
    reviewing WBA forms, 1241–1243
    stakes, 1240–1241
    tracking, 1239
Workshops, 60–61
    educators and peers, interaction with, 61
World Directory of Medical Schools, 5
World Federation for Medical Education (WFME), 5
World Federation of Occupational Therapists (WFOT), 1278, 1288, 1290
World Medical Association (WMA), 5, 822
World Organization of Family Doctors (WONCA), 822
Written accounts, 1155
Written assignment, 101–102
Written comment, 1243
Written feedback
    characteristics, 720
    complex interdependencies, 719
    curriculum, 735
    definition, 720
    factors, 728–731
    guidelines on, 724–735
    mode of, 720–724
    structuring, 736–738
Written self-report questionnaires, 1155

X
XR, 744

Y
YouTube, 753

Z
Zahnbrecher, 257
Zene Artzney, 255
Zone of proximal development (ZPD), 369, 426, 876, 1361
Zwisch model, 924